LEXICON MEDICUM;

OR

MEDICAL DICTIONARY;

CONTAINING AN EXPLANATION OF THE TERMS IN

ANATOMY,	MINERALOGY,
BOTANY,	PHARMACY,
CHEMISTRY,	PHYSIOLOGY,
MATERIA MEDICA,	PRACTICE OF PHYSIC,
MIDWIFERY,	SURGERY,

AND THE VARIOUS BRANCHES OF

NATURAL PHILOSOPHY CONNECTED WITH MEDICINE

SELECTED, ARRANGED, AND COMPILED FROM THE BEST AUTHORS.

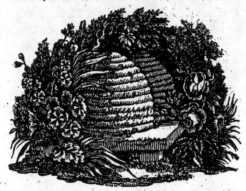

" Nec aranearum sane texus ideo melior, quia ex se fila gignunt, nec
noster vilior quia ex alienis libamus ut apes."
JUST. LIPS. *Monit. Polit.* Lib. i. cap. i.

By ROBERT HOOPER, M.D. F.L.S.

THIRTEENTH AMERICAN, FROM THE LAST LONDON EDITION,
WITH ADDITIONS FROM AMERICAN AUTHORS ON BOTANY, CHEMISTRY, MATERIA MEDICA, MINERALOGY, &c.

By SAMUEL AKERLY, M.D.

FORMERLY PHYSICIAN TO THE NEW-YORK CITY DISPENSARY, RESIDENT PHYSICIAN TO THE CITY HOSPITAL,
LATE HOSPITAL SURGEON UNITED STATES' ARMY, PHYSICIAN TO THE NEW-YORK INSTITUTION
FOR THE INSTRUCTION OF THE DEAF AND DUMB, &c. &c.

IN TWO VOLUMES.
VOL. II.

Willow Bend Books
Westminster, Maryland
2000

Willow Bend Books

65 East Main Street
Westminster, Maryland 21157-5026
1-800-876-6103

Source books, early maps, CDs—Worldwide

For our listing of thousands of titles offered
by hundreds of publishers see our website
<www.WillowBend.net>

Visit our retail store

International Standard Book Number: 1-58549-155-1

Printed in the United States of America

A NEW
MEDICAL DICTIONARY.

K

K AATH. See *Acacia catechu.*

KÆMPFER, ENGELBERT, was born in 1651 at Lippe, in Westphalia. He was educated in Sweden, and being eager to travel, accompanied the Swedish ambassador, Fabricius, to Persia, as secretary: on whose departure from Ispahan, after two years, he obtained the appointment of chief surgeon to the Dutch East India Company; and was thus enabled to penetrate as far as Siam and Japan, and cleared up the geography of these countries, which was very imperfectly known before. On his return to Europe, in 1694, he graduated at Leyden, and settled in his own country; he was afterward appointed physician to his sovereign, and continued engaged in practice, and in composing several works, till his death, in 1716. In his inaugural dissertation, among other subjects relating to medicine, he notices a method of curing colic among the Japanese by puncture with a needle. But his great work, entitled "Amænitates Exoticæ," is more especially esteemed for its botanical information, and authentic details, relating to the history and manners of Persia, &c. His History of Japan, of which there is an English translation in folio, is highly valued for its accuracy and fidelity.

KÆMPFE'RIA. (Named after Kæmpfer, the Westphalian naturalist.) The name of a genus of plants. Class, *Monandria;* Order, *Monogynia.*

KÆMPFERIA GALANGA. The plant which affords the greater galangal root.

KÆMPFERIA ROTUNDA. The systematic name of the plant which affords the officinal zedoary. *Zedoaria. Kæmpferia—foliis lanceolatis petiolatis,* of Linnæus. The roots of this plant are brought to us in long pieces, *zedoaria longa,* about the thickness of the little finger, two or three inches in length, bent, rough, and angular; or in roundish pieces, *zedoaria rotunda,* about an inch in diameter, of an ash colour on the outside, and white within. They have an agreeable camphoraceous smell, and a bitterish aromatic taste. Though formerly much esteemed against rheumatic affections, they are at present thought to possess very little medicinal powers, although they had a place in the confectio aromatica of the London Pharmacopœia.

KA'JEPUT OLEUM. See *Melaleuca.*

KA'LI. (An Arabian word.) The vegetable alkali. See *Potassa.*

KALI ACETATUM. See *Potassæ acetas.*

KALI AERATUM. See *Potassæ carbonas.*

KALI ARSENICATUM. A preparation of arsenic, composed of the vegetable alkali and the acid of arsenic.

KALI CITRATUM. See *Potassæ citras.*

KALI PRÆPARATUM. See *Potassæ subcarbonas.*

KALI PURUM. See *Potassæ fusa.*

KALI SULPHURATUM. See *Sulphuretum potassæ.*

KALI TARTARIZATUM. See *Potassæ tartras.*

KALI VITRIOLATUM. See *Potassæ sulphas.*

KARPHOLITE. A yellow mineral which occurs in thin prismatic concretions.

KEEL. See *Carina.*

Keeled leaf. See *Carinatus.*

KEILL, JAMES, was born in Scotland, 1673. After going through the proper studies abroad, and especially attending to anatomy, he was enabled to lecture on that subject with great reputation in both the Eng-

lish universities, and received an honorary degree at Cambridge. During this period he published a Compendium of Anatomy, chiefly from Cowper. In 1703 he settled in practice at Northampton; and three years after sent to the Royal Society an account of the dissection of a man, reputed to have been 130 years of age; which agreed very much with what Harvey found in old Parr. He was well skilled in mathematics, which he applied to the explanation of the laws of the animal economy. In 1708, he published "An Account of Animal Secretion, the Quantity of Blood in the Human Body, and Muscular Motion." To which, in a second edition, he added an Essay on the Force of the Heart. This engaged him in a controversy with Dr. Jurin, which was carried on in the Philosophical Transactions (Dr. Keill being then a member of the Royal Society) till the period of his premature death in 1719, occasioned by a cancer in the mouth, to which he had applied the cautery, but without any relief.

KEI'RI. See *Cheiranthus cheiri*

KELP. Incinerated seaweed.

KENEANGIA. (From κενος, empty, and αγγειον, a vessel.) 1. A state of inaction of the blood or other vessels.

2. A deficiency of blood in the vessels.

KERATE. The third mineral order of Mohs.

KERATO-PHARYNGÆUS. (From κερας, a horn, and φαρυγξ, the pharynx.) A muscle so named from its shape, and insertion in the pharynx.

KE'RMES. (*Chermah,* Arabian.) *Granum tinctorium; Coccus baphica.* Round reddish grains, about the size of peas, found in Spain, Italy, and the south of France, adhering to the branches of the scarlet oak. They are the nidus of a minute red animalcule, called *Coccus quercus ilicis.* The *confectio alkermes,* now obsolete, was prepared with these, which possess corroborant and adstringent virtues.

KERMES MINERALIS. A preparation of antimony, so termed from its resemblance in colour to the insect of that name. It is now disused in medicine, and gives place to the other preparations of antimony. See *Hydrosulphuretum stibii rubrum.*

KERNEL WORT. See *Scrophularia nodosa.*

KE'RVA. (*Kervah,* Arabian.) The *Ricinus communis.*

KETCHUP. The prepared liquor of the mushroom, made by sprinkling salt on that vegetable, and collecting the fluid which escapes.

KEYSER'S PILLS. A once celebrated mercurial medicine, the method of preparing which was purchased by the French government, and has since been published by Richard. The hydrargyrus acetatus is considered as an adequate substitute for the more elaborate form of Keyser. Richard concludes his account of Keyser's pills with observing, that he considers it to be, without exception, the most effectual remedy for the venereal disease hitherto discovered. But further trials of this remedy do not justify the sanguine accounts of its properties; though it may sometimes succeed when some of the other mercurial preparations have failed.

KIBES. A name for chilblains.

KIDRIA TERRESTRIS. Barbadoes tar.

KIDNEY. (*Ren, nis.* m.) An abdominal viscus,

shaped like a kidney-bean, that secretes the urine. There are two kidneys. One is situated in each lumbar region, near the first lumbar vertebra, behind the peritonæum. This organ is composed of three substances; a cortical, which is external, and very vascular; a tubulous, which consists of small tubes; and a papillous substance, which is the innermost. The kidneys are generally surrounded with more or less adipose membrane, and they have also a proper membrane, *membrana propria*, which is closely accreted to the cortical substance. The renal arteries, called also emulgents, proceed from the aorta. The veins evacuate their blood into the ascending cava. The absorbents accompany the blood-vessels, and terminate in the thoracic duct. The nerves of the kidneys are branches of the eighth pair and great intercostal. The excretory duct of this viscus is called the *ureter*. At the middle of the kidney, where the blood-vessels enter it, is a large membraneous bag. called the pelvis, which diminishes like a funnel, and forms a long canal, the ureter, that conveys the urine from the kidney to the bladder, which it perforates obliquely.

Kidney-shaped leaf. See *Reniformis.*

KIFFEKILL. See *Meerschaum.*

KIKEKUNEMALO. A pure resin, very similar to copal, but of a more beautiful whiteness and transparency. It is brought from America, where it is said to be used medicinally, in the cure of hysteria, tetanus, &c. It forms the most beautiful of all varnishes.

KI′KI. (*Kike*, Arabian.) See *Ricinus.*

KI′NA KINA. See *Cinchona.*

KINATE. *Kinas.* A compound of the Kinic acid, with a salifiable base.

KINIC ACID. (*Acidum kinicum;* from *kinia,* the French name of *cinchona,* from which it is obtained.) "A peculiar acid extracted from cinchona. Let a watery extract from hot infusions of the bark in powder be made. Alkohol removes the resinous part of this extract, and leaves a viscid residue, of a brown colour, which has hardly any bitter taste, and which consists of kinate of lime and a mucilaginous matter. This residue is dissolved in water, the liquor is filtered and left to spontaneous evaporation in a warm place. It becomes thick like syrup, and then deposites by degrees crystalline plates, sometimes hexaëdral, sometimes rhomboidal, sometimes square, and always coloured slightly of a reddish-brown. These plates of kinate of lime must be purified by a second crystallization. They are then dissolved in ten or twelve times their weight of water, and very dilute aqueous oxalic acid is poured into the solution, till no more precipitate is formed. By filtration, the oxalate of lime is separated, and the kinic acid being concentrated by spontaneous evaporation, yields regular crystals. It is decomposed by heat. While it forms a soluble salt with lime, it does not precipitate lead or silver from their solutions. These are characters sufficiently distinctive.

The kinates are scarcely known; that of lime consti tutes seven per cent. of *cinchona.*"

KINKI′NA. See *Cinchona.*

KINO. (An Indian word.) *Gummı gambiense; Gummi rubrum adstringens gambiense.* The tree from which this resin is obtained, though not botanically ascertained, is known to grow on the banks of the river Gambia, in Africa. On wounding its bark the fluid kino immediately issues drop by drop, and, by the heat of the sun, is formed into hard masses. It is in appearance very like the resin called *Sanguis draconis;* much redder, more firm, resinous, and adstringent than catechu. It is now in common use, and is one of the most efficacious vegetable adstringents, or strptics, in the materia medica. Its dose is from twenty to thirty grains.

KNEE-HOLLY. See *Ruscus.*

KNEE-PAN. See *Patella.*

KOLLYRITE. A light greasy mineral of a white colour, which adheres to the tongue.

KOLTO. (A Polonese word.) The plica polonica, or plaited hair.

KOUMIS. A vinous liquid which the Tartars make by fermenting mare's milk. Something similar is prepared in the Orkneys and Shetland.

KRAMERIA. (So named in commemoration of two German botanists, who flourished about the middle of the last century.) The name of a genus of plants in the Linnæan system. Class, *Tetrandria;* Order, *Monogynia.*

KRAMERIA TRIANDRIA. The systematic name of the tree, the root of which is called *rhatania,* a substance which has been long known to the manufacturers of port wine; it is the production of Peru, and was long thought to be the root of the cinchona cordifolia. It is described as externally resembling the root of the rubia tinctorum to the taste, being aromatic, bitter, and very astringent; its infusion or decoction turns black with sulphate of iron, and precipitates tannin. The principal virtues appear to reside in the cortical part of the root, which is thick and resinous. An opinion prevails that the substance sold in the shops under the name of foreign extract of bark, is made from this root.

It is well known that the medical virtues of this root are powerfully tonic. In debility of the digestive organs, in chronic rheumatisms, fluor albus, and in intermittent fevers, it has been employed with good effect. While given in doses similar to cinchona, i has the advantage of being only one-third the price of that substance.

KRAMERIC ACID. (*Acidum kramericum;* from *krameria,* the name of the plant from which it is obtained.) An acid obtained by Peschier from the root of the *Krameria triandria*

KYANITE. See *Cyanite.*

KYNA′NCHE. See *Cynanche.*

L

LA′BDANUM. See *Cistus creticus.*

LABELLUM. A little lip. Applied in botany to the barba, or inferior lip, of ringent and personate plants. See *Corolla.*

LABIUM. (*Labium, i. n.*; απο του λαβειν.)
1. The lip of animals.
2. Applied in botany to corolls of plants, which are termed *unilabiate, bilabiate,* &c.; and from their position in certain flowers, *superior, inferior,* &c.

LA′BIUM LEPORINUM. See *Hare-lip.*

LABORATO′RIUM. (From *laboro,* labour.) A place properly fitted up for the performance of chemical operations.

LABRADOR STONE. See *Felspar.*

LA′BYRINTH. *Labyrinthus.* That part of the internal ear which is behind the cavity of the tympanum; it is constituted by the cochlea, vestibulum, and semicircular canals. See *Ear.*

LAC. (*Lac. tis.* n.) 1. Milk. See *Milk.*
2. The name of a vegetable substance. See *Lacca.*

LAC AMMONIACI. See *Mistura ammoniaci.*

LAC AMYGDALÆ. See *Mistura amygdalæ.*

LAC ASSAFŒTIDÆ. See *Mistura assafœtidæ.*

LAC SULPHURIS. See *Sulphur præcipitatum.*

LA′CCA. (From *lakah,* Arabian.) *Gummi laccæ.* Stick-lac; Gum-lac; Seed-lac; Shell-lac. The improper name of gum-lac is given to a concrete brittle substance, of a dark red colour, brought from the East Indies, incrustated on the twigs of the *Croton lacciferum; foliis ovatis tomentosis serrulatis petiolatis, calycibus tomentosis,* of Linnæus, where it is deposited by a small insect, at present not scientifically known. It is found in very great quantities on the uncultivated mountains on both sides the Ganges, and is of great use to the natives in various works of art, as varnish, painting, dying, &c. When the resinous matter is broken off the wood into small pieces or grains, it is

4

termed *seed-lac*, and when melted and formed into flat plates, *shell-lac*. This substance is chiefly employed for making sealing-wax. A tincture of it is recommended as an antiscorbutic to wash the gums.

LA'CHRYMA. A tear. A limpid fluid secreted by the lachrymal gland, and flowing on the surface of the eye. See *Tear*.

LACHRYMA ABIEGNA. See *Terebinthina argentoratensis*.

LACHRYMAL. *Lachrymalis.* Of or belonging to tears, or parts near where they are secreted.

LACHRYMAL BONE. See *Unguis os*.

LACHRYMAL DUCT. *Ductus lachrymalis.* The excretory duct of the lachrymal gland, which opens upon the internal surface of the upper eyelid.

LACHRYMAL GLAND. *Glandula lachrymalis.* A glomerate gland, situated above the external angle of the orbit, in a peculiar depression of the frontal bone. It secretes the tears, and conveys them to the eye by its excretory ducts, which are six or eight in number.

LACHRYMAL NERVE. The fifth pair of nerves from the head is divided into several branches, the first of which is called the orbitary branch; this is divided into three more, the third of which is called the *lachrymal branch*; it goes off chiefly to the lachrymal gland.

LACCIC ACID. (*Acidum laccicum;* from *lacca*, the substance in which it exists.) "Dr. John made a watery extract of powdered stick-lac, and evaporated it to dryness. He digested alcohol on this extract, and evaporated the alkoholic extract to dryness. He then digested this mass in ether, and evaporated the ethereal solution; when he obtained a syrupy mass of a light yellow colour, which was again dissolved in alkohol. On adding water to this solution, a little resin fell. A peculiar acid united to potassa and lime remains in the solution, which is obtained free, by forming with acetate of lead an insoluble lacoate, and decomposing this with the equivalent quantity of sulphuric acid. Laccic acid crystallizes; it has a wine-yellow colour, a sour taste, and is soluble, as we have seen, in water, alkohol, and ether. It precipitates lead and mercury white; but it does not affect lime, barytes, or silver, in their solutions. It throws down the salts of iron white. With lime, soda, and potassa, it forms deliquescent salt, soluble in alkohol."

LACINIATUS. Laciniate, fringe-like: cut into numerous irregular portions; applied to leaves, petals, &c.; as the leaves of the *Ranunculus parviflorus*, and *Geranium columbinum*, the petals of the *Reseda*.

LACO'NICUM. (Because they were much used by the people of Laconia.) A stove, or sweating-room.

LACQUER. A solution of lac in alkohol.

LACTATE. *Lactas.* A definite compound, formed by the union of the acid of sour whey, or lactic acid, with salifiable bases; thus lactate of potassa, &c.

LACTATION. (*Lactatio;* from *lacteo*, to suckle.) The giving suck.

LACTEAL. (*Lacteus;* from *lac*, milk; because the fluid they absorb looks like milk.)

1. Milky.

2. In anatomy, this term is applied to the *vasa lactea*. The absorbents of the mesentery, which originate in the small intestines, and convey the chyle from thence to the thoracic duct. They are very tender and transparent vessels, possessed of an infinite number of valves, which, when distended with chyle, a milky or lacteal fluid, give them a knotty appearance. They arise from the internal surface of the villous coat of the small intestine, perforate the other coats, and form a kind of net-work, while the greater number unite one with another between the muscular and external coats. From thence they proceed between the laminæ of the mesentery to the conglobate glands. In their course they constitute the greater part of the gland through which they pass, being distributed through them several times, and curled in various directions. The lacteals having passed these glands, go to others, and at length seek those nearest the mesentery. From these glands, which are only four or five, or perhaps more, the lacteals pass out and ascend with the mesenteric artery, and unite with the lymphatics of the lower extremities, and those of the abdominal viscera, and then form a common trunk, the *thoracic duct*, which, in some subjects, is dilated at its origin, forming the *receptaculum chyli*. See *Nutrition*.

LACTESCENS. (From *lac*, milk.) Lactescent or milky.

LACTIC ACID. (*Acidum lacticum;* from *lac*, milk.) "By evaporating sour whey to one-eighth, filtering, precipitating with lime-water, and separating the lime by oxalic acid, Scheele obtained an aqueous solution of what he supposed to be a peculiar acid, which has accordingly been termed the *lactic*. To procure, it separate, he evaporated the solution to the consistence of honey, poured on it alkohol, filtered this solution, and evaporated the alkohol. The residuum was an acid of a yellow colour, incapable of being crystallized, attracting the humidity of the air, and forming deliquescent salts with the earths and alkalies.

Bouillon Lagrange since examined it more narrowly, and from a series of experiments concluded, that it consists of acetic acid, muriate of potassa, a small portion of iron probably dissolved in the acetic acid, and an animal matter.

This judgment of Lagrange was afterward supported by the opinions of Fourcroy and Vauquelin. But since then, Berzelius has investigated its nature very fully, and has obtained, by means of a long and often-repeated series of different experiments, a complete conviction that Scheele was in the right, and that the lactic acid is a peculiar acid, very distinct from all others.

The lactic acid, purified, has a brown-yellow colour, and a sharp sour taste, which is much weakened by diluting it with water. It is without smell in the cold, but emits, when heated, a sharp sour smell, not unlike that of sublimed oxalic acid. It cannot be made to crystallize, and does not exhibit the slightest appearance of a saline substance; but dries into a thick and smooth varnish, which slowly attracts moisture from the air. It is very easily soluble in alkohol. Heated in a gold spoon over the flame of a candle, it first boils, and then its pungent acid smell becomes very manifest, but extremely distinct from that of the acetic acid; afterward it is charred, and has an empyreumatic, but by no means an animal, smell. A porous charcoal is left behind, which does not readily burn to ashes. When distilled, it gives an empyreumatic oil, water, empyreumatic vinegar, carbonic acid, and inflammable gases. With alkalies, earths, and metallic oxides, it affords peculiar salts; and these are distinguished by being soluble in alkohol, and in general by not having the least disposition to crystallize, but drying into a mass like gum, which slowly becomes moist in the air.

LA'CTICA. The Arabian name for the fever which the Greeks call *Typhos*.

LACTIFUGA. (From *lac*, milk, and *fugo*, to drive away.) A medicine or other means which dispel milk.

LACTU'CA. (From *lac*, milk; named from the milky juice which exudes upon its being wounded.) 1. The name of a genus of plants in the Linnæan system. Class, *Syngenesia;* Order, *Polygamia æqualis*. The lettuce.

2. The pharmacopœial name of the garden-lettuce, the *Lactuca sativa*.

LACTUCA GRAVEOLENS. See *Lactuca virosa*.

LACTUCA SATIVA. The systematic name of the lettuce. It is esteemed as a wholesome, aperient, bitter anodyne, easy of digestion, but affording no nutriment. Lettuces appear to agree better with hot, bilious, melancholic temperaments, than the phlegmatic. The seeds possess a quantity of oily substance, which, triturated with water, forms an emulsion esteemed by some in ardor urinæ, and some diseases of the urinary passages. Lettuce was famous for the cure of the emperor Augustus, and formed the opiate of Galen, in his old age; a proof that, in the warmer climates, it must acquire an exaltation of its virtues above what is met with in this country.

LACTUCA SCARIOLA. *Lactuca sylvestris; Scariola; Scariola gallorum.* This species possesses a stronger degree of bitterness than the *Lactuca sativa*, and is said to be more aperient and laxative. It is nearly similar, in virtue as in taste, to endive unblanched.

LACTUCA SYLVESTRIS. See *Lactuca scariola*.

LACTUCA VIROSA. The systematic name of the opium, or strong-scented lettuce. *Lactuca graveolens. Lactuca-foliis horizontalibus carino aculeatis dentatis*, of Linnæus. A common plant in our hedges and ditches. It has a strong, ungrateful smell, resembling that of opium, and a bitterish acrid taste: it abounds with a milky juice, in which its sensible qualities seem to reside, and which appears to have been noticed by Dioscorides, who describes the odour

5

and taste of the juice as nearly agreeing with that of the white poppy. Its effects are also said, according to Haller, to be powerfully narcotic. Dr. Collin, at Vienna, first brought the lactuca virosa into medical repute, and its character has lately induced the College of Physicians at Edinburgh, to insert it in the catalogue of the materia medica. More than twenty-four cases of dropsy are said, by Collin, to have been successfully treated by employing an extract prepared from the expressed juice of this plant, which is stated not only to be powerfully diuretic, but, by attenuating the viscid humours to promote all the secretions, and to remove visceral obstructions. In the more simple cases, proceeding from debility, the extract, in doses of eighteen to thirty grains a-day, proved sufficient to accomplish a cure; but when the disease was inveterate, and accompanied with visceral obstructions, the quantity of extract was increased to three drachms; nor did larger doses, though they excited nausea, ever produce any other bad effect; and the patient continued so strong under the use of this remedy, that it was seldom necessary to employ any tonic medicines. Though Dr. Collin began his experiments with the lactuca at the Pazman hospital, at the time he was trying the arnica, 1771, yet very few physicians, even at Vienna, have since adopted the use of this plant. Plenciz, indeed, has published a solitary instance of its efficacy, while Quarin informs us that he never experienced any good effect from its use; alleging, that those who were desirous of supporting its character, mixed it with a quantity of extractum scillæ. Under these circumstances we shall only say, that the recommendation of this medicine by Dr. Collin will be scarcely thought sufficient to establish its use in England.

["LACTUCA ELONGATA. This is a tall, lactescent, native plant. It is substituted for the *Lactuca virosa* of Europe, which it somewhat resembles in its properties, though of inferior strength. I have no personal experience with this plant, but am informed by physicians who have tried it, that it is anodyne, and promotes the excretion of the skin and kidneys. An extract made by inspissating the expressed juice may be given in doses of from five to fifteen grains. The concrete, lactescent juice would probably be found much stronger."—*Big. Mat. Med.* A.]

["LACTUCARIUM. Common garden-lettuce, like many plants of its class, exudes a milky juice on being wounded after it is fully grown. This juice concretes on exposure to the air, into a brownish, bitter substance, resembling opium in some of its characters. It is most abundant when the plant is in flower, and east so while the leaves are young, or when they are etiolated by heading. Lactucarium has the colour, and in some degree the taste and odour, of opium, for which it has been proposed as a substitute by Dr. Coxe and Dr. Duncan. It has been said to contain morphia in addition to its other component parts. It acts as a soporific, and has been thought useful in phthisis as a palliative. Dose, one or two grains."—*Big. Mat. Med.* A.]

LACTUCE'LLA. (Diminutive of *lactuca*, the lettuce; so named from its milky juice.) The sow-thistle. The *Sonchus arvensis.*

LACTUCI'MINA. (From *lacteo*, to suckle: so called because they happen chiefly to children while at the breast.) The thrush, and little ulcers, or crusty scabs on the skin, which happen during the time the child is at the breast.

LACTU'MEN. (From *lac*, milk; so named because it is covered with a white crust.) The achor, or scald-head; also a little crusty scab on the skin, affecting children at the breast.

LACU'NA. (From *lacus* a channel.) The mouth or opening of the excretory duct of a muciparous gland, as those of the urethra, and other parts.

LA'DANUM. (From *ladon*, Arab.) See *Cistus creticus.*

Ladies' bed-straw. See *Galium.*
Ladies' mantle. See *Alchemilla.*
Ladies' smock. See *Cardamine.*

LÆTIFICA'NTIA. (From *lætifico*, to make glad.) This term has been applied to many compositions under the intention of cordials; but both the medicines and distinctions are now quite disused.

LÆVIS. Smooth and even. Applied to stems of plants, and is opposed to all roughness and inequality whatever.

LÆVITAS INTESTINORUM. A name of the lientery. See *Diarrhœa.*

LA'GAROS. (Λαγαρος, lax; so named from its comparative laxity.) The right ventricle of the heart.

LAGENÆFORMIS. Bottle-shaped. Applied to the gourd; as in *Cucurbita lagenaria.*

LAGNESIS. (From λαγνης, libidinous.) The name of a genus of diseases. Class, *Genetica*; Order, *Orgastica*; in Good's Nosology: lust. It embraces two species, viz. *Lagnesis salacitas*, and *L. furor.*

LAGOPHTHA'LMIA. (From λαγωος, a hare, and οφθαλμος, an eye; because it is believed that hares sleep with their eyes open.) *Lagophthalmos.* The hare's eye. A disease in which the eye cannot be shut. The following complaints may arise from it: a constant weeping of the organ, in consequence of the interruption of the alternate closure and opening of the eyelids, which motions so materially contribute to propelling the tears into the nose; blindness in a strong light, in consequence of the inability to moderate the rays which fall on the eye; on the same account, the sight becomes gradually very much weakened; incapacity to sleep where there is any light; irritation, pain, and redness of the eye, from this organ being exposed to the extraneous substances in the atmosphere, without the eyelids having the power of washing them away in the natural manner.

An enlargement or protrusion of the whole eye, or a staphyloma, may obviously produce lagophthalmos. But affections of the upper eyelids are the common causes. Heister says, he has seen the complaint originate from a disease of the lower one. Now and then lagophthalmos depends on paralysis of the orbicularis muscle. A cicatrix after a wound, ulcer, or burn, is the most frequent cause.

LAGOPO'DIUM. (From λαγωος, a hare, and πους, a foot: so called because it has narrow hairy leaves, like the foot of a hare.) The herb hare's-foot trefoil.

LAGO'STOMA. (From λαγωος, a hare, and ςομα, the mouth: so called because the upper lip is divided in the middle like that of a hare.) See *Hare-lip.*

LAKEWEED. See *Polygonum hydropiper.*

LALLANS. See *Lallatio.*

LALLATIO. That species of vicious pronunciation in which the letter *l* is rendered unduly liquid, or substituted for an *r*. The Greeks denominated it *lambdacismus*, from the letter λ, *lambda.*

LA'MAC. Gum-arabic.

LAMBDACI'SMUS. A defect in speech, which consists in an inability to pronounce certain consonants; or that stammering or difficulty of speech when the letter *l* is pronounced too liquid, and often in the place of *r*. See *Psellismus lallans.*

LAMBDOIDAL. (*Lambdoidalis*; from Λ, and ειδος, resemblance, because it is shaped like the letter Λ.) Belonging to the suture so called.

LAMBDOIDAL SUTURE. (*Sutura lambdoidalis*; because it is shaped like the letter Λ.) Occipital suture. The suture that unites the occipital bone to the two parietal bones.

LAMBITIVUM. (From *lambo*, to lick up.) A linctus or medicine to be licked up.

LAME'LLA. (Dim. of *lamina*, a plate of metal.) 1. A thin plate of metal.

2. The parallel gills or plates in the inferior surface of the agaric family only

LA'MINA. (From ελαω, to beat off.) A bone, or membrane, or any substance resembling a thin plate of metal.

2. The lap of the ear.

3. The parts of the corolla of a polypetalous flower, are named the *unguis*, or claw, and *lamina*, or border.

LAMINABILITY. A property possessed by some bodies of being extended in dimensions by a gradually-applied pressure. See *Ductility.*

LA'MIUM. (From *Lamium*, a mountain of Ionia, where it grew; or from *lama*, a ditch, because it usually grows about ditches and neglected places.) The name of a genus of plants in the Linnæan system. Class, *Didynamia*; Order, *Gymnospermia.* The nettle.

LAMIUM ALBUM. *Urtica mortua; Archangelica; Galeobdolon; Stachys fœtida; Urtica iners magna fœtidissima.* Dead nettle; White archangel nettle. Uterine hæmorrhages and fluor albus are said to be relieved by infusions of this plant, from whose sensible qualities very little benefit can be expected.

LAMPIC ACID. (*Acidum lampeicum* from λαμπω

to shine) "Sir H. Davy, during his admirable researches on the nature and properties of flame, announced the singular fact, that combustible bodies might be made to combine rapidly with oxygen, at temperatures below what were necessary to their *visible* inflammation. Among the phenomena resulting from these new combinations, he remarked the production of a peculiar acid and pungent vapour from the slow combustion of ether; and from its obvious qualities he was led to suspect, that it might be a product yet new to the chemical catalogue. Faraday, in the 3d volume of the Journal of Science and the Arts, has given some account of the properties of this new acid; but from the very small quantities in which he was able to collect it, was prevented from performing any decisive experiments upon it.

In the 6th volume of the same Journal, we have a pretty copious investigation of the properties and compounds of this new acid, by Daniell. From the slow combustion of ether during six weeks, by means of a coil of platina wire sitting on the cotton wick of the lamp, he condensed with the head of an alembic, whose beak was inserted in a receiver, a pint and a half of the lampic acid liquor.

When first collected, it is a colourless fluid, of an intensely sour taste, and pungent odour. Its vapour, when heated, is extremely irritating and disagreeable, and, when received into the lungs, produces an oppression at the chest very much resembling the effect of chlorine. Its specific gravity varies according to the care with which it has been prepared, from less than 1.000 to 1.008. It may be purified by careful evaporation; and it is worthy of remark, that the vapour which rises from it is that of alkohol, with which it is slightly contaminated, and not of ether. Thus rectified, its specific gravity is 1.015. It reddens vegetable blues, and decomposes all the earthy and alkaline carbonates, forming neutral salts with their bases, which are more or less deliquescent."—*Ure's Chem. Dict.*

["Lamp, safety. The safety-lamp as recommended for general use by Sir H. Davy, is a cylinder of wire gauze with a double top, securely and carefully fastened. The whole is protected and rendered convenient for carrying by a frame and ring. If the cylinder be of twilled wire-gauze the wire should be at least of the thickness of one-fortieth of an inch, and of iron or copper, and 30 in the warp, and 16 or 18 in the weft. If of plain wire-gauze the wire should not be less than one-sixtieth of an inch in thickness, and from 28 to 30 both warp and woof.

The operation of this lamp may be shown on a small scale by suspending it in a glass jar, and then admitting a sufficient stream of coal gas to render the enclosed atmosphere explosive. The flame of the lamp first enlarges, and is then extinguished, the whole of the cage being filled with a lambent blue light; on turning off the supply of the gas this appearance gradually ceases and the wick becomes rekindled, when the atmosphere returns to its natural state."—*Web. Man. of Chem.* A.]

LA'MPSANA. See *Lapsana.*

LANA. Wool. In botany, applied to a species of hairy pubescence, consisting of white, long, somewhat crisp hair, like wool. It is applied to stems, leaves, seeds, &c.

Lana philosophica. The snowy flakes of white oxide, which rise and float in the air from the combustion of zinc.

LANATUS. Woolly. Applied to the stems, leaves, seeds, &c. of plants. The Verbascum thapsus is a good example of the *Caulis lanatus;* the Stachys lanata of the leaves; and the Gossypium of the seed.

LANCEOLATUS. Lanceolate, lance-shaped. Applied to leaves, petals, seeds, &c. of a narrow, oblong form, tapering towards each end; as the *leaves* in Plantago lanceolata, and *petals* of Narcissus minor, and *seeds* of the Fraxinus.

LANCE'TTA. (Dim. of *lancea,* a spear.) A lancet. An instrument used for bleeding and other purposes.

LANCISI, John Maria, was born at Rome, in 1654. He was intended for the church, but a taste for natural history led him to the study of medicine, which he pursued with great ardour, and took his degree at the age of 18. After some minor appointments, which enabled him to display his talents and acquirements, he was appointed professor of anatomy in 1684; and continued his duties for 13 years, with great reputation

He was made physician to three succeeding popes, and attained the age of 65. He had great knowledge of mankind, with very engaging manners; and his zeal for the advancement of medicine was extreme and unceasing. He collected a library of above 20,000 volumes, which he devoted to the use of the public, and particularly of medical students: it was opened four years before his death. He left a considerable number of works, several of which were printed, others remain in manuscript in that library. His more important publications are, a treatise, "De Subitaneis Mortibus;" "The Anatomical Plates of Eustachius, with a Preface and Notes, in folio;" and a dissertation, "De Noxiis Paludum Effluviis," referring intermittents to the marsh miasmata, printed in 1717. After his death, a treatise, "De Motu Cordis et Aneurysmatibus," and a collection of cases from his manuscript, were given to the public.

LANGRISH, Browne, a physician of the last century, distinguished himself as an advocate for the mechanical theories of physiology and medicine, which he supported by numerous experiments. He had the merit of ascertaining several interesting facts in respect to the nature of the circulating powers. He died in London, in 1759. His publications are, "A New Essay on Muscular Motion, &c.;" "Modern Theory of Physic;" "Physical Experiments upon Brutes;" and "Croonian Lectures on Muscular Motion."

Lao'nica curatio. A method of curing the gout, by evaporating the morbid matter by topical applications.

LAPA'CTICA. (From λαπαζω, to evacuate.) Purgative medicines.

LA'PARA. (From λαπαζω, to empty; so named from its concave and empty appearance.) The flank.

LAPAROCE'LE. (From λαπαρα, the flank, and κηλη, a rupture.) A rupture through the side of the belly.

LA'PATHUM. (From λαπαζω, to evacuate: so named because it purges gently.) The dock. See *Rumex.*

Lapathum acetosum. See *Rumex acetosa.*

Lapathum acutum. See *Rumex acutus.*

Lapathum aquaticum. See *Rumex hydrolapathum.*

Lapide'llum. (From *lapis,* a stone.) *Lapidellus.* The name of a kind of spoon, formerly used to take out small stones and fragments from the bladder.

LAPIDEUS. Stony. Applied to seeds of plants; as those of the *Lithospermum* and *Osteosperma.*

La'pides cancrorum. See *Cancer.*

Lapi'lli cancrorum. See *Cancer.*

LA'PIS. (*Lapis, idis.* m.; of uncertain deriva tion.) A stone.

Lapis ageratus. See *Ageratus.*

Lapis bezoar. See *Bezoar.*

Lapis cæruleus. See *Lapis lazuli.*

Lapis calaminaris. See *Calamine.*

Lapis calcareus. A carbonate of lime.

Lapis cyanus. See *Lapis lazuli.*

Lapis hæmatites. See *Hæmatites.*

Lapis hibernicus. *Tegula hibernica. Ardesia hibernica. Hardesia.* Irish slate. A kind of slate, or very hard stone, found in different parts of Ireland, in a mass of a bluish-black colour, which stains the hands. When dried and powdered, it is pale, or of a whitish blue, and, by keeping, grows black. In the fire it yields a sulphureous gas, and acquires a pale red colour, with additional hardness. It is occasionally powdered by the common people, and taken in spruce beer, against inward bruises.

Lapis hystricis. See *Bezoar hystricis.*

Lapis infernalis. An old name for the caustic potassa. See *Potassa fusa.*

Lapis lazuli. *Lapis cyanus.* Azure stone. A combination of 46 silica, 28 lime, 14.5 alumina, 3 oxide of iron, 6.5 sulphate of lime, and 2 water, according to Klaproth. This singular mixture forms a stone, of a beautiful azure blue, which it preserves in a strong heat, and does not suffer any alteration by the contact of air. The finest specimens come from China Persia, and Great Bucharia. It was formerly exhibited as a purgative and vomit, and given in epilepsy.

Lapis malacensis. See *Bezoar hystricis.*

Lapis ollaris. Potstone.

Lapis porcinus. See *Bezoar hystricis.*

Lapis simiæ. See *Bezoar simiæ.*

LAPPA. (*Lappa, απο τυ λαβειν,* from its seizing the garments of passengers.) See *Arctium lappa.*

LAPPA MAJOR. See *Arctium lappa.*

LA'PSANA. (*Λαψανη,* from *Lampsacus,* the town near which it flourished; or from *λαπαζω,* to evacuate; because it was said to relax the bowels.) The name of a genus of plants. Class, *Syngenesia;* Order, *Polygamia æquales.*

LAPSANA COMMUNIS. *Lampsana; Napium; Papillaris herba.* Dock-cresses. Nipplewort. This plant is a lactescent bitter, and nearly similar in virtues to the cichory, dandelion, and endive. It has been employed chiefly for external purposes, against wounds and ulcerations, whence the name of nipplewort and papillaris.

LA'QUES GUTTURIS. A malignant inflammation of the tonsils, in which the patient appears as if he were suffocated with a noose.

LARCH. See *Pinus larix.*

LARD. The English name of hog's fat, when melted down. See *Adeps suilla.*

[**LARKSPUR.** See *Delphinium.* A.]

LARYNGISMUS. The name of a genus of diseases, Class, *Pneumatica;* Order, *Pneumonica,* in Good's Nosology. Laryngic suffocation. It has only one species, *stridulus,* the spasmodic croup.

LARYNGOTOMY. (*Laryngotomia;* from *λαρυγξ,* the larynx, and *τεμνω,* to cut.) See *Bronchotomy.*

LARYNX. (*Larynx, gis.* f.; a Greek primitive.) A cartilaginous cavity, situated behind the tongue, in the anterior part of the fauces, and lined with an exquisitely sensible membrane. It is composed of the annular or cricoid cartilage, the scutiform or thyroid, the epiglottis and two arytænoid cartilages. The superior opening of the larynx is called the *glottis.* The *laryngeal arteries* are branches of the external carotids. The *laryngeal veins* evacuate their blood into the external jugulars. The nerves of the larynx are from the eighth pair. The use of the larynx is to constitute the organ of voice, and to serve also for respiration.

LASCI'VUS. (From *lacio,* to ensnare; upon account of its irregular motions.)

1. Lascivious.

2. An epithet used by Paracelsus for the chorea sancti viti.

LA'SER. (A term used by the Cyrenians.) The herb laserwort, or assafœtida.

LASERPI'TIUM. (*Lac serpitium,* alluding to its milky juice.) The name of a genus of plants in the Linnæan system; Class, *Pentandria;* Order, *Digynia.*

LASERPITIUM CHIRONIUM. *Panax.* Hercules' all-heal, or woundwort. The seeds and roots of this plant are warm, and similar in flavour and quality to those of the parsnip. The roots and stalks have a much stronger smell, which resembles that of opoponax; and Boerhaave relates, that, on wounding the plant in the summer, he obtained a yellow juice, which, being inspissated a little in the sun, agreed perfectly in both respects with that exotic gum resin.

LASERPITIUM LATIFOLIUM. The systematic name of the white gentian. *Gentiana alba.* The root of this plant, *Laserpitium foliis cordatis, inciso-serratis,* of Linnæus, possesses stomachic, corroborant, and deobstruent virtues. It is seldom used.

LASERPITIUM SILER. The systematic name of the heartwort. *Seseli; Siler montanum.* Sermountain. The seeds and roots of this plant, which grows in the southern parts of Europe, are directed as officinals. They have an agreeable smell, and a warm, glowing, aromatic taste; and though neglected in this country, do not appear to be deservedly so.

LATERAL. (*Lateralis;* from *latus,* the side.) On the side. A term in general use, applied to parts of the body, operations, and to flower-stalks, when situated on the side of a stem or stalk; as in *Erica vagans.*

LATERAL OPERATION. A name given to an operation. One mode of cutting for the stone, because it is performed on the side of the pelvis. See *Lithotomy.*

LATERAL SINUS. See *Sinus.*

LATERITIOUS. (*Lateritius;* from *later,* a brick.) A term applied to the brick-like sediment occasionally deposited in the urine of people afflicted with fever.

LA'TEX. (*Latex, quod in venis terræ lateat.*)

Water, or juice. A term sometimes applied to the blood, as being the spring or source of all the humours.

LA'THYRIS. (From *λαθω,* to forget; because it was thought to affect the memory.) A term given by some author to a species of tithymal or spurge, commonly known by the name of *Tithymalus latifolius,* the broad-leaved spurge, and called by some also *Cataputia.*

LA'THYRUS. (A name adopted from Theophrastus, whose *λαθυμος,* appears evidently to be like ours, something of the pea or vetch kind, though it is impossible precisely to determine what.) The name of a genus of plants in the Linnæan system. Class, *Diadelphia;* Order, *Decandria.* The vetch.

LATI'BULUM. (From *lateo,* to lie hid.) The fomes or hidden matter of infectious diseases.

LATI'SSIMUS. A term applied to a muscle from its great breadth.

LATISSIMUS COLLI. See *Platysma myoides.*

LATISSIMUS DORSI. *Aniscalptor,* of Cowper. *Dorsi-lumbo sacro humeral,* of Dumas. A muscle of the humerus, situated on the posterior part of the trunk. It is a very broad, thin, and, for the most part, fleshy muscle, which is placed immediately under the skin except where it is covered by the lower extremity of the trapezius. It arises tendinous from the posterior half of the upper edge of the spine of the os ilium, from the spinous processes of the os sacrum and lumbar vertebræ, and from five or six, and sometimes from seven, and even eight, of the lowermost ones of the back; also tendinous and fleshy from the upper edges and external surface of the four inferior false ribs, near their cartilages, by as many distinct slips. From these different origins the fibres of the muscle run in different directions; those from the ilium and false ribs run almost perpendicularly upwards; those from the sacrum and lumbar vertebræ, obliquely upwards and forwards; and those from the vertebræ of the back, transversely outwards and forwards, over the inferior angle of the scapula, where they receive a small thin bundle of fleshy fibres, which arise tendinous from that angle, and are inserted with the rest of the muscle, by a strong, flat, and thin tendon, of about two inches in length, into the forepart of the posterior edge of the groove observed between the two tuberosities of the os humeri, for lodging the tendon of the long head of the biceps. In dissection, therefore, this muscle ought not to be followed to its insertion, till some of the other muscles of the os humeri have been first raised. Its use is to pull the os humeri downwards and backwards, and to turn it upon its axis. Riolanus, from its use on certain occasions, gave it the name of *ani tersor.* When we raise ourselves upon our hands, as in rising from off an arm-chair, we may easily perceive the contraction of this muscle. A *bursa mucosa* is found between the tendon of this muscle and the os humeri, into which it is inserted.

LAUCA'NIA. (From *λαυω,* to receive: so called because it receives and conveys food.) The œsophagus.

LAU'DANUM. (From *laus,* praise: so named from its valuable properties.) See *Tinctura opii.*

LAUMONITE. Diprismatic zeolite.

LAUREL. See *Laurus.*

Laurel, cherry. See *Prunus laurocerasus.*

Laurel, spurge. See *Daphne laureola.*

LAURE'OLA. (Dim. of *laurus,* the laurel: named from its resemblance to the laurel.) See *Daphne laureola.*

LAURO-CERASUS. (From *laurus,* the laurel, and *cerasus,* the cherry-tree: so called because it has leaves like the laurel.) See *Prunus laurocerasus.*

LAURO'SIS. (So called from Mount Laurus, where there were silver mines.) The spodium of silver.

LAU'RUS. (From *laus,* praise; because it was usual to crown the heads of eminent men with branches of it.) 1. The name of a genus of plants in the Linnæan system. Class, *Enneandria;* Order, *Monogynia.* The laurel.

2. The pharmacopœial name of the sweet bay. See *Laurus nobilis.*

LAURUS CAMPHORA. The systematic name of the camphire-tree. *Laurus—foliis triplinerviis lanceolato-ovatis.* It affords the substance called *Camphora; Camphura; Caf; Cafar; Ligatura veneris; Caphora; Capur; Alkosor; Altesor.* Camphire, or camphor, is a peculiar concrete substance prepared by distillation

The tree is indigenous and grows abundantly. The camphire is found to lodge everywhere in the interstices of the fibres of the wood, pith, and knots of the tree. The crude camphire, exported from Japan, appears in small grayish pieces, and is intermixed with various extraneous matters; in this state it is received by the Dutch, and purified by a second sublimation; it is then formed into loaves, in which state it is sent to England.

"Purified camphor is a white concrete crystalline substance, not brittle, but easily crumbled, having a peculiar consistence resembling that of spermaceti, but harder. It has a strong lively smell, and an acrid taste; is so volatile as totally to exhale when left exposed in a warm air; is light enough to swim on water; and is very inflammable, burning with a very white flame and smoke, without any residue.

The roots of zedoary, thyme, rosemary, sage, the inula hellenium, the anemone, the pasque flower or pulsatilla, and other vegetables, afford camphor by distillation. It is observable, that all these plants afford a much larger quantity of camphor, when the sap has been suffered to pass to the concrete state by several months' drying. Thyme and peppermint, slowly dried, afford much camphor; and Achard has observed that a smell of camphor is disengaged when volatile oil of fennel is treated with acids.

Kind, a German chemist, endeavouring to incorporate muriatic acid gas with oil of turpentine, by putting this oil into the vessels in which the gas was received when extricated, found the oil change, first yellow, then brown, and, lastly, to be almost wholly coagulated into a crystalline mass, which comported itself in every respect like camphor. Tromsdorf and Boullay confirm this. A small quantity of camphor may be obtained from oil of turpentine by simple distillation at a very gentle heat. Other essential oils, however, afford more. By evaporation in shallow vessels, at a heat not exceeding 57° F., Proust obtained from oil of lavender .25, of sage .21, of marjoram .1014, of rosemary .0625. He conducted the operation on a pretty large scale.

Camphor is not soluble in water in any perceptible degrees, though it communicates its smell to that fluid, and may be burned as it floats on its surface. It is said, however, that a surgeon at Madrid has effected its solution in water by means of the carbonic acid.

Camphor may be powdered by moistening it with alkohol, and triturating it till dry. It may be formed into an emulsion by previous grinding with near three times its weight of almonds, and afterward gradually adding the water. Yelk of egg and mucilages are also effectual for this purpose; but sugar does not answer well.

It has been observed by Romieu, that small pieces of camphor floating on water have a rotatory motion.

Alkohol, ethers, and oils, dissolve camphor.

The addition of water to the spirituous or acid solutions of camphor, instantly separates it.

Hatchett has particularly examined the action of sulphuric acid on camphor. A hundred grains of camphor were digested in an ounce of concentrated sulphuric acid for two days. A gentle heat was then applied, and the digestion continued for two days longer. Six ounces of water were then added, and the whole distilled to dryness. Three grains of an essential oil, -aving a mixed odour of lavender and peppermint, came over with the water. The residuum being treated twice with two ounces of alkohol each time, fifty-three grains of a compact coal in small fragments remained undissolved. The alkohol, being evaporated in a water-bath, yielded forty-nine grains of a blackish-brown substance, which was bitter, astringent, had the smell of caromel, and formed a dark brown solution with water. This solution threw down very dark brown precipitates, with sulphate of iron, acetate of lead, muriate of tin, and nitrate of lime. It precipitated gold in the metallic state. Isinglass threw down the whole of what was dissolved in a nearly black precipitate.

When nitric acid is distilled repeatedly in large quantities from camphor, it converts it into a peculiar acid." See *Camphoric acid*.

The use of this important medicine, in different diseases, is very considerable. It has been much employed, with great advantage, in fevers of all kinds,

particularly in nervous fevers, attended with delirium and much watchfulness. The experienced Werlhoff has witnessed its utility in several inflammatory diseases, and speaks highly in favour of its refrigerant qualities. The benefit derived from it in putrid fevers, where bark and acids are contra-indicated, is remarkable. In spasmodic and convulsive affections it is also of much service, and even in epilepsy. In chronic diseases this medicine is likewise employed; and against rheumatism, arthritis, and mania, we have several accounts of its efficacy. Nor is it less efficacious when applied externally in certain diseases: it dissipates inflammatory tumours in a short time; and its antiseptic quality, in resisting and curing gangrene, is very considerable. Another property peculiar to this medicine, must not, however, be omitted; the power it possesses of obviating the strangury that is produced by cantharides, when sprinkled over a blister. The preparations of camphor are, *spiritus camphoræ, linimentum camphoræ, tinctura camphoræ composita*, and the *mistura camphoræ*. Camphor, dissolved in acetic acid with some essential oils, forms the aromatic vinegar.

LAURUS CASSIA. *Cassia lignea; Canella malabarica; Cassia lignea malabarica; Xylocassia; Canella malabarica et javensis; Karva; Canella cubana; Arbor judaica; Cassia canella; Canellifera malabarica; Cinnamomum malabaricum; Calihacha canela.* Wild cinnamon-tree; Malabar cinnamon-tree, or castia lignea-tree. Cassia lignea is the bark of the *Laurus* tree, the *foliis triplinerviis lanceolatis*, of Linnæus. The leaves are called *folia malabathri* in the shops. The bark and leaves abound with the flavour of cinnamon, for which they may be substituted; but in much larger doses, as they are considerably weaker.

LAURUS CINNAMOMUM. The systematic name of the cinnamon-tree. *Cinnamomum*. This tree affords the true cinnamon, which is its inner bark. Jacquin describes the tree thus: *Laurus cinnamomum; foliis trinerviis ovato-oblongis; nervis versus apicem evanescentibus.* Cinnamon bark is one of the most grateful of the aromatics; of a fragrant smell, and a moderately pungent, glowing, but not fiery taste, accompanied with considerable sweetness, and some degree of astringency. It is one of the best cordial carminative and restorative spices we are in possession of, and is generally mixed with the diet of the sick. The essential oil, on account of its high price, is seldom used: a tincture, simple and spirituous water, are directed to be kept in the shops. The watery infusion of cinnamon is given with advantage to relieve nausea and check vomiting.

LAURUS CULILAWAN. The systematic name of the plant, the bark of which is called *cortex culilawan* in the shops. *Cullitlawan; Cortex caryophylloides. Laurus—foliis triplinerviis oppositis*, of Linnæus This bark very much resembles cinnamon in appearance and properties.

LAURUS NOBILIS. The systematic name of the sweet bay-tree. *Laurus—foliis venosis lanceolatis perennantibus, floribus quadrifidis*, of Linnæus. This tree is a native of Italy, but cultivated in our gardens and shrubberies, as a handsome evergreen. The leaves and berries possess the same medicinal qualities, both having a sweet fragrant smell, and an aromatic adstringent taste. The laurus of honorary memory, the distinguished favourite of Apollo, may be naturally supposed to have had no inconsiderable fame as a medicine; but its pharmaceutical uses are so limited in the practice of the present day, that this dignified plant is now rarely employed, except in the way of enema, or as an external application: thus the leaves are directed in the *decoctum pro fomento*, and the berries in the *emplastrum cumini.*

LAURUS PERSEA. This species affords the *Avigato pear*, which, when ripe, melts in the mouth like marrow, which it greatly resembles in flavour. It is supposed to be the most nutritious of all the tropical fruits, and grows in vast abundance in the West Indies and New Spain. The unripe fruit have but little taste; yet, being very salubrious, are often eaten with salt and pepper. The sailors, when they arrive at the Havana, and those parts, purchase them in great quantities; and, chopping them into small pieces, with green capsicums, and a little salt, regale themselves heartily with them. They are esteemed also for their antidysenteric qualities, and are prepared in a variety of ways for the tables of the rich.

LAURUS SASSAFRAS. The systematic name of the sassafras-tree. *Sassafras; Cornus mas odorata; Lignum pavanum; Anhuiba.* The wood of this tree, *Laurus—foliis trilobis integrisque,* of Linnæus, is imported from North America, in long straight pieces, very light, and of a spongy texture, and covered with a rough, fungous bark. It has a fragrant smell, and a sweetish, aromatic, subacrid taste; the root, wood, and bark agree in their medicinal qualities, and are all mentioned in the pharmacopœias; but the bark is the most fragrant, and thought to be more efficacious than the woody part; and the branches are preferred to the large pieces. The medical character of this drug was formerly held in great estimation, and publications were professedly written on the subject. It is now, however, thought to be of little importance, and seldom used but in conjunction with other medicines, as a corrector of the fluids. It is an ingredient in the *decoctum sarsaparillæ compositum,* or *decoctum lignorum;* but the only officinal preparation of it is the essential oil, which is carminative and stimulant, and which may be given in the dose of two drops to ten.

LAVA. The cinders or product of volcanoes.

LAVA'NDULA. See *Lavendula.*

LAVENDER. See *Lavendula.*

Lavender, French. See *Lavendula stæchas.*

LAVE'NDULA. (From *lavo,* to wash: so called, because, on account of its fragrancy, it was used in baths.) 1. The name of a genus of plants in the Linnæan system. Class, *Didynamia;* Order, *Gymnospermia.* Lavender.

2. The pharmacopœial name of the common lavender. See *Lavendula spica.*

LAVENDULA SPICA. The systematic name of the common lavender. *Nardus italica. Lavendula—foliis sessilibus lanceolato-linearibus margine revolutis, spica interrupta nuda,* of Linnæus. A native of the southern parts of Europe, but cultivated in our gardens on account of the fragrance of its flowers. Their taste is bitter, warm, and somewhat pungent; the leaves are weaker and less grateful. The essential oil, obtained by distillation, is of a bright yellow colour, of a very pungent taste, and possesses, if carefully distilled, the fragrance of the lavender in perfection. Lavender has been long recommended in nervous debilities, and various affections proceeding from a want of energy in the animal functions. The College directs an essential oil, a simple spirit, and a compound tincture, to be kept in the shops.

LAVENDULA STŒCHAS. The systematic name of the French lavender. *Stæchas; Stæchas arabica; Spica hortulana; Stucadore.* This plant is much less grateful in smell and flavour than the common lavender, to which it is allied in its properties.

LA'VER. (From *lavo,* to wash: so named because it is found in brooks, where it is constantly washed by the stream.)

1. The brook-lime.

2. The English name of a species of fucus which is eaten as a delicacy.

LAVIPE'DIUM. (From *lavo,* to wash, and *pes,* the foot.) A bath for the feet.

LAWSONIA. (After Mr. Lawson, a Scotchman, who published an excellent account of his voyage to Carolina, containing much information concerning the plants of that country.) The name of a genus of plants in the Linnæan system. Class, *Octandria;* Order, *Monogynia.*

LAWSONIA INERMIS. The systematic name of the true alkanna. *Alkanna vera; alkanna orientalis.* An oriental plant; the *Lawsonia—ramis inermibus,* of Linnæus; principally employed, in its native place, as a dye. The root is the officinal part; which, however, is rarely met with in the shops. It possesses astringent properties, and may be used as a substitute for the *anchusa.*

LAXATI'VA. (From *laxo,* to loosen.) Gentle purgatives.

LAXA'TOR. (From *laxo,* to loosen: so called from its office to relax.) A name applied to muscles, the office of which is to relax parts into which they are inserted.

LAXATOR TYMPANI. *Externus mallei,* of Albinus; *Anterior mallei,* of Winslow; *Obliquus auris,* of Douglas; *Externus auris vel laxator internus* of

10

Cowper; and *Sphem salpingo mallien,* of Dumas. A muscle of the internal ear, that draws the malleus obliquely forwards towards its origin; consequently the membrana tympani is made less concave, or is relaxed.

LAXUS. Lax or diffused. Applied by botanists in opposition to *rectus* and *strictus;* as in the stem of the *Bunias cakile,* or sea rocket, the stem of which is described as *caulis laxus.*

LAZULITE. See *Azurite.*

LA'ZULUS. (From *azul,* Arabian.) A precious stone, of a blue colour. See *Lapis lazuli.*

LEAD. *Plumbum.* A metal found in considerable quantity in many parts of the earth, in different states, seldom, if at all, in the metallic state. It is found in that of oxide, *red lead ore,* mixed with a portion of iron, clay, and other earths. The colour of this ore is aurora red, resembling red arsenic. It is found in small lumps, of an indeterminate figure, and also crystallized in four-sided rhomboidal prisms.

Combined with carbonic acid, it forms the *sparry lead ore,* so called because it has the texture and crystallization of certain spars. There are a great many varieties of this kind. It is found also united with sulphuric phosphoric, arsenic, molybdic, and chromic acids. Lastly, lead is found mineralized by sulphur, forming what is called *galena (sulphuret of lead),* which is by far its most abundant ore. This ore, which is very common, is found both in masses and crystals. The primitive form of its crystals is a cube. Its colour is of a bluish lead gray. It has a considerable metallic lustre, its texture is foliated. It stains the fingers, and often feels greasy. It contains in general a minute quantity of silver.

Properties of Lead.—Lead is of a bluish-white colour, and very brilliant when fresh cut. It is malleable. It soon tarnishes in the atmosphere. It may easily be cut with a knife, and stains the fingers bluish-gray when rubbed. It fuses at 612° Fahr. and renders other more refractory metals fusible. It becomes vitrified in a strong and continued heat, and vitrifies various other metals. It is the least elastic of all the metals. It is very laminable, but it possesses very little ductility. Its specific gravity is 11.435. It crystallizes by cooling in small octahedra. When fused in contact with air, its surface first becomes yellow, and then red. It unites by fusion with phosphorus and sulphur. The greater part of the acids act upon it. The sulphuric acid requires the assistance of a boiling heat. Nitric acid is decomposed by it. Muriatic acid acts very weakly on it. Acetic acid dissolves it. Fluoric acid attacks it by heat, and slightly in the cold. It combines with other metals, but few of its alloys are applied to any use. When combined with mercury, it forms a crystallizable alloy which becomes fluid when triturated with that of bismuth.

Method of obtaining Lead.—In order to obtain lead in a great way, the ore is picked from among the extraneous matter with which it was naturally mixed. It is then pulverized and washed. It is next roasted in a reverberatory furnace, in which it is to be agitated, in order to bring the whole in contact with the air. When the external parts begin to soften, or assume the form of a paste, it is covered with charcoal, the mixture is stirred, and the heat increased gradually; the lead then runs on all sides, and is collected at the bottom of the furnace, which is perforated so as to permit the metal to flow into a receptacle defended by a lining of charcoal.

The scoriæ remaining above in the furnace still retain a considerable proportion of lead; in order to extract it, the scoriæ must be fused in a blast furnace. The lead is by that means separated, and cast into iron moulds, each of which contains a portion called a *pig of lead.* These pigs are sold under the name of *ore lead.*

In order to obtain perfectly pure lead, the lead of commerce may be dissolved in pure nitric acid, and the solution be decomposed by adding to it, gradually, a solution of sulphate of soda, so long as a precipitate ensues. This precipitate, which is sulphate of lead, must then be collected on a filter, washed repeatedly in distilled water, and then dried. In order to reduce it to its metallic state, let it be mixed with two or three times its weight of black flux, introduce the mixture into a crucible, and expose it briskly to a red heat.

"There are certainly two, and perhaps three oxides of lead:—

1. The powder precipitated by potassa from the solution of the nitrate of lead, being dried, forms the yellow protoxide. When somewhat vitrified, it con-

stitutes litharge, and combined with carbonic acid, white-lead or ceruse.

2. When massicot has been exposed for about 48 hours to the flame of a reverberatory furnace, it becomes red-lead, or minium.

3. If upon 100 parts of red-lead we digest nitric acid of the sp. gr. 1.26, 92.5 parts will be dissolved, but 7.5 of a dark brown powder will remain insoluble. This is the peroxide of lead.

Chloride of lead is formed, either by placing lead in chlorine, or by exposing the muriate to a moderate heat. It is a semi-transparent, grayish-white mass, somewhat like horn, whence the old name of *plumbum corneum.*

The iodide is easily formed, by heating the two constituents. It has a fine yellow colour. It precipitates when we pour hydriodate of potassa into a solution of nitrate of lead.

The salts of lead have the protoxide for their base, and are distinguishable by the following general characters :—

1. The salts which dissolve in water, usually give colourless solutions, which have an astringent sweetish taste.

2. Placed on charcoal they all yield, by the blowpipe, a button of lead.

3. Ferroprussiate of potassa occasions in their solutions a white precipitate.

4. Hydrosulphuret of potassa, a black precipitate.

5. Sulphuretted hydrogen, a black precipitate.

6. Gallic acid, and infusion of galls, a white precipitate.

7. A plate of zinc, a white precipitate, or metallic lead.

Most of the acids attack lead. The sulphuric does not act upon it, unless it be concentrated and boiling. Sulphurous acid gas escapes during this process, and the acid is decomposed. When the distillation is carried on to dryness, a saline white mass remains, a small portion of which is soluble in water, and is the sulphate of lead; it affords crystals. The residue of the white mass is an insoluble sulphate of lead.

Nitric acid acts strongly on lead.

The nitrate solution, by evaporation, yields tetrahedral crystals, which are white, opaque, and possess considerable lustre.

A *subnitrate* may be formed in pearl-coloured scales, by boiling in water equal weights of the nitrate and protoxide.

Muriatic acid acts directly on lead by heat, oxidizing it, and dissolving part of its oxide.

The acetic acid dissolves lead and its oxides: though probably the access of air may be necessary to the solution of the metal itself in this acid, *white-lead,* or *ceruse,* is made by rolling leaden plates spirally up, so as to leave the space of about an inch between each coil, and placing them vertically in earthen pots, at the bottom of which is some good vinegar. The pots are to be covered, and exposed for a length of time to a gentle heat in a sand-bath, or by bedding them in dung. The vapour of the vinegar, assisted by the tendency of the lead to combine with the oxygen which is present, corrodes the lead, and converts the external portion into a white substance which comes off in flakes, when the lead is uncoiled. The plates are thus treated repeatedly, until they are corroded through. Ceruse is the only white used in oil paintings. Commonly it is adulterated with a mixture of chalk in the shops. It may be dissolved without difficulty in the acetic acid, an affords a crystallizable salt, called *sugar of lead,* from its sweet taste. This, like all the preparations of lead, is a deadly poison. The common sugar of lead is an acetate; and Goulard's extract, made by boiling litharge in vinegar, a subacetate. The power of this salt, as a coagulator of mucus, is superior to the other. If a bit of zinc be suspended by brass or iron wire, or a thread, in a mixture of water and the acetate of lead, the lead will be revived and form an arbor saturni.

The acetate, or sugar of lead, is usually crystallized in needles, which have a silky appearance.

The subacetate crystallizes in plates. The sulphuret, sulphate, carbonate, phosphate, arseniate, and chromate of lead are found native.

When lead is alloyed with an equal weight of tin, or perhaps even less, it ceases to be acted on by vinegar. Acetate and subacetate of lead in solution, has been used as external applications to inflamed sur-

faces, and scrofulous sores, and as eye-washes. In some extreme cases of hæmorrhagy from the lungs and bowels, and uterus, the former salt has been prescribed, but rarely, and in minute doses, as a corrugant or astringent. The colic of the painters, and that formerly prevalent in certain counties of England, from the lead used in the cider presses, show the very deleterious operation of the oxide, or salts of this metal, when habitually introduced into the system in the minutest quantities at a time. Contraction of the thumbs, paralysis of the hand, or even of the extremities, have not unfrequently supervened. A course of sulphuretted hydrogen waters, laxatives, of which sulphur, castor oil, sulphate of magnesia, or calomel, should be preferred, a mercurial course, the hot sea-bath, and electricity, are the appropriate remedies.

Dealers in wines have occasionally sweetened them, when acescent, with litharge or its salts. This deleterious adulteration may be detected by sulphuretted hydrogen water, which will throw down the lead in the state of a dark brown sulphuret. Or, subcarbonate of ammonia, which is a very delicate test, may be employed to precipitate the lead in the state of a white carbonate ; which, on being washed and digested with sulphuretted hydrogen water, will instantly become black. If the white precipitate be gently heated, it will become yellow, and, on charcoal before the blowpipe, it will yield a globule of lead. Chromate of potassa will throw down from saturnine solutions, a beautiful orange-yellow powder. Burgundy wine, and all such as contain tartar, will not hold lead in solution, in consequence of the insolubility of the tartrate.

The proper counter-poison for a dangerous dose of sugar of lead, is a solution of Epsom or Glauber salt, liberally swallowed ; either of which medicines instantly converts the poisonous acetate of lead into the inert and innoxious sulphate. The sulphuret of potassa, so much extolled by Navier, instead of being an antidote, acts itself as a poison on the stomach.

Oils dissolve the oxide of lead, and become thick and consistent; in which state they are used as the basis of plasters, cements for water-works, paints, &c.

Sulphur readily dissolves lead in the dry way, and produces a brittle compound, of a deep gray colour and brilliant appearance, which is much less fusible than lead itself ; a property which is common to all the combinations of sulphur with the more fusible metals.

The phosphoric acid, exposed to heat together with charcoal and lead, becomes converted into phosphorus, which combines with the metal. This combination does not greatly differ from ordinary lead : it is malleable, and easily cut with a knife ; but it loses its brilliancy more speedily than pure lead ; and when fused upon charcoal with the blowpipe, the phosphorus burns, and leaves the lead behind.

Litharge fused with common salt decomposes it ; the lead unites with the muriatic acid, and forms a yellow compound, used as a pigment. The same decomposition takes place in the humid way, if common salt be macerated with litharge ; and the solution will contain caustic alkali.

Lead unites with most of the metals. Gold and silver are dissolved by it in a slight red heat. Both these metals are said to be rendered brittle by a small admixture of lead, though lead itself is rendered more ductile by a small quantity of them. Platina forms a brittle compound with lead ; mercury amalgamates with it ; but the lead is separated from the mercury by agitation, in the form of an impalpable black powder, oxygen being at the same time absorbed. Copper and lead do not unite but with a strong heat. If lead be heated so as to boil and smoke, it soon dissolves pieces of copper thrown into it ; the mixture, when cold, is brittle. The union of these two metals is remarkably slight ; for, upon exposing the mass to a heat no greater than that in which lead melts, the lead almost entirely runs off by itself. This process is called eliquation. The coarser sorts of lead, which owe their brittleness and granulated texture to an admixture of copper, throw it up to the surface on being melted by a small heat. Iron does not unite with lead, as long as both substances retain their metallic form. Tin unites very easily with this metal, and forms a compound, which is much more fusible than lead by itself, and is, for this reason, used as a solder for lead. Two parts of lead and one of tin, form an alloy more fusible than either metal alone : this is the solder of the plumbers

Bismuth combines readily with lead, and affords a metal of a fine close grain, but very brittle. A mixture of eight parts bismuth, five lead, and three tin, will melt in a heat which is not sufficient to cause water to boil. Antimony forms a brittle alloy with lead. Nickel, cobalt, manganese, and zinc, do not unite with lead by fusion."

The preparations of lead used in medicines are:—

1. Plumbi subcarbonas. See *Plumbi subcarbonas.*
2. Oxidum plumbi rubrum. See *Minium.*
3. Oxidum plumbi semivitreum. See *Lithargyrus.*
4. Acetas plumbi. See *Plumbi acetas.*
5. Liquor plumbi acetatis. See *Plumbi acetatis liquor.*
6. Liquor plumbi acetatis dilutus. See *Plumbi acetatis liquor dilutus.*

Lead, white. See *Plumbi subcarbonas.*

LEAF. *Folium.* A laminar expansion of a plant generally of a green colour.

It is difficult, however, to define this universal and important organ of vegetables.

They are considered as the respiratory organs of plants.

Leaves are, for the most part, remarkable for their expanded form; their colour is almost universally green, their internal substance pulpy and vascular, sometimes very succulent, and their upper and under surfaces differ commonly in hue, as well as in kind or degree of roughness.

In discriminating the species of plants, a knowledge of the various forms of leaves is of the utmost importance. Botanists, therefore, have paid particular attention to their names, which are derived either from their origin, distribution, situation, direction, insertion, form, base, point, margin, surface, distribution of its vessels, nerves, expansion, substance, duration, composition, &c.

A leaf consists of a thin and expanded part, which, in common language, is named the leaf, and a stalk called the *petiole* or *petiolus.* The surface of a leaf, *superficies,* or *pagina,* is distinguished into the upper part, or face, and the under part, or back, of the leaf. The *base,* or *origin* of the leaf, is that part next the stem or branch; the *apex* is the termination of the leaf; the *margin,* or edge, the circumference; the *disk,* *discum,* is the middle part of the surfaces within the margin.

From their *origin,* we have the following terms:—

1. *Seminal; folia seminalia,* which are the first leaves of the majority of plants, proceeding from seeds that have more than one seed-lobe; they are seen in Raphanus sativus, and Cannabis sativa.
2. *Radical,* which spring directly from the root; as in Leontodon taraxacum, and Viola odorata.
3. *Cauline,* or stem-leaf. The *Valeriana phu* has its radical leaves undivided, and the cauline leaves pinnate.
4. *Ramial,* or branch-leaf, which are only described when they differ from those of the stem. The *Sison ammi* has its radical leaves, linear; its cauline, setous; and its branch leaves, tripinnate.
5. *Axillary,* when seated on joints or axillæ; as in Parthenium integrifolium.
6. *Floral,* when next the flower, and like the other leaves; as in Lonicera caprifolium.

From their *distribution* on the stem and branches, leaves are named,

7. *Alternate,* when not in pairs, and are given off in various directions, one after another; as in Malva rotundifolia.
8. *Opposite,* when they appear directly on opposite sides of the stem, in pairs; as in Lamium album, and Urtica dioica.
9. *Two-ranked; folia disticha,* which implies that they spread in two directions, and yet are not regularly opposite at their insertion; as in Cupressus disticha, Taxus baccata, Pinus picea, and Lonicera symphoricarpos.
10. *Bifarial,* that is, two-ranked, but given off from the side only of the branch; as in Carpinus betulus, and Fagus sylvatica.
11. *Unilateral,* looking to one side only; as in Convallaria multiflora.
12. *Scattered,* irregular or without any order; as in Reseda luteola, and Sedum reflexum.
13. *Decussate,* crossing each other in pairs; crosslike; as in Euphorbia lathyris, and Crassula tetragona.

14. *Imbricate,* like tiles upon a house; as in Cupressus sempervirens, and Aloe spiralis.
15. *Fasciculate,* or tufted, when several spring from the same point; as in Pinus larix, and Berberis vulgaris.
16. *Stellate,* star-leaved, whirled; several leaves growing in a circle round the stem, without any reference to the precise number; as in Rubia tinctorum, Lilium martagon, Asperula odorata. In large natural genera it is necessary to mention the number; as in Galium.
17. *Remote,* when at an unusual distance from each other.
18. *Clustered;* crowded together; as in Antirrhinum linaria, and Trientalis europea.
19. *Binal,* when there is only two on a plant; as in Galanthus nivalis, Scilla bifolia, and Convallaria magalis.
20. *Ternal,* three together; as in Verbena triphylla.
21. *Quaternal, Quinal,* &c., when four, five, or more are situated together; as in various species of Erica.

From their determinate *direction,* leaves are distinguished into,

22. *Close-pressed; adpressa;* when their upper surface is close to the stem; as in Thlaspi campestris, and Xeranthemum sesamoides.
23. *Erect,* when nearly perpendicular, or forming a very acute angle with the stem; as in Juncus articulatis, and Bryum unquiculatum.
24. *Spreading,* forming a moderately acute angle with the stem; as in Atriplex portulacoides, Nerium oleander, and Veronica beccabunga.
25. *Horizontal,* spreading in the greatest possible degree; as in Gentiana campestris, and Pelargonium patulum.
26. *Ascending,* rising gently, so as to be somewhat arched; as in Geranium nitifolium.
27. *Recurved,* reflexed, curved backward; as in Erica retorta, and Bryum pellucidum.
28. *Reclined,* depending, hanging downward towards the earth; as in Cichorium intybus, and Leonurus cardiaca.
29. *Oblique,* twisted, so that one part is vertical, the other horizontal; as Allium obliquum, and Fritallaria obliqua.
30. *Adverse,* the upper surface turned to the meridian, not the sky; as in Lactuca scariola.
31. *Resupinate,* or reversed, when the upper surface is turned downward; as in Alstromeria pelegrina, and Stœbe prostrata.
32. *Revolute,* having a spiral apex; as Dianthus carthusianorum, and barbatus.
33. *Rooting,* sending rootlets into the earth; as Asplenium rhizophylla.
34. *Floating* on the surface of the water; as in Potamogeton natans, and Nymphæa alba.
35. *Submersed,* demersed, immersed, under water; as Hottonia palustris, and Ranunculus aquatilis.

From their *insertion,* into,

36. *Petiolate,* leaves on footstalks; as Prunus cerasus, and Verbascum nigrum.
37. *Sessile,* without footstalk, lying immediately on the stem; as in Saponaria officinalis, and Pinguicula vulgaris.
38. *Adnate,* the upper surface adhering a little way to the branch; as in Xeranthemum vestitum.
39. *Decurrent,* when a lamellar part of the leaf runs down the stem, or branch; as in Carduus spinosus, and Verbascum thapsus.
40. *Connate,* when two opposite leaves embrace, and are united at their bases; as in Cerastium perfoliatum, and Dipsacus laciniatus.
41. *Connato-perfoliate,* when the union is in the whole or nearly the whole breadth of the leaves, so as to give the two leaves the appearance of being united into but one leaf; as in Eupatorium perfoliatum, and Lonicera dioica. Connate leaves are, in some instances, united by a membrane, which, stretching from the margins of the opposed leaves, near the base, forms a kind of pitcher around the stem, in which the rain is retained; as in Dipsacus fullonium.
42. *Embracing,* clasping the stem with their bases; as in Carduus marianus, and Papaver somniferum.
43. *Vaginate,* sheathing the stem at their bases, as in Canna indica, and Polygonum bistorta.
44. *Peltate,* when the footstalk is inserted, not into

12

the basis, but into the disk of the leaf, as in Drosera peltata, and Tropæolum majus.

45. *Perfoliate*, when the stem runs through the leaf; as in Bupleurum rotundifolium, and Uvularia perfoliata.

46. *Articulate*, one leaf growing out of the apex of another; as Cactus opuntia, and Cactus ficus indica. From the *basis* of the leaf, it is called,

47. *Cordate*, heart-shaped, or ovate, hollowed out at the base; as Arctium lappa, and Tamus communis.

48. *Arrow-shaped*, triangular, hollowed out very much at the base; as Rumex acetosa, and Sagittaria sagittifolia.

49. *Hastate*, halberd-shaped, triangular, hollowed out at the base and sides, but with spreading lobes; as in Arum maculatum, and Rumex acetosella.

50. *Reniform*, kidney shaped, a short, broad, round ish leaf, the base of which is hollowed out; as Asarum europeum, and Glecoma hederacea.

51. *Auricled*, furnished at its base with a pair of leaflets, properly distinct, but occasionally joined with it; as in Citrus aurantium.

Linnæus uses the term *appendiculatum*, which is correct.

52. *Unequal*, the basis larger on one side than the other; as in Tilia europea, and Piper tuberculatum.

The form of the *apex* of a leaf, gives rise to the following names.

53. *Acute*, sharp, ending in an acute angle, which is common to a great number of plants; example in Linum angustifolium, and Campanula trachelium.

54. *Acuminate*, pointed, having a taper, or awl-shaped point; as Arundo phragmitis, and Syringa vulgaris.

55. *Cuspidate*, or *mucronate*, sharp pointed, tipped with a rigid spine, as in the thistles, and Ficus religiosa.

56. *Obtuse*, blunt, terminating in a segment of a circle: as Rumex obtusifolius, and Hypericum quadrangulum.

57. *Retuse*, ending in a broad, shallow notch; as in Ervum ervilia, and Rumex digynus.

58. *Præmorse*, jagged pointed, as if bitten off; very blunt, with various irregular notches; as in Hibiscus præmorsus, and Swartz's genus Aëride.

59. *Truncate*, an abrupt leaf, with the extremity cut off, as it were, by a transverse line; as in Liriodendron tulipifora.

60. *Dedaleous*, with a broad, incised, and crisp apex; as in Asplenium scolopendrum.

61. *Emarginate*, nicked, having a small notch at the summit; as Hydrocotile vulgaris, and Euphorbia tuberosa.

62. *Summit-cut,—folia apice incisa*; as in Glinko biloba.

63. *Cirrhose*, tipped with a tendril; as in Lathyrus articulatus, and Gloriosa superba.

64. *Tridentate*, three-toothed; an obtuse point, beset with three teeth; as in Buchera æthiopica, and Genista tridentata.

65. *Ascidiate*, or pitcher-leaf, a cylindrical tube, filled with water; as in Nepenthes distillatoria, and Saracenia.

The names derived from the *margin* of the leaf, are,

66. *Entire*, not divided; as in Tragopogon pratense, and porrifolium.

67. *Very entire, integerrima*, the margin void of irregularity; as Citrus aurantium.

68. *Undulate*, when the disk near the margin is waved obtusely up and down; as in Panicum hirtellum, and Reseda lutea.

69. *Crenate*, notched, when the teeth are rounded, and not directed towards either end of the leaf; as in Betonica officinalis, and Scutellaria galericulata.

70. *Doubly crenate*, the greater teeth, notched with smaller ones; as in Salvia sclara, and Ranunculus auricomus.

71. *Serrate*, when the teeth are sharp, and resemble those of a saw, pointing towards the extremity of the leaf; as in Sedum telephium.

72. *Acutely serrate*; as in Thymus acines.

73. *Obtusely serrate*; as in Ballota nigra.

74. *Doubly serrate*, having a series of smaller serratures intermixed with the larger; as in Rubus fruticosus, and Campanula trachelium.

75. *Dentate*, toothed, beset with projecting, horizontal, rather distant, teeth of its own substance; as the

lower leaves of the Centaurea cyanus, and Campanula trachelium.

76. *Jagged*, irregularly cut or notched, especially when otherwise also divided; as in Salvia æthiopia, and Senecio squalidus.

77. *Cartilaginous-edged*, hard, and hoary: as in Saxifraga callosa, and Yucca gloriosa.

78. *Prickle-edged*, beset with prickles; as in Carduus lanceolatus, and Ilex aquifolium.

79. *Fringed*, bordered with soft parallel hairs; as in Sempervivum tectorum, and Galium cruciatum.

From the *openings*, or *sinuses*, in the margin.

80. *Sinuated*, cut as it were into rounded, or wide openings; as in Quercus robur, and Alcea rosea.

81. *Repand*, wavy, bordered with numerous angles and segments of circles, alternately; as in Menyanthes nymphoidoo, and Erysimum alliaria.

82. *Pinnatifid*, cut transversely into several oblong parallel segments; as in Centaurea calcitrapa, and Scabiosa arvensis.

83. *Bipinnatifid*, doubly pinnatifid; as in Papaver argemone.

84. *Lyrate*, lyre-shaped, cut into several tranverse segments, gradually larger towards the extremity of the leaf, which is rounded; as in Geum urbanum, and Erysimum barbarea.

85. *Panduriform*, fiddle-shaped, oblong, broad at the two extremities, and contracted in the middle; as in Rumex pulcher, and Convolvulus panduratus.

86. *Runcinate*, lion-toothed, cut into several transverse, acute, segments, pointing backwards; as in Leontodon taraxacum, and Erysimum officinale.

87. *Laciniate*, cut into numerous irregular portions; as in Ranunculus parviflorus, and Geranium columbinum, and Cotyledon laciniata.

88. *Squarrose*, the margin beset with a rough fringe; as in Centaurea calcitrapa, and Carduus marianus.

89. *Partite*, deeply divided nearly to the basis; as in Helleborus viridis; *bipartite*, *tripartite*, and *multipartite*, according to the number of the divisions.

90. *Trifid*, divided into three; as in Bidens tripartita.

91. *Quinquifid*, divided into five; as in Geranium maculatum.

92. *Multifid*, the margin of round leaves cut from the apex almost to the base, without leaving any great intermediate sinuses; as in Aconitum napellus, and Cucumis colocynthis.

From the *angles* in the margin of the leaf,

93. *Rounded*, the margin not having any angle.

94. *Angulate*, the margin having acute angles.

a. *Triangular*; as in Chenopodium bonus henricus, and Atriplex hortensis.

b. *Quinqueangular*; as in Geranium peltatum.

c. *Septangular*; as in Hibiscus abelmoschus.

95. *Rhomboid, trapeziform*, or approaching to a square; as in Chenopodium vulvaria, and Trapa natans.

96. *Quadrangular*, with four angles; as in Liriodendron tulipifera.

97. *Deltoid*, trowel-shaped, having three angles, of which the terminal one is much farther from the base, than the lateral ones; as in Mesembryanthemum deltoideum, and Populus nigra.

98. *Lobate*, when the margins of deep segments are rounded, hence:

a. *Two-lobed*; as in Bauhinia porresta.

b. *Three-lobed*; as in Anemone hepatica.

c. *Five-lobed*; as in Humulus lupulus, and Acer pseudo-platanus.

99. *Palmate*, cut into several oblong, nearly equal segments, about half way, or rather more, towards the base, leaving an entire space like the palm of the hand; as in Passiflora cœrulea, and Alcea ficifolia.

From the *figure of the circumference*, are derived the following names:

100. *Orbiculate*, circular, the length and breadth of which are equal, and the circumference in an even circular line; as in Cotyledon orbiculata and Hydrocotyle vulgaris.

101. *Subrotund*, roundish; as in Pyrola, and Malva rotundifolia.

102. *Oblong*, three or four times longer than broad; as in Musa sapientum, and Elæagnus orientalis.

103. *Ovate*, of the shape of an egg, cut length wise, the base being rounded, and broader than the extremity; as in Origanum vulgare, and Inula helenium.

104. *Obovate*, of the same figure, with the broader end uppermost; as in Primula veris, and Samulus valerandi.

104*. *Oval*, ovate, but each end has the same roundness; as in Rhus catinus, and Mammea americana.

105. *Elliptical*, oval, the longitudinal diameter being greater than the transverse.

106. *Parabolic*, oblong, the summit narrow and round; as in Marrubium pseudodictamnus.

107. *Cuneiform*, wedge-shaped, broad and abrupt at the summit, and tapering down to the base; as Saxifraga cuneifolia, and Iberis semperflorens.

108. *Spatulate*, of a roundish figure, tapering to an oblong base; as in Cotyledon spuria, and Cucubalus otites.

109. *Lanceolate*, of a narrow, oblong form, tapering towards each end; as in Plantago lanceolata.

110. *Linear*, narrow, with parallel sides; as in Senecio linifolius.

111. *Capillary*, long, fine, and flexible, resembling a hair; as in Anethum fœniculum, and Graveolens.

112. *Setaceous*, bristly; as in Asparagus officinalis, and Scirpus setaceus.

113. *Acerose*, needle-shaped, linear, and evergreen, generally acute and rigid; as in Pinus sylvestris, and Juniperus communis.

From the difference of the *surface* of leaves:

114. *Glabrous*, smooth, without roughness; as the leaves of most plants.

115. *Nitid*, smooth and shining; as in Laurus nobilis, and Canna indica.

116. *Lucid*, as if covered with a varnish; as in Angelica lucida, and Royena lucida.

117. *Viscid*, covered with a clammy juice; as in Senecio viscosus, and Erygeron viscosum.

118. *Naked*, without bristles, or hairs; as the leaves of many plants.

119. *Scabrous*, or *asperous*, with little roughness visible, as well as tangible; as in Morus nigra, and Humulus lupulus.

120. *Punctuate*, dotted, perforated with little holes; as in Hypericum perforatum.

121. *Pertuse*, bored, naturally having large perforations; as in Dracontium pertusum.

122. *Maculate*, spotted; as in Orchis maculata, and Pulmonaria officinalis.

123. *Coloured*, being of any other than a green colour; as in Amaranthus tricolor, and Atriplex hortensis rubra.

124. *Hoary*, having a whitish mealy surface; as in Populus alba.

125. *Lineate*, having superficial lines: as in Scirpus maritimus.

126. *Striate*, marked with coloured lines; as in Phalaris arundinacea.

127. *Sulcate*, furrowed, having broad and deep furrows; as in Digitalis ferruginea.

128. *Rugose*, rugged; as in Salvia sclara.

129. *Bullate*, blistered, a greater degree of the last; as in Brassica oleracea.

130. *Papulous*, or *vesiculous*, covered with hollow vesicles; as in Mesembryanthemum crystallinum.

131. *Papillose*, or *Varicose*, covered with solid wartlike tubercles; as in Aloe margaritifera.

132. *Glandular*, covered with small glandiform bodies; as in Salix alba, and Prunus padus.

From the *distributions of the vessels on the surface* of the leaf,

Nerves are white, elevated chords, which originate from the base of the leaf.

A *rib* is the middle nerve, thick, and extending from the basis to the apex of the leaf.

Veins are anastomosing vessels which are given off from the costa or rib.

The greater clusters of vessels are generally called *nervi* or *costæ*, nerves or ribs, and the smaller *venæ*, whether they are branched or reticulate, simple or otherwise.

133. A *nervous* or *ribbed* leaf is where they extend in simple lines from the base to the point; as in the *Convallariæ*, and *Helianthus annuus*. The Laurus camphora is an example of a trinerve; the Smilax tetragona has five nerves; the Dioscorea septemloba, seven.

134. When a pair of large ribs branch off from the main one above the base, and run in a straight line towards the apex, as in Helianthus tuberosus, the leaf is said to be *triple nerved*.

135. When two go from the base and four from the costa in a straight line, it is termed *folium quintuplinervum*.

136. *Venous*, veiny, when the vessels by which the leaf is nourished are branched, subdivided, and more or less prominent, forming a net-work over either, or both its surfaces; as in Clusia venosa, and Verbascum lychritis.

137. *Avenial*, or veinless, when without veins; as in Clusia alba, and rosea.

138. *Enervous*, ribless, when no nerve is given off from the base; as in Asperula levigata.

The terms from the *expansion* of the leaves are,

139. *Flat*, as most leaves are.

140. *Concave*, hollow, depressed in the middle; as in Saxifraga stolonifera.

141. *Convex*, the reverse of the former; as in Ocymum basilicum majus.

142. *Canaliculate*, channelled, having a longitudinal furrow; as in Plantago maritima.

143. *Cucullate*, hooded, when the edges meet in the lower parts, and expand in the upper; as in Geranium cucullatum, and that curious genus Saracenia.

144. *Plicate*, plaited, when the disk of the leaf, especially towards the margin, is acutely folded up and down; as in the Malvas, and Alchemilla vulgaris.

145. *Undulate*, waved, when the disk near the margin is waved obtusely up and down; as in Reseda lutea, and Ixia undulata.

146. *Crisp*, curled, when the border of the leaf becomes more expanded than the disk, so as to grow elegantly, curled, and twisted; as in Malva crispa.

From the *internal substance*:

147. *Membranaceous*, when there is scarcely any pulp between the external membranes of the leaf; as in Citrus aurantium, and the leaves of many plants.

148. *Thick*, the membranes being rather more than usually firm; as in Sedum telephium.

149. *Carneous*, fleshy, of a thick substance, as in all those called succulent plants; as Crassula lactea, and Sempervivum tectorum.

150. *Pulpy*, very thick, and of the consistence of a plumb; as in Mesembryanthemum verruculatum.

151. *Tubular*, hollow within; as in Allium cepa. The leaf of the Lobelia dortmanna is very peculiar, in consisting of a double tube.

152. *Compact*, not hollow.

153. *Rigid*, easily broken on being bent; as in Stapelia.

The thick leaves, *folia crassa*, afford the following distinctions:

154. *Gibbous*, swelling on one side, or both, from excessive abundance of pulp; as in Crassula cotyledon, and Aloe retusa.

155. *Round*, cylindrical; as in Allium schœnoprasum, and Salsola sativa.

156. *Subulate*, awl-shaped, tapering from a thickish base to a point; as in Allium ascalonicum, and Narcissus jonquilla.

157. *Compressed*, flattened laterally; as in Cacalia ficoides.

158. *Depressed*, flattened vertically; as in Crassula tetragona.

159. *Triquetral*, thick and triangular; as in Butomus umbellatus.

160. *Tetragonal*, quadrangular and awl-shaped; as in Gladiolus tristis.

161. *Lingulate*, tongue-shaped, a thick, oblong, blunt figure, and a little convex on its inferior surface; as in Mesembryanthemum linguiforme.

162. *Ancipital*, two-edged; as in Typha latifolia.

163. *Ensiform*, sword-shaped, two edges tapering to a point, slightly convex on both surfaces, neither of which can properly be called upper or under; as in Iris germanica, and Gladiolus communis.

164. *Carinate*, keeled, when the bark is longitudinally prominent; as in Allium carinatum, and Narcissus biflorus.

165. *Acinaciform*, scimitar-shaped, compressed with one thick and straight edge, the other thin and curved; as in Mesembryanthemum acinaciforme.

166. *Dolabriform*, hatchet-shaped, compressed with a very prominent dilated keel, and a cylindrical base; as in Mesembryanthemum dolabriforme.

167. *Uncinate*, hooked, flat above, compressed at its sides, and turned back at the apex, forming a hook.

When the shape of membranaceous leaves is

14

imperfect, the particle *sub* is attached, as *sub-sessile, sub-*ovate, *sub-*pilous, &c.

When the shape is *reversed*, by the ¦prefixing the preposition *ob*, as *ob-*cordate, when the point is inserted into the petiole, *ob-*ovate, &c.

From the *coadunation*, leaves are designated by prefixing the prominent shape, as *lanceolato-ovate;* as in Nicotiana tabacum : and ovato-lanceolate, lanceolate, but swelling out in the middle; as in Saponaria officinalis.

From their *duration*, leaves are termed,

168. *Deciduous*, falling off at the approach of winter, as in most European trees and shrubs.

169. *Caducous*, falling off in the middle of summer.

170. *Perennial*, green the whole year, and falling off as the new ones appear.

171. *Persistant*, lasting many years, and always green; as in Pinus and Taxus.

All the foregoing terms belong to *simple leaves*, or those which have one leaf only on the petiole or footstalk.

The following regard *compound leaves*, or such as consist of two or any greater number of *foliola*, or leaflets, connected by a common footstalk.

172. *Digitate*, fingered, when several leaflets proceed from the summit of a common footstalk; as in Trifolium pratense.

173. *Pinnate*, when several leaflets proceed laterally from one footstalk, instead of being supported at the top; as in Acacia pseudacacia.

A digitate leaf is called, after its *mode of digitation*,

174. *Conjugate*, or yoked, when there is one pair of leaflets, or *pinnæ*; as in Zygophillum fabago.

175. *Binate*, when the pair of leaflets unite somewhat at their base; as in Lathyrus sylvestris.

176. *Ternate*, where there are three leaflets; as in Trifolium pratensis, and Oxalis acetosella.

177. *Quinate*, there being five leaflets; as in Potentilla reptans,¦and Lupinus albus.

178. *Septenate*, with seven; as in Æsculus hippocastanum.

179. *Novenate*, nine; as in Sterculia fœtida.

180. *Pedate*, a peculiar kind of leaf, being ternate, with its lateral leaflets compounded in their forepart; or a leaf with a bifid footstalk, divided into two diverging branches, with an intermediate leaflet, and each supporting two or more lateral leaflets on their anterior edge; as in Helleborus niger.

181. *Articulate*, jointed, when one, or a pair of leaflets, grows out of the summit of another, with a sort of joint; as in Cactus ficus indica, and Fagara tragodes.

Pinnate leaves are called from their number of *pinnæ*,

182. *Bipinnate*, or *duplicato-pinnate*, doubly pinnate; as in Tanacetum vulgare.

183. *Tripinnate*, or *triplicato-pinnate*, three pinnate; as in Scandix odorata.

From the *number of pairs*, pinnate leaves are termed,

184. *Biguga;* as in Mimosa nodosa.

185. *Triguga;* as in Cassia emarginata.

186. *Quadriguga;* as in Cassia longisiliqua.

187. *Quinquiguga;* as in Cassia occidentalis.

188. *Multiguga;* as in Cassia javanica.

The difference in the *termination* of a pinnate leaf,

189. *Impari-pinnate*, with an odd or terminal leaflet; as Rosa centifolia.

190. *Abrupti-pinnate*, with a terminal leaflet, as in Orobus tuberoüs.

191. *Cirrhosi-pinnate*, when furnished with a tendril in place of an odd leaflet; as in the pea and vetch tribe.

From the mode of *adhesion of the leaflets* arise,

192. *Oppositely-pinnate*, when the leaflets are opposite, or in pairs. as in Sium angustifolium.

193. *Alternately-pinnate*, when alternate; as in Vicia sativa.

194. *Interruptedly-pinnate*, when the principal leaflets are arranged alternately with an intermediate series of smaller ones; as in Spiræa ulmaria.

195. *Decurrently-pinnate*, when the leaflets are decurrent; as in Eryngium campestre.

196. *Jointedly-pinnate*, with apparent joints in the common footstalk; as in Fagara tragodes.

197. *Petiolato-pinnate*, the leaflets on footstalks; as in Robinia pseudacacia.

198. *Alate-pinnate*, when the footstalk has little wings between the leaflets.

199. *Sessile-pinnate*, with leaflets within any petiole.

200. *Conjugate-pinnate*, confluent: the leaflets growing somewhat together at their margins.

From their *bipinnation*, pinnate leaves are,

201. *Bigeminate*, two-paired; as in Mimosa unguis cate.

202. *Trigeminate*, or *triplicato-geminate*, thrice-paired; as in Mimosa tergemina.

From the *tripinnation*,

203. *Doubly-ternate*, or *duplicato-ternate*, when the common footstalk supports tnese secondary petioles on its apex, and each of these supports three leaflets; as in Epimedium alpinum.

204. *Triternate*, or *triplicato-ternate*, when the common petiole supports on its apex three secondary footstalks, each of which supports three ternary one and every one of these three leaflets; as in Aquilegia vulgaris, and Fumaria enneaphylla.

205. *Multiplicato-pinnate*, there being more than three orders; as in Ruta hortensis.

Pinnæ are the leaflets of pinnate leaves.

206. *Pinullæ*, the leaflets of the double and triple range of pinnate leaves.

LEÆ'NA. (From λεαινα, a lioness.)

1. The lioness

2. The name of a plaster, so called from its great power.

LEAKE, John, was born in Cumberland, and, after qualifying himself as a surgeon in London, travelled to Portugal and Italy. On his return he settled in the metropolis, and published a dissertation on the Lisbon Diet Drink. He not long after became a licentiate of the College of Physicians, and began to lecture on Midwifery. In 1765, he originated the plan for the Westminster Lying-in Hospital, and purchased a piece of ground for the purpose. His death occurred in 1792. He published a volume of "Practical Observations on Child-bed Fever;" "Medical Instructions, concerning the Diseases of Women;" in two volumes, which passed through several editions; and some other works.

LE CLERC, Daniel, was born at Geneva, in 1652. His father being professor in the Greek language, instructed him in the rudiments of knowledge, and gave him a taste for researches into antiquity. He afterward studied at different universities, and took his medical degree at Valence, at the age of 20. Returning to his native city, he soon got into considerable practice; which he at length relinquished in 1704, on being appointed a member of the council of state, and that he might complete his various literary undertakings, which had already greatly distinguished him His death occurred in 1728. He had published, in conjunction with Mangets, a "Bibliotheca Anatomica," in two volumes, 1685. But his most celebrated work is the "Histoire de la Médécine," from the earliest times to that of Galen. which evinces immense erudition. He afterward added a plan for continuing it to the middle of the 17th century. But Dr. Freind has completed this part of the task on a much better method. Le Clerc also published an account of certain worms occurring in men and animals.

LE DRAN, Henry Francis, was born at Paris, in 1685, and educated under his father, who had acquired reputation as an operator, particularly in removing cancers of the breast. The young surgeon turned his attention principally to lithotomy, which he performed in the lateral method, and made some valuable improvements; which he communicated to the public in 1730, giving an accurate description of the parts: the work was favourably received, has been frequently reprinted, and translated into most modern languages. His surgical observations contain also much valuable practical matter: and his Treatise on Gun-shot Wounds is remarkable for the bold and successful measures which he adopted. He published likewise a Treatise on Operations, another called Surgical Consultations, and sent several papers of considerable merit to the academy of surgeons, which appear in their memoirs. He died in 1770.

LE'DUM. (A name adopted from the Greeks, whose ληδον is generally believed to be a species of *Cistus*.) The name of a genus of plants in the Linnæan system. Class. *Decandria;* Order, *Monogynia*

15

LEDUM PALUSTRE. The systematic name of the *Rosmarinus sylvestris,* and *Cistus ledon* of the shops. The plant has a bitter substringent taste, and was formerly used in Switzerland in the place of hops. Its medicinal use is confined to the Continent, where it is occasionally given in the cure of hooping-cough, sore throat, dysentery, and exanthematous diseases.

["LEE, ARTHUR, M. D. was a native of Virginia, and brother to Richard Henry Lee the celebrated patriot of the revolution. Dr. Lee received his classical education at Edinburgh, and afterward studied medicine in that University. As soon as he was graduated he returned to his native state, and settled at Williamsburgh, where he practised medicine for several years; but afterward abandoned the profession, went to England, and commenced the study of the law in the Temple.

He soon after entered into political life, and rendered important services to his country during the Revolutionary war. To the abilities of the statesman, he is said to have united the acquisitions of the scholar. In the year 1775, Dr. Lee was in London as the agent of Virginia, and he presented in August the second petition to the king. All his exertions were now directed to the good of his country. He was appointed minister to France in 1776; and he was for many subsequent years engaged in the affairs of the public until the close of life, which, after a short illness, took place December 14th, 1792, at Urbanna, in Middlesex county, Virginia.

He was a man of uniform patriotism, of sound understanding, of great probity, of plain manners and strong passions. During his residence in England for a number of years he was indefatigable in his exertions to promote the interests of his country. He was a member of the American Philosophical Society. He published the Monitor's Letters in vindication of the colonial rights in 1769; Extracts from a letter to the President of Congress in answer to a libel by Silas Deane, 1780; and observations on certain commercial transactions in France laid before Congress, 1780." — *Thach. Med. Biog.* A.]

LEECH. *Hirudo.* A genus of insects of the order *Vermes.* The body moves either forward or backward. There are several species, principally distinguished by their colour; but that most known to medical men is the *hirudo medicinalis,* or medicinal leech, which grows to the length of two or three inches. The body is of a blackish-brown colour, marked on the back with six yellow spots, and edged with a yellow line on each side; but both the spots and lines grow faint, and almost disappear at some seasons. The head is smaller than the tail, which fixes 'tself very firmly to any thing the creature pleases. It is viviparous, and produces but one young one at a time, which is in the month of July. It is an inhabitant of clear running waters, and is well known for its use in bleeding. The species most nearly approaching this, and which it is necessary to distinguish, is the *hirudo sanguisuga,* or horse-leech. This is larger than the former; its skin is smooth and glossy; the body is depressed, the back is dusky; and the belly is of a yellowish-green, having a yellow lateral margin. It inhabits stagnant waters.

The leech's head is armed with a sharp instrument that makes three wounds at once. They are three sharp tubercles, strong enough to cut through the skin of a man, or even of an ox, or horse. The mouth is, as it were, the body of the pump, and the tongue, or fleshy nipple, the sucker. By the working of this piece of mechanism, the blood is made to rise up to the conduit which conveys it to the animal's stomach, which is a membranaceous skin, divided into twenty-four small cells. The blood which is sucked out is there preserved for several months, almost without coagulating, and proves a store of provision for the animal. The nutritious parts, absorbed after digestion by animals, need not in this to be disengaged from the heterogeneous substances; nor indeed is there an anus discoverable in the leech; mere transpiration seems to be all that it performs, the matter fixing on the surface of the body, and afterward coming off in small threads. Of this, an experiment may be tried, by putting a leech into oil, where it keeps alive for several days; upon being taken out, and put into water, there appears to loosen from its body a kind of slough, shaped like the creature's body. The organ of respiration though unascertained, seems to be situated in the mouth; for if, like an insect, it drew breath through vent-holes, it

would not subsist in oil, as, by it, these would be stopped up.

The *hirudo medicinalis* is the only species used in medicine; being applied to the skin in order to draw off blood. With this view they are employed to bleed young children, and for the purposes of topical bleeding, in cases of inflammation, fullness or pain. They may be employed in every case where topical bleedings are thought necessary, or where venesection cannot be performed. If the leech does not fasten, a drop of sugared milk is put on the spot it is wished to fix on; or a little blood is drawn by means of a slight puncture, after which it immediately settles. The leech, when fixed, should be watched, lest it should find its way into the anus, when used for the hæmorrhoids, or penetrate into the œsophagus, if employed to draw the gums; otherwise it might fix upon the stomach, or intestines. In such a case, the best and quickest remedy is to swallow some salt; which is the method practised to make it loose its hold, when it sucks longer than is intended. Vegetable or volatile alkali, pepper, or acids, also make it leave the part on which it was applied. Cows and horses have been known to receive leeches, when drinking, into the throat; and the usual remedy is to force down some salt, which makes them fall off. If it is intended that the leech shall draw a larger quantity of blood, the end of the tail is cut off; and it then sucks continually, to make up the loss it sustains. The discharge occasioned by the puncture of a leech after the animal falls off, is usually of more service than the process itself. When too abundant, it is easily stopped with brandy, vinegar, or other styptics, or with a compress of dry linen rags, bound strongly on the bleeding orifice. They are said to be very restless before a change of weather, if confined in glasses, and to fix themselves above the water on the approach of a fine day.

As these little animals are depended on for the removal of very dangerous diseases, and as they often seem capriciously determined to resist the endeavours made to cause them to adhere, the following directions are added, by which their assistance may, with more certainty, be obtained.

The introducing a hand, to which any ill-flavoured medicine adheres, into the water in which they are kept, will be often sufficient to deprive them of life; the application of a small quantity of any saline matter to their skin, immediately occasions the expulsion of the contents of their stomach; and what is most to our purpose, the least flavour of any medicament that has been applied remaining on the skin, or even the accumulation of the matter of perspiration, will prevent them from fastening. The skin should, therefore, previous to their application, be very carefully cleansed from any foulness, and moistened with a little milk. The method of applying them is by retaining them to the skin by a small wine-glass, or the bottom of a large pill-box, when they will, in general, in a little time, fasten themselves to the skin. On their removal, the rejection of the blood they have drawn may be obtained by the application of salt externally: but it is to be remarked, that a few grains of salt are sufficient for this purpose; and that covering them with it, as is sometimes done, generally destroys them.

LEEK. See *Allium porrum.*

LE'GNA. (From λεγνον, a fringed edge.) The extremities of the pudenda muliebria.

LEGU'MEN. (From *lego,* to gather: so called because they are usually gathered by the hand.) A legume. A peculiar solitary fruit of the pea kind formed of two oblong valves, without any longitudina. partition, and bearing the seeds along one of its margins only.

From the figure, the legumen is called,

1. *Teres,* round; as in *Phaseolus radialus.*
2. *Lineare;* as in *Phaseolus vexillatus.*
3. *Compressum;* as in *Pisum sativum.*
4. *Capitatum;* as in *Phaseolus mungo.*
5. *Aciniforme;* as in *Phaseolus lunatus*
6. *Ovatum;* as in *Lotus hirsutus,* and *græcus.*
7. *Inflatum,* a cavity filled with air; as in *Astragalus vesicarius,* and *exscapus.*
8. *Cochleatum,* spiral; as in *Medicago polymorpha,* and *marina.*
9. *Lunatum;* as in *Medicago falcata.*
10. *Obcordatum;* as in *Polygala.*
11. *Contortum;* as in *Medicago sativa.*

Quadrangulatum; as in *Dolychos tetragonolo-bus.*

13. *Canaliculatum,* the upper suture deeply hollowed; as in *Lathyrus sativus.*

14. *Isthmis interceptum;* as in *Coronilla.*

15. *Echinatum;* as in *Glycyrrhiza echinata.*

16. *Rhombeum;* as in *Cicer arietinum.*

From its insertion,

1. *Pendulum;* as in *Phaseolus vulgaris.*

2. *Pedicellatum;* as in *Viscia sæpium.*

From its substance,

1. *Membranaceum;* as in *Phaseolus vulgaris.*

2. *Carnosum;* as in *Cynometra cauliflora.*

3. *Coriaceum,* dry and fleshy; as in *Ceratonia siliqua,* and *Lupinus.*

From the number of seeds,

1. *Monospermum;* as in *Medicago lupulina*

2. *Dispermum;* as in *Glycine tomentosá.*

3. *Trispermum;* as in *Trifolium reflexum.*

4. *Tetraspermum;* as in *Trifolium repens.*

5. *Polyspermum;* as in *Trifolium lupinaster.*

[" *Legumine* is a particular vegetable principle, obtained by M. H. Braconnot, from pease. When well washed it resembled paste; exposed to heat it liquefied without coagulating. Iodine, mixed with it in water, appeared to dissolve. It was insoluble in boiling water, and produced a deep blue colour with starch."—*Web. Man. of Chem.* A.]

LEGUMINOUS. Appertaining to a legume.

LEI'CHEN. See *Lichen.*

LEIENTE'RIA. See *Lienteria.*

LEIPOSY'CHIA. (From λειπω, to leave, and ψυχη, life.) A swoon. See *Syncope.*

LEIPOPY'RIA. (From λειπω, to leave, and πυρ, heat.) An ardent fever, in which the internal parts are much heated, while the external parts are cold.

LEIPOTHY'MIA. (From λειπω, to leave, and θυμος, the mind.) See *Lipothymia.*

LE'ME. (From λα, much, and μυω, to wink.) A constant winking of the eyes.

LEMERY, NICHOLAS, was born at Rouen in 1645, and brought up to the business of pharmacy. He went to Paris at the age of 21 to improve himself, particularly in chemistry; and then travelled for some years: after which, in 1672, he began to give chemical lectures at Paris, and became very popular. Three years after he published his "Cours de Chymie," which passed rapidly through numerous editions; and so great was his reputation, that he acquired a fortune by the sale of his preparations, some of which he kept secret. In 1681, he was interdicted from lecturing on account of his religious principles, and took shelter in this country; but shortly after obtained the degree of doctor of physic at Caen, and got considerable practice in the French metropolis; the revocation of the edict of Nantes, however, forbidding this employment also, he was reduced to such difficulties, that he at length adopted the Catholic religion. He then flourished again, and in 1697 published his "Pharmacopée Universelle," followed the year after by his "Dictionnaire Universel des Drogues simples," which, though with many imperfections, proved of considerable utility. On the re-establishment of the Academy of Sciences, he was made associate chemist, and read before that body his papers on antimony, which were printed in 1707. He died in 1715.

LEMERY, LOUIS, son of the preceding, was born at Paris in 1677, and intended for the law, but adopted such a partiality for his father's pursuits, that he was allowed to indulge it, and graduated in his native city in 1696. Two years after, he was admitted into the Academy of Sciences; and in 1708 began to lecture on chemistry, in the royal garden: he was appointed physician to the Hôtel Dieu in 1710; and twelve years after purchased the office of King's physician, which soon led him to the appointment of consulting physician to the Queen of Spain. In 1731 he was appointed professor of chemistry in the royal garden; and subsequently communicated several papers to the Academy of Sciences, which appeared in their Memoirs. He published also "Traité des Aliments," which was frequently reprinted; "A Dissertation on the Nourishment of Bones, refuting the Idea of its being effected by the Marrow; and "Three Letters on the Generation of Worms." He died in 1743.

LEMITHOCHO'RTON. See *Corallina corsicana.*

LE'MMA. (From λεπω, to decorticate.)

1. The bark of a tree.

2. The skin.

LE'MNIUS. (From *Lemnos,* whence it is brought.) See *Bole.*

LEMON. See *Citrus.*

Lemon scurvy-grass. See *Cochlearia officinalis*

LENIE'NTIA. (From *lenio,* to assuage.) Medicines which abate irritation.

LENITIVE. (From *lenis,* gentle.) Medicines which gently palliate diseases. A gentle purgative.

Lenitive electuary. A preparation composed chiefly of senna and some aromatics, with the pulp of tama rinds. See *Confectio sennæ.*

LENS. (A *lentore;* from its glutinous quality.) 1 The lentil. See *Ervum lens.*

2. See *Crystalline lens.*

LENTI'CULA. (Dim. of *lens,* a lentil.)

1. A smaller sort of lentil.

2. A freckle, or small pustule, resembling the seeds of lentil.

LENTICULAR. (*Lenticularis;* from *lenticulaire,* doubly convex.) A surgical instrument employed for removing the jagged particles of bone from the edge of the perforation made in the cranium with the trephine

LENTICULA'RIA. (From *lenticula.*) A species of lentil.

LENTI'GO. (From *lens,* a lentil: so named from its likeness to lentil-seeds.) A freckle on the skin.

LENTIL. An annual vegetable of the pulse kind, much used for improving the flavour of soups. See *Ervum lens.*

LENTI'SCUS. (From *lentesco,* to become clammy; so called from the gumminess of its juice.) The mastich-tree.

LE'NTOR. (From *lentus,* clammy.) A viscidity to siziness of any fluid.

LEONI'NUS. (From *leo,* the lion.) An epithet of that sort of leprosy called leontiasis.

LEONTI'ASIS. (From λεων, a lion: so called because it is said lions are subject to it.) A species of leprosy resembling the elephantiasis.

LEO'DONTON. (From λεων, the lion, and οδους, a tooth: so called from its supposed resemblance.) The name of a genus of plants in the Linnæan system. Class, *Syngenesia;* Order, *Polygamia æqualis.* The dandelion.

LEONTODON TARAXACUM. *Dens leonis.* The dandelion or pissabed. *Leontodon—caule squamis inferne reflexis, foliis runcinatis, denticulatis, lævibus,* of Linnæus. The young leaves of this plant in a blanched state have the taste of endive, and make an excellent addition to those plants eaten early in the spring as salads; and Murray informs us, that at Goëttingin, the roots are roasted and substituted for coffee by the poorer inhabitants, who find that an infusion prepared in this way, can hardly be distinguished from that of the coffee-berry. The expressed juice of dandelion is bitter and somewhat acrid; but that of the root is bitterer, and possesses more medicinal power than any other part of the plant. It has been long in repute as a detergent and aperient, and its diuretic effects may be inferred from the vulgar name it bears in most of the European languages, *quasi lecti minga et urinaria herba dicitur;* and there are various proofs of its efficacy in jaundice, dropsy, consumption, and some cutaneous disorders. The leaves, roots, flowers, stalks, and juice of dandelion, have all been separately employed for medical purposes, and seem to differ rather in degree of strength than in any essential property; therefore the expressed juice, or a strong decoction of the roots have most commonly been prescribed, from one ounce to four, two or three times a-day. The plant should be always used fresh; even extracts prepared from it appear to lose much of their power by keeping.

LEONTOPO'DIUM. (From λεων, a lion, and πους, a foot: so named from its supposed resemblance.) The herb lion's foot, or *Filago leontopodium.*

LEONU'RUS. (From λεων, a lion, and ουρα, a tail: so named from its likeness.) 1. The name of a genus of plants in the Linnæan system. Class, *Didynamia;* Order, *Gymnospermia.* Lion's tail.

2. The name, in some pharmacopœias, for the lion's tail. See *Leonurus cardiaca.*

LEONURUS CARDIACA. The mother-wort. *Agripalma gallis; Marrubium; Cardiaca crispa; Leonur—foliis caulinis lanceolatis, trilobis,* of Linnæus.

The leaves of this plant have a disagreeable smell and a bitter taste, and are said to be serviceable in disorders of the stomachs of children, to promote the uterine discharge, and to allay palpitation of the heart.

Leopard's bane. See *Arnica montana.*

LEPI'DIUM. (From λεπις, a scale: so named from its supposed usefulness in cleansing the skin from scales and impurities.) The name of a genus of plants in the Linnæan system. Class *Tetradynamia ;* Order, *Siliculosa.*

LEPIDIUM IBERIS. *Iberis ; Cardamantica.* Sciatica cresses. This plant possesses a warm, penetrating, pungent taste, like unto other cresses, and is recommended as an antiscorbutic, antiseptic, and stomachic.

LEPIDIUM SATIVUM. *Nasturtium hortense.* Dittander. This plant possesses warm, nervine, and stimulating qualities, and is given as an antiscorbutic antiseptic, and stomachic, especially by the lower orders.

LEPIDOSARCO'MA. (From λεπις, a scale, and σαρξ, flesh.) A scaly tumour.

LEPIDOSES. (From λεπις-δος, *squama,* a scale.) The name of a genus of diseases Class, *Eccritica ;* Order, *Acrotica ;* in Good's Nosology. Scale-skin. It contains four species, *Lepidosis pityriasis, lepriasis, psoriasis, icthyasis.*

LE'PISMA. (From λεπιζω, to decorticate.) Decortication. A peeling off of the skin.

LEPORINUS. (From *lepus,* a hare.) Leporine or hare-like. Applied to some malformations, diseases, and parts, from their resemblance to *labium leporinum,* &c.

LE'PRA. (From λεπρος, *scaber, vel asper ex squammatis decedentibus ;* named from its appearance.) The leprosy. A disease in the class *Cachexia,* and order *Impetigines,* of Cullen. Dr. Willan describes this disease as characterized by scaly patches, of different sizes, but having always nearly a circular form. In this country, three varieties of the disease are observed, which he has described under the names of *Lepra vulgaris, Lepra alphos, Lepra nigricans.*

1. The *Lepra vulgaris,* exhibits first small distinct elevations of the cuticle, which are reddish and shining, but never contain any fluid ; these patches continue to enlarge gradually, till they nearly equal the dimensions of a crown-piece. They have always an orbicular, or oval form ; are covered with dry scales, and surrounded by a red border. The scales accumulate on them, so as to form a thick prominent crust, which is quickly reproduced, whether it fall off spontaneously, or may have been forcibly detached. This species of lepra sometimes appears first at the elbow, or on the forearm ; but more generally about the knee. In the latter case, the primary patch forms immediately below the patella ; within a few weeks, several other scaly circles appear along the fore part of the leg and thigh, increasing by degrees till they come nearly into contact. The disease is then often stationary for a considerable length of time. If it advance farther, the progress is towards the hip and loins ; afterward to the sides, back, and shoulders, and about the same time to the arms and hands. In the greater number of cases, the hairy scalp is the part last affected ; although the circles formed on it remain for some time distinct, yet they finally unite, and cover the whole surface on which the hair grows with a white scaly incrustation. This appearance is attended, more especially in hot weather, with a troublesome itching, and with a watery discharge for several hours, when any portion of the crust is detached, which takes place from very slight impressions. The pubes in adults is sometimes affected in the same manner as the head : and if the subject be a female, there is usually an internal *pruritus pudendi.* In some cases of the disorder, the nails, both of the fingers and toes, are thickened, and deeply indented longitudinally. When the lepra extends universally, it becomes highly disgusting in its appearance, and inconvenient from the stiffness and torpor occasioned by it in the limbs. The disease, however, even in this advanced stage, is seldom disposed to terminate spontaneously. It continues nearly in the same state for several years, or sometimes during the whole life of the person affected, not being apparently connected with any disorder of the constitution.

2. *Lepra alphos.* The scaly patches in the alphos are smaller than those of the lepra vulgaris, and also differ from them in having their central parts depressed or indented. This disorder usually begins about the elbow, with distinct, eminent asperities, of a dull red colour, and not much longer than papillæ. These, in a short time, dilate to nearly the size of a silver penny. Two or three days afterward, the central part of them suffers a depression, within which small white powdery scales may be observed. The surrounding border, however, still continues to be raised, but retains the same size, and the same red colour as at first. The whole of the forearm, and sometimes the back of the hand, is spotted with similar patches : they seldom become confluent, excepting round the elbow, which in that case, is covered with a uniform crust. This affection appears in the same manner upon the joint of the knee, but without spreading far along the thigh or leg. Dr. Willan has seldom seen it on the trunk of the body, and never on the face. It is a disease of long duration, and not less difficult to cure than the foregoing species of lepra : even when the scaly patches have been removed by persevering in the use of suitable applications, the cuticle still remains red, tender, and brittle, very slowly recovering its usual texture. The alphos, as above described, frequently occurs in this country.

3. The *Lepra nigricans* differs little from the lepra vulgaris, as to its form and distribution. The most striking difference is in the colour of the patches, which are dark and livid. They appear first on the legs and forearms, extending afterward to the thighs, loins, neck, and hands. Their central part is not depressed, as in the alphos. They are somewhat smaller in size than the patches of the lepra vulgaris, and not only is the border livid or purplish, but the livid colour of the base likewise appears through the scaly incrustation, which is seldom very thick. It is further to be observed, that the scales are more easily detached than in the other forms of lepra, and that the surface remains longer excoriated, discharging lymph, often with an intermixture of blood, till a new incrustation forms, which is usually hard, brittle, and irregular. The lepra nigricans, affects persons whose occupation is attended with much fatigue, and exposes them to cold or damp, and to a precarious or improper mode of diet, as soldiers, brewers, labourers, butchers, stage-coachmen, scullermen, &c.; some women are also liable to it, who are habituated to poor living and constant hard labour.

LEPRA GRÆCORUM. The lepra vulgaris, alphos, and nigricans have all been so denominated. See *Lepra.*

LEPRIASIS. (From λεπρος, *scaber.*) The specific name of a species of *leprosis* in Good's Nosology, which embraces the several kinds of leprosy.

LEPROSY. See *Lepra.*

LEPTU'NTICA. (From λεπτος, thin.) Attenuating medicines.

LEPTY'SMUS. (From λεπτος, slender.) Attenuation, or the making a substance less solid.

LEPUS. The name of a genus of animals of the order *Glires,* in the class *Mammalia.* The hare.

LEPUS CUNICULUS. The systematic name of the rabbit, the flesh of which, when young and tender, is easy of digestion.

LEPUS TIMIDUS. The systematic name of the common hare ; the flesh of which is considered as a delicacy, and easy of digestion.

LE'ROS. (From ληρεω, to trifle.) A slight delirium.

LETHARGY. (*Lethargus ;* from ληθη, forgetfulness : so called because with it the person is forgetful.) A heavy and constant sleep, with scarcely any intervals of waking ; when awakened, the person answers, but ignorant or forgetful of what he said, immediately sinks into the same state of sleep. It is considered as an imperfect apoplexy, and is mostly symptomatic.

LETHE'A. The name of the poppy

LETTUCE. See *Lactuca.*

LEUCACA'NTHA. (From λευκος, white, and ακανθα, a thorn : so named from its white blossom.) The cotton-thistle.

LEUCA'NTHEMUM. (From λευκος, white, and ανθεμος, a flower : so called from its white floret.) See *Chrysanthemum leucanthemum.*

LEUCASMUS. (Λευκασμος, whiteness : so named from its appearance.) The specific name, *Epichrosis leucasmus,* veal skin, in Good's Nosology, for the *Vitiligo* of Willan.

LEUCE. (Λευκος, white.) A species of leprosy See *Alphus.*

LEUCELE'CTRUM. (From λευκος, white, and ηλεκτρον, amber.) White amber.

LEUCINE (From λευκος, white; from its appearance.) The name given by Braconnot to a white pulverulent matter obtained by digesting equal parts of beef fibre and sulphuric acid together, and after separating the fat, diluting the acid mixture, and saturating with chalk, filtering and evaporating. A substance tasting like ozmazome is thus procured, which is to be boiled in different portions of alkohol. The alkoholic solutions, on cooling, deposite the white pulverulent matter, or *leucine*.

LEUCOLA'CHANUM. (From λευκος, white, and λαχανον, an herb: so named from its colour.) The *Valeriana sylvestris*.

LEUCO'MA. (From λευκος, white.) Leucoma and albugo are often used synonymously, to denote a white opacity of the cornea of the eye. Both of them, according to Scarpa, are essentially different from the nebula, for they are not the consequence of chronic ophthalmy, attended with varicose veins, and an effusion of a milky serum into the texture of the delicate continuation of the conjunctiva over the cornea, but are the result of violent acute ophthalmy. In this state, a dense coagulating lymph is extravasated from the arteries; sometimes superficially, at other times deeply, into the substance of the cornea. On other occasions, the disease consists of a firm callous cicatrix on this membrane, the effect of an ulcer, or wound, with loss of substance. The term *albugo*, strictly belongs to the first form of the disease; *leucoma*, to the last, more particularly when the opacity occupies the whole, or the chief part, of the cornea.

LEUCONYMPHÆ'A. (From λευκος, white, and νυμφαια, the water-lily.) See *Nymphœa alba*.

LEUCOPHA'GIUM. (From λευκος, white, and φαγω, to eat.) A medicated white food.

LEUCOPHLEGMA'SIA. (From λευκος, white, and φλεγμα, phlegm.) Leuco-phlegmatic. A tendency in the system to a dropsical state known by a pale colour of the skin, a flabby condition of the solids, and a redundancy of serum in the blood.

LEUCO'PIPER. (From λευκος, white, and πεπερι, pepper.) White pepper. See *Piper nigrum*.

LEUCORRHŒ'A. (From λευκος, white, and ρεω, to flow.) *Fluor albus.* The whites. A secretion of whitish or milky mucus from the vagina of women, arising from debility and not from the venereal virus. This disease is marked by the discharge of a thin white or yellow matter from the uterus and vagina, attended likewise with some degree of fœtor, smarting in making water, pains in the back and loins, anorexia and atrophy. In some cases, the discharge is of so acrid a nature, as to produce effects on those who are connected with the woman, somewhat similar to venereal matter, giving rise to excoriations about the glans penis and præputium, and occasioning a weeping from the urethra.

To distinguish leucorrhœa from gonorrhœa, it will be very necessary to attend to the symptoms. In the latter the running is constant, but in a small quantity; there is much ardor urinæ, itching of the pudenda, swelling of the labia, increased inclination to venery, and very frequently an enlargement of the glands in the groin; whereas, in the former the discharge is irregular, and in considerable quantities, and is neither preceded by, nor accompanied with, any inflammatory affection of the pudenda.

Immoderate coition, injury done to the parts by difficult and tedious labours, frequent miscarriages, immoderate flowings of the menses, profuse evacuations, poor diet, an abuse of tea, and other causes, giving rise to general debility, or to a laxity of the parts more immediately concerned, are those which usually produce the whites, vulgarly so called, from the discharge being commonly of a milky white colour.

Fluor albus, in some cases, indicates that there is a disposition to disease in the uterus, or parts connected with it, especially where the quantity of the discharge is very copious, and its quality highly acrimonious. By some the disease has been considered as never arising from debility of the system, but as being always a primary affection of the uterus. Delicate women, with lax fibres, who remove from a cold climate to a warm one, are very apt to be attacked with it, without the parts having previously sustained any kind of injury

The disease shows itself by an irregular discharge from the uterus and vagina of a fluid which, in different women, varies much in colour, being either of a white, green, yellow, or brown hue. In the beginning, it is, however, most usually white and pellucid, and in the progress of the complaint acquires the various discolorations, and different degrees of acrimony, from whence proceeds a slight degree of smarting in making water. Besides the discharge, the patient is frequently afflicted with severe and constant pains in the back and loins, loss of strength, failure of appetite, dejection of spirits, paleness of the countenance, chilliness, and languor. Where the disease has been of long continuance, and very severe, a slow fever, attended with difficult respiration, palpitations, faintings, and swellings of the lower extremities, often ensues.

A perfect removal of the disorder will at all times be a difficult matter to procure; but it will be much more so in cases of long standing, and where the discharge is accompanied with a high degree of acrimony. In these cases, many disorders, such as prolapsus uteri, ulcerations of the organ, atrophy, and dropsy, are apt to take place, which in the end prove fatal.

Where the disease terminates in death, the internal surface of the uterus appears, on dissection, to be pale, flabby, and relaxed; and where organic affections have arisen, much the same appearances are to be met with as have been noticed under the head of menorrhagia.

LEUCO'RRHOIS. (From λευκος, white, and ρεω, to flow.) A discharge of mucus from the urethra or vagina.

LEVA'TOR. (From *levo*, to lift up.) A muscle, the office of which is to lift up the part to which it is attached.

LEVATOR ANGULI ORIS. *Abducens labiorum*, of Spigelius; *Elevator labiorum communis*, of Douglas. *Caninus*, of Winslow, and *Sus maxillo labial*, of Dumas. A muscle situated above the mouth, which draws the corner of the mouth upwards, and makes that part of the cheek opposite to the chin prominent, as in smiling. It arises thin and fleshy from the hollow of the superior maxillary bone, between the root of the socket of the first grinder and the foramen infra orbitarium, and is inserted into the angle of the mouth and under lip, where it joins with its antagonist.

LEVATOR ANI. *Levator magnus, seu internus*, of Douglas; *Pubo coccigi annulaire*, of Dumas. A muscle of the rectum. It arises from the os pubis, within the pelvis, as far up as the upper edge of the foramen thyroideum, and joining of the os pubis with the os ischium, from the thin tendinous membrane that covers the obturator internus and coccygeus muscles, and from the spinous process of the ischium. From these origins all round the inside of the pelvis, its fibres run down like rays from the circumference to a centre, to be inserted into the sphincter ani, acceleratores urinæ, and anterior part of the two last bones of the os coccygis, surrounding the extremity of the rectum, neck of the bladder, prostrate gland, and part of the vesiculæ seminales. Its fibres, joining with those of its fellow, form a funnel-shaped hole, that draws the rectum upwards after the evacuation of the fæces, and assists in shutting it. The levatores ani also sustain the contents of the pelvis, and assist in ejecting the semen; urine, and contents of the rectum, and perhaps, by pressing upon the veins, contribute greatly to the erection of the penis.

LEVATOR LABII INFERIORIS. A muscle of the mouth situated below the lips. *Levator menti*, of Albinus. *Incisivus inferior*, of Winslow. *Elevator labii inferioris proprius*, of Douglas. It arises from the lower jaw, at the roots of the alveoli of two incisor teeth and the cuspidatus, and is inserted into the under lip and skin of the chin.

LEVATOR LABII SUPERIORIS ALÆQUE NASI. *Elevator labii superioris proprius*, of Douglas; *Incisivus lateralis et pyramidalis*, of Winslow. A muscle of the mouth and lips, that raises the upper lip towards the orbit, and a little outwards; it serves also to draw the skin of the nose upwards and outwards, by which the nostril is dilated. It arises by two distinct origins; the first, broad and fleshy, from the external part of the orbitar process of the superior maxillary bone, immediately above the foramen infra orbitarium; the second, from the nasal process of the superior maxillary bone, where it joins the os frontis. The first portion is inserted into the upper lip and orbicularis muscle, the second into the upper lip and outer part of the ala nasi.

LEVATOR LABII SUPERIORIS PROPRIUS. *Musculus incisivus.* A muscle of the upper lip. It arises under the edge of the orbit, and is inserted into the middle of the lip.

LEVATOR OCULI. See *Rectus superior oculi.*

LEVATOR PALATI. A muscle situated between the lower jaw and the os hyoides laterally. *Levator palati mollis,* of Albinus; *Petrosalpingo-staphilinus, vel salpingo-staphilinus internus,* of Winslow; *Salpingo-staphilinus,* of Valsalva; *Pterigo-staphilinus externus vulgo,* of Douglas; *Spheno-staphilinus,* of Cowper. It arises tendinous and fleshy from the extremity of the petrous portion of the temporal bone, where it is perforated by the Eustachian tube, and also from the membraneous part of the same tube, and is inserted into the whole length of the velum pendulum palati, as far as the root of the uvula, and unites with its fellow. Its use is to draw the velum pendulum palati upwards and backwards, so as to shut the passage from the fauces into the mouth and nose.

LEVATOR PALATI MOLLIS. See *Levator palati.*

LEVATOR PALPEBRÆ SUPERIORIS. *Aperiens palpebrarum rectus; Apertor oculi.* A proper muscle of the upper eyelid, that opens the eyes, by drawing the eyelid upwards. It arises from the upper part of the foramen opticum of the sphenoid bone, above the rectus superior oculi, near the trochlearis, and is inserted by a broad thin tendon into the cartilage that supports the upper eyelid.

LEVATOR PARVUS. See *Transverus perinei.*

LEVATOR SCAPULÆ. A muscle situated on the posterior part of the neck, that pulls the scapula upwards and a little forwards. This name, which was first given to it by Riolanus, has been adopted by Albinus. Douglas calls it *elevator seu musculus patientia;* and Winslow, *angularis, vulgo levator proprius.* It is a long muscle, nearly two inches in breadth, and is situated obliquely under the anterior edge of the trapezius. It arises tendinous and fleshy from the transverse processes of the four and sometimes five superior vertebræ colli, by so many distinct slips, which soon unite to form a muscle that runs obliquely downwards and outwards, and is inserted by a flat tendon into the upper angle of the scapula. Its use is to raise the scapula upwards and a little forwards.

LEVIGATION. (*Lævigatio;* from *lævigo,* to make smooth.) The reduction of a hard substance, by triture, to an impalpable powder.

LEVISTICUM. (From *levo,* to assuage: so called from the relief it gives in painful flatulencies.) See *Ligusticum levisticum.*

LEVRET, ANDREW, a French surgeon and accoucheur, was admitted into the Royal Academy of Surgery, at Paris, in 1742. He obtained considerable reputation by the improvements which he made in some of the instruments used in difficult cases, and by the great number of pupils whom he instructed. He was employed and honoured with official appointments by all the female branches of the royal family. He published several works, which went through various editions and translations, mostly on obstetrical subjects; but there is one on the Radical Cure of Polypi in different parts of the body.

LEXIPHA'RMACA. (From λην γω, to terminate, and φαρμακον, poison.) Medicines which resist or destroy the power of poison.

LEXIPY'RETA. (From ληγω, to make cease, and πυρετος, a fever.) Febrifuge medicines.

LIBA'DIUM. (From λιβαζω, to make moist: so called because it grows in watery places.) The less centaury. See *Chironia centaurium.*

LIBANO'TIS. (From λιβανος, frankincense: so called from its resemblance in smell to frankincense.) Rosemary.

LI'BANUS. (From *Libanon,* a mountain in Syria, where it grows.) 1. The *Pinus cedrus,* or cedar of Lebanon.

2. The frankincense tree, or *Pinus abies.*

LIBER. Bark. Immediately under the cuticle of plants and trees is a succulent cellular substance, for the most part of a green colour, at least of the leaves and branches, called by Du Hamel *enveloppe cellulaire,* and by Mirbel *tissue herbacé.* Under this is the bark, consisting of but one layer in plants or branches only one year old. In the older branches and trunks of

20

trees, it consists of as many layers as they are years old, the innermost being called the *liber;* and it is this layer only that the essential vital functions are carried on for the time being, after which it is pushed outwards with the cellular integument, and becomes, like that, a lifeless crust.—*Smith.*

LI'BOS. (From λειβω, to distil.) A rheum or defluxion from the eyes, or nose.

LIBU'RNUM. (From *Liburnia,* the country where it flourished.) The mealy-tree. See *Viburnum lantana.*

LICETO, FORTUNIO, was son of a Genoese physician, and born in 1577. After prosecuting with diligence the requisite studies, he settled at Pisa at the age of twenty-two, and soon obtained the professorship of philosophy there; and in 1609 he received a similar appointment at Padua. Thence, after twenty-seven years, he removed to Bologna, being disappointed of the medical chair; but on a vacancy occurring in 1645, he was induced, by the pressing invitations made to him, to accept the office, in which he continued till his death in 1657. He was a very copious writer, having published above fifty treatises on different subjects, and displayed much erudition; but no great acuteness or originality. His treatise, "De Monstrorum Causis, Natura, et Differentiis," is best known, and shews him to have been very credulous; which appears farther from his belief, that the ancients had a method of making lamps, which should burn for ever without a fresh supply of fuel, and that such had been found in sepulchres.

LI'CHANUS. (From λειχω, to lick: so called because it is commonly used in licking up any thing.) The forefinger.

LI'CHEN. (Λειχην, or λιχην, a tetter, or ringworm.) Tetter, or ringworm.

1. The name of a disease, defined, by Dr. Willan, an extensive eruption of papulæ affecting adults, connected with internal disorder, usually terminating in scurf, recurrent, not contagious. The varieties of lichen he considers under the denominations of *Lichen simplex, Lichen agrius, Lichen pilaris, Lichen lividus,* and *Lichen tropicus.*

The *Lichen simplex* usually commences with headache, flushing of the face, loss of appetite, general languor, and increased quickness of the pulse. Distinct red papulæ arise first about the cheeks and chin, or on the arms; and, in the course of three or four days, the same appearance takes place on the neck, body, and lower extremities, accompanied with an unpleasant sensation of tingling, which is somewhat aggravated during the night. In about a week, the colour of the eruption fades, and the cuticle begins to separate; the whole surface is at length covered with scurvy exfoliations, which are particularly large, and continue longest in the flexures of the joints. The duration of the complaint is seldom in any two cases alike; ten, fourteen, seventeen, or sometimes twenty days intervene between the eruption and the renovation of the cuticle. The febrile state, or rather the state of irritation at the beginning of this disorder, is seldom considerable enough to confine the patient to the house. After remaining five or six days, it is generally relieved on the appearance of the eruption. This, as well as some other species of the lichen, occurs about the beginning o. summer, or in autumn, more especially affecting persons of a weak and irritable habit; hence women are more liable to it than men. Lichen simplex is also a frequent sequel of acute diseases, particularly fever and catarrhal inflammation, of which it seems to produce a crisis. In these cases the eruption has been termed, by medical writers, scabies critica. Many instances of it are collected under that title by Sauvages, Nosol. Method. Class x. Order 5. *Impetigines.*

The *Lichen agrius* is preceded by nausea, pain in the stomach, headache, loss of strength, and deep-seated pains in the limbs, with fits of coldness and shivering; which symptoms continue several days, and are sometimes relieved by the papulous eruption. The papulæ are distributed in clusters, or often in large patches, chiefly on the arms, the upper part of the breast, the neck, face, back and sides of the abdomen, they are of a vivid red colour, and have a redness, or some degree of inflammation, diffused round them to a considerable extent, and attended with itching, heat, and a painful tingling. Dr. Willan has observed, in one or two cases where it was produced from imprudent exposure to cold, that an acute disease ensued, with great quickness of the pulse, heat, thirst, pains of the bowels, frequent vomiting, headache, and delirium. After these symptoms had continued ten days, or somewhat longer, the patient recovered, though the eruption did not return. The diffuse redness connecting the papulæ, and the tendency to become pustular, distinguish the lichen agrius from the lichen simplex, and the other varieties of this complaint, in which the inflammation does not extend beyond the basis of the papulæ, and terminates in scurf, or scales.

Lichen pilaris. This is merely a modification of the first species of lichen, and, like it, often alternates with complaints of the head, or stomach, in irritable habits. The peculiarity of the eruption is, that the small tubercles or asperities appear only at the roots of the hairs of the skin, being probably occasioned by an enlargement of their bulbs, or an unusual fulness of the blood-vessels distributed to them. This affection is distinguishable from the cutis anserina, by its permanency, by its red papulæ, and by the troublesome itching or tingling which attends it. If a part thus affected be violently rubbed, some of the papulæ enlarge to the size of wheals, but the tumour soon subsides again. The eruption continues more or less vivid for about ten days, and terminates, as usual, in small exfoliations of the cuticle, one of which surrounds the base of each hair. This complaint, as likewise the lichen agrius, frequently occurs in persons accustomed to drink largely of spirituous liquors undiluted.

Lichen lividus. The papulæ characterizing this eruption are of a dark red, or livid hue, and somewhat more permanent than in the foregoing species of lichen. They appear chiefly on the arms and legs, but sometimes extend to other parts of the body. They are finally succeeded, though at very uncertain periods, by slight exfoliations of the cuticle, after which a fresh eruption is not preceded or attended by any febrile symptoms. It principally affects persons of a weak constitution, who live on a poor diet, and are engaged in laborious occupations. Young persons, and often children living in confined situations, or using little exercise, are also subject to the lichen lividus; and in them, the papulæ are generally intermixed with petechiæ, or larger purple spots, resembling vibices. This circumstance points out the affinity of the lichen lividus with the purpura, or land scurvy, and the connexion is further proved by the exciting causes, which are the same in both complaints. The same method of treatment is likewise successful in both cases. They are presently cured by nourishing food, moderate exercise in the open air, along with the use of Peruvian bark and vitriolic acid, or the tincture of muriated steel.

Lichen tropicus. By this term is expressed the prickly heat, a papulous eruption, almost universally affecting Europeans settled in tropical climates. The prickly heat appears without any preceding disorder of the constitution. It consists of numerous papulæ, about the size of a small pin's head, and elevated so as to produce a considerable roughness on the skin. The papulæ are of a vivid red colour, and often exhibit an irregular form, two or three of them being in many places united together; but no redness or inflammation extends to the skin in the interstices of the papulæ.

2. The name of a genus of plants (applied by the Romans to a plant which was supposed by them to cure the lichen, or tetter,) in the Linnæan system. Class, *Cryptogamia;* Order, *Algæ.* There are several species, some of which are used in medicine.

LICHEN APHTHOSUS. *Muscus camatilis.* This plant is said to have a decided good effect in some complaints of the intestines, but is not used in the practice of this country.

LICHEN CANINUS. The systematic name of the ash-coloured ground liverwort. *Lichen cinereus terrestris; Muscus caninus.* This cryptogamous plant has a weak, faint smell, and a sharpish taste. It was for a long time highly extolled as a medicine of singular virtue, in preventing and curing that dreadful disorder which is produced by the bite of rabid animals, but it is now deservedly forgotten.

LICHEN CINEREUS TERRESTRIS. See *Lichen caninus.*
LICHEN COCCIFERUS. See *Lichen pyxidatus.*

LICHEN ISLANDICUS. The medicinal qualities of this plant have lately been so well established at Vienna, that it is now admitted into the materia medica of the London pharmacopœia. It is extremely mucilaginous, and to the taste bitter, and somewhat astringent. Its bitterness, as well as the purgative quality which it manifests in its recent state, are in a great measure dissipated on drying, or may be extracted by a slight infusion in water, so that the inhabitants of Iceland convert it into a tolerably grateful and nutritive food. An ounce of this lichen, boiled a quarter of an hour in a pint of water, yielded seven ounces of a mucilage as thick as that procured by the solution of one part of gum-arabic in three of water.

The medical virtues of this lichen were probably first learned from the Icelanders, who employ it in its fresh state as a laxative; but when deprived of this quality, and properly prepared, we are told that it is an efficacious remedy in consumptions, coughs, dysenteries, and diarrhœas. Scopoli seems to have been the first who, of late years, called the attention of physicians to this remedy in consumptive disorders: and further instances of its success are related by Herz, Cramer, Tromsdorff, Ebeling, Paulisky, Stoll, and others, who bear testimony to its efficacy in most of the other complaints above mentioned. Dr. Herz says, that since he first used the lichen in dysentery, he found it so successful, that he never had occasion to employ any other remedy; it must be observed, however, that cathartics and emetics were always repeatedly ad ministered before he had recourse to the lichen, to which he also occasionally added opium. Dr. Crichton informs us, that during seven months' residence at Vienna, he had frequent opportunities of seeing the lichen islandicus tried in phthisis pulmonalis at the general hospitals, and confesses, "that it by no means answered the expectation he had formed of it." He adds, however, "from what I have seen, I am fully convinced in my own mind, that there are only two species of this disease where this sort of lichen promises a cure. The two species I hint at are the phthisis hæmoptoica, and the phthisis pituitosa, or mucosa. In several cases of these, I have seen the patients so far get the better of their complaints as to be dismissed the hospital cured, but whether they remained long so or not, I cannot take upon me to say." That this lichen strengthens the digestive powers, and proves extremely nutritious, there can be no doubt; but the great medicinal efficacy attributed to it at Vienna, will not readily be credited at London. It is commonly given in the form of a decoction: an ounce and a half of the lichen being boiled in a quart of milk. Of this, a teacupful is directed to be drank frequently in the course of the day. If milk disagree with the stomach, a simple decoction of the lichen in water is to be used. Care ought to be taken that it be boiled over a slow fire, and not longer than a quarter of an hour.

LICHEN PLICATUS. The systematic name of the *muscus arboreus.* This plant, we are informed by the great botanist Linnæus, is applied by the Laplanders to parts which are excoriated by a long journey. It is slightly astringent, and is applied with that intention to bleeding vessels.

LICHEN PULMONARIUS. The systematic name of the officinal *muscus pulmonarius quercinus. Pulmonaria arborea.* This subastringent and rather acid plant was once in high estimation in the cure of diseases of the lungs, especially coughs, asthmas, and catarrhs. Its virtues are similar, and in no way inferior, to those of the lichen islandicus.

LICHEN PYXIDATUS. The systematic name of the cup-moss. *Muscus pyxidatus; Musculus pyxoides terrestris; Lichen pyxidatus major.* These very common little plants, *Lichen cocciferus,* and *pyxidatus,* of Linnæus, for both are used indifferently, are employed by the common people in this country in the cure of hooping-cough, in the form of decoction.

LICHEN ROCCELLA. The systematic name of the roccella of the shops. *Roccella.* It has been employed medicinally with success in allaying the cough attendant on phthisis, and in hysterical coughs. The principal use is as a blue dye. It is imported to us as it gathered: those who prepare it for the use of the dyer, grind it between stones, so as thoroughly to bruise, but not to reduce it into powder, and then moisten it occasionally with a strong spirit of urine, or urine itself mixed with quicklime: in a few days it acquires a purplish-red, and at length a blue colour; in the first state it is called archil, in the latter lacmus or litmus.

Litmus is used in chemistry as a test, either staining paper with it, or by infusing it in water, when it is very commonly, but with great impropriety, called *tincture of turnsole.* The persons by whom this article was prepared formerly, gave it the name of turnsole, pretending that it was extracted from the turnsole *heliotropium tricoccum,* in order to keep its true source a secret. The tincture should not be too strong, otherwise it will have a violet tinge, which, however, may be removed by dilution. The light of the sun turns it red even in close vessels. It may be made with spirit instead of water. This tincture, or paper stained with it, is presently turned red by acids; and if it be first reddened by a small quantity of vinegar, or some weak acid, its blue colour will be restored by an alkali.

LICHEN SAXATILIS. The systematic name of the *muscus cranii humani. Usnea.* This moss, when growing on the human skull, was formerly in high estimation, but is now deservedly forgotten.

LI'EN. (From λειος, soft, or smooth.) The spleen. See *Spleen.*

LIEN SINARUM. The Faba ægyptia. See *Nymphæa nelumbo.*

LIENTE'RIA. (From λειος, smooth, and εντερον, the intestine.) Lientery. See *Diarrhæa.*

LIEUTAUD, JOSEPH, was born at Aix, in Provence, in 1703. A taste for botany induced him to travel into the countries which Tournefort had visited: and he brought back many plants unnoticed by that distinguished botanist: this gained him great applause, and he obtained the reversion of the chairs of Botany and Anatomy, which his maternal uncle had long filled. He was also appointed physician to the hospital at Aix, which led him to turn his attention chiefly to anatomy. His audience soon became numerous, and in 1742 he published a syllabus, entitled, "Essais Anatomiques," which was many times reprinted, with improvements. He communicated also several papers on morbid anatomy, and on physiology, to the Academy of Sciences, of which he was elected a corresponding member. In 1749 he went to Versailles, Senac having obtained for him the appointment of physician to the Royal Infirmary; which act of friendship is ascribed to a liberal private communication of some errors committed by Senac. He there continued his investigations with great zeal, and was soon elected assistant anatomist to the Royal Academy, which he presented with many valuable memoirs. He also printed a volume, "Elementa Physiologiæ," composed for his class at Aix. In 1755 he was nominated physician to the royal family, and 20 years after, first physician to Louis XVI. In 1759 his "Précis de la Médecine Pratique," appeared, which went through several editions; and seven years after, his "Précis de la Matière Médicale." But his most important work, which still ranks high in the estimation of physicians, is entitled, "Historia Anatomico-Medica," in 2 vols. quarto, 1767, containing numerous dissections of morbid bodies. His death occurred in 1780.

LIEVRITE. *Yenite.* A blackish green-coloured mineral, composed of silica, alumina, lime, oxide of iron, and oxide of manganese, found in primitive limestone, along with epidote, quartz, &c. in the isle of Elba.

LI'FE. A peculiar condition, or mode of existence, of living beings. Surrounding matter is divided into two great classes, living and dead. The latter is subject to physical laws, which the former also obeys in a great degree. Living matter exhibits also physical properties, which are found equally in dead matter. But living bodies are endowed likewise with a set of properties altogether different from these, and contrasting with them in a very remarkable way; these are called vital properties, actions, powers, faculties, or forces. These animate living matter so long as it continues alive, and are the source of the various phenomena which constitute the functions of the living animal body, and which distinguish its history from that of dead matter. The study of life is the object of the science of physiology which includes an inquiry into the properties that characterize living matter, and an investigation of the functions which the various organs, by virtue of these properties, are enabled to execute. The vital principle diffused throughout these organs induces a mode of union in the elements, widely differing from that which arises from the common laws of chemical affinity. By the aid of this principle, nature produces the animal fluids, as blood, bile, semen, and the rest, which can never be produced by the art of chemistry. But if, in consequence of death, the laws of vital attraction, or affinity, cease to operate, then the elements, recovering their physical properties, become again obedient to the common laws of chemical affinity, and enter into new combinations, from which new principles, in the process of putrefaction, are produced. Thus the hydrogen, combining itself with the azote, forms volatile alkali; and the carburetted hydrogen, with the azote, putrid air, into which the whole body is converted. It also appears from hence, why organized bodies alone, namely, animal and vegetable, are subject to putridity; to which inorganic or mineral substances are in no degree liable, the latter not being compounded according to the laws of vital affinity, but only according to those of chemical affinity. For the fatiscence, or resolution of pyrites, or sulphuret of iron, in atmospheric air, is not putrefaction, but only the oxygen, furnished by the air, combining with the sulphur, and forming iron and sulphate of iron.

The life of an animal body appears to be threefold.

1. *Its chemical life,* which consists in that attraction of the elements, by which the vital principle, diffused through the solids and fluids, defends all the parts of the body from putrefaction. In this sense it may be said, that every atom of our body lives *chemically,* and that life is destroyed by putrefaction alone.

2. *Its physical life,* which consists in the irritability of the parts. This physical property remains for some time after death. Thus the heart or intestines removed from the body, while still warm, contract themselves on the application of a stimulus. In like manner the serpent or eel, being cut into pieces, each part moves and palpitates for a long time afterward. Hence these parts may be said to live physically, as long as they are warm and soft.

3. *Its physiological life,* consists in the action of inorganic parts proper to each, as the action of the heart and vessels; so that these actions ceasing, the body is said to be physiologically dead. The physiological life ceases first, next the physical, and finally the chemical perishes.

LIGAMENT. (*Ligamentum;* from *ligo,* to bind.) An elastic and strong membrane connecting the extremities of the moveable bones. Ligaments are divided into *capsular,* which surround joints like a bag, and *connecting* ligaments. The use of the capsular ligaments is to connect the extremities of the moveable bones, and prevent the efflux of synovia; the external and internal connecting ligaments strengthen the union of the extremities of the moveable bones.

LIGAMENTUM ANNULARE. The angular ligament. A strong ligament on each ankle and each wrist.

LIGAMENTUM ARTERIOSUM. The ductus arteriosus of the fœtus becomes a ligament after birth, which is so called.

LIGAMENTUM CILIARE. Behind the uvea of the human eye, there arise out of the choroid membrane, from the ciliary circle, white complicated striæ, covered with a black matter. The fluctuating extremities of these striæ are spread abroad even to the crystalline lens, upon which they lie, but are not affixed. Taken together, they are called *ligamentum ciliare.*

LIGAMENTUM DENTICULATUM. A small ligament supporting the spinal marrow.

LIGAMENTUM FALLOPII. The round ligament of the uterus has been so called. See also *Ligamentum pouparti.*

LIGAMENTUM INTEROSSEUM. The ligament uniting the radius and ulna, and also that between the tibia and fibula.

LIGAMENTUM LATUM. The broad ligament of the liver, and that of the uterus. See *Liver* and *Uterus.*

LIGAMENTUM NUCHÆ. A strong ligament of the neck, which proceeds from one spinous process to an other.

LIGAMENTUM OVARII. The thick, round portion of the broad ligament of the uterus, by which the ovarium is connected with the uterus.

LIGAMENTUM POUPARTI. Fallopian ligament. Pou part's ligament. A ligament extending from the anterior superior spinous process of the ilium to the crista of the os pubis.

LIG

LIG

LIGAMENTUM ROTUNDUM. The round ligament of the uterus. See *Uterus.*

LIGATURE. (*Ligatura;* from *ligo,* to bind.) A thread, or silk, of various thickness, covered with white wax, for the purpose of tying arteries, or veins, or other parts. Ligatures should be round and very firm, so as to allow their being tied with some force, without risk of breaking.

The immediate effect of a tight ligature on an artery is to cut through its middle and internal coats, a circumstance that tends very much to promote the adhesion of the opposite sides of the vessel to each other. Hence the form and mode of applying a ligature to an artery should be such as are most certain of dividing the above coats of the vessel in the most favourable manner. A broad flat ligature does not promise to answer the purpose in the best manner; because it is scarcely possible to tie it smoothly round the artery, which is very likely to be thrown into folds, or to be puckered by it, and consequently to have an irregular bruised wound made in its middle and internal coats. A ligature of an irregular form is likely to cut through these coats more completely at some parts than at others; and if it does not perfectly divide them no adhesion can take place, and secondary hæmorrhage will follow. A fear of tying, the ligature too tight may often lead to the same consequences.

LIGHT. *Lux.* The nature of light has occupied much of the attention of philosophers, and numerous opinions have been entertained concerning it. It has been sometimes considered as a distinct substance, at other times as a quality; sometimes as a cause, frequently as an effect; by some it has been considered as a compound, by others as a simple substance. Philosophers of the present day are mostly agreed as to the independent existence of light, or the cause by which we see.

Nature of light.—Light is that which proceeds from any body producing the sensation of vision, or perception of other bodies, by depicting an image of external objects on the retina of the eye. Hence it announces to animals the presence of the bodies which surround them, and enables them to distinguish these bodies into transparent, opaque, and coloured. These properties are so essentially connected with the presence of light, that bodies lose them in the dark, and become undistinguishable.

Light is regarded by philosophers as a substance consisting of a vast number of exceedingly small particles, which are actually projected from luminous bodies, and which probably never return again to the body from which they were emitted.

It is universally expanded through space. It exerts peculiar actions, and is obedient to the laws of attraction, and other properties of matter.

Explanation of certain terms of light.—In order to facilitate the doctrine of light, we shall shortly explain a few terms made use of by philosophers when treating of it; namely,

A *ray of light* is an exceedingly small portion of light as it comes from a luminous body.

A *medium* is a body which affords a passage for the rays of light.

A *beam of light* is a body of parallel rays.

A *pencil of rays* is a body of diverging or converging rays.

Converging rays are rays which tend to a common point.

Diverging rays are those which come from a point, and continually separate as they proceed.

The rays of light are *parallel,* when the lines which they describe are so.

The *radiant point* is the point from which diverging rays proceed.

The *focus* is the point to which the converging rays are directed.

Sources of light.—Light is emitted from the sun the fixed stars, and other luminous bodies. It is produced by percussion, during electrization, combustion, and in various other chemical processes.

Why the sun and stars are constantly emitting light, is a question which probably will for ever baffle human understanding.

The light emitted during combustion exists previously, either combined with the combustible body, or with the substance which supports the combustion. The light liberated during chemical action, formed a constituent part of the bodies which act on each other

Chemical properties of light.—The chemical effects of light have much engaged the attention of philosophers. Its influence upon animal, vegetable, and other substances, is as follows:

1. *On vegetables.*—Every body knows that most of the discous flowers follow the sun in his course; that they attend him to his evening retreat, and meet his rising lustre in the morning with the same unerring law. It is also well known that the change of position in the leaves of plants, at different periods of the day, is entirely owing to the agency of light, and that plants which grow in windows, in the inside of houses, are, as it were, solicitous to turn their leaves towards the light. Natural philosophers have long been aware of the influence of light on vegetation. It was first observed that plants growing in the shade, or darkness, are pale and without colour. The term *etiolation* has been given to this phenomenon, and the plants, in which it takes place, are said to be *etiolated,* or *blanched.* Gardeners avail themselves of the knowledge of this fact, to furnish our tables with white and tender vegetables. When the plants have attained a certain height, they compress the leaves, by tying them together, and by these means (or by laying earth over them,) deprive them of the contact of light: and thus it is that our white celery, lettuce, cabbages, endive, &c. are obtained. For the same reason, wood is white under the green bark; and roots are less coloured than plants; some of them alter their taste, &c.; they even acquire a deleterious quality when suffered to grow exposed to light. Potatoes are of this kind. Herbs that grow beneath stones, or in places utterly dark, are white, soft, aqueous, and of a mild and insipid taste. The more plants are exposed to the light, the *more colour* they acquire. Though plants are capable of being nourished exceedingly well in the dark, and in that state grow much more rapidly than in the sun, (provided the air that surrounds them is fit for vegetation,) they are colourless and unfit for use.

Professor Davy found, by experiment, that red rose-trees, carefully excluded from light, produce roses almost white. He likewise ascertained that this flower owes its colour to light entering into its composition; that pink, orange, and yellow flowers imbibe a smaller portion of light than red ones, and that white flowers contain no light. But vegetables are not only indebted to the light for their colour: taste and odour are likewise derived from the same source.

Light contributes greatly to the maturity of fruits and seeds. This seems to be the cause why, under the burning sun of Africa, vegetables are in general more odoriferous, of a stronger taste, and more abounding with resin. From the same cause it happens, that hot climates seem to be the native countries of perfumes, odoriferous fruits, and aromatic resins.

The action of light is so powerful on the organs of vegetables, as to cause them to pour forth torrents of pure air from the surface of their leaves into the atmosphere, while exposed to the sun; whereas, on the contrary, when in the shade, they emit an air of a noxious quality. Take a few handfuls of fresh-gathered leaves of mint, cabbage, or any other plant; place them in a bell-glass, filled with fresh water, and invert it into a basin with the same fluid. If the whole be then exposed to the direct rays of the sun, small air bubbles will appear on the surface of the leaves, which will gradually grow larger, and at last detach them selves and become collected at the surface of the wa ter. This is oxygen gas, or vital air.

All plants do not emit this air with the same facility; there are some which yield it the moment the sun acts upon them; as the jacobœa or ragwort, lavender, peppermint, and some other aromatic plants. The leaves afford more air when attached to the plant than when gathered; the quantity is also greater, the fresher and sounder they are, and if full grown and collected during dry weather. Green plants afford more air than those which are of a yellowish or white colour. Green fruits afford likewise oxygen gas; but it is not so plentifully furnished by those which are ripe. Flowers in general render the air noxious. The Nasturtium indicum, in the space of a few hours, gives out more air than is equal to the bulk of all its leaves. On the contrary, if a like bell-glass, prepared in the same manner, be kept in the dark, another kind of air will be disengaged, of an opposite quality.

There is not a substance which, in well-closed glass

23

vessels, and exposed to the sun's light, does not experience some alteration.

Camphor, kept in glass bottles, exposed to light, crystallizes into the most beautiful symmetrical figures, on that side of the glass which is exposed to the light.

Yellow wax, exposed to the light, loses its colour and becomes bleached. Gum guaiacum, reduced to powder, becomes green on exposure to light. Vegetable colours, such as those of saffron, logwood, &c. become pale, or white, &c.

2 *On animals.*—The human being is equally dependent on the influence of light. Animals in general droop when deprived of light, they become unhealthy, and even sometimes die. When a man has been long confined in a dark dungeon (though well aired), his whole complexion becomes sallow; pustules, filled with aqueous humours, break out on his skin; and the person, who has been thus deprived, of light, becomes languid, and frequently dropsical. Worms, grubs, and caterpillars, which live in the earth, or in wood, are of a whitish colour; moths, and other insects of the night, are likewise distinguishable from those which fly by day by the want of brilliancy in their colour. The difference between those insects, in northern and southern parts, is still more obvious.

The parts of fish which are exposed to light, as the back, fins, &c. are uniformly coloured, but the belly, which is deprived of light, is white in all of them.

Birds which inhabit the tropical countries have much brighter plumage than those of the north. Those parts of the birds which are not exposed to the light are uniformly pale. The feathers on the belly of a bird are generally pale, or white; the back, which is exposed to the light, is almost always coloured; the breast, which is particularly exposed to light in most birds, is brighter than the belly.

Butterflies, and various other animals of equatorial countries, are brighter coloured than those of the polar regions. Some of the northern animals are even darker in summer and paler in winter.

3. *On other substances.*—Certain metallic oxides become combustible when exposed to light; and acids, as the nitric, &c. are decomposed by its contact, and various other substances change their nature.

Light carbonated hydrogen. See *Carburetted hydrogen gas.*

LIGNEUS. Woody. Applied in botany to pods, barks, &c. which are of a hard membraneous, or woody texture; as the strobilus of the *Pinus sylvestris.*

LI'GNUM. Wood.

LIGNUM AGALLOCHI VERI. See *Lignum aloes.*

LIGNUM ALOES. *Lignum agallochi veri; Agalluge; Agallugum; Lignum aquilæ; Lignum calambac; Lignum aspalathi; Xylo aloes; Agallochum; Calambac.* Aloes wood. The tree, the wood of which bears this name, is not yet scientifically known. It is by some supposed to be the *Excæaria agallocha,* the bark as well as the milk of which is purgative. It is imported from China in small, compact, ponderous pieces, of a yellow rusty brown colour, with black or purplish veins, and sometimes of a black colour. It has a bitterish resinous taste, and a slight aromatic smell. It is used to fumigate rooms in eastern countries.

LIGNUM AQUILÆ. See *Lignum aloes.*

LIGNUM ASPALATHI. See *Lignum aloes.*

LIGNUM CALAMBAC. See *Lignum aloes.*

LIGNUM CAMPECHENSE. (*Campechensis:* so called because it was brought from Campeachy, in the bay of Honduras. See *Hæmatoxylon campechianum.*

LIGNUM INDICUM. See *Guaiacum.*

LIGNUM MOLUCCENSE. See *Croton tiglium.*

LIGNUM NEPHRITICUM. See *Guilandina moringo.*

LIGNUM PAVANÆ. See *Croton tiglium.*

[LIGNUM QUASSIÆ. See *Quassia amara.* A.]

LIGNUM RHODIUM. See *Aspalathus Canariensis.*

LIGNUM SANCTUM. See *Guaiacum.*

LIGNUM SANTALI RUBRI. See *Pterocarpus santalinus*

LIGNUM SAPPAN. See *Hæmatoxylon campechianum.*

LIGNUM SERPENTUM. See *Ophioxylum serpentinum.*

[" LIGNUM VITÆ. The tree which produces this wood grows in the West Indies and tropical parts of America. It attains to the height of forty feet, and its trunk is four or five feet in circumference.

Lignum vitæ is brought in logs or masses, consisting of a dark greenish heart, covered with a yellowish al-

burnum. It is exceedingly hard, sinks in water, has little smell except when heated, and possesses a bitter and pungent taste.

The medicinal properties of the wood are principally derived from its resinous particles. It is, however, used as an ingredient in some decoctions, to which it imparts a certain portion of extractive matter of a tonic and stimulating nature. It was formerly much celebrated as an antisyphilitic. The hardness and solidity of lignum vitæ render it of great importance in the mechanic arts."—*Big. Mat. Med.* A.]

LIGULA. (*Ligula,* a strap.) 1. The clavicle.

2. The glottis.

3. The name of a measure and a weight.

3. A genus of the Mollusca order.

5. The small transparent membrane on the margin of the sheath and base of the leaves of grasses.

LIGULATUS. Shaped like a straw or ribband; a term applied to a kind of floret of a compound flower, which is so shaped; as those of the *Tragopogon* and *Taraxacum.*

LIGUSTICUM. (Λιγυστικον of Dioscorides; so called from *Liguria,* in Italy, its native country.) The name of a genus of plants. Class *Pentandria;* Order, *Digynia.*

LIGUSTICUM LEVISTICUM. The systematic name of lovage. *Levisticum.* The odour of this plant, *Ligusticum—foliis multiplicibus, foliolis superne incisis,* of Linnæus, is very strong, and particularly ungrateful; its taste is warm and aromatic. It abounds with a yellowish gummy resinous juice, very much resembling opoponax. Its virtues are supposed to be similar to those of angelica and masterwort, in expelling flatulencies, exciting sweat, and opening obstructions; therefore it is chiefly used in hysterical disorders and uterine obstructions. The leaves, eaten in salad, are accounted emmenagogue. The root, which is less ungrateful than the leaves, is said to possess similar virtues, and may be employed in powder.

LIGUSTRUM. (From *ligo,* to bind: so named from its use in making bands.)

1. The name of a genus of plants in the Linnæan system. Class, *Diandria;* Order, *Monogynia.*

2. The pharmacopœial name of the herb privet The *Ligustrum vulgare.*

LI'LALITE. The mineral lipidolite.

LILIACEUS. (From *lilium,* a lily.) Liliaceous, or resembling the lily.

LILIACEÆ. The name of an order of plants in Linnæus's Fragments of a Natural Method, consisting of such as have liliaceous corollæ, and a three-lobed stigma; as colchicum, lilium, crocus, &c.

LILIA'GO. (Diminutive of *lilium,* the lily : so named from the resemblance of its flower to that of a lily.) *Liliastrum.* Spiderwort. The *Anthericum liliastrum* of Linnæus, formerly said to be alexipharmic and carminative.

LI'LIUM. (From λειος, smooth, graceful: so named from the beauty of its leaf.) The name of a genus of plants in the Linnæan system. Class, *Hexandria;* Order, *Monogynia.* The lily.

LILIUM ALBUM. The white lily. See *Lilium candidum.*

LILIUM CANDIDUM. The systematic name of the white lily. *Lilium album. Lilium—foliis sparsis, corollis campanulatis, intus glabris,* of Linnæus. The roots are directed by the Edinburgh pharmacopœia; they are extremely mucilaginous, and chiefly used, boiled in milk and water, in emollient and suppurating cataplasms, to inflammatory tumours. These lily-roots afford a good substitute, in times of scarcity, for bread. The distilled water has been sometimes used as a cosmetic.

LILIUM CONVALLIUM. See *Convallaria majalis.*

LILIUM MARTAGON. The martagon lily. Linnæus tells us that the root of this plant forms a part of the ordinary food of the Siberians.

LILY. See *Lilium* and *Nymphæa.*

Lily, May. See *Convallaria majalis.*

Lily, water. See *Nymphæa alba,* and *Nymphæa lutea.*

Lily, white. See *Lilium candidum.*

Lily of the valley. See *Convallaria majalis.*

LIMATU'RA. (From *lima,* a file.) File dust or powder.

LIMATURA FERRI. Steel filings are considered as possessing stimulating and strengthening qualities, and are exhibited in worm cases, ataxia, leucorrhœa, diarrhœa, chlorosis, &c.

LI′MAX. (From *limus*, slime: so named from its sliminess.) *Cochlea terrestris.* The snail. This animal .abounds with a viscid slimy juice, which is readily given out by boiling, to milk or water, so as to render them thick and glutinous. These decoctions are apparently very nutritious and demulcent, and are recommended in consumptive cases and emaciations.

LIMBUS. The brim or border. Applied to a part of the corolla in botany. See *Corolla.*

LIME. *Calx.* 1. The oxide of calcium, one of the primitive earths. It is found in great abundance in nature, though never pure, or in an uncombined state. It is always united to an acid, and very frequently to the carbonic acid, as in chalk, common lime-stone, marble, calcareous spar, &c. It is contained in the waters of the ocean; it is found in vegetables; and is the basis of the bones, shells, and other hard parts of animals. Its combination with sulphuric acid is known by the name of sulphate of lime (*gypsum*, or plaster of Paris). Combined with flouric acid it constitutes fluate of lime, or Derbyshire spar.

Properties.—Lime is in solid masses, of a white colour, moderately hard, but easily reducible to powder. Its taste is bitter, urinous, and burning. It changes blue cabbage juice to a green. It is unalterable by the heat of our furnaces. It splits and falls into powder in the air, and loses its strong taste. It is augmented in weight and in size by slowly absorbing water and carbonic acid from the atmosphere. Its specific gravity is 2.3. It combines with phosphorus by heat. It unites to sulphur both in the dry and humid way. It absorbs sulphuretted hydrogen gas. It unites with some of the metallic oxides. Its slaking by water is attended with heat, hissing, splitting, and swelling up, while the water is partly consolidated and partly converted into vapour; and the lime is reduced into a very voluminous dry powder, when it has been sprinkled with only a small quantity of water. It is soluble when well prepared in about 450 parts of water. It unites to acids. It renders silex and alumine fusible, and more particularly these two earths together.

Method of obtaining Lime.—Since the carbonic acid may be separated from the native carbonate of lime, this becomes a means of exhibiting the lime in a state of tolerable purity. For this purpose, introduce into a porcelain, or earthen retort, or rather into a tube of green glass, well coated over with lute, and placed across a furnace, some powdered Carara marble, or oyster-shell powder. Adapt to its lower extremity a bent tube of glass, conveyed under a bell. If we then heat the tube, we obtain carbonic acid gas; and lime will be found remaining in the tube or retort.

The burning of lime in the large way, depends on the disengagement of the carbonic acid by heat; and, as lime is infusible in our furnaces, there would be no danger from too violent a heat, if the native carbonate of lime were perfectly pure; but as this is seldom the case, an extreme degree of heat produces a commencement of vitrification in the mixed stone, and enables it to preserve its solidity, and it no longer retains the qualities of lime, for it is covered with a sort of crust, which prevents the absorption of the water when it is attempted to be slaked. This is called over-burnt lime.

In order to obtain lime in a state of great purity, the following method may be had recourse to.

Take Carara marble, or oyster-shells; reduce them to powder, and dissolve the powder in pure acetic acid; precipitate the solution by carbonate of ammonia. Let the precipitate subside, wash it repeatedly in distilled water, let it dry, and then expose it to a white heat for some hours.

The acetic acid, in this operation, unites to the lime, and forms acetate of lime, disengaging at the same time the carbonic acid, which flies off in the gaseous state: on adding to the acetate of lime carbonate of ammonia, acetate of ammonia, and an artificial carbonate of lime are formed; from the latter the carbonic acid is again expelled, by exposure to heat, and the lime is left behind in a state of perfect purity. See *Calx.*

2. A fruit like a small lemon, the juice of which is a very strong acid, and very much used in the making of punch. Externally, the same acid is applied in the cutaneous affections of warm climates, and also as a remedy against the pains that precede the appearance of yaws. See *Tilia.*

LIME, CHLORIDE OF. The bleaching salt or bleaching powder, sold under the name of oxymuriate of lime.

LIMESTONE. A genus of minerals which Professor Jameson divides into the four following species:
1. Rhombspar. 2. Dolomite. 3. Limestone. 4. Arragonite.

Limestone has twelve sub-species.

1. *Foliated limestone.* Of this there are two kinds, calcareous spar, and foliated granular limestone.

2. *Compact limestone*, of which there are three kinds, common compact limestone, blue Vesuvian, and rosestone.

3. *Chalk.*

4. *Agaric-mineral*, or *Rock milk.*

5. *Fibrous limestone*, to which belong the satin spar and the fibrous calc-sinter.

6. *Tufaceous limestone*, or *calc-tuff.*

7. *Pisiform limestone*, or *peastone.*

8. *Slatespar.*

9. *Aphrite.*

10. *Luculite*, of which there are three kinds, compact, prismatic, and foliated.

11. *Marle*, of which there are two species, the earthy and compact.

12. *Bituminous marle slate.*

Limestone, bituminous. See *Bituminous limestone.*

• **LIME-TREE.** See *Tilia.*

Lime-water. See *Calcis liquor.*

LI′MON. (Hebrew.) See *Citrus medica*

LIMO′NIUM. (From λειμων, a green field; so called from its colour.) This name has been applied to,
1. The *Valeriana rubra.*
2. The *Polygonum fagopyrum.*
3. The *Pyroli rotundifolia.*
4. More commonly to the sea-lavender, or *Statice limonium*, of Linnæus, which is said to possess astringent properties.

LIMO′NUM. (From λειμων, a green field: so called from the colour of its unripe fruit.) The lemontree. See *Citrus medica.*

LIMOSIS. (From λιμος, hunger.) The name of a genus of diseases in Good's Nosology. Class, *Cæliaca*; Order, *Enterica.* Morbid appetite. It has seven species, viz. *Limosis avens, expers, pica, cardialgia, flatus, emesis, dyspepsia.*

LINACRE, THOMAS, was born at Canterbury, about the year 1460. After studying at Oxford, he travelled to Italy, where he acquired a perfect knowledge of the Latin and Greek languages; and afterward devoted his attention to medicine and natural philosophy at Rome. On his return, he graduated at Oxford, and gave lectures there on physic, as well as taught the Greek language. His reputation soon became so high, that he was called to court by Henry VII. who not only intrusted him with the education of his children, but also appointed him his physician; which office he likewise enjoyed under his successor Henry VIII. He appears in this monarch's reign to have stood, above all rivalship, at the head of his profession; and evinced his attachment to its interests, as well as to the public good, by founding medical lectures at the two universities, and obtaining the institution, in 1518, of the royal college of physicians in London. The practice of medicine was then occupied by illiterate monks and empirics, who were licensed by the bishops, whence much mischief must have arisen. A corporate body of regularly bred physicians was therefore established, in whom was vested the sole right of examining and admitting persons to practice, as well as of examining apothecaries' shops. Linacre was the first president, which office he retained during the remainder of his life; and, at his death, in 1524, bequeathed his house to the college. He had relinquished practice, and entered into holy orders, about five years before, being greatly afflicted with the stone, which was the cause of his dissolution. In his literary character, Linacre stands eminently distinguished, having been one of the first to introduce the learning of the ancients into this country. He translated several of the most valuable works of Galen into Lat'n; and his style is remarkable for its purity and elegance; he had indeed devoted great time to Latin composition, on which he published a large philosoph.:.-.

treatise. His professional skill was universally allowed among his contemporaries, as well as the honour and humanity with which he exercised the medical art; and the celebrated Erasmus has bestowed upon him the highest commendation. He was buried in St. Paul's Cathedral, where a monument was afterward erected to his memory, with a Latin inscription, by Dr. Caius.

LINAGRO'STIS. (From λινον, cotton, and αγρωϛις, grass: so called from the softness of its texture.) Cotton-grass. The *Eriophorum* of Linnæus, four species of which are found in Britain.

LINANGI'NA. (From *linum*, flax, and *ango*, to strangle: so called because, if it grows among flax or hemp, it twists round it, and chokes it.) The herb *dodder*. The *Cuscuta europæa* of Linnæus.

LINA'RIA. (From *linum*, flax: named from the resemblance of its leaves to those of flax.) See *Antirrhinum linaria*.

LI'NCTUS. (*Linctus, us.* m.; from *lingo*, to lick.) *Lohoc ; Eclegma; Elexis ; Elegma; Eclectos ;. Ecleitos ; Illinctus*. A loch, a lambative. A term in pharmacy, that is generally applied to a soft and somewhat oily substance, of the consistence of honey, which is licked off the spoon, it being too solid and adhesive to be taken otherwise.

LI'NÆA. (From *linum*, a thread.) This term is applied to some parts which have a thread or line-like appearance, as the long tendinous appearance of the muscles in the abdomen, &c.

LINEA ALBA. *Linea centralis.* An aponeurosis that extends from the scrobiculus cordis straight down to the navel, and from thence to the pubes. It is formed by the tendinous fibres of the internal oblique ascending and the external oblique descending muscles, and the transversalis, interlaced with those of the opposite side.

LINEÆ SEMILUNARES. The lines which bound the outer margin of the recti muscles, formed by the union of the abdominal tendons.

LINEÆ TRANSVERSÆ. The lines which cross the *recti* muscles of the abdomen.

LINEARIS. Linear. Applied to leaves, petals, leaf-stalks, seeds, &c. of plants, which are narrow, with parallel sides, as the leaves of most grasses, those of the *Narcissus, Pseudo-narcissus*, and the petals of the *Tussilago farfara*, leaf-stalk of the *Citrus medica*, and seeds of the *Crucianella*.

LINEATUS. Lineate. See *Linearis*.

LI'NGUA. (From *lingo*, to lick up.) The tongue. See *Tongue*.

LINGUA AVIS. The seeds of the *Fraxinus*, or ash, are so called, from their supposed resemblance to a bird's tongue.

LINGUA CANINA. So called from the resemblance of its leaves to a dog's tongue. See *Cynoglossum*.

LINGUA CERVINA. See *Asplenium Scolopendrium*.

LINGUA'LIS. (From *lingua*; the tongue.) *Basioglossus*, of Cowper. A muscle of the tongue. It arises from the root of the tongue laterally, and runs forward between the hyo-glossus and genio-glossus, to be inserted into the tip of the tongue, along with part of the stylo-glossus. Its use is to contract the substance of the tongue, and to bring it backwards.

LINGUIFORMIS. See *Lingulatus*.

LINGULATUS. (From *lingua*, a tongue.) Tongue-shaped. A term applied to a leaf of a thick, oblong, blunt figure, generally cartilaginous at the edges: as in the *Mesembryanthemum linguiforme*.

LINIMENT. See *Linimentum*.

LINIME'NTUM. (From *lino*, to anoint.) A liniment. An oily substance of a mediate consistence, between an ointment and oil, but so thin as to drop. The following are some of the most approved forms.

LINIMENTUM ÆRUGINIS. Liniment of verdigris, formerly called oxymel æruginis, mel ægyptiacum, and unguentum ægyptiacum:—Take of verdigris, powdered, an ounce; vinegar, seven fluid ounces; clarified honey, fourteen ounces. Dissolve the verdigris in the vinegar, and strain it through a linen cloth; having added the honey, gradually boil it down to a proper consistence.

LINIMENTUM AMMONIÆ FORTIUS. Strong liniment of ammonia.—Take of solution of ammonia, a fluid ounce; olive oil, two fluid ounces. Shake them together until they unite. A more powerful stimulating application than the former, acting as a rubefacient

In pleurodynia, indolent tumours, stiffness of the joints, and anthritic pains, it is to be preferred to the milder one.

LINIMENTUM AMMONIÆ SUBCARBONATIS. Liniment of subcarbonate of ammonia, formerly called linimentum ammoniæ and linimentum volatile.—Take of solution of subcarbonate of ammonia, a fluid ounce; olive oil, three fluid ounces. Shake them together until they unite. A stimulating liniment, mostly used to relieve rheumatic pains, bruises, and paralytic numbness.

LINIMENTUM AQUÆ CALCIS. Liniment of lime-water. Take of lime-water, olive oil, of each eight ounces; rectified spirit of wine, one ounce. Mix. This has been long in use as an application to burns and scalds.

LINIMENTUM CAMPHORÆ. Camphor liniment. Take of camphor, half an ounce; olive oil, two fluid ounces. Dissolve the camphor in the oil. In retentions of urine, rheumatic pains, distentions of the abdomen from ascites, and tension of the skin from abscess, this is an excellent application.

LINIMENTUM CAMPHORÆ COMPOSITUM. Compound camphor liniment. Take of camphor, two ounces; solution of ammonia, six fluid ounces; spirit of lavender, a pint. Mix the solution of ammonia with the spirit in a glass retort; then, by the heat of a slow fire, distil a pint. Lastly, in this distilled liquor dissolve the camphor. An elegant and useful stimulant application in paralytic, spasmodic, and rheumatic diseases. Also, for bruises, sprains, rigidities of the joints, incipient chilblains, &c. &c.

LINIMENTUM HYDRARGYRI. Mercurial liniment. Take of strong mercurial ointment, prepared lard, of each four ounces, camphor an ounce; rectified spirit, fifteen minims; solution of ammonia, four fluid ounces. First powder the camphor, with the addition of the spirit, then rub it with the mercurial ointment and the lard; lastly, add gradually the solution of ammonia, and mix the whole together. An excellent formula for all surgical cases, in which the object is to quicken the action of the absorbents, and gently stimulate the surfaces of parts. It is a useful application for diminishing the indurated state of particular muscles, a peculiar affection every now and then met with in practice; and it is peculiarly well calculated for lessening the stiffness and chronic thickening often noticed in the joints. If it be frequently or largely applied, it affects the mouth more rapidly than the mercurial ointment.

LINIMENTUM OPIATUM. A resolvent anodyne embrocation, adapted to remove indolent tumours of the joints, and those weaknesses which remain after strains and chilblains before they break.

LINIMENTUM SAPONIS COMPOSITUM. Compound soap liniment. *Linimentum saponis*. Take of hard soap, three ounces; camphor, an ounce; spirit of rosemary, a pint. Dissolve the camphor in the spirit, then add the soap, and macerate in the heat of a sand-bath, until it be melted. The basis of this form was first proposed by Riverius, and it is now commonly used under the name of opodeldoc. This is a more pleasant preparation, to rub parts affected with rheumatic pains, swellings of the joints, &c. than any of the foregoing, and at the same time not inferior, except where a rubefacient is required.

LINIMENTUM SAPONIS CUM OPIO. Soap liniment, with opium. Take of compound soap liniment, six ounces; tincture of opium, two ounces. Mix. For dispersing indurations and swellings, attended with pain, but no acute inflammation.

LINIMENTUM TEREBINTHINÆ. Turpentine liniment. Take of resin cerate, a pound; oil of turpentine, half a pint. Add the oil of turpentine to the cerate, previously melted, and mix. This liniment is very commonly applied to burns, and was first introduced by Mr. Kentish, of Newcastle.

LINIMENTUM TEREBINTHINÆ VITRIOLICUM. Vitriolic liniment of turpentine. Take of olive oil, ten ounces; oil of turpentine, four ounces; vitriolic acid, three drachms. Mix. This preparation is said to be efficacious in chronic affections of the joints, and in the removal of long-existing effects of sprains and bruises.

Liniment of ammonia. See *Linimentum ammoniæ*
Liniment of camphire. See *Linimentum camphoræ*
Liniment of mercury. See *Linimentum hydrargyri*

26

Liniment of turpentine. See *Linimentum terebinthinæ.*

Liniment of verdigris. See *Linimentum æruginis.*

LINNÆ'A. (So named in honour of Linnæus.) The name of a genus of plants in the Linnæan system. Class, *Didynamia;* Order, *Angiospermia.*

LINNÆA BOREALIS. The systematic name of the plant named in honour of the immortal Linnæus, which has a bitter, subastringent taste, and is used in some places in the form of fomentation, to rheumatic pains, and an infusion with milk is much esteemed in Switzerland in the cure of sciatica.

LINNÆUS, CHARLES, was born in Sweden, in 1707. He derived at a very early age from his father, that attachment to the study of nature, by which he afterward so eminently distinguished himself. He was intended for the church, but made so little improvement in the requisite learning, that this was soon abandoned for the profession of medicine. He appears to have had a singular inaptitude for learning languages; though he was sufficiently versed in Latin. His scanty finances much embarrassed his progress at first; but his taste for botany at length having procured him the patronage of Dr. Celsius, professor of divinity at Upsal, he was enabled to pursue his studies to more advantage. In 1730, he was appointed to give lectures in the botanic garden, and began to compose some of those works, by which he rendered his favourite science more philosophical, and more popular than it had ever been before. Two years afterward he was commissioned to make a tour through Lapland, of which he subsequently published an interesting account; and having learned the art of assaying metals, he gave lectures on this subject also on his return. In 1735, he took his degree in physic at Harderwyck, and in his inaugural dissertation advanced a strange hypothesis, that intermittent fevers are owing to particles of clay, taken in with the food, obstructing the minute arteries. Soon after this, his Systema Naturæ first appeared; which was greatly enlarged and improved in numerous successive editions. In Holland, he fortunately obtained the support of a Mr. Clifford, an opulent banker, whereby he was enabled to visit England also; but his great exertions afterward impaired his health, and being attacked with a severe intermittent, he could not resist the desire, when somewhat recovered, of returning to his native country. Arriving there in 1738, he settled at Stockholm, where his reputation soon procured him some medical practice, and the appointment of physician to the navy, as well as lecturer on botany and mineralogy; a literary society was also established, of which he was the first president, and by which numerous volumes of transactions have since been published. In 1740, he was chosen professor of medicine at Upsal, having been admitted a member of that academy on his return to Sweden; he also shared with Dr. Rosen the botanical duties, and considerably improved the garden; he was afterward made secretary, and on some public occasions did the honours of the university. He received likewise marks of distinction from several foreign societies. About the year 1746, he was appointed Archiater; and it became an object of national interest to make additions to his collection from every part of the world. A systematic treatise on the Materia Medica was published by him in 1749; and two years after his Philosophia Botanica, composed during a severe fit of the gout, in which he supposed himself to have derived great benefit from taking a large quantity of wood strawberries. This was soon followed by his great work, the Species Plantarum; after which he was honoured with the order of the Polar Star, never before conferred for literary merit; and having declined a splendid invitation to Spain, he was raised to the rank of nobility. In 1763 his son was allowed to assist him in the botanical duties. About this time he published his Genera Morborum, and three years after his Clavis Medicinæ. His medical lectures, though too theoretical, were very much esteemed; but he had declined general practice on his establishment at Upsal. As he advanced in life, the fatiguing occupations in which he was engaged impaired his health, notwithstanding his temperate and regular habits; and at length brought on his dissolution in 1778. This was regarded as a loss to the nation, and even to the world. About ten years after, a society, adopting his name, was formed in this country, which has published many valuable volumes of

transactions, and the president purchased Linnæus's collections of his widow; similar institutions have also been established in other parts of the world.

LINNÆAN SYSTEM. This name is applied particularly to that arrangement of plants, which Linnæus has founded on the fructification or sexes of plants. See *Sexual system of plants.*

LINOSPE'RMUM. (From λινον, flax, and σπερμα, seed.) See *Linum usitatissimum.*

LINOZOSTRIS. A name given by the ancient Greek writers to two plants, very different from one another. The one is the *Mercurialis,* or British mercury; the other the *Epilinum,* or dodder.

LINSEED. See *Linum usitatissimum.*

LINT. See *Linteum.*

LI'NTEUM. Lint. A soft, woolly substance, made by scraping old linen cloth, and employed in surgery as the common dressing in all cases of wounds and ulcers, either simply or covered with different unctuous substances.

LI'NUM. (From λειος, soft, smooth: so called from its soft, smooth texture.) 1. The name of a genus of plants in the Linnæan system. Class, *Pentandria.* Order, *Pentagynia.*

2. The pharmacopœial name of the common flax. See *Linum usitatissimum.*

LINUM CATHARTICUM. *Linum minimum; Chamælium.* Purging flax, or mill-mountain. This small plant, *Linum—foliis oppositis ovato-lanceolatis, caule dichotomo, corollis acutis,* of Linnæus, is an effectual and safe cathartic. It has a bitterish and disagreeable taste. A handful infused in half a pint of boiling water is the dose for an adult.

LINUM USITATISSIMUM. The systematic name of the common flax, *Linum sylvestre. Linum—calycibus capsulisque mucronatis, petalis crenatis, foliis lanceolatis alternis, caule subsolitario,* of Linnæus. The seeds of this useful plant, called linseed, have an unctuous, mucilaginous, sweetish taste, but no remarkable smell; on expression they yield a large quantity of oil, which, when carefully drawn without the application of heat, has no particular taste or flavour: boiled in water, they yield a large proportion of strong flavourless mucilage, which is in use as an emollient or demulcent in cough, hoarseness, and pleuritic symptoms, that frequently prevail in catarrhal affections and it is likewise recommended in nephritic pains and stranguries. The meal of the seeds is also much used externally, in emollient and maturating cataplasms. The expressed oil is an officinal preparation, and is supposed to be of a more healing and balsamic nature than the other oils of this class: it has, therefore, been very generally employed in pulmonary complaints, and in colics and constipations of the bowels. The cake which remains after the expression of the oil, contains the farinaceous part of the seed, and is used in fattening cattle under the name of oil-cake.

Lion-toothed leaf. See *Runcinatus.*

LI'PARIS. (From λιπος, fat: so named from its unctuous quality.) See *Pinguicula.*

LIPAROCE'LE. (From λιπος, fat, and κηλη, a tumour.) That species of sarcocele in which the substance constituting the disease very much resembles fat.

LIPO'MA. (From λιπος, fat.) A solitary, soft, unequal, indolent tumour, arising from a luxuriancy of adeps in the cellular membrane. The adipose structure forming the tumour is sometimes diseased towards its centre, and more fluid than the rest. At other times it does not appear to differ in any respect from adipose membrane, except in the enlargement of the cells containing the fat. These tumours are always many years before they arrive at any size.

LIPOPSY'CHIA. (From λειπω, to leave, and ψυχη the soul, or life.) A swoon, or fainting. See *Syncope*

LIPOTHY'MIA. (From λειπω, to leave, and θυμος the mind.) Fainting. See *Syncope.*

LIPPITU'DO. (From *lippus,* blear-eyed.) *Epiphora; Xerophthalmia.* Blear-eyedness. An exudation of a puriform humour from the margin of the eyelids. The proximate cause is a deposition of acrimony on the glandulæ meibomianæ in the margin of the eyelids. This humour in the night glues the tarsi of the eyelids together. The margins of the eyelids are red and tumefy, are irritated, and excite pain. An opthalmia, fistula lachrymalis, and sometimes an ectropium, are the consequences. The species of the lippitudo are,

1. *Lippitudo infantum*, which is familiar to children, particularly of an acrimonious habit. The lippitudo of infants is mostly accompanied with tinea, or some scabby eruption, which points out that the disease originates, not from a local, but general or constitutional affection.

2. *Lippitudo adultorum*, or *senilis*. This arises from various acrimonies, and is likewise common to hard drinkers.

3. *Lippitudo venerea*, which arises from a suppressed gonorrhœa, or fluor albus, and is likewise observed of children born of parents with venereal complaints.

4. *Lippitudo scrophulosa*, which accompanies other scrofulous symptoms.

5. *Lippitudo scorbutica*, which affects the scorbutic.

LIPY'RIA. (From λειπω, to leave, and πυρ, heat.) A sort of fever, where the heat is drawn to the inward parts, while the externals are cold.

LIQUIDA'MBAR. (From *liquidum*, fluid, and *ambar*, a fragrant substance, generally taken for ambergris; alluding to the aromatic liquid gum which distils from this tree.) The name of a genus of plants in the Linnæan system. Class, *Monœcia ;* Order, *Polyandria*.

LIQUIDAMBAR STYRACIFLUA. The systematic name of the tree which affords both the liquid amber and *storax liquida*, or liquid storax. The liquid amber is a resinous juice of a yellow colour, inclining to red, at first about the consistence of turpentine, by age hardened into a solid brittle mass. It is obtained by wounding the bark of this tree, which is described by Linnæus the *Liquidambar—foliis palmato-angulatis ; foliis indivisis, acutis*. The juice has a moderately pungent, warm, balsamic taste, and a very fragrant smell, not unlike that of the *Styrax calamita* heightened by a little ambergris. It is seldom used medicinally. The *Styrax liquida* is also obtained from this plant by boiling. There are two sorts distinguished by authors ; the one the purer part of the resinous matter, that rises to the surface in boiling, separated by a strainer, of the consistence of honey, tenacious like turpentine, of a reddish or ash-brown colour, moderately transparent, of an acrid unctuous taste and a fragrant smell, faintly resembling that of the solid styrax, but somewhat disagreeable. The other, the more impure part, which remains on the strainer, untransparent, and in smell and taste much weaker than the former. Their use is chiefly as stomachics, in the form of plaster.

LIQUIFACTION. A chemical term, in some instances synonymous with *fusion*, in others with the word *deliquescence*, and in others with the word *solution*.

LIQUIRI'TIA. (From *liquor*, juice, or from *elikoris*, Welsh.) See *Glycyrrhiza*.

LI'QUOR. A liquor. This term is applied in the last editions of the London Pharmacopœia to some preparations, before improperly called waters ; as the *aqua ammoniæ*, &c.

LIQUOR ACETATIS PLUMBI. See *Plumbi acetatis liquor*.

LIQUOR ACETATIS PLUMBI DILUTUS. See *Plumbi acetatis liquor dilutus*.

LIQUOR ÆTHEREUS VITRIOLICUS. See *Æther sulphuricus*.

LIQUOR ALUMINIS COMPOSITUS. Compound solution of alum. Take [of alum, sulphate of zinc, of each half an ounce ; boiling water two pints. Dissolve at the same time the alum and sulphate of zinc in the water, and then strain the solution through paper. This water was long known in our shops under the title of *Aqua aluminosa batcana*. It is used for cleansing and healing ulcers and wounds, and for removing cutaneous eruptions, the part being bathed with it hot three or four times a-day. It is sometimes likewise employed as a collyrium ; and as an injection in fluor albus and gonorrhœa, when not accompanied with virulence.

LIQUOR AMMONIÆ. See *Ammonia*.

LIQUOR AMMONIÆ ACETATIS. See *Ammoniæ acetatis liquor*.

LIQUOR AMMONIÆ CARBONATIS. See *Ammoniæ subcarbonatis liquor*.

LIQUOR AMMONIÆ SUBCARBONATIS. See *Ammoniæ subcarbonatis liquor*.

Liquor of ammonia. See *Ammonia*.

LIQUOR AMNII. All that fluid which is contained in the membranaceous ovum surrounding the fœtus in utero, is called by the general name of the waters, the water of the amnion, or ovum, or liquor amnii. The

quantity, in proportion to the size of the different parts of the ovum, is greatest by far in early pregnancy. At the time of parturition, in some cases, it amounts to or exceeds four pints ; and, in others, it is scarcely equal to as many ounces. It is usually in the largest quantity when the child has been some time dead, or is born in a weakly state. This fluid is generally transparent, often milky, and sometimes of a yellow or light-brown colour, and very different in consistence ; and these alterations seem to depend upon the state of the constitution of the parent. It does not coagulate with heat, like the serum of the blood, and chemically examined, it is found to be composed of phlegm, earthy matter, and sea-salt, in different proportions in different subjects, by which the varieties in its appearance and consistence are produced. It has been supposed to be excrementitious ; but it is generally thought to be secreted from the internal surface of the ovum, and to be circulatory as in other cavities. It was formerly imagined that the fœtus was nourished by this fluid, of which it was said to swallow some part frequently ; and it was then asserted, that the qualities of the fluid were adapted for its nourishment. But there have been many examples of children born without any passage to the stomach ; and a few of children in which the head was wanting, and which have nevertheless arrived at the full size. These cases fully prove that this opinion is not just, and that there must be some other medium by which the child is nourished, besides the waters. The incontrovertible uses of this fluid are, to serve the purpose of affording a soft bed for the residence of the fœtus, to which it allows free motion, and prevents any external injury during pregnancy ; and enclosed in the membranes, it procures the most gentle, yet efficacious, dilatation of the os uteri, and soft parts, at the time of parturition. Instances have been recorded, in which the waters of the ovum are said to have been voided so early as in the sixth month of pregnancy, without prejudice either to the child or parent. The truth of these reports seems to be doubtful ; because when the membranes are intentionally broken, the action of the uterus never fails to come on, when all the water is evacuated. A few cases have occurred to me, says Dr. Denman, in practice, which might have been construed to be of this kind ; for there was a daily discharge of some colourless fluid from the vagina, for several months before delivery ; but there being no diminution of the size of the abdomen, and the waters being regularly discharged at the time of labour, it was judged that some lymphatic vessel near the os uteri had been ruptured, and did not close again till the patient was delivered. He also met with one case, in which, after the expulsion of the placenta, there was no sanguineous discharge, but a profusion of lymph, to the quantity of several pints, in a few hours after delivery ; but the patient suffered no inconvenience except from surprise.

LIQUOR ANTIMONII TARTARIZATI. See *Antimonii tartarizati liquor*.

LIQUOR ARSENICALIS. See *Arsenicalis liquor*.

LIQUOR CALCIS. See *Calcis liquor*.

LIQUOR CUPRI AMMONIATI. See *Cupri ammoniati liquor*.

LIQUOR FERRI ALKALINI. See *Ferri alkalini liquor*.

LIQUOR HYDRARGYRI OXYMURIATIS. See *Hydrargyri oxymurias*.

LIQUOR MINERALIS ANODYNUS HOFFMANNI. Hoffmann's anodyne liquor. See *Spiritus ætheris sulphurici compositi*.

LIQUOR POTASSÆ. See *Potassæ liquor*.

LIQUOR SUBCARBONATIS POTASSÆ. See *Potassæ subcarbonatis liquor*.

LIQUOR VOLATILIS CORNU CERVI. This preparation of the fluid volatile alkali, commonly termed hartshorn is in common use to smell at in faintings, &c. See *Ammoniæ subcarbonas*.

LIQUORICE. See *Glycyrrhiza*.

Liquorice, Spanish. See *Glycyrrhiza*.

LIRELLA. (A diminutive of *lire*, a ridge between two furrows.) Acharius's name for the black letter like receptacles of the genus *Opegrapha*.

LISTER, MARTIN, was born about 1638, of a Yorkshire family, settled in Buckinghamshire, which produced many medical practitioners of reputation ; and his uncle Sir Matthew Lister, was physician to Charles I. and president of the college. After studying at Cambridge, where he was made fellow of St. John's

28

college, by royal mandate, he travelled to the Continent for improvement. On his return, in 1670, he settled at York, where he practised for many years with considerable success. Having communicated many papers on the natural history and antiquities of the north of England to the Royal Society, he was elected a fellow of that body ; and he likewise enriched the Ashmolean Museum at Oxford. He came by the solicitation of his friends to London in 1684, having received a diploma at Oxford ; and soon after was admitted a fellow of the College of Physicians. In 1698 he accompanied the embassy to France, and published an account of this journey on his return. He was made physician to Queen Anne about three years before his death, which happened in the beginning of 1712. He wrote on the English medicinal waters, on small-pox, and some other diseases; but his writings, though containing some valuable practical observations, are marked by too much hypothesis and attachment to ancient doctrines ; and he particularly condemned the cooling plan of treatment in febrile diseases, introduced by the sagacious Sydenham. His reputation is principally founded on his researches in natural history and comparative anatomy, on which he published several separate works, as well as nearly forty papers in the Philosophical Transactions.

LITHAGO'GA (From λιθος, a stone, and αγω, to bring away.) Medicines which expel the stone.

LITHARGE. See Lithargyrus.

Litharge plaster. See Emplastrum lithargyri.

LITHA'RGYRUS. (From λιθος, a stone, and αργυρος, silver.) Lithargyrum. Litharge. An oxide of lead, in an imperfect state of vitrification. When silver is refined by cupellation with lead, this latter metal, which is scorified, and causes the scorification of the imperfect metals alloyed with the silver, is transformed into a matter composed of small, semitransparent, shining plates, resembling mica; which is litharge. Litharge is more or less white or red, according to the metals with which the silver is alloyed. The white is called litharge of silver; and the red has been improperly called litharge of gold. See Lead, and Plumbi subacetatis liquor.

LITHIA. (Lithia, from λιθειος, lapideus.) Lithion; Lithina. 1. A new alkali. It was discovered by Arfredson, a young chemist of great merit, employed in the laboratory of Berzelius. It was found in a mineral from the mine of Uten in Sweden called petalite by D'Andrada, who first distinguished it. Sir H. Davy demonstrated by Voltaic electricity, that the basis of this alkali is a metal, to which the name of lithium has been given.

Berzelius gives the following simple process as a test for lithia in minerals :—

A fragment of the mineral, the size of a pin's head, is to be heated with a small excess of soda, on a piece of platinum foil, by a blowpipe for a couple of minutes. The stone is decomposed, the soda liberates the lithia, and the excess of alkali preserving the whole fluid at this temperature, it spreads over the foil, and surrounds the decomposed mineral. That part of the platinum near to the fused alkali becomes of a dark colour, which is more intense, and spreads over a larger surface, in proportion as there is more lithia in the mineral. The oxidation of the platinum does not take place beneath the alkali, but only around it, where the metal is in contact with both air and lithia. Potassa destroys the reaction of the platinum on the lithia, if the lithia be not redundant. The platina resumes its metallic surface, after having been washed and heated.

Caustic lithia has a very sharp, burning taste. It destroys the cuticle of the tongue like potassa. It does not dissolve with great facility in water, and appears not to be much more soluble in hot than in cold water. In this respect it has an analogy with lime. Heat is evolved during its solution in water.

When exposed to the air it does not attract moisture but absorbs carbonic acid, and becomes opaque. When exposed for an hour to a white heat in a covered platinum crucible, its bulk does not appear to be diminished : but it has absorbed a quantity of carbonic acid.

2. The name of a genus of diseases in Good's Nosology. Class, Eccritica ; Order, Catotica. Urinary calculus.

LI'THIAS. A lithiate, or salt, formed by the union of the lithic acid or acid of the stone sometimes found in the bladder of animals with salifiable bases; thus lithiate of ammonia, &c.

LITHI'ASIS. (From λιθος, a stone.)
1. The formation of stone or gravel.
2. A tumour of the eyelid, under which is a hard concretion resembling a stone.

LITHIC ACID. (Acidum lithicum; from λιθος, a stone, because it is obtained from the stones of the bladder.) Acidum uricum. This was discovered in analyzing human calculi, of many of which it constitutes the greater part, and of some, particularly that which resembles wood in appearance, it forms almost the whole. It is likewise present in human urine, and in that of the camel. It is found in those arthritic concretions commonly called chalkstones. It is often called uric acid.

The following are the results of Scheele's experiments on calculi, which were found to consist almost wholly of this acid.

1. Dilute sulphuric acid produced no effect on the calculus, but the concentrated dissolved it; and the solution, distilled to dryness, left a black coal, giving off sulphurous acid fumes. 2. The muriatic acid, either diluted or concentrated, had no effect on it even with ebullition. 3. Dilute nitric acid attacked it cold ; and with the assistance of heat, produced an effervescence and red vapour, carbonic acid was evolved, and the calculus was entirely dissolved. The solution was acid, even when saturated with the calculus, and gave a beautiful red colour to the skin in half an hour after it was applied; when evaporated, it became of a blood-red, but the colour was destroyed by adding a drop of acid ; it did not precipitate muriate of barytes, or metallic solutions, even with the addition of an alkali ; alkalies rendered it more yellow, and if superabundant, changed it by a strong digesting heat to a rose colour ; and this mixture imparts a similar colour to the skin, and is capable of precipitating sulphate of iron black, sulphate of copper green, nitrate of silver gray, superoxygenated muriate of mercury, and solutions of lead and zinc, white. Lime-water produced in the nitric solution a white precipitate, which dissolved in the nitric and muriatic acids without effervescence, and without destroying their acidity. Oxalic acid did not precipitate it. 4. Carbonate of potassa did not dissolve it, either cold or hot, but a solution of perfectly pure potassa dissolved it even cold. The solution was yellow; sweetish to the taste; precipitated by all the acids, even the carbonic; did not render lime-water turbid; decomposed and precipitated solution of iron brown, of copper gray, of silver black, of zinc, mercury, and lead, white; and exhaled a smell of ammonia. 5. About 200 parts of lime-water dissolved the calculus by digestion, and lost its acrid taste. The solution was partly precipitated by acids. 6. Pure water dissolved it entirely, but it was necessary to boil for some time 360 parts with one of the calculus in powder. This solution reddened tincture of litmus, did not render lime-water turbid, and on cooling deposited in small crystals almost the whole of what it had taken up. 7. Seventy-two grains distilled in a small glass retort over an open fire, and gradually brought to a red heat, produced water of ammonia mixed with a little animal oil, and a brown sublimate, weighing 28 grains, and 12 grains of coal remained, which preserved its black colour on red-hot iron in the open air. The brown sublimate was rendered white by a second sublimation; was destitute of smell, even when moistened by an alkali ; was acid to the taste; dissolved in boiling water, and also in alkohol, but in less quantity ; did not precipitate lime-water ; and appeared to resemble succinic acid.

Fourcroy has found, that this acid is almost entirely soluble in 2000 times its weight of cold water, when the powder is repeatedly treated with it. From his experiments he infers, that it contains azote, with a considerable portion of carbon, and but little hydrogen, and little oxygen.

Of its combinations with the basis we know but little.

Much additional information has been obtained within these few years on the nature and habitudes of the lithic acid. Dr. Henry wrote a medical thesis, and afterward published a paper on the subject, in the second volume of the new series of the Manchester memoirs, both of which contain many important facts. He procured the acid in the manner above described by Fourcroy. It has the form of white shining plates, which are denser than water. Has no taste nor smell. It dissolves in about 1400 parts of boiling water. It reddens the infusion of litmus. When dissolved in nitric acid, and evaporated to dryness, it leaves a pink sediment. The dry acid is not acted on nor dissolved by the alkaline carbonates, or sub-carbonates. It decomposes soap when assisted by heat; as it does also the alkaline sulphurets and hydrosulphurets. No acid acts on it, except those that occasion its decomposition. It dissolves in hot solutions of potassa and soda, and likewise in ammonia, but less readily. The lithates may be formed, either by mutually saturating the two constituents, or we may dissolve the acid in an excess of base, and we may then precipitate by carbonate of ammonia. The lithates are all tasteless, and resemble in appearance lithic acid itself. They are not altered by exposure to the atmosphere. They are very sparingly soluble in water. They are decomposed by a red heat, which destroys the acid. The lithic acid is precipitated from these salts by all the acids, except the prussic and carbonic. They are decomposed by the nitrates, muriates, and acetates of barytes, strontites, lime, magnesia, and alumina. They are precipitated by all the metallic solutions except that of gold. When lithic acid is exposed to heat, the products are carburetted hydrogen, and carbonic acid, prussic acid, carbonate of ammonia, a sublimate, consisting of ammonia combined with a peculiar acid, which has the following properties:—

Its colour is yellow, and it has a cooling, bitter taste. It dissolves readily in water, and in alkaline solutions, from which it is not precipitated by acids. It dissolves also sparingly in alkohol. It is volatile, and when sublimed a second time, becomes much whiter. The watery solution reddens vegetable blues, but a very small quantity of ammonia destroys this property. It does not cause effervescence with alkaline carbonates. By evaporation it yields permanent crystals, but ill defined, from adhering animal matter. These redden vegetable blues. Potassa, when added to these crystals, disengages ammonia. When dissolved in nitric acid, they do not leave a red stain, as happens with uric acid; nor does their solution in water decompose the earthy salts, as happens with alkaline lithates (or urates). Neither has it any action on the salts of copper, iron, gold, platinum, tin, or mercury. With nitrates of silver, and mercury, and acetate of lead, it forms a white precipitate, soluble in an excess of nitric acid. Muriatic acid occasions no precipitate in the solution of these crystals in water. These properties show, that the acid of the sublimate is different from the uric, and from every other known acid. Dr. Austin found, that by repeated distillations lithic acid was resolved into ammonia, nitrogen, and prussic acid.

When lithic acid is projected into a flask with chlorine, there is formed, in a little time, muriate of ammonia, oxalate of ammonia, carbonic acid, muriatic acid, and malic acid; the same results are obtained by passing chlorine through water, holding this acid in suspension.

LITHIUM. The metallic basis of lithia. See *Lithia*.

LITHOIDES. (From λιθος, a stone, and ειδος, a likeness: so called from its hardness.) The petrous portion of the temporal bone.

LITHO'LABUM. (From λιθος, a stone, and λαμβανω, to seize.) An instrument for extracting the stone from the bladder.

LITHO'LOGY. (*Lithologia;* from λιθος, a stone, and λογος, a discourse.) A discourse, or treatise on stones.

LITHOMA'RGA. See *Lithomarge.*

LITHOMARGE. Stone-marrow. A mineral, of which there are two kinds, the friable and the indurated.

LITHONTRIPTIC. (*Lithontripticus;* from λιθος, a stone, and τριβω, to bear away.) Lithontryptic. From the strict sense and common acceptation of the word, this class of medicine should comprehend such as possess a power of dissolving calculi in the urinary passages. It is, however, doubted by many, whether there be in nature any such substances. By this term, then, is meant those substances which possess a power of removing a disposition in the body to the formation of calculi. The researches of modern chemists have proved, that these calculi consist mostly of a peculiar acid, named the lithic or uric acid. With this sub

stance, the alkalies are capable of uniting, and forming a soluble compound; and these are, accordingly, almost the sole lithontriptics. From the exhibition of alkaline remedies, the symptoms arising from stone in the bladder are very generally alleviated; and they can be given to such an extent that the urine becomes very sensibly alkaline, and is even capable of exerting a solvent power on these concretions. Their administration, however, cannot be continued to this extent for any length of time, from the irritation they produce on the stomach and urinary organs. The use, therefore, of the alkalies, as solvents, or lithontriptics, is now scarcely ever attempted; they are employed merely to prevent the increase of the concretion, and to palliate the painful symptoms, which they do apparently by preventing the generation of lithic acid, or the separation of it by the kidneys; the urine is thus rendered less irritating, and the surface of the calculus is allowed to become smooth.

When the alkalies are employed with this view, they are generally given neutralized, or with excess of carbonic acid. This renders them much less irritating It at the same time, indeed, diminishes their solvent power; for the alkaline carbonates exert no action on urinary calculi; but they are still capable of correcting that acidity in the primæ viæ, which is the cause of the deposition of the lithic acid from the urine, and, therefore, serve equally to palliate the disease. And when their acrimony is thus diminished, their use can be continued for any length of time.

It appears, from the experiments of Fourcroy and others, that some other ingredients of calculi, as well as the lithic acid, are dissolved by the caustic alkali, and various experiments have shown, that most calculi yield to its power. It is obvious, however, that what is taken by the mouth is subject to many changes in the alimentary canal, and also the lymphatic and vascular systems; and in this way it must be exceedingly diffi cult to get such substances (even were they not liable to alterations) in sufficient quantity into the bladder. Indeed, there are very few authenticated cases of the urine being so changed as to become a menstruum for the stone. Excepting the case of Dr. Newcombe, recorded by Dr. Whytt, the instance of Mr. Home is almost the only one. Though lithontriptics, however, may not in general dissolve the stone in the bladder, yet it is an incontrovertible fact, that they frequently mitigate the pain: and to lessen such torture as that of the stone in the bladder, is surely an object of no little importance. Lime was long ago known as a remedy for urinary calculi, and different methods were employed to administer it. One of these plans fell into the hands of a Mrs. Steevens, and her success caused great anxiety for the discovery of the secret. At last Parliament bought the secret for the sum of 5000l. In many instances, stones which had been unquestionably felt, were no longer to be discovered; and as the same persons were examined by surgeons of the greatest skill and eminence, both before and after the exhibition of her medicines, it was no wonder that the conclusion was drawn, that the stones really were dissolved. From the cessation of such success, and from its now being known that the stones are occasionally protruded between the fasciculi of the muscular fibres of the bladder, so as to be lodged in a kind of cyst on the outside of the muscular coat, and cause no longer any grievances, surgeons of the present day are inclined to suspect that this must have happened in Mrs. Steevens's cases. This was certainly what happened in one of the cases on whom the medicine had been tried. It is evident that a stone, so situated, would not any longer produce irritation, but would also be quite indiscoverable by the sound, for, in fact, it is no longer in the cavity of the bladder.

As soap was, with reason, supposed to increase the virtues of the lime, it led to the use of caustic alkali, taken in mucilage, or veal broth. Take of pure potassa, ℥ viij; of quick-lime, ℥ iv; of distilled water, lbij. Mix them well together in a large bottle, and let them stand for twenty-four hours. Then pour off the ley, filter it through paper, and keep it in well-stopped vials for use. Of this, the dose is from thirty drops to ℈ ij, which is to be repeated two or three times a-day, in a pint of veal broth, early in the morning, at noon, and in the evening. Continue this plan for three or four months, living, during the course, on such things as least counteract the effect of the medicine.

The common fixed alkalies, or carbonated alkali, and the acidulous soda-water, have of late been used as lithontriptics. Honey has also been given; and Mr. Home, surgeon at the Savoy, has recorded its utility in his own and in his father's cases. Bitters have likewise been tried.

Dismissing all theories, lime-water, soap, acidulous soda-water, caustic, alkali, and bitters, are useful in cases of stone. Of the soap, as much may be taken as the stomach will bear, or as much as will prove gently laxative; but of the lime-water, few can take more than a pint daily.

The acidulous soda-water may be taken in larger quantities, as it is more agreeable.

There is a remedy celebrated in Holland, under the name of liquor lithontriptica Loosii, which contains, according to an accurate analysis, muriate of lime. This, professor Hufeland recommends in the following form:

R. Calcis muriate 3 j.
Aquæ distillatæ, ℥ ij. ft. solutio.

Thirty drops are to be taken four times a-day, which may be increased as far as the stomach will bear.

For curing stone patients, little reliance can be placed in any lithontriptics hitherto discovered, though they may rationally be given, with a confident hope of procuring an alleviation of the fits of pain attending the presence of stone in the bladder. After all, the only certain method of getting rid of the calculus is the operation. See *Lithotomy.*

["LITHONTRIPTOR. (From λιθος, a stone, and Spvπτω, to break.) The name of an instrument, invented by Dr. Civiale of Paris, for reducing calculi in the bladder into small particles or a powder, which is voided with the urine, and lithotomy thus rendered unnecessary. The lithontriptor consists of a straight silver catheter, of considerable diameter, and enclosing another of steel, the lower extremity of which consists of three branches, calculated to grasp the stone on withdrawing the steel catheter a short way within the outer one, when they become approximated. The cavity of the inner catheter is capable of admitting a steel rod, to which may be affixed, at the surgeon's option, a simple quadrangular drill, or a strawberry-shaped file, or a trephine. By means of a spring, the latter part of the apparatus is pressed evenly inwards, and it is made to revolve with velocity through the medium of a bow, after the manner of a common hand drill."—*Coop. Sur. Dic.* A.]

LITHONTRY'PTIC. (From λιθος, a stone, and Spvπ]ω, to break.) See *Lithontriptic.*

LITHOSPE'RMUM. (From λιθος, a stone, and σπερμα, seed; named from the hardness of its seed.) 1. The name of a genus of plants in the Linnæan system. Class, *Pentandria;* Order, *Monogynia.*

2. The pharmacopœial name of common gromwell. See *Lithospermum officinale.*

LITHOSPERMUM OFFICINALE. The systematic name of the officinal gromwell. The seeds of this officinal plant, *Lithospermum—seminibus lævibus, corollis vix calycem superantibus, foliis lanceolatis,* of Linnæus, were formerly supposed, from their stony hardness, to be efficacious in calculous and gravelly disorders. Little credit is given to their lithontriptic character, yet they are occasionally used as diuretic for clearing the urinary passages, and for obviating strangury, in the form of emulsion.

LITHO'TOMY. (*Lithotomia;* from λιθος, a stone, and τεμνω, to cut.) *Cystomia.* The operation of cutting into the bladder, in order to extract a stone. Several methods have been recommended for performing this operation, but there are only two which can be practised with any propriety. One is, where the operation is to be performed immediately above the pubes, in that part of the bladder which is not covered with peritonæum, called the *high operation.* The other, where it is done in the perinæum, by laying open the neck and lateral part of the bladder, so as to allow of the extraction of the stone, called the *lateral operation,* from the prostate gland of the neck of the bladder being laterally cut.

LITMUS. The beautiful blue prepared from a white lichen. See *Lichen roccello.*

LI'TRON. See *Nitre.*

LI'TUS. A liniment.

LI'VER. (*Hepar, ἡπαρ.*) A large viscus, of a deep red colour of great size and weight, situated under the diaphragm, in the right hypochondrium, its smaller portion occupying part of the epigastric region. In the human body, the liver is divided into two principal lobes, the right of which is by far the greatest. They are divided on the upper side by a broad ligament, and on the other side by a considerable depression or fossa. Between and below these two lobes is a smaller lobe, called *lobulus spigelii.* In describing this viscus, it is necessary to attend to seven principal circumstances:— its ligaments; its surfaces; its margins; its tubercles; its fissure; its sinus; and the pori biliarii.

The *ligaments* of the liver are five in number, all arising from the peritonæum. 1. *The right lateral ligament,* which connects the thick right lobe with the posterior part of the diaphragm. 2. *The left lateral ligament,* which connects the convex surface and margin of the left lobe with the diaphragm, and, in those of whom the liver is very large, with the œsophagus and spleen. 3. *The broad or middle suspensory ligament,* which passes from the diaphragm into the convex surface, and separates the right lobe of the liver from the left. It descends from above through the large fissure to the concave surface, and is then distributed over the whole liver. 4. *The round ligament,* which in adults consists of the umbilical vein, indurated into a ligament. 5. *The coronary ligament.*

The liver has two *surfaces,* one superior, which is convex and smooth, and one inferior, which is concave, and has holes and depressions to receive, not only the contiguous viscera, but the vessels running into the liver.

The *margins* of the liver are also two in number; the one, which is posterior and superior is obtuse, the other, situated anteriorly and inferiorly, is acute.

The *tubercles* of the liver are likewise two in number, viz. *lobulus anonymus,* and *lobulus caudatus,* and are found near the vena portæ.

Upon looking on the concave surface of this viscus, a considerable fissure is obvious, known by the name of the *fissure of the liver.*

In order to expose the *sinus,* it is necessary to remove the gall-bladder, when a considerable sinus, before occupied by the gall-bladder, will be apparent.

The *blood-vessels* of the liver are the hepatic artery, the vena portæ, and the vena cavæ hepaticæ, which are described under their proper names. The *absorbents* of the liver are very numerous. The liver has *nerves,* from the great intercostal and eighth pair, which arise from the hepatic plexus, and proceed along with the hepatic artery and vena portæ into the substance of the liver. With regard to the substance of the liver, various opinions have been entertained. It is, however, now pretty well ascertained to be a large gland, composed of lesser glands connected together by cellular structure. The small glands which thus compose the substance of the liver, are termed penicilli, from the arrangement of the minute ramifications of the vena portæ composing each gland, resembling that of the hairs of a pencil. The chief use of this large viscus is to supply a fluid, named bile, to the intestines, which is of the utmost importance in chylification. The small penicilli perform this function by a specific action on the blood they contain, by which they secrete in their very minute ends the fluid termed *hepatic bile;* but whether they pour it into what is called a follicle, or not, is yet undecided, and is the cause of the difference of opinion respecting the substance of the liver. If it be secreted into a follicle, the substance is truly glandular, according to the notion of the older anatomists: but if it be secreted merely into a small vessel, called a biliary pore (the existence of which can be demonstrated) corresponding to the end of each of the penicilli, without any intervening follicle, its substance is then, in their opinion, vascular. According to our notions in the present day, in either case, the liver is said to be glandular; for we have the idea of a gland when any arrangement of vessels performs the office of separating from the blood a fluid or substance different in its nature from the blood. The small vessels which receive the bile secreted by the penicilli, are called *pori biliarii;* these converge together throughout the substance of the liver towards its under surface, and, at length, form one trunk, called *ductus hepaticus,* which conveys the bile into either the *ductus communis choledochus,* or *ductus cysticus.* See *Gall-bladder.*

Liver, inflammation of. See *Hepatitis.*

Liver of sulphur. See *Potassæ sulphuretum.*

LIVERWORT. See *Marchantia polymorpha.*

Liverwort, ash-coloured. See *Lichen caninus.*

Liverwort, ground. See *Lichen caninus.*

Liverwort, Iceland. See *Lichen islandicus.*

Liverwort, noble. See *Marchantia polymorpha.*

LI'VOR. (From *liveo,* to be black and blue.) Lividness. A black mark, from a blow. A dark circle under the eye.

LIX. (From λιξ, light.) - Woodash.

LIX'IVIAL. Salts are so called which are extracted by lixiviation.

LIXIVIATION. (*Lixivialis;* from *lix,* woodash.) *Lessive.* The process employed by chemists of dissolving, by means of warm water, the saline and soluble particles of cinders, the residues of distillation and combustion, coals, and natural earths. Salts thus obtained are called *Lixivial salts.*

LIXI'VIUM. (From *lix,* woodash.) The liquor in which saline and soluble particles of the residues of distillation and combustion are dissolved.

LIXIVIUM SAPONARIUM. See *Potassæ liquor.*

LIXIVIUM TARTARI. See *Potassæ subcarbonatis liquor.*

LOBATUS. (From *lobus,* a lobe.) Lobed. Applied to leaves which have the margins of the segments lobed, as in *Anemone hepatica,* and to such as are lobed like the vine thistle, and many geraniums.

LOBB, THEOPHILUS, practised as a physician in London with considerable reputation, and left several works on medical topics. He died in 1763, in the 85th year of his age. He wrote on fevers, small-pox, and some other diseases; but his most celebrated publication was, "A Treatise on Solvents of the Stone, and on curing the Stone and the Gout by Aliments," which passed through several editions, and was translated into Latin and French; he considered the morbid matter of an alkaline nature, and vegetable acids as the remedy. He was author also of "A Compendium of the Practice of Physic," and of several papers in the Gentleman's Magazine.

Lobed leaf. See *Lobatus.*

LOBE'LIA. (Named in honour of Lobel, a botanist.) 1. The name of a genus of plants in the Linnæan system. Class, *Syngenesia;* Order, *Monogamia.*

2. The pharmacopœial name of the blue lobelia. See *Lobelia syphilitica.*

LOBELIA SYPHILITICA. The systematic name of the blue lobelia of the pharmacopœias. The root is the part directed by the Edinburgh Pharmacopœia for medicinal use; in taste it resembles tobacco, and is apt to excite vomiting. It derived the name of *syphilitica* from its efficacy in the cure of syphilis, as experienced by the North American Indians, who considered it as a specific in that disease, and with whom it was long an important secret, which was purchased by Sir William Johnson, and since published by different authors. The method of employing this medicine is stated as follows: a decoction is made of a handful of the roots in three measures of water. Of this half a measure is taken in the morning fasting, and repeated in the evening; and the dose is gradually increased, till its purgative effects become too violent, when the decoction is to be intermitted for a day or two, and then renewed, until a perfect cure is effected. During the use of this medicine, a proper regimen is to be enjoined, and the ulcers are also to be frequently washed with the decoction, or if deep and foul, to be sprinkled with the powder of the inner bark of the New-Jersey teatree, *Ceanothus americanus.* Although the plant thus used is said to cure the disease in a very short time, yet it is not found that the antisyphilitic powers of the lobelia have been confirmed in any instance of European practice.

[LOBELIA INFLATA. See *Indian tobacco.* A.]

LO'BULUS. (Dim. of *lobus,* a lobe.) A small lobe, as *lobulus spigelii.*

LOBULUS ACCESSORIUS. See *Lobulus anonymus.*

LOBULUS ANONYMUS. *Lobulus accessorius anteriorquadratus.* The anterior point of the right lobe of the liver. Others define it to be that space of the great lobe between the fossa of the umbilical vein and gall-bladder, and extending forward from the fossa for the lodgment of the vena portæ, to the anterior margin of the liver.

LOBULUS CAUDATUS. *Processus caudatus.* A tail-like process of the liver, stretching downward from the

middle of the great right lobe to the lobulus spigelii. It is behind the gall-bladder, and between the fossa venæ portarum, and the fissure for the lodgment of the vena cava.

LOBULUS SPIGELII. *Lobulus posterior; Lobulus posticus papillatus.* A lobe of the liver between the two greater lobes, but rather belonging to the right great lobe. From its situation deep behind, and from its having a perpendicular papilla-like projection, it is called lobulus posterior, or papillatus. To the left side it has the fissure for the lodgment of the ductus venosus; on the right, the fissure for the vena cava; and above, it has the great transverse fissure of the liver for the lodgment of the cylinder of the porta; obliquely to the right, and upwards, it has a connexion with the lower concave surface of the great lobe, by the processus caudatus, which Winslow calls one of the roots of the lobulus spigelii. It is received into the bosom of the less curve of the stomach.

LOCA'LES. (*Locales,* the plural of *localis.*) The fourth class of Cullen's Nosology, which comprehends morbid affections that are partial, and includes eight orders, viz. dysæsthesiæ, dysorexiæ, dyscinesiæ, apocenoses, epischeses, tumores, ectopia, and dialyses.

LOCA'LIS. Local. Belonging to a part and not the whole. A common division of diseases is into general and local.

Localis membrana. The pia mater.

LO'CHIA. (From λοχευω, to bring forth.) The cleansings. The serous, and for the most part green-coloured, discharge that takes place from the uterus and vagina of women, during the first four days after delivery.

LOCHIORRHŒ'A. (From λοχια, and ρεω, to flow.) An excessive discharge of the lochia.

LOCKED-JAW. See *Tetanus.*

LOCULAMENTUM. In botany means the space or cell between the valves and partitions of a capsule, distinguished from their number into unilocular, bilocular, &c. See *Capsula.*

LOCUSTA. A term sometimes applied to the spikelet of grasses. See *Spicula.*

LOGWOOD. See *Hæmatoxylon campechianum.*

LOMENTACEÆ. (From *lomentum;* in allusion to the pulse-like nature of the plants in question, so as to keep in view their analogy with the *papilionaceæ.*) The name of an order of plants in Linnæus's Fragments of a Natural Method, consisting of such as have a bivalve pericarpium or legume, and not papilionaceous corolls; as Cassia, Fumaria, Ceretonia, &c.

LOMENTUM. 1. A word used by old writers on medicine, to express a meal made of beans, or bread made of this meal, and used as a wash.

2. A bivalve pericarpium, divided into cells by very small partitions, never lateral like those of the legume. From its figure it is termed,

1. *Articulatum,* when the partitions are visible externally; as in Hedysarum argenteum.

2. *Moniliforme,* necklace-like, consisting of a number of little globules; as in Hedysarum moliferum.

3. *Aculeatum;* as in Hedysarum onobrychis.

4. *Crystatum;* as in Hedysarum caput galli.

5. *Isthmis interceptum,* when the cells are much narrower than the joints; as in Hippocrepis.

6. *Corticosum,* the external bark being woody, and the inside pulpy; as in Cassia fistula.

LOMMIUS, JODOCUS, was born in Guelderland, about the commencement of the 16th century. Having received from his father a good classical education, he turned his attention to medicine, which he studied chiefly at Paris. He practised for a considerable time at Tournay, where he was pensionary physician in 1557; and, three years after, he removed to Brussels. The period of his death is not known. He left three small works, which are still valued from the purity and elegance of their Latinity; a Commentary on Celsus; Medicinal Observations, in three books; and a Treatise on the Cure of Continued Fevers; the two latter having been several times reprinted and translated.

LOMONITE. Diphrismatic zeolite.

LONCHI'TIS. (From λογχη, a lance: so named because the leaves resemble the head of a lance.) The herb spleenwort. The Ceterach officinalis.

LONGA'NUM. (From *longus,* long: so named from its length.) The intestinum rectum.

LONGING. A desire peculiar to the female, and

only during pregnancy, and those states in which the uterine discharge is suppressed.

LONGISSIMUS. The longest. Parts are so named from their length, compared to that of others; as *longissimus dorsi*, &c.

LONGISSIMUS DORSI. *Lumbo dorso trachelien*, of Dumas. This muscle, which is somewhat thicker th n the sacrolumbalis, greatly resembles it, however, in its shape and extent, and arises, in common with that muscle, between it and the spine. It ascends upwards along the spine, and is inserted by small double tendons into the posterior and inferior part of all the transverse processes of the vertebræ of the back, and sometimes of the last vertebra of the neck. From its outside it sends off several bundles of fleshy fibres, interspersed with a few tendinous filaments, which are usually inserted into the lower edge of the ten uppermost ribs, not far from their tubercles. In some subjects, however, they are found inserted in a less number, and in others, though more rarely, into every one of the ribs. Towards the upper part of this muscle is observed a broad and thin portion of fleshy fibres, which cross and intimately adhere to the fibres of the longissimus dorsi. This portion arises from the upper and posterior part of the transverse processes of the five or six uppermost vertebræ of the back, by as many tendinous origins, and is usually inserted by six tendinous and fleshy slips, into the transverse processes of the six inferior vertebræ of the neck. This portion is described, by Winslow and Albinus, as a distinct muscle; by the former under the name of *transversalis major colli*, and by the latter under that of *transversalis cervices*. But its fibres are so intimately connected with those of the longissimus dorsi, that it may very properly be considered as an appendage to the latter. The use of this muscle is to extend the vertebræ of the back, and to keep the trunk of the body erect; by means of its appendage, it likewise serves to turn the neck obliquely backwards, and a little to one side

LONGISSIMUS MANUS. See *Flexor tertii internodii pollicis*.

LONGISSIMUS OCULI. See *Obliquus superior oculi*.

LONGITUDINAL. *Longitudinalis*. Parts are so named from their direction.

LONGITUDINAL SINUS. Longitudinal sinus of the dura mater. A triangular canal, proceeding in the falciform process of the dura mater, immediately under the bones of the skull, from the crista galli to the tentorium, where it branches into the lateral sinuses. The longitudinal sinus has a number of trabeculæ or fibres crossing it. Its use is to receive the blood from the veins of the pia mater, and convey it into the lateral sinuses, to be carried through the internal jugulars to the heart.

LONGUS. Long. Some parts are so named from their comparative length; as *longus colli*, &c.

LONGUS COLLI. *Præ dorso cervical*, of Dumas. This is a pretty considerable muscle, situated close to the anterior and lateral part of the vertebræ of the neck. Its outer edge is in part covered by the rectus internus major. It arises tendinous and fleshy within the thorax, from the bodies of the three superior vertebræ of the back, laterally; from the bottom and forepart of the transverse processes of the first and second vertebræ of the back, and of the last vertebræ of the neck: and likewise from the upper and anterior points of the transverse processes of the sixth, fifth, fourth, and third vertebræ of the neck, by as many small distinct tendons; and is inserted tendinous into the forepart of the second vertebra of the neck, near its fellow. This muscle, when it acts singly, moves the neck to one side; but when both act, the neck is brought directly forwards.

LONICERA. The name of a genus of plants in the Linnæan system. Class, *Pentandria*; Order, *Monogynia*.

LONICERA DIERVILLA. The systematic name of a species of honeysuckle. *Diervilla*. The young branches of this species, *Lonicera—racemis terminalibus, foliis serratis*, of Linnæus, are employed in North America as a certain remedy in gonorrhœa and suppression of urine. It has not yet been exhibited in Europe.

LONICERA PERICLIMENUM. Honeysuckle. This beautiful and common plant was formerly used in the cure of asthma, for cleansing sordid ulcers, and re-

moving diseases of the skin, virtues it does not now appear to possess.

LOOSENESS. See *Diarrhœa*.

LOPEZ. *Radix lopeziana; Radix indica lopeziana.* The root of an unknown tree, growing, according to some, at Goa. It is met with in pieces of different thickness, some at least of two inches diameter. The woody part is whitish, and very light; softer, more spongy, and whiter next the bark, including a denser, somewhat reddish, medullary part. The bark is rough, wrinkled, brown, soft, and, as it were, woolly, pretty thick, covered with a thin paler cuticle. Neither the woody nor cortical part has any remarkable smell or taste, nor any appearance of resinous matter. It appears that this medicine has been remarkably effectual in stopping colliquative diarrhœas, which had resisted the usual remedies. Those attending the last stage of consumptions were particularly relieved by its use. It seemed to act, not by an astringent power, but by a faculty of restraining and appeasing spasmodic and inordinate motions of the intestines. Dr. Gaubius, who gives this account, compares its action to that of Simarouba, but thinks it more efficacious than this medicine.

LOPEZ root. See *Lopez*.

LOPEZIANA RADIX. See *Lopez*.

LOPHADIA. (From λοφος, the hinder part of the neck.) *Lophia*. The first vertebra of the neck.

LORDOSIS. (From λορδος, curved, bent.) An affection af the spine, in which it is bent inwards.

LORICA. (From *lorico*, to crust over.) A kind of lute, with which vessels are coated before they are put into the fire.

LORICATION. Coating. Nicholson recommends the following composition for the coating of glass vessels, to prevent their breaking when exposed to heat. Take of sand and clay, equal parts; make them into a thin paste, with fresh blood, prevented from coagulating by agitation, till it is cold, and diluted with water; add to this some hair, and powdered glass; with a brush, dipped in this mixture, besmear the glass; and when this layer is dry, let the same operation be repeated twice, or oftener, till the coat applied is about one-third part of an inch in thickness.

LORRY, ANNE-CHARLES, was born near Paris, in 1725. He studied and practised as a physician, with unremitting zeal and peculiar modesty, and obtained a high reputation. At 23, he was admitted doctor of medicine at Paris, and subsequently became doctor-regent of the faculty. He was author of several works, some of which still maintain their value; particularly his Treatise on Cutaneous Diseases, which combines much erudition and accurate observation, with great clearness of arrangement, and perspicuity of language. He died in 1783.

LOTION. (*Lotio*; from *lavo*, to wash.) An external fluid application. Lotions are usually applied by wetting linen in them, and keeping it on the part affected.

LOTUS. (From λω, to desire.) 1. A tree, the fruit of which was said to be so delicious as to make those who tasted it forsake all other desires; hence the proverb, Λωτον εϕαγον, *lotum gustavi:* I have tasted lotus.

2. The name of a genus of plants in the Linnæan system. Class, *Diadelphia*; Order, *Decandria*.

LOUIS, ANTHONY, was born at Metz, in 1723. He attained great reputation as a surgeon, and was honoured with numerous appointments, and marks of distinction, as well in his own as in foreign countries. He wrote the surgical part of the "Encyclopédie," and presented several interesting papers to the Royal Academy of Surgery, of which he was secretary: besides which, he was author of several works on anatomical, medical, and other subjects. In a memoir, on the legitimacy of retarded births, he maintains that the detention of the fœtus, more than ten days beyond the ninth month, is physically impossible.

LOVAGE. See *Ligusticum levisticum*.

LOVE-APPLE. See *Solanum lycopersicum*.

LOWER, RICHARD, was born in Cornwall, about the year 1631. He graduated at Oxford, and having materially assisted the celebrated Dr. Willis, in his dissections, he was introduced into practice by that physician. In 1665, he published a defence of Willis's work on Fevers, displaying much learning and ingenuity. But his most important performance was entitled, "Tractatus de Corde, item de motu et calore Sanguinis, et Chyli in eum transitu," printed four years after. He demonstrated the dependence of the motions of the heart upon the nervous influence, and referred the red colour of arterial blood to the action of the air in the lungs; he also gave an account of his experiments, made at Oxford in February, 1665, on the transfusion of blood from one living animal to another, of which an abstract had before appeared in the Philosophical Transactions. He afterward practised this upon an insane person, before the Royal Society, of which he was admitted a fellow in 1667, as well as of the College of Physicians. The reputation acquired by these, and some other minor publications, procured him extensive practice, particularly after the death of Dr. Willis; but his political opinions brought him into discredit at court, and he declined considerably before the close of his life, in 1691. The operation of transfusion was soon exploded, experience having shown that it was attended with pernicious consequences.

LOXA'RTHROS. (From λυξος, oblique, and αρθρον, a joint.) *Loxarthrus.* An obliquity of the joint, without spasm or luxation.

LOXIA. (From λυξος, oblique.) The specific name in the genus *Entasia* of Good's Nosology, for wry neck. ["Also, in Ornithology, the name of a genus of birds, including the Grosbeaks, or Crossbills, of which there are numerous species." A.]

LUCULLITE. A species of limestone.

LU'DUS HELMONTII. *Ludus paracelsi.* The waxen vein. A stony matter said to be serviceable in calculus.

LUDWIG, CHRISTIAN THEOPHILUS, was born in Silesia in 1709, and educated for the medical profession. Having a strong bias towards natural history, he went on an expedition to the north of Africa : and soon after his return, in 1733, he became professor of medicine at Leipsic. The first thesis defended there under his presidency related to the manner in which marine plants are nourished; which he showed not to be by the root, as is the case in the generality of the vegetable kingdom. He afterward published several botanical works, in which he finds many objections to the Linnæan arrangement, rather preferring that of Rivinus; but on very unsatisfactory grounds. Elementary works were likewise written by him on the different branches of medical knowledge. A more important work is entitled "Adversaria Medico-practica," in three octavo volumes. He has given an account of his trials of Stramonium and Belladonna in epilepsy, by no means favourable to either. He died in 1773.

LU'ES. (*Lues, is.* f.; from λυω, to dissolve, because t produces dissolution.) A pestilence, poison, plague.

LUES DEIFICA. One of the many pompous names formerly given to epilepsy.

LUES NEURODES. A typhus fever.

LUES VENEREA. The plague of Venus, or the venereal disease. See *Syphilis.*

LUISINUS, LOUIS, was born at Udina, where he obtained considerable reputation about the middle of the 16th century. He translated Hippocrates's aphorisms into Latin hexameters: and published a treatise on regulating the affections of the mind by moral philosophy and the medical art : but his most celebrated work is entitled "Aphrodisiacus," printed at Venice, in two folio volumes: the first containing an account of preceding treatises on syphilis, the second comprehended principally the manuscript works on the subject which had not then been committed to the press.

LU'JULA. (Corrupted or contracted from *Allelujah, Praise the Lord;* so called from its many virtues.) See *Oxalis ascetosella.*

LUMBA'GO. (From *lumbus,* the loin.) A rheumatic affection of the muscles about the loins. See *Rheumatismus.*

LUMBAR. *Lumbalis.* Belonging to the loins.

LUMBAR ABSCESS. *Psoas abscess.* A species of arthropuosis, that receives its name from the situation in which the matter is found, namely, upon the side of the psoas muscle, or between that and the iliacus internus. Between these muscles, there lies a quantity of loose cellular membrane, in which an inflammation often takes place, either spontaneously or from mechanical injuries. This terminates in an abscess that can procure no outlet but by a circuitous course in which it generally produces irreparable mischief, without any violent symptoms occurring to alarm the

34

patient. The abscess sometimes forms a swelling above Poupart's ligament: sometimes below it; and frequently the matter glides under the fascia of the thigh. Occasionally, it makes its way through the sacro-ischiatic foramen, and assumes rather the appearance of a fistula in ano. The uneasiness in the loins, and the impulse communicated to the tumour by coughing, evince that the disease arises in the lumbar region; but it must be confessed, that we can hardly ever know the existence of the disorder, before the tumour, by presenting itself externally, leads us to such information. The lumbar abscess is sometimes connected with diseased vertebræ, which may either be a cause or effect of the collection of matter. The disease, however, is frequently unattended with this complication.

The situation of the symptoms of lumbar abscess renders this affection liable to be mistaken for some other, viz. lumbago and nephritic pains, and, towards its termination, for crural or femoral hernia. The first, however, is not attended with the shivering that occurs here; and nephritic complaints are generally discoverable by attention to the state of the urine. The distinction from crural hernia is more difficult. In both, a soft inelastic swelling is felt in the same situation; but in hernia, it is attended with obstructed fæces, vomiting, &c. and its appearance is always sudden, while the lumbar tumour is preceded by various complaints before its appearance in the thigh. In a horizontal posture, the abscess also totally disappears, while the hernia does not.

Lumbar regions. The loins.

LUMBARIS EXTERNUS. See *Quadratus lumborum.*

LUMBARIS INTERNUS. See *Psoas magnus.*

LUMBRICA'LIS. (*Lumbricalis musculus;* from its resemblance to the *lumbricus,* or earth worm.) A name given to some muscles from their resemblance t a worm.

LUMBRICALIS MANUS. *Fidicinales. Flexor primi in ternodii digitorum manus, vel perforatus lumbricalis,* of Cowper; *Anuli tendino-phalangiens,* of Dumas. The small flexors of the fingers which assist the bending the fingers when the long flexors are in full action. They arise thin and fleshy from the outside of the tendons of the flexor profundus, a little above the lowe edge of the carpal ligaments, and are inserted by long slender tendons into the outer sides of the broad ten dons of the interosseal muscles, about the middle of th first joints of the fingers.

LUMBRICALES PEDIS. *Plantitendino-phalangien,* o' Dumas. Four muscles like the former, that increas the flexion of the toes, and draw them inwards.

LUMBRI'CUS. (*A Lubricitate;* from its slipper ness.) *Ascaris lumbricoides; Lumbricus teres* The long round worm. A species of worm which inhabit occasionally the human intestines. It has three nip ples at its head, and a triangular mouth in its middle Its length is from four to twelve inches, and its thick ness, when twelve inches long, about that of a goose quill. They are sometimes solitary, at other time very numerous. See *Worms.*

LUMBRICUS TERRESTRIS. *Vermis terrestris.* Th earth worm. Formerly given internally when dries and pulverized as a diuretic.

LU'MBUS VENERIS. See *Achillea millefolium.*

LU'NA. (*Luna, æ.* f.; à *lucendo.*) 1. The moo 2. The old alchemistical name of silver.

LUNA CORNEA. Muriate of silver.

LUNA PLENA. A term used by the old alchemists the transmutation of metals.

Lunar caustic. See *Argenti nitras.*

LUNA'RE OS. One of the bones of the wrist.

LUNARIA REDIVIVA. Bulbonach of the German Satin and honesty. It was formerly esteemed as warm diuretic.

LUNA'TICUS. (From *luna* the moon; so called because the malady returns, or is aggravated, or influ enced by the moon.)

1. A lunatic.

2. A disease which appears to be influenced by the moon.

LUNG. *Pulmo.* The lungs are two viscera situated in the chest, by means of which we breathe. The lung in the right cavity of the chest is divided into three lobes, that in the left cavity into two. They hang in the chest, attached at their superior part to the neck, by means of the trachea, and are separated by the mediastinum. They are also attached to the heart by means of the pulmonary vessels. The substance of the lungs is of four kinds, viz. vesicular, vascular, bronchial, and parenchymatous. The vesicular substance is composed of the air-cells. The vascular invests those cells like a net-work. The bronchial is formed by the ramifications of the bronchia throughout the lungs, having the air-cells at their extremities ; and the spongy substance that connects these parts is termed the *parenchyma.* The lungs are covered with a fine membrane, a reflection of the pleura, called *pleura pulmonalis.* The internal surface of the air-cells is covered with a very fine, delicate, and sensible membrane, which is continued from the larnyx through the trachea and bronchia. The arteries of the lungs are the bronchial, a branch of the aorta, which carries blood to the lungs for their nourishment; and the pulmonary, which circulates the blood through the air-cells to undergo a certain change. The pulmonary veins return the blood that has undergone this change, by four trunks, into the left auricle of the heart. The bronchial veins terminate in the vena azygos. The nerves of the lungs are from the eighth pair and great intercostal. The absorbents are of two orders ; the superficial, and deep-seated : the former are more readily detected than the latter. The glands of these viscera are called bronchial. They are muciparous, and situated about the bronchia. See *Respiration.*

LUNG WORT. See *Pulmonaria officinalis.*

LUNULATUS. Crescent-shaped, or half-moon-like : a term applied to leaves, pods, &c. which are so shaped, whether the points are directed towards the stalk, or from it ; as in the leaves of *Passiflora lunata,* and legumen of *Medicago foliata.*

LU'PIA. (From λυπεω, to molest.)

1. A genus of disease, including encysted tumours, the contents of which are very thick, and sometimes solid ; as *meliceris, atheroma, steatoma,* and *ganglion.*

2. (From *lupus,* a wolf: so called because it does not cease to destroy the part it seizes.) A malignant ulcer which eats away the soft parts on which it appears, laying bare the bones and cartilages, and which is equally fatal with the cancer.

LUP'INUS. (So called by Pliny and other ancient writers. Professor Martin says the word owes its origin to *Lupus,* a wolf, because plants of this genus ravage the ground by overrunning it, after the manner of that animal. It is also derived from λυπη, grief: whence Virgil's epithet, *tristes lupini;* from the fanciful idea of its acrid juices, when tasted, producing a sorrowful appearance on the countenance.) The name of a genus of plants. Class, *Diadelphia,* Order, *Decandria.*

2. Under this term the white lupin is directed in some pharmacopœias.

LUPINUS ALBUS. The systematic name of the white lupin. The seed, the ordinary food of mankind in the days of Galen and Pliny, is now forgotten. Its farinaceous and bitter'meal is occasionally exhibited to remove worms from the intestines, and made into poultices to resolve indolent tumours.

LUPULIN. Lupuline. The name given by Dr. Ives, of New York, to an impalpable yellow powder, in which he believes the virtue of the hop to reside, and which may be obtained by beating and sifting the hops used in brewing. It appears to be peculiar to the female plant, and is probably secreted by the nectaria. In preserving beer from the acetous fermentation, and in communicating an agreeable flavour to it, lupulin was found to be equivalent to ten times its weight of hop leaves.

LU'PULUS. (From λυπη, dislike: so named from its bitterness.) See *Humulus.*

LU'PUS. 1. The wolf, so named from its rapacity.

2. The cancer is also so called, because it eats away the flesh like a wolf.

LURID Æ. The name of an order of plants in Linnæus's Fragments of a Natural Method, consisting of those which prove some deadly poison ; the corolla mostly monopetalous ; as *Datura, Solanum, Nicotiana.*

LUSTRA'GO. (From *lustro,* to expiate : so called because it was used in the ancient purifications.) Fiat or base vervain.

LUSUS. A sport.

LUSUS NATURÆ. A sport of nature ; a monster. See *Monster.*

LUTE. See *Lutum.*

LU'TEA CORPORA. See *Corpus luteum.*

LUTE'OLA. (From *lutum,* mud ; because it grows in muddy places, or is of the colour of mud.) See *Reseda luteola.*

LU'TUM. (From λυτος, soluble.) *Cæmentum.* Mud. Lute. A composition with which chemical vessels are covered, to preserve them from the violence of the fire, and to close exactly their joinings to each other, to retain the substances which they contain when they are volatile and reduced to vapour.

LUXATION. (*Luxatio;* from *luxo,* to put out of joint.) A dislocation of a bone from its proper cavity.

LYCA'NCHE. (From λυκος, a wolf, and αγχω, to strangle.) A species of quincy, in which the patient makes a noise like the howling of a wolf.

LYCANTHRO'PIA. (From λυκος, a wolf, and ανθρωπος, a man.) A species of insanity, in which the patients leave their houses in the night, and wander about like wolves, in unfrequented places.

LY'CHNIS. (From λυχνος, a torch; because the ancients used its leaves rolled up for torches.) 1. A name of several vegetable productions.

2. The name of a genus of plants. Class, *Decandria;* Order, *Pentagynia.*

LYCHNIS SEGETUM. See *Agrostemma githago.*

LYCHNOIDES. (From *lychnis,* the name of a plant, and ειδος, resemblance.) Like the herb *lychnis.*

LYCHNOIDES SEGETUM. See *Agrostemma githago.*

LYCO'CTONUM. (From λυκος, a wolf, and κτεινω, to slay : so called because it was the custom of hunters to secrete it in raw flesh, for the purpose of destroying wolves.) The *Aconitum lycoctonum.*

LYCOPE'RDON. (From λυκος, a wolf, and περδω, to break wind : so named because it was supposed to spring from the dung of wolves.) 1. The name of a genus of plants in the Linnæan system. Class, *Cryptogamia;* Order, *Fungi.*

2. The pharmacopœial name of the puff-ball. See *Lycoperdon bovista.*

LYCOPERDON BOVISTA. The systematic name of the puff-ball. *Crepitus lupi.* A round or egg-shaped fungus, the *Lycoperdon; subrotundum, laceato dehiscens,* of Linnæus; when fresh, of a white colour, with a very short, or scarcely any pedicle, growing in dry pasture grounds. When young, it is sometimes covered with tubercles on the outside, and is pulpy within. By age it becomes smooth externally, and dries internally into a very fine, light, brownish dust, which is used by the common people to stop hæmorrhages. See *Lycoperdon.*

LYCOPERDON TUBER. The systematic name of the truffle. *Tuber cibarium,* of Dr. Withering. A solid fungus of a globular figure, which grows under the surface of the ground without any roots or the access of light, and attains a size from a pea to the largest potato. It has a rough, blackish coat, and is destitute of fibres. Cooks are well acquainted with its use and qualities. It is found in woods and pastures in some parts of Kent, but is not very common in England. In France and Spain, truffles are very frequent, and grow to a much larger size than they do here. In these places the peasants find it worth their while to search for them, and they train up dogs and swine for this purpose, who, after they have been inured to their smell by their masters frequently placing them in their way, will readily scrape them up as they ramble the fields and woods.

LYCOPE'RSICUM. (From λυκος, a wolf, and περσικον, a peach : so called from its exciting a violent degree of lust.) *Lycopersicon.* Wolf's peach. Love apple. See *Solanum lycopersicon.*

LYCOPO'DIUM. (From λυκος, a wolf, and πους, a foot: so called from its supposed resemblance.) 1. The name of a genus of plants in the Linnæan system. Class, *Cryptogamia;* Order, *Musci.*

2. The pharmacopœial name of the club-moss. See *Lycopodium clavatum.*

LYCOPODIUM CLAVATUM. The systematic name of the club-moss. Wolf's claw. *Muscus clavatus.* This plant affords a great quantity of pollen, which is much esteemed in some places to sprinkle on young children, to prevent, and in the curing parts which are fretting. A decoction of the herb is said to be a specific in the cure of the plica polonica.

LYCOPODIUM SELAGO. The systematic name of the upright club-moss. *Muscus erectus.* The decoction of this plant acts violently as a vomit and a purgative, and was formerly on that account employed to produce abortions.

LYCO'PSIS. (From λτκος, a wolf, and οψις, an aspect: so called from its being of the colour of a wolf, or from the circumstance of the flowers being ringent, and having the appearance of a grinning mouth. The herbage is also furnished, says Ambrosinus, with a sort of rigid hairiness similar to the coat of a wolf.) 1. The name of a genus of plants. Class, *Pentandria*; Order, *Monogynia*.

2. The pharmacopœial name of the Wall-bugloss, *Echium ægyptiacum*, the *Asperugo agyptiaca* of Wildenow.

LY'COPUS. (From λυκος, a wolf, and πους, a foot: so named from its likeness.) The name of a genus of plants in the Linnæan system. Class, *Diandria*; Order, *Monogynia*. Wolf's-claw, or water hoarhound.

LYCOPUS EUROPEUS. This plant is sometimes used as an astringent.

[LYCOPUS VIRGINICA. See *Bugle weed*. A.]

Lydian stone. A flinty slate.

LYGI'SMUS. (From λυγιζω, to distort.) A dislocation.

LY'GUS. (From λυγιζω, to bend: so called from its flexibility.) The agnus castus.

LYMPH. *Lympha.* The liquid contained in the lymphatic vessels. Two processes may be employed to procure lymph. One is to lay bare a lymphatic vessel, divide it, and receive the liquid that flows from it; but this is a method difficult to execute, and besides, as the lymphatic vessels are not always filled with lymph, it is uncertain: the other consists in letting an animal fast during four or five days, and then extracting the fluid contained in the thoracic duct.

The liquid obtained in either way has at first a slightly opaline rose colour. It has a strong spermatic odour; a salt taste; it sometimes presents a slight yellow tinge, and at other times a red madder colour.

But lymph does not long remain liquid; it congeals. Its rose colour becomes more deep, an immense number of reddish filaments are developed, irregularly arborescent, and very analogous in appearance to the vessels spread in the tissue of organs.

When we examine carefully the mass of lymph thus coagulated, we find it formed of two parts; the one solid, and forming a great many cells, in which the other remains in a liquid state. If the solid part be separated, the liquid congeals again.

The quantity of lymph procured from one animal is but small; a dog of a large size scarcely yields an ounce. Its quantity appears to increase according to the time of fasting.

The solid part of the lymph, which may be called clot, has much analogy with that of the blood. It becomes scarlet-red by the contact of oxygen gas, and purple when plunged in carbonic acid.

This specific gravity of lymph is to that of distilled water as 1022·28: 1000·00.

Chevreuil analyzed the lymph of the dog:

Water,	926·4
Fibrin,	004·2
Albumen,	61·0
Muriate of Soda,	6.1
Carbonate of Soda,	1·8
Phosphate of Lime,	} 0·5
Phosphate of Magnesia,	
Carbonate of Lime,	
Total	1000·0

Its specific gravity is greater than water; in consistence, it is thin and somewhat viscid. The quantity in the human body appears to be very great, as the system of the lymphatic vessels forms no small part of it. Its constituent principles appear to be albuminous water and a little salt. The lymphatic vessels absorb this fluid from the tela cellulosa of the whole body, from all the viscera and the cavities of the viscera; and convey it to the thoracic duct, to be mixed with the chyle.

The use of the lymph is to return the superfluous nutritious jelly from every part, and to mix it with the chyle in the thoracic duct, there to be further converted into the nature of the animal; and, lastly, it has mixed with it the superfluous aqueous vapour, which

36

is effused into the cavities of the cranium, thorax, abdomen, &c.

LYMPHATIC. (*Lymphaticus;* from *lympha,* lymph.) 1. Of the nature of lymph.

2. An absorbent vessel, that carries a transparent fluid, or lymph. The lymphatic vessels of the human body are small and transparent, and originate in every part of the body. With the lacteal vessels of the intestines, they form what is termed the *absorbent system.* Their termination is in the thoracic duct. See *Absorbent, Lacteal,* and *Thoracic duct.*

Lymphatics of the head and neck.—Absorbents are found on the scalp and about the viscera of the neck, which unite into a considerable *branch,* that accompanies the jugular vein. Absorbents have not been detected in the human brain: yet there can be no doubt of there being such vessels: it is probable that they pass out of the cranium through the canalis caroticus and foramen lacerum in basi cranii, on each side, and join the above *jugular branch,* which passes through some glands as it proceeds into the chest to the angle of the subclavian and jugular veins.

The absorbents from the right side of the head and neck, and from the right arm, do not run across the neck, to unite with the great trunk of the system; they have an equal opportunity of dropping their contents into the angle between the right subclavian and the jugular vein. These vessels then uniting, form a trunk, which is little more than an inch, nay, sometimes not a quarter of an inch, in length, but which has nearly as great a diameter as the proper trunk of the left side.

This vessel lies upon the right subclavian vein, and receives a very considerable number of lymphatic vessels; not only does it receive the lymphatics from the right side of the head, thyroid gland, neck, &c. and the lymphatics of the arm, but it receives also those from the right side of the thorax and diaphragm, from the lungs of this side, and from the parts supplied by the mammary artery. Both in this and in the great trunk, there are many valves.

Of the upper extremities.—The absorbents of the upper extremities are divided into superficial and deepseated. The *superficial absorbents* ascend under the skin of the hand in every direction to the wrist, from whence a *branch* proceeds upon the posterior surface of the fore-arm, to the head of the radius, over the internal condyle of the humerus, up to the axilla, receiving several branches as it proceeds. Another *branch* proceeds from the wrist along the anterior part of the fore-arm, and forms a *net-work,* with a *branch* coming over the ulna from the posterior part, and ascends on the inside of the humerus to the glands of the axilla. The *deep seated absorbents* accompany the larger blood-vessels, and pass through two glands about the middle of the humerus, and ascend to the glands of the axilla. The superficial and deep-seated absorbents having passed through the axillary glands, form *two trunks,* which unite into *one,* to be inserted with the jugular absorbents into the thoracic duct, at the angle formed by the union of the subclavian with the jugular vein.

Lymphatics of the inferior extremities.—These are also superficial and deep-seated. The *superficial ones* lie between the skin and muscles. Those of the toes and foot form a *branch,* which ascends upon the back of the foot, over the tendon of the cruræus anticus, forms with other branches a *plexus* above the ankles, then proceeds along the tibia over the knee, sometimes passes through a gland, and proceeds up the inside of the thigh, to the subinguinal glands. The *deep-seated* absorbents follow the course of the arteries, and accompany the femoral artery, in which course they pass through some glands in the leg and above the knee, and then proceed to some deep-seated subinguinal glands. The absorbents from about the external parts of the pubes, as the penis and perineum, and from the external parts of the pelvis, in general, proceed to the inguinal glands. The subinguinal and inguinal glands send forth several branches, which pass through the abdominal ring into the cavity of the abdomen.

Of the abdominal and thoracic viscera.—The absorbents of the lower extremities accompany the external iliac artery, where they are joined by many branches from the *uterus, urinary bladder, spermatic chord,* and some branches accompanying the internal iliac artery; they then ascend to the sacrum, where they form a *plexus*, which proceeds over the psoas muscles, and meeting with the lacteals of the mesentery, form the thoracic duct, or trunk of the absorbents, which is of a serpentine form, about the size of a crow-quill, and runs up the dorsal vertebræ, through the posterior opening of the diaphragm, between the aorta and vena azygos, to the angle formed by the union of the left subclavian and jugular veins. In this course it receives:—the *absorbents of the kidneys*, which are superficial and deep-seated, and unite as they proceed towards the thoracic duct: and *the absorbents of the spleen*, which are upon its peritoneal coat, and unite with those of the pancreas:—a *branch* from the plexus of vessels passing above and below the duodenum, and formed by the absorbents of the *stomach*, which come from the less and greater curvature, and are united about the pylorus with those of the pancreas and liver, which converge from the external surface and internal parts towards the portæ of the liver, and also by several branches from the *gall-bladder*.

Use of lymphatics.—The office of these vessels is to take up substances which are applied to their mouths; thus the vapour of circumscribed cavities, and of the cells of the cellular membrane, are removed by the lymphatics of those parts; and thus mercury and other substances are taken into the system when rubbed on the skin.

The principle by which this absorption takes place, is a power inherent in the mouths of absorbing vessels, a vis insita, dependent on the high degree of irritability of their internal membrane by which the vessels contract and propel the fluid forwards. Hence the use of this function appears to be of the utmost importance, viz. to supply the blood with chyle; to remove the superfluous vapour of circumscribed cavities, otherwise dropsies, as hydrocephalus, hydrothorax, hydrocardia, ascites, hydrocele, &c. would constantly be taking place: to remove the superfluous vapour from the cells of the cellular-membrane dispersed throughout every part of the body, that anasarca may not take place: to remove the hard and soft parts of the body, and to convey into the system medicines which are applied to the surface of the body.

LYMPHATIC GLANDS. *Glandulæ lymphaticæ.* See *Conglobate gland.*

LYPO'MA. See *Lipoma.*

LY'RA. (From λυρα, a lyre, or musical instrument.) *Psalterium.* The triangular medullary space between the posterior crura of the fornix of the cerebrum, which is marked with prominent medullary fibres that give the appearance of a lyre.

LYRATUS. (From *lyra*, a musical instrument.) Lyrate or lyre-shaped. A leaf is so named which is cut into transverse segments, generally longer towards the extremities of the leaf, which is rounded as in *Erysimum barbaria.*

LY'RUS. (From *lyra*, the lyre: so called because its leaves are divided like the strings of a lyre.) See *Arnica montana.*

LYSIGY'IA. (From λυω, to loosen, and γυιον, a member.) The relaxation of limbs.

LYSIMA'CHIA. (From *Lysimachus*, who first discovered it.) The name of a genus of plants in the Linnæan system. Class, *Pentandria*; Order, *Monogynia.*

LYSIMACHIA NUMULARIA. The systematic name of the money-wort. *Nummularia; Hirundinaria; Centimorbia.* Money-wort. This plant is very common in our ditches. It was formerly accounted vulnerary; and was said to possess antiscorbutic and restringent qualities. Boerhaave looks upon it as similar to a mixture of scurvy-grass with sorrel.

LYSIMACHIA PURPUREA. See *Lythrum salicaria.*

LYSSA. (Λυσσα, *rabies.*) The specific name in Good's Nosology for hydrophobia. *Entasia lyssa.*

LYSSODE'CTUS. (From λυσσα, canine madness, and δακνυμι, to bite.) One who is mad in consequence of having been bitten by a mad animal.

LYTHRODES. See *Scapolite.*

LY'THRUM. (From λυθρον, blood: so called from its resemblance in colour.) The name of a genus of plants in the Linnæan system. Class, *Dodecandria*; Order, *Digynia.*

LYTHRUM SALICARIA. *Lysimachia purpurea.* The systematic name of the common or purple willow-herb. The herb, root, and flowers possess a considerable degree of astringency, and are used medicinally in the cure of diarrhœas and dysenteries, fluor albus, and hæmoptysis.

LYTTA. (The name of a genus of insects.) See *Cantharis.*

M

M. This letter has two significations. When herbs, flowers, chips, or such-like substances are ordered in a prescription, and M. follows them, it signifies *manipulus*, a handful; and when several ingredients have been directed, it is a contraction of *misce*; thus, *m. f. haust.* signifies mix and let a draught be made.

MACA'NDON. (Indian.) A tree growing in Malabar, the fruit of which is roasted and eaten as a cure for dysenteries, and in cholera morbus, and other complaints.

MACAPA'TLI. Sarsaparilla.

MACAXOCOTLI'FERA. The name of a tree in the West Indies, the fruit of which is sweet and laxative. A decoction of the bark of this tree cures the itch, and the powder thereof heal ulcers.

MACBRIDE, DAVID, was born in the county of Antrim, of an ancient Scotch family, in 1726. After serving his apprenticeship to a surgeon, he went into the navy, where he remained some years. At this period he was led to investigate particularly the treatment of scurvy, upon which he afterward published a treatise. After the peace of Aix-la-Chapelle, he attended the lectures in Edinburgh and London; and about the end of 1749, settled in Dublin as a surgeon and accoucheur, but his youth and modesty greatly retarded his advancement at first. In 1764, he published his Experimental Essays, which were every where received with great applause; and the University of Glasgow conferred on him a Doctor's degree. For several years after this he gave private lectures on physic; which he published in 1772: this work displayed great acuteness of observation, and very philo-

sophical views of pathology; and contained a new arrangement of diseases, which appeared to Dr. Cullen of sufficient importance to be introduced into his system of nosology. His merit being thus displayed, he go into very extensive practice; indeed, he was so much harassed, that he suffered for some time an almost total incapacity for sleep; when an accidental cold brough up his high fever and delirium, which terminated his existence towards the close of 1778.

MACE. See *Myristica moschata.*

Macedonian parsley. See *Bubon macedonicum.*

MACEDONI'SIUM SEMEN. See *Smyrnium olusatrum*

MA'CER. (From *masa*, Hebrew.) Grecian macer or mace. The root which is imported from Barbary by this name, and is supposed to be the simarouba, and is said to be anti-dysenteric.

MACERA'TION. (*Maceratio*; from *macero*, to soften by water.) In a pharmaceutical sense, this term implies an infusion either with or without heat, wherein the ingredients are intended to be almost wholly dissolved in order to extract their virtues.

MACERO'NA. See *Smyrnium olusatrum.*

MACHÆ'RION. *Machæris.* The amputating knife.

MACHA'ON. The proper name of an ancien physician, said to be one of the sons of Æsculapius whence some authors have fancied to dignify their own inventions with his name, as particularly a collyrium, described by Scribonius, intituled, *Asclepias Machaonis*; and hence also, medicine in general is by some called *Ars Machaonia.*

MACHINAME'NTUM ARISTIONIS. A machine for reducing dislocation.

3*

MA'CIES. Emaciation. See *Atrophy* and *Tabes.*

MA'CIS. Mace. See *Myristica.*

MACKAREL. This delicious fish is the *Scomber scomber* of Linnæus. When fresh it is of easy digestion, and very nutritious. Pickled and salted, it becomes hard and difficult for the stomach to manage.

[The Scomber genus forms a family of fish, most of which are remarkable for their beauty and elegance, as well as for their qualities of being generally good food. The New-York markets are supplied with abundance of mackarel in their season. There are eight species frequenting the ocean and waters adjacent to this city, and they are all eatable; some of them, however, are more abundant than others. We have the following, viz

> Scomber grex,
> ..   vernalis,
> ..   plumbeus,
> ..   ductor,
> ..   crysos,
> ..   maculatus,
> ..   zonatus, and
> ..   sarda.—A.]

MACQUER, Joseph, was born at Paris, in 1710, where he became doctor of medicine, professor of pharmacy, and censor royal. He was likewise a member of some foreign academies, and conducted the medical and chemical department of the Journal des Sçavans. He pursued chemistry, not so much with a view of multiplying pharmaceutical preparations, as had been mostly the case before, but, rather as a branch of natural philosophy; and gained a considerable reputation by publishing several useful and popular works on the subject. The most laborious of these was a dictionary in two octavo volumes; subsequently translated into English by Keir, with great improvements. He published also "Formulæ Medicamentorum Magistralium," and had a share in the composition of the Pharmacopœia Parisiensis of 1758. His death occurred in 1784.

MACROCE'PHALUS. (From μακρος, long, and κεφαλη, the head.) The name of a whale fish. See *Physeter macrocephalus.*

MACROPHYSOCE'PHALUS. (From μακρος, long, φυσις, nature, and κεφαλη, the head, so called from the length of the head.) One who has a head unnaturally long and large. This word, according to Turton, is only used by Ambrose Paré.

MACRO'PIPER. (From μακρος, long, and πεπερι, pepper.) See *Piper longum.*

MACROPNŒ'A. (From μακρος, long, and πνεω, to breathe.) A difficulty of breathing, where the inspirations are at long intervals.

MA'CULA. A spot, a permanent discoloration of some portion of the skin, often with a change of its texture, but not connected with any disorder of the constitution.

MACULA MATRICIS. A mother's mark. See *Mævus maternus.*

MACULATUS. Spotted: applied in botany to stems, petals, &c. as the stem of the common hemlock, *Conium maculatum;* the *petals* of the *Digitalis purpurea,*

Mad-apple. See *Solanum melongena.*

MADARO'SIS. (From μαδος, bald, without hair.) A defect or loss of eyebrows or eyelashes, causing a disagreeable deformity, and painful sensation of the eyes, in a strong light.

MADDER. See *Rubia.*

MADNESS. See *Melancholia,* and *Mania.*

Madness, canine. See *Hydrophobia.*

MA'DOR. Moisture. A sweating.

MADREPORA. *Madrepore.* 1. A genus in natural history, of the class, *Vermes;* and order, *Zoophyta.* An animal resembling a Medusa.

2. A species of coral. It consists of carbonate of lime, and a little animal membraneous substance.

MAGATTI, Cæsar, was born in 1579, in the dutchy of Reggio. He distinguished himself by his early proficiency in philosophy and medicine at Bologna, where he graduated in his 18th year; and afterward went to Rome. Returning at last to his native country, he soon acquired so much reputation in his profession, that he was invited, as professor of surgery, to Ferrara; and after greatly distinguishing himself in that capacity, he was induced, during a severe illness, to enter into the fraternity of Capuchins. He still continued,

however, to practise, and acquired the confidence of persons of the first rank, especially the duke of Modena. But suffering severely from the stone, he underwent an operation at Bologna in 1647, which he did not long survive. He was author of a considerable improvement in the art of surgery, by his work entitled, "De rara Medicatione Vulnerum," condemning the use of tents, and recommending a simple, easy method of dressing, without the irritation of frequently cleansing and rubbing the tender granulations: and in an appendix he refutes the notion of gun-shot wounds being envenomed, or attended with cauterization. He afterward published a defence of this work against some objections of Sennertus.

MAGDA'LEON. (From μασσω, to knead.) A mass of plaster, or other composition, reduced to a cylindrical form.

MAGELLA'NICUS CORTEX. See *Wintera aromatica.*

MA'GISTERY. (*Magisterium;* from *magister,* a master.) An obsolete term used by ancient chemists to signify a peculiar and secret method of preparing any medicine, as it were, by a masterly process. The term was also long applied to all precipitates.

MAGISTRA'LIA. (From *magister,* a master.) Applied, by way of eminence, to such medicines as are extemporaneous, or in common use.

MAGISTRA'NTIA. (From *magistro,* to rule: so called, by way of eminence, as exceeding all others in virtue.) See *Imperatoria.*

MA'GMA. (From μασσω, to blend together.) *Ecpiesma.* 1. A thick ointment.

2. The fæces of an ointment after the thinner parts are strained off.

3. A confection.

MA'GNES. (From *Magnes,* its inventor.) The magnet, or loadstone. A muddy iron ore, in which the iron is modified in such a manner as to afford a passage to a fluid called the magnetic fluid. The magnet exhibits certain phenomena; it is known by its property of attracting steel filings, and is found in Auvergne, in Biscay, in Spain, in Sweden, and Siberia.

MAGNES ARSENICALIS. Arsenical magnet. It is a composition of equal parts of antimony, sulphur, and arsenic, mixed and melted together, so as to become a glassy body.

MAGNES EPILEPSIÆ. An old and obsolete name of native cinnabar.

MAGNE'SIA. 1. The ancient chemists gave this name to such substances as they conceived to have the power of attracting any principle from the air. Thus an earth which, on being exposed to the air, increased in weight, and yielded vitriol, they called *magnesia vitriolata;* and later chemists, observing in their process for obtaining magnesia, that nitrous acid was separated, and an earth left behind, supposing it had attracted the acid, called it *magnesia nitri,* which, from its colour, soon obtained the name of *magnesia alba.*

2. The name of one of the primitive earths, having a metallic basis, called magnesium. It has been found native in the state of hydrate.

Magnesia may be obtained by pouring into a solution of its sulphate a solution of subcarbonate of soda, washing the precipitate, drying it, and exposing it to a red heat. It is usually procured in commerce, by acting on magnesian limestone with the impure muriate of magnesia, or bittern of the sea-salt manufactories. The muriatic acid goes to the lime, forming a soluble salt, and leaves behind the magnesia of both the bittern and limestone. Or the bittern is decomposed by a crude subcarbonate of ammonia, obtained from the distillation of bones in iron cylinders. Muriate of ammonia and subcarbonate of magnesia result. The former is evaporated to dryness, mixed with chalk, and sublimed. Subcarbonate of ammonia is thus recovered, with which a new quantity of bittern may be decomposed; and thus, in ceaseless repetition, forming an elegant and economical process. 100 parts of crystallized Epsom salt, require for complete decomposition 56 of subcarbonate of potassa, or 44 dry subcarbonate of soda, and yield 16 of pure magnesia after calcination.

Magnesia is a white, soft powder. Its sp. gr. is 2.3 by Kirwan. It renders the syrup of violets, and infusion of red cabbage, green, and reddens turmeric. It is infusible, except by the hydroxygen blow-pipe. It has scarcely any taste, and no smell. It is nearly insoluble in water; but it absorbs a quantity of that liquid with the production of heat. And when it is thrown down from the sulphate by a caustic alkali, it is combined with water constituting a hydrate, which, however, separates at a red heat. It contains about one fourth its weight of water.

When magnesia is exposed to the air, it very slowly attracts carbonic acid. It combines with sulphur, forming a sulphuret.

The metallic basis, or magnesium, may be obtained in the state of amalgam with mercury by electrization.

When magnesia is strongly heated in contact with 2 volumes of chlorine, this gas is absorbed, and 1 volume of oxygen is disengaged. Hence it is evident that there exists a combination of magnesium and chlorine, or a true chloride. The salt called muriate of magnesia, is a compound of the chloride and water. When it is acted on by a strong heat, by far the greatest part of the chlorine unites to the hydrogen of the water, and rises in the form of muriatic acid gas; while the oxygen of the decomposed water combines with the magnesium to form magnesia.

Magnesia is often associated with lime in minerals, and their perfect separation becomes an interesting problem in analysis.

Properties. Pure magnesia does not form with water an adhesive ductile mass. It is in the form of a very white spongy powder, soft to the touch, and perfectly tasteless. It is very slightly soluble in water. It absorbs carbonic acid gradually from the atmosphere. It changes very delicate blue vegetable colours to green. Its attraction to the acids is weaker than those of the alkalies. Its salts are partially decomposed by ammonia, one part of the magnesia being precipitated, and the other forming a triple compound. Its specific gravity is about 2.3. It is infusible even by the most intense heat; but when mixed with some of the other earths it becomes fusible. It combines with sulphur. It does not unite to phosphorus or carbon. It is not dissolved by alkalies in the humid way. When heated strongly, it becomes phosphorescent. With the dense acids it becomes ignited. With all the acids it forms salts of a bitter taste, mostly very soluble.

The magnesia of the present London Pharmacopœia was formerly called *Magnesia calcinata; usta; pura.* It is directed to be made thus:—Take of carbonate of magnesia, four ounces; burn it in a very strong fire, for two hours, or until acetic acid being dropped in, extricates no bubbles of gas. It is given as an absorbent, antacid, and eccoprotic, in cardialgia, spasms, convulsions, and tormina of the bowels of infants; pyrosis, flatulencies, and other diseases of the primæ viæ; obstipation, leucorrhœa, rickets, scrofula, crusta lactea, and podagra. The dose is from half a drachm to a drachm.

MAGNESIA CALCINATA. See *Magnesia.*

MAGNESIA, HYDRATE OF. A mineral found in New Jersey, consisting of magnesia and water.

["The structure of this new and interesting mineral is very distinctly foliated; and the foliæ frequently radiate from a centre. Their lustre is more or less shining and pearly; and they are somewhat elastic.

The laminæ when separate are transparent; in the mass only semi-transparent; and by exposure to the weather, their surface becomes dull and opaque.

It is soft, and may be scratched by the finger nail, like talc. It slightly adheres to the tongue; and its sp. gr. is 2.13. Its colour is white, often tinged with green; its powder is a pure white.

It becomes opaque and friable before the blow-pipe, and its weight is diminished. In diluted sulphuric acid, it nearly dissolves without effervescence, and yields a limpid solution extremely bitter to the taste. According to Prof. Bruce, to whom we are indebted for a knowledge of this mineral, it is composed of pure magnesia 70, water 30.

It is sufficiently distinguished from talc by its solubility in acids.

It is found at Hoboken, New-Jersey, in veins, a few lines to two inches in thickness; that traverse serpentine in various directions; and, near the sides of the veins, the serpentine is sometimes intermixed with the foliæ of the magnesia."—*Cleav. Min.*

Specimens of this hydrate, or native magnesia, have also been found in the veins of the serpentine at Hoboken, and on Staten Island, in a pulverulent form, and

when collected has the appearance of the magnesia alba of the shops, a specimen of which is in my possession. A.]

MAGNESIA USTA. See *Magnesia.*

MAGNESIA VITRIOLATA. See *Magnesia sulphas.*

MAGNESIÆ SUBCARBONAS. *Magnesiæ carbonas; Magnesia alba.* Subcarbonate of Magnesia. The London College direct it to be made as follows:—Take of sulphate of magnesia, a pound ; subcarbonate of potassa, nine ounces; water, three gallons. Dissolve the subcarbonate of potassa in three pints of the water, and strain; dissolve also the sulphate of magnesia separately in five pints of the water, and strain; then add the rest of the water to this latter solution, apply heat, and when it boils, pour in the former solution, stirring them well together; next, strain through a linen cloth; lastly, wash the powder repeatedly with boiling water, and dry it upon bibulous paper, in a heat of 200°. It is in form of very fine powder, considerably resembling flour in its appearance and feel; it has no sensible taste on the tongue; it gives a faint greenish colour to the tincture of violets, and converts turnsole to a blue. It is employed medicinally as an absorbent, antacid, and purgative, in doses from half a drachm to two drachms.

MAGNESIÆ SULPHAS. *Sulphas magnesiæ; Sulphas magnesiæ purificata; Magnesia vitriolata; Sal catharticus amarus. Sal catharticum amarum.* Sulphate of magnesia. Epsom salt. Bitter purging salt. The sulphate of magnesia exists in several minera. springs, and in sea-water.

It is from these saline solutions that the salt is obtained ; the method generally adopted for obtaining it is evaporation, which causes the salt to crystallize in tetrahedral prisms. It has a very bitter taste, and is soluble in its own weight of water at 60°, and in three-fourths of its weight of boiling water. Sulphate of magnesia, when perfectly pure, effloresces; but that of commerce generally contains foreign salts, such as the muriate of magnesia, which renders it so deliquescent, that it must be kept in a close vessel or bladder. By the action of heat it undergoes the watery fusion, and loses its water of crystallization, but does not part with its acid. One hundred parts of crystallized sulphate of magnesia consist of 29.35 parts of acid, 17 of earth, and 53.65 of water. The alkalies, strontian, barytes, and all the salts formed by these salifiable bases, excepting the alkaline muriates, decompose sulphate of magnesia. It is also decomposed by the nitrate, carbonate, and muriate of lime.

Epsom salt is a mild and gentle purgative, operating with sufficient efficacy, and in general with ease and safety, rarely occasioning any gripes, or the other inconveniences of resinous purgatives. Six or eight drachms may be dissolved in a proper quantity of common water ; or four, five, or more in a pint or quart of the purging mineral waters. These solutions may likewise be so managed, in small doses, as to produce evacuation from the other emunctories; if the patient be kept warm, they increase perspiration, and by moderate exercise in the cool air, the urinary discharge. Some allege that this salt has a peculiar effect in allaying pain, as in colic, even independently of evacuation.

It is, however, principally used for the preparation of the subcarbonate of magnesia.

[MAGNESIAN LIMESTONE. This is a magnesian carbonate of lime, of which there are two varieties; common magnesian limestone, or bitter-spar, and dolomite ; both of which have been found in abundance in Pennsylvania, New-York, and Connecticut. Some of the quarries supplying this limestone may hereafter become important in the manufacture of Epsom salts, or sulphate of magnesia. A.]

MAGNESITE. A yellowish gray or white mineral, composed of magnesia, carbonic acid, alumina, a ferruginous manganese, lime, and water, found in serpentine rocks, in Moravia.

MAGNESIUM. The metallic basis of magnesia. See *Magnesia.*

MAGNET. See *Magnes.*

MAGNETISM. The property which iron possesses of attracting or repelling other iron, according to circumstances, that is, similar poles of magnets repel, but opposite poles attract each other.

MAGNETISM, ANIMAL. A sympathy lately supposed, by some persons, to exist between the magnet and the human body; by means of which the former became capable of curing many diseases in an unknown way, somewhat resembling the performances of the old magicians. Animal magnetism is now entirely exploded.

MAGNUM OS. The third bone of the lower row of bones of the carpus, reckoning from the thumb towards the little finger.

MAGNUS. The term is applied to parts from their relative size; and to diseases and remedies from their importance; as *magnum os, magnus morbus, magnum dei donum,* &c.

MAGNUM DEI DONUM. So Dr. Mead calls the Peruvian bark.

MAGNUS MORBUS. The great disease. So Hippocrates calls the epilepsy.

MAGY'DARIS. The root of the laserwort·

Mahagoni. See *Swietenia.*

MAHALEB. A species of *Prunus.*

MAHMOU'DY. *Scammonium.*

MAIDENHAIR. See *Adianthum.*

Maidenhair, Canada. See *Adianthum pedatum.*

Maidenhair, common. See *Asplenium trichomanes.*

Maidenhair, English. See *Adianthum.*

Maidenhair, golden. See *Polytrichum.*

MAIDENHAIR-TREE. *Ginan itsio.* The *Ginko biloba.* In China and Japan, where this tree grows, the fruit acquires the size of a damask plumb, and contains a kernel resembling that of our apricot. These kernels always make part of the dessert at all public feasts and entertainments. They are said to promote digestion, and to cleanse the stomach and bowels. The oil is used at the table.

MAJANTHEMUM. See *Convallaria majalis.*

MAJORA'NA. (*Quod mense Maio floreat,* because it flowers in May.) See *Origanum majorana.*

MAJORANA SYRIACA. See *Teucrium marum.*

MA'LA. (From *malus,* an apple: so called from its roundness.) A prominent part of the cheek. See *Jugale os.*

MALA ÆTHIOPICA. A species of love-apple. See *Solanum lycopersicum.*

MALA ASSYRIA. The citron.

MALA AURANTIA. See *Citrus aurantium.*

MALA COTONEA. The quince.

MALA INSANA NIGRA. See *Solanum melongena.*

Malabar plum. See *Eugenia jambos.*

MALABATHRI OLEUM. Oil of cassia.

MALABA'THRINUM. (From μαλαβαθρον, malabathrum.) Ointment of malabathrum. It is compounded of myrrh, spikenard, malabathrum, and many other aromatic ingredients.

MALABA'THRUM. (Μαλαβαθρον: from *Malabar,* in India, whence it was brought, and *betre,* a leaf, Ind.) See *Laurus cassia.*

MA'LACA RADIX. See *Sagittaria alexipharmaca.*

Malacca bean. See *Avicennia tomentosa.*

MA'LACHE. (*Malache,* es. f.; from μαλακος, soft: so called from the softness of its leaf.) The mallow. See *Malva.*

. MALACHITE. (From μαλαχη, the mallow: from its resemblance in colour to the mallow.) Mountain blue, a carbonate of copper ore found in Siberia.

MALACHOLITE. See *Sahlite.*

MALA'CIA. (From μαλαχιον, a ravenous fish.) Depraved appetite, when such things are coveted as are not proper for food. See *Pica.*

MALACO'STEON. (From μαλακος, soft, and οςεον, bone.) A softness of the bones. *Mollities ossium.* A disease of the bones, wherein they can be bent without fracturing them, in consequence either of the inordinate absorption of the phosphate of lime, from which their natural solidity is derived, or else of this matter not being duly secreted and deposited in their fabric. In rickets, the bones only yield and become distorted by slow degrees; but in the present disease they may be at once bent in any direction. The mollities ossium is rare, and its causes not well understood. All the cases of mollities ossium yet on record have proved fatal, and no means of cure are yet known. On dissection of those who have died, all the bones, except the teeth, have been found unusually soft, so that scarcely any of them could resist the knife, the periosteum has been found thicker than usual, and the bones have been found to contain a great quantity of oily matter and little earth.

MALA'CTICA. (From μαλασσω, to soften.) Emollient medicines.

40

MALAGFUE'TTA. Grains of paradise.

MALAGUETTA. Grains of paradise.

MALA'GMA. (From μαλασσω, to soften) A poultice.

MALAMIRIS. A species of *Piper.*

MALA'RIA. The name in Italy of an endemic intermittent, which attacks people in the neighbourhood of Rome, and especially about the Pontine marshes, which have often been drained to carry off the decomposing animal and vegetable materials that spread their *Aria cattiva,* as it is called, over the whole of the campagna.

[The Malaria of Rome is an *infected atmosphere* arising from *marsh-miasmata,* producing an endemic disease. We have, in the United States, many similar instances of malaria producing also local and endemic diseases. The Pontine marshes in the neighbourhood of Rome are very extensive, and infect the atmosphere over a large tract of country. Lancisi has ably described the condition and effects of the *marsh-miasma* of Rome, in his work *De noxiis paludum effluviis.* The Malaria returns annually during the height of the warm season, and is destroyed with the approach of winter, producing in this country what we call a *seasonable disease.* The term *marsh-miasma,* has become rather unfashionable, as perhaps its meaning is too indefinite, but it is not more so than Malaria. In fact, they both mean the same thing, or the same state of the atmosphere, both producing seasonable, and local or endemic diseases. One is an Italian word, meaning *bad air,* or a sickening state of the atmosphere. *Miasma* is a Greek word, from μιαινω, to infect, importing a polluted, corrupted, or infected state of the atmosphere. A.]

MALARUM OSSA. See *Jugale os.*

MA'LATE. *Malas.* A salt formed by the union of the malic acid, or acid of apples with salifiable bases; thus *malate of copper, malate of lead,* &c.

MA'LE. The arm-pit.

Male fern. See *Polypodium filix mas.*

Male orchis. See *Orchis mascula.*

Male speedwell. See *Veronica officinalis.*

MALIC ACID. *Acidum malicum.* This acid is obtained by saturating the juice of apples with alkali, and pouring in the acetous solution of lead, until it occasions no more precipitate. The precipitate is then to be edulcorated and sulphuric acid poured on it, until the liquor has acquired a fresh acid taste, without any mixture of sweetness. The whole is then to be filtered, to separate the sulphate of lead. The filtered liquor is the malic acid, which is very pure, remains always in a fluid state, and cannot be rendered concrete. See *Sorbic acid.*

MALIASMUS. (From μαλις, cutaneous vermination.) Breeding animalcules on the skin, as the louse, flea, tick, &c.

MALI'GNANT. (*Malignus;* from *malus.*) A term which may be applied to any disease, the symptoms of which are so aggravated as to threaten the destruction of the patient. It is frequently used to signify a dangerous epidemic.

Malignant fever. See *Typhus.*

Malignant sore throat. See *Cynanche maligna.*

MA'LIS. (Μαλις, and μαλιασμος, are Greek nouns composing cutaneous vermination.) The name of a genus of diseases in Good's Nosology. Class, *Ecentica,* Order, *Acrotica.* Cutaneous vermination. It has six species, vix. *Malis pediculi; pulicis; acari; filariæ, æstri; gordii.*

MALLEABILITY. (*Malleabilitas;* from *malleus,* a hammer.) The property which several metals possess of being extended under the hammer into thin plates, without cracking. The thin leaves of silver and gold. are the best examples of malleability. See *Ductility.*

MALLEAMOTHE. *Pavette; Pavate; Erysipelas cu rans arbor.* A shrub which grows in Malabar. The leaves, boiled in palm oil, cure the impetigo; the root, powdered and mixed with ginger, is diuretic.

MALLEATIO. A species of St. Vitus's dance, in which the person has a convulsive action of one or both hands, which strike the knee like a hammer.

MALLEI ANTERIOR. See *Laxator tympani.*

MALLEI EXTERNUS. See *Laxator tympani.*

MALLEI INTERNUS. See *Tensor tympani.*

MALLE'OLUS. (Dim. of *malleus,* a mallet: so called from its supposed resemblance to a mallet.)

The ankle, distinguished into external and internal, or *malleolus externus* and *internus*.

MA′LLEUS. (*Malleus quasi molleus;* from *mollio*, to soften; a hammer.) A bone of the internal ear is so termed from its resemblance. It is distinguished into a head, neck, and manubrium. The *head* is round, and incrusted with a thin cartilage, and annexed to another bone of the ear, the incus, by ginglymus. Its *neck* is narrow, and situated between the head and manubrium, or handle; from which a long slender process arises, adheres to a furrow in the auditory canal, and is continued as far as the fissure in the articular cavity of the temporal bone. The *manubrium* is terminated by an enlarged extremity, and connected to the membrana tympani by a short conoid process.

MALLOW. See *Malva*.
Mallow, round-leaved. See *Malva rotundifolia.*
Mallow, vervain. See *Malva alcea.*

MALOGRANA′TUM. (From *malum*, an apple, and *granum*, a grain: so named from its grain-like seeds.) The pomegranate.

MALPIGHI, MARCELLO, was born near Bologna, in 1628. He went through his preliminary studies with great eclat, and especially distinguished himself by his zealous pursuit of anatomy. His merit procured him, in 1653, the degree of doctor in medicine, and, three years after, the appointment of professor of physic, at Bologna; but he was soon invited to Pisa, by the Grand Duke of Tuscany. However, the air of this place injuring his health, which was naturally delicate, he was obliged, in 1659, to return to his office at Bologna. Three years after, he was tempted by the magistrates of Messina to accept the medical professorship there; but his little deference to ancient authorities involved him in controversies with his colleagues, which forced him to return again to Bologna, in 1666. His reputation rapidly extended throughout Europe, as a philosophical inquirer, and he was chosen a member of the Royal Society of London, which afterward printed his works at their own expense. In 1691, Pope Innocent XII., on his election, chose Malpighi for his chief physician and chamberlain, when he removed to Rome; but, three years after, he was carried off by an apoplectic stroke. He joined, with an indefatigable pursuit of knowledge, a remarkable degree of candour and modesty; and ranks very high among the philosophers of the physiological age in which he lived. He was the first to employ the microscope in examining the circulation of the blood; and the same instrument assisted him in exploring the minute structure of various organs, as is evident from his first publication on the lungs, in 1661; and this was followed by successive treatises on many other parts. In 1669, his essay, "De Formatione Pulli in Ovo," was printed at London, with his remarks on the silkworm, and on the conglobate glands: much light was thrown by these investigations on the obscure subject of generation, and other important points of physiology. He was thence led to the consideration of the structure and functions of plants, and evinced himself an original, as well as a very profound observer. His "Anatome Plantarum" was published by the Royal Society, in 1675 and 1679, with some observations on the incubation of the egg. His only medical work, "Consultatiorum Medicinalium Centuria Prima," did not appear till 1713: he was not distinguished as a practitioner, but deserves praise for pointing out the mischief of bleeding, in the malignant epidemics which prevailed in Italy in his time.

MALPI′GHIA. (So named in honour of Malpighi, the celebrated vegetable anatomist.) The name of a genus of plants in the Linnæan system. Class, *Decandria;* Order, *Trigynia.*

MALPIGHIA GLABRA. The systematic name of a tree which affords an esculent cherry.

MALT. Grain which has become sweet, from the conversion of its starch into sugar, by an incipient growth or germination, artificially induced, called malting.

MA′LTHA. (From μαλασσω, to soften.) *Malthacodes.* 1. A medicine softened and tempered with wax.
2. The name of the mineral tallow of Kirwan, which resembles wax, and is said to have been found on the coast of Finland.

MALTHA′OTICA. (From μαλθακιζω, to soften.) Emollient medicines.

MALTHEORUM. Common salt.

MA′LUM. 1. A disease.
2. An apple.

MALUM MORTUUM. A disease that appears in the form of a pustule, which soon forms a dry, brown, hard, and broad crust. It is seldom attended with pain, and remains fixed for a long time before it can be detached. It is mostly observed on the tibia and os coccygis, and sometimes the face.

MALUM PILARE. See *Plica.*

MA′LUS. See *Pyrus malus.*

MALUS INDICA. *Bilumbi biting-bing*, of Bontius. The *Malus indica—fructu pentagono*, of Europeans. It is carefully cultivated in the gardens of the East Indies, where it flowers throughout the year. The juice of the root is cooling, and drank as a cure for fevers. The leaves, boiled and made into a cataplasm with rice, are famed in all sorts of tumours, and the juice of the fruit is used in almost all external heats, dipping linen rags in it, and applying them to the parts. It is drank, mixed with arrack, to cure diarrhœas; and the dried leaves, mixed with betel leaves, and given in arrack, are said to promote delivery. The ripe fruit is eaten as a delicacy, and the unripe made into a pickle for the use of the table.

MA′LVA. (*Malva quasi molva;* from *mollis*, soft: named from the softness of its leaves.) 1. The name of a genus of plants in the Linnæan system. Class, *Monadelphia;* Order, *Polyandria.*
2. The pharmacopœial name of the common mallow. See *Malva sylvestris.*

MALVA ALCEA. *Malva verbenaca.* The vervain mallow. This plant is distinguished from the common mallow by its leaves being jagged, or cut in about the edges. It agrees in virtues with the other mallows, but it is the least mucilaginous of any. This, like to the other mallows, abounds with a mucilage, and is good for pectoral drinks.

MALVA ARBOREA. See *Alcea rosea.*

MALVA ROTUNDIFOLIA. Round-leaved mallow. The whole herb and root possess similar virtues to the common mallow. See *Malva sylvestris.*

MALVA SYLVESTRIS. The systematic name of the common mallow. *Malva vulgaris; Malva—caule erecto herbaceo, foliis septemlobatis acutis, pedunculis petiolisque pilosis.* This indigenous plant has a strong affinity to the althæa, both in a botanical and a medical respect. See *Althæa.* The leaves and flowers are principally used in fomentations, cataplasms, and emollient enemas. The internal use of the leaves seems to be wholly superseded by the radix althæa.

MALVA VERBENACA. See *Malva alcea.*

MALVA VULGARIS. See *Malva sylvestris.*

MALVAVI′SCUS. (From *malva*, the mallow, and *viscus*, glue: so named from its viscidity.) See *Althæa officinalis.*

MALVERN. The village of Great Malvern has, for many years, been celebrated for a spring of remarkable purity, which has acquired the name of the holy well, from the reputed sanctity of its waters, and the real and extensive benefit long derived in various cases from its use.

The holy well water, when first drawn, appears quite clear and pellucid, and does not become sensibly turbid on standing. It possesses somewhat of an agreeable pungency to the taste; but this is not considerable. In other respects it does not differ in taste from pure well water.

The contents of Malvern holy well are:—some carbonic acid, which is in an uncombined state, capable of acting upon iron, and of giving a little taste to the water; but the exact quantity of which has not been ascertained:—a very small portion of earth, either lime or magnesia, united with the carbonic and marine acids; perhaps a little neutral alkaline salt, and a very large proportion of water:—for we may add, that, the carbonic acid perhaps excepted, the foreign matter is less than that of any spring-water which we use. No iron or metal of any kind is found in it, though there are chalybeates in the neighbourhood.

It is singular that, notwithstanding its apparent purity, this water is said not to keep well, and soon acquires a fœtid smell, by standing in open vessels.

Malvern water, like many others, was at first only employed as an external application; and this, indeed, is still its principal use, though it is extended, with some advantage, to a few internal diseases. It has been found highly efficacious in painful and deep ulcerations, the consequence of a scrofulous habit of body, and which are always attended with much local irritation, and often general fever. Applied to the sore, it moderates the profuseness of the discharge, corrects the fœtor, which so peculiarly marks a caries of the bone, promotes the granulating process, and a salutary exfoliation of the carious part; and by a long perseverance in this course, very dangerous and obstinate cases have at last been cured. Inflammation of the eye, especially the ophthalmia, which is so troublesome in scrofulous habits, often yields to this simple application, and we find, that, for a great number of years, persons afflicted with sore eyes have been in the habit of resorting to Malvern holy well. Another order of external diseases, for which this water is greatly celebrated, is cutaneous eruptions; even those obstinate cases of dry desquamations, that frequently follow a sudden application of cold in irritable habits, are often cured by this remedy. Where the skin is hot and dry, it remarkably relieves the intolerable itching of herpetic disorders, and renders the surface of the body more cool and perspirable. It appears, however, from a nice observation of Dr. Wall, that this method of treatment is not so successful in the cutaneous eruptions of very lax leucophlegmatic habits, where the extremities are cold and the circulation languid; but that it succeeds best where there is unusual irritation of the skin, and where it is apt to break in painful fissures, that ooze out a watery acrid lymph. On the first application of this water to an inflamed surface, it will often, for a time, increase the pain and irritation, but these effects go off in a few days.

The great benefit arising from using Malvern waters as an external remedy, in diseases of the skin and surface of the body, has led to its employment in some internal disorders, and often with considerable advantage. Of these, the most important are painful affections of the kidneys and bladder, attended with the discharge of bloody, purulent, or fœtid urine, the hectic fever, produced by scrofulous ulceration of the lungs, or very extensive and irritating sores on the surface of the body, and also fistulas of long standing, that have been neglected, and have become constant and troublesome sores.

The Malvern water is in general a perfectly safe application, and may be used with the utmost freedom, both as an external dressing for sores, and as a common drink.

The internal use of Malvern waters is sometimes attended at first with a slight nausea, and not unfrequently, for the first day or two, it occasions some degree of drowsiness, vertigo, or slight pain of the head, which comes on a few minutes after drinking it. These symptoms go off spontaneously, after a few days, or may readily be removed by a mild purgative. The effects of this water on the bowels are not at all constant; frequently it purges briskly for a few days, but it is not uncommon for the body to be rendered costive by its use, especially, as Dr. Wall observes, with those who are accustomed to malt liquors. In all cases, it decidedly increases the flow of urine, and the general health of the patient. The duration of a course of Malvern waters must vary very considerably on account of the different kinds of disease for which this spring is resorted to.

MAME'I. The mammoe, momin, or toddy-tree. This tree is found in different parts of the West Indies, but those on the Island of Hispaniola are the best. From incisions made in the branches, a copious discharge of pellucid liquor is obtained, which is called momin, or toddy-wine. It must be drank very sparingly, because of its very diuretic quality. It is esteemed as an effectual preservative from the stone, as also a solvent of it when generated. There are two species.

MAMI'LLA. (Diminutive of *mamma*, the breast.)
1. The breast of man.
2. The nipple of the male and female breasts.

MAMI'RA. It is said, by Paulus Ægineta, to be the root of a plant which is of a detergent quality. Some think it is the root of the doronicum; but what it really is cannot be ascertained.

MA'MMA. See *Breast*.

MA'MMARY. Belonging to the breast.

MAMMARY ARTERY. *Arteria mammillaris*. The internal mammary artery is a branch of the subclavian,

and gives off the mediastinal, thymal, and pericardial arteries. The external mammary is a branch of the axillary artery.

MAMMARY VEIN. *Vena mamillaris*. These vessels accompany the arteries, and evacuate their blood into the subclavian vein.

MAMMEA. (So called from its vernacular appellation in the West Indies, *mamei*; and allowed by Linnæus, because of its affinity to *mamma*, a breast, alluding to the shape of its fruit.) The name of a genus of plants. Class, *Polyandria*; Order *Monogynia*.

MAMMEA AMERICANA. The systematic name of a tree, which affords a delicious fruit called *mammea*. It has a very grateful flavour when ripe, and is much cultivated in Jamaica, where it is generally sold in the markets for one of the best fruits of the island.

MAN. *Homo*. Man is compounded of solids, fluids, a vital principle, and, what distinguishes him from every other animal, a soul. See *Animal*.

MA'NCORON. According to Oribasius, a kind of sugar found in a sort of cane.

MANCURA'NA. See *Origanum vulgare*.

MANDI'BULA. (From *mando*, to chew.) The jaw. See *Maxilla inferior*.

MANDRA'GORA. (From ηανδρα, a den, and αγειρω, to collect; because it grows about caves and dens of beasts; or from the German *man dragen*, bearing man.) See *Atropa mandragora*.

MANDRAGORI'TES. (From μανδραγορα, the mandrake.) Wine, in which the roots of the male mandrake are infused.

MANDRAKE. See *Atropa mandragora*.

MANDUCA'TOR. (From *manduco*, to chew, A muscle which assists in the action of chewing.

MA'NGA. (Indian.) The mango-tree.

MANGANESE. This metallic substance seems after iron, to be the most frequently diffused meta through the earth; its ores are very common. As a peculiar metal, it was first noticed by Gahn and Schoele, in the years 1774 and 1777. It is always found in the state of an oxide, varying in the degree of oxidisement. La Peyrouse affirmed that he had found manganese in a metallic state; but there was probably some mistake in his observation. The ores are distinguished into *gray oxide of manganese, black oxide of manganese, reddish white oxide of manganese*, and *carbonate of manganese*. All these combinations have an earthy texture; they are very ponderous; they occur both amorphous and crystallized; and generally contain a large quantity of iron. Their colour is black, blackish-brown, or gray, seldom white. They soil the fingers like soot. They are sometimes crystallized in prisms, tetrahedral, rhomboidal, or striated.

Properties.—Manganese is of a whitish gray colour. Its fracture is granulated, irregular, and uneven. It is of a metallic brilliancy, which it, however, soon loses in the air. Its specific gravity is about 8. It is very hard, and extremely brittle. It is one of the most refractory metals, and most difficult to fuse, requiring at least 160° of Wedgwood's pyrometer. Its attraction of oxygen is so rapid, that exposure to the air is sufficient to render it red, brown, black, and friable, in a very short time; it can, therefore, only be kept under water, oil, or ardent spirits. It is the most combustible of all the metals. It decomposes water by means of heat, very rapidly, as well as the greater part of the metallic oxides. It decomposes sulphuric acid. It is soluble in nitric acid. It is fusible with earths, and colours them brown, violet, or red, according to its state of oxidisement. It frees from colour glasses tinged by iron. It does not readily unite with sulphur. It combines with phosphorus. It unites with gold, silver, and copper, and renders them brittle. It unites to arsenic in close vessels, but does not enter into union with mercury.

Manganese, heated in oxygen or chlorine, takes fire and forms an oxide or chloride. It has been thought difficult to decide on the oxides of manganese.

According to Sir H. Davy there are two oxides only, the olive and the black; Mr. Brande has three, the olive, dark red, and black; Thenard has four, the green, the white (in the state of hydrate), the chesnut-brown, and the black; Berzelius has five, the first gray the second green, the third and fourth are not well defined, and the fifth is the black.

Two oxides, however, are well defined.

1. The first oxide may be obtained by dissolving com

mon black manganese in sulphuric or nitric acid, adding a little sugar, and precipitating by solution of potassa. A white powder is obtained, which being heated to redness out of the contact of air, becomes yellow, puce-coloured, and, lastly, red-brown. To be preserved, it should be washed in boiling water, previously freed from air, and then dried by distilling off the moisture in a retort filled with hydrogen. The dark olive oxide, when examined in large quantities, appears almost black; but when spread upon white paper, its olive tint is apparent. It takes fire when gently heated, increases in weight, and acquires a browner tint. It slowly absorbs oxygen from the air, even at common temperatures. It dissolves in acids without effervescence. The white powder obtained above, is the hydrated protoxide. The different tints which it assumes by exposure to air, are supposed by Sir H. Davy to depend on the formation of variable quantities of the black-brown oxide, which probably retains the water contained in the white hydrate, and is hence deep puce-coloured.

2. The black *peroxide*. Its sp. gr. is 4. It does not combine with any of the acids. It yields oxygen when heated; and by intense ignition passes in a great measure into the protoxide.

Method of obtaining Manganese.—This metal is obtained by mixing the black oxide, finely powdered, with pitch; making it into a ball, and putting this into a crucible, with powdered charcoal, one-tenth of an inch thick at the sides, and one-fourth of an inch deep at the bottom. The empty space is then to be filled with powdered charcoal; a cover is to be luted on; and the crucible exposed, for an hour, to the strongest heat that can be raised. Or, digest the black oxide of manganese repeatedly, with the addition of one-sixteenth of sugar, in nitric acid; dilute the mixture with three times its bulk of water; filter it, and decompose it by the addition of potassa; collect the precipitate, form it into a paste with oil, and put it into a crucible, well lined with charcoal. Expose the crucible for at least two hours to the strongest heat of a forge.

MANGANESIC ACID. (*Acidum manganesium*; from *manganese*, its base.) Chevillott and Edwards have ascertained that the carnelion mineral, which is formed by igniting a mixture of the black oxide of manganese and nitre, has the property of making a neutral manganesate of potassa.

MANGEL WURSEL. The root of scarcity. The *Beta hybrida* of Linnæus. A plant of great importance, as a substitute for bread in periods of famine. It is cultivated here as green food for cattle, especially milch cows. It has not, however, succeeded so well in this country as in Germany.

MANGET, JOHN JAMES, was born at Geneva in 1652. He originally studied for the clerical profession, but, after five years' labour, his inclination to medical pursuits prevailed, and he made such progress, without the aid of any teacher, that he was admitted to the degree of doctor at Valence in 1678. He then commenced practice in his native city, and obtained considerable reputation, and refused many invitations to go to other countries. In 1699 he was appointed chief physician to Frederick III. afterward first King of Prussia. In his literary labours he was indefatigable even to the end of his life, which terminated in his 91st year. Among the numerous works of compilation, executed by him, originality is not to be expected; nor are they remarkable for judgment or accuracy, though still sometimes useful for reference. He published ample collections on almost every subject connected with medicine, besides improved editions of the works of others; but the most important of his productions is entitled " Bibliotheca Scriptorum Medicorum veterum et recentiorum," at which he laboured when at least eighty years of age.

MANGI'FERA. (From *mango*, the name of the fruit which it bears.) The name of a genus of plants in the Linnæan system. Class *Pentandria*; Order, *Monogynia*. The Mango-tree.

MANGIFERA INDICA. The systematic name of the mango-tree, which is cultivated all over Asia. Mangoes, when ripe, are juicy, of a good flavour, and so fragrant as to perfume the air to a considerable distance. They are eaten either raw or preserved with sugar. Their taste is so luscious, that they soon pall the appetite. The unripe fruits are pickled in the milk of the cocoa-nut, that has stood until sour, with salt,

capsicum, and garlick. From the expressed juice is prepared a wine; and the remainder of the kernel can be reduced to an excellent flour for the making of bread

MANGO. See *Mangifera indica*.

MANGOSTANA. See *Garcinia mangostana*.

MANGOSTEEN. See *Garcinia mangostana*.

MANIA. (From μαινομαι, to rage.) Raving or furious madness. A genus of disease in the class *Neuroses;* and order *Vesaniæ*, of Cullen. The definition of mania is delirium, unaccompanied with fever; but this does not seem altogether correct, as a delirium may prevail without any frequency of pulse or fever; as happens sometimes with women in the hysteric disease. In mania, the mind is not perfectly master of all its functions; it receives impressions from the senses, which are very different from those produced in health; the judgment and memory are both lost, or impaired, and the irritability of the body is much diminished, being capable, as is supposed, of resisting the usual morbid effects of cold, hunger, and watching, and being likewise less susceptible of other diseases than before.

Mania may be said to be a false perception of things, marked by an incoherence, or raving, and a resistance of the passions to the command of the will, accompanied, for the most part, with a violence of action, and furious resentment at restraint.

There are two species of madness, viz. the melancholic and furious.

Madness is occasioned by affections of the mind, such as anxiety, grief, love, religion, terror, or enthusiasm; the frequent and uncurbed indulgence in any passion, or emotions, and by abstruse study. In short, it may be produced by any thing that affects the mind so forcibly as to take off its attention from all other affairs. Violent exercise, frequent intoxication, a sedentary life, the suppression of periodical and occasional discharges and secretions, excessive evacuations, and paralytic seizures, are likewise enumerated as remote causes Certain diseases of the febrile kind have been found to occasion madness, where their action has been very violent. In some cases it proceeds from an hereditary predisposition. Two constitutions are particularly the victims of madness; the sanguine and melancholic: by the difference of which its appearance is somewhat modified. Each species of mania is accompanied with particular symptoms. Those which attend on the melancholic are sadness, dejection of spirits, and its attendants. Those which accompany an attack of furious madness, are severe pains in the head, redness of the face, noise in the ears, wildness of the countenance, rolling and glistening of the eyes, grinding of the teeth, loud roaring, violent exertion of strength, absurd incoherent discourse, unaccountable malice to certain persons, particularly to the nearest relatives and friends, a dislike to such places and scenes as formerly afforded particular pleasure, a diminution of the irritability of the body, with respect to the morbid effects of cold, hunger, and watching, together with a full, quick pulse.

Mania comes on at different periods of life; but, in the greater number of cases, it makes its attack between thirty and forty years of age. Females appear to be more subject to mania than males.

Dissections of maniacal cases, Dr. Thomas observes, most generally show an effusion of water into the cavities of the brain; but in some cases, we are able to discover evident marks of previous inflammation, such as thickening and opacity of the tunica arachnoides and pia mater. In a few instances, a preternatual hardness of the substance of the brain.

From Dr. Greding's observations, it appears that the skulls of the greater number of such persons are com monly very thick. Some he found of a most extraordinary degree of thickness; but it appears that the greater number of insane people die of atrophy and hydrothorax.

The treatment of madness is partly corporeal, partly mental. The leading indications under the first head are: to diminish vascular or nervous excitement when excessive, as in mania; to increase them when defective, as in melancholia; at the same time guarding against the several exciting causes, and removing any obvious fault in the constitution, or in particular parts by which the brain may be sympathetically affected. Among the most powerful means of lessening excitement is the abstraction of blood, which, freely practised

43

has been often an effectual remedy in recent cases and robust habits; but repeated small bleedings are rather likely to confirm the disease; and in those who have long laboured under it, the object should merely be to obviate dangerous accumulation in the head, by occasionally withdrawing the requisite quantity locally. Purging is much more extensively applicable: where the strength will admit, it may be useful to make very large evacuations in this way; and in all cases it should be a rule to procure regular discharges from the bowels, which are generally torpid. Calomel is mostly proper, as it may evacuate bile more freely, and have other beneficial effects; but it usually requires the assistance of other cathartics. The application of cold to the head is materially serviceable under increased excitement, and some have advised it to the body generally; at any rate, the accumulation of heat should be avoided, and the antiphlogistic regimen steadily observed. Emetics have sometimes had a good effect, especially as influencing the mind of the patient; but to diminish excitement, and induce diaphoresis, it will generally be better to give merely nauseating doses; and occasionally their operation may be promoted by the tepid bath; even the hot bath has been found useful, producing great relaxation, and rendering the patient more tractable. Digitalis may be employed with advantage from its sedative power, exerted especially on the circulation, pushing it till some obvious effect is produced. Narcotics, particularly opium, have been much used, but certainly are not indiscriminately proper; where there is fulness of the vessels of the head, they may even do mischief; and where organic disease exists, they will probably only palliate: whenever resorted to, the dose should be large, such as may induce sleep, and if no mitigation of the disease appear, it may be better not to persevere in them. Camphor has been sometimes decidedly useful carried gradually to a very considerable extent. Blisters and other means of lessening fulness and irritation in the brain, should not be neglected, where circumstances indicate their use.— In the melancholic, on the other hand, where there is rather a deficiency of excitement, it is necessary to direct a more generous diet, nutritious and easy of digestion, as the stomach is usually weak, with a moderate quantity of some fermented liquor, and medicines of a tonic or even stimulant nature, especially ammonia, to relieve flatulence and acidity. Attention should be paid to the bowels, and to maintain the function of the skin, &c. The utility of the cold bath seems questionable in melancholics; though it may occasionally arrest a paroxysm of mania. Regular exercise may contribute materially to improve the health; and even hard labour has been often signally useful in a convalescent state, particularly to those accustomed to it. If the mental derangement supervened on the stoppage of any evacuation, or the metastasis of any other disorder; or appear connected with a scrofulous or syphilitic taint; proper remedies to restore the former, or remove the latter, should be exhibited : and in some instances trepanning has relieved the brain from local irritation. In the management of the insane, it is necessary to inspire a certain degree of awe from a conviction of superior power, and at the same time seek to gain their confidence and affection by steadiness and humanity. Some restraint is often necessary for the security of the patient, or of others, carefully watching, or even confining them, if they threaten the lives of their attendants. When they refuse to take food, or medicine, or any thing which appears absolutely necessary, coercion is proper, or sometimes these caprices may be overcome by stratagem; or exciting uneasy sensations by the motion of a swing, whirling chair, &c. In order to remove any deranged association of ideas, it will be right to endeavour to occupy their minds with some agreeable and regular train of thought, cheerful music, poetry, narrative, the elementary parts of geometry, &c. according to their previous inclinations; to lead them gradually to their former habits, and the society of their friends, engage them in rural sports, take them to public amusements, the watering places, &c. but with as little appearance of design as possible.

MANIGUETTA. See *Amomum granum Paradisi.*

MA′NIHOT. See *Jatropha manihot.*

MANI′PULUS. (*Quod manum impleat,* because it fills the hand.) A handful.

MANJAPU′MERAM. A common tree in the West

Indies, the flowers of which are distilled, and the waters used against inflammation of the eyes.

MA′NNA. (From *mano,* a gift, Syrian; it being the food given by God to the children of Israel in the wilderness; or from *mahna,* what is it? an exclamation occasioned by their wonder at its appearance.) See *Fraxinus ornus.*

MANNA BRIGANTIACA. A species of manna brought from the neighbourhood of Brianconois, in Dauphiny.

MANNA CALABRINA. Calabrian manna.

MANNA CANULATA. Flaky manna, or manna concreted on straw, or chips.

MANNA THURIS. A coarse powder of olibanum.

MANNIFERA ARBOR. (From *manna,* and *fero,* to bear.) See *Fraxinus ornus.*

MANSO′RIUS. (From *mando,* to chew.) The masseter muscle.

MANTI′LE. The name of a bandage.

MANUS. The hand. This consists of the carpus, metacarpus, and fingers.

MA′NUS DEI. 1. A name of a resolvent plaster, described by Lemery.

2. An old name of opium.

MAPLE. See *Acer pseudoplatanus,* and *acer saccharinum.*

MARA′NDA. A species of myrtle, growing in the island of Ceylon, a decoction of the leaves of which is said to be excellent against the venereal disease.

MARA′NTA. 1. The name of a genus of plants in the Linnæan system. Class, *Monandria ;* Order, *Monogynia.*

2. The name of the Indian arrow-root, of which there are three species, the *Arundinacea, Galanga,* and *Comesa,* all of them herbaceous, perennial exotics of the Indies, kept here in hot-houses for curiosity; they have thick, knotty, creeping roots, crowned with long, broad, arundinaceous leaves, ending in points, and upright stalks half a yard high, terminated by bunches of monopetalous, ringent, five-parted flowers. They are propagated by parting the roots in spring, and planting them in pots of light rich earth, and then plunging them in the bark-bed.

MARANTA ARUNDINACEA. The root of this species, commonly called arrow-root, is used by the Indians to extract the virus communicated by their poisoned arrows, from whence it has obtained its name. It is cultivated in gardens and provision-grounds in the West Indies; and the starch is obtained from it by the following process:—The roots, when a year old, are dug up, well washed in water, and then beaten in a large deep wooden mortar, to a pulp; this is thrown into a large tub of clean water: the whole is then well stirred, and the fibrous part wrung out by the hands, and thrown away. The milky liquor being passed through a hair sieve, or coarse cloth, is suffered to settle, and the clear water drained off. At the bottom of the vessel is a white mass, which is again mixed with clean water, and drained : lastly, the mass is dried on sheets in the sun, and is pure starch.

Arrow-root contains, in small bulk, a greater proportion of nourishment than any other yet known. The powder, boiled in water, forms a very pleasant transparent jelly, very superior to that of sago or tapioca, and is much recommended as a nutritious diet for children and invalids. The jelly is made in the following manner :—to a dessert spoonful of powder, add as much cold water as will make it into a paste ; then pour on half a pint of boiling water : stir it briskly, and boil it a few minutes, when it will become a clear smooth jelly ; a little sugar and sherry wine may be added for debilitated patients, but for infants a drop or two of essence of caraway-seeds or cinnamon, is preferable, wine being very liable to become acescent in the stomachs of infants, and thus disagree with the bowels. Fresh milk, either alone or diluted with water, may be substituted for the water. For very debilitated frames, and especially for ricketty children, this jelly, blended with an animal jelly, as that of the stag's horn (*rasuræ cornu cervi*), affords a more nutritious diet than arrow-root alone, which may be done in the following manner :—Boil half an ounce of stag's horn shavings, in a pint of water, for fifteen minutes; then strain and add two dessert-spoonfuls of arrow-root powder previously well-mixed with a tea-cupful of water; stir them briskly together, and boil them for a few minutes. If the child should be much troubled with flatulency, two or three drops of essence of caraway-seeds, or a

44

little grated nutmeg may be added; but for adults, port wine, or brandy, will answer best.

MARANTA GALANGA. The smaller galangal. The roots of this plant are used medicinally; two kinds of galangal are mentioned in the pharmacopœias; the greater galangal obtained from the *Kæmpferia galanga* of Linnæus, and the smaller galangal, the root of the *Maranta galanga; caulino simplici foliis lanceolatis subsessilibus* of Linnæus. The dried root is brought from China, in pieces from an inch to two in length, scarcely half so thick, branched, full of knots and joints, with several circular rings of a reddish-brown colour on the outside, and brownish within. It has an aromatic smell, not very grateful, and an unpleasant, bitterish, hot, biting r ste. It was formerly much used as a warm stomachic bitter, and generally ordered in bitter infusions. It is now, however, seldom employed.

MARA'SMUS. (From μαραινω, to grow lean.) Emaciation. 1. A wasting away of the flesh, without fever or apparent disease. See *Atrophia*.

2. The name of a genus of diseases in Good's Nosology. Class, *Hæmatica;* Order, *Dysthetica.* Emaciation. It embraces four species, viz. *Marasmus atrophia, climactericus, tabes, phthisis.*

MARATHRI'TES. (From μαραθρον, fennel.) A vinous infusion of fennel; or wine impregnated with fennel.

MARATHROPHY'LLUM. (From μαραθρον, fennel, and φυλλον, a leaf: so named because its leaves resemble those of the common fennel. See *Peucedanum officinale.*

MARA'THRUM. (From μαραινω, to wither: so called because its stalk and flowers wither in the autumn.) See *Anethum fœniculum.*

MARATHRUM SYLVESTRE. See *Peucedanum officinale.*

MARBLE. A species of limestone or carbonate of lime. Powdered marble is used in pneumatic medicine, to give out carbonic acid gas.

MARCASITE. See *Bismuth.*

MARCESCENS. Withering, decaying: applied to the perianths of the *Pyrus communis,* and *Mespilus germanica.*

MARCHANTIA. (Named after Marchant, who wrote several Essays on the Memoirs of the Academy of Science, 1713.) The name of a genus of plants. Class, *Cryptogamia;* Order, *Algæ.*

MARCHANTIA POLYMORPHA. The systematic name of the liverwort. *Hepatica terrestris; Jecoraria.* A plant very common in this country. It has a penetrating though mild pungency, and bitter taste, sinking, as it were, into the tongue. It is recommended as an aperient, resolvent, and antiscorbutic; and, though seldom used in this country, appears to be a plant of no inconsiderable virtue.

MARCO'RES. (*Marcores,* pl. of *marcor;* from *marceo,* to become lean.) Universal emaciation. The first order in the class *Cachexiæ,* of Cullen's Nosology.

MARESTAIL. See *Hippuris vulgaris.*

MARGARI'TA. (From *margalith,* Rab.) The pearl. 1. The pearl. *Perla ; Unio.* A small, calcareous concretion, of a bright transparent whiteness, found on the inside of the shell, *Concha margaritifera* of Linnæus, or mother-of-pearl fish. Pearls are very highly prized. They consist of alternating concentric layers of membrane and carbonate of lime. They were formerly exhibited as antacids.

2. A tumour upon the eye resembling a pearl.

MARGARITIC ACID. (*Acidum margariticum; from margarita,* the pearl: so called from its pearly appearance.) Margaric acid. When we immerse soap made of pork-grease and potassa in a large quantity of water, one part is dissolved, while another part is precipitated in the form of several brilliant pellets. These are separated, dried, washed in a large quantity of water, and then dried on a filter. They are now dissolved in boiling alkohol, sp. gr. 0.820, from which, as it cools, the pearly substance falls down pure. On acting on this with dilute muriatic acid, a substance of a peculiar kind, which Chevreuil, the discoverer, calls margarine, or margaric acid, is separated. It must be well washed with water, dissolved in boiling alkohol, from which it is recovered in the same crystalline pearly form, when the solution cools.

Margaric acid is pearly white, and tasteless. Its smell is feeble, and a little similar to that of melted wax. Its specific gravity is inferior to water. It melts at 134° F. ir to a very limpid, colourless liquid, which crystallizes, on cooling, into brilliant needles of the finest white. It is insoluble in water, but very soluble in alkohol, sp. gr. 0.800. Cold margaric acid has no action on the colour of litmus; but when heated so as to soften without melting, the blue was reddened. It combines with the salifiable bases, and forms neutral compounds. Two orders of margarates are formed, the *margarates* and the *supermargarates,* the former being converted into the latter, by pouring a large quantity of water on them. Other fats besides that of the hog yield this substance.

That of man is obtained under three different forms. 1. In very fine long needles, disposed in flat stars. 2 In very fine and very short needles, forming waved figures, like those of the margaric acid of carcasses. 3. In very large brilliant crystals disposed in stars, similar to the margaric acid of the hog. The margaric acids of man and the hog resemble each other; as do those of the ox and the sheep; and of the goose and the jaguar The compounds, with the bases, are real soaps. The solution in alkohol affords the transparent soap of this country.

MARIGOLD. See *Calendula officinalis.*

Marigold, marsh. See *Caltha palustris.*

MARINE. (*Marinus ;* from *mare,* the sea.) Appertaining to the sea.

Marine acid. See *Muriatic acid.*

Marine salt. See *Sodæ murias.*

MARIPE'NDAM. A plant in the island of St. Do mingo: a distilled water from the tops is held in great esteem against pains in the stomach.

MARI'SCA. An excrescence about the anus, or the piles in a state of tumefaction.

MARI'SICUM. The *Mercurialis fruticosa.*

MARJORAM. See *Origanum.*

MARJORA'NA. See *Origanum.*

MARLE. See *Limestone.*

MARMALADE. The pulp of quinces, or any other fruit, boiled into a consistence with honey.

MARMARY'GÆ. (From μαρμαιρω, to shine.) An appearance of sparks, or coruscations, flashing before the eyes.

MARMOLA'RIA. (From *marmor,* marble : so named because it is spotted like marble). See *Acanthus mollis.*

MARMOR. Marble.

MARMOR METALICUM. Native sulphate of barytes.

MARMORA'TA AURIUM. (From *marmor,* marble.) The wax of the ear.

MARMO'REUS TARTARUS. The hardest species of *human calculus.*

MARMORIGE. An affection of the eyes, in which sparks and flashes of fire are supposed to present themselves.

MAROCO'STINUM. A purgative extract made of the marum and costus; originally made by Mindererus.

MARROW. *Medulla.* The fat substance secreted by the small arteries of its proper membrane; and contained in the medullary cavities of the long cylindrical bones. See *Bone.*

Marrow, spinal. See *Medulla spinalis.*

MARRUBIA'STRUM. The *Balote nigra,* or stinking hoarhound.

MARRUBIUM. (From *marrob,* a bitter juice, Heb.) Hoarhound. 1. The name of a genus of plants in the Linnæan system. Class, *Didynamia;* Order *Gymnospermia.*

2. The pharmacopœial name of the common hoarhound. See *Marrubium vulgare.*

MARRUBIUM ALBUM. See *Marrubium vulgare.*

MARRUBIUM ALYSSON. *Alyssum.* Galen's madwort. It is supposed to be diaphoretic.

MARRUBIUM AQUATICUM. Water hoarhound; opening, corroborant.

MARRUBIUM HISPANICUM, or Spanish hoarhound See *Marrubium verticillatum.*

MARRUBIUM NIGRUM FŒTIDUM. The black, stinking hoarhound, or *Balote nigra.*

MARRUBIUM VERTICILLATUM. *Marrubium hispanicum.* The *Sideritis syriaca,* or base hoarhound.

MARRUBIUM VULGARE. The systematic name of the common hoarhound. *Marrubium album; Marrubium—dentibus calycinis, setaceis uncinatis* of Linnæus. The leaves of this indigenous plant have a moderately strong smell of the aromatic kind, but not agreeable; which, by drying, is improved; and in keeping for some months is, in great part, dissipated; their taste is very bitter, penetrating, diffusive, and durable in the mouth. That hoarhound possesses some share of medicinal power, may be inferred from its sensible qualities; but its virtues do not appear to be clearly ascertained. It is a favourite remedy with the common people in coughs and asthmas. The usual dose is from half an ounce to an ounce, in infusion, two or three times a day. The dose of the extract is from gr. x. to 3 ss.

MARS The mythological and alchemistical name of iron.

MARS ALKALIZATUS. One of the alkalies with an admixture of iron.

MARS SACCHARATUS. Iron mixed with starch and melted sugar.

MARS SOLUBILIS. Ferrum tartarizatum.

MARS SULPHURATUS. Iron filings, and sulphur deflagrated.

Marseilles hart-wort. See *Seseli tortuosum.*

Marsh-mallow. See *Althæa officinalis.*

Marsh trefoil. See *Menyanthes trifoliata.*

MARSUPIA'LIS. (From *marsupium,* a purse: so named from its resemblance.) See *Obturator internus.*

Martagon lily. See *Lilium martagon.*

MARTIAL. (*Martialis;* from *Mars,* iron.) Sometimes used to express preparations of iron, or such as are impregnated therewith; as the *Martial Regulus* of antimony, &c.

Martial ethiops. The protoxide of iron.

Martial salts. Salts of iron.

MARTIA'TUM UNGUENTUM. Soldiers' ointment. Ointment of laurel, rue, marjoram, &c.

MA'RTIS LIMATURA PRÆPARATA. Purified filings of iron.

MARTYN, JOHN, was born in 1699. His father, being in a mercantile station in London, he was intended to succeed in this, which he does not appear to have neglected; but his taste for literature led him to devote much of the night to study. His partiality, however, was particularly directed to botany, and he made many experiments on the germination of seeds, &c. When about 22 years of age, he became secretary of a botanical society, and proved one of its most active members: three years after, he was admitted into the Royal Society, and many of his papers appeared in the Philosophical Transactions, of which he subsequently took a part in the abridgment. At what period he changed to the medical profession is not known. In 1726, he published his tables of officinal plants, disposed according to Ray's system. Having given public lectures on botany in London with much approbation, he was thought qualified to teach that science at Cambridge; and accordingly, in the following year, he delivered the first course ever heard in that university. In 1730, he entered at Emanuel college, with an intention of graduating in physic; but this was soon abandoned on his marriage, and from the necessary attendance to his profession in London. On the death of the botanical professor at Cambridge, Mr. Martyn was appointed to succeed him in the beginning of 1733; but he continued lecturing only two or three years, owing to the want of sufficient encouragement, and especially of a botanic garden there. In 1741, he published a splendid quarto addition of Virgil's Georgics, in which much new light was thrown on the natural history of that author. Dr. Halley having assisted him in the astronomical part; this was followed by the Bucolics, on the same plan. In 1752, he retired from practice, and about nine years after resigned his professorship in favour of his son, the Rev. Thomas Martyn; in consequence of whose election he presented his botanical library, of above 200 volumes, with his drawings, herbarium, &c. to the university. He died in 1768.

MA'RUM. (From *mar,* Hebrew for bitter: so named from its taste.) Several species of teucrium were so named.

MARUM CRETICUM. See *Teucrium marum.*

MARUM SYRIACUM. (From *mar,* bitter, Hebrew.) See *Teucrium marum.*

MARUM VERUM. See *Teucrium marum.*

MARUM VULGARE. See *Thymus mastichina.*

46

MA RVISUM. Malmsey wine.

MA'SCHALE. Μασχαλη. The armpit.

MASCHALI'STER. (From μασχαλιςηρ.) The second vertebra of the back.

MASCULUS. There are two sexes of animals and vegetables, the male and the female. The male of animals is distinguished by his peculiar genital organs, and the analogy is carried to vegetables. A flower is called a male flower, which has stamina only, which are reckoned by the sexualists to be the male organ.

MA'SLACH. A medicine of the opiate kind, in use among the Turks.

MASPETUM. The leaf of the asafœtida plant.

MA'SSA. (From μασσω, to blend together.) A mass. A term generally applied to the compound out of which pills are to be formed.

MASSA CARNEA JACOBI SYLVII. See *Flexor longus digitorum pedis.*

MA'SSALIS. An old name for mercury.

MASSE'TER. (From μασσαομαι, to chew; because it assists in chewing.) *Zigomato-maxillaire,* of Dumas. A muscle of the lower jaw, situated on the side of the face. It is a short, thick muscle, which arises, by fleshy and tendinous fibres, from the lower edge of the malar process of the maxillary bone, the lower horizontal edge of the os malæ, and the lower edge of the zygomatic process of the temporal bone, as far backwards as the eminence belonging to the articulation of the lower jaw. From some little interruption in the fibres of this muscle, at their origin, some writers describe it as arising by two, and others by three, distinct portions, or heads. The two layers of fibres, of which it seems to be composed, cross each other as they descend, the external layer extending backwards, and the internal one slanting forwards. It is inserted into the basis of the coronoid process, and into all that part of the lower jaw which supports the coronoid and condyloid processes. Its use is to raise the lower jaw, and, by means of the above-mentioned decussation, to move it a little forwards and backwards in the act of chewing.

MASSICOT. The yellow oxide of lead.

MA'SSOY CORTEX. See *Cortex massoy.*

MASTERWORT. See *Imperatoria.*

MASTIC. See *Pistachia lentiscus.*

MASTICATION. (*Masticatio;* from *mastico,* to chew.) Chewing. A natural function. It embraces the seizing, catching, or taking the food, the chewing and the insalivation. The organs for taking in food are the superior extremities and the mouth.

The mouth is the oval cavity formed above, by the palate and the upper jaw; below, by the tongue and the lower jaw; on the sides, by the cheeks; behind, by the *velum* of the palate and the pharynx; and in front by the lips.

The dimensions of the mouth are variable in different persons, and are susceptible of an enlargement in every direction; downwards, by lowering the tongue and separating the jaws; transversely, by the distention of the cheeks, and from the front backward, by the motion of the lips, and of the *velum* of the palate.

The jaws determine most particularly the form and dimensions of the mouth; the superior jaw makes an essential part of the face, and moves only along with the head; on the contrary, the inferior possesses a very great mobility.

The jaws are furnished with small, very hard bodies, called teeth.

The edge of the socket is covered with a thick layer, fibrous, resisting, denominated gum.

We ought to consider in the parts that contribute to the apprehension of aliments, the muscles that move the jaws, and particularly the inferior. The same thing takes place with the tongue, the numerous motions of which have a great influence on the dimensions of the mouth.

Mechanism of the taking of food.—Nothing is simpler than the taking in of aliments: it consists in the introduction of alimentary substances into the mouth For this purpose the hands seize the aliments, and divide them into small portions susceptible of being contained in the mouth, and introduce them into it either directly or by means of proper instruments.

But, in order to their being received into this cavity, the jaws must separate; in other words, the mouth opens.

In many cases, when the food is introduced into the

mouth, the jaws come together to retain it, and assist in mastication, or deglutition; but frequently the elevation of the inferior jaw contributes to the taking of the food. We have an example of it when one bites into fruit: then the incisors are thrust into the alimentary substance in opposite directions, and, acting as the blades of scissors, they detach a portion of the mass.

This motion is produced, principally by the contraction of the elevated muscles of the lower jaw, which represents a lever of the third kind, the *power* of which is at the insertion of the elevating muscles, the *point of support* at the articulation temporo-maxillary, and the resistance in the substance upon which the teeth act. The volume of the body placed between the incisors has an influence upon the force by which it may be pressed. If it is small, the power will be much greater, for all the elevating muscles are inserted perpendicularly to the jaw, and the whole of their force is employed in moving the lever that it represents; if the volume of the body is such that it can hardly enter the mouth, though it presents very little resistance, the incisors will not enter it, for the *masseter*, the temporal, and the internal *pterygoid* muscles, are inserted very obliquely into the jaw, whence results the loss of the greater part of the force that they develope in contracting. When the efforts of the muscles of the jaws are not sufficient to detach a portion of the alimentary mass, the hand so acts upon it as to separate it from the portion retained by the teeth. On the other hand, the posterior muscles of the neck draw the head strongly back, and from the combination of these efforts results the separation of a portion of the food which remains in the mouth. In this mode the incisors and eye teeth are generally employed; the grinders are rarely used. By the succession of these motions of taking food the mouth is filled, and on account of the suppleness of the cheeks, and the easy depression of the tongue, a considerable quantity of food may be accumulated in it.

When the mouth is full, the *velum* of the palate is lowered, its inferior edge is applied upon the most distant part of the base of the tongue, so that all communication is intercepted between the mouth and the pharynx.

Independently of what we have said of the mouth, in respect to taking the food, to conceive its uses in mastication and insalivation, it is useful to remark that fluids abound in the mouth proceeding from different sources. First, the mucous membrane which covers its sides secretes an abundant mucosity; numerous isolated, or agglomerated follicles that are observed in the interior of the cheeks, at the junction of the lips with the gums, upon the back of the tongue, on the anterior aspect of the *velum* and the uvula, pour continually the liquid that they form into the internal surface of the mouth. The same thing takes place with mucous glands, which exist in great number in the interior of the cheeks and palate.

Lastly, there is poured into the mouth, the saliva secreted by six glands, three on each side, and which bear the name of *parotid*, *sub-maxillary*, and *sub-lingual*. The first, placed between the external ear and the jaw, have each a secreting canal which opens on the level of the second small superior grinder; each maxillary gland has one which terminates on the sides of the ligaments of the tongue, near which those of the sub-lingual glands open.

These fluids are probably variable in their physical and chemical properties according to the organs by which they are formed; but the distinction has not yet been established by chemistry by direct experiments: the mixture under the name of saliva has been exactly analyzed.

Among the alimentary substances deposited in the mouth, the one sort only traverse this cavity without suffering any change; the others, on the contrary, remain a considerable time in it, and undergo important modifications. The first are the soft sorts of food, or nearly liquid, of which the temperature is little different from that of the body; the second are the aliments, which are hard, dry, fibrous, and those whose temperature is more or less different from what is proper for the animal economy. They are both in common, however, appreciated by the organs of taste in passing through the mouth.

We may attribute to three principal modifications the changes that the food undergoes in the mouth: 1st,

change of temperature; 2d, mixture with the fluids that are poured into the mouth, and sometimes dissolution in these fluids; 3d, pressure more or less strong, and very often division, which bruising destroys the cohesion of their parts. It is besides easily and frequently transported from one part of this cavity to another. These three modes of change do not take place successively, but simultaneously, by mutually favouring each other.

The change of temperature of the food retained in the mouth is evident; the sensation which it excites in it is sufficient to prove this. If it has a low temperature, it produces a vivid impression of cold, which continues until it has absorbed the caloric necessary to bring it near to the temperature of the sides of the mouth; the contrary takes place if the temperature is higher than that of the mouth.

It is the same with our judgment on this occasion, as with that which relates to the temperature of bodies which touch the skin; we join to it, unknown to us, a comparison with the temperature of the atmosphere and with that of the bodies which have been previously in contact with the mouth; so that a body preserving the same degree of heat will appear to us alternately hot or cold, according to the temperature of the bodies formerly in the mouth.

The change of temperature that the food undergoes in the mouth is only an accessary phenomenon; its trituration and its mixture more or less intimate with the fluids poured into this cavity, are what merit particular attention.

As soon as an aliment is introduced into the mouth, it is pressed by the tongue, applying it against the palate, or against some other part of the sides of the mouth. If the aliment is soft, if its parts cohere but little, this simple pressure is enough to break it; if the alimentary substance is composed of liquid and solid, the liquid is expressed by this pressure, and the solid part only remains in the mouth. The tongue produces the effect, of which we speak, so much better in proportion as its membrane is muscular, and as a great number of muscles are destined to move it.

It might astonish us that the tongue, which is so soft, could be capable of breaking a body offering even small resistance; but, on the one hand, it hardens in contracting, like all the muscles, and, besides, it presents under the mucous membrane which covers its superior aspect, a dense and thick fibrous layer.

Such are the phenomena that take place if the food has but little resistance; but if it presents a considerable resistance, it then undergoes the action of the masticating organs.

The essential agents of mastication are the muscles that move the jaws, the tongue, the cheeks, and the lips: the *maxillary* bones and the teeth serve only as simple instruments.

Though the motions of both jaws may contribute to mastication, it is produced almost always by those of the inferior one. This bone may be lowered, raised, and pressed strongly against the upper jaw; carried forward, backward, and even directed a little towards the sides. These different motions are produced by the numerous muscles which are attached to the jaw.

But the jaws could never have produced the necessary effect in mastication if they had not been furnished with teeth, the physical properties of which are particularly suited to this digestive action.

[There are exceptions to all rules, and although teeth are absolutely necessary in general, yet it is within our knowledge that a man, who has followed the coasting trade from New-York, never had any teeth, and could eat crackers, ship-bread, or any hard substance, breaking and chewing it with his gums, as well as any one with teeth. A.]

Mechanism of mastication.—For the commencement of mastication, the inferior jaw must be lowered, an effect which is produced by the relaxation of its elevating, and the contraction of its depressing muscles. The food must then be placed between the dental arches, either by the tongue or some other agent; the inferior jaw is then raised by the masseter, internal pterygoid, and temporal muscles, the intensity of whose contraction depends upon the resistance of the food. This being pressed between two unequal surfaces whose asperities fit into each other, is divided into small portions, the number of which is in proportion to the facility with which they have given way.

But a motion of this kind reaches only a part of the food contained in the mouth, and it must be all equally divided. This takes place by the successive motions of the inferior jaw, and by the contraction of the muscles of the cheeks, of those of the tongue and lips, which bring the food between the teeth successively and promptly during the separation of the jaws, that it may be bruised when they come together.

When the alimentary substances are soft and easily bruised, two or three masticatory motions are sufficient to divide all that is in the mouth; the three kinds of teeth are employed in it. A longer continued mastication is necessary when the substances are more resisting, fibrous, or tough: in this case we chew only with the *molares*, and often only with one side at a time, to allow the other to rest. In employing the grinders there is an advantage of shortening the arm of the lever represented by the jaw, and by so doing of rendering it more advantageous for the power that moves it.

In the mastication, the teeth have sometimes to support very considerable efforts, which would inevitably shake, or else displace them, were it not for the extreme solidity of their articulation with the jaws. Each root acts like a wedge, in transmitting to the sides of the sockets the force by which it is pressed.

The advantage of the conical form of the roots is not doubtful. By reason of this form, the force by which the tooth is pressed, and which tends to thrust it into the jaw, is decomposed; one part tends to separate the sides of the sockets, the other to lower them; and the transmission, instead of being carried to the extremity of the root, which could not have failed to take place in a cylindric form, is distributed over all the surface of the socket. The grinders that have more considerable efforts to sustain, have a number of roots, or at least one very large. The incisors and eye teeth, that have only one small root, have never any great pressure to support.

If the gums had not presented a smooth surface and a dense tissue, placed as they are round the neck of the teeth and filling their intervals, they would have been torn every instant; for, in the mastication of hard and irregular substances, they are constantly exposed to the pressure of their edges and angles. This inconvenience happens whenever their tissue becomes soft, as in scorbutic affections.

During the time of mastication the mouth is shut behind by the curtain of the palate, the anterior surface of which is pressed against the base of the tongue; the food is retained before by the teeth and the lips.

Insalivation of the aliments.—Whenever we have an appetite, the view of food determines a considerable afflux of saliva into the mouth; in some people it is so strong as to be projected to the distance of several feet.

While the aliments are bruised and triturated by the masticating organs, they imbibe, and are penetrated completely by the fluids that are poured into the mouth, and particularly by the saliva. It is easy to conceive that the division of the food and the numerous displacements that it suffers during mastication, singularly favour its mixture with the mucous and salivary juices.

Most of the alimentary substances submitted to the action of the mouth are dissolved or suspended wholly or in part in the saliva, and immediately they become proper for being introduced into the stomach, and are forthwith swallowed.

On account of its viscosity, the saliva absorbs air, by which it is swept in the different motions necessary for mastication; but the quantity of air absorbed in this circumstance is inconsiderable, and has been generally exaggerated.

Of what use is the trituration of food and its mixture with the saliva? Is it a simple division which renders the aliments more proper for the alterations which they undergo in the stomach, or do they suffer the first degree of animalization in the mouth? On this point there is nothing certain known.

Let us remark that mastication and insalivation change the savour and odour of the food; that mastication, sufficiently prolonged, generally renders digestion more quick and easy; that, on the contrary, people who do not chew their food, have often on this account very painful and slow digestion.—*Magendie's Physiology.*
48

MASTICATORY. (*Masticatorium; from mastico* to chew.) A medicine intended for chewing.

MA'STICHE. (From μασσω, to express.) See *Pistacia lentiscus.*

Mastich-herb. See *Thymus mastichina.*

Mastich, Syrian. See *Teucrium marum.*

Mastich-tree. See *Pistacia lentiscus.*

Mastich wood. See *Pistacia lentiscus.*

MASTICHE'UM. (From μαϛιχη, mastich, and ελαιον, oil.) Oil of mastich.

MASTI'CHINA. (Diminutive of *mastiche.*) See *Thymus mastichina.*

Masticot. See *Massicot.*

MA'STIX. See *Pistacia lentiscus.*

MASTODY'NIA. (From μαϛος, a breast, and οδυνη, pain.) *Nacta.* Phlegmon of the breast of women. This disease may take place at any period of life, but it most commonly affects those who give suck. It is characterized by tumefaction, tension, heat, redness, and pain; and comes sometimes in both breasts, but most commonly in one. Pyrexia generally attends the disease. It is sometimes very quickly formed, and in general without any thing preceding to show it; but now and then a slight shivering is the forerunner. This disease terminates either in resolution, in suppuration, or scirrhus. If the disease is left to itself, it generally terminates in suppuration.

The causes which give rise to this disease, are those which give rise to most of the phlegmasiæ, as cold, violent blows, &c. In women who are lying-in, or giving suck, it mostly arises either from a suppression of the lochia, or a retention of milk. Mastodynia is often of long continuance; it is a very painful disease, but is seldom fatal, unless when absolutely neglected, when it may run into scirrhus, and finally cancer. The termination of the disease by gangrene is never to be apprehended, at least few, if any, have seen the disease terminate in this way.

MASTOID. (*Mastoideus;* from μαϛος, a breast, and ειδος, resemblance.) 1. Those processes of bones are so named that are shaped like the nipple of the breast, as the mastoid process of the temporal bone, &c.

2. The name of a muscle. See *Sterno-cleido-mastoideus.*

Mastoid foramen. A hole in the temporal bone of the skull.

MASTOIDEUS LATERALIS. A name for the complexus muscle.

MATALI'STA RADIX. A root said to be imported from America, where it is given as a purgative, its action being rather milder than that of jalap.

MA'TER. (Ματηρ, a mother: so called by the Arabians, who thought they gave origin to all other membranes of the body.) 1. Two membranes of the brain had this epithet given them. See *Dura mater,* and *Pia mater.*

2. A name of the herb mugwort, because of its virtue in disorders of the womb.

MATER HERBARUM. Common mugwort. See *Artemisia vulgaris.*

MATER METALLORUM. Quicksilver.

MATER PERLARUM. See *Margarita.*

MATE'RIA. A term given to a substance that is selected for a particular experiment or purpose, which is expressed by adding the name of that purpose; hence *materia medica, materia chemica,* &c.

MATERIA MEDICA. By this term is understood a general class of substances, both natural and artificial, which are used in the cure of diseases.

Cartheuser, Newman, Lewis, Gleditsch, Linnæus, Vogel, Alston, Bergius, Cullen, Murray, Paris, in his excellent work on pharmacology, and other writers on the Materia Medica, have been at much labour to contrive arrangements of these articles. Some have disposed them according to their natural resemblances; others according to their real or supposed virtues; others according to their active constituent principles. These arrangements have their peculiar advantages. The first may be preferred by the natural historian, the second by the physiologist, and the last by the chemist The pharmacopœias, published by the Colleges of Physicians of London, Dublin, and Edinburgh, have the articles of the Materia Medica arranged in alphabetical order; this plan is also adopted by almost all the continental pharmacopœias

MATERIA MEDICA.

Dr. Cullen has arranged the Materia Medica as follows:—

- NUTRIMENTS, which are
  - Food,
  - Drinks,
  - Condiments;
- MEDICINES which act on the
  - Solids,
    - Simple, as
      - Astringents,
      - Tonics,
      - Emollients,
      - Corrosives;
    - Living, as
      - Stimulants,
      - Sedatives,
        - Narcotics,
        - Refrigerants,
      - Antispasmodics.
  - Fluids,

Producing a change of fluidity,
  - Attenuants,
  - Inspissants.

Mixture,
  - Correctors of Acrimony
    - Demulcents,
    - Antacids,
    - Antalkalines,
    - Antiseptics.

Evacuants; viz.
  - Errhines,
  - Sialagogues,
  - Expectorants,
  - Emetics,
  - Cathartics,
  - Diuretics,
  - Diaphoretics,
  - Emmenagogues

The following is a list of articles which come under the preceding classes:—

I. NUTRIMENTS.
α FRUITS.

a. *Fresh, sweet, acidulous,* as
Prunes
Oranges
Lemons
Raspberries
Red and black currants
Mulberries
Grapes, &c.

b. *Dried, sweet, acidulous,* as
Raisins
Currants
Figs.

β. OLERACEOUS HERBS.
Water-cresses
Dandelion
Parsley
Artichoke.

γ. ROOTS.
Carrot
Garlick
Satyrion.

δ. SEEDS and NUTS.
Almonds, sweet and bitter
Walnuts
Olives.

II. MEDICINES.
1. ASTRINGENTS.
Red rose
Cinquefoil
Tormentil
Madder
Sorrel
Water-dock
Bistort
Fern
Pomegranate
Oak-bark
Galls
Logwood
Quince
Mulberry
Sloe
Gum-arabic
Catechu
Dragon's blood
Alkanet
Balaustine flower
St. John's wort
Millefoil
Plantain
Convallaria
Bear's berry.

2. TONICS.
Gentian
Lesser centaury
Quassia
Simarouba
Marsh trefoil
Fumitory
Camomile
Tansy

Wormwood
Southernwood
Sea-wormwood
Water-germander
Virginian snake-root
Leopard's bane
Peruvian bark.

3. EMOLLIENTS.
Columniferous,
Marsh mallow
Mallow.
Farinaceous,
Quince-seeds
Fænugreek-seed
Linseed
Various emollients,
Pellitory
Verbascum
White lily.

4. CORROSIVES.

5. STIMULANTS.
Verticellated,
Lavender
Balm
Marjoram
Sweet marjoram
Syrian herb mastich
Rosemary
Hyssop
Ivy
Mint
Peppermint
Pennyroyal
Thyme
Mother of thyme
Sage.
Umbellated,
Fennel
Archangel
Anise
Caraway
Coriander
Cumin
Dill
Saxifrage.
Siliquose,
Horseradish
Watercress
Mustard
Scurvy-grass.
Alliaceous,
Garlick.
Coniferous,
Fir
Juniper.
Balsamics,
Venice turpentine
Common turpentine
Canada balsam
Copaiba balsam
Tolu balsam
Balm of Gilead.
Resinous,
Guaiacum
Ladanum
Storax

Benzoin.
Aromatics,
Cinnamon
Nutmeg
Mace
Clove
Allspice
Canella
Cascarilla
Black pepper
Long pepper
Indian pepper
Ginger
Lesser cardamom
Zedoary
Virginian snake-root
Ginseng
Aromatic reed.
Acrids,
Wake-robin
Pellitory
Stavesacre.

6. NARCOTICS.
Rhœadaceous,
White poppy
Red poppy.
Umbellated,
Hemlock
Water hemlock.
Solanaceous,
Belladonna
Henbane
Tobacco
Bitter-sweet
Stramonium
Varia,
Laurel
Camphor
Saffron
Wine.

7. REFRIGERANTS.
Fruits of plants
Acidulous herbs and roots.

8. ANTISPASMODICS.
Fœtid herbs,
Wormwood
Fœtid goosefoot
Cumin
Pennyroyal
Rue
Savine.
Fœtid gums,
Asafœtida
Galbanum
Opoponax
Valerian.

9. DILUENTS.
Water.

10. ATTENUANTS.
Alkalies
Sugar
Liquorice
Dried fruits.

11. INSPISSANTS.
Acids

Farinaceous and mucilaginous demulcents
12. DEMULCENTS.
Mucilaginous,
Gum arabic
—— tragacanth.
Farinaceous,
as
Starch
Bland oils.
13. ANTACIDS.
Alkalies and earths.
14. ANTALKALINES.
Acids.
15. ANTISEPTICS.
Acid parts of plants
Acescent herbs
Sugar
Siliquose plants
Alliaceous plants
Astringents
Bitters
Aromatics
Essential oils
Camphor
Gum resins
Saffron
Contrayerva
Valerian
Opium
Wine.
16. ERRHINES.
Asarabacca
White hellebore
Water iris
Pellitory.
17. SIALAGOGUES
Archangel
Cloves
Masterwort
Tobacco
Pepper
Pellitory.
18. EXPECTORANTS
Ivy
Hoarhound
Pennyroyal
Elecampane
Florentine orris-root
Tobacco
Squill
Coltsfoot
Benzoin
Storax
Canada balsam
Tolu balsam.
19. EMETICS.
Asarabacca
Ipecacuan
Tobacco
Squill
Mustard
Horseradish
Bitters.
20. CATHARTICS.
Milder,

L l

49

Mild acid fruits	Castor oil	Bitter-sweet[1]	Contrayerva
Cassia pulp	Senna	Wake-robin	Serpentaria
Tamarind	Black hellebore	Asarabacca	Sage
Sugar	Jalap	Foxglove	Water germander
Manna	Scammony	Tobacco	Guaiacum
Sweet roots	Buckthorn	Rue	Sassafras
Bland oils	Tobacco	Savine	Seneka
Damask rose	White hellebore	Snakeroot	Vegetable acids
Violet	Coloquintida	Squill	Essential oil
Polypody	Elaterium.	Bitters	Wine
Mustard	21 DIURETICS.	Balsamics	Diluents.
Bitters	Parsley	Siliquosæ	23. EMMENAGOGUES
Balsamics.	Carrot	Alliaceæ.	Aloes
Acrid,	Fennel	22. DIAPHORETICS	Fœtid gums
Rhubarb	Pimpinel	Saffron	Fœtid plants
Seneka	Eryngo	Bitter-sweet	Saffron.
Broom	Madder	Opium	
Elder	Burdock	Camphor	

The following is the arrangement of the Materia Medica, according to J. Murray, in his Elements of Materia Medica and Pharmacy.

A. General stimulants.

    a. Diffusible { Narcotics / Antispasmodics.

    b. Permanent { Tonics / Astringents.

B Local stimulants.   Emetics
    Cathartics
    Emmenagogues
    Diuretics
    Diaphoretics
    Expectorants
    Sialagogues
    Errhines
    Epispastics.

C Chemical remedies.   Refrigerants
    Antacids
    Lithontriptics
    Escharotics.

D. Mechanical remedies. Anthelmintics
    Demulcents
    Diluents
    Emollients.

Under the head of NARCOTICS are included—
Alkohol. Ether. Camphor. Papaver somniferum. Hyoscyamus niger. Atropa belladonna. Aconitum napellus. Conium maculatum. Digitalis purpurea. Nicotiana tabacum. Lactuca virosa. Datura stramonium. Rhododendron chrysanthemum. Rhus toxicodendron. Arnica montana. Strychnos nux vomica. Prunus lauro-cerasus.

Under the second class, ANTISPASMODICS, are included—Moschus. Castoreum. Oleum animale empyreumaticum. Petroleum. Ammonia. Ferula asafœtida. Sagapenum. Bubon galbanum. Valeriana officinalis. Crocus sativus. Melaleuca leucadendron.

Narcotics used as Antispasmodics—
Ether. Camphor. Opium.

Tonics used as Antispasmodics—
Cuprum. Zincum. Hydrargyrus. Cinchona.

The head of TONICS embraces—
1. From the *mineral* kingdom,
Hydrargyrus. Ferrum. Zincum. Cuprum. Arsenicum. Barytes. Calx. Acidum nitricum. Oxymurias potassæ.

2. From the *vegetable* kingdom,
Cinchona officinalis. Cinchona caribæna. Cinchona floribunda. Cusparia. Aristolochia serpentaria. Dorstenia contrayerva. Croton eleutheria. Calumba. Quassia excelsa. Quassia simarouba. Swietenia febrifuga. Swietenia mahagoni. Gentiana lutea. Anthemis nobilis. Artemisia absinthum. Chironia centaurium. Marrubium vulgare. Menyanthes trifoliata. Centaurea benedicta. Citrus aurantium. Citrus medica. Laurus cinnamomum. Laurus cassia. Canella alba. Acorus calamus. Amomum zinziber. Kænipferia rotunda. Santalum album. Pterocarpus santalinus. Myristica moschata. Caryophyllus aromaticus. Capsicum annuum. Piper nigrum. Piper longum. Piper cubeba. Myrtus pimenta. Amomum repens. Carum carui. Coriandrum sativum. Pimpinella anisum. Anethum fæniculum. Anethum graveolens. Cuminum cyminum. Angelica archangelica. Mentha piperita. Mentha viridis. Mentha pulegium. Hysopus officinalis.

The class of ASTRINGENTS comprehends the following:—

1. From the *vegetable* kingdom,
Quercus robur. Quercus cerris. Tormentilla erecta. Polygonum bistorta. Anchusa tinctoria. Hæmatoxylon campechianum. Rosa gallica. Arbutus uva ursi. Mimosa catechu. Kino. Pterocarpus draco. Ficus indica. Pistachia lentiscus.

2. From the *mineral* kingdom,
Acidum sulphuricum. Argilla. Supersulphas argillæ et potassæ. Calx. Carbonas calcis. Plumbum. Zincum. Ferrum. Cuprum.

The articles which come under the head of EMETICS, are
1. From the *vegetable* kingdom,
Calliocca ipecacuanha. Scilla maritima. Anthemis nobilis. Sinapis alba. Asarum europæum. Nicotiana tabacum.

2. From the *mineral* kingdom.
Antimonium. Sulphas zinci. Sulphas cupri. Sub acetas cupri. Ammonia. Hydro-sulphuretum ammoniæ.

CATHARTICS include
Laxatives. Manna. Cassia fistula. Tamarindus indica. Ricinus communis. Sulphur. Magnesia.
Purgatives. Cassia senna. Rheum palmatum Convolvulus jalapa. Helleborus niger. Bryonia alba Cucumis colocynthis. Momordica elaterium. Rhamnus catharticus. Aloe perfoliata. Convolvulus scammonia. Gambojia gutta. Submurias hydrargyri Sulphas magnesiæ. Sulphas sodæ. Sulphas potassæ Supertartras potassæ. Tartras potassæ et sodæ. Murias sodæ. Terebinthina veneta. Nicotiana tabacum

The medicines arranged under EMMENAGOGUES, are
1. From the class of Antispasmodics.
Castoreum. Ferula asafœtida. Bubon galbanum.
2. From the class of tonics.
Ferrum. Hydrargyrus. Cinchona officinalis.
3. From the class of Cathartics.
Aloe. Helleborus niger. Sinapis alba. Rosmarinus officinalis. Rubia tinctorum. Ruta graveolens. Juniperus sabina.

The class of DIURETICS includes,
1. Saline diuretics.
Supertartras potassæ. Nitras potassæ. Murias ammoniæ. Acetas potassæ. Potassa.
2. From the *vegetable* kingdom,
Scilla maritima. Digitalis purpurea. Nicotiana tabacum. Solanum dulcamara. Lactuca virosa. Colchicum autumnale. Gratiola officinalis. Spartium scoparium. Juniperus communis. Copaifera officinalis. Pinus balsamea. Pinus larix.
3. From the *animal* kingdom,
Meloe vesicatorius.

Under the class DIAPHORETICS, are,
Ammonia. Murias ammoniæ. Acetas ammoniæ. Citras ammoniæ. Submurias hydrargyri. Antimonium. Opium. Camphor. Guaiacum officina e. Daphne mezereum. Smilax sarsaparilla. Laurus sassafras. Cochlearia armoracia. Salvia officinalis.

The class EXPECTORANTS comprehends,
Antimonium. Ipecacuanha. Nicotiana tabacum Digitalis purpurea. Scilla maritima. Allium sativum. Polygala senega. Ammoniacum. Myrrha. Styrax benzoin. Styrax officinalis. Toluifera balsamum. Myroxylon peruiferum. Amyris gileadensis.

The articles of the class SIALAGOGUES are Hydrargyrus. Anthemis pyrethrum. Arum maculatum. Amomum zinziber. Daphne mezereum. Nicotiana tabacum.

The class of ERRHINES are, Iris florentina. Æscu

MATERIA MEDICA.

lus hippocastanum. Origanum majorana. Lavendula spica. Assarum europæum. Veratrum album. Nicotiana tabacum. Euphorbia officinalis.

In the class Epispastics, and Rubefacients are Meloe vesicatorius. Ammonia Pix Burgundica. Sinapis alba. Allium sativum.

Refrigerants are constituted by the following articles. Citrus aurantium. Citrus medica. Tamarindus indica. Acidum acetosum. Supertartras potassæ. Nitras potassæ. Boras sodæ.

The list of articles that come under the class Antacids are, Potassa. Soda. Ammonia. Calx. Carbonas calcis. Magnesia.

In the class Lithontriptics are, Potassa. Carbonas potassæ. Soda. Carbonas sodæ. Sapo albus Calx.

In the class Escharotics are, Acida mineralia. Potassa. Nitras argenti. Murias antimonii. Sulphas

cupri. Acetas cupri. Murias hydrargyri. Subnitras hydrargyri. Oxydum arsenici album. Juniperus sabina.

In the class Anthelmintics are, Dolichos pruriens. Ferri limatura. Stannum pulveratum. Olea europæa. Artemisia santonica. Spigelia marilandica. Polypodium filix mas. Tanacetum vulgare. Geoffrœa inermis. Gambojia gutta. Submurias hydrargyri.

Demulcents are, Mimosa nilotica. Astragalus tragacanthus. Linum usitatissimum. Althæa officinalis. Malva sylvestris. Glycyrrhiza glabra. Cycas circinalis. Orchis mascula. Maranta arundinacea. Triticum hybernum. Ichthyocolla. Olea europæa. Amygdalus communis. Sevum ceti. Cera.

Water is the principal article of the class Diluents; and as for the last class, Emollients, heat conjoined with moisture is the principal, though all unctuous applications may be included.

The New London Pharmacopœia presents us with the following list for the Materia Medica:—

Abietis resina
Absinthium
Acaciæ gummi
Acetosæ folia
Acetosella
Acetum
Acidum aceticum fortius
Acidum citricum
Acidum sulphuricum
Aconiti folia
Adeps
Ærugo
Allii radix
Aloes spicatæ extractum
Althææ folia et radix
Alumen
Ammoniacum
Ammoniæ murias
Amygdala amara et dulcis
Amylum
Anethi semina
Anisi semina
Anthemidis floris
Antimonii sulphuretum
Antimonii vitrum
Argentum
Armoraciæ radix
Arsenicum album
Asara folia
Asafœtidæ gummi resina
Avenæ semina
Aurantii baccæ
Aurantii cortex
Balsamum peruvianum
Balsamum tolutanum
Belladonnæ folia
Benzoinum
Bismuthum
Bistorta radix
Cajuputi oleum
Calamina
Calami radix
Calumba
Camphora
Canellæ cortex
Cantharis
Capsici baccæ
Carbo ligni
Cardamines flores
Cardamomi semina
Caricæ fructus
Carui semina
Caryophilli
Caryophyllorum oleum
Cascarillæ cortex
Cassiæ pulpa
Castoreum
Catechu extractum
Centaurii cacumina
Cera alba
Cera flava
Cerevisiæ fermentum
Cetaceum
Cinchonæ lancifoliæ, cordifoliæ et oblongifoliæ cortex
Cinnamomi cortex
Cinnamomi oleum

Coccus
Colchici radix et semina
Colocynthidis pulpa
Conii folia et semina
Contrayerva radix
Copaiba
Coriandri semina
Cornua
Creta
Croci stigmata
Cubeba
Cumini semina
Cupri sulphas
Cuspariæ cortex
Cydoniæ semina
Dauci radix
Dauci semina
Digitalis folia et semina
Dolichi pubes
Dulcamaræ caulis
Elaterii pepones
Elemi
Euphorbiæ gummi resina
Farina
Fœniculi semina
Ferrum
Filicis radix
Fucus
Galbani gummi resina
Gallæ
Gentianæ radix
Glycyrrhizæ radix
Granati cortex
Guaiaca resina et lignum
Hæmatoxyli lignum
Helenium
Hellebori fœtidi folia
Hellebori nigri radix
Hordei semina
Humuli strobili
Hydrargyrum
Hyoscyami folia et semina
Ipecacuanhæ radix
Jalapæ radix
Juniperi baccæ et semina
Kino
Krameriæ radix
Lactuca
Lavendulæ flores
Lauri baccæ et folia
Lichen
Limones
Limonum cortex et oleum
Linum catharticum
Lini usitatissimi semina
Magnesiæ subcarbonas
Magnesiæ sulphas
Malva
Manna
Marmor album
Marrubium
Mastiche
Mel
Mentha piperita
Mentha viridis
Menyanthes
Mezerei cortex

Mori baccæ
Moschus
Myristicæ nuclei et oleum expressum
Myrrha
Olibanum
Olivæ oleum
Opium
Opopanacis gummi resina
Origanum
Ovum
Papaveris capsulæ
Petroleum
Pimentæ baccæ
Piperis longi fructus
Piperis nigri baccæ
Pix abietina
Pix liquida
Pix nigra
Plumbi subcarbonas
Plumbi oxydum semivitreum
Porri radix
Potassa impura
Potassæ nitras
Potassæ sulphas
Potassæ supertartras
Pruna
Pterocarpi lignum
Pulegium
Pyrethri radix
Quassiæ lignum
Quercûs cortex
Resina flava
Rhamni baccæ
Rhei radix
Rhœados petala
Ricini semina et oleum
Rosæ caninæ pulpa
Rosæ centifoliæ petala
Rosæ gallicæ petala
Rosmarini cacumina
Rubiæ radix
Rutæ folia
Sabinæ folia
Saccharum
——————— purificatum
Salicis cortex
Sagapenum
Sambuci flores
Sapo durus et mollis
Sarsaparillæ radix
Sassafras lignum et radix
Scammoneæ gummi resina
Scillæ radix
Senegæ radix
Sennæ folia
Serpentariæ radix
Sevum
Simaroubæ cortex
Sinapis semina
Sodæmurias
Sodæ subboras
Sodæ sulphas
Soda impura
Spartii cacumina
Spigeliæ radix
Spiritus rectificatus et tenuior
Spongia

L 2

51

Stramonii folia et semina
Stannum
Staphisagriæ semina
Styracis balsamum
Succinum
Sulphur et sulphur sublimatum
Tabaci folia
Tamarindi pulpa
Taraxaci radix

Tartarum
Terebinthina Canadensis
———— Chia
———— vulgaris
Terebinthinæ oleum
Testæ
Tiglii oleum
Tormentillæ radix
Toxicodendri folia

Tragacantha
Tussilago
Valerianæ radix
Veratri radix
Ulmi cortex
Uvæ passæ
Uvæ ursi folia
Zincum
Zingiberis radix.

MATERIA PERLATA. If, instead of crystallizing the salts contained in the liquor separated from diaphoretic antimony, an acid be poured into it, a white precipitate is formed, which is nothing else but a very refractory calx of antimony.

MATERIATU'RA. Castellus explains *morbi materiaturæ* to be diseases of intemperance.

MATLOCK. A village in Derbyshire. It affords a mineral water of the acidulous class: which issues from a limestone rock, near the banks of the Derwent. Several of the springs possess a temperature of 66°. Matlock water scarcely differs from common good spring water, in sensible properties. It is extremely transparent, and exhales no vapour, excepting in cold weather. It holds little or no excess of aërial particles; it curdles soap when first taken up, but it loses this effect upon long keeping, perhaps from the deposition of its calcareous salts; it appears to differ very little from good spring water when tasted: and its effects seem referrible to its temperature. It is from this latter circumstance that it forms a proper tepid bath for the nervous and irritable, and those of a debilitated constitution; hence it is usually recommended after the use of Bath and Buxton waters, and as preparatory to sea-bathing.

MATRICA'LIA. (*Matricalis ;* from *matrix,* the womb.) Medicines appropriated to disorders of the uterus.

MATRICA'RIA. (From *matrix,* the womb: so called from its uses in disorders of the womb.) 1. The name of a genus of plants in the Linnæan system. Class, *Syngenesia ;* Order, *Polygamia superflua.*

2. The pharmacopœial name of the Matricaria parthenium. See *Matricaria parthenium.*

MATRICARIA CHAMOMILLA. *Chamæmelum vulgare ; Chamomilla nostras ; Leucanthemum* of Dioscorides. Common wild corn, or dog's camomile. The plant directed under this name in the pharmacopœias, is the *Matricaria—receptaculis conicis radiis patentibus ; squamis calycinis, margine æqualibus,* of Linnæus. Its virtues are similar to those of the *parthenium,* but in a much inferior degree.

MATRICARIA PARTHENIUM. The systematic name of the fever-few. *Parthenium febrifuga.* Common fever-few, or febrifuge, and often, but very improperly, feather-few. Mother's wort. The leaves and flowers of this plant, *Matricaria—foliis compositis, planis ; foliolis ovatis, incisis ; pedunculis ramosis,* have a strong, not agreeable smell, and a moderately bitter taste, both which they communicate by warm infusion, to water and rectified spirit. The watery infusions, inspissated, leave an extract of considerable bitterness, and which discovers also a saline matter, both to the taste, and in a more sensible manner by throwing up to the surface small crystalline efflorescences in keeping. The peculiar flavour of the matricaria exhales in the evaporation, and impregnates the distilled water, on which also a quantity of essential oil is found floating. The quantity of spirituous extract, according to Cartheuser's experiments, is only about one-sixth the weight of the dry leaves, whereas the watery extract amounts to near one-half. This plant is evidently the *Parthenium* of Dioscorides, since whose time it has been very generally employed for medical purposes. In natural affinity, it ranks with camomile and tansy, and its sensible qualities show it to be nearly allied to them in its medicinal character. Bergius states its virtues to be tonic, stomachic, resolvent, and emmenagogue. It has been given successfully as a vermifuge, and for the cure of intermittents; but its use is most celebrated in female disorders, especially in hysteria; and hence it is supposed to have derived the name of matricaria. Its smell, taste, and analysis, prove it to be a medicine of considerable activity; we may, therefore, say, with Murray—*Rarius hodie præscribitur, quam debetur.*

MATRISY'LVA. See *Asperula.*

MA'TRIX. (Matηρ.) 1. The womb See *Uterus.*
2. The earthy or stony matter which accompanies ores, or envelopes them in the earth.

MATRONA'LIS. (From *matrona,* a matron : so called because its smell is grateful to women.) The violet.

MATTHIOLUS, PETER ANDREW, was born at Sienna in 1501. He went to study the law at Padua; but disliking that pursuit, he turned his attention to medicine. His father's death interrupted him in his progress; but having conciliated the good opinion of the professors, the degree of doctor was conferred upon him before his departure. He speedily found ample employment in his native place, but afterward went to Rome, and in 1527 to the court of the prince bishop of Trent. During his residence of fourteen years there, he acquired such general esteem, that on his removal, men, women, and children, accompanied him, calling him their father and benefactor. At Gorizia, where he then settled as public physician, he likewise experienced a signal mark of gratitude; a fire having consumed all his furniture, the people flocked to him next day with presents, which more than compensated his loss, and the magistrates advanced him a year's salary. After twelve years, he accepted an invitation to the Imperial court, where he was highly honoured, and created aulic counsellor: but finding the weight of age pressing upon him, he retired to Trent, where he shortly died of the plague in 1577. He left several works, chiefly relating to the virtues of plants: and that, by which he principally distinguished himself, was a Commentary on the writings of Dioscorides. This was first published in Italian, afterward translated by him into Latin, with plates, and passed through numerous editions. He certainly contributed much to lay the foundation of botanical science, though he was not sufficiently scrupulous in consulting the original sources, and examining the plants themselves.

MATURA'NTIA. (*Maturans ;* from *maturo,* to ripen.) Medicines which promote the suppuration of tumours.

MATURATION. (*Maturatio ;* from *maturo,* to make ripe.) A term in surgery, signifying that process which succeeds inflammation, by which pus is collected in an abscess.

MAUDLIN. See *Achillea ageratum.*

MAURICEAU, FRANCIS, was born at Paris, where he studied surgery with great industry for many years, especially at the Hôtel-Dieu. He had acquired so much experience in midwifery, before he commenced public practice, that he rose almost at once to the head of his profession. His reputation was farther increased by his writings, and maintained by his prudent conduct during a series of years ; after which he retired into the country, and died in 1709. He published several works, relating to the particular branch of the art which he practised, containing a great store of useful facts, though not well arranged, nor free from the false reasoning prevalent in his time.

MAURO-MARSON. See *Marrubium.*

Maw-worm. See *Ascaris.*

MAXI'LLA. (From ησσσαω, to chew.) The jaw, both upper and lower.

MAXILLARE INFERIUS os. *Maxilla inferior. Mandibula.* The maxilla inferior, or lower jaw, which, in its figure, may be compared to a horse-shoe, is at first composed of two distinct bones ; but these, soon after birth, unite together at the middle of the chin, so as to form only one bone. The superior edge of this bone has, like the upper jaw, a process, called the *alveolar* process. This, as well as that of the upper jaw, to which it is in other respects a good deal similar, is like wise furnished with cavities for the reception of the teeth. The posterior part of the bone, on each side, rises perpendicularly into two processes, one of which is called the *coronoid,* and the other the *condyloid* process. The first of these is the highest: it is thin and pointed; and the temporal muscle, which is attached to it, serves to elevate the jaw. The condyloid process is narrower, thicker, and shorter than the other, terminating in an oblong, rounded head, which is formed for a moveable articulation with the cranium, and is received into the forepart of the fossa described in the temporal bone. In this joint there is a moveable cartilage, which, being more closely connected to the condyle than to the cavity, may be considered as belonging to the former. This moveable cartilage is connected with both the articulating surface of the temporal bone and the condyle of the jaw, by distinct ligaments arising from its edges all round. These attachments of the cartilage are strengthened, and the whole articulation secured, by an external ligament, which is common to both, and which is fixed to the temporal bone, and to the neck of the condyle. On the inner surface of the ligament, which attaches the cartilage to the temporal bone, and backwards in the cavity, is placed what is commonly called the gland of the joint; at least the ligament is there found to be much more vascular than at any other part. At the bottom of each coronoid process, on its inner part, is a foramen, or canal, which extends under the roots of all the teeth, and terminates at the outer surface of the bone near the chin. Each of these foramina affords a passage to an artery, vein, and nerve, which send off branches to the several teeth.

This bone is capable of a great many motions. The condyles, by sliding from the cavity towards the eminences on each side, bring the jaw horizontally forwards, as in the action of biting; or the condyles only may be brought forwards, while the rest of the jaw is tilted backwards, as is the case when the mouth is open. The condyles may also slide alternately backwards and forwards from the cavity to the eminence, and *vice versâ;* so that while one condyle advances, the other moves backwards, turning the body of the jaw from side to side, as in grinding the teeth. The great use of the cartilages seems to be that of securing the articulation, by adapting themselves to the different inequalities in these several motions of the jaw, and to prevent any injuries from friction. This last circumstance is of great importance where there is so much motion, and, accordingly, this cartilage is found in the different tribes of carnivorous animals, where there is no eminence and cavity, nor other apparatus for grinding.

The alveolar processes are formed of an external and internal plate, united together by thin bony partitions, which divide the processes at the forepart of the jaw, into as many sockets as there are teeth. But, at the posterior part, where the teeth have more than one root, each root has a distinct cell. These processes in both jaws, begin to be formed with the teeth, accompany them in their growth, and disappear when the teeth fall. So that the loss of the one seems constantly to be attended with the loss of the other.

MAXILLARE SUPERIUS OS. *Maxilla superior.* The superior maxillary bones constitute the most considerable portion of the upper jaw, are two in number, and generally remain distinct through life. Their figure is exceedingly irregular, and not easily to be described. On each of these bones are observed several eminences. One of these is at the upper and forepart of the bone, and, from its making part of the nose, is called the *nasal* process. Internally, in the inferior portion of this process, is a fossa, which, with the os unguis, forms a passage for the lachrymal duct. Into this nasal process, likewise, is inserted the short round tendon of the *musculus orbicularis palpebrarum.* Backwards and outwards, from the root of the nasal process, the bone helps to form the lower side of the orbit, and this part is therefore called the *orbitar* process. Behind this orbitar process, the bone forms a considerable tuberosity, and, at the upper part of this tuberosity, is a channel, which is almost a complete hole. In this channel passes a branch of the fifth pair of nerves, which, together with a small artery, is transmitted to the face through the external orbitar foramen, which opens immediately under the orbit. Where the bone on each side is joined to the os malæ, and helps to form the cheeks, is observed what is called the *malar* process. The lower and anterior parts of the bone make a kind of circular sweep, in which are the *alveoli,* or sockets for the teeth; this is called the *alveolar* pro-

cess. This alveolar process has posteriorly a considerable tuberosity on its internal surface. Above this alveolar process, and just behind the fore-teeth, is an irregular hole, called the *foramen incisivum,* which, separating into two, and sometimes more holes, serves to transmit small arteries and veins, and a minute branch of the fifth pair of nerves to the nostrils. There are two horizontal lamellæ behind the alveolar process, which, uniting together, form part of the root of the mouth, and divide it from the nose. This partition, being seated somewhat higher than the lower edge of the alveolar process, gives the roof of the mouth a considerable hollowness. Where the ossa maxillaria are united to each other, they project somewhat forwards, leaving between them a furrow, which receives the inferior portion of the septum nasi. Each of these bones is hollow, and forms a considerable sinus under its orbitar part. This sinus, which is usually, though improperly, called *antrum Highmorianum,* is lined with the pituitary membrane. It answers the same purposes as the other sinuses of the nose, and communicates with the nostrils by an opening, which appears to be a large one in the skeleton, but which, in the recent subject, is much smaller. In the fœtus, instead of these sinuses, an oblong depression only is observed at each side of the nostrils, nor is the tuberosity of the alveolar process then formed. On the side of the palate, in young subjects, a kind of fissure may be noticed, which seems to separate the portion of the bone which contains the dentes incisores from that which contains the dentes canini. This fissure is sometimes apparent till the sixth year, but after that period it in general wholly disappears.

The ossa maxillaria not only serve to form the cheeks, but likewise the palate, nose, and orbits; and, besides their union with each other, they are connected with the greatest part of the bones of the face and cranium, viz. with the ossa nasi, ossa malarum, ossa unguis, ossa palati, os frontis, os sphenoides, and os ethmoides.

MAXILLARIS. (From *maxilla;* the jaw.) Maxillary: appertaining to the jaw.

MAXILLARY ARTERY. *Arteria maxillaris.* A branch of the external carotid. The *external maxillary* is the fourth branch of the carotid; it proceeds anteriorly, and gives off the facial or mental, the coronary of the lips, and the angular artery. The *internal maxillary* is the next branch of the carotid; it gives off the sphenomaxillary, the inferior alveolar, and the spinous artery.

MAXILLARY GLAND. *Glandula maxillaris.* The gland so called is conglomerate, and situated under the angles of the lower jaw. The excretory ducts of these glands are called Warthouian, after their discoverer.

MAXILLARY NERVE. *Nervus maxillaris.* The superior and inferior maxillary nerves are branches of the fifth pair, or trigemini. The former is divided into the sphenopalatine, posterior alveolar, and the infra-orbital nerve. The latter is divided into two branches, the internal lingual, and one, more properly, called the inferior maxillary.

[*May-apple.* See *Podophyllum peltatum.* A.]
May-lily. See *Convallaria majalis.*
May-weed. See *Anthemis cotula.*

MAYERNE, SIR THEODORE TURQUET DE, BARON D'AUBONNE, was born at Geneva in 1573, and graduated at Montpelier. He then went to Paris, and, by the influence of Riverius, was appointed in 1600 to attend the Duke de Rohan, in his embassy to the diet at Spire; and also one of the physicians in ordinary to Henry IV. On his return, he settled in Paris as physician, and gave lectures in anatomy and pharmacy, in which he strongly recommended various chemical remedies: this drew on him the ill-will of the faculty, and he was anonymously attacked as an enemy to Hippocrates and Galen; whence in his "Apologia," he cleared himself from this imputation, making also some severe strictures on his opponents. They consequently issued a decree against consulting with him; but the esteem of the king supported him against this persecution, and he would have been appointed first physician, had he not refused to embrace the Catholic religion. After the assassination of Henry IV. in 1610, he received an invitation from James I. of England, to whom he had been introduced three years before: he accepted the office of his first physician, and passed the remainder of his life in this country. He was admitted to the degree of doctor in both universities, and into the College of Physicians, and met with very general respect. He incurred some obloquy, indeed, on the death of the Prince of Wales, having differed in opinion from the other physicians, but his conduct obtained the written approbation of the king and council. He was knighted in 1624, and honoured with the appointment of physician to the two succeeding monarchs; and accumulated a large fortune by his extensive practice. He died in 1655, and bequeathed his library to the College of Physicians. Several papers, written by him, were published after his death: among which are the cases of many of his distinguished patients, well drawn up.

MAYOW, John, was born in Cornwall in 1645. He studied at Oxford, and took a degree in civil law, but afterward changed to medicine, which he practised chiefly at Bath, but he died in London at the age of 34. These are the only records of the life of a man, who went before his age in his views of chemical physiology, and anticipated, though obscurely, some of the most remarkable discoveries in pneumatic chemistry, which have since been made. He published at Oxford in 1669 two tracts, one on Respiration, the other on Rickets; which were reprinted five years after with three additional dissertations, one on the Respiration of the Fœtus in Utero et Ovo, another on Muscular Motion and the Animal Spirits, and the remaining one on Saltpetre and the Nitro-aërial Spirit. On this latter his claim above-mentioned chiefly rests, the existence of the nitro-aërial spirit being proved by many ingenious experiments, as a constituent of air, and of nitre, the food of life and flame, agreeing with the oxygen of modern chemists. Much vague speculation, indeed, occurs in the work: but he clearly maintains that this spirit is absorbed by the blood in the lungs, and proves the source of the animal heat, as also of the nervous energy and of muscular motion, He likewise anticipated the mode of operating with aërial fluids in vessels inverted over water, and transferring them from one to another.

Mays, Indian. See *Zea mays.*

MEAD. 1. The name of a physician, Dr. Richard, born near London in 1673. After studying some time at Leyden, and in different parts of Italy, he graduated at Padua in 1695. Then returning to his native country, he settled in practice, and met with considerable success. His first publication, "A Mechanical Account of Poisons," appeared in 1702, and displayed much ingenuity; though he afterward candidly retracted some of his opinions, as inadequate to explain the functions of a living body. He was soon after elected a member of the Royal Society, and in the following year physician to St. Thomas's Hospital. In 1704, he published a treatise, maintaining the influence of the sun and moon on the human body, arguing from the Newtonian theory of the tides, and the changes effected by those bodies in the atmosphere. In 1707, he received a diploma from Oxford, and about four years after he was appointed to read the anatomical lectures at Surgeons' Hall, which he continued for some time with great applause. In 1714, on the death of his patron Dr. Radcliffe, he took his house, and being then a fellow of the College of Physicians, and having been called into consultation, in the last illness of Queen Anne, when he displayed superior judgment, he seems to have been regarded among the first of the profession, and soon after, from his extensive engagements, resigned his office at St. Thomas's Hospital. The plague raging at Marseilles in 1719, he was officially consulted on the means of prevention, which led to a publication by him, in the following year, decidedly maintaining its infectious nature, which had been questioned in France, and recommending suitable precautions: this work passed rapidly through many editions. In 1721, he superintended the experiment of innoculating the small-pox in the persons of some criminals; and his report being favourable, the practice was rapidly diffused. He was soon after engaged in a controversy with Dr. Middleton, concerning the condition of physicians among the Romans, which was, however, carried on in a manner honourable to both parties. About the same period Dr. Freind having been committed to the Tower for his political sentiments, Dr. Mead obtained his liberation in a spirited manner, and presented him a considerable sum, received from his patients during his imprisonment. In 1727, he was appointed physician in ordinary to George II. and his professional occupations became so extensive, that he had no leisure for writing. It was

not till 20 years after, therefore, that he printed his treatise on Small-pox and Measles, written in a pure Latin style, with a translation in the same language of Rhazes' Commentary on the former disease. In 1749, he published a treatise on the Scurvy, ascribing the disease to moisture and putridity, and recommending Mr. Sutton's ventilator, which was, in consequence of his interposition, received into the navy. His "Medicina Sacra," appeared in the same year, containing remarks on the diseases montioned in the Scripture His last work was a summary of his experience, entitled "Monita et Præcepta Medica," in 1751; it was frequently reprinted, and translated into English. His life terminated in 1754; and a monument was erected to him in Westminster Abbey. He distinguished himself, not only in his profession, but he was the greatest patron of science and polite literature of his time; and he made an ample collection of scarce and valuable books, manuscripts, and literary curiosities; to which all respectable persons had free access.

2. An old English liquor made from the honey-combs, from which honey has been drained out by boiling in water, and then fermenting. This is often confounded with metheglin.

Meadow crowfoot. See *Ranunculus acris.*
Meadow, queen of the. See *Spiræa ulmaria.*
Meadow saffron. See *Colchicum.*
Meadow saxifrage. See *Peucedanum silaus.*
Meadow sweet. See *Spiræa ulmaria.*
Meadow thistle, round leaved. See *Cnicus oleraceus.*

MEASLES. See *Rubeola.*

MEASURE. The English measures of capacity, are according to the following table:

One gallon, wine measure, } four quarts.
 is equal to - - - }
One quart, - - - - two pints.
One pint, - - - - 28.875 cubic inches.

The pint is subdivided by chemists and apothecaries into 16 ounces

MEA'TUS. An opening which leads to a canal or duct.

MEATUS AUDITORIUS EXTERNUS. The external passage of the ear is lined with the common integuments, under which are a number of glands, which secrete the wax. The use of this duct is to admit the sound to the tympanum, which is at its extremity.

MEATUS AUDITORIUS INTERNUS. The internal auditory passage is a small bony canal, beginning internally by a longitudinal orifice at the posterior surface of the petrous portion of the temporal bone, running towards the vestibulum and cochlea, and there being divided into two less cavities by an eminence. The superior and smaller of these is the orifice of the aqueduct of Fallopius, which receives the portio dura of the auditory nerve: the other inferior and larger cavity is perforated by many small holes, through which the portio mollis of the auditory nerve passes into the labyrinth.

MEATUS CÆCUS. A passage in the throat to the ear, called Eustachian tube.

MEATUS CUTICULARES. The pores of the skin.

MEATUS CYSTICUS. The gall-duct.

MEATUS URINARIUS. In women, this is situated in the vagina, immediately below the symphisis of the pubes, and behind the nymphæ. In men, it is at the end of the glans penis.

Mecca balsam. See *Amyris gileadensis.*

MECHOACAN. See *Convolvulus mechoacanna.*

MECHOACA'NNA. (From *Mechoacan,* a province in Mexico, whence it is brought.) See *Convolvulus mechoacanna.*

MECHOACANNA NIGRA. See *Convolvulus jalapa.*

ME'CON. (From μηκος, bulk: so named from the largeness of its head.) The papaver, or poppy.

MECONIC ACID. (*Acidum meconicum;* so called from μηκων, the poppy, from which it is procured.) This acid is a constituent of opium. It was discovered by Sertuerner, who procured it in the following way: After precipitating the *morphia,* from a solution of opium, by ammonia, he added to the residual fluid a solution of the muriate of barytes. A precipitate is in this way formed, which is supposed to be a quadruple compound of barytes, morphia, extract, and the meconic acid. The extract is removed by alkohol, and the barytes by sulphuric acid; when the meconic acid is left, merely in combination with a portion of the morphia; and from this it is purified by successive solutions and evaporations. The acid, when sublimed, forms long colourless needles; it has a strong affinity for the oxide of iron, so as to take it from the muriatic solution, and form with it a cherry-red precipitate. It forms a crystallizable salt with lime, which is not decomposed by sulphuric acid; and what is curious, it seems to possess no particular power over the human body, when received into the stomach. The essential salt of opium, obtained in Derosne's original experiments, was probably the meconiate of morphia.

Robiquet has made a useful modification of the process for extracting meconic acid. He treats the opium with magnesia, to separate the morphia, while meconiate of magnesia is also formed. The magnesia is removed by adding muriate of barytes, and the barytes is afterward separated by dilute sulphuric acid. A larger proportion of meconic acid is thus obtained.

ME'CONIS. (From μηκων, the poppy: so called because its juice is soporiferous, like the poppy.) The lettuce.

MECO'NIUM. (From μηκων, the poppy.) 1. The inspissated juice of the poppy. ⊕pium.

2. The green excrementitious substance that is found in the large intestines of the fœtus.

MEDIAN. *Medianus.* This term is applied to vessels, &c. from their situation between others.

MEDIAN NERVE. The second branch of the brachial plexus.

MEDIAN VEIN. The situation of the veins of the arms is extremely different in different individuals. When a branch proceeds near the bend of the arm, inwardly from the basilic vein, it is termed the *basilic median;* and when a vein is given off from the cephalic in the like manner, it is termed the *cephalic median.* When these two veins are present, they mostly unite just below the bend of the arm, and the common trunk proceeds to the cephalic vein.

MEDIA'NUM. The *Mediastinum.*

MEDIASTI'NUM. (*Quasi in medio stans,* as being in the middle.) The membraneous septum, formed by the duplicature of the pleura, that divides the cavity of the chest into two parts. It is divided into an anterior and posterior portion.

MEDIASTINUM CEREBRI. The falciform process of the dura mater.

ME'DICA. (*Modicus;* from *medico,* to heal.) 1. Belonging to medicine.

2. (From Media, its native soil.) A sort of trefoil.

MEDICA'GO. (So called by Tourneforte; from *medica,* which is indeed the proper name of the plant— μηδικη, of Dioscorides.) The name of a genus of plants in the Linnæan system. Class, *Diadelphia;* Order, *Decandria.* The herb trefoil.

MEDICAMENTA'RIA. Pharmacy, or the art of making and preparing medicines.

MEDICAME'NTUM. (From *medico,* to heal.) A medicine.

MEDICA'STER. A pretender to the knowledge of medicine: the same as quack.

MEDICI'NA. (From *medico,* to heal.) Medicine.
1. The medical art: applied to the profession generally.

2. Any substance that is exhibited with a view to cure or allay the violence of a disease. It is also very frequently made use of to express the healing art, when it comprehends anatomy, physiology, and pathology.

MEDICINA DIÆTETICA. That department of medicine which regards the regulation of regimen, or the non-naturals.

MEDICINA DIASOSTICA. That part of medicine which preserves health.

MEDICINA GYMNASTICA. That part of medicine which relates to exercise.

MEDICINA HERMETICA. The application of chemical remedies.

MEDICINA PROPHYLACTICA. That part of medicine which relates to preservation of health.

MEDICINA TRISTITIÆ. Common saffron.

MEDICINAL. (*Medicinalis;* from *medicina.*) Medicinal, having a power to restore health, or remove disease.

MEDICINAL DAYS. Such days were so called by some writers, wherein the crisis or change is expected, so as to forbid the use of medicines, in order to wait nature's effort, and require all the assistance of art to help forward, or prepare the humours for such a crisis:

but it is most properly used for those days wherein purging, or any other evacuation, is most conveniently complied with.

MEDICINAL HOURS. Are those wherein it is supposed that medicines may be taken to the greatest advantage, commonly reckoned in the morning fasting, about an hour before dinner, about four hours after dinner, and at going to bed; but in acute cases, the times are to be governed by the symptoms and aggravation of the distemper.

MEDINA. A species of ulcer, mentioned by Paracelsus.

MEDINE'NSIS VENA. (*Medinensis;* so cal'ed because it is frequent at Medina, and improperly called *vena* for *vermis;* and sometimes *nervus medinensis,* and no one knows why.) *Dracunculus; Gordius medinensis,* of Linnæus. The muscular hair worm. A very singular animal, which, in some countries, inhabits the cellular membrane between the skin and muscles. See *Dracunculus.*

MEDITU'LLIUM. (From *medius,* the middle.) See *Diploë.*

ME'DIUS VENTER. The middle venter, the thorax, or chest.

MEDLAR. See *Mespilus.*

MEDU'LLA. (*Quasi in medio ossis.*) 1. The marrow. See *Marrow.*

2. The pith or pulp of vegetables. The centre or heart of a vegetable within the wood. "This," says Dr. E. Smith, "in parts most endowed with life, as roots and young growing stems or branches, is a tolerably firm juicy substance, of a uniform texture, and commonly a pale green or yellowish colour. In many annual stems the petal, abundant and very juicy while they are growing, becomes little more than a web, lining the hollow of the complete stem; as in some thistles. Concerning the nature and functions of this part various opinions have been held. Du Hamel considered it as merely cellular substance, connected with what is diffused through the whole plant, combining its various parts, but not performing any remarkable office in the vegetable economy. Linnæus, on the contrary, thought it the seat of life, and source of vegetation; that its vigour was the main cause of the propulsion of the branches, and that the seeds were more especially formed from it. This latter hypothesis is not better founded than his idea of the pith adding new layers to the wood. In fact, the pith in soon obliterated in the trunk of many trees; which, nevertheless, keep increasing for a long series of years, by layers of wood, added every year from the bark, even after the heart of the tree is become hollow from decay.

Some considerations have led Sir James Smith to hold a medium opinion between these two extremes. There is in certain respects, he observes, an analogy between the medulla of plants and the nervous system of animals. It is no less assiduously protected than the spinal marrow or principal nerve. It is branched off and diffused through the plant, as nerves are through the animal; hence it is not absurd to presume that it may, in like manner, give life and vigour to the whole, though by no means any more than nerves, the organ or source of nourishment.

It is certainly most vigorous and abundant in young and growing branches, and must be supposed to be subservient, in some way or other, to their increase.

Mr. Lindsay, of Jamaica, thought he demonstrated the medulla in the leafstalk of the *Mimosa pudica,* or sensitive plant.

Knight supposes the medulla may be a reservoir of moisture, to supply the leaves whenever an excess of perspiration renders such assistance necessary, but it should be recollected that all the moisture in the medulla of a whole plant is, in some cases, too little to supply one hour's perspiration of a single leaf, and it is not found that the moisture of the medulla varies, let the leaves be ever so flaccid

3. The white substance of the brain is called medulla, or the medullary part, to distinguish it from the cortical.

MEDULLA CASSIÆ. The pulp of the cassiæ fistularis. See *Cassia fistularis.*

MEDULLA OBLONGATA. *Cerebrum elongatum.* The medullary substance that lies within the cranium, upon the basillary process of the occipital bone. It is formed by the connexion of the crura cerebri and crura cerebelli, and terminates in the spinal marrow. It has several eminences, viz. pons varolii, corpora pyramidalia, and corpora olivaria.

MEDULLA SPINALIS. *Cerebrum elongatum Æon.* The spinal marrow. A continuation of the medulla oblongata, which descends into the specus vertebralis from the foramen magnum occipitale, to the third vertebra of the loins, where it terminates in a number of nerves, which, from their resemblance, are called *cauda equina.* The spinal marrow is composed, like the brain, of a cortical and medullary substance; the former is placed internally. It is covered by a continuation of the dura mater, pia mater, and tunica arachnoidea. The use of the spinal marrow is to give off, through the lateral or intervertebral foramina, thirty pairs of nerves, called cervical, dorsal, lumbar, and sacral nerves.

MEDULLARY. (*Medullaris;* from *medulla,* marrow.) Like unto marrow.

MEDULLARY SUBSTANCE. The white or internal substance of the brain is so called. See *Cerebrum.*

MEDELLIN. The name given by Dr. John to the porous pith of the sun-flower.

MEERSCHAM. *Kessecil* of Kirwan. A mineral composed of silica, magnesia ,lime-water, and carbonic acid, of a yellowish and grayish white colour, and greasy feel, and soft when first dry. It lathers like soap, and is used by the Tartars for washing. In Turkey they make tobacco pipes from meerschaum, dug in Natolia and near Thebes.

MEGALOSPLA'NCHNUS. (From μεγας, great, and σπλαγχνον, a bowel.) Having some of the viscera enlarged.

ME'GRIM. A species of headache; a pain generally affecting one side of the head, towards the eye, or temple, and arising from the state of the stomach.

MEIBOMIUS, HENRY, was born at Lubeck in 1638. After studying in different universities, he graduated at Angers, and afterward was appointed professor of medicine at Helmstadt, where he continued till his death in 1700. He published several works, and commentaries on those of others. That which chiefly illustrates his name is entitled "De Vasis Palpebrarum novis," printed in 1666. He seems to have contemplated a history of medicine, and published a letter on the subject, which indeed his father had begun; but the difficulties which he met with in investigating the medicine of the Arabians, arrested his progress.

MEIBOMIUS'S GLANDS. *Meibomii glandulæ.* The small glands which are situated between the conjunctive membrane of the eye and the cartilage of the eyelid, first described by Meibomius.

MEIONITE. Prismatico-pyramidal felspar. This mineral occurs along with ceylanite, and nepheline, in granular limestone, at Monte Somna, near Naples.

MEL. *Honey.* A substance collected by bees from the nectary of flowers, resembling sugar in its elementary properties. It has a white or yellowish colour, a soft and grained consistence, and a saccharine and aromatic smell. It is supposed to consist of sugar, mucilage, and an acid. Honey is an excellent food, and a softening and slightly aperient remedy: mixed with vinegar, it forms *oxymel,* and is used in various forms, in medicine and pharmacy. It is particularly recommended to the asthmatic, and those subject to gravel complaints, from its detergent nature. Founded upon the popular opinion of honey, as a pectoral remedy, Dr. Hill's balsam of honey, a quack medicine, was once in demand; but this, besides honey, contained balsam of Tolu, or gum benjamin, in solution.

MEL ACETATUM. See *Oxymel.*

MEL BORACIS. Honey of borax.—Take of borax, powdered, a drachm; clarified honey, an ounce. Mix. This preparation is found very useful in aphthous affections of the fauces.

MEL DESPUMATUM. Clarified honey. Melt honey in a water bath, then remove the scum.

MEL ROSÆ. Rose honey.—Take of red-rose petals, dried, four ounces; boiling water, three pints; clarified honey, five pounds. Macerate the rose petals in the water for six hours, and strain; then add the honey to the strained liquor, and, by means of a water-bath, boil it down to a proper consistence. An admirable preparation for the base of various gargles and collutories. It may also be employed with advantage, mixed with extract of bark, or other medicines, for children who have a natural disgust to medicines.

MEL SCILLÆ. See *Oxymel scillæ*

ME'LA. (From μαω, to search.) A probe.

MELÆ'NA. (From μελας, black.) The black vomit. The black disease. Μελαινα νουσος, of the Greeks. Hippocrates applies this name to two diseases. In the first, the patient vomits black bile, which is sometimes bloody and sour; sometimes he throws up a thin saliva; and at others a green bile, &c. In the second, the patient is as described in the article *Morbus niger.* See *Morbus niger.*

[The Malaria which produces intermittent, remittent, and other fevers, occasionally becomes so powerful, or produces such a corrupted, or infected state of the atmosphere, as to induce black vomiting, and yellow fevers, as was long since noticed by Hippocrates.

"The morbus regius, or Icterus, of the first section of his Coan Prognostics, is undoubtedly febrile yellowness, and not idiopathic jaundice. The epithet οξυς, acute, is repeatedly applied by Hippocrates to denote a febrile jaundice, which soon destroys life, in contradistinction to the other kinds, which are of a more chronic type, and less fatal. The like interpretation is to be put upon the sixty-third aphorism of the third book, which declares a yellowness (ικτεροι) supervening in fevers, *on* the seventh, ninth, or fourteenth day, to be a good symptom, provided there is no hardness in the region of the liver. In the sixty-second aphorism, he clearly means to be understood in the same manner, when he says that yellowness (ικτεροι again) appearing in fevers *before* the seventh day, is an unfavourable symptom. A similar meaning must be intended in the ninth section of his book on Crises, where it is laid down as a maxim, that ' *in burning fevers, a yellowness* (ικτερος) *breaking out on the fifth day, and accompanied by hiccough, is a fatal sign.*' (Εν τοισι καυσοισιν εαν επιγενηται ικτερος και λυξη πεμπταιω εοντι, θανατωδες υποστροφαι λαμβανονται.)

Let this sentence be particularly considered. In the whole catalogue of diseases, there is none but *that* commonly called yellow fever to which this aphorism can properly be applied. And it would be exceedingly difficult, in so few words, to give a more expressive delineation of the disease in question. In the third section of the same book, he declares that yellowness appearing on, or after the seventh day, denotes a critical sweating. In contradistinction to all which is the case mentioned in the forty-second aphorism of the sixth book, in which it is stated, that an indurated liver following a yellowness, is an unfavourable occurrence, because it is a case of idiopathic jaundice, connected with a very morbid condition of that important viscus. Yellowness, as a symptom of fever, is mentioned in other places. I shall mention but one more, and that bears so direct an application to the subject, that it is impossible to mistake its meaning. It is from his book *De Ratione Victus in Morbis acutis. In a bilious* fever, yellowness coming on with shivering before the seventh day, terminates the fever; but if it come on abruptly (or unseasonably) without shivering, it is mortal. (Εν πυρετω χολωδει, προ της εβδομης, ρε'[α ριγεος ικτερος επιγενομενος, λυει τον πυρετον; ανευ δε ριγεος ην επιγενη]αι, εξω των καιρων, ολιθριον.)

It will not appear strange that Hippocrates should have been acquainted with the disease called yellow fever, if we attend to the following account of the Phasians, delivered in his book on *air, water,* and *situation.*

"As to the inhabitants of Phasis, their country is *marshy, hot, watery, woody,* and subject to many violent *showers* at all seasons. They also live in the marshes, in houses or huts, built in the water, of wood and reeds; seldom walk to the city or the market, but pass from place to place, as they have many canals and ditches, in boats cut out of one piece of timber. The waters they drink are hot and stagnant, corrupted by the sun, and supplied by the rain. The river *Phasis* itself is the most stagnant of all rivers, and the stream the gentlest. The fruits they have there never come to perfection, but are cramped in their growth, and, as it were, effeminated by the vast quantity of water. The air of the country is also thick, and misty from so much water. For these reasons the Phasians differ in their appearance from other people; for they are large and thick to a prodigy, without any sign of joint or vessel. Their colour is a pale yellow like that in a jaundice." Την δε χροιην ωχρην εχουσιν, ωσπερ υπο ικτερου εχομενοι.

Having found these facts in the works of the father

of physic, I turned over his pages with a view of finding whether he knew any thing of black vomiting. I soon found the phrases μελαινα χολη, black bile, μελανα εμετον, black vomit, and μελανων εμε]ον, the vomiting of black matter. In the twelfth section of his prognostics, he affirms, that if the matter vomited be of a livid or black colour, it betokens ill. So in the first section of the first book of his *Coan Prognostics*, he enumerates black vomiting among a number of the most desperate symptoms. And also in the fourth section of the same book, he considers leek-green, livid, and black vomiting, as omens of sad import. (Ει δη ειη το ευμευμενον πρασοειδες, η πηλιον, η μελαν, αν η του]εων των χρωμα των, νομιζειν χεη πονηρον ειται.) The passage in the eleventh paragraph of the first book of his *Predictions* indicates strongly the unfavourable issue of a fever after black vomiting. The connexion between black vomiting and death is noticed likewise in the third paragraph of the second section of his *Coan Prognostics*. The same symptom is mentioned in the first paragraph of the first section of the same book. And you will find the like to occur in the fourth paragraph of the third section.

I have confined myself in citing the works of Hippocrates to some of the passages which contain pointed facts and opinions, relative to a yellowness of the skin, and a vomiting of dark or black matter in fevers. My object is, to show that these are by no means new symptoms: that they existed in the days of Artaxerxes, certainly among the Greeks, and probably among the Persians; that they had been observed more than 2000 years ago by one of the most careful of men in the southern parts of Europe; and of course, since they existed so long before the voyage of Columbus, there is no need of resorting to the stale and delusive notion that the fevers with these symptoms are of modern existence, and imported solely from America. Unfortunately, fevers with these accompaniments were long, long before, found to prostrate the strength and shorten the life of man. This subject may be further illustrated by recollecting that Hippocrates practised physic, for a considerable portion of his life, in parts of Greece, situated nearly in the same parallel of latitude with those in North America where the yellow fever has exhibited its greatest ravages," and where it has always been a seasonable and local disease and not contagious.—*Med. Repos.* A.]

MELAINA NOSOS. See *Melæna*.

MELALEU'CA. (From μελας, black, and λευκος, white: so named by Linnæus, because the principal, and indeed original, species was called *leucadendron*, and *arbor alba;* words synonymous with its appellation in the Malay tongue, *Caja-puti*, or white tree, but it is not known why the idea of black was associated with white.) The name of a genus of plants in the Linnæan system. Class, *Polyandria;* Order, *Icosandria*.

MELALEUCA LEUCADENDRON. The systematic name of the plant which is said to afford the cajeput oil. *Oleum cajeputæ; Oleum Wittnebianum; Oleum volatile melaleucæ; Oleum cajeput*. Thunberg says cajeput oil has the appearance of inflammable spirit, is of a green colour, and so completely volatile, that it evaporates entirely, leaving no residuum; its odour is of the camphoraceous kind, with a terebinthinate admixture. Goetz says it is limpid, or rather yellowish. It is a very powerful medicine, and in high esteem in India and Germany, in the character of a general remedy in chronic and painful diseases: it is used for the same purposes for which we employ the officinal æthers, to which it seems to have a considerable affinity; the cajeput, however, is more potent and pungent; taken into the stomach, in the dose of five or six drops, it heats and stimulates the whole system, proving, at the same time, a very certain diaphoretic, by which probably the good effects it is said to have in dropsies and intermittent fevers, are to be explained. For its efficacy in various convulsive and spasmodic complaints, it is highly esteemed. It has also been used both internally and externally, with much advantage, in several other obstinate disorders: as palsies, hypochondriacal, and hysterical affections, deafness, defective vision, toothache, gout, rheumatism, &c. The dose is from two to six, or even twelve drops. The tree which affords this oil, by distillation of its leaves, generally was supposed to be the *Melaleuca leucadendron* of Linnæus, but it appears from the specimens of the tree

producing the true oil, sent home from India, by Christopher Smith, that it is another species, which is therefore named *Melaleuca cajaputi*.

MELAMEMA. (From μελας, black, and αιμα, blood.) A term applied to blood when it is of a morbidly dark colour.

MELAMPHY'LLUM. (From μελας, black, and φυλλον, a leaf: so named from the blackness of its leaf.) See *Acanthus mollis*.

MELAMPO'DIUM. (From *Melampus*, the shepherd who first used it.) Black hellebore. See *Helleborus niger*.

MELANAGO'GA. (From μελας, black, and αγω, to expel.) Medicines which purge off black bile.

MELANCHLO'RUS. Μελαγχλωρος. I. A livid colour of the skin.

2. The black jaundice.

MELANCHO'LIA. (From μελας, black, and χολη, bile; because the ancients supposed that it proceeded from a redundance of black bile.) Melancholy madness. A disease in the class *Neuroses*, and order *Vesaniæ*, of Cullen, characterized by erroneous judgment, but not merely respecting health, from imaginary perceptions, or recollection influencing the conduct and depressing the mind with ill-grounded fears; not combined with either pyrexia or comatose affections; often appearing without dyspepsia, yet attended with costiveness, chiefly in persons of rigid fibres and torpid insensibility. See *Mania*.

MELANITE. A velvet-black coloured mineral in roundish or crystallized grains, found in a rock at Frascate near Rome.

MELANO'MA. (From μελας, black.) *Melanosis*. A rare disease which is found under the common integuments, and in the viscera, in the form of a tubercle, of a dark soot-black colour.

MELANO'PIPER. (From μελας, black, and πεπερι pepper.) See *Piper nigrum*.

MELANORRHIZON. (From μελας, black, and ριζα, a root.) A species of hellebore with black roots. See *Helleborus niger*.

MELANO'SIS. See *Melanoma*.

MELANTE'RIA. (From μελας, black: so called because it is used for blacking leather.) Green vitriol, or sulphate of iron.

MELANTHELÆ'UM. (From μελας, black, and ελαιον, oil.) Oil expressed from the black seeds of the Nigella sativa.

MELA'NTHIUM. (From μελας, black: so named from its black seed.) The Nigella sativa, or herb fennel flower.

ME'LAS. (From μελας, black.) *Vitiligo nigra*, *Morphæ nigra; Lepra maculosa nigra*. A disease that appears upon the skin in black or brown spots, which very frequently penetrate deep, even to the bone, and do not give any pain, or uneasiness. It is a disease very frequent in, and endemial to, Arabia, where it is supposed to be produced by a peculiar miasma.

MELA'SMA. (From μελας, black.) *Melasmus*. A disease that appears not unfrequently upon the tibia of aged persons, in form of a livid black spot, which, in a day or two, degenerates into a very foul ulcer.

MELASPE'RMUM. (From μελας, black, and σπερμα, seed.) See *Nigella sativa*.

MELASSES. Treacle. The black empyreumatic syrup which exists in raw sugar.

MELASSIC ACID. The acid present in melasses, which has been thought a peculiar acid by some; by others, the acetic.

ME'LCA. (From αμελγω, to milk.) Milk. A food made of acidulated milk.

ME'LE. (From μαω, to search.) A probe.

MELEA'GRIS. (From *Meleager*, whose sisters were fabled to have been turned into this bird.) 1 The guinea fowl.

2. A species of *fritillaria:* so called because its flowers are spotted like a guinea-fowl.

MELEGE'TA. Grains of paradise.

MELEGUETTA. Grains of paradise. See *Amomum granum paradisi*.

MELEI'OS. (From *Melos*, the island where it is made.) A species of alum.

MELI. Μελι. Honey. See *Mel*.

MELICERIA. See *Meliceris*.

MELI'CERIS. (From μελι, honey, and κερος, wax.

Meliceria. An encysted tumour, the contents of which resemble honey in consistence and appearance.

MELI'CRATON. (From μελι, honey, and κεραννυμι, to mix.) Wine impregnated with honey.

MELIGEI'ON. (From μελι, honey.) A fœtid humour, discharged from ulcers attended with a caries of the bone, of the consistence of honey.

MELILOT. See *Melilotus.*

MELILO'TUS. (From μελι, honey, and λωτος, the lotus: so called from its smell, being like that of honey.) See *Trifolium melilotus officinalis.*

MELIME'LUM. (From μελι, honey, and μηλον, an apple: so named from its sweetness.) Paradise apple, the produce of a dwarf wild apple-tree.

MELI'NUM. (From μελον, an apple.) Oil made from the flowers, or the fruit of the apple-tree.

MELIPHY'LLUM. (From μελι, honey, and φυλλον, a leaf: so called from the sweet smell of its leaf, or because bees gather honey from it.) See *Melissa.*

MELI'SSA. (From μελισσα, a bee; because bees gather honey from it.) The name of a genus of plants in the Linnæan system. Class, *Didynamia;* Order, *Gymnospermia.* Balm.

MELISSA CALAMINTHA. The systematic name of the common calamint. *Calamintha; Calamintha vulgaris; Calamintha officinarum; Melissa—pedunculis axillaribus, dichotomis, longitudine foliorum,* of Linnæus. This plant smells strongly like wild mint, though more agreeable; and is often used by the common people, in form of tea, against weakness of the stomach, flatulent colic, uterine obstructions, hysteria, &c.

MELISSA CITRINA. See *Melissa officinalis.*

MELISSA GRANDIFLORA. The systematic name of the mountain calamint. *Calamintha magno flore; Calamintha montana.* This plant has a moderately pungent taste, and a more agreeable aromatic smell than the common calamint, and appears to be more eligible as a stomachic.

MELISSA NEPETA. Field calamint. Spotted calamint. *Calamintha anglica; Calamintha pulegii odore; Nepeta agrestis.* It was formerly used as an aromatic.

MELISSA OFFICINALIS. The systematic name of balm. *Citrago; Citraria; Melissophyllum; Mellitis; Cedronella; Apiastrum; Melissa citrina; Erotion.* A native of the southern parts of Europe, but very common in our gardens. In its recent state, it has a roughish aromatic taste, and a pleasant smell of the lemon kind. It was formerly much esteemed in nervous diseases, and very generally recommended in melancholic and hypochondriacal affections; but, in modern practice, it is only employed when prepared as tea, as a grateful diluent drink in fevers, &c.

MELISSA TURCICA. See *Dracocephalum moldavica.*

MELISSOPHY'LLUM. (From μελισσα, baum, and φυλλον, a leaf.) A species of melittis, with leaves resembling baum. See *Melittis melissophyllum.*

MELITI'SMUS. (From μελι, honey.) A linctus, prepared with honey.

MELI'TTIS. (From μελιτ7α, which, in the Attic dialect, is the name of a bee; so that this word is, in fact, equivalent to *Melissa,* and was adopted by Linnæus, therefore, for the bastard balm.) The name of a genus of plants. Class, *Didynamia;* Order, *Gymnospermia.* Bastard balm.

MELITTIS MELISSOPHYLLUM. The systematic name of the mountain balm, or nettle. *Sophyllum.* This elegant plant is seldom used in the present day; it is said to be of service in uterine obstructions and calculous diseases.

MELITTO'MA. (From μελι, honey) A confection made with honey. Honey-dew.

MELIZO'MUM. (From μελι, honey, and ζωμος, broth.) Honey-broth. A drink prepared with honey, like mead.

MELLA'GO. (From *mel,* honey.) Any medicine which has the consistence and sweetness of honey.

MELLATE. A compound of mellitic acid, with salifiable bases.

MELLICERIS. See *Meliceris.*

MELLILO'TUS. See *Melilotus.*

MELLI'NA. (From *mel,* honey.) Mead. A sweet drink prepared with honey.

MELLI'TA. (From *mel,* honey.) Preparations of honey.

MÉLLITE. Mellilite. Honey-stone. A mineral of a honey-yellow colour, slightly resino-electric

by friction, hitherto found only at Atern, in Thuringia.

MELLITIC ACID. (*Acidum melliticum;* from *mellilite,* the honey-stone, from which it is obtained.) "Klaproth discovered in the mellilite, or honey-stone, what he conceives to be a peculiar acid of the vegetable kind, combined with alumina. This acid is easily obtained by reducing the stone to powder, and boiling it in about seventy times its weight of water; when the acid will dissolve, and may be separated from the alumina by filtration. By evaporating the solution, it may be obtained in the form of crystals. The follow ing are its characters :—

It crystallizes in fine needles or globules by the union of these, or small prisms. Its taste is at first a sweetish-sour, which leaves a bitterness behind. On a plate of hot metal it is readily decomposed, and dissipated in copious gray fumes, which affect not the smell, leaving behind a small quantity of ashes, that do not change either red or blue tincture of litmus. Neutralized by potassa it crystallizes in groups of long prisms: by soda, in cubes, or triangular laminæ, sometimes in groups, sometimes single; and by ammonia, in beautiful prisms with six planes, which soon lose their transparency, and acquire a silver-white hue. If the mellitic acid be dissolved in lime-water, and a solution of calcined strontian or barytes be dropped into it, a white precipitate is thrown down, which is redissolved on adding muriatic acid. With a solution of acetate of barytes, it produces likewise a white precipitate, which nitric acid redissolves. With solution of muriate of barytes, it produces no precipitate, or even cloud; but, after standing some time, fine trans parent needly crystals are deposited. The mellitic acid produces no change in a solution of nitrate of silver. From a solution of nitrate of mercury, either hot or cold, it throws down a copious white precipi tate, which an addition of nitric acid immediately redissolves. With nitrate of iron, it gives an abundant precipitate of a dun-yellow colour, which may be re dissolved by muriatic acid. With a solution of ace tate of lead, it produces an abundant precipitate, immediately redissolved on adding nitric acid. With acetate of copper, it gives a grayish-green precipitate; but it does not affect a solution of muriate of copper. Lime-water, precipitated by it, is immediately redissolved on adding nitric acid."—*Ure's Chem. Dict.*

ME'LO. See *Cucumis melo.*

MELOCA'RPUS. (From μηλον, an apple, and καρπος, fruit: from its resemblance to an apple.) The fruit of the aristolochia, or its roots.

ME'LOE. An insect called the blossom-eater. A genus of the order *Coleoptera.* Some of its species were formerly used medicinally.

MELOE VESICATORIUS. See *Cantharis.*

[MELOE VITTATA, or potato-fly. See *Cantharides vittata.* A.]

MELON. See *Cucumis melo.*

Melon, musk. See *Cucumis melo.*

Melon, water. See *Cucurbita citrullus.*

ME'LON. Μηλον. A disorder of the eye, in which the ball of the eye is pressed forward from the socket.

MELO'NGENA. *Mala insana. Solanum pomiferum.* Mad-apple. The Spaniards and Italians eat it in sauce and in sweetmeats. The taste somewhat resembles citron. See *Solanum melongena.*

MELO'SIS. Μηλωσις. A term which frequently occurs in Hippocrates, De Capitis Vulneribus, for that search into wounds which is made by surgeons with the probe.

MELO'TIS. Μηλωτις. A little probe, and that particular instrument contrived to search or cleanse the ear with, commonly called *Auriscalpium.*

MELO'THRIA. (A name borrowed by Linnæus in his *Hortus Cliffortianus;* from the μηλωθρον, of Dioscorides.) The name of a genus of plants. Class, *Triandria;* Order, *Monogynia.*

MELOTHRIA PENDULA. The systematic name of the small creeping cucumber plant. The American bry ony. The inhabitants of the West Indies pickle the berries of this plant, and use them as we do capers.

MELYSSOPHYLLUM. (From μελισσα, balm, and φυλλον, a leaf.) See *Melittis.*

MEMBRANA. See *Membrane.*

MEMBRANA HYALOIDEA. *Membrana arachnoidea* The transparent membrane which includes the vitre ous humour of the eye.

MEMBRANA PUPILLARIS. *Velum pupillæ.* A very delicate membrane of a thin and vascular texture, and an ash colour, arising from the internal margin of the iris, and totally covering the pupil in the fœtus before the sixth month.

MEMBRANA RUYSCHIANA. The celebrated anatomist Ruysch discovered that the choroid membrane of the eye was composed of two laminæ. He gave the name of membrana ruyschiana to the internal lamina, leaving the old name of choroides to the external.

MEMBRANA SCHNEIDERIANA. The very vascular pituitary membrane which lines the nose and its cavities; secretes the mucus of that cavity, and is the bed of the olfactory nerves.

MEMBRANA TYMPANI. The membrane covering the cavity of the drum of the ear, and separating it from the meatus auditorius externus. It is of an oval form, convex below the middle, towards the hollow of the tympanum, and concave towards the meatus auditorius, and convex above the meatus, and concave towards the hollow of the tympanum. According to the observations of anatomists, it consists of six laminæ; the first and most external, is a production of the epidermis; the second is a production of the skin lining the auditory passage; the third is cellular membrane, in which the vessels form an elegant net-work; the fourth is shining, thin, and transparent, arising from the periosteum of the meatus; the fifth is cellular membrane, with a plexus of vessels like the third; and the sixth lamina, which is the innermost, comes from the periosteum of the cavity of the tympanum. This membrane, thus composed of several laminæ, has lately been discovered to possess muscular fibres.

MEMBRANACEUS. Membranaceous: Applied to leaves, pods, &c. of a thin and pliable texture, as the leaf of the Magnolia purpurea, and several capsules, ligaments, &c.

MEMBRANOLO'GIA. (From *membrana*, a membrane, and λογος, a discourse.) Membranology. That which relates to the common integuments and membranes.

MEMBRANE. *Membrana.* 1. In anatomy. A thin expanded substance, composed of cellular texture, the elastic fibres of which are so arranged and woven together, as to allow of great pliability. The membranes of the body are various, as the skin, peritoneum, pleura, dura mater, &c. &c.

2. In botany. See *Testa.*

MEMBRANO'SUS. See *Tensor vaginæ femoris.*

MEMBRA'NUS. See *Tensor vaginæ femoris.*

MEMO'RIÆ OS. See *Occipital bone.*

MEMORY. *Memoria.* The brain is not only capable of perceiving sensations, but it possesses the faculty of reproducing those it has already perceived. This cerebral action is called remembrance, when the ideas are reproduced which have not been long received: it is called recollection when the ideas are of an older date. An old man who recalls the events of his youth, has recollection; he who recalls the sensations which he had last year, has memory, or remembrance.

Reminiscence is an idea produced which one does not remember having had before.

In childhood and youth, memory is very vivid as well as sensibility: it is therefore at this age, that the greatest variety of knowledge is acquired, particularly that sort which does not require much reflection; such as history, languages, the descriptive science, &c. Memory afterward weakens along with age: in adult age it diminishes; in old age it fails almost completely. There are, however, individuals who preserve their memory to a very advanced age; but if this does not depend on great exercise, as happens with actors, it exists often only to the detriment of the other intellectual faculties.

The sensations are recalled with ease in proportion as they are vivid. The remembrance of internal sensations is almost always confused; certain diseases of the brain destroy the memory entirely.

MENACHANITE. A mineral of a grayish black colour, found accompanied with fine quartz sand in the bed of a rivulet, which enters the valley of Manaccan, in Cornwall.

MENAGOGUE. See *Emmenagogue.*

MENDO'SUS. (From *mendax*, counterfeit.) This term is used, by some, in the same sense as spurious, or illegitimate; *Mendosæ costæ* false or spurious ribs;

Mendosa sutura, the squamous suture, or bastard suture of the skull.

MENILITE. A sub-species of indivisible quartz. It is of two kinds, the brown and the gray.

MENINGO'PHYLAX. (From μηνιγξ, a membrane, and φυλασσω, to guard.) An instrument to guard the membranes of the brain, while the bone is cut, or rasped, after the operation of the trepan.

ME'NINX. (From μενω, to remain.) Before the time of Galen, meninx was the common term for all the membranes of the body, afterward it was appropriated to those of the brain. See *Dura mater*, and *Pia mater.*

MENISPERMIC ACID. (*Acidum menispermicum;* from *menispermum,* the name of the plant in the berries of which it exists.) The seeds of *Menispermum oogoulua* being macerated for 24 hours in 5 times their weight of water, first cold, and then boiling hot, yield an infusion, from which solution of subacetate of lead throws down a menispermate of lead. This is to be washed and drained, diffused through water, and decomposed by a current of sulphuretted hydrogen gas. The liquid, thus freed from lead, is to be deprived of sulphuretted hydrogen by heat, and then forms solution of menispermic acid. By repeated evaporations and solutions in alkohol, it loses its bitter taste, and becomes a purer acid. It occasions no precipitate with lime-water; with nitrate of barytes it yields a gray precipitate; with nitrate of silver, a deep yellow; and with sulphate of magnesia, a copious precipitate.

MENISPE'RMUM. (From μηνη, the moon, and σπερμα, seed, in allusion to the crescent-like form of the seed.) Moon-seed. The name of a genus of plants. Class, *Diœcia;* Order, *Dodecandria.*

MENISPERMUM COCCULUS. The systematic name of the plant, the berries of which are well known by the name of *Cocculus indicus.* Indian berries, or Indian cockles; *Coccus indicus; Cocculæ officinarium; Cocci orientales.* The berry, the produce of the *Menispermum—foliis cordatis, retusis, mucronatis; caule lacero,* of Linnæus, is rugous and kidney-shaped, and contains a white nucleus. It is brought from Malabar and the East Indies. It is poisonous if swallowed, bringing on nausea, fainting, and convulsions. The berries possess an inebriating quality; and are supposed to impart that power to most of the London porter. While green, they are used by the Indians to catch fish, which they have the power of intoxicating and killing. In the same manner they catch birds, making the berry into a paste, forming it into small seeds, and putting these in places where they frequent. A peculiar acid called *menispermic,* is obtained from these berries.

By recent chemical analysis, this seed is found to contain, 1st, about one-half of its weight of a concrete fixed oil; 2d, an albuminous vegeto-animal substance; 3d, a peculiar colouring matter; 4th, one-fiftieth of picrotoxia; 5th, one-half its weight of fibrous matter; 6th, bimalate of lime and potassa; 7th, sulphate of potassa; 8th, muriate of potassa; 9th, phosphate of lime; 10th, a littleiron and silica. It is poisonous; and is frequently employed to intoxicate or poison fishes. The deleterious ingredient is the Picrotoxia.

The poisonous principle called *picrotoxia,* is obtained in the following way: "To the filtered decoction of these berries, add acetate of lead, while any precipitate falls. Filter and evaporate the liquid cautiously to the consistence of an extract. Dissolve in alkohol of 0.817, and evaporate the solution to dryness. By repeating the solutions and evaporations, we at last obtain a substance equally soluble in water and alkohol. The colouring matter may be removed by agitating it with a little water. Crystals of pure picrotoxia now fall, which may be washed with a little alkohol.

The crystals are four-sided prisms, of a white colour, and intensely bitter taste. They are soluble in 25 times their weight of water, and are not precipitable by any known reagent. Alkohol, sp. gr. 0.810, dissolves one-third of its weight of picrotoxia. Pure sulphuric ether dissolves two-fifths of its weight.

Strong sulphuric acid dissolves it, but not when much diluted. Nitric acid converts it into oxalic acid. It dissolves and neutralizes in acetic acid, and falls when this is saturated with an alkali. It may, therefore be regarded as a vegeto-alkali itself. Aqueous potassa dissolves it, without evolving any smell of ammonia. It acts as an intoxicating poison.

Sulphate of picrotoxia must be formed by dissolving picrotoxia in dilute sulphuric acid, for the strong acid chars and destroys it. The solution crystallizes on cooling. The sulphate of picrotoxia dissolves in 120 times its weight of boiling water. The solution gradually lets fall the salt in fine silky filaments disposed in bundles, and possessed of great beauty.

Nitrate of picrotoxia. Nitric acid, of the specific gravity 1.38, diluted with twice its weight of water, dissolves when assisted by heat, the fourth of its weight of picrotoxia. When this solution is evaporated to one-half, it becomes viscid, and on cooling is converted into a transparent mass, similar to a solution of gum-arabic. In this state the nitrate of picrotoxia is acid, and exceedingly bitter.

Muriate of picrotoxia. Muriatic acid, of the specific gravity 1.145, has little action on picrotoxia. It dissolves it when assisted by heat, but does not become entirely saturated. Five parts of this acid, diluted with three times its weight of water, dissolve about one part of picrotoxia at a strong boiling temperature. The liquor, on cooling, is converted into a grayish crystalline mass, composed of confused crystals. When these crystals are well washed, they are almost destitute of taste, and feel elastic under the teeth.

Acetate of picrotoxia. Acetic acid dissolves picrotoxia very well, and may be nearly saturated with it by the assistance of a boiling heat. On cooling, the acetate precipitates in well-defined prismatic needles. This acetate is soluble in fifty times its weight of boiling water.

MENORRHA'GIA. (From μηνια, the menses, and ρηγνυμι, to break out.) *Hæmorrhagia uterina.* Flooding. An immoderate flow of the menses, or uterine hæmorrhage. A genus of diseases in the class *Pyrexia*, and order *Hæmorrhagiæ*, of Cullen, characterized by pains in the back, loins, and belly, similar to those of labour, attended with a preternatural flux of blood from the vagina, or a discharge of menses, more copious than natural. He distinguishes six species:—

1. *Menorrhagia rubra;* bloody, from women neither with child nor in child-birth.

2. *Menorrhagia alba,* serous; the fluor albus. See *Leucorrhœa.*

3. *Menorrhagia vitorium,* from some local disease.

4. *Menorrhagia lochialis,* from women after delivery. See *Lochia.*

5. *Menorrhagia abortus.* See *Abortion.*

6. *Menorrhagia nabothi,* when there is a serous discharge from the vagina in pregnant women.

This disease seldom occurs before the age of puberty, and is often an attendant on pregnancy. It is in general a very dangerous disease, more particularly if it occur at the latter period, as it is then often so rapid and violent as to destroy the female in a very short time, where proper means are not soon adopted. Abortions often give rise to floodings, and at any period of pregnancy, but more usually before the fifth month than at any other time. Moles, in consequence of an imperfect conception, becoming detached, often give rise to a considerable degree of hæmorrhage.

The causes which most frequently give rise to floodings, are violent exertions of strength, sudden surprises and frights, violent fits of passion, great uneasiness of mind, uncommon longings during pregnancy, over fulness of blood, profuse evacuations, general weakness of the system, external injuries, as blows and bruises, and the death of the child, in consequence of which the placenta becomes partially or wholly detached from the uterus, leaving the mouths of the vessels of the latter, which anastomosed with those of the former, perfectly open. It is necessary to distinguish between an approaching miscarriage and a common flooding, which may be readily done by inquiring whether or not the hæmorrhage has proceeded from any evident cause, and whether it flows gently or is accompanied with unusual pains. The former usually arises from some fright, surprise, or accident, and does not flow gently and regularly but bursts out of a sudden, and again stops all at once, and also is attended with severe pains in the back and the bottom of the belly; whereas the latter is marked with no such occurrence. The further a woman is advanced in pregnancy, the greater will be the danger if floodings take place, as the mouths of the vessels are much enlarged during the last stage of pregnancy, and of course a quantity will be discharged in a short time.

The treatment must differ according to the particular causes of the disease, and according to the different states of constitution under which it occurs. The hæmorrhage is more frequently of the active kind, and requires the antiphlogistic plan to be strictly enforced, especially obviating the accumulation of heat in every way, giving cold acidulated drink, and using cold local applications; the patient must remain quiet in the horizontal posture; the diet be of the lightest and least stimulant description; and the bowels kept freely open by cooling laxatives, as the neutral salts, &c. It may be sometimes advisable in robust, plethoric females, particularly in the pregnant state, to take blood at an early period, especially where there is much pain with a hard pulse; digitalis and antimonials in nauseating doses would also be proper under such circumstances. But where the discharge is rather of a passive character, tonic and astringent medicines ought to be given: rest and the horizontal position are equally necessary, costiveness must be obviated, and cold astringent applications may be materially useful, or the escape of the blood may be prevented mechanically. In alarming cases, perhaps the most powerful internal remedy is the superacetate of lead, combined with opium; which latter is often indicated by the irritable state of the patient. A nourishing diet, with gentle exercise in a carriage, and the prudent use of the cold bath, may contribute to restore the patient, when the discharge has subsided.

ME'NSA. The second lobe of the liver was so called by the ancients.

ME'NSES. (From *mensis*, a month.) See *Menstruation.*

Menses, immoderate flow of the. See *Menorrhagia.*

Menses, interruption of. See *Amenorrhœa.*

Menses, retention of. See *Amenorrhœa.*

MENSIS PHILOSOPHICUS. A philosophical, or chemical month. According to some, it is three days and nights; others say it is ten; and there are who reckon it to be thirty or forty days.

MENSTRUATION. (*Menstruatio;* from *menses.*) From the uterus of every healthy woman who is not pregnant, or who does not give suck, there is a discharge of a red fluid, at certain periods, from the time of puberty to the approach of old age; and from the periods or returns of this discharge being monthly, it is called *Menstruation.* There are several exceptions to this definition. It is said that some women never menstruate; some menstruate while they continue to give suck; and others are said to menstruate during pregnancy; some are said to menstruate in early infancy, and others in old age; but such discharges, Dr. Denman is of opinion, may, with more propriety, be called morbid, or symptomatic; and certainly the definition is generally true.

At whatever time of life this discharge comes on, a woman is said to be at puberty: though of this state it is a consequence, and not a cause. The early or late appearance of the menses may depend upon the climate, the constitution, the delicacy or hardness of living, and upon the manners of those with whom young women converse. In Greece, and other hot countries, girls begin to menstruate at eight, nine, and ten years of age; but, advancing to the northern climates, there is a gradual protraction of the time till we come to Lapland, where women do not menstruate till they arrive at maturer age, and then in small quantities, at long intervals, and sometimes only in the summer. But, if they do not menstruate according to the genius of the country, it is said they suffer equal inconveniences as in warmer climates, where the quantity discharged is much greater, and the periods shorter. In this country, girls begin to menstruate from the fourteenth to the eighteenth year of their age, and sometimes at a later period, without any signs of disease; but if they are luxuriously educated, sleeping upon down beds, and sitting in hot rooms, menstruation usually commences at a more early period.

Many changes in the constitution and appearance of women are produced at the time of their first beginning to menstruate. Their complexion is improved, their countenance is more expressive and animated, their attitudes graceful, and their conversation more intelligent and agreeable; the tone of their voice becomes more harmonious, their whole frame, but particularly their breasts, are expanded and enlarged, and their minds are no longer engaged in childish pursuits and amusements.

Some girls begin to menstruate without any preceding indisposition; but there are generally appearances or symptoms which indicate the change which is about to take place. These are usually more severe at the first than in the succeeding periods; and they are similar to those produced by uterine irritation from other causes, as pains in the back and inferior extremities, complaints of the viscera, with various hysteric and nervous affections. These commence with the first disposition to menstruate, and continue till the discharge comes on, when they abate, or disappear, returning however with considerable violence in some women, at every period during life. The quantity of fluid discharged at each evacuation, depends upon the climate, constitution, and manner of living; but it varies in different women in the same climate, or in the same woman at different periods; in this country it amounts to about five or six ounces.

There is also a great difference in the time required for the completion of each period of menstruation. In some women the discharge returns precisely to a day, or an hour, and in others there is a variation of several days without inconvenience. In some it is finished in a few hours, and in others it continues from one to ten days; but the intermediate time, from three to six days, is most usual.

There has been an opinion, probably derived from the Jewish legislature, afterward adopted by the Arabian physicians, and credited in other countries, that the menstruous blood possessed some peculiar malignant properties. The severe regulations which have been made in some countries for the conduct of women at the time of menstruation; the expression used, Isaiah, chap. xxx. and in Ezekiel: the disposal of the blood discharged, or of any thing contaminated with it;—the complaints of women attributed to its retention :—and the effects enumerated by grave writers, indicate the most dreadful apprehensions of its baneful influence. Under peculiar circumstances of health, or states of the uterus, or in hot climates, if the evacuation be slowly made, the menstruous blood may become more acrimonious or offensive than the common mass, or any other secretion from it; but in this country and age no malignity is suspected, the menstruous woman mixes in society as at all other times, and there is no reason for thinking otherwise than that this discharge is of the most inoffensive nature.

At the approach of old age, women cease to menstruate; but the time of cessation is commonly regulated by the original early or late appearance of the menses. With those who began to menstruate at ten or twelve years of age, the discharge will often cease before they arrive at forty; but if the first appearance was protracted to sixteen or eighteen years of age, independently of disease, such women may continue to menstruate till they have passed the fiftieth, or even approach the sixtieth year of their age. But the most frequent time of the cessation of the menses in this country, is between the forty-fourth and forty-eighth year; after which women never bear children. By this constitutional regulation of the menses, the propagation of the species is in every country confined to the most vigorous part of life; and had it been otherwise, children might have become parents, and old women might have had children when they were unable to supply them with proper or sufficient nourishment. See *Catamenia.*

ME'NSTRUUM. Solvent. All liquors are so called which are used as dissolvents, or to extract the virtues of ingredients by infusion, decoction, &c. The principal *menstrua* made use of in *Pharmacy,* are water, vinous spirits, oils, acid, and alkaline liquors. Water is the *menstruum,* of all salts, of vegetable gums, and of animal jellies. Of the first it dissolves only a determinate quantity, though of one kind of salt more than of another; and being thus saturated, leaves any additional quantity of the same salt untouched. It is never saturated with the two latter, but unites readily with any proportion of them, forming, with different quantities, liquors of different consistencies. It takes up likewise, when assisted by trituration, the vegetable gummy resins, as ammoniacum and myrrh; the solutions of which, though imperfect, that is, not transparent, but turbid and of a milky hue, are nevertheless applicable to valuable purposes in medicine. Rectified

spirit of wine is the *menstruum* of the essential oils and resins of vegetables; of the pure distilled oils of animals, and of soaps, though it does not act upon the expressed oil, and fixed alkaline salt, of which soap is composed. Hence, if soap contains any superfluous quantity of either the oil or salt, it may, by means of this *menstruum,* be excellently purified therefrom. It dissolves, by the assistance of heat, volatile alkaline salts, and more readily the neutral ones, composed either of fixed alkali and the acetic acid, as the sal diureticus, or of volatile alkali and the nitric acid. Oils dissolve vegetable resins and balsams, wax, animal fats, mineral bitumens, sulphur, and certain metallic substances, particularly lead. The expressed oils are, for most of these bodies, more powerful *menstrua* than those obtained by distillation; as the former are more capable of sustaining, without injury, a strong heat, which is, in most cases, necessary to enable them to act. All acids dissolve alkaline salts, alkaline earths, and metallic substances. The different acids differ greatly in their action upon these last: one dissolving some particular metals, and another others. The vegetable acids dissolve a considerable quantity of zinc, iron, copper, and tin; and extract so much from the metallic part of antimony as to become powerfully emetic; they likewise dissolve lead, if previously calcined by fire; but more copiously if corroded by their steam. The muriatic acid dissolves zinc, iron, and copper; and though it scarcely acts on any other metallic substance in the common way of making solutions, it may nevertheless be artfully combined with them all. The corrosive sublimate and antimonial caustic of the shops, are combinations of it with the oxides of mercury and antimony, effected by applying the acid in the form of fume, to the subjects at the same time strongly heated. The nitric acid is the common *menstruum* of all metallic substances, except gold and antimony, which are soluble only in a mixture of the nitric and muriatic. The sulphuric acid easily dissolves zinc, iron, and copper; and may be made to corrode or imperfectly dissolve most of the other metals. Alkaline lixivia dissolve oils, resinous substances, and sulphur. Their power is greatly promoted by the addition of quicklime, instances of which occur in the preparation of soap and in the common caustic. Thus assisted, they reduce the flesh, bones, and other solid parts of animals, into a gelatinous matter. Solutions made in water and spirit of wine, possess the virtue of the body dissolved: while oils generally sheathe its activity, and acids and alkalies vary its quality. Hence watery and spirituous liquors are the proper *menstrua* of the native virtues of vegetable and animal matters. Most of the foregoing solutions are easily effected, by pouring the *menstruum* on the body to be dissolved, and suffering them to stand together for some time, exposed to a suitable warmth. A strong heat is generally requisite to enable oils and alkaline liquors to perform their office; nor will acids act on some metallic bodies without its assistance. The action of watery and spirituous *menstrua* is likewise expedited by a moderate heat, though the quantity which they afterward keep dissolved, is not, as some suppose, by this means increased. All that heat occasions these to take up, more than they would do in a longer time in the cold, will, when the heat ceases, subside again. The action of acids on the bodies which they dissolve, is generally accompanied with heat, effervescence, and a copious discharge of fumes. The fumes which arise during the dissolution of some metals, in the sulphuric acid, prove inflammable; hence, in the preparation of the artificial vitriols of iron and zinc, the operator ought to be careful, especially where the solution is made in a narrow-mouthed vessel, lest, by the imprudent approach of a candle, the exhaling vapour be set on fire. There is another species of solution in which the moisture of air is the *menstruum.* Fixed alkaline salts, and those of the neutral kind, composed of alkaline salts and certain vegetable acids, or of alkaline earths, and any acid except the sulphuric; and some metallic salts, on being exposed for some time to a moist air, gradually attract its humidity, and at length become liquid. Some substances, not dissoluble in water in its grosser form, as the butter of antimony, are easily liquefied by this slow action of the aërial moisture. This process is termed *Deliquation.* The cause of solution assigned by some naturalists, namely, the admission of the fine particles of one body into the pores of another, whose figure fits them for their reception, is not just, or adequate, but hypothetical and ill-presumed; since it is found that some bodies will dissolve their own quantity of others, as water does of Epsom salt, alkohol of essential oils, mercury of metals, one metal of another, &c. whereas the sum of the pores or vacuities of every body must be necessarily less than the body itself, and consequently those pores cannot receive a quantity of matter equal to the body wherein they reside.

How a *menstruum* can suspend bodies much heavier than itself, which very often happens, may be conceived by considering, that the parts of no fluids can be so easily separated, but they will a little resist or retard the descent of any heavy bodies through them; and that this resistance is, *cæteris paribus*, still proportional to the surface of the descending bodies. But the surfaces of bodies do by no means increase or decrease in the same proportion as their solidities do: for the solidity increases as the cube, but the surface only as the square of the diameter; wherefore it is plain, very small bodies will have much larger surfaces, in proportion to their solid contents, than larger bodies will, and consequently, when grown exceeding small, may easily be buoyed up in the liquor.

MENTA'GRA. (From *mentum*, the chin, and αγρα, a prey.) An eruption about the chin, forming a tenacious crust, like that on scald heads.

ME'NTHA. (From *Minthe*, the harlot who was changed into this herb.) *Hedyosmus* of the Greeks. The name of a genus of plants in the Linnæan system. Class, *Didynamia*; Order, *Gymnospermia*. Mint.

MENTHA AQUATICA. *Menthastrum; Sisymbrium menthrastrum; Mentha rotundifolia palustris.* Watermint. This plant is frequent in most meadows, marshes, and on the banks of rivers. It is less agreeable than the spearmint, and in taste bitterer and more pungent. It may be used with the same intentions as the spearmint, to which, however, it is much inferior.

MENTHA CATARIA. See *Nepeta cataria.*

MENTHA CERVINA. The systematic name of the hart's pennyroyal. *Pulegium cervinum.* This plant possesses the virtues of pennyroyal in a very great degree; but is remarkably unpleasant. It is seldom employed but by the country people, who substitute it for pennyroyal.

MENTHA CRISPA. *Colymbifera minor; Achillea ageratum.* This species of mentha has a strong and fragrant smell, its taste is warm, aromatic, and slightly bitter. In flatulence of the primæ viæ, hypochondriacal and hysterical affections, it is given with advantage.

MENTHA PIPERITA. The systematic and pharmacopœial name of peppermint. *Mentha piperitis; Mentha—floribus capitatis, foliis ovatis petiolatis, staminibus corolla brevioribus,* of Linnæus. The spontaneous growth of this plant is said to be peculiar to Britain. It has a more penetrating smell than any of the other mints; a strong pungent taste, glowing like pepper, sinking, as it were, into the tongue, and followed by a sense of coolness. The stomachic, antispasmodic, and carminative properties of peppermint, render it useful in flatulent colics, hysterical affections, retchings, and other dyspeptic symptoms, acting as a cordial, and often producing an immediate relief. Its officinal preparations are an essential oil, a simple water, and a spirit.

MENTHA PIPERITIS. See *Mentha piperita.*

MENTHA PULEGIUM. The systematic name of the pennyroyal. *Pulegium; Pulegium regale; Pulegium latifolium glechon.* Pudding-grass. *Mentha—floribus verticillatis, foliis ovatis obtusis subcrenatis, caulibus subteretibus repentibus,* of Linnæus. This plant is considered as a carminative, stomachic, and emmenagogue; and is in very common use in hysterical disorders. The officinal preparations of pennyroyal are, a simple water, a spirit, and an essential oil.

MENTHA SARACENICA. See *Tanacetum balsamita.*

MENTHA SATIVA. See *Mentha viridis.*

MENTHA SPICATA. See *Mentha viridis.*

MENTHA VIRIDIS. Spearmint. Called also *Mentha vulgaris; Mentha spicata; Mentha—spicis oblongis, foliis lanceolatis nudis serratis sessilibus, staminibus corolla longioribus,* of Linnæus. This plant grows wild in many parts of England. It is not so warm to the taste as peppermint, but has a more agreeable flavour, and is therefore preferred for culinary purposes. Its medicinal qualities are similar to those of pepper-

mint; but the different preparations of the former though more pleasant, are, perhaps, less efficacious. The officinal preparations of spearmint are an essential oil, a conserve, a simple water, and a spirit.

MENTHA'STRUM. (Diminutive of *mentha.*) See *Mentha aquatica.*

ME'NTI LEVATOR. See *Levator labii inferioris.*

ME'NTULA. (From *matah*, a staff, Heb.) The penis.

MENTULA'GRA. (From *mentula*, the penis, and αγρα, a prey.) A disorder of the penis, induced by a contraction of the erectores musculi, and causing im potence.

MENYA'NTHES. The name of a genus of plants in the Linnæan system. Class, *Pentandria*; Order, *Monogynia.*

MENYANTHES TRIFOLIATA. The systematic name of the buck-bean. *Trifolium paludosum: Trifolium aquaticum; Trifolium fibrinum; Menyanthes.* Water trefoil, or buck-bean. *Menyanthes—foliis ternatis,* of Linnæus. The whole plant is so extremely bitter, that in some countries it is used as a substitute for hops, in the preparation of malt liquor. It is sometimes employed in country places as an active eccoprotic bitter in hydropic and rheumatic affections. Cases are related of its good effects in some cutaneous diseases of the herpetic and seemingly cancerous kind.

MEPHITIC. Having a disagreeable noxious smell or vapour.

Mephitic acid. The carbonic acid.

Mephitic air. See *Nitrogen.*

MEPHI'TIS. (From *mephuhith*, a blast, Syr.) A poisonous exhalation.

MERCURIALI, GIROLAMO, was born at Torli, in Romagna, in 1530. After taking the requisite degrees, he settled as a physician in his native town; and was delegated, at the age of 32, on some public business to Pope Pius IV. at Rome. He evinced so much talent on this occasion, that he was particularly invited to remain there; which he accepted, chiefly as it enabled him to pursue his favourite studies to more advantage. He produced, in 1569, a learned and elegant work, "De Arte Gymnastica," which was many times reprinted; and the reputation of this procured him the appointment to the first medical chair at Padua. In 1573, he was called to Vienna to attend the emperor Maximilian II., and was so successful, that he returned loaded with valuable presents, and honoured with the dignities of a knight and count palatine. In 1587, he removed to Bologna, which is ascribed to a degree of self-accusation, in consequence of an error of judgment, into which he had been led, in pronouncing a disease, about which he was consulted at Venice, not contagious, whence much mischief had arisen. His reputation, however, does not appear to have materially suffered from this; and he was invited, in 1599, by the grand duke of Tuscany, to Pisa; but shortly after, a severe calculous affection prevented the execution of his duties, and he retired to his native place, where his death happened in 1606. He was a voluminous writer, and, among many other publications, edited a classified collection of the works of Hippocrates, with a learned commentary; but he was too much bigoted to ancient authority and hypothesis. He wrote on the diseases of the skin, those peculiar to women and children, on poisons, and several other subjects.

MERCURIA'LIS. (From *Mercurius*, its discoverer.)

1. The name of a genus of plants in the Linnæan system. Class, *Diœcia*; Order, *Enneandria.*

2. The pharmacopœial name of the French mercury See *Mercurialis annua.*

MERCURIALIS ANNUA. The systematic name of the French mercury. The leaves of this plant have no remarkable smell, and very little taste. It is ranked among the emollient oleraceous herbs, and is said to be gently aperient. Its principal use has been in clysters.

MERCURIALIS MONTANA. See *Mercurialis perennis.*

MERCURIALIS PERENNIS. The systematic name of dog's mercury. *Cynocrambe; Mercurialis montana sylvestris.* A poisonous plant, very common in our hedges. It produces vomiting and purging, and the person then goes to sleep, from which he does not often awake.

MERCURIALIS SYLVESTRIS. See *Mercurialis perennis.*

MERCURIUS. (So called from some supposed relation it bears to the planet of that name.) Mercury. See *Mercury.*

MERCURIUS ACETATUS. See *Hydrargyrus acetatus.*

MERCURIUS ALKALIZATUS. See *Hydrargyrum cum creta.*

MERCURIUS CALCINATUS. See *Hydrargyri oxydum rubrum.*

MERCURIUS CHEMICORUM. Quicksilver.

MERCURIUS CINNABARINUS. See *Sulphuretum hydrargyri rubrum.*

MERCURIUS CORROSIVUS. See *Hydrargyri oxymurias.*

MERCURIUS CORROSIVUS RUBER. See *Hydrargyri nitrico-oxydum.*

MERCURIUS CORROSIVUS SUBLIMATUS. See *Hydrargyri oxymurias.*

MERCURIUS DULCIS SUBLIMATUS. See *Hyrdargyri submurias.*

MERCURIUS EMETICUS FLAVUS. See *Hydrargyrus vitriolatus.*

MERCURIUS MORTIS. See *Mercurius vitæ.*

MERCURIUS PRÆCIPITATUS ALBUS. See *Hydrargyrum præcipitatum album.*

MERCURIUS PRÆCIPITATUS DULCIS. See *Hydrargyri submurias.*

MERCURIUS PRÆCIPITATUS RUBER. See *Hydrargyri nitrico-oxydum.*

MERCURY. *Hydrargyrum; Hydrargyrus ; Mercurius.* A metal found in five different states in nature. 1. Native, (*native mercury,*) adhering in small globules to the surface of cinnabar ores, or scattered through the crevices, or over the surfaces of different kinds of stones. 2. It is found united to silver, in the ore called *amalgam of silver,* or *native amalgam of silver.* This ore exhibits thin places, or grains; it sometimes crystallizes in cubes, parallelopipeda, or pyramids. Its colour is of a silver white, or gray ; its lustre is considerably metallic. 3. Combined with sulphur, it constitutes *native cinnabar,* or sulphuret of mercury. This ore is the most common. It is frequently found in veins, and sometimes crystallized in tetrahedra, or three-sided pyramids. Its colour is red. Its streak metallic. 4. Mercury oxidized, and united either to muriatic or sulphuric acid, forms the ore called *horn quicksilver,* or corneous mercury. These ores are, in general, semi-transparent, of a gray or white colour, sometimes crystallized, but more frequently in grains. 5. United to oxygen, it constitutes the ore called *native oxide of mercury.* Mercurial ores particularly abound in Spain, Hungary, China, and South America.

Properties.—Mercury, or quicksilver, is the only one of the metals that remains fluid at the ordinary temperature of the atmosphere, but when its temperature is reduced to —40 degrees below 0 on Fahrenheit's thermometer; it assumes a solid form. This is a degree of cold, however, that only occurs in high northern latitudes, and, in our climate, mercury cannot be exhibited in a solid state, but by means of artificial cold. When rendered solid, it possesses both ductility and malleability. It crystallizes in octahedra, and contracts strongly during congelation. It is divisible into very small globules. It presents a convex appearance in vessels to which it has little attraction, but is concave in those to which it more strongly adheres. It becomes electric and phosphorescent by rubbing upon glass, and by agitation in a vacuum. It is a very good conductor of caloric, of electricity, and of galvanism. The specific gravity of mercury is 13.563. Although fluid, its opacity is equal to that of any other metal, and its surface, when clean, has considerable lustre. Its colour is white, similar to silver. Exposed to the temperature of somewhat above 600° Fah. it is volatilized. When agitated in the air, especially in contact with viscous fluids, it becomes converted into a black oxide. At a temperature nearly the same as that at which it boils, it absorbs about 14 or 15 per cent. of oxygen, and then becomes changed into a red crystallizable oxide, which is spontaneously reducible by light and caloric at a higher temperature. The greater number of the acids act upon mercury, or are at least capable of combining with its oxides. It combines with sulphur by trituration, but more intimately by heat. It is acted on by the alkaline sulphurets. It combines with many of the metals; these compounds are brittle, or soft, when the mercury is in large pro-

portion. There is a slight union between mercury and phosphorus. It does not unite with carbon, or the earths.

Method of obtaining Mercury.—Mercury may be obtained pure by decomposing cinnabar, by means of iron filings. For that purpose, take two parts of red sulphuret of mercury (cinnabar), reduce it to powder, and mix it with one of iron filings, put the mixture into a stone retort, direct the neck of it into a bottle, or receiver, filled with water, and apply heat. The mercury will then be obtained in a state of purity. In this process, the sulphuret of mercury, which consists of sulphur and mercury, is heated in contact with iron, the sulphur quits the mercury and unites to the iron, and the mercury becomes disengaged ; the residue in the retort is a sulphuret of iron.

Mercury is a very useful article both in the cure of diseases and the arts. There is scarcely a disease against which some of its preparations are not exhibited ; and over the venereal disease it possesses a specific power. It is considered to have first gained repute in curing this disease, from the good effects it produced in eruptive diseases. In the times immediately following the venereal disease, practitioners only attempted to employ this remedy with timorous caution, so that, of several of their formulæ, mercury scarcely composed a fourth part, and few cures were effected. On the other hand, empirics who noticed the little efficacy of these small doses, ran into the opposite extreme, and exhibited mercury in such large quantities, and with such little care, that most of their patients became suddenly attacked with the most violent salivations, attended with dangerous consequences. From these two very opposite modes of practice, there originated such uncertainty respecting what could be expected from mercury, and such fears of the consequences which might result from its employment, that every plan was eagerly adopted which offered the least chance of cure without having recourse to this mineral. A medicine, however, so powerful, and whose salutary effects were seen by attentive practitioners, amid all its inconveniences, could not sink into oblivion. After efforts had been made to discover a substitute for it, and it was seen how little confidence those means deserved on which the highest praises had been lavished, the attempts to discover its utility were renewed. A medium was pursued, between the too timid methods of those physicians who had first administered it, and the inconsiderate boldness of the empirics. Thus the causes from which both parties failed were avoided; the character of the medicine was revived in a more durable way, and from this period its reputation has always been maintained.

It was about this epoch that mercury began to be internally given : hitherto it had only been externally employed, which was done in three manners. The first, was in the form of liniment, or ointment ; the second, as a plaster; and the third, as a fumigation. Of the three methods just described, only the first is at present much in use, and even this is very much altered. Mercurial plasters are now only used as topical discutient applications to tumours and indurations. Fumigations, as anciently managed, were liable to many objections, particularly from its not being possible to regulate the quantity of mercury to be used, and from the effect of the vapour on the organs of respiration frequently occasioning trembling, palsies, &c. Frictions with ointment have always been regarded as the most efficacious mode of administering mercury.

Mercury is carried into the constitution in the same way as other substances, either by being absorbed from the surface of the body, or that of the alimentary canal. It cannot, however, in all cases, be taken into the constitution in both ways, for sometimes the absorbents of the skin will not readily receive it; at least no effect is produced, either on the disease or constitution, from this mode of application. On the other hand, the internal absorbents will, sometimes, not take up the medicine, or, at least, no effect is produced either on the disease or constitution. In many persons, the bowels can hardly bear mercury at all ; and it should then be given in the mildest form possible, conjoined with such medicines as will lessen or correct its violent effects, although not its specific ones, on the constitution. When mercury can be thrown into the constitution with propriety, by the external method, it is preferable to the internal plan ; because the skin is not nearly so essential to life as the stomach, and is therefore in itself capable of bearing much more than the stomach. The constitution is also less injured. Many courses of mercury would kill the patient if the medicine were only given internally, because it proves hurtful to the stomach and intestines, when given in any form, or joined with the greatest correctors.

Mercury has two effects: one as a stimulus on the constitution and particular parts, the other as a specific on a diseased action of the whole body, or of parts. The latter action can only be computed by the disease disappearing.

In giving mercury in the venereal disease, the first attention should be to the quantity, and its visible effects in a given time; which, when brought to a proper pitch, are only to be kept up, and the decline of the disease to be watched; for by this we judge of the invisible or specific effects of the medicine, and know what variation in the quantity may be necessary. The visible effects of mercury affect either the whole constitution, or some parts capable of secretion. In the first, it produces universal irritability, making it more susceptible of all impressions. It quickens the pulse, increases its hardness, and occasions a kind of temporary fever. In some constitutions it operates like a poison. In some it produces a hectic fever; but such effects commonly diminish on the patient becoming accustomed to the medicine.

Mercury often produces pains like those of rheumatism, and nodes of a scrofulous nature. The quantity of mercury to be thrown in for the cure of any venereal complaint, must be proportioned to the violence of the disease. A small quantity used quickly, will have equal effects to those of a large one employed slowly; but if these effects are merely local, that is, upon the glands of the mouth, the constitution at large not being equally stimulated, the effects upon the diseased parts must be less, which may be known by the local disease not giving way in proportion to the effects of mercury on some particular part. If it be given in very small quantities, and increased gradually, so as to steal insensibly on the constitution, a vast quantity at a time may at length be thrown in, without any visible effects at all.

The constitution, or parts, are more susceptible of mercury at first than afterward.

Mercury occasionally attacks the bowels, and causes violent purging, even of blood. This effect is remedied by intermitting the use of the medicine, and exhibiting opium. At other times, it is suddenly determined to the mouth, and produces inflammation, ulceration, and an excessive flow of saliva. To obtain relief in this circumstance, purgatives, nitre, sulphur, gum-arabic, lime-water, camphor, bark, sulphuret of potassa, blisters, &c. have been advised. Pearson, however, does not place much confidence in the efficacy of such means; and, the mercury being discontinued for a time, he recommends the patient to be freely exposed to cold air, with the occasional use of cathartics, mineral acids, Peruvian bark, and the assiduous application of astringent gargles. The most material objection (says Pearson) which I foresee against the method of treatment I have recommended, is the hazard to which the patient will be exposed of having the saliva suddenly checked, and of suffering some other disease in consequence of it.

The hasty suppression of a ptyalism may be followed by serious inconveniences, as violent pains, vomiting, and general convulsions.

Cold liquids taken into the stomach, or exposure of the body to the cold air, must be guarded against during a course of mercury. Should a suppression of the ptyalism take place, from any act of indiscretion, a quick introduction of mercury should be had recourse to, with the occasional use of the warm bath.

Mercury, when it falls on the mouth, sometimes produces inflammation, which now and then terminates in mortification. The ordinary operation of mercury does not permanently injure the constitution; but, occasionally, the impairment is very material; mercury may even produce local diseases, and retard the cure of chancres, buboes, and certain effects of the lues venerea, after the poison has been destroyed. Occasionally mercury acts on the system as a poison, quite unconnected with its agency as a remedy, and neither proportionate to the inflammation of the mouth

nor actual quantity of the mineral absorbed. Pearson has termed this morbid state of the system erethismus it is characterized by great depression of strength, a sense of anxiety about the præcordia, irregular action of the heart, frequent sighing, trembling, a small, quick, and sometimes intermitting pulse, occasional vomiting, a pale contracted countenance, a sense of coldness; but the tongue is seldom furred, and neither the natural nor vital functions are much disturbed. When this effect of mercury takes place, the use of mercury should be discontinued, whatever may be the stage, extent, or violence of the venereal disease. The patient should be exposed to a dry and cool air, in such a way as not to give fatigue; in this way, the patient will often recover in ten or fourteen days. In the early stage, the erethismus may often be averted by leaving off the mercury, and giving camphor mixture with volatile alkali. Occasionally, the use of mercury brings on a peculiar eruption, which has received the names of mercurial rash, eczema mercuriale, lepra mercurialis, mercurial disease, and erythema mercuriale.

In order that mercury should act on the human body, it is necessary that it should be oxidised, or combined with an acid. The mercury contained in the unguentum hydrargyri, is an oxide. This, however, is the most simple and least combined form of all its preparations, and hence (says Mr. S. Cooper), it not only operates with more mildness on the system, but with more specific effect on the disease. Various salts of mercury operate more quickly when given internally than mercurial frictions; but few practitioners of the present day confide in the internal use of mercury alone; particularly when the venereal virus has produced effects in consequence of absorption. Rubbing in mercurial ointment is the mode of affecting the system with mercury in the present day; and, as a substitute for this mode of applying mercury, Mr. Abernethy recommends the mercurial fumigation, where the patient has not strength to rub in ointment, and whose bowels will not bear the internal exhibition of it.

The preparations of mercury now in use are,

1. Nitrico-oxydum hydrargyri.
2. Oxydum hydrargyri cinereum.
3. Oxydum hydrargyri rubrum.
4. Oxy-murias hydrargyri.
5. Submurias hydrargyri.
6. Sulphuretum hydrargyri rubrum et nigrum.
7. Hydrargyrum cum creta.
8. Hydrargyrum precipitatum album.
9. Hydrargyrum purificatum.

Mercury, dog's. See *Mercurialis.*
Mercury, English. See *Chenopodium bonus henricus*
Mercury, French. See *Mercurialis.*

MEROBA′LANUM. (From μερος, a part, and βαλανειον a bath.) A partial bath.

MEROCE′LE. (From μερος, the thigh, and κηλη, a tumour.) A femoral hernia. See *Hernia.*

ME′RON. Μηρος. The thigh.

MERRET, CHRISTOPHER, was born at Winchcombe in 1614. After graduating at Oxford, he settled in London, became a fellow of the College of Physicians, and one of the original members of the Philosophical Society, which, after the Restoration, was called the Royal Society. He appears to have had a considerable practice, and reached his 81st year. His first publication was a Collection of Acts of Parliament, &c. in proof of the exclusive Rights of the College, printed in 1660; which afforded the basis of Dr. Goodall's history: this was followed nine years after by "A Short View of the Frauds of Apothecaries," which involved him in much controversy. He published also a Catalogue of the Natural Productions of this Island, of which the botanical part is best executed; and he communicated several papers to the Royal Society.

ME′RUS. Applied to several things in the same sense as genuine, or unadulterated; as *merum vinum*, neat wine.

MERY, JOHN, was born at Vatau, in France, in 1645. His father being a surgeon, he determined upon the same profession, and went accordingly to the Hôtel Dieu at Paris, where he studied with extraordinary ardour, even passing the night in dissection in his bedroom. In 1681 he was appointed to the office of queen's surgeon; and two years after, surgeon-major to the invalids. Soon after this he was chosen to attend the Queen of Portugal, who died, however, before his arrival; and he refused very advantageous offers to detain him at that, as well as the Spanish court. He was now received into the Academy of Sciences, and shortly after sent on a secret journey to England; then chosen to attend upon the Duke of Burgundy, who was a child. But these occupations were irksome to him, and he even shunned private practice, and general society, devoting himself to the duties of the hospital of Invalids, and to the dissecting-room. In 1700, he was appointed first surgeon to the Hôtel Dieu, which gratified his utmost ambition; and he declined repeated solicitations to give lectures there on anatomy. He procured, however, the erection of a theatre for the students, where they might have more regular instruction. It was a great part of the labour of his life to form an anatomical museum, yet he did not estimate these researches too highly, and was very slow in framing, or in receiving, new theories concerning the animal economy. About the age of 75, he suddenly lost the use of his legs, after which his health declined, and he died in 1722. Besides many valuable communications to the Academy of Sciences, he published a description of the ear; Observations on Frère Jacques's Method of Cutting for the Stone, the general principle of which he approved; a tract on the Fœtal Circulation, controverting the received opinion, that part of the blood passes from the right to the left ventricle, through the foramen ovale, and even assigning it an opposite course; and physical problems, concerning the connexion of the fœtus with the mother, and its nutrition.

MESARÆ'UM. (From μεσος, the middle, and αραια, the belly.) The mesentery.

MESEMBRYA'NTHEMUM. (So called from the circumstance of its flowers expanding at midday. The name of a vast genus of plants. Class, *Icosandria*; Order, *Pentagynia*.

MESEMBRYANTHEMUM CRYSTALLINUM. The juice of this plant, in a dose of four spoonfuls every two hours, it is asserted, has removed an obstinate spasmodic affection of the neck of the bladder, which would not yield to other remedies.

MESENTERIC. *Mesentericus*. Belonging to the mesentery. See *Mesentery*.

MESENTERIC ARTERY. *Arteria mesenterica*. Two branches of the aorta in the abdomen are so called. The superior mesenteric is the second branch; it is distributed upon the mesentery, and gives off the superior or right colic artery. The inferior mesenteric is the fifth branch of the aorta; it sends off the internal hæmorrhoidal.

MESENTERIC GLANDS. *Glandulæ mesentericæ*. These are conglobate, and are situated here and there in the cellular membrane of the mesentery. The chyle from the intestines passes through these glands to the thoracic duct.

MESENTERIC NERVES. *Nervorum plexus mesentericus*. The superior, middle, and lower mesenteric plexuses of nerves are formed by the branches of the great intercostal nerves.

MESENTERIC VEINS. *Venæ mesentericæ*. They all run into one trunk, that evacuates its blood into the vena portæ. See *Vena portæ*.

MESENTERI'TIS. (From μεσεντερον, the mesentery.) An inflammation of the mesentery. See *Peritonitis*.

ME'SENTERY. (*Mesenterium*; from μεσος, the middle, and εντερον, an intestine.) A membrane in the cavity of the abdomen attached to the vertebræ of the loins, and to which the intestines adhere. It is formed of a duplicature of the peritonæum, and contains within it adipose membrane, lacteals, lymphatics, lacteal glands, mesenteric arteries, veins, and nerves. Its use is to sustain the intestines in such a manner that they possess both mobility and firmness; to support and conduct with safety the blood-vessels, lacteals, and nerves; to fix the glands, and give an external coat to the intestines.

It consists of three parts: one uniting the small intestines, which receives the proper name of mesentery; another connecting the colon, termed mesocolon; and a third attached to the rectum, termed mesorectum.

MESERAIC. The same as mesenteric.

MESE'RION. See *Daphne mezereum*.

MESE'RE. A disorder of the liver, mentioned by Avicenna, accompanied with a sense of heaviness, tumour, inflammation, pungent pain, and blackness of the tongue.

MESOCO'LON. (From μεσος, the middle, and κωλον, the colon.) The portion of the mesentery to which the colon is attached. The mesentery and mesocolon are the most important of all the productions of the peritonæum. In the pelvis, the peritonæum spreads itself shortly before the rectum. But where that intestine becomes loose, and forms the semilunar curve, the peritonæum there rises considerably from the middle iliac vessels, and region of the psoas muscle, double, and with a figure adapted for receiving the bol low colon. But above, on the left side, the colon is connected with almost no intermediate loose production to the peritonæum, spread upon the psoas muscle, as high as the spleen, where this part of the peritonæum, which gave a coat to the colon, being extended under the spleen, receives and sustains that viscus in a hollow superior recess.

Afterward the peritonæum, from the left kidney from the interval between the kidneys, from the large vessels, and from the right kidney, emerges forwards under the pancreas, and forms a broad and sufficiently long continuous production, called the transverse mesocolon, which, like a partition, divides the upper part of the abdomen, containing the stomach, liver, spleen, and pancreas, from the lower part. The lower plate of this transverse production is continued singly from the right mesocolon to the left, and serves as an external coat to a pretty large portion of the liver, and descending part of the duodenum. But the upper plate, less simple in the course, departs from the lumbar peritonæum at the kidney, and region of the vena cava, farther to the right than the duodenum, to which it gives an external membrane, not quite to the valve of the pylorus; and beyond this intestine, and beyond the colon, it is joined with the lower plate, so that a large part of the duodenum lies within the cavity of the mesocolon. Afterward, in the region of the liver, the mesocolon is inflected, and descending over the kidney of the same side much shorter, it includes the right of the colon, as far as the intestinum cæcum, which rests upon the iliac muscle and the appendix, which is provided with a peculiar long curved mesentery. There the mesocolon terminates, almost at the bifurcation of the aorta.

The whole of the mesocolon and of the mesentery is hollow, so that the air may be forced in between its two laminæ, in such a manner as to expand them into a bag. At the place where it sustains the colon, and also from part of the intestinum rectum, the mesocolon, continuous with the outer membrane of the intestine, forms itself into small slender bags, resembling the omentum, for the most part in pairs, with their loose extremities thicker and bifid, and capable of admitting air blown in between the plates of the mesocolon.

MESOCRA'NIUM. (From μεσος, the middle, and κρανιον, the skull.) The crown of the head, or vertex.

MESOGA'STRIUM. (From μεσος, the middle, and γαςηρ, the stomach.) The concave part of the stomach, which attaches itself to the adjacent parts.

MESOGLO'SSUS. (From μεσος, the middle, and γλωσσα, the tongue.) A muscle inserted in the middle of the tongue.

MESOME'RA. (From μεσος, the middle, and μηρος, the thigh.) The parts between the thighs.

MESOMPHALIUM. (From μεσος, the middle, and ομφαλος, the navel.) The middle of the navel.

MESO'PHRYUM. (From μεσος, the middle, and οφρυα, the eyebrows.) The part between the eyebrows.

MESOPLEU'RUM. (From μεσος, the middle, and πλευρον, a rib.) The space or muscles between the ribs.

MESORE'CTUM. (From μεσος, the middle, and rectum, the straight gut.) The portion of peritonæum which connects the rectum of the pelvis.

MESO'THENAR. (From μεσος, the middle, and θεναρ, the palm of the hand.) The muscle situated in the middle of the palm of the hand.

MESOTICA. (From μεσος, *medius*.) The name of an order of diseases in the class *Eccritica*, in Good's Nosology. Diseases affecting the parenchyma. Its genera are the following: *Polysarcia*; *Emphyma*; *Parostia*; *Cyrtosis*; *Osthexia*.

MESOTYPE. Prismatic zeolite. A species of the genus zeolite.

ME'SPILUS. (Οτι εν τω μεσω πιλος, because it

has a cap or crown in the middle of it.) 1. The name of a genus of plants in the Linnæan system. Class, *Icosandria*; Order, *Pentagynia*.

2. The pharmacopœial name of the medlar. See *Mespilus germanica.*

MESPILUS GERMANICA. The systematic name of the medlar-tree. This fruit, and also its seeds, have been used medicinally. The immature fruit is serviceable in checking diarrhœas; and the seeds were formerly esteemed in allaying the pain attendant on nephritic diseases.

MESUE, one of the early physicians among the Arabians, was born in the province of Khorasan, and flourished in the beginning of the ninth century. His father was an apothecary at Nisaboar. He was educated in the profession of physic by Gabriel, the son of George Backtishua, and through his favour was appointed physician to the hospital of his native city. Although a Christian, he was in great favour with several successive Caliphs, being reputed the ablest scholar and physician of his age. When Haroun al Raschid appointed his son viceroy of Khorasan, Mesue was nominated his body physician, and was placed by him at the head of a college of learned men, which he instituted there. When Almammon succeeded to the throne in 813, he brought Mesue to Bagdad, and made him a professor of medicine there, as well as superintendent of the great hospital, which offices he filled a great number of years. He was also employed in transferring the science of the Greeks to his own country, by translating their works. He is supposed by Freind to have written in the Syriac tongue. He was author of some works, which are cited by Rhazes, and others, but appear to have perished; for those now extant in his name do not correspond with these citations, nor with the character given of them by Haly Abbas, besides that Rhazes is quoted in them, who lived long after Mesue: they probably belonged to another physician of the same name, who is mentioned by Leo Africanus, and died in the beginning of the eleventh century.

META′BASIS. (From μεταβαινω, to digress.) *Metabole.* A change of remedy, of practice, or disease; or any change from one thing to another, either in the curative indications, or the symptoms of a distemper.

META′BOLE. See *Metabasis.*

METACARPAL. Belonging to the metacarpus.

METACARPAL BONES. The five longitudinal bones that are situated between the wrist and the fingers; they are distinguished into the metacarpal bone of the thumb, forefinger, &c.

META CA′RPUS. (From μετα, after, and καρπος, the wrist.) *Metacarpium.* That part of the hand which is between the wrist and the fingers.

METACA′RPEUS. A muscle of the carpus. See *Adductor metacarpi minimi digiti manus.*

METACERA′SMA. (From μετα, after, and κεραννυμι, to mix.) *Cerasma.* A mixture tempered with any additional substance.

METACHEIRI′XIS. (From μεταχειριζω, to perform by the hand.) Surgery, or any manual operation.

METACHORE′SIS. (From μεταχωρεω, to digress.) The translation of a disease from one part to another.

METACINE′MA. (From μετα, and κινεω, to remove.) A distortion of the pupil of the eye.

METACO′NDYLUS. (From μετα, after, and κονδυλος, a knuckle.) The last joint of a finger, which contains the nail.

META′LLAGE. (From μεταλλατ7ω, to change. A change in the state or treatment of a disease.

META′LLURGIA. (From μεταλλον, a metal, and εργον, work, labour.) That part of chemistry which concerns the operations of metals.

METALS. The most numerous class of undecompounded chemical bodies, distinguished by the following general characters:—

1. They possess a peculiar lustre, which continues in the streak, and in their smallest fragments.

2. They are fusible by heat; and in fusion retain their lustre and opacity.

3. They are all, except selenium, excellent conductors, both of electricity and caloric.

4. Many of them may be extended under the hammer, and are called malleable; or under the rolling press, and are called laminable; or drawn into wire, and are called ductile. This capability of extension depends, in some measure, on a tenacity peculiar to the metals, and which exists in the different species with very different degrees of force.

5. When their saline combinations are electrized, the metals separate at the resino-electric or negative pole.

6. When exposed to the action of oxygen, chlorine, or iodine, at an elevated temperature, they generally take fire; and, combining with one or other of these three elementary dissolvents in definite proportions, are converted into earthy or saline-looking bodies, devoid of metallic lustre and ductility, called oxides, chlorides or iodides.

7. They are capable of combining in their melted state with each other, in almost every proportion, constituting the important order of metallic alloys; in which the characteristic lustre and tenacity are preserved.

8. From this brilliancy and opacity conjointly, they reflect the greater part of the light which falls on their surface, and hence form excellent mirrors.

9. Most of them combine in definite proportions with sulphur and phosphorus, forming bodies frequently of a semi-metallic aspect: and others unite with hydrogen, carbon, and boron, giving rise to peculiar gaseous or solid compounds.

10. Many of the metals are capable of assuming, by particular management, crystalline forms; which are, for the most part, either cubes or octohedrons.

The relations of the metals of the various objects of chemistry, are so complex and diversified, as to render their classification a task of peculiar difficulty.

The first 12 are malleable; and so are the 31st and 32d, in their congealed state.

The first 16 yield oxides, which are neutral salifiable bases.

The metals 17, 18, 19, 20, 21, 22, and 23, are acidifiable by combination with oxygen. Of the oxides of the rest, up to the 30th, little is known. The remaining metals form, with oxygen, the alkaline and earthy bases.

All the metals are found in the bowels of the earth, though sometimes they are on the surface. They are met with in different combinations with other matters, such as sulphur, oxygen, and acids; particularly with the carbonic, muriatic, sulphuric, and phosphoric acids. They are also found combined with each other, and sometimes, though rarely, in a pure metallic state, distinguishable by the naked eye.

In their different states of combination, they are said to be mineralized, and are called *ores*. The ores of metals are, for the most part, found in nature in mountainous districts; and always in such as form a continued chain. There are mountains which consist entirely of iron ore, but, in general, the metallic part of a mountain bears a very inconsiderable proportion to its bulk. Ores are also met with in the cavities or crevices of rocks, forming what are termed *veins*, which are more easily discovered in these situations than when they lie level in plains.

The metallic matter of ores is very generally incrusted, and intermingled with some earthy substance, different from the rock in which the vein is situated; which is termed its *matrix*. This, however, must not be confounded with the mineralizing substance with which the metal is combined, such as sulphur, &c

General Table of the Metals.

NAMES.	Sp. gr.	Precipitants.	Colour of Precipitates by			
			Ferroprussiate of potassa	Infusion of galls.	Hydrosulphurets.	Sulphuretted hydrogen.
1 Plantinum	21.47	Mur. Ammon.	0	0		Black met. powd.
2 Gold	19.30	Sulph. iron / Nitr. mercury	Yellowish white	Green; met.	Yellow	Yellow
3 Silver	10.45	Common salt	White	Yellow-brown	Black	Black
4 Palladium	11 8	Prus. mercury	Deep orange		Blackish-brown	Black-brown
5 Mercury	13.6	Common salt / Heat	White passing to yellow	Orange-yellow	Brownish-black	Black
6 Copper	8.9	Iron	Red brown	Brown	Black	Do.
7 Iron	7.7	Succin. soda with perox.	Blue, or white passing to blue	Protox. 0. Perox. black	Black	0
8 Tin	7.29	Cor. sublim.	White	0	Protox. black Perox. yellow	Brown
9 Lead	11.35	Sulph. soda	Do.	White	Black	Black
10 Nickel	8.4	Sulph. potassa ?	Do.	Gray-white	Do.	
11 Cadmium	8.6	Zinc	Do.	0	0	0
12 Zinc	6.9	Alk. carbonates	Do.	0	Orange-yellow	Orange-yellow
13 Bismuth	9.88	Water	Do.	Yellow	White	Yellowish-white
14 Antimony	6.70	Water / Zinc	With dilute solutions white	White from water	Black-brown	Black-brown
15 Manganese	8.	Tatr. pot.	White	0	Orange	Orange
16 Cobalt	8.6	Alk. carbonates	Brown-yellow	Yellow-white	White	Milkiness
17 Tellurium	6.115	Water / Antimony	0	Yellow	Black Blackish	0
18 Arsenic	8.35 ? / 5.76 ?	Nitr. lead	White		Yellow	Yellow
19 Chromium	5.90	Do. ?	Green	Brown	Green	
20 Molybdenum	8.6	Do. ?	Brown	Deep brown		Brown
21 Tungsten	17.4	Mur. lime ?	Dilute acids			
22 Columbium	5.6 ?	Zinc or inf. galls	Olive	Orange	Chocolate	
23 Selenium	4.3 ?	Iron / Sulphite amm.				
24 Osmium	?	Mercury		Purple passing to deep blue		
25 Rhodium	10.65	Zinc ?	0		0	
26 Iridium	18.68	Do. ?	0	0		
27 Uranium	9.0	Ferropr. pot.	Brown-red	Chocolate	Brown-yellow	0
28 Titanium	?	Inf. galls.	Grass-green	Red-brown	Grass-green	0
29 Cerium	?	Oxal. amm.	Milk-white	0	White	0
30 Potassium	0.865	Mur. plat. / Tart. acid.	0	0	0	0
31 Sodium	0.972					
32 Lithium						
33 Calcium						
34 Barium						
35 Strontium						
36 Magnesium						
37 Yttrium						
38 Glucinum						
39 Aluminum						
40 Thorinum						
41 Zirconium						
42 Silicium						

METAMORPHO'PSIA. (From μεταμορφωσις, a change, and οψις, sight.) *Visus defiguratus.* Disfigured vision. It is a defect in vision, by which persons perceive objects changed in their figures. The species are,

1. *Metamorphopsia acuta,* when objects appear much larger than their size.

2. *Metamorphopsia diminuta,* when objects appear diminished in size, arising from the same causes as the former.

3. *Metamorphopsia mutans,* when objects seem to be in motion: to the vertiginous and intoxicated persons, every thing seems to stagger.

4. *Metamorphopsia tortuosa seu flexuosa,* when objects appear tortuous, or bending.

5. *Metamorphopsia inversa,* when all objects appear inverted.

6. *Metamorphopsia imaginaria,* is the vision of a thing not present, as may be observed in the delirious, and in maniacs.

7. *Metamorphopsia from a remaining impression:* it happens to those who attentively examine objects, particularly in a great light, for some time after to perceive the impression.

METAPE'DIUM. (From μετα, after, and πους, the foot.) The metatarsus.

META'PHRENUM. (From μετα, after, and φρενες, the diaphragm.) That part of the back which is behind the diaphragm.

METAPOROPOIE'SIS. (From μετα, πορος, a duct, and ποιεω, to make.) A change in the pores of the body.

METAPTO'SIS. (From μεταπιπτω, to digress.) A change from one disease to another.

META'STASIS. (From μεθιστημι, to change, to translate.) The translation of a disease from one place to another.

METASY'NCRICIS. (From μετασυγκρινω, to transmute.) Any change of constitution.

METATARSAL. Belonging to the metatarsus.

METATARSAL BONES. The five longitudinal bones between the tarsus and the toes; they are distinguished into the metatarsal bone of the great-toe, fore-toe, &c.

META'RSUS. (From μετα, after, and ταρσος, the tarsus.) That part of the foot between the tarsus and toes.

METE'LLA NUX. See *Strychnos nux vomica.*

METEORISMUS. (From μετεωρος, a vapour.) 1. A dropsy of the belly, accompanied by a considerable distention from wind in the bowels.

2. A tympanitic state of the abdomen, that takes place in acute diseases suddenly and unexpectedly, as does the appearance of a meteor in the heavens.

METEOROLITE. Meteoric stone. A peculiar solid compound of earthy and metallic matters, of singular aspect and composition, which occasionally descends from the atmosphere; usually from the bosom of a luminous meteor.

METEO'ROS. (Μετεωρος; from μεῖα, and αειρω, to elevate.) Elevated, suspended, erect, sublime, tumid. Galen expounds pains of this sort, as being those which affect the peritonæum, or other more superficial parts of the body: these are opposed to the more deep seated ones.

METHE'GLIN. A drink prepared from honey by fermentation. It is often confounded with mead. It is made in the following way. Honey, one hundred weight; boiling water, enough to fill a thirty-two gallon cask, or half a hogshead; stir it well for a day or two, then add yeast and ferment. Some boil the honey in water with one ounce of hops to each gallon, for an hour or two, but this boiling hinders its fermentation.

METHEMERI'NUS. (From μετα, and ημερα, a day.) A quotidian fever.

METHO'DIC MEDICINE. That practice which was conducted by rules, such as are taught by Galen and his followers, in opposition to the empirical practice

ME'THODUS. (From μετα, and οδος, a way.) The method, or ratio, by which any operation or cure is conducted.

METO'PION. Μετωπιον. 1. American sumach, a species of *Rhus*.

2. A name of the bitter almond.

3. An oil, or an ointment, made by Dioscorides, which was thus called because it had galbanum in it, which was collected from a plant called *Metopium*.

METO'PIUM. Μετωπιον. An ointment made of galbanum.

METO'PUM. (From μετα, after, and ωψ, the eye.) The forehead.

METO'SIS. A kind of amaurosis, from an excess of short-sightedness.

ME'TRA. (From μητηρ, a mother.) The womb. See *Uterus*.

METRE'NCHYTA. (From μητρα, the womb, and εγχυω, to pour into.) Injections into the womb.

METRE'NCHYTES. (From μητρα, the womb, and εγχυω, to pour in.) A syringe to inject fluids into the womb.

METRI'TIS. (From μητρα, the womb.) Inflammation of the womb. See *Hysteritis*.

METROCE'LIS. (*Metrocelis, idis.* f.; from μητηρ, a mother, and κηλις, a blemish.) A mole, or mark, impressed upon the child by the mother's imagination.

METROMA'NIA. A rage for reciting verses. In the Acta Societatis Medicæ Havniensis, published 1779, is an account of a tertian attended with remarkable symptoms; one of which was the *metro-mania*, by which the patient spoke verses extempore, having never before had the least taste for poetry ; when the fit was off, the patient became stupid, and remained so till the return of the paroxysm, when the poetical powers returned again.

METROPTO'SIS. (From μητρα, the uterus, and πιπ7ω, to fall down.) *Prolapsus uteri.* The descent of the uterus through the vagina.

METRORRHA'GIA. (From μητρα, the womb, and ρηγνυμι, to break out.) An excessive discharge from the womb.

ME'U. See *Æthusa meum*.

ME'UM. (From μειων, less: so called, according to Minshew, from its diminutive size.) See *Æthusa meum*.

MEUM ATHAMANTICUM. See *Æthusa meum*.

Mexico seed. See *Ricinus*.

Mexico tea. See *Chenopodium ambrosioides*.

MEZEREON. See *Daphne mezereum*.

MEZE'REUM. (A word of some barbarous dialect.) Mezereon. See *Daphne mezereum*.

MEZEREUM ACETATUM. Thin slices of the bark of fresh mezereon root are to be steeped for twenty-four hours in common vinegar. Some practitioners direct this application to issues, when a discharge from them cannot be encouraged by the common means. It generally answers this purpose very effectually in the course of one night, the pea being removed, and a small portion of the bark applied over the opening. See *Daphne gnidium*.

MIA'SMA. (*Miasma, tis.* n.; from μιαινω, to infect.) Miasma is a Greek word, importing pollution, corruption, or defilement generally ; and contagion a Latin word, importing the application of such miasm or corruption to the body by the medium of touch. There is, therefore, says Dr. Good, neither parallelism nor antagonism, in their respective significations ; there is nothing that necessarily connects them either disjunctively, or conjunctively. Both equally apply to the animal and vegetable worlds, or to any source whatever of defilement or touch ; and either may be predicated of the other ; for we may speak correctly of the miasm of contagion, or of contagion produced by miasm. See *Contagion*.

MICA. A species of mineral which Professor Jameson subdivides into ten sub-species, viz. mica, pinite, lepidolite, chlorite, green earth, talc, nacrite, potstone, steatite, and figure stone.

Mica comes in abundance from Siberia, where it is used for window glass.

MICROCO'SMIC BEZOAR. See *Calculus*.

MICROCOSMIC SALT. A triple salt of soda, ammonia, and phosphoric acid obtained from urine, and much used in assays with the blow-pipe.

MICROLEUCONYMPHÆ'A. (From μικρος, small, λευκος,

white, and νυμφαια, the water-lily.) The small white water-lily.

MICRONYMPHÆ'A. (From μικρος, small, and νυμφαια, the water-lily.) The smaller water-lily.

MICRO'RCHIS. (From μικρος, small, and ορχις, a testicle.) One whose testicles are unusually small.

MICROSPHY'XIA. (From μικρος, small, and σφυξις, the pulse.) A debility and smallness of the pulse.

[MIDDLETON, PETER, M.D. This gentleman, a native of Scotland, flourished in the profession of medicine in the city of New-York about the middle of the last century, and was one of the very few medical men of this country, who, at that early period, were distinguished equally for various and profound learning and great professional talents. He, with Dr. J Bard, in 1750, dissected a human body, and injected the blood-vessels, which was the first attempt of the kind to be found on medical record in America, and in 1767 he proffered his services for carrying into effect the establishment of a new medical school in the city of New-York, of which he was appointed first professor of Physiology and Pathology, and afterward was the instructer in Materia Medica.

In his profession he was learned and liberal, and his whole life was a practical illustration of his doctrines. He wrote an able letter on the croup, addressed to Dr. Richard Bayley, which was published in the Medical Repository, Volume IX. He was also author of a Medical Discourse, or Historical Inquiries into the ancient and present state of Medicine, the substance of which was delivered at the opening of the Medical School of New-York ; it was published in 1769, and is an honourable specimen of his talents and attainments.

This highly respectable man, for a considerable period, struggled with an impaired state of health, induced by the toils of a laborious practice, and after enduring the severest bodily suffering for more than ten months, from a stricture and scirrhous state of the pylorus, died in the city of New-York, in 1781."— *Thach. Med. Biog.* A.]

MIDRIFF. See *Diaphragma*.

MIEMITE. A mineral found at Miemo in Tuscany, and other places. There are two kinds, the granular and prismatic.

MI'GMA. (From μιγνυω, to mix.) A confection, or ointment.

MIGRA'NA. A corruption of hemicrania.

MILFOIL. See *Achillea millefolium*.

MILIA'RIA. (From *milium*, millet: so called because the small vesicles upon the skin resemble millet-seed.) Miliary fever. A genus of disease in the class *Pyrexiæ*, and order *Exanthemata*, of Cullen, characterized by synochus ; cold stage considerable: hot stage attended with anxiety and frequent sighing ; perspiration of a strong and peculiar smell ; eruption, preceded by a sense of pricking, first on the neck and breast, of small red pimples, which in two days become white vesicles, desquamate, and are succeeded by fresh pimples. Miliary fever has been observed to affect both sexes, and persons of all ages and constitutions: but females, of a delicate habit, are most liable to it, particularly in child-bed. Moist variable weather is most favourable to its appearance, and it occurs most usually in the spring and autumn. It is by some said to be a contagious disease, and has been known to prevail epidemically.

Very violent symptoms, such as coma, delirium, and convulsive fits, now and then attend miliary fever, in which case it is apt to prove fatal. A numerous eruption indicates more danger than a scanty one. The eruption being steady is to be considered as more favourable than its frequently disappearing and coming out again, and it is more favourable when the places covered with the eruption appear swelled and stretched than when they remain flaccid. According to the severity of the symptoms, and depression of spirits, is the danger greater. See also *Sudamina*.

MILI'OLUM. (Diminutive of *milium*, millet.) A small tumour on the eyelids, resembling in size a millet-seed.

MILITA'RIS. (From *miles*, a soldier: so called from its efficacy in curing fresh wounds.) See *Achillea millefolium*.

MILITARIS HERBA. See *Achillea millefolium*.

MI'LIUM. (From *mille*, a thousand. An ancien name for a sort of corn or grass, remarkable for the abundance of its seeds.) The name of a genus of plants in the Linnæan system. Class, *Triandria.* Order, *Digynia.*

2. (From *milium,* a millet-seed.) A very white and hard tubercle, in size and colour resembling a millet-seed. Its seat is immediately under the cuticle, so that, when pressed, the contents escape appearing of an atheromatous nature.

MILIUM SOLIS. See *Lithospermum.*

MILK. *Lac.* A fluid secreted by peculiar glands, and designed to nourish animals in the early part of their life. It is of an opaque white colour, a mild saccharine taste, and a slightly aromatic smell. It is separated immediately from the blood, in the breasts or udders of female animals. Man, quadrupeds, and cetaceous animals, are the only creatures which afford milk. All other animals are destitute of the organs which secrete this fluid. Milk differs greatly in the several animals.

The following are the general *Properties* of animal and human milk:—

Milk separates spontaneously into *cream, cheese,* and *serum of milk ;* and that sooner in a warm situation than in a cold one. In a greater temperature than that of the air, it acesces and coagulates, but more easily and quicker by the addition of acid salts, or coagulating plants. *Lime-water* coagulates milk imperfectly. It is not coagulated by pure *alkali ;* which indeed dissolves its caseous part. With carbonated *alkali* the caseous and cremoraceous parts of milk are changed into a liquid soap, which separates in the form of white flakes; such milk, by boiling, is changed into a yellow and then into a brown colour. Milk, distilled to dryness, gives out an insipid water, and leaves a whitish brown extract, called the *extract of milk ;* which, dissolved in water, makes a milk of less value. Milk fresh drawn, and often agitated in a warm place, by degrees goes into the vinous fermentation, so that alkohol may be drawn over by distillation, which is called *spirit of milk.* It succeeds quicker if yest be added to the milk. Mares' milk, as it contains the greatest quantity of the sugar of milk, is best calculated for vinous fermentation.

The *Principles* of milk, or its integral parts, are,

1. The *Aroma,* or odorous volatile principle, which flies off from fresh-drawn milk in the form of visible vapour.

2. *Water,* which constitutes the greatest part of milk. From one pound eleven ounces of water may be extracted by distillation. This water, with the sugar of milk, forms the *serum of the milk.*

3. *Bland oil,* which, from its lightness, swims on the surface of milk after standing, and forms the *cream of milk.*

4. *Cheese,* separated by coagulating milk, falls to the bottom of the vessel, and is the animal gluten.

5. *Sugar,* obtained from the serum of milk by evaporation. It unites the caseous and butyraceous part with the water of the milk.

6. Some *neutral salts,* as the muriate of potassa and muriate of lime, which are accidental, not being found at all times, nor in every milk. These principles of milk differ widely in respect to quantity and quality, according to the diversity of the animals.

The *aroma* of the milk is of so different an odour, that persons accustomed to the smell, and those whose olfactory nerves are very sensible, can easily distinguish whether milk be that of the cow, goat, mare, ass, or human. The same may be said of the serum of the milk, which is properly the seat of the aroma. The *serum* of milk is thicker and more copious in the milk of the sheep and goat, than in that of the ass, mare, or human milk. The *butter* of goats' and cows' milk is easily separated, and will not again unite itself with the butter-milk. Sheep's butter is soft, and not of the consistence of that obtained from the cow and goat. Asses', mares', and human butter, can only be separated in the form of cream ; which cream, by the assistance of heat, is with ease again united to the milk from which it is separated. The *cheese* of cows' and goats' milk is solid and elastic, that from asses and mares soft, and that from sheep's milk almost as soft as gluten. It is never separated spontaneously from the milk of a woman but only by art, and is wholly fluid. The *serum* abounds most in human, asses', and mares' milk. The milk of the cow and goat contain ess, and that of the sheep least of all. The *sugar* of

milk is in the greatest quantity in the mares' and asses', and somewhat less in the human milk.

When milk is left to spontaneous decomposition, at a due temperature, it is found to be capable of passing through the vinous, acetous, and putrefactive fermentations. It appears, however, probably on account of the small quantity of alkohol it affords, that the vinous fermentation lasts a very short time, and can scarcely be made to take place in every part of the fluid at once, by the addition of any ferment. This seems to be the reason why the Tartars, who make a fermented liquor, or wine, from mares' milk, called *koumiss,* succeed by using large quantities at a time, and agitating it very frequently. They add, as a ferment, a sixth part of water, and an eighth part of the sourest cow's milk they can get, or a smaller portion of koumiss already prepared: cover the vessel with a thick cloth, and let it stand in a moderate warmth for 24 hours: then beat it with a stick, to mix the thicker and thinner parts, which have separated ; let it stand again 24 hours, in a high narrow vessel, and repeat the heating, till the liquor is perfectly homogeneous. This liquor will keep some months, in close vessels, and a cold place ; but must be well mixed by beating, or shaking, every time it is used. They sometimes extract a spirit from it by distillation. The Arabs prepare a similar liquor by the name of *leban,* and the Turks by that of *yaourt.* Eaton informs us, that, when properly prepared, it may be left to stand till it becomes quite dry : and in this state it is kept in bags, and mixed with water when wanted for use.

The saccharine substance, upon which the fermenting property of milk depends, is held in solution by the whey, which remains after the separation of the curd in making cheese. This is separated by evaporation in the large way, for pharmaceutical purposes, in various parts of Switzerland. When the whey has been evaporated by heat, to the consistence of honey, it is poured into proper moulds, and exposed to dry in the sun. If this crude sugar of milk be dissolved in water, clarified with whites of eggs, and evaporated to the consistence of syrup, white crystals, in the form of rhomboidal parallelopipedons, are obtained.

Sugar of milk has a faint saccharine taste, and is soluble in three or four parts of water. It yields by distillation the same products that other sugars do, only in somewhat different proportions. It is remarkable, however, that the empyreumatic oil has a smell resembling flowers of benzoin. It contains an acid frequently called the *saccolactic ;* but as it is common to all mucilaginous substances, it is more generally termed mucic. See *Mucic acid.*

Milk, according to Berzelius, consists of,

Water	928.75
Curd, with a little cream	28.00
Sugar of milk	35.00
Muriate of potassa	1.70
Phosphate of potassa	0.25
Lactic acid, acetate of potassa, with a trace of lactate of iron	6.00
Earthy phosphates	0.30
	1000.00

MILK, 'ASSES'. Asses' milk has a very strong resemblance to human milk in colour, smell, and consistence. When left at rest for a sufficient time, a cream forms upon its surface, but by no means in such abundance as on women's milk. Asses' milk differs from cows' milk, in its cream being less abundant and more insipid ; in its containing less curd ; and in its possessing a greater proportion of sugar.

MILK, COWS'. The milk of women, mares, and asses, nearly agree in their qualities ; that of cows goats, and sheep, possess properties rather different Of these, cows' milk approaches nearest to that yielded by the female breast, but differs very much in respect to the aroma ; it contains a larger proportion of cream and cheese, and less serum than human milk ; also less sugar than mares' and asses' milk.

Cows' milk forms a very essential part of human sustenance, being adapted to every state and age of the body ; but particularly to infants, after being weaned.

MILK, EWES'. This resembles almost precisely that of the cow ; its cream, however, is more abundant and yields a butter not so consistent as cows' milk butter. It makes excellent cheese.

MILK, GOATS'. It resembles cows', except in its greater consistence : like that milk, it throws up abundance of cream, from which butter is easily obtained.

MILK, HUMAN. The white, sweetish fluid, secreted by the glandular fabric of the breasts of women. The *secretory organ* is constituted by the great conglomerate glands situated in the fat of both breasts, above the musculus pectoralis major. From each acinus, composing a mammary gland, there arises a radical of a *lactiferous* or *galactiferous* duct. All these canals, gradually converging, are terminated without anastomosis, in the papillæ of the breasts, by many orifices, which, upon pressure, pour forth milk. The smell of fresh-drawn milk is peculiar, animal, fatuous, and not disagreeable. Its taste sweetish, soft, bland, agreeable. The specific gravity is greater than that of water, but it is lighter than blood; hence it swims on it. Its colour is white and opaque. In consistence it is oily and aqueous. A drop, put on the nail, flows slowly down, if the milk be good.

Time of Secretion.—The milk most frequently begins to be secreted in the last months of pregnancy; but, on the third day after delivery, a serous milk, called *Colostrum*, is separated; and at length pure milk is secreted very copiously into the breasts, that, from its abundance often spontaneously drops from the nipples.

If the secretion of milk be daily promoted by suckling an infant, it often continues many years, unless a fresh pregnancy supervene. The quantity usually secreted within twenty-four hours, by nurses, is various, according as the nourishment may be more or less chylous. It appears that not more than two pounds of milk are obtained from five or six pounds of meat. But there have been known nurses who have given from their breasts two, or even more than three pounds, in addition to that which their child has sucked. That the origin of the milk is derived from chyle carried with the blood of the mammary arteries into the glandular fabric of the breasts, is evident from its more copious secretion a little after meals; its diminished secretion from fasting; from the smell and taste of food or medicines in the secreted milk; and, lastly, from its occasional spontaneous *acescence*; for humours perfectly animal become putrid.

The *milk of a woman* differs: 1. In respect to *food*. The milk of a woman who suckles, living upon vegeto-animal food, never acesces nor coagulates spontaneously, although exposed for many weeks to the heat of a furnace. But it evaporates gradually in an open vessel, and the last drop continues thin, sweet, and bland. The reason appears to be, that the caseous and cremoraceous parts cohere together by means of the sugar, more intimately than in the milk of animals, and do not so easily separate; hence its acescence is prevented. It does *acesce*, if mixed or boiled with vinegar, juice of lemons, supertartrate of potassa, dilute sulphuric acid, or with the human stomach. It is *coagulated* by the acid of salt, or nitre, and by an acid gastric juice of the infant; for infants often vomit up the coagulated milk of the nurse. The milk of a suckling woman, who lives upon vegetable food only, like cows' milk, easily and of its own accord acesces, and is acted upon by all coagulating substances like the milk of animals. 2. In respect *of the time of digestion*. During the first hours of digestion, the chyle is crude, and the milk less subacted; but towards the twelfth hour after eating, the chyle is changed into blood, and then the milk becomes yellowish and nauseous, and is spit out by the infant. Hence the best time for giving suck is about the fourth or fifth hour after meals. 3. In respect *of the time after delivery*. The milk secreted immediately after delivery is serous, purges the bowels of the infant, and is called *colostrum*. But in the following days it becomes thicker and more pure, and the longer a nurse suckles, the thicker the milk is secreted; thus new-born infants cannot retain the milk of a nurse who has given suck for a twelvemonth, on account of its spissitude. 4. In respect *of food and medicines*. Thus, if a nurse eat garlic, the milk becomes highly impregnated with its odour, and is disagreeable. If she indulge too freely in the use of wine or beer, the infant becomes ill. From giving a purging medicine to a nurse, the child

also is purged; and, lastly, children affected with tormina of the bowels, arising from acids, are often cured by giving the nurse animal food. 5. In respect of the *affections of the mind*. There are frequent examples of infants being seized with convulsions, from sucking mothers irritated by anger. An infant of one year old, while he sucked milk from his enraged mother, on a sudden was seized with a fatal hæmorrhage, and died. Infants at the breast in a short time pine away, if the nurse be afflicted with grievous care; and there are also infants who, after every coition of the mother, or even if she menstruate, are taken ill.

The use of the mother's milk is, 1. It affords the natural *aliment* to the new-born infant, as milk differs little from chyle. Those children are the strongest who are nourished the longest by the mother's milk. 2. The *colostrum* should not be rejected; for it relaxes the bowels, which, in new-born infants, ought to be open, to clear them of the *meconium*. 3. *Lactation* defends the mother from a dangerous reflux of the milk into the blood, whence lacteal metastasis, and leucorrhœa, are so frequent in lying-in women, who do not give suck. The motion of the milk also being hastened through the breast by the sucking of the child, prevents the very common induration of the breast, which arises in consequence of the milk being stagnated. 4. *Men* may *live*, upon milk, unless they have been accustomed to the drinking of wine. For all nations, the Japanese alone excepted, use milk, and many live upon it alone.

MILK, MARES'. This is thinner than that of the cow, but scarcely so thin as human milk. Its cream cannot be converted into butter by agitation. The whey contains sugar.

MILK-BLOTCHES. An eruption of white vesicles, which assume a dark colour, resembling the blackening of the small-pox, and are succeeded by scabs producing an ichorous matter, attended with considerable itching. It generally appears on the forehead and scalp, extending half over the face, and at times even proceeding farther. The period of its attack is the time of teething; and it is probably the same disease as the *crusta lactea*.

Milk-fever. See *Puerperal fever.*
Milk-teeth. See *Teeth.*
Milk-thistle. See *Carduus marianus.*
MILK-VETCH. See *Astragalus excapus*
MILK-WORT. See *Polygala vulgaris.*
Milk-wort, rattle-snake root. See *Polygala senega.*

MILLEFO'LIUM. (From *mille*, a thousand, and *folium*, a leaf: named from its numerous leaves.) See *Achillea millefolium.*

MILLEMO'RBIA. (From *mille*, a thousand, and *morbus*, a disease: so called from its use in many diseases.) See *Scrophularia nodosa.*

MILLE'PEDÆ. See *Oniscus asellus.*

MILLE'PES. (From *mille*, a thousand, and *pes*, a foot: named from their numerous feet.) See *Oniscus asellus.*

[MILLER, EDWARD, M.D., was a native of Dover, in the state of Delaware. He was born on the 9th of May, 1760. Dr. Miller, in the year 1784, commenced the practice of medicine in the village of Frederica, a short distance from his native town, in Delaware; but soon afterward removed to Somerset county, in Maryland. Here also his stay was short. In 1786 he returned to Dover, and entered on the practice of his profession in his native place.

In 1796 he removed from Dover to the city of New-York. Here he soon conciliated the esteem and confidence of his medical brethren; and notwithstanding the many disadvantages under which a stranger engages in the competition for medical practice in a great city, he succeeded beyond his most sanguine expectations. His business, in a few months, became such as to afford him an ample support, and continued to become more and more extensive until his death.

In a few weeks after his removal to New-York, Dr Miller, in connexion with his friends, Dr. Mitchill and the late Dr. Elihu H. Smith, formed the plan of a periodical publication to be devoted to medical science. Their prospectus was issued in November of that year (1796); and in the month of August, 1797, the first number of the work appeared under the title of the "*Medical Repository*." The commencement of this publication undoubtedly forms an era in the literary and medical history of our country. No work of a similar kind had ever appeared in the United States. Its influence in exciting and recording medical inquiries, and in improving medical science, soon became apparent. It led to the establishment of other similar works in different parts of our own country as well as of Europe; and may thus, with great truth, be said to have contributed more largely, than any other single publication, to that taste for medical investigation and improvement, which has been for a number of years so conspicuously and rapidly advancing on this side of the Atlantic. Dr. Miller lived to see the fifteenth volume of this work nearly brought to a close, and rejoiced in the generous competition which it had been so evidently the means c exciting.

At the close of the season of 1805, in his official character as resident physician, he addressed to his excellency Governor Lewis a report of the rise, progress, and termination of the yellow fever. To this detail he added an exhibition and defence of the doctrine concerning the origin of yellow fever, which, after much inquiry and long experience, he had adopted. This report was shortly afterward laid before the public; and has been pronounced by good judges to be one of the most luminous, forcible, comprehensive, and satisfactory defences of the doctrine which it supports, that ever appeared, within the same compass, in any language.

He fell a victim to an inflammatory attack upon the lungs, which, after symptoms of convalescence, degenerated into a typhus fever, which put an end to his valuable life on the 17th day of March, 1812, in the 52d year of his age.

Dr. Miller's published writings were not numerous. A few of them were originally printed in detached pamphlets; but the greater part first appeared in the Medical Repository. Since his decease they have been collected and reprinted in one large octavo volume.

The moral and social qualities of Dr. Miller were worthy of no less praise than his talents, learning, and professional skill. His humanity and practical beneficence were no less conspicuous. These were manifested throughout his professional life, and especially in his attendance on the poor and friendless, to an extent truly rare.

His delicacy in conversation has been seldom equalled, perhaps never exceeded. Nothing ever escaped from his lips, even in his most unreserved moments, to which the most refined and scrupulous might not listen without offence.

Nor was his temperance less conspicuous than his delicacy. He not only avoided the use of ardent spirits, with a scrupulousness which to some might appear excessive, but he was unusually sparing, and even abstemious, in the use of every kind of drink stronger than water. He rejected the use of tobacco in every form, not only as an odious and unhealthy practice, but also as a most insidious provocation to the love of drinking.—*Thach. Med. Biog.* A.]

MILLET. See *Panicum miliaceum.*

Millet, Indian. See *Panicum italicum.*

MILL-MOUNTAIN. See *Linum catharticum.*

MILPHO′SIS. Μιλφωσις. A baldness of the eyebrows.

MI′LTOS. Μιλτος. Red-lead.

MILTWASTE. See *Asplenium ceterach.*

MILZADE′LLA. (From *milza,* the Spanish for the spleen: so called from its supposed virtues in diseases of the spleen.) The herb archangel. See *Angelica archangelica.*

MIMO′SA. (From *mimus,* an actor, or imitator, meaning a sort of imitative plant, the motions of which mimic the sensibility of animal life.) The name of a genus of plants in the Linnæan system. Class, *Polygamia;* Order, *Monœcia.* The sensitive plant.

MIMOSA CATECHU. The former name of the tree which affords catechu. See *Acacia catechu.*

MIMOSA NILOTICA. See *Acacia vera.*

MIMOSA SENEGAL. The systematic name of the tree from which the gum senegal exudes. The gum is brought from the country through which the river Senegal runs, in loose or single drops, much larger than gum-arabic. It is similar in virtue and quality to the gum-arabic, and the gum which exudes in this climate from the cherry-tree. See *Acacia vera.*

Mindererus spirit. See *Ammoniæ acetatis liquor.*

MINERAL. (*Mineralis;* from *mina,* a mine of metal.) A substance which does not possess organiza-tion, or is not produced by an organized body, belongs to the division of the production of nature called minerals. Among this varied class of materials, which require the attention of the chemist and manufacturer, many are compounded of such principles, and formed under such circumstances and situations in the earth, that it is difficult to distinguish them without having recourse to the test of experiment; several are formed with considerable regularity as to the proportion of their principle, their fracture, their colour, specific gravity, and figure of crystallization.

Mineral bodies which enter into the composition of the globe, are classed by mineralogists under four heads:—1. Earths. 2. Salts. 3. Inflammable fossils; and, 4. Metals and their ores. Under the term earths, are arranged stones and earths, which have no taste, and do not burn when heated with contact of air.

Under the second, salts, or those saline substances which melt in water and do not burn, they require, according to Kirwan, less than two hundred times their weight of water to dissolve them.

By inflammable fossils are to be understood all those minerals not soluble in water, and exhibiting a flame more or less evident when exposed to fire in contact with air.

The fourth class, or ores, are compound bodies. Nature has bestowed their proper metallic appearance on some substances, and when this is the case, or they are alloyed with other metals, or semi-metals, they are called native metals. But such as are distinguished, as they commonly are, in mines, in combination with some other unmetallic substances, are said to be mineralized. The substance that sets them in that state, is called the mineralizer, and the compound of both an ore. For example, in the common ore of copper, this metal is found oxidized, and the oxide combined with sulphur. The copper may be considered as mineralized with oxygen and sulphur, and the compound of the three bodies forms an ore of copper.

[MINERALS, ARRANGEMENT OF. The systematic arrangement of minerals by writers on the subject differs very materially. The only elementary work on mineralogy published in this country is by Parker Cleaveland, professor in Bowdoin College, State of Maine. As it is a work highly creditable to the author, and much approved as a standard work, we give a tabular view of his arrangement.

TABULAR VIEW.*

CLASS. 1.—*Substances not metallic, composed entirely, or in part, of an Acid.*

This class contains four orders. In the first order, the acid is free or not combined; in the second, it is combined with an alkali; in the third, with an earth or earths; and in the fourth, with both an alkali and an earth. Hence the presence of an acid, provided it be not united to a metallic base, characterizes this class.

ORDER I.—*Acids not combined.*

The base of the acid determines the genus. All the species in this order have oxygen, as a common ingredient, so combined with a base, as to produce an acid

GENUS I

SPEC. 1. Sulphuric acid.
    2. *Sulphurous acid.*
GENUS II.
SPEC. 1. *Muriatic acid.*
GENUS III.
    1. *Carbonic acid.*
GENUS IV.
    1. Boracic acid.
ORDER II.—*Alkaline salts.*

These salts are composed of an alkali, united to an acid. Hence an alkali, so combined as to form a salt, characterizes this order. Each alkali designates a genus.

GENUS I.—*AMMONIA.*
SPEC. 1. Sulphate of Ammonia.
    2. Muriate of Ammonia.
GENUS II.—*POTASH.*
    1. Nitrate of Potash.

* In the tabular view, *subspecies* are distinguished from *varieties* by their position in the column. A number of species, recently discovered, and concerning which little is yet known, are alphabetically arranged in an appendix to the earthy class. Those species which have never been analyzed, are marked by an asterisk. Those species which are printed in Italics, have not hitherto been observed in crystals, nor even with a crystalline structure.

GENUS III.—*SODA.*
Spec. 1. Sulphate of Soda.
    2. Muriate of Soda.
    3. Carbonate of Soda.
    4. Borate of Soda.
ORDER III.—*Earthy Salts.*
These consist of an earth, or of earths, united to an acid. Hence an earth, so combined as to form a salt, characterizes this order. Each genus is determined by the earth it contains.

GENUS I.—*Barytes.*

SUBSPECIES AND VARIETIES
Spec. 1. Sulphate of Barytes.
    lamellar
    columnar
    radiated
    fibrous
    concreted
    granular
    compact
    earthy
    fetid
  2. Carbonate of Barytes.

GENUS II.—*STRONTIAN.*
Spec. 1. Sulphate of Strontian.
    foliated
    fibrous
    calcareous
  2. Carbonate of Strontian.

GENUS III.—*LIME.*
Spec. 1. Arseniate of Lime.
    2. Nitrate of Lime.
    3. Phosphate of Lime.
    Apatite.
    Asparagus stone.
    fibrous
    amorphous
    siliceous
  4. Fluate of Lime.
    Fluor spar.
    compact
    earthy
    argillaceous
  5. Sulphate of Lime.
    Selenite.
    massive
    Gypsum.
    fibrous
    granular
    compact
    branchy
    snowy
    earthy
    Plaster stone.
  6. Anhydrous Sulphate of Lime.
    sparry
    compact
    silico-anhydrous
  7. Carbonate of Lime.
    calcareous spar
    crystallized
    laminated
    granular
    fibrous
    compact
    coarse grained
    Chalk.
    Agaric Mineral.
    Fossil Farina.
    concreted
    Pisolite.
    Oolite.
    calcareous sinter.
    Tufa.
    Argentine.
    Silvery chalk.
    magnesian
    common
    Dolomite.
    siliceous
    Madreporite.
    Calp.
    fetid
    bituminous
    ferruginous
    Brown spar.

SUBSPECIES AND VARIETIES
Spec.
    Marl.
    indurated
    common
    Bituminous marlite.
  8. Arragonite.
    fibrous
    coralloidal
  9. Siliceous Borate of Lime.
    Botryolite.

GENUS IV.—*MAGNESIA.*
Spec. 1. Sulphate of Magnesia.
    2. Carbonate of Magnesia.
    3 Borate of Magnesia.
    4. Fluate of Magnesia.

GENUS V.—*ALUMINE.*
Spec. 1. Mellate of Alumine.
ORDER IV.—*Salts with an alkaline and earthy base.*
Spec. 1. Alkaline sulphate of Alumine.
    2. Fluate of Soda and Alumine.
    3. Glauberite.

CLASS II.—*Earthy compounds, or stones.*
The minerals which belong to this class, are composed chiefly of earths, combined with each other: they frequently contain some metallic oxide, and sometimes an alkali, or acid.

Alumine, silex and fluoric acid. — Spec. 1. Topaz.
    Pycnite.
    2. Sapphire.
    perfect
    blue
    violet
Alumine nearly pure.
    red
    yellow
    limpid
    Corundum.
    Adamantine spar
    Emery.
Alumine and water. — 3. Disaspore.
    4. Wavellite.
Alumine and magnesia. — 5. Spinelle.
    Ruby.
    Ceylanite.
Alumine and silex. — 6. Fibrolite.
    7. Cyanite.
    8. Staurotide.
Alumine, silex and lime. — 9. Chrysoberyl.
Alumine, silex and zinc. — 10. Gahnite.
Ittria & silex. — 11. Gadolinite.
Zirconia and silex. — 12. Zircon.
    Jargon,
    Hyacinth.
  13. Quartz.
    common
    limpid
    smoky
    yellow
    blue
    rose red
    irrsed
    aventurine
    milky
    greasy
    radiated
    tabular
    granular
    arenaceous
    pseudomorphous
    Amethyst.
    Prase.
    ferruginous
    yellow
    red
    greenish
    fetid
    Cat's eye.
Silex nearly pure. — Chalcedony.
    common
    Cacholong
    Carnelian.
    Sardonyx.
    Plasma.

SUBSPECIES AND VARIETIES.

Hyalite.
Heliotrope.
Chrysoprase.
Opal.
  precious
  common
  Hydrophane.
Girasole.
  Semi-opal.
Flint.
  swimming
Hornstone.
Silicicalce.
Buhrstone.
Jasper.
  common
  striped
  Egyptian
SPEC. 14. *Tripoli.*
15. *Porcellanite.*
16. *Siliceous Slate.*
  Basanite.
17. *Petrosilex.*
18. *Clinkstone.*
19. *Pumice.*
20. *Obsidian*
  vitreous
  Pearlstone.
21. *Pitchstone.*
22. Spodumen.
23. Lepidolite.
24. Mica.
  laminated
  lamellar
  prismatic
25. Leucite.
26. Fettstein.
27. Lapis Lazuli.
  Lazulite.
28. Schor.
  common
  Tourmaline.
  Indicolite.
  Rubellite.
29. Andaluzite.
30. Feldspar.
  common
  Adularia.
  opalescent
  aventurine
  Petuntze.
  granular
  compact
31. *Jade.*
  Nephrite.
  Saussurite.
  Axestone.
32. Emerald.
  precious
  Beryl.
33. Euclase.
34. *Basalt.*
  columnar
  tabular
  globular
  amorphous
35. *Wacke.*
36. Dipyre.
37. Scapolite.
38. Wernerite.
39. Axinite.
40. Garnet.
  precious
  Pyrope.
  common
  Melanite.
  manganesian
41. Aplome.
42. Epidote.
  Zoisite.
  Skorza.
  manganesian
43. Cinnamon Stone.
44. Allochroite.
45. Idocrase.
46. *Meionite.

Side labels (left column): Silex, alumine, and alkali — Silex, alumine, lime, and alkali. — Silex, alumine, and glucine. — Silex, alumine, and lime.

SUBSPECIES AND VARIETIES.

SPEC. 47. Byssolite.
48. Prehnite.
  crystallized
  Koupholite.
  fibrous
49. Ædelite.
50. Stilbite.
51. Zeolite.
  mealy
  Crocalite.
  Needlestone.
52. *Laumonite.
53. *Melilite.
54. Sodalite.
55. Natrolite.
56. Analcime.
57. *Bildstein.*
58. Nacrite.
59. Chabasie.
60. Allenite.
61. Yenite.
62. Schaalstein.
63. Ichthyophthalmite
64. Harmotome.
65. Chrysolite.
  common
  Olivine.
66. Labrador Stone.
67. Tremolite.
  common
  fibrous
  Baikalite.
68. Asbestus.
  Amianthus
  common
  Mountain Cork.
  ligniform
  compact
69. Diopside.
70. Sahlite.
71. Amianthoide.
72. Augite.
  common
  Coccolite.
73. Hornblende.
  common
  Basaltic
  lamellar
  fibrous
  slaty
  Actynolite.
  common
  acicular
74. Diallage.
  granular
  resplendent
  Bronzite.
75. *Macle.
76. Native Magnesia.
77. *Magnesite.*
  Keffekil.
  Argillo-murite.
78. *Serpentine.*
  precious
  common
79. Steatite.
  common
  Potstone
80. Talc.
  common
  indurated
81. Chlorite.
  common
  slaty
  foliated
  Green earth
82. Sommite.
83. Anthophyllite.
84. Pinite.

Side labels (right column): Silex, alumine, lime, and water — Silex, alumine, soda, and muriatic acid. — Silex, alumine, alkali, and water. — Silex, lime, and cerium. — Silex, lime, and iron. — Silex, lime, and water. — Silex, barytes, alumine, and water. — Magnesia and silex. — Silex, magnesia, & lime. — Silex, magnesia, alumine, and lime. — Silex, magnesia, and alumine. — Silex & alumine.

SUBSPECIES
AND VARIETIES.

SPEC. 85. *Argillaceous Slate.*

Argillite.
Shale.
Novaculite.
Aluminous Slate.
graphic

86. *Claystone.*
87. *Clay.*

Native Argill.
Collyrite.
Kaolin.
Cimolite.
adhesive
Potter's
Lithomarge.
Fuller's Earth.
Bole.
Reddle.
Yellow Earth.
Umber.

88. *Alum-stone.*
Appendix.
89. *Bergmanite.*
90. *Chusite.*
91. *Fuscite.*
92. *Gabronite.*
93. *Haüyene.*
94. *Iolite.*
95. *Petalite.*
96. *Pseudo-sommite.*
97. *Sideroclepte.*
98. *Spinellane.*
99. *Spinthere.*

CLASS III.—*Combustibles.*

SPEC. 1. *Hydrogen Gas.*

carburetted
sulphuretted

2. Sulphur.
3. *Bitumen.*

Naptha.
Petrolium.
Maltha.
elastic
Asphaltum.
Retinasphaltum.

4. *Amber.*
5. Diamond.
6 Anthracite.

slaty
granular
conchoidal
columnar

7. Graphite.

foliated
granular

8. *Coal.*

cannel
slaty
coarse

9 *Lignite.*

Jet.
brittle
Bituminous Wood.
brown
earthy

10. *Peat.*

fibrous
compact

CLASS IV.—*Ores.*
GENUS I.—*GOLD.*
SPEC. 1. Native Gold.
GENUS II.—*PLATINA.*
SPEC. 1. Native Platina.
GENUS III.—*SILVER.*
SPEC. 1. Native silver.

auriferous

2. Antimonial Silver.
3. Arsenical Silver.
4. Sulphuret of Silver.
5. Sulphuretted Antimonial Silver.

brittle

6. *Black Silver*
7. *Carbonate of Silver.*
8. Muriate of Silver.

argillaceous

74

SUBSPECIES
AND VARIETIES.

GENUS IV —*MERCURY.*
SPEC. 1. *Native Mercury.*
2. Argental Mercury.
3. Sulphuret of Mercury.

common
fibrous
bituminous

4. Muriate of Mercury.

GENUS V.—*COPPER.*
SPEC. 1. Native Copper.
2. Sulphuret of Copper.

pseudomorphou

3. Pyritous Copper.

variegated

4. Gray Copper.

arsenical
antimonial

5. Red Oxide of Copper.

foliated
capillary
compact
ferruginous

6. Azure Carbonate of Copper.

earthy

7. Green Carbonate of Copper.

fibrous
compact
earthy
ferruginous

8. Dioptase.
9. Muriate of Copper.

sandy

10. Sulphate of Copper.
11. Phosphate of Copper.
12. Arseniate of Copper.

obtuse octaedral
acute octaedral
foliated
prismatic
fibrous
ferruginous

GENUS VI.—*IRON.*
SPEC. 1. Native Iron.
2. Arsenical Iron.

argentiferous

3. Sulphuret of Iron.

common
radiated
hepatic
magnetic
arsenical

4. Magnetic Oxide of Iron.

Native magnet
Iron sand.

5. Specular Oxide of Iron.

micaceous

6. Red Oxide of Iron.

scaly
Hematite.
compact
ochrey

7 Brown Oxide of Iron.

scaly
Hematite.
compact
ochrey

8. *Argillaceous Oxide of Iron.*

columnar
granular
lenticular
nodular
common
Bog ore

9. Carbonate of Iron.
10. Sulphate of Iron.
11. Phosphate of Iron.

foliated
earthy
Green iron earth.

12. Arseniate of Iron.
13. Chromate of Iron.

crystallized
granular
amorphous

	SUBSPECIES AND VARIETIES.

GENUS VII.—LEAD.

Spec. 1. *Native Lead.*
2. Sulphuret of Lead.
    - common
    - compact
    - fibrous
    - antimonial
    - argento-antimonial
    - argento-bismuthal
3. *Oxide of Lead.*
    - earthy
4. Carbonate of Lead.
    - crystallized
    - acicular
    - columnar
    - compact
    - black
5. Carbonated Muriate of Lead.
6. Sulphate of Lead.
7. Phosphate of Lead.
    - acicular
    - arseniated
    - bluish
8. Arseniate of Lead.
9. Chromate of Lead.
10. Molybdate of Lead.

GENUS VIII.—TIN.

Spec. 1. Oxide of Tin.
    - fibrous
2. *Pyritous Tin.*

GENUS IX.—ZINC.

Spec. 1. Sulphuret of Zinc.
    - yellow
    - brown
    - black
    - fibrous
2. Red Oxide of Zinc.
3. Siliceous Oxide of Zinc.
    - foliated
    - common
4. Carbonate of Zinc.
5. Sulphate of Zinc.

GENUS X.—NICKEL.

Spec. 1. Native Nickel.
2. *Arsenical Nickel.*
3. *Oxide of Nickel.*

GENUS XI.—COBALT.

Spec. 1. Arsenical Cobalt.
    - dull
2. Gray Cobalt.
3. *Sulphuret of Cobalt.*
4. *Oxide of Cobalt.*
    - black
    - brown
    - yellow
5. Sulphate of Cobalt.
6. Arseniate of Cobalt.
    - acicular
    - earthy
    - argentiferous

GENUS XII.—MANGANESE.

Spec. 1. Oxide of Manganese.
    - radiated
    - compact
    - earthy
    - ferruginous
2. Sulphuret of Manganese.
3. Carbonate of Manganese.
4. Phosphate of Manganese.

GENUS XIII.—ARSENIC.

Spec. 1. Native Arsenic.
    - concreted
    - specular
    - amorphous
2. Sulphuret of Arsenic.
    - Realgar.
    - Orpiment.
Oxide of Arsenic.

	SUBSPECIES AND VARIETIES

GENUS XIV.—BISMUTH.

Spec. 1. Native Bismuth.
2. Sulphuret of Bismuth.
3. *Oxide of Bismuth.*

GENUS XV.—ANTIMONY.

Spec. 1. Native Antimony.
    - arsenical
2. Sulphuret of Antimony.
    - radiated
    - foliated
    - compact
    - plumous
3. Oxide of Antimony.
    - earthy
4. Sulphuretted Oxide of Antimony.

GENUS XVI.—TELLURIUM.

Spec. 1. Native Tellurium.
    - auro-argentiferous.
    - auro-plumbiferous.

GENUS XVII.—CHROME.

GENUS XVIII.—MOLYBDENA.

Spec. 1. Sulphuret of Molybdena.

GENUS XIX.—TUNGSTEN.

Spec. 1. Calcareous Oxide of Tungsten.
2. Ferruginous Oxide of Tungsten.

GENUS XX.—TITANIUM.

Spec. 1. Red Oxide of Titanium.
2. Ferruginous Oxide of Titanium.
    - Menachanite.
    - Nigrine.
    - Iserine.
3. Silico-calcareous Oxide of Titanium
4. Octaedral Oxide of Titanium.

GENUS XXI.—URANIUM

Spec. 1. Black Oxide of Uranium.
2. Green Oxide of Uranium.
    - crystallized
    - earthy

GENUS XXII.—COLUMBIUM.

Spec. 1. Oxide of Columbium.
    - ferruginous
    - Ittrious

GENUS XXIII.—CERIUM.

Spec. 1. *Oxide of Cerium.*
Mineral caoutchouc. See *Caoutchouc.*
Mineral oil. Petroleum.
Mineral pitch. Bitumen.
Mineral poisons. See *Poisons.*
Mineral salts. See *Salts.*

MINERAL WATERS. *Aquæ minerales. Aquæ medicinales.* Waters holding minerals in solution are called *mineral waters.* But as all water, in a mineral state, is impregnated, either more or less, with some mineral substances, the name *mineral waters,* should be confined to such waters as are sufficiently impregnated with mineral matters to produce some sensible effects on the animal economy, and either to cure or prevent some of the diseases to which the human body is liable. On this account, these waters might be with much more propriety called *medicinal waters,* were not the name by which they are commonly known too firmly established by long use.

The mineral waters which are the most esteemed, and consequently the most resorted to for the cure of diseases, are those of,

1. Aix.	13. Malvern.
2. Barege.	74. Matlock.
3. Bath.	15. Moffat.
4. Bristol.	16. Pyrmont.
5. Buxton.	17. Scarborough.
6. Borset.	18. Spa.
7. Cheltenham.	19. Seidlitz.
8. Carlsbad.	20. Sea-water.
9. Epsom.	21. Seltzer.
10. Harrowgate.	22. Tunbridge.
11. Hartfell.	23. Vichy, and others of
12. Holywell.	less note.

For the properties and virtues of these, consult their respective heads.

A SYNOPTICAL TABLE, showing the Composition of MINERAL WATERS.

CLASS.	NAME.	Highest Temperature. Fahrenheit.	Contained in an English Wine Pint of 28.875 Cubic Inches.						
			Azotic Gas. Cubic Inches.	Carbonic Acid Gas. Cubic Inches.	Sulphuretted Hydrogen. Cubic Inches.	Carbonated Soda. Grains.	Neutral Purging Salts. Grains.	Selenite and Earthy Carbonates. Grains.	Oxide of Iron. Grains.
Simple cold {	Malvern			uncertain	none	none	uncertain	uncertain	none
	Holywell				none	none	uncertain	uncertain	none
Simple thermal {	Bristol	74°	uncertain	3.75	none	none	2.81	3.16	none
	Matlock	66°		uncertain	none	none	uncertain	uncertain	none
	Buxton	82°	0.474	uncertain	none	none	0.25	1.625	none
Simple saline {	Seidlitz			1.	none	none	185.6	8.68	none
	Epsom				none	none	40.?	8.?	none
	Sea				none	none	237.5	6.	none
Highly carbonated alkaline	Seltzer			17.	none	4.	17.5	8.	none
Simple carbonated chalybeate	Tunbridge		0.675	1.325	none	none	0.344	0.156	0.125
Hot carbonated chalybeate	Bath	116°	1.?	1.?	none	none	10.?	10.?	uncertain
Highly carbonated chalybeate {	Spa			12.79	none	1.47	4.632	1.47	0.56
	Pyrmont		uncertain	26.	none	none	7.13	23.075	0.56
Saline, carbonated chalybeate {	Cheltenham			5.687	uncertain	none	62.125	6.85	0.625
	Scarborough			uncertain	none	uncertain	20.	10.	uncertain
Hot, saline, highly-carbonated chalybeate {	Vichy	130°?		uncertain	none	uncertain		uncertain	uncertain
	Carlsbad	165°		uncertain	none	11.76	47.04	4.15	uncertain
Vitriolated chalybeate	Hartfell				none	none	none	none	4.815*
Cold sulphureous {	Harrowgate		0.875	1	2.375	none	91.25	3.	none
	Moffat		0.5	0.625	1.25	none	4.5	none	none
Hot, alkaline, sulphureous {	Aix	143°		uncertain	uncertain	12.	5.	4.75	none
	Borset	132°		uncertain	uncertain	uncertain	uncertain		none
	Barege	120°		uncertain	uncertain	2.5	0.5	uncertain	none

* That is, 2.94 contained in the sulphate of iron, (this salt when crystallized, containing 28 per cent. of oxide of iron, according to Kirwan,) and 1.875 additional of oxide of iron.

Fourcroy divides all mineral and medicinal waters into nine orders, viz.

1. Cold acidulous waters.
2. Hot or thermal acidulous waters.
3. Sulphuric saline waters.
4. Muriatic saline waters.
5. Simple sulphureous waters.
6. Sulphurated gaseous waters.
7. Simple ferruginous waters.
8. Ferruginous and acidulous waters.
9. Sulphuric ferruginous waters.

Dr. Saunders arranges mineral waters into the following classes:

1. Simple cold.
2. .. thermal.
3. .. saline.
4. Highly carbonated alkaline.
5. Simple carbonated chalybeate.
6. Hot carbonated chalybeate.
7. Highly carbonated chalybeate.
8. Saline carbonated chalybeate.
9. Hot saline highly carbonated chalybeate.
10. Vitriolated chalybeate.
11. Cold, sulphureous.
12. Hot, alkaline, sulphureous.

In order to present the reader, under one point of view, with the most conspicuous features in the composition of the mineral waters of this and some other countries, the preceding Synoptical Table has been subjoined, from Dr. Saunders's work on mineral waters.

The reader will please to observe, that under the head of *Neutral Purging Salts*, are included the sulphates of soda and magnesia, and the muriates of lime, soda, and magnesia. The power which the earthy muriates may possess of acting on the intestinal canal, is not quite ascertained, but, from their great solubility, and from analogy with salts, with similar component parts, we may conclude that this forms a principal part of their operation.

The reader will likewise observe, that where the spaces are left blank, it signifies that we are ignorant whether any of the substance at the head of the column is contained in the water; that the word *none*, implies a certainty of the absence of that substance: and the term *uncertain*, means that the substance is contained, but that the quantity is not known.

Dr. Henry, in his epitome of chemistry, gives the following concise and accurate account for the analysis of mineral waters:

Water is never presented by nature in a state of complete purity. Even when collected as it descends in the form of rain, chemical tests detect in it foreign ingredients. And when it has been absorbed by the earth, has traversed its different strata, and is returned to us by springs, it is found to have acquired various impregnations. The readiest method of judging of the contents of natural waters, is by applying what are termed tests, or reagents, *i. e.* substances which, on being added to a water, exhibit by the phenomena they produce, the nature of the saline and other ingredients. For example, if, on adding an infusion of litmus to any water, its colour is changed to red, we infer that the water contains an uncombined acid; if this change ensue even after the water has been boiled, we judge that the acid is a fixed and not a volatile one; and if, on adding the muriate of barytes, a precipitate falls down, we safely conclude that the peculiar acid present in the water is either entirely or in part the sulphuric acid. Dr. Henry first enumerates the tests generally employed in examining mineral waters, and describes their application, and afterward indicates by what particular tests the substances generally found in waters may be detected.

A. *Infusion of Litmus. Syrup of Violets, &c.*

As the infusion of litmus is apt to spoil by keeping, some solid litmus should be kept. The infusion is prepared by steeping this substance, first bruised in a mortar, and tied up in a thin rag, in distilled water, which extracts its blue colour. If the colour of the infusion tends too much to purple, it may be amended by a drop or two of pure ammonia; but of this no more should be added than what is barely sufficient, lest the delicacy of the test should be impaired. The syrup of violets is not easily obtained pure. The genuine syrup may be distinguished from the spurious by a solution of corrosive sublimate, which changes the former to green, while it reddens the latter. When it can be

procured genuine, it is an excellent test of acids, and may be employed in the same manner as the infusion of litmus. Paper stained with the juice of the marsh violet, or with that of radishes, answers a similar purpose. In staining paper for the purpose of a test, it must be used unsized; or, if sized, it must previously be washed with warm water; because the alum which enters into the composition of the size will otherwise change the vegetable colour to a red.

Infusion of litmus is a test of most uncombined acids.

If the infusion redden the unboiled but not the boiled water under examination, or if the red colour occasioned by adding the infusion to a recent water, return to blue on boiling, we may infer that the acid is a volatile one, and most probably the carbonic acid. Sulphuretted hydrogen gas, dissolved in water, also reddens litmus, but not after boiling. To ascertain whether the change be produced by carbonic acid, or sulphuretted hydrogen, when experiment shows that the reddening cause is volatile, add a little lime-water. This, if carbonic acid be present, will occasion a precipitate, which will dissolve with effervescence, on adding a little muriatic acid. Sulphuretted hydrogen may also be contained in the same water, which will be ascertained by the tests hereafter to be described.

Paper tinged with litmus is also reddened by the presence of carbonic acid, but regains its blue colour by drying. The mineral and fixed acids redden it permanently. That these acids, however, may produce their effect, it is necessary that they should be present in a sufficient proportion.

Infusion of litmus reddened by vinegar—Spirituous tincture of Brazil-wood—Tincture of turmeric and paper stained with each of these three substances—Syrup of violets. All these different tests have one and the same object.

1. Infusion of litmus reddened by vinegar, or litmus paper reddened by vinegar, has its blue colour restored by alkalies and pure earths, and by carbonated alkalies and earths.

2. Turmeric paper and tincture are changed to a reddish brown by alkalies, whether pure or carbonated, and by pure earths; but not by carbonated earths.

3. The red infusion of Brazil-wood, and paper stained with it, become blue by alkalies and earths, and even by the latter, when dissolved by an excess of carbonic acid. In the last-mentioned case, however, the change will either cease to appear or be much less remarkable, when the water has been boiled.

4. Syrup of violets, when pure, is by the same causes turned green, as also paper stained with the juices of violets, or radishes.

B. *Tincture of Galls.*

Tincture of galls is the test generally employed for discovering iron, with all the combinations of which it produces a black tinge, more or less intense, according to the quantity of iron. The iron, however, in order to be detected by this test, must be in the state of red oxide, or, if oxidated in a less degree, its effects will not be apparent, unless after standing some time in contact with air. By applying this test before and after evaporation or boiling, we may know whether the iron be held in solution by carbonic acid, or a fixed acid; for,

1. If it produce its effects before the application of heat, and not afterward, carbonic acid is the solvent.

2. If after, as well as before, a mineral acid is the solvent.

3. If, by the boiling, a yellowish powder be precipitated, and yet galls continue to strike the water black afterward, the iron, as often happens, is dissolved both by carbonic acid and a fixed acid. A neat mode of applying the gall test was used by Klaproth, in his analysis of the Carlsbad water. A slice of the gall-nut was suspended by a silken thread, in a large bottle of the recent water; and so small was the quantity of iron, that it could only be discovered in water fresh from the spring.

C. *Sulphuric Acid.*

1. Sulphuric acid discovers, by a slight effervescence, the presence of carbonic acid, whether uncombined or united with alkalies, or earths.

2. If lime be present, whether pure or uncombined the addition of sulphuric acid, occasions, after a few days, a white precipitate.

77

3. Barytes is precipitated instantly in the form of a white powder.

4. Nitrous and muriatic salts, on adding sulphuric acid and applying heat, are decomposed; and if a stopper, moistened with pure ammonia, be held over the vessel, white clouds appear. For distinguishing whether nitric or muriatic acid be present, rules will be given hereafter.

Nitric and Nitrous Acid.

These acids, if they occasion effervescence, give the same indications as the sulphuric. The nitrous acid has been recommended as a test distinguishing between hepatic waters that contain sulphuret of potassa, and those that only contain sulphuretted hydrogen gas. In the former case a precipitate ensues on adding nitrous acid, and a very fœtid smell arises; in the latter, a slight cloudiness only appears, and the smell of the water becomes less disagreeable.

D. Oxalic Acid and Oxalates.

This acid is a most delicate test of lime, which it separates from all its combinations.

1. If a water which is precipitated by oxalic acid, becomes milky on adding a watery solution of carbonic acid gas, or by blowing air through it by means of a quill, or glass tube, we may infer that pure lime (or barytes, which has never yet been found pure in water) is present.

2. If the oxalic acid occasion a precipitate before but not after boiling, the lime is dissolved by an excess of carbonic acid.

3. If, after boiling, by a fixed acid: a considerable excess of any of the mineral acids, however, prevents the oxalic acid from occasioning a precipitate, even though lime be present; because some acids decompose the oxalic, and others, dissolving the oxalate of lime, prevent it from appearing.

The oxalates of ammonia, or of potassa, (which may easily be formed by saturating their respective carbonates with a solution of oxalic acid,) are not liable to the above objections, and are preferable, as reagents, to the uncombined acid. Yet even these oxalates fail to detect lime when supersaturated with muriatic or nitric acids; and if such an excess be present, it must be saturated, before adding the test with pure ammonia. Fluate of ammonia is the best test of lime. It is made by adding carbonate of ammonia to diluted fluoric acid.

E. Pure Alkalies and Carbonated Alkalies.

1. The pure fixed alkalies precipitate all earths and metals, whether dissolved by volatile or fixed menstrua, but only in certain states of dilution: for example, sulphate of alumine may be present in water, in the proportion of 4 grains to 500, without being discovered by pure fixed alkalies. As the alkalies precipitate so many substances, it is evident they cannot afford any precise information when employed as reagents. From the colour of the precipitate, as it approaches to pure white, or recedes from it, an experienced eye will judge that the precipitated earth contains less or more of the metallic admixture.

2. Pure fixed alkalies decompose all salts with basis of ammonia, which becomes evident by its smell, and also by the white fumes it exhibits when a stopper is brought near it, moistened with muriatic acid.

3. Carbonates of potassa and soda have similar effects.

4. Pure ammonia precipitates all earthy and metallic salts. Besides this property, it also imparts a deep blue colour to any liquid that contains copper in a state of solution.

Carbonate of ammonia has the same properties, except that it does not precipitate magnesia from its combinations. Hence, to ascertain whether this earth be present in any solution, add the carbonate of ammonia till no further precipitation ensues, filter the liquor, and then add pure ammonia. If any precipitation now occurs, we may infer the presence of magnesia.

F. Lime-Water.

1. Lime-water is applied for the purposes of a test, chiefly for detecting carbonic acid. Let any liquor, supposed to contain this acid, be mixed with an equal bulk of lime-water. If carbonic acid be present, either free or combined, a precipitate will immediately appear, which, on adding a few drops of muriatic acid, will immediately dissolve with effervescence.

2. Lime-water will immediately show the presence of corrosive sublimate, by a brickdust-coloured sediment. If arsenic be present in any liquid, lime-water,

when added, will occasion a precipitate, consisting of lime and arsenic, which is very difficultly soluble in water. This precipitate, when mixed up with oil, and laid on hot coals, yields the well-known garlic smell of arsenic.

G. Pure Barytes, and its Solution in Water.

1. A solution of pure barytes is even more effectual than lime-water, in detecting the presence of carbonic acid, and is much more portable and convenient; since from the crystals of this earth, the solution may at any time be prepared. In discovering fixed air, the solution of barytes is used similarly to lime-water; and, if this acid be present, gives, in like manner, a precipitate soluble with effervescence in muriatic acid.

Pure strontites has similar virtues as a test.

H. Metals.

1. Of the metals, silver and mercury are tests of the presence of sulphurets, and of sulphuretted hydrogen gas. If a little quicksilver be put into a bottle, containing water impregnated with either of these substances, its surface soon acquires a black film, and, on shaking, a blackish powder separates from it. Silver is immediately tarnished from the same cause.

2. The metals also may be used as tests of each other, and on the principle of elective affinity. Thus, for example, a polished iron plate, immersed in a solution of sulphate of copper, soon acquires a coat of this metal, and the same in other similar examples.

I. Sulphate of Iron.

This is the only one of the sulphates, except that of silver, applicable to the purposes of a test. When used in this view, it is generally employed to ascertain the presence of oxygenous gas, of which a natural water may contain a small quantity.

A water suspected to contain this gas, may be mixed with a little recently dissolved sulphate of iron, and kept corked up. If an oxide of iron be precipitated in the course of a few days, the water may be inferred to contain oxygenous gas.

Sulphate, Nitrate, and Acetate of Silver.

These solutions are, in some measure, applicable to the same purpose.

1. They are peculiarly adapted to the discovery of muriatic acid and muriates. For the silver, quitting the nitric or other acid, combines with the muriatic, and forms a flaky precipitate, which at first is white, but, on exposure to the sun's light, acquires a violet colour. This precipitate Dr. Black states to contain, in 1000 parts, as much muriatic acid as would form 425 parts and a half of crystallized muriate of soda, which estimate scarcely differs at all from that of Klaproth. A precipitation, however, may arise from other causes, which it may be proper to state.

2. The solutions of silver in acids are precipitated by carbonated alkalies and earths. The agency of these may be prevented by previously adding a few drops of the same acid in which the silver is dissolved.

3. The nitrate and acetate of silver are decomposed by the sulphuric and sulphurous acids; but this may be prevented by adding previously a few drops of nitrate or acetate of barytes, and after allowing the precipitate to subside, the clear liquor may be decanted, and the solution of silver added. Should a precipitation now take place, the presence of muriatic acid, or some one of its combinations, may be suspected. To obviate uncertainty, whether a precipitation be owing to sulphuric or muriatic acid, a solution of sulphate of silver may be employed, which is affected only by the latter acid.

4. The solutions of silver are precipitated by extractive matters; but in this case also the precipitate is discoloured, and is soluble in nitrous acid.

K. Nitrate and Acetate of Lead.

1. Acetate of lead, the most eligible of these two tests, is precipitated by sulphuric and muriatic acids; but as, of both these, we have much better indicators, it is not necessary to enlarge on its application to this purpose.

2. The acetate is also a test of sulphuretted hydrogen and sulphurets of alkalies, which occasion a black precipitate; and if a paper, on which characters are traced with a solution of acetate of lead, be held over a portion of water containing a sulphuretted hydrogen, they are soon rendered visible.

3. The acetate of lead is employed in the discovery of uncombined boracic acid, a very rare ingredient of waters. To ascertain whether this be present, some

cautions are necessary. The uncombined alkalies and earths (if any be suspected) must be saturated with acetic acid. The sulphates must be decomposed by acetate or nitrate of barytes, and the muriates by acetate or nitrate of silver. The filtered liquor, if boracic acid be contained in it, will give a precipitate soluble in nitric acid of the specific gravity of 1.3.

L. *Nitrate of Mercury, prepared with and without heat.*

This solution, differently prepared, is sometimes employed as a test. But, since other tests answer the same purposes more effectually, it is not absolutely necessary to have these tests.

M. *Muriate, Nitrate, and Acetate of Barytes.*

1. These solutions are all most delicate tests of sulphuric acid, and of its combinations, with which they give a white precipitate, insoluble in dilute muriatic acid. They are decomposed, however, by carbonates of alkalies; but the precipitate occasioned by these is soluble in dilute muriatic and nitric acid with effervescence, and may even be prevented by adding previously a few drops of the acid contained in the barytic salt.

One hundred grains of dry sulphate of barytes (according to Klaproth, p. 168,) contain about 45 one-fifth of sulphuric acid of the specific gravity 1850, according to Clayfield, 33 of acid of sp. gr. 2240; according to Thenard, after calcination about 25. These estimates differ very considerably. From Klaproth's experiments, it appears that 1000 grains of sulphate of barytes indicate 595; desiccated sulphate of soda, or 1415 of the crystallized salt. The same chemist has shown that 100 grains of sulphate of barytes are produced by the precipitation of 71 grains of sulphate of lime.

2. Phosphoric salts also occasion a precipitate with these tests, which is soluble in muriatic acid without effervescence.

N. *Prussiates of Potassa and Lime.*

Of these two the prussiate of potassa is the most eligible. When pure it does not speedily assume a blue colour on the addition of acid, nor does it immediately precipitate muriatic barytes. Prussiate of potassa is a very sensible test of iron, with the solutions of which in acids it produces a Prussian blue precipitate, in consequence of a double elective affinity. To render its effect more certain, however, it may be proper to add previously, to any water suspected to contain iron, a little muriatic acid, with a view to the saturation of uncombined alkalies, or earths, which, if present, prevent the detection of any minute portions of iron.

1. If a water, after boiling and filtration, does not afford a blue precipitate on the addition of prussiate of potassa, the solvent of the iron may be inferred to be a volatile one, and probably the carbonic acid.

2. Should the precipitation ensue in the boiled water, the solvent is a fixed acid, the nature of which must be ascertained by other tests.

O. *Solutions of Soap in Alkohol.*

This solution may be used to ascertain the comparative hardness of waters. With distilled water it may be mixed without producing any change; but, if added to a hard water, it produces a milkiness, more or less considerable as the water is less pure: and from the degree of milkiness, an experienced eye will judge of its quality. The acids, alkalies, and all earthy and metallic salts, decompose soap, and occasion that property in water termed hardness.

Alkohol.

Alkohol, when mixed with any water in the proportion of about an equal bulk, precipitates all the sorts which it is not capable of dissolving.

P. *Hydro-sulphuret of Ammonia.*

This and other sulphurets, as well as water saturated with sulphuretted hydrogen, may be employed in detecting lead and arsenic, with the former of which they give a black, and with the latter a yellowish precipitate. As lead and arsenic, however, are never found in natural waters, these tests are not required.

MINERA'LIA. See *Mineral*

MINERALIZE. Metallic substances are said to be mineralized when deprived of their usual properties by combination with some other substance.

MINERA'LOGY. *Mineralogia.* That part of natural history which relates to minerals.

Minim. See *Minimum.*

MINIMUM. A minim. The sixtieth part of a fluid drachm. An important change has been adopted in the last London Pharmacopœia, for the mensuration of liquids, and the division of the wine pint, to ensure accuracy in the measurement of quantities of liquids below one drachm. The number of drops contained in one drachm has been assumed to be sixty: and taking water as a standard, this number, though by no means accurate, would still be sufficient for ordinary purposes; but when other liquids of less specific gravity are used, a much larger number is required to fill the same measure, as of proof spirit, 140 drops are required to equal the bulk of 60 of water, dropped from the same vessel. If, therefore, in the composition of medicines, measures suited to the standard of water were used occasionally only, and it was generally assumed that 60 drops were equal to one fluid-drachm, and one fluid-drachm was substituted for 60 drops prescribed, twice the dose intended would be given. There are further objections to the use of drops; that their bulk is influenced by the quantity of liquid contained in the bottle from which they fall, by the thickness of the lip, and even by the inequalities on the surface of the lip of the same bottle; that volatile liquids, to which this mode is most commonly applied, are thus exposed with extensive surfaces, and their evaporation promoted; and on all these accounts the adoption of some decisive, convenient, and uniform substitute became necessary. The subdivision of the wine pint has, therefore, been extended to the sixtieth part of the fluid-drachm, which is termed minim: and glass measures expressive of such subdivision, have been adopted by the college.

MI'NIUM. Red oxide of lead. See *Lead.*

MINIUM GRÆCORUM. Native cinnabar

MINT. See *Mentha.*

Mint, pepper. See *Mentha piperita.*

Mint, water. See *Mentha aquatica.*

MISCARRIAGE. See *Abortion.*

MISERE'RE MEI. (Have compassion on me: so called from its unhappy torments.) The iliac passion. See *Iliac passion.*

MISLAW. See *Musa paradisiaca.*

MISLETOE. See *Viscum.*

MISOCHY'MICUS. An enemy to the chemists and their enthusiastic conceits.

MISPICKLE. Common arsenical pyrites. A white, brilliant, granulated iron ore, composed of iron in combination with arsenic.

MISTU'RA. A mixture. A fluid composed of two or more ingredients. It is mostly contracted in prescriptions thus, *mist.* e. g. —*f. mist.* which means, let a mixture be made.

MISTURA AMMONIACI. *Lac ammoniaci.* Mixture of ammoniacum.—Take of ammoniacum, two drachms; of water, half a pint; rub the ammoniacum with the water gradually added, till they are thoroughly mixed

MISTURA AMYGDALÆ. *Lac amygdalæ.* Almond mixture, or emulsion.—Take of almond confection, two ounces; distilled water, a pint: gradually add the water to the almond confection, rubbing them together till properly mixed; then strain.

MISTURA ASAFŒTIDÆ. *Lac asafœtidæ.* Mixture of asafœtida.—Take of asafœtida, two drachms; water, half a pint; rub the asafœtida with the water, gradually added, till they are thoroughly mixed,

MISTURA CAMPHORÆ. Camphor mixture.—Take of camphor, half a drachm; rectified spirit, ten minims; water, a pint. First rub the camphor with the spirit, then with the water gradually added, and strain the liquor. A very elegant preparation of camphor, for delicate stomachs, and those who cannot bear it in substance, as an antispasmodic and nervine. There is a great loss of camphor in making it as directed by the pharmacopœia. Water can only take up a certain quantity. For its virtues, see *Laurus camphora.*

MISTURA CORNU USTI. *Decoctum album.* Decoction of hartshorn. Take of hartshorn, burnt and prepared, two ounces; acacia gum, powdered, an ounce; water, three pints. Boil down to two pints, constantly stirring, and strain. This is a much weaker absorbent than the mistura cretæ, but is much more agreeable to most people. It forms an excellent drink in fevers attended with diarrhœa, and acidities of the primæ viæ.

MISTURA CRETÆ. Chalk mixture.—Take of prepared chalk, half an ounce; refined sugar, three drachms; gum-arabic, powdered, half an ounce; water, a pint. Mix. A very useful and pleasant form of administering chalk as an adstringent and antacid. It is particularly calculated for children, in whom it allays the many deranged actions of the primæ viæ, which are produced by acidities. Dose, one ounce to three, frequently. See *Creta* and *Carbonas calcis.*

MISTURA FERRI COMPOSITA.—Take of myrrh, powdered, a drachm ; subcarbonate of potassa, twenty-five grains ; rose-water, seven fluid ounces and a half ; sulphate of iron, powdered, a scruple ; spirit of nutmeg, half a fluid ounce ; refined sugar, a drachm. Rub together the myrrh, the subcarbonate of potassa and sugar ; and, during the trituration, add gradually, first, the rose-water and spirit of nutmeg, and last, the sulphate of iron. Pour the mixture immediately into a proper glass bottle, and stop it close. This preparation is the celebrated mixture of Dr. Griffiths. A chemical decomposition is effected in forming this mixture, a subcarbonate of iron is formed, and a sulphate of potassa.

MISTURA GUAIACI. Take of guaiacum gum-resin, a drachm and a half ; refined sugar, two drachms ; mucilage of acacia gum, two fluid drachms ; cinnamon water, eight fluid ounces. Rub the guaiacum with the sugar, then with the mucilage ; and, when they are mixed, pour on the cinnamon-water gradually, rubbing them together. For its virtues, see *Guaiacum.*

MISTURA MOSCHI. Take of musk, acacia gum, powdered, refined sugar, of each a drachm : rose-water, six fluid ounces. Rub the musk first with the sugar, then with the gum, and add the rose-water by degrees. An excellent diaphoretic and antispasmodic. It is by far the best way of administering musk, when boluses cannot be swallowed. Dose, one ounce to three, frequently.

Mithridate mustard. See *Thlaspi campestre.*

MITHRIDATIUM The electuary called *Mithridate,* from Mithridates, king of Pontus and Bithynia, who, experiencing the virtues of the simples separately, afterward combined them ; but then the composition consisted of but few ingredients, viz. twenty leaves of rue, two walnuts, two figs, and a little salt : of this he took a dose every morning, to guard himself against the effects of poison.

MITRAL. (*Mitralis ;* from *mitra,* a mitre.) Mitre-like : applied by anatomists to parts which were supposed to resemble a bishop's mitre.

MITRAL VALVES. *Valvulæ mitrales.* The valves of the left ventricle of the heart.

MI'VA. An ancient term for the form of a medicine, not unlike a thick syrup, now called *Marmalade.*

MIXTURE. 1. See *Mistura.*

2. Mixture in chemistry should be distinguished from solution ; in the former, the aggregate particles can again be separated by mechanical means, and the proportion of the different particles determined : but, in solution, no mechanical power whatsoever can separate them.

Mocha stone. A species of agate.

MO'CHILA. (From μοχλος, a lever.) A reduction of the bones from an unnatural to a natural situation.

MO'CHLICA. (From μοχλευω, to move.) Violent purges.

MODI'OLUS. (Diminutive of *Modus,* a measure.) The nucleus, as it were, of the cochlea of the ear is so termed. It ascends from the basis of the cochlea to the apex.

Mofette. See *Nitrogen.*

MOFFAT. A village situated about fifty-six miles southwest of Edinburgh. It affords a cold sulphureous water, of a very simple composition ; when first drawn, it appears rather milky and bluish ; the smell is exactly similar to that of Harrowgate ; the smell is sulphureous and saline, without any thing bitter. It sparkles somewhat on being poured from one glass to another.

According to Dr. Garnett's analysis, a wine gallon of Moffat water contains thirty-six grains of muriate of soda, five cubic inches of carbonic acid gas, four of azotic gas, and ten of sulphuretted hydrogen, making altogether nineteen cubic inches of gas. Moffat water is, therefore, very simple in its composition, and hence it produces effects somewhat similar to those of Harrowgate. It is, perhaps, on this account also that it so soon loses the hepatic gas, on which depends the greatest part of its medicinal power. The only sensible effect of this water is that of increasing the flow of urine ; when it purges, it appears rather to take place from the excessive dose than from its mineral ingredients. This water appears to be useful chiefly in cutaneous eruptions, and as an external application at an

increased temperature, scrofula in its early stage appears to be elevated by it ; it is also used as an external application to irritable ulcers, and is recommended in dyspepsia, and where there is inaction of the alimentary canal.

MOGILA'LIA. (From μογις, difficulty, and λαλεω, to speak.) A difficulty of speech.

MO'LA. (Hebrew.) 1. The knee-pan : so named because it is shaped like a millstone.

2. A mole, or shapeless mass of flesh in the uterus See *Mole.*

MOLA'RIS. (From *molaris,* a grindstone ; because they grind the food.) A double-tooth. See *Teeth.*

MOLARES GLANDULÆ. Molar glands. Two salival glands situated on each side of the mouth, between the masseter and buccinator muscles, the excretory ducts of which open near the last dens molaris.

MOLARES DENTES. See *Teeth.*

MOLASSES. See *Saccharum.*

MOLDA'VICA. See *Dracocephalum.*

MOLE. *Mola.* By this term authors have intended to describe different productions of, or excretions from, the uterus.

By some it has been used to signify every kind of fleshy substance, particularly those which are properly called polypi ; by others, those only which are the consequence of imperfect conception, or when the ovum is in a morbid or decayed state ; and by many, which is the most popular opinion, every coagulum of blood which continues long enough in the uterus to assume somewhat of an organized form, to have only the fibrous part, as it has been called, remaining, is denominated a mole. There is surely much impropriety, says Dr. Denham, in including, under one general name, appearances so contrary and substances so different.

1. For an account of the first kind, see *Polypus.*

2. Of the second kind, which has been defined as an *ovum deforme,* as it is the consequence of conception, it might more justly be arranged under the class of monsters ; for though it has the appearance of a shapeless mass of flesh, if examined carefully with a knife, various parts of a child may be discovered, lying together in apparent confusion, but in actual regularity The pedicle also by which it is connected to the uterus, is not of a fleshy texture, like that of the polypus, but has a regular series of vessels like the umbilical cord, and there is likewise a placenta and membranes containing water. The symptoms attending the formation, growth, and expulsion of this apparently confused mass from the uterus, correspond with those of a well-formed child.

3. With respect to the third sort of mole, an incision into its substance will discover its true nature ; for, although the external surface appears at the first view to be organized flesh, the internal part is composed merely of coagulated blood. As substances of this kind, which mostly occur after delivery, would always be expelled by the action of the uterus, there seems to be no reason for a particular inquiry, if popular opinion had not annexed the idea of mischief to them, and attributed their formation or continuance in the uterus to the negligence or misconduct of the practitioner. Hence the persuasion arose of the necessity of extracting all the coagula of blood out of the uterus, immediately after the expulsion of the placenta, or of giving medicines to force them away : but abundant experience hath proved, that the retention of such coagula is not, under any circumstances, productive of danger, and that they are most safely expelled by the action of the uterus, though at very different periods after their formation.

MO'LLE. Indian mastich.

MOLLIFICA'TIO. A softening: formerly applied to a palsy of the muscles in any particular part.

MOLLI'TIES. (From *mollis,* soft.) A softness applied to bones, nails, and other parts.

MOLLITIES OSSIUM. See *Malacosteon*

MOLLITIES UNGUIUM. A preternatural softness of the nails : it often accompanies chlorosis.

MOLUCCE'NSE LIGNUM. See *Croton tiglium.*

MOLYBDATE. *Molybdas.* A salt formed by the union of the molybdic acid with salifiable bases : thus *molybdate of antimony,* &c.

MOLYBDENUM. (From μολυβδος, lead.) *Molybditis.* A metal which exists mineralized by sulphur in the ore, called *sulphuret of molybdena.* This ore, which is very scarce, is so similar in several of its properties to plumbago, that they were long considered as varieties of the same substance. It is of a light lead-gray colour; its surface is smooth, and feels unctuous; its texture is lamellated; it soils the fingers, and marks paper bluish-black, or silver-gray. It may be cut with a knife. It is generally found in compact masses; seldom in particles, or crystallized. It is met with in Sweden, Spain, Saxony, Siberia, and Iceland. Scheele showed that a peculiar metallic acid might be obtained from it; and later chemists have succeeded in reducing this acid to the metallic state. We are indebted to Hatchett for a full and accurate analysis of this ore.

The native *sulphuret of molybdena*, is the only ore hitherto known which contains this metal.

Properties of molybdena.—Molybdena is either in an agglutinated blackish friable mass, having little metallic brillancy, or in a black powder. The mass slightly united, shows, by a magnifying glass, small, round, brilliant grains. Its weight is about 8. It is one of the most infusible of the metals. It is capable of combining with a number of metals by fusion. It forms with sulphur an artificial sulphuret of molybdena analogous to its ore. It unites also to phosphorus. The affinity of molybdena for oxygen is very feeble, according to Hatchett. The alkalies have no action on molybdena in the moist way, but it enters readily into fusion with potassa and soda. It is oxidisable by boiling sulphuric acid, and acidifiable by the nitric acid. Muriatic acid does not act upon it. It is capable of existing in not less than four different degrees of oxygenation.

Method of obtaining molybdena.—To obtain molybdena is a task of the utmost difficulty. Few chemists have succeeded in producing this metal, on account of its great infusibility. The method recommended in general is the following:—Molybdic acid is to be formed into a paste with oil, dried at the fire, and then exposed to a violent heat in a crucible lined with charcoal. By this means the oxide becomes decomposed; a black agglutinated substance is obtained, very brittle under the finger, and having a metallic brilliancy. This is the metal called molybdena.

MOLYBDIC ACID. (*Acidum, molybdicum;* from *Molybdenum,* its base.) The native sulphuret of molybdenum being roasted for some time, and dissolved in water of ammonia, when nitric acid is added to this solution, the molybdic acid precipitates in fine white scales, which become yellow on melting and subliming them. It changes the vegetable blues to red, but less readily and powerfully than the molybdous acid.

Molybdic acid has a specific gravity of 3.460. In an open vessel it sublimes into brilliant yellow scales; 960 parts of boiling water dissolve one of it, affording a pale yellow solution, which reddens litmus, but has no taste. Sulphur, charcoal, and several metals, decompose the molybdic acid. Molybdate of potassa is a colourless salt. Molybdic acid gives, with nitrate of lead, a white precipitate, soluble in nitric acid; with the nitrates of mercury and silver, a white flaky precipitate; with nitrate of copper, a greenish precipitate; with solutions of the *neutral* sulphate of zinc, muriate of bismuth, muriate of antimony, nitrate of nickel, muriates of gold and platinum, it produces white precipitates. When melted with borax, it yields a bluish colour; and paper dipped in its solution becomes, in the sun, of a beautiful blue.

The neutral alkaline molybdates precipitate all metallic solutions. Gold, muriate of mercury, zinc, and manganese, are precipitated in the form of a white powder; iron and tin, from their solutions in muriatic acid, of a brown colour; cobalt, of a rose colour; copper, blue; and the solutions of alum and quicklime, white. If a dilute solution of recent muriate of tin be precipitated by a dilute solution of molybdate of potassa, a beautiful blue powder is obtained.

The concentrated sulphuric acid dissolves a considerable quantity of the molybdic acid, the solution becoming of a fine blue colour as it cools, at the same time that it thickens; the colour disappears again on the application of heat, but returns again by cooling. A strong heat expels the sulphuric acid. The nitric acid has no effect on it; but the muriatic dissolves it in considerable quantity, and leaves a dark blue residuum when distilled. With a strong heat it expels a portion of sulphuric acid from sulphate of potassa. It also disengages the acid from nitre and common salt by

N n

distillation. It has some action upon the filings of the metals in the moist way.

MOLYBDI'TIS. See *Molybdenum.*

MOLY'BDOS. (Ὅτι νολει εις βαθος; from its gravity.) Lead.

MOLYBDOUS ACID. *Acidum molybdosum.* The deut-oxide of molybdenum is of a blue colour, and possesses acid properties. Triturate 2 parts of molybdic acid, with one part of the metal, along with a little hot water, in a porcelain mortar, till the mixture assumes a blue colour. Digest in 10 parts of boiling water, filter and evaporate the liquid in a heat of about 120°. The blue oxide separates. It reddens vegetable blues, and forms salts with the bases. Air or water, when left for some time to act on molybdenum, convert it into this acid. It consists of about 100 metal to 34 oxygen.

MOLY'ZA. (Diminutive of μωλυ, moly.) Garlic; the head of which, like moly, is not divided into cloves.

MOMISCUS. (From μωμος, a blemish.) That part of the teeth which is next the gums, and which is usually covered with a foul tartareous crust.

MOMO'RDICA. (*Momordica;* from *mordeo,* to bite; from its sharp taste.) The name of a genus of plants in the Linnæan system. Class, *Monœcia;* Order, *Syngenesia.*

MOMORDICA ELATERIUM. The systematic name of the squirting cucumber. *Elaterium; Cucumis agrestis; Cucumis asininus; Cucumis sylvestris; Elaterium officinarum; Boubalios; Charantia; Guarerba orba.* Wild, or squirting cucumber. *Momordica-pomis hispidis cirrhisnullis* of Linnæus. The dried sediment from the juice of this plant is the elaterium of the shops. It has neither smell nor taste, and is the most powerful cathartic in the whole Materia Medica. Its efficacy in dropsies is said to be considerable; it, however, requires great caution in the exhibition. From the eighth to the half of a grain should be given at first, and repeated at proper intervals until it operates. The cathartic power of this substance is derived from a small portion of a very active principle, which Dr. Paris, in his Pharmacologia, has called *Elatin.* From ten grains of elaterium he obtained,

Water	0.4
Extractive	2.6
Fecula	2.8
Gluten	0.5
Woody matter	2.5
Elatin	} 1.2
Bitter principle	
	10.

MONA'RDA. (So called in honour of Nicholas Monardes, a Spanish physician and botanist.) The name of a genus of plants in the Linnæan system. Class, *Diandria;* Order, *Monogynia.*

MONARDA FISTULOSA. The systematic name of the purple monarda. The leaves of this plant have a fragrant smell, and an aromatic and somewhat bitter taste, possessing nervine, stomachic, and deobstruent virtues. An infusion is recommended in the cure of intermittent fevers.

[" The Monarda is a very pungent aromatic, growing native in the United States, with various other species, some of which resemble it in efficacy. In different parts of the country it is known by the names of *mountain-balm* and horsemint. It is a warm diaphoretic, anti-emetic, and carminative; used in flatulent colics, rheumatism, &c. The distilled oil, according to Dr. Atlee, is one of the most powerful rubefacients." —*Big. Mat. Med.* A.]

MONADE'LPHIA. (From μονος, alone, and αδελφια, a brotherhood.) The name of a class of plants in the sexual system of Linnæus, consisting of plants with hermaphrodite flowers, in which all the stamina are united below into one body or cylinder, through which the pistil passes.

MONA'NDRIA. (From μονος, alone, and ανηρ, a husband.) The name of a class of plants in the sexual system of Linnæus, consisting of plants with hermaphrodite flowers, which have only one stamen.

MONE'LLI. A species of *Anagallis.*

MONEY-WORT. See *Lysimachia nummularia.*

MONILIFORMIS. (*Monilo,* an ornament for any

81

part of the body, especially a necklace or collar.)
Moniliform applied to the pod of the *Hedysarum moniliferum* from its necklace appearance.

Monk's rhubarb. See *Rumex alpinus.*

MONKSHOOD. See *Aconitum napellus.*

MONOCOTYLEDON. (From μονος, one, and κοτυληδων, a cotyledon.) Having one cotyledon.

MONOCOTYLEDONES. A tribe of plants which are supposed to have only one cotyledon; as the grass and corn tribe, palms, and the orchis family. See *Cotyledon.*

MONOCULUS (From μονος, one, and *oculus*, an eye.) *Monopia.* 1. A very uncommon species of monstrosity, in which there is but one eye, and that mostly above the root of the nose.

2. *Intestinum monoculum* is the name given to the cæcum, or blind gut, by Paracelsus, because it is perforated only at one end.

[3. A genus of crustacea, to which belongs the great *horse-foot* of America, or the *Monoculus Polyphemus.* A.]

MONŒ'CIA. (From μονος, alone, and οικια, a house.) The name of a class of plants in the sexual system of Linnæus, consisting of those which have male and female organs in separate flowers, but on the same plant.

MONOGY'NIA. (From μονος, alone, and γυνη, a woman, or wife.)—The name of an order of plants in the sexual system of Linnæus. It contains those plants which, besides their agreement in the classic character, have only one style.

MONOHE'MERA. (From μονος, single, and ημερα, a day.) A disease of one day's continuance.

MONOICUS. (From μονος, one, and οικια, a house.) Linnæus calls flowers *monoici*, monœteous, when the stamens and pistils are situated in different flowers, on the same individual plant; because they are confined to one house, as it were, or dwelling; and if the barren and fertile flowers grow from separate roots, *flores dioici*, or diœcious flowers.

MONO'MACHON. The intestinum cæcum.

MONOPE'GIA. (From μονος, single, and πηγνυμι, to compress.) A pain in only one side of the head.

MONOPHYLLUS. (From μονος, one, and φυλλον, a leaf.) One-leafed: having only one leaf applied to the perianthium of flowers; thus the flower-cup of the *Datura stramonium* is monophyllous, or formed of one leaf.

MONO'PIA. (From μονος, single, and ωψ, the eye.) See *Monoculus.*

MONO'RCHIS. (From μονος, one, and ορχις, a testicle.) An epithet for a person that has but one testicle.

MONRO, ALEXANDER, was born in London, of Scotch parents, in 1697. His father, who was an army surgeon, settled afterward at Edinburgh, and took great interest in his education. At a proper age, he sent him to attend Cheselden in London, where he displayed great assiduity, and laid the foundation of his celebrated work on the bones; he then went to Paris, and in 1718 to Leyden, where he received the particular commendation of Boerhaave. Returning to Edinburgh the following year, he was appointed professor and demonstrator of anatomy to the Company of Surgeons, and soon after he began to give public lectures on that subject, Dr. Alston at the same time taking up the Materia Medica and Botany. This may be regarded as the opening of that medical school, which has since extended its fame throughout Europe and even to America. The two lectureships were placed upon the university establishment in 1720, and others shortly added to complete the system of medical education; but an opportunity of seeing practice being still wanting, Dr. Monro pointed out in a pamphlet the advantages of such an institution; the Royal Infirmary was therefore established, and he commenced Clinical Lecturer on Surgery; and Dr. Rutherford afterward extended the plan to Medical cases. None of the new professors contributed so much to the celebrity of this school as Dr. Monro, not only by the diligent and skilful execution of the duties of his office, but also by various ingenious and useful publications. He continued his lectures during upwards of six months annually for nearly forty years, and acquired such reputation, that students flocked to him from the most distant parts of the kingdom. His first and chief work was his "Osteology," in 1726, intended for his pupils; but which

became very popular, passed through numerous editions, and was translated into most European languages: he afterward added a concise description of the nerves, and a very accurate account of the lacteal system and thoracic duct. He was also the father and active supporter of a society, to which the public was indebted for six volumes of "Medical Essays and Observations:" he acted as secretary, and had the chief labour in the publication of these, besides having contributed many valuable papers, especially an elaborate "Essay on the Nutrition of the Fœtus." The plan of the society was afterward extended, and three volumes of "Essays Physical and Literary" were published, in which Dr. Monro has several useful papers. His last publication was an "Account of the Success of Inoculation in Scotland." He left, however, several works in manuscript; of which a short "Treatise on Comparative Anatomy," and his oration "De Cuticula," have been since given to the public. In 1759, Dr. Monro resigned his anatomical chair to his son, but continued his Clinical lectures; he exerted himself also in promoting almost every object of public utility. He was chosen a fellow of the Royal Society of London, and an honorary member of the Royal Academy of Surgery at Paris. He died in 1767.

MONS. A mount, or hill.

MONS VENERIS. The triangular eminence immediately over the os pubis of women, that is covered with hair.

MONSTER. *Lusus naturæ.* Dr. Denman divides monsters into, 1st, Monsters from redundance or multiplicity of parts; 2d, Monsters from deficiency or want of parts; 3d, Monsters from confusion of parts. To these might perhaps be added, without impropriety, another kind, in which there is neither redundance, nor deficiency, nor confusion of parts, but an error of place, as in transposition of the viscera. But children born with diseases, as the hydrocephalus, or their effects, as in some cases of blindness, from previous inflammation, cannot be properly considered as monsters, though they are often so denominated.

Of the first order there may be two kinds; redundance or multiplicity of natural parts, as of two heads and one body, of one head and two bodies, an increased number of limbs, as legs, arms, fingers, and toes; or excrescences or additions to parts of no certain form, as those upon the head and other parts of the body. It is not surprising that we should be ignorant of the manner in which monsters or irregular births are generated or produced; though it is probable that the laws by which these are governed are as regular, both as to cause and effect, as in common or natural productions. Formerly, and indeed till within these few years, it was a generally received opinion, that monsters were not primordial or aboriginal, but that they were caused subsequently, by the power of the imagination of the mother, transferring the imperfection of some external object, or the mark of something for which she longed, and with which she was not indulged, to the child of which she was pregnant; or by some accident which happened to her during her pregnancy. Such opinions, it is reasonable to think, were permitted to pass current, in order to protect pregnant women from all hazardous and disagreeable occupations, to screen them from severe labour, and to procure for them a greater share of indulgence and tenderness than could be granted to them in the common occurrences of life. The laws and customs of every civilized nation have, in some degree, established a persuasion that there was something sacred in the person of a pregnant woman: and this may be right in several points of view; but these only go a little way towards justifying the opinion of monsters being caused by the imagination of the mother. The opinion has been disproved by common observation, and by philosophy, not perhaps by positive proofs, but by many strong negative facts: as the improbability of any child being born perfect, had such a power existed; the freedom of children from any blemish, their mothers being in situations most exposed to objects likely to produce them; the ignorance of the mother of any thing being wrong in the child, till, from information of the fact, she begins to recollect every accident which happened during her pregnancy, and assigns the worst or the most plausible, as the cause; the organization and colour of these adventitious substances; the frequent occurrence of monsters in the brute creation, in which the power of the imagination cannot be great; and the analogous appearances in the vegetable system, where it does not exist in any degree. Judging, however, from appearances, accidents may perhaps be allowed to have considerable influence in the production of monsters of some kinds, either by actual injury upon parts, or by suppressing or deranging the principle of growth, because, when an arm, for instance, is wanting, the rudiments of the deficient parts may generally be discovered.

MONTMARTRITE. A mineral compound of sulphate and carbonate of lime, that stands the weather, which common gypsum does not. It is found at Montmartre, near Paris.

MOONSTONE. A variety of adularia.

["MOORE, WILLIAM, M. D. This ornament of the profession and of Christianity, was born at Newtown, on Long-Island, state of New-York, in 1754. His father Samuel, and his grandfather Benjamin, Moore, were agriculturists. He received the rudiments of a classical education under the tuition of his elder brother, afterward bishop Moore, and president for many years of Columbia college. He attended the lectures on medicine delivered by Drs. Clossey and Samuel Bard. In 1778 he went to London, and thence to Edinburgh. In 1780 he was graduated doctor of medicine, on which occasion he published his dissertation *De Bile.* For more than forty years he continued unremittingly engaged in the arduous duties of an extensive practice, particularly in midwifery, estimating his number of cases at about three thousand. He died in the seventy-first year of his age, in April, 1824.

The medical papers of Dr. Moore may be found in the American Medical and Philosophical Register, the New-York Medical Repository, and the New-York Medical and Physical Journal. For many years Dr. Moore was president of the Medical Society of the county of New-York, and an upright and vigilant trustee of the College of Physicians and Surgeons. On his death the College recorded their testimony to his pre-eminent worth."—*Thach. Med. Biog.* A.]

MORBI'LLI. (Diminutive of *morbus*, a disease.) See *Rubeola.*

MORBUS. A disease.

MORBUS ARQUATUS. The jaundice.

MORBUS ATTONITUS. The epilepsy, and apoplexy.

MORBUS COXARIUS. See *Arthropuosis.*

MORBUS GALLICUS. The venereal disease.

MORBUS HERCULEUS. The epilepsy.

MORBUS INDICUS. The venereal disease.

MORBUS INFANTILIS. The epilepsy.

MORBUS MAGNUS. The epilepsy.

MORBUS NIGER. The black disease. So Hippocrates named it, and thus described it. This disorder is known by vomiting a concrete blood of a blackish red colour, and mixed with a large quanty of insipid acid, or viscid phlegm. This evacuation is generally preceded by a pungent tensive pain, in both the hypochondria; and the appearance of the disease is attended with anxiety, a compressive pain in the præcordia, and fainting, which last is more frequent and violent, when the blood which is evacuated is fœtid and corrupt. The stomach and the spleen are the principal, if not the proper seat of this disease.

MORBUS REGIUS. The jaundice.

MORBUS SACER. The epilepsy.

MORDANT. In dying, the substance combined with the vegetable or animal fibre, in order to fix the dye-stuff.

MOREL. See *Phallus esculentus.*

MORE'TUS. (From *morum*, the mulberry.) A decoction of mulberries.

MORGAGNI, GIAMBATISTA, was born at Forli in 1682. He commenced his medical studies at Bologna, and displayed such ardour and talent, that Valsalva availed himself of his assistance in his researches into the organ of hearing, and in drawing up his memoirs on that subject. He also performed the professorial duties during the temporary absence of Valsalva, and by his skill and obliging manners procured general esteem. He afterward prosecuted his studies at Venice and Padua, and then settled in his native place. He soon, however, perceived that this was too contracted a sphere for his abilities; wherefore he returned to Padua, where a vacancy soon occurring, he was nominated, in 1711, to teach the theory of physic. He had already distinguished himself by the publication five

years before of the first part of his "Adversaria Anatomica," a work remarkable for its accuracy, as well as originality; of which, subsequently, five other parts appeared. He assisted Lancisi in preparing for publication the valuable drawings of Eustachius, which came out in 1714. The following year he was appointed to the first anatomical professorship in Padua; and from that period ranked at the head of the anatomists of his time. He was also well versed in general literature, and other subjects not immediately connected with his profession: and honours were rapidly accumulated upon him from every quarter of Europe. He was distinguished by the particular esteem of three successive Popes, and by the visits of all the learned and great, who came into his neighbourhood; and his native city placed a bust of him in their public hall during his life, with an honorary inscription. Though he had a large family, he accumulated a considerable property by his industry and economy; and by means of a good constitution and regular habits, he attained the advanced age of 90. Besides the Adversaria he published several other works, two quarto volumes of anatomical epistles, an essay on the proper method of acquiring medical science, which appeared on his appointment to the theoretical chair, &c. But that which has chiefly rendered his name illustrious is entitled "De Sedibus et Causis Morborum," printed at Venice in 1760. It contains a prodigious collection of dissections of morbid bodies, made by Valsalva and himself, arranged according to the organs affected. He followed the plan of Bonetus; but the accuracy of his details renders the collection far superior in value to any that had preceded it.

MO'RIA. (From μωρος, foolish.) The name of a genus of diseases in Good's Nosology. Class, *Neurotica;.* Order, *Phrenica.* Idiotism. Fatuity. It has two species, *Moria imbecillis, demens.*

MO'RO. (From *morum*, a mulberry.) A small abscess resembling a mulberry.

MORO'SIS. (From μωρος, foolish.) See *Amentia.*

MOROXYLATE. A compound of moroxylic acid with a salifiable basis.

MOROXYLIC ACID. (*Acidum moroxylicum;* from *morus*, the mulberry-tree, and ξυλον, wood; because it is found on the bark or wood of that tree.) In the botanic garden at Palermo, Mr. Thompson found an uncommon saline substance on the trunk of a white mulberry-tree. It appeared as a coating on the surface of the bark in little granulous drops of a yellowish and blackish-brown colour, and had likewise penetrated its substance. Klaproth, who analyzed it, found that its taste was somewhat like that of succinic acid; on burning coals, it swelled up a little, emitted a pungent vapour scarcely visible to the eye, and left a slight earthy residuum. Six hundred grains of the bark loaded with it were lixiviated with water, and afforded 320 grains of a light salt, resembling in colour a light wood, and composed of short needles united in radii. It was not deliquescent; and though the crystals did not form till the solution was greatly condensed by evaporation, it is not very soluble, since 1000 parts of water dissolve but 35 with heat, and 15 cold.

This salt was found to be a compound of lime and a peculiar vegetable acid, with some extractive matter.

To obtain the acid separate, Klaproth decomposed the calcareous salt by acetate of lead, and separated the lead by sulphuric acid. He likewise decomposed it directly by sulphuric acid. The product was still more like succinic acid in taste; was not deliquescent; easily dissolved both in water and alkohol: and did not precipitate the metallic solutions, as it did in combination with lime. Twenty grains being slightly heated in a small glass retort, a number of drops of an acid liquor first came over; next a concrete salt arose, that adhered flat against the top and part of the neck of the retort in the form of prismatic crystals, colourless and transparent; and a coaly residuum remained. The acid was then washed out, and crystallized by spontaneous evaporation.—This sublimation appears to be the best mode of purifying the salt, but it adhered too strongly to the lime to be separated from it directly by heat without being decomposed.

Not having a sufficient quantity to determine its specific characters, though he conceives it to be a peculiar acid, coming nearest to the succinic both in taste and other qualities, Klaproth has provisionally given it the same of moroxylic, and the calcareous salt containing it, that of moroxylate of lime.

MORPHE′A ALBA. (From μορφη, form.) A species of cutaneous leprosy. See *Lepra alphos.*

MORPHIA. Morphine. A new vegetable alkali, extracted from opium, of which it constitutes the narcotic principle. See *Papaver somniferum.*

MORPHINE. See *Morphia.*

MORSE′LLUS. A lozenge.

MORSULUS. An ancient name for that form of medicine which was to be chewed in the mouth, as a lozenge ; the word signifying a little mouthful.

MO′RSUS DIABOLI. The fimbriæ of the Fallopian tubes.

MO′RTA. See *Pemphigus.*

MORTARI′OLUM. (Dim. of *mortarium,* a mortar.) In chemistry, it is a sort of mould for making cupels with ; also a little mortar. In anatomy, it is the sockets of the teeth.

MORTIFICATION. (*Mortificatio* ; from *mors,* death, and *fio,* to become.) *Gangrena; Sphacelus.* The loss of vitality of a part of the body. Surgeons divide mortification into two species, the one preceded by inflammation, the other without it. In inflammations that are to terminate in mortification, there is a diminution of power joined to an increased action ; this becomes a cause of mortification, by destroying the balance of power and action, which ought to exist in every part. There are, however, cases of mortification that do not arise wholly from that as a cause : of this kind are the carbuncle, and the slough, formed in the small-pox pustule. Healthy phlegmonous inflammation seldom ends in mortification, though it does so when very vehement and extensive. Erysipelatous inflammation is observed most frequently to terminate in gangrene ; and whenever phlegmon is in any degree conjoined with an erysipelatous affection, which it not unfrequently is, it seems thereby to acquire the same tendency, being more difficult to bring to resolution, or suppuration, than the true phlegmon, and more apt to run into a mortified state.

Causes which impede the circulation of the part affected, will occasion mortification, as is exemplified in strangulated hernia, tied polypi, or a limb being deprived of circulation from a dislocated joint.

Preventing the entrance of arterial blood into a limb, is also another cause. Paralysis, conjoined with pressure, old age, and ossification of the arteries, may produce mortification ; also cold, particularly if followed by the sudden application of warmth ; and likewise excessive heat applied to a part.

The symptoms of mortification that take place after inflammation are various, but generally as follows :— the pain and sympathetic fever suddenly diminish, the part affected becomes soft, and of a livid colour, losing at the same time more or less of its sensibility.

When any part of the body loses all motion, sensibility, and natural heat, and becomes of a brown livid or black colour, it is said to be affected with sphacelus. When the part becomes a cold, black, fibrous, senseless substance, it is termed a slough. As long as any sensibility, motion, and warmth continue, the state of the disorder is said to be gangrene. When the part has become quite cold, black, fibrous, incapable of moving, and destitute of all feeling, circulation, and life ; this is the second stage of mortification, termed *sphacelus.*

When gangrene takes place, the patient is usually troubled with a kind of hiccough : the constitution always suffers an immediate dejection, the countenance assumes a wild cadaverous look, the pulse becomes small, rapid, and sometimes irregular ; cold perspirations come on, and the patient is often affected with diarrhœa and delirium.

MORTON, RICHARD, was born in Suffolk, and after taking the degree of Bachelor of Arts at Oxford, officiated for some time as a chaplain : but the intolerance of the times, and his own religious scruples, compelled him to change for the medical profession. He was accordingly admitted to his doctor's degree in 1670, having accompanied the Prince of Orange to Oxford, as physician to his person. He afterward settled in London, became a Fellow of the College, and obtained a large share of the city practice. He died in 1698. His works have had considerable reputation, and evince some acuteness of observation, and acti-

vity of practice. They abound, however, with the errors of the humoral pathology, which then prevailed ; and sanction a method of treatment in acute diseases, which his more able contemporary, Sydenham, discountenanced, and which subsequent experience has generally discarded. His first publication was an attempt to arrange the varieties of consumption, but not very successfully. His "Pyretologia" came out in two volumes, the first in 1691, the other at an interval of three years ; in this work, especially, the stimulant treatment of fevers is carried to an unusual extent, and a more general use of cinchona recommended.

MO′RUM. See *Morus nigra.*

MO′RUS. (From μαυρος, black ; so called from the colour of its fruit when ripe.) The name of a genus of plants in the Linnæan system. Class, *Monœcia;* Order, *Tetrandria.* The mulberry-tree.

MORUS NIGRA. The systematic name of the mulberry-tree. *Morus—foliis cordatis scabris,* of Linnæus. Mulberries abound with a deep violet-coloured juice, which, in its general qualities, agrees with that of the fruits called *acido-dulces,* allaying thirst, partly by refrigerating, and partly by exciting an excretion of mucus from the mouth and fauces ; a similar effect is also produced in the stomach, where, by correcting putrescency, a powerful cause of thirst is removed. The London College directs a *syrupus mori,* which is an agreeable vehicle for various medicines. The bark of the root of this tree is said, by Andrée, to be useful in cases of tænia.

Mosaic gold. See *Aurum musivum.*

MOSCHA′TA NUX. See *Myristica moschata.*

MO′SCHUS. (*Mosch,* Arabian.) Musk. See *Moschus moschiferus.*

MOSCHUS MOSCHIFERUS. The systematic name of the musk animal, a ruminating quadruped, resembling the antelope. An unctuous substance is contained in excretory follicles about the navel of the male animal, the strong and permanent smell of which is peculiar to it. It is contained in a bag placed near the umbilical region. The best musk is brought from Tonquin, in China ; an inferior sort from Agria and Bengal, and a still worse from Russia. It is slightly unctuous, of a black colour, having a strong durable smell and a bitter taste. It yields part of its active matter to water, by infusion ; by distillation the water is impregnated with its flavour ; alkohol dissolves it, its impurities excepted. Chewed, and rubbed with a knife on paper, it looks bright, yellowish, smooth, and free from grittiness. Laid on a red-hot iron, it catches flame and burns almost entirely away, leaving only an exceedingly small quantity of light grayish ashes. If any earthy substances have been mixed with the musk, the impurities will discover them. The medicinal and chemical properties of musk and castor are very similar : the virtues of the former are generally believed to be more powerful, and hence musk is preferred in cases of imminent danger. It is prescribed as a powful antispasmodic, in doses of three grains or upwards, even to half a drachm, in the greater number of spasmodic diseases, especially in hysteria and singultus, and also in diseases of debility. In typhus, it is employed to remove subsultus tendinum, and other symptoms of a spasmodic nature. In cholera, it frequently stops vomiting ; and, combined with ammonia, it is given to arrest the progress of gangrene. It is best given in the form of bolus. To children, it is given in the form of enema, and is an efficacious remedy in the convulsions arising from dentition. It is also given in hydrophobia, and in some forms of mania.

MOSQUI′TA. (From *mosquita,* a gnat, Spanish.) An itching eruption of the skin, produced in hot climates by the bite of gnats.

MOSY′LLUM. Μοσυλλον. The best cinnamon.

Mother of thyme. See *Thymus serpyllum.*

MOTHER-WATER. When sea-water, or any other solution containing various salts, is evaporated, and the crystals taken out, there always remains a fluid containing deliquescent salts, and the impurities, if present. This is called the mother-water.

MOTHERWORT. See *Leonurus cardiaca.*

MOTION. See *Muscular motion.*

Motion, peristaltic. See *Peristaltic motion.*

MOTO′RES OCULORUM. (*Nervi motores oculorum:* so called because they supply the muscles which move the eye.) The third pair of nerves of the brain.

They arise from the crura cerebri, and are distributed on the muscles of the bulb of the eye.

MOTO'RII. See *Motores oculorum*.

MOULD. See *Fontanella*.

Mountain cork. See *Asbestos*.

Mountain green. Common copper green, a carbonate.

Mountain leather. See *Asbestos*.

Mountain parsley, black. See *Athamanta oreoselinum*.

Mountain soap. See *Soap, mountain*.

Mountain wood. See *Asbestos*.

MOUSE-EAR. See *Hieracium pilosella*.

MOUTH. *Os*. The cavity of the mouth is well known. The parts which constitute it are the common integuments, the lips, the muscles of the upper and under jaw, the palate, two alveolar arches, the gums, the tongue, the cheeks, and salival glands. The bones of the mouth are the two superior maxillary, two palatine, the lower jaw, and thirty-two teeth. The arteries of the external parts of the mouth are branches of the infra-orbital, inferior alveolar, and facial arteries. The veins empty themselves into the external jugulars. The nerves are branches from the fifth and seventh pair. The use of the mouth is for mastication, speech, respiration, deglutition, suction, and taste.

MO'XA. A Japanese word. See *Artemisia chinensis*.

MOXA JAPANICA. See *Artemisia chinensis*.

MUCIC ACID. (*Acidum mucicum;* from *mucus*, it being obtained from gum.) "This acid has been generally known by the name of *saccholactic*, because it was first obtained from sugar of milk; but as all the gums appear to afford it, and the principal acid in sugar of milk is the oxalic, chemists in general now distinguish it by the name of *mucic* acid.

It was discovered by Scheele. Having poured twelve ounces of diluted nitric acid on four ounces of powdered sugar of milk in a glass retort on a sand bath, the mixture became gradually hot, and at length effervesced violently, and continued to do so for a considerable time after the retort was taken from the fire. It is necessary, therefore, to use a large retort, and not to lute the receiver too tight. The effervescence having nearly subsided, the retort was again placed on the sand heat, and the nitric acid distilled off, till the mass had acquired a yellowish colour. This exhibiting no crystals, eight ounces more of the same acid were added, and the distillation repeated, till the yellow colour of the fluid disappeared. As the fluid was inspissated by cooling, it was redissolved in eight ounces of water, and filtered. The filtered liquor held oxalic acid in solution, and seven drachms and a half of white powder remained on the filter. This powder was the acid under consideration.

If one part of gum be heated gently with two of nitric acid, till a small quantity of nitrous gas and of carbonic acid is disengaged, the dissolved mass will deposite on cooling the mucic acid. According to Fourcroy and Vauquelin, different gums yield from 14 to 26 hundredths of this acid.

This pulverulent acid is soluble in about sixty parts of hot water, and, by cooling, a fourth part separates in small shining scales, that grow white in the air. It decomposes the muriate of barytes, and both the nitrate and muriate of lime. It acts very little on the metals, but forms with their oxides salts scarcely soluble. It precipitates the nitrates of silver, lead, and mercury. With potassa it forms a salt soluble in eight parts of boiling water, and crystallizable by cooling. That of soda requires but five parts of water, and is equally crystallizable. Both these salts are still more soluble when the acid is in excess. That of ammonia is deprived of its base by heat. The salts of barytes, lime, and magnesia, are nearly insoluble."

MUCILAGE. *Mucilago*. An aqueous solution of gum. See *Gum*.

MUCILAGINOUS. Gummy.

MUCILAGINOUS EXTRACTS. Extracts that readily dissolve in water, scarcely at all in spirits of wine, and undergo spirituous fermentation.

MUCILA'GO. (*Mucilage*.) See *Gum*.

MUCILAGO ACACIÆ. Mucilage of acacia. *Mucilago gummi arabici*.—Take of acacia gum, powdered, four ounces; boiling water, half a pint. Rub the gum with the water, gradually added, until it incorporates into a mucilage. A demulcent preparation, more fre-

quently used to combine medicines, than in any other form.

MUCILAGO AMYLI. Starch mucilage.—Take of starch, three drachms; water, a pint. Rub the starch, gradually adding the water to it; then boil until it incorporates into a mucilage. This preparation is mostly exhibited with opium, in the form of clyster in diarrhœas and dysenteries, where the tenesmus arises from an abrasion of the mucus of the rectum.

MUCILAGO ARABICI GUMMI. See *Mucilago acaciæ*.

MUCILAGO SEMINIS CYDONII. See *Decoctum cydonia*.

MUCILAGO TRAGACANTHÆ. Mucilage of tragacanth, joined with syrup of mulberries, forms a pleasant demulcent, and may be exhibited to children, who are fond of it. This mucilage is omitted in the last London Pharmacopœia, as possessing no superiority over the mucilage of acacia.

MUCOCA'RNEUS. In M. A. Severinus, it is an epithet for a tumour, and an abscess, which is partly fleshy and partly mucous.

MUCOUS. Of the nature of mucus.

MUCOUS ACID. See *Mucic acid*.

MUCOUS GLANDS. *Glandulæ mucosæ*. Mucipalous glands. Glands that secrete mucus, such as the glands of the Schneiderian membrane of the nose, the glands of the fauces, œsophagus, stomach, intestines, bladder, urethra, &c.

MUCRONATUS. (From *mucro*, a sharp point.) Sharp-pointed. See *Cuspidatus*.

MUCUS. (From μυξα, the mucus of the nose.) A name given to the two following substances.

1. *Mucus, animal*. One of the primary fluids of an animal body, perfectly distinct from gelatin, and vegetable mucus. Tannin, which is a delicate test for gelatin, does not affect mucus. "This fluid is transparent, glutinous, thready, and of a salt savour; it reddens paper of turnsole, contains a great deal of water, muriate of potassa and soda, lactate of lime, of soda, and phosphate of lime. According to Fourcroy and Vauquelin, the mucus is the same in all the mucous membranes. On the contrary, Berzelius thinks it variable according to the points from which it is extracted.

The mucus forms a layer of greater or less thickness at the surface of the mucous membranes, and it is renewed with more or less rapidity; the water it contains evaporates under the name of *mucous exhalation;* it also protects these membranes against the action of the air, of the aliment, the different glandular fluids, &c.; it is, in fact, to these membranes nearly what the epidermis is to the skin. Independently of this general use, it has others that vary according to the parts of mucous membranes. Thus, the mucus of the nose is favourable to the smell, that of the mouth gives facility to the taste, that of the stomach and the intestines assists in the digestion, that of the genital and urinary ducts serves in the generation and the secretion of the urine, &c.

A great part of the mucus is absorbed again by the membranes which secrete it; another part is carried outwards, either alone, as in blowing the nose, or spitting, or mixed with the pulmonary transpiration, or else mixed with the excremental matter or the urine, &c.

Animal mucus differs from that obtained from the vegetable kingdom, in not being soluble in water, swimming on its surface, nor capable of mixing oil with water, and being soluble in mineral acids, which vegetable mucus is not.

2. *Mucus, vegetable*. See *Gum*.

MUGWORT. See *Artemisia vulgaris*.

Mugwort, China. See *Artemisia chinensis*.

MU'LÆ. Pustules contracted either by heat or cold.

MULBERRY. See *Morus Nigra*.

MULLEIN. See *Verbascum*.

MU'LSUM. See *Hydromeli*.

MULTI'FIDUS SPINÆ. (From *multus*, many, and *findo*, to divide.) , *Transverso-spinalis lumborum Musculus sacer; Semi-spinalis internus, sive trans verso spinalis dorsi; Semi-spinalis, sive transverso spinalis colli*, *pars interna*, of Winslow. *Transver salis lumborum vulgo sacer; Transversalis dorsi, Transversalis colli*, of Douglas. *Lumbo dorsi spinal*, of Dumas. The generality of anatomical writers have unnecessarily multiplied the muscles of the spine, and hence their descriptions of these parts are confused, and difficult to be understood. Under the name of *multifidus spinæ*, Albinus has, therefore, very properly included those portions of muscular flesh, intermixed with tendinous fibres, which lie close to the posterior part of the spine, and which Douglas and Winslow have described as three distinct muscles, under the names of *transversales*, or *transverso-spinales*, of the loins, back, and neck. The multifidus spinæ arises tendinous and fleshy from the upper convex surface of the os sacrum, from the posterior adjoining part of the ilium, from the oblique and transverse processes of all the lumbar vertebræ, from the transverse processes of all the dorsal vertebræ, and from those of the cervical vertebræ, excepting the three first. From all these origins the fibres of the muscles run in an oblique direction, and are inserted, by distinct tendons, into the spinous processes of all the vertebræ of the loins and back, and likewise into those of the six inferior vertebræ of the neck. When this muscle acts singly, it extends the back obliquely, or moves it to one side ; when both muscles act, they extend the vertebræ backwards.

MULTIFLORUS. Many-flowered. Applied to the flower-stalk of plants, which is so called when it bears many flowers ; as the *Daphne laureola*. See *Pedunculus*.

MULTIFO'RME OS. See *Ethmoid bone*.

MU LTIPES. (From *multus*, many, and *pes*, a foot.)
1. The wood-louse.
2. The polypus.
3. Any animal having more than four feet.

MUMPS. See *Cynanche parotidea*.

MUNDICATI'VA. (From *mundo*, to cleanse.) *Mundificantia*. Medicines which purify and cleanse away foulness.

MUNDIFICA'NTIA. See *Mundicativa*.

MU'NGOS. See *Ophiorrhiza mungos*.

MURA'LIS. (From *murus*, a wall ; so called because it grows upon walls.) Pellitory. See *Parietaria*.

MURA'RIA. (From *murus*, a wall: because it grows about walls.) A species of maiden-hair : the *Asplenium murale*.

MURIACITE. Gypsum.

MU'RIAS. A muriate, or salt, formed by the union of the muriatic acid with salifiable bases ; as *muriate of ammonia*, &c.

MURIAS AMMONIÆ. See *Sal ammoniac*.

MURIAS ANTIMONII. Butter of antimony. Formerly used as a caustic.

MURIAS BARYTÆ. See *Barytes*.

MURIAS CALCIS. See *Calx*.

MURIAS FERRI. *Ferrum salitum; Oleum martis per deliquium*. This preparation of iron is styptic and tonic, and may be given in chlorosis, intermittents, rachitis, &c.

MURIAS FERRI AMMONIACALIS. See *Ferrum ammoniatum*.

MURIAS HYDRARGYRI. There are two muriates of mercury. See *Hydrargyri submurias*, and *Hydrargyri oxymurias*.

MURIAS HYDRARGYRI AMMONIACALIS. See *Hydrargyrum præcipitatum album*.

MURIAS HYDRARGYRI OXYGENATUS. See *Hydrargyri oxymurias*.

MURIAS POTASSÆ. *Alkali vegetabile salitum; Sal digestivus; Sal febrifugus Sylvii*. This salt is exhibited with the same intention as the muriate of soda, and was formerly in high estimation in the cure of intermittents, &c.

MURIAS POTASSÆ OXYGENATUS. Chlorate of potassa. The oxygenated muriate of potassa has lately been extolled in the cure of the venereal disease. It is exhibited in doses of from fifteen to forty grains in the course of a day. It increases the action of the heart and arteries, and is supposed to oxygenate the blood, and prove of great service in scorbutus, asthenia, and cachectic diseases.

MURIAS SODÆ. See *Sodæ murias*.

MURIAS STIBII. See *Murias antimonii*.

MURIATIC. (*Muriaticus ;* from *muria*, brine.) Belonging to sea salt.

MURIATIC ACID. *Acidum muriaticum*. The *Hydrochloric* of the French chemists. Let six parts of pure and well dried sea salt be put into a glass retort, to the beak of which is luted; in a horizontal direction, a long glass tube artificially refrigerated, and containing a quantity of ignited muriate of lime. Upon the salt

pour at intervals five parts of concentrated oil of vitriol, through a syphon funnel, fixed air-tight, in the tubulure of the retort. The free end of the long tube being recurved, so as to dip into the mercury of a pneumatic trough, a gas will issue, which, on coming in contact with the air, will form a visible cloud, or haze, presenting, when viewed in a vivid light, prismatic colours. This gas is muriatic acid.

When received in glass jars over dry mercury, it is invisible, and possesses all the mechanical properties of air. Its odour is pungent and peculiar. Its taste acid and corrosive. Its specific gravity, according to Sir H. Davy, is such, that 100 cubic inches weigh 39 grains, while by estimation, he says, they ought to be 38.4 gr. If an inflamed taper be immersed in it, it is instantly extinguished. It is destructive of animal life ; but the irritation produced by it on the epiglottis scarcely permits its descent into the lungs. It is merely changed in bulk by alterations of temperature ; it experiences no change of state.

When potassium, tin, or zinc, is heated in contact with this gas over mercury, one half of the volume disappears, and the remainder is pure hydrogen. On examining the solid residue, it is found to be a metallic chloride. Hence muriatic acid gas consists of chlorine and hydrogen, united in equal volumes. This view of its nature was originally given by Scheele, though obscured by terms derived from the vague and visionary hypothesis of phlogiston. The French school afterward introduced the belief that muriatic acid gas was a compound of an unknown radical and water; and that chlorine consisted of this radical and oxygen. Sir H. Davy has proved, by decisive experiments, that in the present state of our knowledge, chlorine must be regarded as a simple substance ; and muriatic acid gas, as a compound of it with hydrogen.

Muriatic acid, from its composition, has been termed by Lussac the hydrochloric acid ; a name objected to by Sir H. Davy. It was prepared by the older chemists in a very rude manner, and was called by them spirit of salt.

In the ancient method, common salt was previously decrepitated, then ground with dried clay, and kneaded or wrought with water to a moderately stiff consistence, after which it was divided into balls of the size of a pigeon's egg ; these balls, being previously well dried, were put into a retort, so as to fill the vessel two-thirds full ; distillation being then proceeded upon, the muriatic acid came over when the heat was raised to ignition. In this process eight or ten parts of clay to one of salt are to be used. The retort must be of stoneware well coated, and the furnace must be of that kind called reverberatory.

It was formerly thought, that the salt was merely divided in this operation by the clay, and on this account more readily gave out its acid: but there can be little doubt, that the effect is produced by the silicious earth, which abounds in large proportions in all natural clays, and detains the alkali of the salt by combining with it.

Sir H. Davy first gave the just explanation of this decomposition. Common salt is a compound of sodium and chlorine. The sodium may be conceived to combine with the oxygen of the water in the earth, and with the earth itself, to form a vitreous compound; and the chlorine to unite with the hydrogen of the water, forming muriatic acid gas. 'It is also easy,' adds he, 'according to these new ideas, to explain the decomposition of salt by moistened litharge, the theory of which has so much perplexed the most acute chemists. It may be conceived to be an instance of compound affinity ; the chlorine is attracted by the lead and the sodium combines with the oxygen of the litharge, and with water, to form hydrate of soda, which gradually attracts carbonic acid from the air. When common salt is decomposed by oil of vitriol, it was usual to explain the phenomenon by saying, that the acid, by its superior affinity, aided by heat, expelled the gas, and united to the soda. But as neither muriatic acid nor soda exists in common salt, we must now modify the explanation, by saying that the water of the oil of vitriol is first decomposed, its oxygen unites to the sodium to form soda, which is seized on by the sulphuric acid, while the chlorine combines with the hydrogen of the water, and exhales in the form of muriatic acid gas.'

As 100 parts of dry sea salt are capable of yielding 62 parts by weight of muriatic acid gas, these ought to afford, by economical management, nearly 221 parts of liquid acid, specific gravity 1.142, as prescribed by the London College, or 200 parts of acid sp. gr. 1.160, as directed by the Edinburgh and Dublin Pharmacopœias.

The ancient method of extracting the gas from salt is now laid aside.

The English manufacturers use iron stills for this distillation, with earthen heads: the philosophical chemist, in making the *acid of commerce*, will doubtless prefer glass. Five parts by weight of strong sulphuric acid are to be added to six of decrepitated sea salt, in a retort, the upper part of which is furnished with a tube or neck, through which the acid is to be poured upon the salt. The aperture of this tube must be closed with a ground stopper immediately after the pouring. The sulphuric acid immediately combines with the alkali, and expels the muriatic acid in the form of a peculiar air, which is rapidly absorbed by water. As this combination and disengagement take place without the application of heat, and the aërial fluid escapes very rapidly, it is necessary to arrange and lute the vessels together before the sulphuric acid is added, and not to make any fire in the furnace until the disengagement begins to slacken; at which time it must be very gradually raised. Before the modern improvements in chemistry were made, a great part of the acid escaped for want of water to combine with; but by the use of Wolfe's apparatus the acid air is made to pass through water, in which it is nearly condensed, and forms muriatic acid of double the weight of the water, though the bulk of this fluid is increased one-half only. The acid condensed in the first receiver, which contains no water, is of a yellow colour, arising from the impurities of the salt.

The marine acid in commerce has a straw colour: but this is owing to accidental impurity; for it does not obtain in the acid produced by the impregnation of water with the aëriform acid.

The muriatic acid is one of those longest known, and some of its compounds are among those salts with which we are most familiar.

The *muriates*, when in a state of dryness, are actually chlorides, consisting of chlorine and the metal; yet they may be conveniently treated of under the title muriates.

The *muriate of barytes* crystallizes in tables bevelled at the edges, or in octahedral pyramids applied base to base. It is soluble in five parts of water at 60°, in still less at a boiling heat, and also in alkohol. It is not altered in the air, and but partly decomposable by heat. The sulphuric acid separates its base; and the alkaline carbonates and sulphates decompose it by double affinity. It is best prepared by dissolving the carbonate in dilute muriatic acid; and if contaminated with iron or lead, which occasionally happens, these may be separated by the addition of a small quantity of liquid ammonia, or by boiling and stirring the solution with a little barytes. Goettling recommends to prepare it from the sulphate of barytes; eight parts of which, in fine powder, are to be mixed with two of muriate of soda, and one of charcoal powder. This is to be pressed hard into a Hessian crucible, and exposed for an hour and a half to a red heat in a wind furnace. The cold mass, being powdered, is to be boiled a minute or two in sixteen parts of water, and then filtered. To this liquor muriatic acid is to be added by little and little, till sulphuretted hydrogen ceases to be evolved. It is then to be filtered, a little hot water to be poured on the residuum, the liquor evaporated to a pellicle, filtered again, and then set to crystallize. As the muriate of soda is much more soluble than the muriate of barytes, and does not separate by cooling, the muriate of barytes will crystallize into a perfectly white salt, and leave the muriate of soda in the mother water, which may be evaporated repeatedly till no more muriate of barytes is obtained. This salt was first employed in medicine by Dr. Crawford, chiefly in scrofulous complaints and cancer, beginning with doses of a few drops of the saturated solution twice a day, and increasing it gradually, as far as forty or fifty drops in some instances. In large doses it excites nausea, and has deleterious effects. Fourcroy says it has been found very successful in scrofula in France. It has likewise been recommended as a vermifuge; and it has been given with much apparent advantage even to very young children, where the usual symptoms of worms

occurred, though none were ascertained to be present As a test of sulphuric acid it is of great use.

The *muriate of potassa*, formerly known by the names of *febrifuge salt of Sylvius, digestive salt*, and *regenerated sea salt*, crystallizes in regular cubes, or in rectangular parallelopipedons; decrepitating on the fire, without losing much of their acid, and acquiring a little moisture from damp air, and giving it out again in dry. Their taste is saline and bitter. They are soluble in thrice their weight of cold water, and in but little less of boiling water, so as to require spontaneous evaporation for crystallizing. Fourcroy recommends, to cover the vessel with gauze, and suspend hairs in it, for the purpose of obtaining regular crystals.

It is sometimes prepared in decomposing sea salt by common potassa for the purpose of obtaining soda; and may be formed by the direct combination of its constituent parts.

It is decomposed by the sulphuric and nitric acids. Barytes decomposes it, though not completely; and both silex and alumina decomposed it partially in the dry way. It decomposes the earthy nitrates, so that it might be used in saltpetre manufactories to decompose the nitrate of lime.

Muriate of soda or *common salt*, is of considerable use in the arts, as well as a necessary ingredient in our food. It crystallizes in cubes, which are sometimes grouped together in various ways, and not unfrequently form hollow quadrangular pyramids. In the fire it decrepitates, melts, and is at length volatilized. When pure, it is not deliquescent. One part is soluble in 2½ of cold water, and in little less of hot, so that it cannot be crystallized but by evaporation.

Common salt is found in large masses, or in rocks under the earth, in England and elsewhere. In the solid form it is called *sal gem*, or *rock salt*. If it be pure and transparent, it may be immediately used in the state in which it is found; but if it contain any impure earthy particles, it should be previously freed from them. In some countries it is found in incredible quantities, and dug up like metals from the bowels of the earth. In this manner has this salt been dug out of the celebrated salt mines near Bochnia and Wieliczka, in Poland, ever since the middle of the 13th century, consequently above these 500 years, in such amazing quantities, that sometimes there have been 20,000 tons ready for sale. In these mines, which are said to reach to the depth of several hundred fathoms, 500 men are constantly employed. The pure and transparent salt needs no other preparation than to be beaten to small pieces or ground in a mill. But that which is more impure must be elutriated, purified, and boiled. That which is quite impure, and full of small stones, is sold under the name of rock salt, and is applied to ordinary uses. It may likewise be used for strengthening weak and poor brine-springs.

The waters of the ocean every where abound with common salt, though in different proportions. The water of the Baltic sea is said to contain one sixty-fourth of its weight of salt; that of the sea between England and Flanders contains one thirty-second part; that on the coast of Spain one-sixteenth part; and between the tropics it is said, erroneously, to contain from an eleventh to an eighth part.

The water of the sea contains, besides the common salt, a considerable proportion of muriate of magnesia, and some sulphate of lime, of soda, and potassa. The former is the chief ingredient of the remaining liquid which is left after the extraction of the common salt, and is called the mother water. Sea water, if taken up near the surface, contains also the putrid remains of animal substances, which render it nauseous, and in a long-continued calm cause the sea to stink.

The whole art of extracting salt from waters which contain it, consists in evaporating the water in the cheapest and most convenient manner. In England, a brine composed of sea-water, with the addition of rock salt, is evaporated in large shallow iron boilers; and the crystals of salt are taken out in baskets. In Russia, and probably in other northern countries, the sea-water is exposed to freeze; and the ice, which is almost entirely fresh, being taken out, the remaining brine is much stronger, and is evaporated by boiling. In the southern parts of Europe, the salt-makers take advantage of spontaneous evaporation. A flat piece of ground near the sea is chosen, and banked round, to prevent its being overflowed at high water. The space within the banks is divided by low walls into several compartments, which successively communicate with each other. At flood tide, the first of these is filled with sea-water, which, by remaining a certain time, deposites its impurities, and loses part of its aqueous fluid. The residue is then suffered to run into the next compartment, and the former is again filled as before. From the second compartment, after a due time, the water is transferred into a third, which is lined with clay, well rammed and levelled. At this period, the evaporation is usually brought to that degree, that a crust of salt is formed on the surface of the water, which the workmen break, and it immediately falls to the bottom. They continue to do this until the quantity is sufficient to be raked out, and dried in heaps. This is called *bay salt*.

Besides its use in seasoning our food, and preserving meat both for domestic consumption and during the longest voyages, and in furnishing us with the muriatic acid and soda, salt forms a glaze for coarse pottery, by being thrown into the oven where it is baked; it improves the whiteness and clearness of glass; it gives greater hardness to soap; in melting metals it preserves their surface from calcination, by defending them from the air, and is employed with advantage in some assays; it is used as a mordant, and for improving certain colours, and enters more or less into many other processes of the arts.

The *muriate of strontian* has not long been known. Dr. Hope first distinguished it from muriate of barytes. It crystallizes in very slender hexagonal prisms; has a cool pungent taste, without the austerity of the muriate of barytes, or the bitterness of the muriate of lime; is soluble in 0.75° of water at 60°, and to almost any amount in boiling water; is likewise soluble in alkohol, and gives a blood-red colour to its flame.

It has never been found in nature, but may be prepared in the same way as the muriate of barytes.

The *muriate of lime* has been known by the names of *marine selenite, calcareous marine salt, muria,* and *fixed sal ammoniac*. It crystallizes in hexahedral prisms terminated by acute pyramids. Its taste is acrid, bitter, and very disagreeable. It is soluble in half its weight of cold water, and by heat in its own water of crystallization. It is one of the most deliquescent salts known; and, when deliquesced, has been called *oil of lime*. It exists in nature, but neither very abundantly nor very pure. It is formed in chemical laboratories, in the decomposition of muriate of ammonia; and Homberg found, that if it were urged by a violent heat till it condensed, on cooling into a vitreous mass, it emitted a phosphoric light upon being struck by any hard body, in which state it was called *Homberg's phosphorus*.

Hitherto it has been little used except for frigorific mixtures; and with snow it produces a very great degree of cold. Fourcroy, indeed, says he has found it of great utility in obstructions of the lymphatics, and in scrofulous affections.

The *muriate of ammonia* has long been known by the name of *sal ammonia*, or *ammoniac*. It is found native in the neighbourhood of volcanoes, where it is sublimed sometimes nearly pure, and in different parts of Asia and Africa. A great deal is carried annually to Russia and Siberia from Bucharian Tartary; and we formerly imported large quantities from Egypt, but now manufacture it at home. See *Sal Ammoniac*.

The salt is usually in the form of cakes, with a convex surface on one side, and concave on the other, from being sublimed into large globular vessels; but by solution it may be obtained in regular quadrangular crystals. It is remarkable for possessing a certain degree of ductility, so that it is not easily pulverable. Its is soluble in 3½ parts of water at 60°, and in little more than its own weight of boiling water. Its taste is cool, acrid, and bitterish. Its specific gravity is 1.42. It attracts moisture from the air but very slightly.

Muriate of ammonia has been more employed in medicine than it is at present. It is sometimes useful as an auxiliary to the bark in intermittents; in gargles it is beneficial, and externally it is a good discutient. In dying, it improves or heightens different colours. In tinning and soldering, it is employed to preserve the surface of the metals from oxidation. In assaying, it discovers iron, and separates t from some of its combinations.

The *muriate of magnesia* is extremely deliquescent,
88

soluble in an equal weight of water, and difficultly crystallizable. It dissolves also in five parts of alkohol. It is decomposable by heat, which expels its acid. Its taste is intensely bitter.

With ammonia this muriate forms *a triple salt*, crystallizable in little polyhedrons, which separate quickly from the water, but are not very regularly formed. Its taste partakes of that of both the preceding salts. The best mode of preparing it is by mixing a solution of 27 parts of muriate of ammonia with a solution of 73 of muriate of magnesia; but it may be formed by a semi-decomposition of either of these muriates by the base of the other. It is decomposable by heat, and requires six or seven times its weight of water to dissolve it.

Of the *muriate of glucine* we know but little. I. appears to crystallize in very small crystals; to be decomposable by heat; and, dissolved in alkohol and diluted with water, to form a pleasant saccharine liquor

Muriate of alumina is scarcely crystallizable, as on evaporation it assumes the state of a thick jelly. It has an acid, styptic, acrid taste. It is extremely soluble in water, and deliquescent. Fire decomposes it. It may be prepared by directly combining the muriatic acid with alumina; but the acid always remains in excess.

The *muriate of zircon* crystallizes in small needles which are very soluble, attract moisture, and lose their transparency in the air. It has an austere taste, with somewhat of acrimony. It is decomposable by heat. The gallic acid precipitates from its solution, if it be free from iron, a white powder. Carbonate of ammonia, if added in excess, redissolves the precipitate it had before thrown down.

Muriate of yttria does not crystallize when evaporated, but forms a jelly. It dries with difficulty, and deliquesces.

Fourcroy observes, that when silicious stones, previously fused with potassa, are treated with muriatic acid, a limpid solution is formed, which may be reduced to a transparent jelly by slow evaporation. But a boiling heat decomposes the silicious muriate, and the earth is deposited. The solution is always acid."

This acid possesses active tonic powers. In typhus, or nervous fevers, although employed on the continent with success, it has not proved so beneficial in this country; and when freely used it is apt to determine to the bowels. Externally, the muriatic acid has been applied in the form of a bath, to the feet, in gout. In a late publication, there are accounts of its successful application as a lithontriptic.

MURIATIC ACID, OXYGENIZED. This supposed acid was lately described by Thenard. He saturated common muriatic acid of moderate strength with deutoxide of barium, reduced it into a soft paste by trituration with water. He then precipitated the barytes from the liquid, by adding the requisite quantity of sulphuric acid. He next took his oxygenized muriatic acid, and treated it with deutoxide of barium and sulphuric acid, to oxygenate it anew. In this way he charged it with oxygen as often as 15 times. He thus obtained a liquid acid which contained 32 times its volume of oxygen at the temperature of 68° Fahr. and at the ordinary atmospheric pressure, and only 4½ times its volume of muriatic acid, which gives about 28 equivalent prințes of oxygen to one of muriatic acid.

This oxygenized acid leaves no residuum when evaporated. It is a very acid, colourless liquid, almost destitute of smell, and powerfully reddens turnsole. When boiled for some time, its oxygen is expelled.

We ought, however, to regard this apparent oxygenation of the acid merely as the conversion of a portion of its combined water into deutoxide of hydrogen.

MURICATUS. Sharp-pointed: applied to seeds, as those of the *Ranunculus parviflorus* and *Sida ciliaris*.

MURRAY, John Andrew, was born at Stockholm, of a Scotch family, in 1740. At 16 he was sent to Upsal, and had the benefit of the instructions of Linnæus, for whom he ever after entertained the highest esteem. In 1759 he took a journey through the southern provinces of Sweden, and thence to Copenhagen; and in the following year he went to Gottingen, where his brother was professor of philosophy. In 1763 he took his degree of doctor in medicine, and by a special license from the Hanoverian government, gave lectures in botany: and in the following spring he was appointed extraordinary professor of medicine in that university. From this period his reputation rapidly extended; he was elected a member in the course of a few years of most of the learned societies in Europe. In 1769 he succeeded to the actual professorship of medicine, and was made doctor of the botanic garden. He was still farther honoured by receiving the title of the Order of Vasa from the King of Sweden in 1780 : and two years afterward by being raised to the rank of privy counsellor by his Britannic Majesty. In 1791 he was attacked with a spurious peripneumony, which shortly terminated his existence. He was a man of sound judgment, great activity, and extensive information. He composed a great number of tracts on various subjects in botany, natural history, medicine, pharmacy, and medical literature. His principal work, which occupied a large portion of his time and attention, was on the Materia Medica, under the title of "Apparatus Medicaminum," in six octavo volumes : indeed, he was employed in correcting the last for the press the day before his death. In the Transactions of the Royal Society of Gottingen, there are many valuable papers by him, chiefly botanical; and his descriptions are deemed models of elegance and accuracy.

MU'SA. (This word is corrupted, or rather refined, from *Mauz*, the Egyptian appellation of this valuable plant; and is made classical in the works of Linnæus, by an allusion to *Musa*, a muse; or, with much greater propriety, to *Antonius Musa*, the physician of Augustus, who, having written on some botanical subjects, may justly be commemorated in the above name.) The name of a genus of plants. Class, *Polygamia;* Order, *Monœcia.* The plantain and badana-tree.

MUSA PARADISIACA. *Musa; Palma humilis; Ficus Indica; Bala; Platanus.* The plantain-tree. It grows spontaneously in many parts of India, but has been immemorially cultivated by the Indians in every part of the continent of South America. It is an herbaceous tree, growing to the height of fifteen or twenty feet. The fruit are nearly of the size and shape of ordinary cucumbers, and when ripe, of a pale yellow colour, of a mealy substance, a little clammy, with a sweetish taste, and will dissolve in the mouth without chewing. The whole spike of fruit often weighs forty or fifty pounds. When they are brought to table by way of dessert, they are either raw, fried, or roasted; but, if intended for bread, they are cut before they are ripe, and are then either roasted or boiled. The trees being tall and slender, the Indians cut them down to get at the fruit; and in doing this they suffer no loss, for the stems are only one year's growth, and would die if not cut; but the roots continue, and new stems soon spring up, which in a year produce ripe fruit also. From the ripe plantains they make a liquor called *mistaw.* When they make this, they roast the fruit in their husks, and, after totally beating them to a mash, they pour water upon them, and, as the liquor is wanted, it is drawn off. But the nature of this fruit is such, that they will not keep long without running into a state of putrefaction; and therefore, in order to reap the advantage of them at all times, they make cakes of the pulp, and dry them over a slow fire, and, as they stand in need of mistaw, they mash the cakes in water, and they answer all the purposes of fresh fruit. These cakes are exceedingly convenient to make this liquor in their journeys, and they never fail to carry them for that purpose. The leaves of the tree being large and spacious, serve the Indians for tablecloths and napkins.

MUSA SAPIENTUM. The systematic name of the banana-tree.—*Banana, Bananeira; Ficoides; Ficus indica; Musa fructu cucumerino breviori; Senoria; Pacæira.* This and the plantain-tree are among the most important productions of the earth. The banana-tree is cultivated, on a very extensive scale, in Jamaica; without the fruit of which, Dr. Wright says, the island would scarcely be habitable, as no species of provision would supply their place. Even flour, or bread itself, would be less agreeable, and less able to support the laborious negro, so as to enable him to do his business, or to keep in health. Plantains also fatten horses, cattle, swine, dogs, fowls, and other domestic animals. The leaves, being smooth and soft, are employed as dressings after blisters. The water from the soft trunk is astringent, and employed by some to check diarrhœas. Every other part of the tree is useful in different parts of rural economy. The leaves are used as

napkins and tablecloths, and are food for hogs. The second sort, musa sapientum, or banana-tree, differs from the paradisiaca, in having its stalks marked with dark purple stripes and spots. The fruit is shorter, straighter, and rounder; the pulp is softer, and of a more luscious taste. It is never eaten green; but when ripe, it is very agreeable, either eaten raw or fried in slices, as fritters, and is relished by all ranks of people in the West Indies. Both the above plants were carried to the West Indies from the Canary Islands; whither, it is believed, they had been brought from Guinea, where they grow naturally.

MUSADI. *Sal ammoniac.*

MUSCI'PULA. (From *mus*, a mouse, and *capio*, to take, being originally applied to a mousetrap; afterward to a plant; so called from its viscidity, by which flies are caught as with birdlime.) A species of lychnis.

MUSCLE. *Musculus.* The parts that are usually included under this name consist of distinct portions of flesh, susceptible of contraction and relaxation; the motions of which, in a natural and healthy state, are subject to the will, and for this reason they are called *voluntary* muscles. Besides these, there are other parts of the body that owe their power of contraction to their muscular fibres : thus the heart is a muscular texture, forming what is called a hollow muscle; and the urinary bladder, stomach, intestines, &c. are enabled to act upon their contents, merely because they are provided with muscular fibres; these are called *involuntary* muscles, because their motions are not dependent on the will. The muscles of respiration being in some measure influenced by the will, are said to have a *mixed* motion. The names by which the voluntary muscles are distinguished, are founded on their size, figure, situation, use, or the arrangement of their fibres, or their origin and insertion; but, besides these particular distinctions, there are certain general ones that require to be noticed. Thus, if the fibres of a muscle are placed parallel to each other, in a straight direction, they form what anatomists term a *rectilinear* muscle; if the fibres cross and intersect each other, they constitute a *compound* muscle; when the fibres are disposed in the manner of rays, a *radiated* muscle; when they are placed obliquely with respect to the tendon, like the plume of a pen, a *penniform* muscle. Muscles that act in opposition to each other are called *antagonists;* thus every extensor has a flexor for his antagonist, and *vice versâ.* Muscles that concur in the same action are termed *congeneres.* The muscle being attached to the bones, the latter may be considered as levers, that are moved in different directions by the contraction of those organs. That end of the muscle which adheres to the most fixed part is usually called the *origin;* and that which adheres to the more moveable part, the *insertion* of the muscle. In almost every muscle, two kinds of fibres are distinguished; the one soft, of a red colour, sensible, and irritable, called *fleshy* fibres, see *Muscular Fibre;* the other of a firmer texture, of a white glistening colour, insensible, without irritability or the power of contracting, and named *tendinous* fibres. They are occasionally intermixed, but the fleshy fibres generally prevail in the belly, or middle part of the muscle, and the tendinous ones in the extremities. If these tendinous fibres are formed into a round slender cord, they form what is called the *tendon* of the muscle; on the other hand, if they are spread into a broad flat surface, it is termed an *aponeurosis.*

Each muscle is surrounded by a very thin and delicate covering of cellular membrane, which encloses it as it were like a sheath, and, dipping down into its substance, surrounds the most minute fibres we are able to trace, connecting them to each other, lubricating them by means of the fat which its cells contain in more or less quantity in different subjects, and serving as a support to the blood-vessels, lymphatics, and nerves which are so plentifully distributed through the muscles. This cellular membrane, which in no respect differs from what is found investing and connecting the other parts of the body, has been sometimes mistaken for a membrane, peculiar to the muscles; and hence we often find writers giving it the name of *membrana propria musculosa.* The muscles owe their red colour which so particularly distinguishes their belly part, to an infinite number of arteries, which are every where dispersed through the whole of their reticular substance; for their fibres, after having been macerated in water, are (like all other parts of the body divested of their blood) found to be of a white colour. These arteries usually enter the muscles by several considerable branches, and ramify so minutely through their substance, that we are unable, even with the best microscopes, to trace their ultimate branches. Ruysch fancied that the muscular fibre was hollow, and a production of a capillary artery; but this was merely conjectural. The veins, for the most part, accompany the arteries, but are found to be larger and more numerous. The lymphatics, likewise, are numerous, as might be expected from the great proportion of reticular substance, which is every where found investing the muscular fibres. The nerves are distributed in such abundance to every muscle, that the muscles of the thumb alone are supplied with a greater proportion of nervous influence than the largest viscera, as the liver for instance. They enter the generality of muscles by several trunks, the branches of which, like those of the blood-vessels, are so minutely dispersed through the cellular substance, that their number and minuteness soon elude the eye, and the knife of the anatomist. This has given rise to a conjecture, as groundless as all the other conjectures on this subject, that the muscular fibre is ultimately nervous.

A table of the Muscles.—The generality of anatomical writers have arranged muscles according to their several uses; but this method is evidently defective, as the same muscle may very often have different and opposite uses. The method here adopted is that more usually followed at present; they are enumerated in the order in which they are situated, beginning with those that are placed nearest the integuments, and proceeding from these to the muscles that are more deeply seated.

[The reader will observe, that all the muscles are in pairs, except those marked thus.*]

Muscles of the integuments of the cranium:
1. *Occipito frontalis.**
2. *Corrugator supercilii.*
    Muscles of the eyelids:
3. *Orbicularis palpebrarum.*
4. *Levator palpebræ superioris.*
    Muscles of the eyeball:
5. *Rectus superior.*
6. *Rectus inferior.*
7. *Rectus internus.*
8. *Rectus externus.*
9. *Obliquus superior.*
10. *Obliquus inferior.*
    Muscles of the nose and mouth:
11. *Levator palpebræ superioris alæque nasi.*
12. *Levator labii superioris proprius.*
13. *Levator anguli oris.*
14. *Zygomaticus major.*
15. *Zygomaticus minor.*
16. *Buccinator.*
17. *Depressor anguli oris.*
18. *Depressor labii inferioris.*
19. *Orbicularis oris.**
20. *Depressor labii superioris alæque nasi.*
21. *Constrictor nasi.*
22. *Levator menti vel labii inferioris.*
    Muscles of the external ear:
23. *Superior auris.*
24. *Anterior auris.*
25. *Posterior auris.*
26. *Helicis major.*
27. *Helicis minor.*
28. *Tragicus.*
29. *Antitragicus.*
30. *Transversus auris.*
    Muscles of the internal ear:
31. *Laxator tympani.*
32. *Membrana tympani.*
33. *Tensor tympani.*
34. *Stapedius.*
    Muscles of the lower jaw:
35. *Temporalis.*
36. *Masseter.*
37. *Pterygoideus externus.*
38. *Pterygoideus internus.*
    Muscles about the anterior part of the neck:
39. *Platysma myoides.*
40. *Sterno-cleidomastoideus.*

Muscles between the lower jaw and os hyoides:
41. *Digastricus.*
42. *Mylo-hyoideus.*
43. *Genio-hyoideus.*
44. *Genio-glossus.*
45. *Hyo-glossus.*
46. *Lingualis.*
Muscles situated between the os hyoides and trunk:
47. *Sterno-hyoideus.*
48. *Crico-hyoideus.*
49. *Sterno-thyroideus.*
50. *Thyro-hyoideus.*
51. *Crico-thyroideus.*
Muscles between the lower jaw and os hyoides laterally:
52. *Stylo-glossus.*
53. *Stylo-hyoideus.*
54. *Stylo-pharyngeus.*
55. *Circumflexus.*
56. *Levator palati mollis.*
    Muscles about the entry of the fauces:
57. *Constrictor isthmi faucium.*
58. *Palatopharyngeus.*
59. *Azygos uvulæ.**
Muscles situated on the posterior part of the pharynx:
60. *Constrictor pharyngis superior.*
61. *Constrictor pharyngis medius.*
62. *Constrictor pharyngis inferior.*
    Muscles situated about the glottis:
63. *Crico-arytænoideus posticus.*
64. *Crico-arytænoideus lateralis.*
65. *Thyro-arytænoideus.*
66. *Arytænoideus obliquus.**
67. *Arytænoideus transversus.**
68. *Thyro-epiglottideus.*
69. *Arytæno-epiglottideus.*
Muscles situated about the anterior part of the abdomen:
70. *Obliquus descendens externus.*
71. *Obliquus ascendens internus.*
72. *Transversus abdominis.*
73. *Rectus abdominis.*
74. *Pyramidalis.*
Muscles about the male organs of generation:
75. *Dartos.**
76. *Cremaster.*
77. *Erector penis.*
78. *Accelerator urinæ.*
79. *Transversus perinei.*
    Muscles of the anus:
80. *Sphincter ani.**
81. *Levator ani.**
    Muscles of the female organs of generation:
82. *Erector clitoridis.*
83. *Sphincter vaginæ.*
    Muscles situated within the pelvis:
84. *Obturator internus.*
85. *Coccygeus.*
Muscles situated within the cavity of the abdomen:
86. *Diaphragma.**
87. *Quadratus lumborum.*
88. *Psoas parvus.*
89. *Psoas magnus.*
90. *Iliacus internus.*
Muscles situated on the anterior part of the thorax:
91. *Pectoralis major.*
92. *Subclavius.*
93. *Pectoralis minor.*
94. *Serratus major anticus.*
Muscles situated between the ribs, and within the thorax:
95. *Intercostales externi.*
96. *Intercostales interni.*
97. *Triangularis.*
Muscles situated on the anterior part of the neck, close to the vertebræ:
98. *Longus colli.*
99. *Rectus internus capitis major.*
100. *Rectus capitis internus minor.*
101. *Rectus capitis lateralis.*
Muscles situated on the posterior part of the trunk:
102. *Trapezius.*
103. *Latissimus dorsi.*
104. *Serratus posticus inferior.*
105. *Rhomboideus.*
106. *Splenius.*
107. *Serratus superior posticus.*
108. *Spinalis dorsi.*
109. *Levatores costarum.*

110. *Sacro lumbalis.*
111. *Longissmus dorsi.*
112. *Complexus.*
113. *Trachelo mastoideus.*
114. *Levator scapulæ.*
115. *Semi-spinalis dorsi.*
116. *Multifidus spinæ.*
117. *Semi-spinalis colli.*
118. *Transversalis colli.*
119. *Rectus capitis posticus minor.*
120. *Obliquus capitis superior.*
121. *Obliquus capitis inferior.*
122. *Scalenus.*
123. *Interspinales.*
124. *Intertransversales.*

    Muscles of the superior extremities:

125. *Supra-spinatus.*
126. *Infra spinatus.*
127. *Teres minor.*
128. *Teres major.*
129. *Deltoides.*
130. *Coracobrachialis.*
131. *Subscapularis.*

    Muscles situated on the os humeri:

132. *Biceps flexor cubiti.*
133. *Brachialis internus.*
134. *Biceps extensor cubiti.*
135. *Anconeus.*

    Muscles situated on the forearm:

136. *Supinator radii longus.*
137. *Extensor carpi radialis longior.*
138. *Extensor carpi radialis brevior.*
139. *Extensor digitorum communis.*
140. *Extensor minimi digiti.*
141. *Extensor carpi ulnaris.*
142. *Flexor carpi ulnaris.*
143. *Palmaris longus.*
144. *Flexor carpi radialis.*
145. *Pronator radii teres.*
146. *Supinator radii brevis.*
147. *Extensor ossis metacarpi pollicis manus.*
148. *Extensor primi internodii.*
149. *Extensor secundi internodii.*
150. *Indicator.*
151. *Flexor digitorum sublimis.*
152. *Flexor digitorum profundus.*
153. *Flexor longus pollicis.*
154. *Pronator radii quadratus.*

    Muscles situated chiefly on the hand:

155. *Lumbricales.*
156. *Flexor brevis pollicis manus.*
157. *Opponens pollicis.*
158. *Abductor pollicis manus.*
159. *Adductor pollicis manus.*
160. *Abductor indicis manus.*
161. *Palmaris brevis.*
162. *Abductor minimi digiti manus.*
163. *Abductor minimi digiti.*
164. *Flexor parvus minimi digiti.*
165. *Interossei interni.*
166. *Interossei externi.*

    Muscles of the inferior extremities:

167. *Pectinalis.*
168. *Triceps adductor femoris.*
169. *Obdurator externus.*
170. *Gluteus maximus.*
171. *Gluteus minimus.*
172. *Gluteus medius.*
173. *Pyriformis.*
174. *Gemini.*
175. *Quadratus femoris.*

    Muscles situated on the thigh:

176. *Tensor vaginæ femoris.*
177. *Sartorius.*
178. *Rectus femoris.*
179. *Vastus externus.*
180. *Vastus internus.*
181. *Cruralis.*
182. *Semi-tendinosus.*
183. *Semi-membranosus.*
184. *Biceps flexor cruris.*
185. *Popliteus.*

    Muscles situated on the leg:

186. *Gastrocnemius externus.*
187. *Gastrocnemius internus.*
188. *Plantaris.*
189. *Tibialis anticus.*

190. *Tibialis posticus.*
191. *Peroneus longus.*
192. *Peroneus brevis.*
193. *Extensor longus digitorum pedis.*
194. *Extensor proprius pollicis pedis.*
195. *Flexor longus digitorum pedis.*
196. *Flexor longus pollicis pedis.*

    Muscles chiefly situated on the foot:

197. *Extensor brevis digitorum pedis*
198. *Flexor brevis digitorum pedis.*
199. *Lumbricales pedis.*
200. *Flexor brevis pollicis pedis.*
201. *Abductor pollicis pedis.*
202. *Adductor pollicis pedis.*
203. *Abductor minimi digiti pedis.*
204. *Flexor brevis minimi digiti pedis.*
205. *Transversales pedis.*
206. *Interossei pedis externi.*
207. *Interossei pedis interni.*

MUSCULAR. (*Muscularis ;* from *musculus,* a muscle.) Belonging to a muscle.

MUSCULAR FIBRE. The fibres that compose the body of a muscle are disposed in fasciculi, or bundles, which are easily distinguishable by the naked eye ; but these fasciculi are divisible into still smaller ones ; and these again are probably subdivisible *ad infinitum.* The most minute fibre we are able to trace seems to be somewhat indivisible ; these plaits disappearing when the fibre is put upon the stretch, seem evidently to be the effect of contraction, and have probably induced some writers to assert, that the muscular fibre is twisted or spiral. Various have been the opinions concerning the structure of these fibres, their form, size, position, and the nature of the atoms which compose them. A fibre is essentially composed of *fibrine* and czmazome, receives a great deal of blood, and, at last, one nervous filament. The other suppositions are all of them founded only on conjecture, and therefore we shall mention only the principal ones, and this with a view rather to gratify the curiosity of the reader, than to afford him information. Borelli supposes them to be so many hollow cylinders, filled with a spongy medullary substance, which he compares to the pith of elder, *spongiosa ad instar sambuci.* These cylinders, he contends, are intersected by circular fibres, which form a chain of very minute bladders. This hypothesis has since been adopted by a great number of writers, with certain variations. Thus, for instance, Bellini supposes the vesicles to be of a rhomboidal shape ; whereas Bernouilli contends that they are oval. Cowper went so far as to persuade himself that he had filled these cells with mercury ; a mistake, no doubt, which arose from its insinuating itself into some of the lymphatics. It is observable, however, that Leeuwhenoeck says nothing of any such vesicles. Here, as well as in many other of her works, Nature seems to have drawn a boundary to our inquiries, beyond which no human penetration will probably ever extend. By chemical analysis muscle is found to consist chiefly of fibrine, with albumen, gelatine, extractive, phosphate of soda, phosphate of ammonia, phosphate and carbonate of lime, and sulphate of potassa.

MUSCULAR MOTION. Muscular motions are of three kinds : namely, voluntary, involuntary, and mixed. The *voluntary motions* of muscles are such as proceed from an immediate exertion of the active powers of the will : thus the mind directs the arm to be raised or depressed, the knee to be bent, the tongue to move, &c. The *involuntary motions* of muscles are those which are performed by organs, seemingly of their own accord, without any attention of the mind, or consciousness of its active power : as the contraction and dilatation of the heart, arteries, veins, absorbents, stomach intestines, &c. The *mixed motions* are those which are in part under the control of the will, but which ordinarily act without our being conscious of their acting ; and is perceived in the muscles of respiration, the intercostals, the abdominal muscles, and the diaphragm

When a muscle acts, it becomes shorter and thicker ; both its origin and insertion are drawn towards its middle. The sphincter muscles are always in action : and so likewise are antagonist muscles, even when they seem at rest. When two antagonist muscles move with equal force, the part which they are designed to move remains at rest ; but if one of the antagonist muscles remains at rest, while the other acts, the part is moved towards the centre of motion.

When a muscle is divided, it contracts. If a muscle be stretched to a certain extent, it contracts, and endeavours to acquire its former dimensions, as soon as the stretching cause is removed : this takes place in the dead body ; in muscles cut out of the body, and also in parts not muscular, and is called by the immortal Haller *vis mortua*, and by some *vis elastica*. It is greater in living than in dead bodies, and is called the *tone* of the muscles.

When a muscle is wounded, or otherwise irritated, it contracts independent of the will : this power is called *irritability*, and by Haller *vis insita* ; it is a property peculiar to, and inherent in, the muscles. The parts of our body which possess this property are called irritable, as the heart, arteries, muscles, &c. to distinguish them from those parts which have no muscular fibres. With regard to the degree of this property, peculiar to various parts, the heart is the most iritable, then the stomach and intestines ; the diaphragm, the arteries, veins, absorbents, and at length the various muscles follow ; but the degree of irritability depends upon the age, sex, temperament, mode of living, climate, state of health, idiosyncrasy, and likewise upon the nature of the stimulus.

When a muscle is stimulated, either through the medium of the will or any foreign body, it contracts, and its contraction is greater or less, in proportion as the stimulus applied is greater or less. The contraction of muscles is different according to the purpose to be served by their contraction : thus, the heart contracts with a jerk ; the urinary bladder, slowly and uniformly ; puncture a muscle, and its fibres vibrate ; and the abdominal muscles act slowly in expelling the contents of the rectum. Relaxation generally succeeds the contraction of muscles, and alternates with it.

" Muscular contraction, such as takes place in the ordinary state of life, supposes the free exercise of the brain, of the nerves which enter the muscles, and of the muscles themselves. Every one of these organs ought to receive arterial blood, and the venous blood ought not to remain too long in its tissue. If one of these conditions is wanting, the muscular contraction is weakened, injured, or rendered impossible.

Phenomena of Muscular Contraction.—When a muscle contracts, its fibres shorten, become hard, with more or less rapidity, without any preparatory oscillation or hesitation ; they acquire all at once such an elasticity, that they are capable of vibrating, or producing sounds. The colour of the muscle does not appear to change in the instant of contraction ; but there is a certain tendency to become displaced, which the *aponeuroses* oppose. ●

There have been discussions about the size of a muscle, in its contracted and relaxed state : the question does not seem to be resolved, in which of these states it is most voluminous ; it is happily of small consequence.

The whole of the sensible phenomena of muscular contraction passes in the muscles ; but, to a certainty, no action can take place without the immediate action of the brain and the nerves.

If the brain of a man, or of an animal, is compressed, the faculty of contracting the muscles ceases ; the nerves of a muscle being cut, it loses all power.

What change happens in the muscular tissue during the state of contraction ? This is totally unknown. In this respect there is no difference between muscular contraction and the vital actions, of which no explanation can be given. There is no want of attempts to explain the action of the muscles, as well as that of the nerves and the brain, in muscular contraction ; but none of the proposed hypotheses can be received.

Instead of following such speculations, which can be easily invented or refuted, and which ought to be banished from physiology, it is necessary to study in muscular contraction, 1st, the intensity of the contraction ; 2dly, its duration ; 3dly, its rapidity ; 4thly, its extent.

The intensity of muscular contraction, that is, the degree of power with which the fibres draw themselves together, is regulated by the action of the brain ; it is generally regulated by the will according to certain limits, which are different in different individuals. A particular organization of the muscles is favourable to the intensity of their contraction : this organization is a considerable volume of fibres, strong, of a deep red, and striated transversely. With an equal power

of the will, these will produce much more powerfu effects than muscles whose fibres are fine, colourless, and smooth. However, should a very powerful cerebral influence, or a great exertion of the will, be joined to such fibres, the contraction will acquire great intensity ; so that the cerebral influence, and the disposition of the muscular tissue, are the two elements of the intensity of muscular contraction.

A very great cerebral energy is rarely found united in the same individual, with that disposition of the muscular fibres which is necessary to produce intense contractions ; these elements are almost always in an inverse ratio. When they are united, they produce astonishing effects. Perhaps this union existed in the *athletæ* of antiquity ; in our times it is observed in certain mountebanks.

The muscular power may be carried to a wonderful degree by the action of the brain alone : we know the strength of an enraged person, of maniacs, and of persons in convulsions.

The will governs the duration ɔ the contraction ; it cannot be carried beyond a certa.n time, however it may vary in different individuals. A feeling of weariness takes place, not very great at first, but which goes on increasing until the muscle refuses contraction. The quick developement of this painful feeling depends on the intensity of the contraction and the weakness of the individual.

To prevent this inconvenience, the motions of the body are so calculated that the muscles act in succession, the duration of each being but short : our not being able to rest long in the same position is thus explained, as an attitude which causes the contraction of a small number of muscles cannot be preserved but for a very short time.

The feeling of fatigue occasioned by muscular contraction soon goes off, and in a short time the muscles recover the power of contracting.

The quickness of the contractions are, to a certain degree, subject to cerebral influence : we have a proof of this in our ordinary motions ; but beyond this degree, it depends evidently on habit. In respect of the rapidity of motion, there is an immense difference between that of a man who touches a piano for the first time, and that which the same man produces after several years' practice. There is, besides, a very great difference in persons, with regard to the quickness of contractions, either in ordinary motions or in those which depend on habit.

As to the extent of the contractions, it is directed by the will ; but it must necessarily depend on the length of the fibres, long fibres having a greater extent of contraction than those that are short.

After what has been said, we see that the will has generally a great influence on the contraction of muscles ; it is not, however, indispensable : in many circumstances motions take place, not only without the participation of the will, but even contrary to it ; we find very striking examples of this in the effects of habit, of the passions, and of diseases."

MUSCULAR POWER. See *Irritability*.

MU'SCULUS. (A diminutive of *mus*, a mouse ; from its resemblance to a flayed mouse.) See *Muscle*.

MUSCULUS CUTANEUS. See *Platysma myoides*.

MUSCULUS FASCIÆ LATÆ. See *Tensor vaginæ femoris*.

MUSCULUS PATIENTIÆ. See *Levator scapulæ*.

MUSCULUS STAPEDIUS. See *Stapedius*.

MUSCULUS SUPERCILII. See *Corrugator supercilii*.

MUSCULUS TUBÆ NOVÆ. See *Circumflexus*.

MUSCUS. (*Muscus, i. m.* ; the moss of a tree.) A moss. A cryptogamous plant, which has its fructification contained in a capsule.

Mosses are distinguished, according to the splitting of the capsule, into,

1. *Musci frondosi*, the capsule of which is *operculate*, having a lid and the fronds very small.

2. *Musci hepatici*, liverworts ; the capsules of which split into *valves*, and the herbage is *frondose* and stemless.

The parts of the capsule of frondose mosses, which are distinguished by particular names, are,

1. The *surculus*, which bears the leaves.

2. The *seta*, or fruitstalk, which goes from the surculus, and supports the theca.

3. The *theca*, or capsule ; the dry fructification adhering to the apex of the frondose stem.

4. The *operculum*, or lid, found in the fringe.

5. The *peristoma*, *peristomium*, or fringe, which in most mosses borders the opening of the theca.

6. The *calyptra*, the veil, placed on the capsule like an extinguisher on a candle; as in *Bryum cæspititium*.

7. The *perichætium*, a slender or squamous membrane at the base of the fruitstalk.

8. The *fimbria*, or fringe, a dentate ring of the operculum, by the elastic force of which the operculum is displaced.

9. The *epiphragma*, a slender membrane which shuts the fringe; as in *Polytricum*.

10. The *sphrongidium*, or *columnula;* the last column or filament which passes the middle of the capsule, and to which the seeds are attached.

Mosses are found in the hottest and coldest climates. They are extremely tenacious of life, and, after being long dried, easily recover their health and vigour by moisture. Their beautiful structure cannot be too much admired. Their species are numerous, and difficult to determine.

MU′SCUS. (From μοσχος, tender; so called from its delicate and tender consistence.) Moss.

MUSCUS ARBOREUS. See *Lichen plicatus*.

MUSCUS CANINUS. See *Lichen caninus*.

MUSCUS CLAVATUS. See *Lycopodium*.

MUSCUS CRANII HUMANI. See *Lichen jaxatilis*.

MUSCUS CUMATILIS. See *Lichen apthosus*.

MUSCUS ERECTUS. See *Lycopodium selago*.

MUSCUS ISLANDICUS. Iceland moss. See *Lichen islandicus*.

MUSCUS MARITIMUS. See *Corallina*.

MUSCUS PULMONARIUS QUERCIÑUS. See *Lichen pulmonarius*.

MUSCUS PYXIDATUS. Cup-moss. See *Lichen pyxidatus*.

MUSCUS SQUAMOSUS TERRESTRIS. See *Lycopodium*.

MUSGRAVE, WILLIAM, was born in Somersetshire, 1657. He went to Oxford with the intention of studying the law; but he afterward adopted the medical profession, and became a Fellow of the Royal Society, of which body he was appointed secretary, in 1684. In this capacity he edited the Philosophical Transactions for some time; he likewise communicated several papers on anatomical and physiological subjects. In 1689 he took his doctor's degree, and became a Fellow of the College of Physicians. Not long after this he settled at Exeter, where he practised his profession with considerable success for nearly 30 years, and died in 1721. Beyond the circle of his practice, he made himself known principally by his two treatises on gout, which are valuable works, and were several times reprinted. He was also a distinguished antiquary, and author of several learned tracts on the subjects of his researches in this way.

MUSHROOM. See *Agaricus campestris*.

MU′SIA PATTRÆ. A name for moxa.

MUSK. See *Moschus*.

MUSK, ARTIFICIAL. Let three fluid drachms and a half of nitric acid be gradually dropped on one fluid drachm of rectified oil of amber, and well mixed. Let it stand twenty-four hours, then wash it well, first in cold, and then in hot water. One drachm of this resinous substance, dissolved in four ounces of rectified spirit, forms a good tincture, of which the mean dose is twenty minims. In preparing the above, great attention should be given to the washing the resin, otherwise it is offensive to the stomach.

Musk-cranesbill. See *Geranium moschatum*.

Musk-melon. See *Cucumis melo.*

Musk-seed. See *Hibiscus abelmoschus*.

MUSQUITTO. A variety of our common gnat, the *Culex pipens* of Linnæus, which, in the West Indies, produce small tumours on whatever part they settle and bite, attended with so high a degree of itching and inflammation, that the person cannot refrain from scratching; by a frequent repetition of which he not uncommonly occasions them to ulcerate, particularly if he is of a robust and full habit.

MUSSITE. Diopside.

MUSSENDA. (The vernacular name of the original species, in the island of Ceylon, which, though of barbarous origin, has obtained unusual suffrage.) The name of a genus of plants. Class, *Pentandria;* Order, *Monogynia.*

MUSSENDA PONDOSA. Ray attributes a cooling property to an infusion or decoction of this plant, which the Indians drink by the name of *beleson*.

MUST. The juice of the grape, composed of water, sugar, jelly, gluten, and bitartrite of potassa. By fermentation it forms wine.

MUSTARD. See *Sinapis*.

Mustard, hedge. See *Erysimum alliaria*.

Mustard, mithridrate. See *Thlaspi*.

Mustard, treacle. See *Thlaspi*.

Mustard, yellow. See *Sinapis*.

MUTICUS. (From *mutilus*, without horns.) Beardless, as applied to the arista or awn of plants. *Glumæ muticæ*, beardless husks. See *Gluma.*

MU′TITAS. (From *mutus*, dumb.) Dumbness. A genus of disease in the class *Locales*, and order, *Dyscinesiæ* of Cullen, which he defines an inability of articulation. He distinguishes three species, viz.

1. *Mutitas organica*, when the tongue is removed or injured.

2. *Mutitas atonica*, arising from an affection of the nerves of the organ.

3. *Mutitas surdorum*, depending upon being born deaf, or becoming so in their infantile years.

MUYS, WYER-WILLIAM, was born at Steenwyk, in 1682. His father being a physician, he was led to follow the same profession, and at 16 commenced his studies at Leyden, whence he went to Utrecht, and took his degree of doctor in 1701. He settled at first in his native town, and afterward removed to Arnheim, where he practised with reputation. In 1709, he was elected to the mathematical chair at Franeker, where he subsequently filled also those of medicine, chemistry and botany. The House of Orange afterward retained him as consulting physician, with a considerable salary, which he received to the end of his life in 1744. He had been five times rector of the university of Franeker, and was a member of the Royal Academy of Sciences of Berlin. His writings were partly medical, partly philosophical. Of the former kind was a dissertation, highly commending the use of sal ammoniac in intermittents: also a very elaborate investigation of the structure of muscles, comprehending an account of all that had been previously discovered on the subject.

MU′ZA. See *Musa.*

MYACA′NTHA. (From μυς, a mouse, and ακανθα, a thorn: so called because its prickly leaves are used to cover whatever is intended to be preserved from mice.) See *Ruscus.*

MYA′GRO. See *Myagrum.*

MYA′GRUM. (From μυια, a fly, and αγρευω, to seize, because flies are caught by its viscidity.) A species of wild mustard.

MY′CE. (From μυω, to wink, shut up, or obstruct.) 1. A winking, closing, or obstruction. An obsolete term, formerly applied to the eyes, to ulcers, and to the viscera, especially the spleen, where it imports obstructions.

2. In surgery, it is a fungus, such as arises in ulcers and wounds.

3. Some writers speak of a yellow vitriol, which is called *Myce.*

MYCHTHI′SMOS. (From ιυζω, to mutter, or groan.) In Hippocrates, it is a sort of sighing, or groaning during respiration, while the air is forced out of the lungs.

MYCONO′IDES. (From μυκη, a noise, and ειδος, a likeness.) Applied to an ulcer full of mucus, and which upon pressure emits a wheezing sound.

MY′CTER. The nose.

MYCTE′RES. Μυκτηρες. The nostrils.

MYDE′SIS. (From μυδαω, to abound with moisture.) It imports, in general, a corruption of any part from a redundant moisture. But Galen applies it particularly to the eyelids.

MY′DON. (From μυδαω, to grow putrid.) Fungus or putrid flesh in a fistulous ulcer.

MYDRI′ASIS. (From μυδαω, to abound in moisture: so named because it was thought to originate in redundant moisture.) A disease of the iris. Too great a dilatation of the pupil of the eye, with or without a defect of vision. It is known by the pupil always appearing of the same latitude or size in the light. The species of mydriasis are,

1. *Mydriasis amaurotica*, which, for the most part, but not always, accompanies an amaurosis.

2. *Mydriasis hydrocephalica*, which owes its origin to a hydrocephalus internus, or dropsy of the ventricles of the cerebrum. It is not uncommon among children, and is the most certain diagnostic of the disease.

3. *Mydriasis verminosa*, or a dilatation of the pupil from saburra and worms in the stomach or small intestines.

4. *Mydriasis a synechia*, or a dilatation of the pupil, with a concretion of the uvea with the capsula of the crystalline lens.

5. *Mydriasis paralytica*, or a dilated pupil, from a paralysis of the orbicular fibres of the iris: it is observed in paralytic disorders, and from the application of narcotics to the eye.

6. *Mydriasis spasmodica*, from a spasm of the rectilineal fibres of the iris, as often happens in hysteric and spasmodic diseases.

7. *Mydriasis*, from atony of the iris, the most frequent cause of which is a large cataract distending the pupil in its passing when extracted. It vanishes in a few days after the operation, in general; however, it may remain so from over and long-continued distention.

MYLA'CRIS. (From μυλη, a grindstone: so called from its shape.) The patella, or knee-pan.

MY'LE. Μυλη. 1. The knee-pan.
2. A mole in the uterus.

MY'LO. (From μυλη, a grinder tooth.) Names compounded with this word belong to muscles, which are attached near the grinders; such as,

MYLO-GLOSSI. Small muscles of the tongue.

MYLO-HYOIDEUS. *Mylo-hyoidien*, of Dumas. This muscle, which was first described by Fallopius, is so called from its origin near the *dentes molares*, and its insertion into the os hyoides. It is a thin, flat muscle, situated between the lower jaw and the os hyoides, and is covered by the anterior portion of the digastricus. It arises fleshy, and a little tendinous, from all the inner surface of the lower jaw, as far back as the insertion of the pterygoideus internus, or, in other words, from between the last dens molaris and the middle of the chin, where it joins its fellow, to form one belly, with an intermediate tendinous streak, or *linea alba*, which extends from the chin to the os hyoides, where both muscles are inserted into the lower edge of the basis of that bone. This has induced Riolanus, Winslow, Albinus, and others, to consider it as a single penniform muscle. Its use is to pull the os hyoides upwards, forwards, and to either side.

MYLO-PHARYNGEUS. See *Constrictor pharyngis superior.*

MY'LON. See *Staphyloma.*

MYOCE'PHALUM. (From μυια, a fly, and κεφαλη, a head: from its resemblance to the head of a fly.) A tumour in the uvea of the eye.

MYOCOILI'TIS. (From μυς, a muscle, and κοιλια, a belly.) Inflammation of the muscles of the belly.

MYODESOPSIA. (From μυια, a fly, ειδος, resemblance, and οψις, vision.) A disease of the eyes, in which the person sees black spots, an appearance of flies, cobwebs, or black wool, before his eyes.

MYOLOGY. (*Myologia;* from μυς, a muscle, and λογος, a discourse.) The doctrine of the muscles. See *Muscle.*

MYO'PIA. (From μυω, to wink, and ωψ, the eye.) Near-sighted, purblind. The myopes are considered those persons who cannot see distinctly above twenty inches. The myopia is likewise adjudged to all those who cannot see at three, six, or nine inches. The proximate cause is the adunation of the rays of light in a focus before the retina. The species are,

1. *Myopia*, from too great a convexity of the cornea. The cause of this convexity is either from nativity, or a greater secretion of the aqueous humour: hence, on one day there shall be a greater myopia than on another. An incipient hydrophthalmia is the origin of this myopia.

2. *Myopia*, from too great a longitude of the bulb. This length of the bulb is native, or acquired from a congestion of the humours in the eye; hence artificers occupied in minute objects, as the engravers of seals, and persons reading much, frequently after puberty become myopes.

3. *Myopia*, from too great a convexity of the anterior superficies of the crystalline lens. This is likewise from birth. The image will so much sooner be formed

94

as the cornea or lens is more convex. This perfectly accounts for short-sightedness; but an anterior too great convexity of the cornea is the most common cause.

4. *Myopia*, from too great a density of the cornea, or humours of the eye. Optics teach us, by so much sooner the rays of light are forced into a focus, as the diaphanous body is denser.

5. *Myopia*, from mydriasis, or too dilated a pupil

6. *Myopia infantilis.* Infants, from the great convexity of the cornea, are often myopes; but by degrees, as they advance in years, they perceive objects more remotely, by the cornea becoming less convex.

MY'OPS. (From μυω, to wink, and ωψ, the eye.) One who is near-sighted.

MYO'SIS. Μυωσις. A disease of the eye which consists in a contraction or too small perforation of the pupil. It is known by viewing the diameter of the pupil, which is smaller than usual, and remains so in an obscure place, where, naturally, if not diseased, it dilates. It occasions weak sight, or a vision that remains only a certain number of hours in the day; but, if wholly closed, total blindness. The species of this disorder are,

1. *Myosis spasmodica*, which is observed in the hysteric, hypochondriac, and in other spasmodic and nervous affections; it arises from a spasm of the or bicular fibres of the iris.

2. *Myosis paralytica* arises in paralytic disorders.

3. *Myosis inflammatoria*, which arises from an inflammation of the iris or uvea, as in the internal oph thalmia, hypopium, or wounded eye.

4. *Myosis*, from an accustomed contraction of the pupil. This frequently is experienced by those who contemplate very minute objects; by persons who write; by the workers of fine needlework; and by frequent attention to microscopical inquiries.

5. *Myosis*, from a defect of the aqueous humour, as after extraction.

6. *Myosis nativa*, with which infants are born.

7. *Myosis naturalis*, is a coarctation of the pupil by light, or from an intense examination of the minutest objects. These coarctations of the pupil are temporary, and spontaneously vanish.

MYOSI'TIS. (From μυς, a muscle.) Inflammation of a muscle. It is the term given by Sagar to acute rheumatism.

MYOSO'TIS. (Μυς, a muscle, and ους, ωτος, an ear: so called because its leaves are hairy, and grow longitudinally like the ear of a mouse.) See *Hieracium pilosella.*

MYOTOMY. (*Myotomia;* from μυς, a muscle, and τεμνω, to cut.) The dissection of the muscles.

MY'RICA. (A name borrowed from the ancient Greeks, whose μυρικη, however, appears to be the *Tamarix gallica.*) The name of a genus or family of plants. Class, *Diœcia;* Order, *Tetrandria.*

MYRICA GALE. The systematic name of the Dutch myrtle or sweet willow. *Myrtus brabantica; Myrtus anglica; Myrtifolia belgica; Gale; Gagel; Rus sylvestris; Acaron; Eleagnus; Eleagnus cordo: Chamœleagnus; Dodonœo.* The leaves, flowers, and seeds of this plant, have a strong, fragrant smell, and a bitter taste. They are said to be used among the common people for destroying moths and cutaneous insects, and the infusion is given internally as a stoma chic and vermifuge.

[MYRICA CERIFERA. See *Cera vegetabilis.* A.]

MYRICIN. The ingredient of wax which remains after digestion in alkohol. It is insoluble also in water and æther; but very soluble in fixed and volatile oils.

MYRIOPHY'LLON. (From μυριος, infinite, and φυλλον, a leaf, named from the number of its leaves.) The milfoil plant, a species of Achilleæ. See *Achillea millefolium.*

MYRI'STICA. The name of a genus of plants in the Linnæan system. Class, *Diœcia;* Order, *Monadelphia.*

MYRISTICA AROMATICA. Swart's name of the nutmeg-tree.

MYRISTICA MOSCHATA. The systematic name of the tree which produces the nutmeg and mace.

1. The nutmeg, *Myristicæ nucleus; Nux moschata; Nucista; Nux myristica; Chrysobalanus Galeni; Unguentaria; Assala; Nux aromatica.* The seed, or kernel, of the *Myristica—foliis lanceolatis, fructu glabro,* of Linnæus. It is a spice that is well known,

and has been long used both for culinary and medical purposes. Distilled with water they yield a large quantity of essential oil, resembling in flavour the spice itself; after the distillation, an insipid sebaceous matter is found swimming on the water; the decoction, inspissated, gives an extract of an unctuous, very slightly bitterish taste, and with little or no astringency. Rectified spirit extracts the whole virtue of nutmegs, by infusion, and elevates very little of it in distillation; hence the spirituous extract possesses the flavour of the spice in an eminent degree. Nutmegs, when heated, yield to the press a considerable quantity of limpid, yellow. oil. There are three kinds of unctuous substances, called oil of mace, though really expressed from the nutmeg. The best is brought from the East Indies, in stone jars; this is of a thick consistence, of the colour of mace, and has an agreeable fragrant smell; the second sort, which is paler-coloured, and much inferior in quality, comes from Holland, in solid masses, generally flat, and of a square figure; the third, which is the worst of all, and usually called common oil of mace, is an artificial composition of suet, palm-oil, and the like, flavoured with a little genuine oil of nutmeg. The medicinal qualities of nutmeg are supposed to be aromatic, anodyne, stomachic, and astringent; and hence it has been much used in diarrhœas and dysenteries. To many people, the aromatic flavour of nutmeg is very agreeable; they, however, should be cautioned not to use it in large quantities, as it is apt to affect the head, and even to manifest an hypnotic power in such a degree as to prove extremely dangerous. Bontius speaks of this as a frequent occurrence in India; and Dr. Cullen relates a remarkable instance of this soporific effect of nutmeg, which fell under his own observation: and hence concludes that, in apoplectic and paralytic cases, this spice may be very improper. The officinal preparations of nutmeg are a spirit and an essential oil, and the nutmeg, in substance, roasted to render it more astringent: both the spice itself and the essential oil enter several compositions, as the *confectio aromatica, spiritus ammoniæ aromaticus,* &c.

2. *Mace* is the middle bark of the nutmeg. A thick, tough, reticulated, unctuous membrane, of a lively, reddish-yellow colour, approaching to that of saffron, which envelopes the shell of the nutmeg. The mace, when fresh, is of a blood-red colour, and acquires its yellow hue in drying. It is dried in the sun, upon hurdles fixed above one another, and then, it is said, sprinkled with sea-water, to prevent its crumbling in carrying. It has a pleasant, aromatic smell, and a warm, bitterish, moderately pungent taste. It is in common use as a grateful spice, and appears to be in its general qualities nearly similar to the nutmeg. The principal difference consists in the mace being much warmer, more bitter, less unctuous, and sitting easier on weak stomachs. Mace possesses qualities similar to those of nutmeg, but is less astringent, and its oil is supposed to be more volatile and acrid.

MYRISTICA NUX. See *Myristica moschata.*

MYRME'CIA. (From μυρμηξ, a pismire.) A small painful wart, of the size and shape of a pismire. See *Myrmecium.*

MYRME'CIUM. A moist soft wart about the size of a lupine, with a broad base, deeply rooted, and very painful. It grows on the palms of the hands and soles of the feet.

MYRO'COPUM. (From μυρον, an ointment, and κοπος, labour.) An unguent to remove lassitude.

MYROBA'LAN. See *Myrobalanus.*

MYROBA'LANUS. (From μυρος, an unguent, and βαλανος, a nut: so called because it was formerly used in ointments.) A myrobalan. A dried fruit of the plum kind, brought from the East Indies. - All the myrobalans have an unpleasant, bitterish, very austere taste, and strike an inky blackness with a solution of steel. They are said to have a gently purgative as well as an astringent and corroborating virtue. In this country they have been long expunged from the pharmacopœias. Of this fruit there are several species.

MYROBALANUS BELLIRICA. The belliric myrobalan. The fruit is of a yellowish-gray colour, and an irregular roundish or oblong figure, about an inch in length, and three quarters of an inch thick.

MYROBALANUS CHEBULA. The chebule myrobalan. This resembles the yellow in figure and ridges, but is larger, of a darker colour, inclining to brown or blackish, and has a thicker pulp.

MYROBALANUS CITRINA. Yellow myrobalan. This fruit is somewhat longer than the belliric, with generally five large longitudinal ridges, and as many smaller between them, somewhat pointed at both ends.

MYROBALANUS EMBLICA. The emblic myrobalan is of a dark blackish-gray colour, roundish, about half an inch thick, with six hexagonal faces, opening from one another.

MYROBALANUS INDICA. The Indian or black myrobalan, of a deep black colour, oblong, octangular, differing from all the others in having no stone, or only the rudiments of one, from which circumstance they are supposed to have been gathered before maturity.

MY'RON. (From μυρω, to flow.) An ointment, medicated oil, or unguent.

MYROPHY'LLUM. *Millefolium aquaticum.* Water fennel. It is said to be vulnerary.

MYRO'XYLON. (From μυρον, an ointment, and ξυλον, wood.) The name of a genus of plants in the Linnæan system. Class, *Diandria;* Order, *Monogynia.*

MYROXYLON PERUIFERUM. The systematic name of the tree which gives out the Peruvian balsam. *Balsamum peruvianum; Putzochill; Indian, Mexican,* and *American balsam; Carbareiba,* is the name of the tree from which, according to Piso and Ray, it is taken. It is the *Myroxylon peruiferum,* of Linnæus, which grows in the warmest provinces of South America, and is remarkable for its elegant appearance. Every part of the tree abounds with a resinous juice; even the leaves being full of transparent resinous points, like those of the orange-tree.

Balsam of Peru is of three kinds: or rather, it is one and the same balsam, having three several names: 1. The balsam of incision; 2. The dry balsam; 3. The balsam of lotion. The virtues of this balsam, as a cordial, pectoral, and restorative, stimulant, and tonic, are by some thought to be very great. It is given with advantage from 5 to 10 or 15 drops for a dose, in dyspepsia, atonic gout, in consumptions, asthmas, nephritic complaints, obstructions of the viscera, and suppressions of the menses. It is best taken dropped upon sugar. The yelk of an egg, or mucilage of gum-arabic, will, indeed, dissolve it; it may, by that way, be made into an emulsion; and it is less acrid in that form than when taken singly. It is often made an ingredient in boluses and electuaries, and enters into two of the officinal compositions; the tinctura balsami Peruviani composita, and the trochisci glycyrrhizæ. Externally, it is recommended as a useful application to relaxed ulcers, not disposed to heal.

MY'RRHA. (A Hebrew word. Also called *stacte,* and the worst sort *ergasma.*) A botanical specimen of the tree which affords this gum resin has not yet been obtained; but from the account of Bruce, who says it very much resembles the *Acacia vera* of Linnæus, there can be little doubt in referring it to that genus, especially as it corresponds with the description of the tree given by Dioscorides. The tree that affords the myrrh, which is obtained by incision, grows on the eastern coast of Arabia Felix, and in that part of Abyssinia which is situated near the Red Sea, and is called by Bruce, *Troglodyte.* Good myrrh is of a turbid black-red colour, solid and heavy, of a peculiar smell, and bitter taste. Its medicinal effects are warm, corroborant, and antiseptic; it has been given as an emmenagogue in doses from 5 to 20 grains: it is also given in cachexies, and applied externally as an antiseptic and vulnerary. In doses of half a drachm. Dr. Cullen remarks that it heated the stomach, produced sweat, and agreed with the balsams in affecting the urinary passages. It has lately come more into use as a tonic in hectical cases, and is said to prove less heating than most other medicines of that class. Myrrh dissolves almost totally in boiling water, but as the liquor cools, the resinous matter subsides. Rectified spirit dissolves less of this concrete than water; but extracts more perfectly that part in which its bitterness, virtues, and flavour reside; the resinous matter which water leaves undissolved is very bitter, but the gummy matter which spirit leaves undissolved is insipid, the spirituous solution containing all the active part of the myrrh: it is applied to ulcers, and other external affections of a putrid tendency; and also as a wash, when diluted, for the teeth and gums. There are several preparations of this drug in the London and Edinburgh Pharmacopœis.

MYRRHI'NE. (From μυρρα, myrrh: so called because it smells like myrrh.) The common myrtle. See *Myrtus communis.*

MY'RRHIS. (From μυρρα, myrrh: so named from its myrrh-like smell.) Sweet cicely See *Scandix odorata.*

MYRSINELÆ'UM. (From μυρσινη, the myrtle, and ελαιον, oil.) Oil of myrtle.

MYRTACA'NTHA. (From μυρτος, a myrtle, and ακανθα, a thorn: so called from its likeness to myrtle, and from its prickly leaves.) Butcher's broom. See *Ruscus.*

MYRTI'DANUM. (From μυρτος, the myrtle.) An excrescence growing on the trunk of the myrtle, and used as an astringent.

Myrtiform caruncles. See *Carunculæ myrtiformes.*
Myrtiform glands. See *Carunculæ myrtiformes.*

MYRTI'LLUS. See *Vaccinium myrtillus.*

MYRTLE. See *Myrtus.*

Myrtle, Dutch. See *Myrica gale.*

MYRTO CHEILIDES. (From μυρτον, the clitoris, and χειλος, a lip.) The nymphæ of the female pudenda.

MY'RTON. The clitoris.

MY'RTUM. (From μυρτος, a myrtle.) A little prominence in the pudenda of women, resembling a myrtle-berry. It also means the clitoris.

MY'R'TUS. (From μυρρα, myrrh, because of its smell, or from *Myrrha,* a virgin, who was fabled to have been turned into this tree.) 1. The name of a genus of plants in the Linnæan system. Class, *Icosandria;* Order, *Monogynia.*

2. The pharmacopœial name of the myrtle. See *Myrtus communis.*

MYRTUS BRABANTICA. See *Myrica gale.*

MYRTUS CARYOPHYLLATA. The systematic name of the tree which affords the clove bark. *Cassia caryophyllata.* The bark of this tree, *Myrtus—pedunculis trifido-multifloris, foliis ovatis,* of Linnæus, is a warm aromatic, of the smell of clove spice, but weaker, and with a little admixture of the cinnamon flavour. It may be used with the same views as cloves, or cinnamon.

MYRTUS COMMUNIS. The systematic name of the common myrtle.

MYRTUS COMMUNIS ITALICA. *Oxymyrrhine; Oxymyrsine.* The berries of this plant are recommended in alvine and uterine fluxes, and other disorders from relaxation and debility. They have a roughish, and not unpleasant taste, and appear to be moderately astringent and corroborant, partaking also of aromatic qualities.

MYRTUS PIMENTA. The systematic name of the tree which bears the Jamaica pepper, or allspice. *Pimento; Piper caryophyllatum; Cocculi Indi aromatici; Piper chiapæ; Amomum pimenta; Caryophyllus aromaticus; Caryophyllus americanus; Piper odoratum jamaicense. Myrtus—floribus trichotoma-paniculatis, foliis oblongo-lanceolatis,* of Linnæus. This spice, which was first brought over for dietetic uses, has been long employed in the shops as a succedaneum to the more costly oriental aromatics: it is moderately warm, of an agreeable flavour, somewhat resembling that of a mixture of cloves, cinnamon, and nutmegs. Both pharmacopœias direct an aqueous and spirituous distillation to be made from these berries; and the Edinburgh College orders the *Oleum essentiale piperi-jamaicensis.*

MY'STAX. The hair which forms the beard in man, on each side the upper lip. See *Capillus.*

MYC'RUS. An epithet for a sort of sinking pulse, when the second stroke is less than the first, the third than the second, &c. Of this there are two kinds: the first is when the pulse so sinks as not to rise again; the other, when it returns again, and rises in some degree. Both are esteemed bad presages.

MYXOSARCO'MA. (From μυξα, mucus, and σαρξ, flesh.) *Mucocarneus.* A tumour which is partly fleshy and partly mucous.

MY'XTER. (From μυξα, the mucus of the nose.) The nose or nostril.

N

N. In prescriptions this letter is a contraction for *numero,* in number.

NACRITE. See *Talcite.*

NA'CTA. An abscess of the breast.

NADLESTEIN. An ore of Titanium.

NA'DUCEM. A uterine mole.

NÆ'VUS. (*Nævus, i. m.*) A natural mark, spot, or blemish.

NÆ'VUS MATERNUS. *Macula matricis; Stigma, Metrocelis.* A mother's mark. A mark on the skin of children, which is born with them, and which is said to be produced by the longing of the mother for particular things, or her aversion to them; hence these marks resemble mulberries, strawberries, grapes, pines, bacon, &c.

NA'I CORONA. A name of the cowage.

NAIL. See *Unguis.*

NA'KIR. According to Schenkius this means wandering pains of the limbs.

NANCEIC ACID. *Acidum nanceicum.* Zumic acid. "An acid called by Braconnot, in honour of the town of Nancy, where he lives. He discovered it in many acescent vegetable substances; in sour rice; in putrefied juice of beet-root; in sour decoction of carrots, pease, &c. He imagines that this acid is generated at the same time as vinegar in organic substances, when they become sour. It is without colour, does not crystallize, and has a very acid taste.

He concentrates the soured juice of the beet-root till it becomes almost solid, digests it with alkohol, and evaporates the alkoholic solution to the consistence of syrup. He dilutes this with water, and throws into it carbonate of zinc till it be saturated. He passes the liquid through a filter, and evaporates till a pellicle appears. The combination of the new acid with oxide of zinc crystallizes. After a second crystallization, he redissolves it in water, pours in an excess of water of barytes, decomposes by sulphuric acid the barytic salt formed, separates the deposite by a filter, and obtains, by evaporation, the new acid pure.

It forms with alumina a salt resembling gum, and with magnesia one unalterable in the air, in little granular crystals, soluble in 25 parts of water at 66° Fahr.; with potassa and soda it forms uncrystallizable salts, deliquescent and soluble in alkohol; with lime and strontites, soluble granular salts; with barytes, an uncrystallizable nondeliquescent salt, having the aspect of gum; with white oxide of manganese, a salt which crystallizes in tetrahedral prisms, soluble in 12 parts of water at 66°; with oxide of zinc, a salt crystallizing in square prisms, terminated by summits obliquely truncated, soluble in 50 parts of water at 66°; with iron, a salt crystallizing in slender four-sided needles, of sparing solubility, and not changing in the air; with red oxide of iron, a white noncrystallizing salt; with oxide of tin, a salt crystallizing in wedge-form octahedrons; with oxide of lead, an uncrystallizable salt, not deliquescent, and resembling a gum; with black oxide of mercury, a very soluble salt, which crystallizes in needles."

NAPE'LLUS. (A diminutive of *napus:* so called because it has a bulbous root like that of the napus.) See *Aconitum.*

NA'PHÆ FLORES. Orange flowers are sometimes so called. See *Citrus aurantium.*

NA'PHTHA. (*Naptha, æ. f.; ναφθα.*) A native combustible liquid of a yellowish white colour, perfectly fluid and shining. It feels greasy, and exhales an agreeable bituminous smell. It occurs in considerable springs on the shores of the Caspian Sea, in Sicily, and Italy. It is used instead of oil, and differs from petroleum obtained by distilling coal only by its greater purity and lightness. This fluid has been used as an external application for removing old pains, nervous disorders, such as cramps, contractions of the limbs, paralytic affections, &c.

NAPHTHA VITRIOLI. See *Æther sulphuricus.*

NAPIFO'LIA. Bore cole. See *Brassica.*

NA'PIUM. See *Lapsana communis.*

["NAPTHALINE This substance is one of the products of the decomposition of coal. If the distillation be conducted at a very gentle heat, naptha, from its greater volatility, first passes over, and afterward *napthaline* rises in vapour, and condenses in the neck of the retort, as a white crystalline solid.

"Pure napthaline is heavier than water, has a pungent aromatic taste, and a peculiar odour not unlike that of the narcissus. It is smooth and unctuous to the touch, is perfectly white, and has a silvery lustre. It fuses at 180° Fah., volatilizes slowly at common temperatures, and boils at 410° Fah. It is not very readily inflamed, but when set on fire it burns rapidly, and emits a large quantity of smoke. It is soluble in cold, and dissolves very sparingly in hot water. Its proper solvents are alkohol and ether.

"Sulphuric acid enters into direct combination with napthaline, and forms a new and peculiar acid, which Mr. Faraday has described under the name of *sulphonapthalic acid.*

"Napthaline, according to Dr. Thompson, is a *sesquicarburet of hydrogen*, that is, a compound of 9, or an a om and a half, of carbon, and 1 atom of hydrogen." —*Webs. Man. Chem.* A.]

NA'PUS. See *Brassica napus.*

NAPUS DULCIS. See *Brassica rapa.*

NAPUS SYLVESTRIS. See *Brassica rapa.*

NARCA'PHTHUM. A name of the cordial confection.

NARCI'SSUS. A genus of plants in the Linnæan system. Class, *Hexandria;* Order, *Monogynia.*

NARCO'SIS. (From ναρκοω, to stupify.) Stupefaction, stupor, numbness.

NARCOTIC. (*Narcotictis;* from ναρκοω, to stupify.) A medicine which has the power of procuring sleep. See *Anodyne.*

NARCOTINE. The active principle of narcotic vegetables. See *Opium.*

NARD. See *Valeriana celtica.*

Nard, Indian. See *Andropogon nardus.*

NARDO'STACHYS. (From ναρδος, spikenard, and ςαχυς, sage.) A species of wild sage resembling spikenard in its leaves and smell.

NA'RDUS. (From *nard*, Syrian.) Spikenard.

NARDUS CELTICA. *Valeriana celtica.*

NARDUS INDICA. See *Andropogon nardus.*

NARDUS ITALICA. The lavendula spica of Linnæus.

NARDUS MONTANA. An old name of asarabacca. See *Asarum europeum.*

NARDUS RUSTICA. An old name of the asarabacca. See *Asarum europeum.*

NARIFUSO'RIA. (From *nares*, the nostrils, and *fundo* to pour.) Medicines dropped into the nostrils.

NA'RIS. The nostril. The cavity of the nostrils is of a pyramidal figure, and is situated under the anterior part of the cranium, in the middle of the face. The two nostrils are composed of fourteen bones, viz. the frontal, two maxillary, two nasal, two lachrymal, two inferior spongy, the sphenoid, the vomer, the ethmoid, and two palatine bones, which form several eminences and cavities. The eminences are the septum narium, the cavernous substance of the ethmoid bone, called the superior conchæ, and the inferior spongy bones. The cavities are three pair of pituitary sinuses, namely, the frontal, sphenoid, and maxillary; the anterior and posterior foramina of the nostrils; the ductus nasalis, the sphenopalatine foramina, and anterior palatine foramina. All these parts are covered with periosteum, and a pituitary membrane which secretes the mucus of the nostrils. The arteries of this cavity are branches of the internal maxillary. The veins empty themselves into the internal jugulars. The nerves are branches of the olfactory, ophthalmic, and superior maxillary. The use of the nostrils is for smelling, respiration, and speech.

NARIS COMPRESSOR. See *Compressor naris.*

NA'RTA. (Napra, *ex nardi odore,* from its smell.) A plant used in ointments.

NARTHE'CIA. (From *Narthecis,* the island where t flourished.) *Narthex.* A kind of fennel.

NASALIS. (From *nasus*, the nose.) Appertaining to the nose.

NASALIS LABII SUPERIORIS. See *Orbicularis oris*

NASA'RIUM. (From *nasus*, the nose.) The mucus of the nose.

NASCA'LE. (From *nasus*, the nose.) A wood or cotton pessary for the nose.

NASCA'PHTHUM. Cordial confection.

NASI DEPRESSOR. See *Depressor labii superioris alæque nasi.*

NASI OSSA. The two small bones of the nose that are so termed from the bridge of the nose. In figure they are quadrangular and oblong.

NASTU'RTIUM. (*Quod nasum torqueat,* because the seed, when bruising, irritates the nose.) The name of a genus of plants in the Linnæan system. Class, *Tetradynamia ;* Order, *Siliquosa.*

NASTURTIUM AQUATICUM. See *Sisymbrium nasturtium.*

NASTURTIUM HORTENSE. See *Lepidium sativum.*

NASTURTIUM INDICUM. See *Tropæolum majus.*

NA'SUS. The nose.

NA'TA. *Natta.* A species of wen with slender pendent neck. Linnæus speaks of it as rooted in a muscle.

NATANS. (From *nato,* to swim.) Floating on the surface of the water: applied to leaves, in opposition to those which are naturally under, and different, and are called demersed, immersed, and submersed; as in *Potamogeton natans.*

NA'TES. (From *nato,* to flow; because the excrements are discharged from them.) 1. The buttocks, or the fleshy parts upon which we sit.

2. Two of the eminences, called turbercula quadrigemina, of the brain, are so named from their resemblance.

NATES CEREBRI. See *Tubercula quadrigemina.*

NATROLITE. A subspecies of prismatic zeolite or mesotype.

["This substance has usually occurred in small, reniform, rounded, or irregular masses, composed of very minute fibres. The fibres are divergent, or even radiate from a centre; and are sometimes so very minute and close, that the fracture appears almost or quite compact. It has little or no lustre. Sometimes also it presents minute crystals, especially on the surface of its masses, whose forms appear to be similar to those of the Zeolite.

Before the blow-pipe it easily melts into a white glass, which often contains small bubbles. In nitric acid it is reduced, in the course of a few hours, without effervescence, into a jelly somewhat thick. It contains silex 48.0, alumine 24.25, soda 16.5, water 9.0, oxide of iron 1.75;=99.5 (according to Klaproth). This result is very similar to that obtained by Smithson Tennant, from the Zeolite.—*Cleav. Min.* A.]

NA'TRON. (So called from *Natron,* a lake in Judæa, where it was produced.) *Natrum.* 1. The name formerly given to the alkali, now called soda. See *Soda.*

2. A native salt, which is found crystallized in Egypt, in the lake called Natron, and in the other hot countries, in sands surrounding lakes of salt water. It is an impure subcarbonate of soda, and there are two kinds of it, the common and the radiated.

3. The name of an impure subcarbonate of soda, obtained by burning various marine plants. See *Soda.*

NATRON MURIATUM. See *Sodæ murias.*

NATRON PRÆPARATUM. See *Sodæ subcarbonas.*

NATRON TARTARISATUM. See *Soda tartarizata.*

NATRON VITRIOLATUM. See *Sodæ sulphas.*

NA'TULÆ. (Diminutive of *nates*, the buttocks: so called from their resemblance.) The two uppermost of four small eminences of the brain. See *Tubercula quadrigemina.*

NATURAL. Appertaining to nature.

NATURAL ACTIONS. Those functions by which the body is preserved; as hunger, thirst, &c. See *Actions.*

NATURAL HISTORY. A description of the natural products of the earth, water, or air; *ex. gr.* beasts, birds, fish, insects, worms, plants, metals, minerals, and fossils; together with such extraordinary phenomena as at any time appear in the material world, as meteors, monsters, &c.

NATURAL ORDERS. A division or arrangement of plants, from their external habits or characters. They are

1. *Coniferæ.*	3. *Compositæ.*
2. *Amentaceæ.*	4. *Aggregatæ.*

5. *Conglomeratæ.*	31. *Columniferæ.*
6. *Umbellatæ.*	32. *Gruinales.*
7. *Hederaceæ.*	33. *Caryophyllæ.*
8. *Sarmentaceæ.*	34. *Colycanthemæ*
9. *Stellatæ.*	35. *Ascirodeæ.*
10. *Cymosæ.*	36. *Coadunatæ.*
11. *Cucurbitaceæ.*	37. *Dumosæ.*
12. *Luridæ.*	38. *Trihilatæ.*
13. *Campanaceæ.*	39. *Tricoccæ.*
14. *Contortæ.*	40. *Oleraceæ.*
15. *Rotaceæ.*	41. *Scabridæ.*
16. *Sepiaciæ.*	42. *Vapiculæ.*
17. *Bicornes.*	43. *Pipiritæ.*
18. *Asperifoliæ.*	44. *Scetamineæ.*
19. *Verticillatæ.*	45. *Liliaceæ.*
20. *Personatæ.*	46. *Ensatæ.*
21. *Rhoeadeæ.*	47. *Tripetaloideæ.*
22. *Putamineæ.*	48. *Orchideæ.*
23. *Siliquosæ.*	49. *Culmariæ.*
24. *Papilionaceæ*	50. *Gramina.*
25. *Tomentaceæ.*	51. *Palmæ.*
26. *Multisiliquæ.*	52. *Filices.*
27. *Senticosæ.*	53. *Musci.*
28. *Pomaceæ.*	54. *Algæ.*
29. *Hesperidæ.*	55. *Fungi.*
30. *Succulentæ.*	

NATURAL PHILOSOPHY. Physics. The science which considers the properties of natural bodies, and their mutual actions on one another, being contrasted with moral philosophy or ethics, which treat of the phenomena of mind and rules of morality.

NATURA'LIA. (From *natura,* nature.) The parts of generation.

NATURE. *Natura;* from *nascor, natus.*) A term variously used.

1. It is most frequently employed to express the system of the world, the assemblage of all created beings, and in this case is synonymous with *world,* or *universe.*

2. That power which is said to be diffused throughout the creation, moving and acting in all bodies, and giving them certain properties. In this last sense, when a personified being is meant, nature is nothing else but God, acting himself, and according to certain laws which he himself has fixed. According to the supposition of some, however, the principle called nature is a power delegated by the Creator; as it were, a middle being between God and created things, which has been styled *Anima mundi;* but it does not appear that there is any foundation for this hypothesis, or that any thing is explained by referring the whole series of second causes to an intermediate principle, instead of to one universal agent.

3. In medical writings, the expression *nature* is usually taken for the aggregate of powers belonging to any body, especially a living one; as when physicians say that, in such a disease nature, left to herself, will perform the cure. It may be proper here to observe, with regard to this phrase of leaving the cure to nature, that there is a wide difference between suspending for a time all interference with the vital processes, and *neglecting* a disease; although to those who are ignorant of the principles of medicine, these appear to be the same thing.

It would be the perfection of this science to ascertain upon what causes healthy and diseased actions depend, and to what extent either can be affected by human agency: but at present the judicious physician never aims at a cure independently of the original powers of the system, but rather seeks to call them into action, or, at most, to assist when the inherent elasticity of the vital functions is insufficient to recover them from the oppression of disease. As, for example, when we allow a wound to heal by the first intention, or restore the digestive functions by obliging a man to attend to the rules of diet and exercise, &c. upon which health depends; we call upon the restorative powers of Nature, because art, that is to say, human ingenuity, can supply nothing equivalent. Or, again, when, in the treatment of a diseased joint, rest is enjoined at one period on account of inflammation, and perhaps motion is ordered at another, to keep up the proper uses of the part, we show the importance of alternately interfering and looking on, as we judge it proper to check the tendency of vital actions, or to trust entirely to them. While to those who are ignorant of these principles, the practitioner, when really exercising his greatest skill, is supposed to be idle.

NAU'SEA. (Ναυσεα; from ναυς, a ship: because it is a sensation similar to that which people experience upon sailing in a ship.) *Nausiosis; Nautia.* An inclination to vomit without effecting it; also a disgust of food approaching to vomiting. It is an attendant on cardialgia, and a variety of other disorders, pregnancy, &c. occasioning an aversion for food, an increase of saliva, disgusted ideas at the sight of various objects, loss of appetite, debility, &c.

NAUSIO'SIS. See *Nausea.*

NAU'TIA. See *Nausea.*

NAU'TICUS. (*Nauticus,* a sailor: so called from the use which sailors make of it in climbing ropes.) A muscle of the leg, exerted in climbing up.

NAVEW. See *Brassica rapa.*

Navew, garden. See *Brassica rapa.*

Navew, sweet. See *Brassica rapa.*

NAVICULA'RE OS. *Naviformis; Navicularis; Os scaphoides; Cymba.* A bone of the carpus and tarsus is so called, from its supposed resemblance to a boat.

NAVICULA'RIS. (From *navicula,* a little boat.) See *Naviculare os.*

NAVIFO'RMIS. See *Naviculare os.*

NEAPOLITAN. (From *Neapolis,* or *Naples,* because it was said to have been first discovered at Naples, when the French were in possession of it.) The venereal disease was once so called.

NE'BULA. (From νεφελη.) 1. A cloudy spot in the cornea of the eye.

2. The cloud-like appearance in the urine, after it has been a little time at rest.

NECK. *Collum.* The parts which form the neck are divided into external and internal. The external parts are the common integuments, several muscles, eight pair of cervical nerves, the eighth pair of nerves of the cerebrum, and the great intercostal nerve; the two carotid arteries, the two external jugular veins, and the two internal; the glands of the neck, viz. the jugular, submaxillary, cervical, and thyroid. The internal parts are the fauces, pharynx, œsophagus, larynx, and trachea. The bones of the neck are the seven cervical vertebræ.

NECRO'SIS. (From νεκρ̱ω, to destroy.) This word, the strict meaning of which is only mortification, is, by the general consent of surgeons, confined to an affection of the bones. The death of parts of bones was not distinguished from caries, by the ancients. However, necrosis and caries are essentially different; for in the first, the affected part of the bone is deprived of the vital principle; but this is not the case when it is simply carious. Caries is very analogous to ulceration, while necrosis is exactly similar to mortification of the soft parts.

NECROSIS USTILAGINEA. A painful convulsive contraction of the limbs. See *Raphania.*

NE'CTAR. Νεκταρ. A wine made of honey.

NECTA'RIUM. The nectary. An accidental part of a flower which does not come under the description of any of its organs. It may be defined that part of the corolla which contains or which secretes honey, though it is not necessary to a nectary that honey be present.

Scarce a flower can be found that has not more or less honey, though it is far from being universally, or even generally formed, by an apparatus separate from the petals.

In monopetalous flowers, as the Lamium album, the dead nettle, the tube of the corolla contains, and probably secretes, the honey without any evident nectary.

Sometimes the part under consideration is a production or elongation of the corolla, as in the violet: sometimes indeed of the calyx, as in the garden nasturtium, Tropæolum, the coloured calyx of which partakes much of the nature of the petals.

Sometimes it is distant from both, either resembling the petals; as in Aquilegia; or more different, as in Epimedium, Aconitum, Helleborus, Delphinium. Such at least is the mode in which Linnæus and his followers understand the four last numbered flowers.

The most indubitable of all nectaries, as actually secreting honey, are those of a glandular kind. In the natural order of cruciform plants, composing the class Tetradynamia, there are generally four green glands at the base of the stamens, as in Dentaria, and Sisymbrium; while in Pelargonium, the nectary is a tube running down one side of the flower-stalk. The ele gant Parnassia has a most elaborate apparatus or nectary.—*Smith.*

From the figure of the nectary it is said to be,

1. *Calcurate*, or spur-like; as in Aquilegia vulgaris, Delphinium ajax, and Antirrhinum linaria.

2. *Cucullate*, hooded; as in Impatiens balsamina, Aconitum, and Asclepias vincetoxicum.

3. *Foveate*, a little depression in the claw of the petal, as in Fritillaria imperialis.

4. *Campanulate;* as in Narcissus jonquilla and Pseudonarcissus.

5. *Crown-like;* as in Passiflora cærulea.

6. *Pedicellate*, resting on a partial flower-stalk; as in Aconitum napellus.

7. *A bilabiate tube;* as in Helleborus fœtidus, and Nigella.

8. *Poriform*, there being three pores in the germen; as in the Hyacinths.

9. *Squamate*, a little scale in the claw; as in Ranunculus.

10. *Glandular*, little nectiferous glands between the stamens and pistils; as in Sinapis alba.

11. *Stellate*, a double star covering the internal organs; as in Stapelia.

12. *Pilous*, fine hairy fascicles at the base of the stamina; as in Parnassia palustris.

13. *Bearded;* as in Iris germanica.

14. *Forniciform*, arched; small prolongations at the opening of the corolla, and covering the internal organs; as in Symphatum officinale, and Myosotis scorpioides.

15. *Bristle-like*, fine horn-like filaments around the internal organs; as in Periploca græca.

16. *Rotate;* as in Cissampelos.

17. *Scrotiforme*, behind the flower; as in Satyrium.

18. *Horn-like*, behind the flower; as in Orchis.

19. *Sandaliform*, slipper-like; as in Cypripedium calceolus.

20. *Globose*, inverting the germen; as in Mirabilis jalappa.

21. *Cyathiform*, cup-like; as in Urtica urens.

22. *Conical;* as in Utricularia foliosa.

23. *Acidiforme*, pitcher-like, a membraneous tube, containing water, and behind the flower; as in Ascium and Ruyschia.

24. *Calycine*, adhering to the calyx, by a spur; as in Tropæolum majus.

NEDY′IA. (*Nedys;* from νηδυς, the belly.) The intestines.

NEEDLE ORE. Acicular bismuth glance.

Needle-shaped leaf. See *Acerosus.*

Needle zeolite. See *Zeolite.*

NEGRO CACHEXY. *Cachexia africana.* A propensity for eating earth, common to males as well as females, in the West Indies and Africa.

NELE′RA. (From νειαρος, furthermost.) The lower part of the belly.

NEMORO′SA. (From *nemus*, a grove: so called because it grows in woods.) A species of wind-flower, the *Anemone nemerosa*, of Linnæus.

NEP. See *Nepeta.*

NE′PA THEOPHRASTI. See *Spartium scoparium.*

NEPE′NTHOS. (From νη, neg. and πενθος, grief: so called from their exhilarating qualities.) 1. A preparation of opium.

2. A kind of bugloss.

NE′PETA. (From *nepte*, German.) The name of a genus of plants in the Linnæan system. Class, *Didynamia;* Order, *Gymnospermia.*

NEPETA CATARIA. The systematic name of the catmint. *Herba felis; Mentha felina; Calamintha; Nepetella; Mentha cataria.* The leaves of this plant, *Nepeta—floribus spicatis; verticillis; subpedicellatis; foliis petiolatis, cordatis, dentato-serratis*, of Linnæus, have a moderately pungent aromatic taste, and a strong smell, like an admixture of spearmint and pennyroyal. The herb is recommended in uterine disorders, dyspepsia, and flatulency

NEPETE′LLA. (Dim. of *nepeta.*) The lesser catmint.

NE′PHELA. (Dim. of νεφος, a cloud.) A cloud-like spot on the cornea of the eye.

NEPHELOI′DES. (From νεφελη, a cloud, and ειδος, a likeness.) Cloudy. Applied to the urine.

NEPHRA′LGIA. (From νεφρος, the kidney, and αλγος, pain.) Pain in the kidney.

NEPHRELINE. Rhomboidal felspar. This occurs in drusy cavities along with ceylanite, vesuvian, and meionite, at Monte Somma, near Naples, in drusy cavities in granular limestone.

NEPHRITE. Of this mineral there are two species, common nephrite, and axe-stone. The former is of a leek-green colour, and occurs in granite and gneiss, in Switzerland. The most beautiful come from Persia and Egypt. See *Axe-stone.*

NEPHRITIC. (*Nephriticus;* from νεφρος, the kidney.) Of or belonging to the kidney.

2. Medicine is so termed that is employed in the cure of diseases of the kidneys.

Nephritic wood. See *Guilandina moringa.*

NEPHRITICA AQUA. Spirituous distillation of nut meg and hawthorn flowers.

NEPHRITICUM LIGNUM. See *Guilandina moringa.*

NEPHRI′TIS. (*Nephritis, idis.* f.; from νεφρος, a kidney.) Inflammation of the kidney. A genus of disease in the class *Pyrexiæ* and order *Phlegmasiæ*, of Cullen; known by pyrexia, pain in the region of the kidneys, and shooting along the course of the ureter; drawing up of the testicles; numbness of the thigh; vomiting; urine high-coloured, and frequently discharged; costiveness, and colic pains. Nephritis is symptomatic of calculus, gout, &c.

This inflammation may be distinguished from the colic by the pain being seated very far back, and by the difficulty of passing urine, which constantly attends it; and it may be distinguished from rheumatism, as the pain is but little influenced or increased by motion.

Nephritis is to be distinguished from a calculus in the kidney or ureter, by the symptoms of fever accompanying, or immediately following the attack of pain, and these continuing without any remarkable intermission; whereas, in a calculus of the kidney or ureter, they do not occur until a considerable time after violent pain has been felt. In the latter case, too, a numbness of the thigh, and a retraction of the testicle on the affected side, usually takes place.

The causes which give rise to nephritis are external contusions, strains of the back, acrids conveyed to the kidneys in the course of the circulation, violent and severe exercise, either in riding or walking, calculous concretions lodged in the kidneys or ureters, and exposure to cold. In some habits there is an evident predisposition to this complaint, particularly the gouty, and in these there are often translations of the matter to the kidneys, which very much imitate nephritis.

An inflammation of the kidney is attended with a sharp pain on the affected side, extending along the course of the ureter; and there is a frequent desire to make water, with much difficulty in making it. The body is costive, the skin is dry and hot, the patient feels great uneasiness when he endeavours to walk, or sit upright; he lies with most ease on the affected side, and is generally troubled with nausea and frequent vomiting.

When the disease is protracted beyond the seventh or eighth day, and the patient feels an obtuse pain in the part, has frequent returns of chillness and shiverings, there is reason to apprehend that matter is forming in the kidney, and that a suppuration will ensue.

Dissections of nephritis show the usual effects of inflammation on the kidney; and they likewise often discover the formation of abscesses, which have destroyed its whole substance. In a few instances, the kidney has been found in a scirrhous state.

The disease is to be treated by bleeding, general and local, the warm bath, or fomentations to the loins, emollient clyster, mucilaginous drinks, and the general antiphlogistic plan. The bowels should be effectually cleared at first by some sufficiently active formula; but the saline cathartics are considered not so proper, as they may add to the irritation of the kidney. Calomel with antimonial powder, followed by the infusion of senna, or the ol ricini, may be given in preference, and repeated occasionally. It will be right also to endeavour to promote diaphoresis, by moderate doses of antimonials especially. Blisters are inadmissible in this disease; but the linimentum ammoniæ, or other rubefacient application, may in some measure supply their place. Opium will often prove useful, particularly where the symptoms appear to originate from calculi given in the form of clyster, or by the mouth; in which latter mode of using it, however, it will be much better joined with other remedies, which may obviate its heating effect, and determine it rather to pass off by the skin. A decoction of the dried leaves of the peach tree is said to have been serviceable in many cases of this disease. In affections of a more chronic nature where there is a discharge of mucus or pus, by urine in addition to suitable tonic medicines, the uva ursi in moderate doses, or some of the terebinthinate remedies may be given with probability of relief.

NE'PHROS. (From νεω, to flow, and φερω, to bear; as conveying the urinary fluid.) The kidney. See *Kidney.*

NEPHRO'TOMY. (*Nephrotomia ;* from νεφρος, a kidney, and τεμνω, to cut.) The operation of extracting a stone from the kidney. A proceeding which, perhaps, has never been actually put in practice. The cutting into the kidney, the deep situation of this viscus, and the want of symptoms by which the lodgment of a stone in it can be certainly discovered, will always be strong objections to the practice.

NE'RIUM. (From νηρος, humid: so called because it grows in moist places.) The name of a genus of plants in the Linnæan system. Class, *Pentandria ;* Order, *Monogynia.*

NERIUM ANTIDYSENTERICUM. The systematic name of the tree which affords the Codaga pala bark. *Conessi cortex ; Codaga pala ; Cortex Bela-aye ; Cortex profluvii.* The bark of the *Nerium ;—foliis ovatis, acuminatis, petiolatis,* of Linnæus. It grows on *the coast of Malabar. It is of a dark black colour externally, and generally covered with a white moss, or scurf. It is very little known in the shops; has an austere, bitter taste ; and is recommended in diarrhœas, dysenteries, &c. as an astringent.

NERIUM TINCTORIUM. This tree grows in Hindostan, and, according to Dr. Roxburg, affords indigo.

NE'ROLI OLEUM. Essential oil of orange flowers. See *Citrus aurantium.*

NERVA'LLI OSSA. (From *nervus,* a nerve.) The bones through which the nerves pass.

NERVE. (*Nervus, i.* m. from νεῦρον.)

A. In *anatomy.* Formerly it meant a sinew. This accounts for the opposite meanings of the word *nervous,* which sometimes means strong, sinewy, and sometimes weak and irritable. Nerves are long, white, medullary cords, that serve for sensation. They originate from the brain and spinal marrow; hence they are distinguished into cerebral and spinal nerves, and distributed upon the organs of sense, the viscera, vessels, muscles, and every part that is endowed with sensibility. The cerebral nerves are the olfactory, optic, motores oculorum, pathetici, or trochleatores, trigemini, or divisi, abducent, auditory, or acoustic, par vagum, and lingual. Heister has drawn up the use of these nerves in the two following verses:

Olfaciens, cernens, oculosque movens, patiensque,
Gustans, abducens, audiensque, vagansque, lo-
*   quensque.*

The spinal nerves are thirty pairs, and are divided into eight pair of cervical, twelve pair of dorsal, five pair of lumbar, and five of sacral nerves. In the course of the nerves there are a number of knots: these are called *ganglions ;* they are commonly of an oblong shape, and of a grayish colour, somewhat inclining to red, which is perhaps owing to their being extremely vascular. Some writers have considered these little ganglions as so many little brains. Lancisi fancied he had discovered muscular fibres in them; but they certainly are not of an irritable nature. A late writer (Dr. Johnson) imagines they are intended to deprive us of the power of the will over certain parts, as the heart, for instance; but if this hypothesis were well founded, they should be met with only in nerves leading to involuntary muscles; whereas it is certain that the voluntary muscles receive nerves through ganglions. Dr. Monroe, from observing the accurate intermixture of the minute nerves which compose them, considers them as new sources of nervous energy. The nerves, like the blood-vessels, in their course through the body, communicate with each other, and each of these communications constitutes what is called a *plexus,* from whence branches are again detached to different parts of the body. The use of the nerves is to convey impressions to the brain from all parts of the system, and the principles of motion and sensibility from the brain to every part of the system. The manner in which this operation is effected is not yet determined. The inquiry has been a constant source of hypothesis in all ages, and has produced some ingenious ideas, and many erroneous positions, but without having hitherto afforded much satisfactory information. Some physiologists have considered a trunk of nerves as a solid cord, capable

of being divided into an infinite number of filaments, by means of which the impressions of feeling are conveyed to the common sensorium. Others have supposed each fibril to be a canal, carrying a volatile fluid, which they term the *nervous fluid.* Those who con tend for their being solid bodies, are of opinion that feeling is occasioned by vibration; so that, for instance, according to this hypothesis, by pricking the finger, a vibration would be occasioned in the nerve distributed through its substance; and the effects of this vibration, when extended to the sensorium, would be an excital of pain; but the inelasticity, the softness, the connexion, and the situation of the nerves, are so many proofs that vibration has no share in the cause of feeling.

A Table of the Nerves.

CEREBRAL NERVES.

1. The *first pair,* called *olfactory.*
2. The *second pair,* or *optic nerves.*
3. The *third pair,* or *oculorum motores.*
4. The *fourth pair,* or *pathetici.*
5. The *fifth pair,* or *trigemini,* which gives off,
  a. The *ophthalmic,* or *orbital nerve,* which sends,
    1. A *branch* to unite with one from the sixth
      pair, and form the great intercostal nerve.
    2. The *frontal nerve.*
    3. The *lachrymal.*
    4. The *nasal.*
  b. The *superior maxillary,* which divides into,
    1. The *spheno-palatine* nerve.
    2. The *posterior alveolar.*
    3. The *infra orbital.*
  c. The *inferior maxillary* nerve, from which arise,
    1. The *internal lingual.*
    2. The *inferior maxillary,* properly so called.
6. The *sixth pair,* or *abducentes,* which send off,
    1. A *branch* to unite with one from the fifth, and
      form the great intercostal.
7. The *seventh pair,* or *auditory nerves :* these arise by two separate beginnings, viz.
  The *portio dura,* a nerve going to the face.
  The *portio mollis,* which is distributed on the
    ear.
  The *portio dura,* or *facial* nerve, gives off the
    chorda tympani, and then proceeds to the face.
8. The *eighth pair,* or *par vagum,* arise from the medulla oblongata, and join with the accessory of Willis. The par vagum gives off,
    1. The *right* and *left recurrent nerve.*
    2. Several branches in the chest, to form the *car-*
      diac plexus.
    3. Several branches to form the *pulmonic plexus.*
    4. Several branches to form the *œsophageal*
      plexus.
    5. It then forms in the abdomen the *stomachic*
      plexus.
    6. The *hepatic plexus.*
    7. The *splenic plexus.*
    8 The *renal plexus,* receiving several branches
      from the great intercostal, which assists in
      their formation.
9. The *ninth pair,* or *lingual nerves,* which go from the medulla oblongata to the tongue.

SPINAL NERVES.

Those nerves are called *spinal,* which pass' out through the lateral or intervertebral foramina of the spine.

They are divided into *cervical, dorsal, lumbar,* and *sacral* nerves.

CERVICAL NERVES.

The *cervical nerves* are *eight* pairs.

The *first* are called the *occipital :* they arise from the beginning of the spinal marrow, pass out between the margin of the occipital foramen and atlas, form a ganglion on its transverse process. and are distributed about the occiput and neck.

The *second* pair of cervical nerves send a branch to the accessory nerve of Willis, and proceed to the parotid gland and external ear.

The *third* cervical pair supply the integuments of the scapula, the cucullaris, and triangularis muscles, and send a branch to form, with others, the diaphragmatic nerve.

The *fourth, fifth, sixth, seventh,* and *eighth* pair all converge to form the *brachial plexus,* from which arise the six following

Nerves of the upper Extremities.

1 The *axillary* nerve, which sometimes arises from the radial nerve. It runs backwards and outwards around the neck of the humerus, and ramifies in the muscles of the scapula.

2. The *external cutaneal*, which perforates the caraco-brachialis muscle, to the bend of the arm, where it accompanies the median vein as far as the thumb, and is lost in its integuments.

3. The *internal cutaneal*, which descends on the inside of the arm, where it bifurcates. From the bend of the arm the anterior branch accompanies the basilic vein, to be inserted into the skin of the palm of the hand; the posterior branch runs down the internal part of the forearm, to vanish in the skin of the little finger.

4. The *median* nerve, which accompanies the brachial artery to the cubit, then passes between the brachialis internus, pronator rotundus, and the perforatus and perforans, under the ligament of the wrist to the palm of the hand, where it sends off branches in every direction to the muscles of the hand, and then supplies the digital nerves, which go to the extremities of the thumb, fore, and middle fingers.

5. The *ulnar* nerve, which descends between the brachial artery and basilic vein, between the internal condyle of the humerus, and the olecranon, and divides in the forearm into an *internal* and *external* branch. The former passes over the ligament of the wrist and sesamoid bone, to the hand, where it divides into three branches, two of which go to the ring and little finger, and the third forms an arch towards the thumb, in the palm of the hand, and is lost in the contiguous muscles. The latter passes over the tendon of the extensor carpi ulnaris and back of the hand, to supply also the two last fingers.

6. The *radial* nerve which sometimes gives off the axillary nerve. It passes backwards, about the os humeri, descends on the outside of the arm, between the brachialis externus and internus muscles to the cubit: then proceeds between the supinator longus and brevis, to the superior extremity of the radius, giving off various branches to adjacent muscles. At this place it divides into two branches; *one* goes along the radius, between the supinator longus and radialis internus to the back of the hand, and terminates in the interosseous muscles, the thumb and first three fingers; the *other* passes between the supinator brevis and head of the radius, and is lost in the muscles of the fore-arm.

Dorsal Nerves.

The *Dorsal* nerves are twelve pairs in number. The first pair gives off a branch to the brachial plexus. All the dorsal nerves are distributed to the muscles of the back, intercostals, serrati, pectoral, abdominal muscles, and diaphragm. The five inferior pairs go to the cartilages of the ribs, and are called *costal*.

Lumbar nerves.

The five pairs of Lumbar nerves are bestowed about the loins and muscles, skin of the abdomen and loins, scrotum, ovaria, and diaphragm. The second, third, and fifth pairs unite and form the *obturator nerve*, which descends over the psoas muscle into the pelvis, and passes through the foramen thyroideum to the obturator muscle, triceps, pectineus, &c.

The third and fourth, with some branches of the second pair, form the *crural nerve*, which passes under Poupart's ligament with the femoral artery, sends off branches to the adjacent parts, and descends in the direction of the sartorius muscle to the internal condyle of the femur, from whence it accompanies the saphena vein to the internal ankle, to be lost in the skin of the great toe.

The fifth pair is joined to the first pair of the sacral nerves.

Sacral Nerves.

There are five pairs of *sacral* nerves, all of which arise from the *cauda equina*, or termination of the medulla spinalis, so called from the nerves resembling the tail of a horse. The first four pairs give off branches to the pelvic viscera, and are afterward united to the last lumbar, to form a large *plexus*, which gives off

The *ischiatic nerve*, the largest in the body. The ischiatic nerve, immediately at its origin, sends off branches to the bladder, rectum, and parts of generation; proceeds from the cavity of the pelvis through the ischiatic notch, between the tuberosity of the ischium and great trochanter, to the ham, where it is called the *popliteal nerve*. In the ham it divides into two branches.

1. The *peroneal*, which descends on the fibula, and distributes many branches to the muscles of the leg and back of the foot.

2. The *tibial*, which penetrates the gastrocnemii muscles to the internal ankle, passes through a notch in the os calcis to the sole of the foot, where it divides into an *internal* and *external plantar* nerve, which supply the muscles and aponeurosis of the foot and the toes.

Physiology of the Nervous system.

The nervous system, as the organ of sense and motion, is connected with so many functions of the animal economy, that the study of it must be of the utmost importance, and a fundamental part of the study of the whole economy. The nervous system consists of the medullary substance of the brain, cerebellum, medulla oblongata, and spinalis; and of the same substance continued into the nerves by which it is distributed to many different parts of the body. The whole of this system seems to be properly distinguished into these four parts.

1. The medullary substance contained in the cranium and vertebral cavity; the whole of which seems to consist of distinct fibres, but without the smaller fibres being separated from each other by any evident enveloping membranes.

2. Connected with one part or other of this substance are, the nerves, in which the same medullary substance is continued; but here more evidently divided into fibres, each of which is separated from the others by an enveloping membrane, derived from the pia mater

3. Parts of the extremities of certain nerves, in which the medullary substance is divested of the enveloping membranes from the pia mater, and so situated as to be exposed to the action of certain external bodies, and perhaps so framed as to be affected by the action of certain bodies only; these are named the *sentient extremities* of the nerves.

4. Certain extremities of the nerves, so framed as to be capable of a peculiar contractility; and, in consequence of their situations and attachments to be, by their contraction, capable of moving most of the solid and fluid parts of the body. These are named the *moving extremities* of the nerves.

These several parts of the nervous system are every where the same continuous medullary substance, which is supposed to be the vital solid of animals, so constituted in living animals, and in living systems only, as to admit of motions being readily propagated from any one part to every other part of the nervous system, so long as the continuity and naturally living state of the medullary substance remains. In the living man there is an immaterial thinking substance, or *mind*, constantly present, and every phenomenon of thinking is to be considered as an affection or faculty of the mind alone. But this immaterial and thinking part of man is so connected with the material and corporeal part of him, and particularly with the nervous system, that motions excited in this give occasion to thought, and thought, however occasioned, gives occasion to new motions in the nervous system. This mutual communication, or influence, is assumed with confidence as a fact: but the mode of it we do not understand, nor pretend to explain; and therefore are not bound to obviate the difficulties that attend any of the suppositions which have been made concerning it. The phenomena of the nervous system appear commonly in the following order: The impulse of external bodies acts upon the sentient extremities of the nerves; and this gives occasion to perception or thought, which, as first arising in the mind, is termed *sensation*. This sensation, according to its various modifications, gives occasion to *volition*, or the willing of certain ends to be obtained by the motion of certain parts of the body; and this volition gives occasion to the contraction of muscular fibres, by which the motion of the part required is produced. As the impulse of bodies on the sentient extremities of a nerve does not occasion any sensation, unless the nerve between the sentient extremity and the brain be free; and as, in like manner, violition does not produce any contraction of muscles, unless the nerve between the brain and muscle be also free; it is concluded from both these facts that sensation and volition, so far as they are connected with corporeal motions, are functions of the brain alone; and it is presumed that sensation arises only in consequence of external impulse producing motion in the sentient extremities of the nerves, and of that motion being thence propagated along the nerves of the brain ; and, in like manner, that the will operating in the brain only, by a motion begun there, and propagated along the nerves, produces the contraction of muscles. From what is now said, we perceive more distinctly the different functions of the several parts of the nervous system. 1. The sentient extremities seem to be particularly fitted to receive the impressions of external bodies; and according to the difference of these impressions, and of the condition of the sentient extremity itself, to propagate along the nerves motions of a determined kind, which communicated to the brain, give occasion to sensation. 2. The brain seems to be a part fitted for, and susceptible of, those motions with which sensation, and the whole consequent operations of thought, are connected : and thereby is fitted to form a communication between the motions excited in the sentient, and those in consequence arising in the moving extremities of the nerves, which are often remote and distant from each other. 3. The moving extremities are so framed as to be capable of contraction, and of having this contraction excited by motion propagated from the brain, and communicated to the contractile fibre. 4. The nerves, more strictly so called, are to be considered as a collection of medullary fibres, each enveloped in its proper membrane, and thereby so separated from every other, as hardly to admit of any communication of motion from any one to the others, and to admit only of motion along the continuous medullary substance of the same fibre, from its origin to the extremities, or contrarywise. From this view of the parts of the nervous system, of their several functions and communication with each other, it appears that the beginning of motion in the animal economy is generally connected with sensation : and that the ultimate effects of such motion are chiefly actions depending immediately upon the contraction of moving fibres, between which and the sentient extremities, the communication is by means of the brain.

B. In *botany* : the term *nerve* is applied to a cluster of vessels that runs like a rib or chord on certain leaves ; as that of the *Laurus cinnamomum*, and *Arctium lappa*.

NE'RVEA SPONGIOSA. The cavernous part of the penis.

NERVINE. (*Nervinus ;* from *nervus,* a nerve.) Neurotic. That which relieves disorders of the nerves. All the antispasmodics, and the various preparations of bark and iron

NERVO'RUM RESOLUTIO. Apoplexy and palsy have been so considered.

NERVOSUS. Nervous. 1. Applied, *in medicine,* to fevers and affections of the nervous system

2. In *anatomy :* to the structure of parts being composed of, or resembling a nerve.

3. In *botany :* to leaves which have nervelike cords.

NERVOSUM os. The occipital bone.

NERVOUS. See *Nervosus.*

Nervous consumption. See *Atrophia.*

Nervous diseases. See *Neuroses.*

Nervous fever. See *Febris nervosa.*

Nervous headache. See *Cephalalgia.*

NERVOUS FLUID. Nervous principle. The vascularity of the cortical part of the brain, and of the nerves themselves, their softness, pulpiness, and natural humid appearance, give reason to believe that between the medullary particles of which they are principally composed, a fine fluid is constantly secreted which may be fitted to receive and transmit, even more readily than other fluids do, all impressions which are made on it. It appears to exhale from the extremities of the nerves. The lassitude and debility of *muscles* from too great exercise, and the dulness of the sensorial organs from excessive use, would seem to prove this. It has no *smell* nor *taste ;* for the cerebrine medulla is insipid and inodorous. Nor has it any *colour,* for the cerebrum and nerves are white. It is of so subtile a *consistence,* as never to have been detected. Its *mobility* is stupendous, for in less than a moment, with the consent of the mind, it is conveyed from the cerebrum to the muscles, like the electric matter. Whether the nervous fluid be carried from the organ of sense in the *sensorial* nerves to the cerebrum, and from thence in the *motory* nerves to the muscles, cannot be positively affirmed. The *constituent principles* of this liquid are perfectly unknown, as they cannot be rendered visible by art, or proved by experiment.

102

Upon making a ligature upon a nerve, the motion of the fluid is interrupted, which proves that something corporeal flows through it. It is therefore a weak argument to deny its existence because we cannot see it; for who has seen the matter of heat, oxygen, azote, and other elementary bodies, the existence of which, no physician in the present day doubts ? The *electric matter,* whose action on the nerves is very great, does not appear to constitute the nervous fluid ; for nerves exhibit no signs of spontaneous electricity; nor can it be the *magnetic matter,* as the experiment of Gavian with the magnet demonstrates: nor is it *oxygen,* nor *hydrogen,* nor *azote ;* for the first very much irritates the nerves, and the other two suspend their action. The nervous fluid, therefore, is an *element* sui generis, which exists and is produced in the nerves only ; hence, like other elements, it is only to be known by its effects. The pulpous softness of some nerves, and their lax situation, does not allow them and the brain to act on the body and soul only by *oscillation.* Lastly, a tense chord, although tied, oscillates. The *use* of the nervous fluid is, 1. It appears to be an intermediate substance between the body and the soul, by means of which the latter thinks, perceives, and moves the muscles subservient to the will. Hence, the body acts upon the soul, and the soul upon the body. 2. It appears to differ from the *vital principle;* for parts live and are irritable which want nerves, as bones, tendons plants, and insects.

Nervous principle. See *Nervous fluid.*

NE'STIS. (From νη, neg. and εσθιω, to eat; so called because it is generally found empty.) The jejunum.

NETTLE. See *Urtica.*

Nettle, dead. See *Lamium album*

Nettle-rash. See *Urticaria.*

NEURALGIA. (From νευρον, a nerve, and αλγος, pain.) 1. A pain in a nerve.

2. The name of a genus of diseases, in Good's Nosology. Class, *Neurotica:* Order, *Æsthetica ;* nerveache. It has three species, *Neuralgia faciei, pedis, mammæ.*

NEUROCHONDRO'DES. (From νευρον, a sinew, χονδρος, a cartilage, and ειδος, resemblance.) A hard substance between a sinew and a cartilage.

NEUROLOGY. (*Neurologia;* from νευρον, a nerve, and λογος, a discourse.) The doctrine of the nerves.

NEUROME'TORES. (From νευρον, a nerve, and μητρα, a matrix.) The psoas muscles are so called by Fallopius, as being the repository of many small nerves.

NEURO'SES. (The plural of *neurosis ;* from νευρον, a nerve.) Nervous diseases. The second class of Cullen's Nosology is so called ; it comprehends affections of sense and motion disturbed; without either idiopathic pyrexia, or topical diseases.

NEUROTICA. (From νευρον, a nerve.) The name of a class of diseases in Good's Nosology. Diseases of the nervous system. It comprehends four orders, viz. *Phrenica ; Æsthetica ; Cinetica ; Systatica.*

NEURO'TICA. (From νευρον, a nerve.) Nervous medicines.

NEURO'TOMY. (*Neurotomia ;* from νευρον, a nerve, and τεμνω, to cut.) 1. A dissection of the nerves.

2. A puncture of a nerve.

NEUTRAL. A term applied to saline compounds of an acid and an alkali, which are so called, because they do not possess the characters of acid or alkaline salts; such are Epsom salts, nitre, and all the compounds of the alkalies with the acids.

NEUTRALIZATION. When acid and alkaline matter are combined in such proportions, that the compound does not change the colour of litmus or violets, they are said to be neutralized.

NE'XUS. (From *necto,* to wind.) A complication of substances in one part, as the membrane which involves the fœtus.

NICHOLS, FRANK, was born in London, where his father was a barrister, in 1699. After passing through the usual academical exercises at Oxford with great assiduity, he chose medicine for his profession ; and pursued a course of dissections with so much diligence and perseverance, as to render himself highly skilful in this branch of his art. Hence he was chosen reader of anatomy in the university, where he used his utmost endeavours to introduce a zeal for this pursuit, and obtained a high reputation. At the close of his course he made a short trial of practice in Cornwall, and sub sequently paid a visit to the principal schools of France and Italy. On his return he resumed his anatomical and physiological lectures in London, which were frequented, not only by students from the universities, but also by many surgeons, apothecaries, and others. In 1728 he was chosen a fellow of the Royal Society, to which he communicated several papers; and shortly after he received his doctor's degree at Oxford, and became a fellow of the College of Physicians. In 1734, he was appointed to read the Gulstonian lectures, and chose the Heart and Circulation, for his subjects. In 1743, he married one of the daughters of the celebrated Dr. Mead. About five years after he was appointed lecturer on surgery to the college, and began his course with a learned and elegant dissertation on the " Anima Medica," which was afterward published. On the death of Sir Hans Sloane in 1753, Dr. Nichols was appointed his successor as one of the King's physicians; which office he held till the death of his Majesty, seven years after. To a second edition of the treatise, " De Anima Medica," in 1772, he added a dissertation, " De Motu Cordis et Sanguinis in Homine nato et non nato." Weary at length with his profession, and wishing to superintend the education of his son at Oxford, he removed to that city: and when the study of the law recalled his son to London, the Doctor took a house at Epsom, where he passed the remainder of his life in literary retirement. He died in 1778.

Nicked leaf. See *Emarginatus.*

NICKEL. A metal discovered by Cronstedt in 1751. though the substance from which he extracted it was known in the year 1694. Nickel is found in nature generally in the metallic state, more rarely in that of an oxide. Its ores have a coppery-red colour, generally covered more or less with a greenish-gray efflorescence. The most abundant ore is that termed *sulphuret of nickel*, or *kupfernickel*, which is a compound of nickel, arsenic, sulphuret of iron, and sometimes cobalt and copper. This ore occurs either massive, or disseminated, but never crystallized; it is of a copper colour, sometimes yellowish, white, or gray. It exists also combined with oxygen, and a little carbonic acid, in what is called *native oxide of nickel (nickel ochre);* it then has an earthy appearance, and is very friable; it is found coating *kupfernickel*, and seems to originate from the decomposition of this ore. It is found contaminated with iron in the mineral substance called *martial nickel;* this native combination, when fresh broken, has a lamellated texture; when exposed to the air, it soon turns black, and sometimes exhibits thin rhomboidal plates placed irregularly over each other. It is also found united to arsenic, cobalt, and alumine in the ore, called *arseniate of nickel.*

Nickel is a metal of great hardness, of a uniform texture, and of a colour between silver and tin; very difficult to be purified, and magnetical. It even acquires polarity by the touch. It is malleable, both cold and redhot; and is scarcely more fusible than manganese. Its oxides, when pure, are reducible by a sufficient heat without combustible matter; and it is little more tarnished by heating in contact with air, than platina, gold, and silver. Its specific gravity, when cast, is 8.279 ; when forged, 8.666.

Nickel is commonly obtained from its sulphuret, the kupfernickel of the Germans, in which it is generally mixed also with arsenic, iron, and cobalt. This is first roasted, to drive off the sulphur and arsenic, then mixed with two parts of black flux, put into a crucible, covered with muriate of soda, and heated in a forge furnace. The metal thus obtained, which is still very impure, must be dissolved in dilute nitric acid, and then evaporated to dryness; and after this process has been repeated three or four times, the residuum must be dissolved in a solution of ammonia, perfectly free from carbonic acid. Being again evaporated to dryness, it is now to be well mixed with two or three parts of black flux, and exposed to a violent heat in a crucible for half an hour or more.

There are two oxides of nickel; the dark ash-gray, and the black. If potassa be added to the solution of the nitrate or sulphate, and the precipitate dried, we obtain the protoxide. The peroxide was formed by Thenard, by passing chlorine through the protoxide diffused in water. A black insoluble peroxide remains at the bottom.

Little is known of the chloride, iodide sulphuret, or phosphuret of this metal.

The salts of nickel possess the following general characters. They have usually a green colour, and yield a white precipitate with ferroprussiate of potassa. Ammonia dissolves the oxide of nickel. Sulphuretted hydrogen and infusion of galls occasion no precipitate: The hydrosulphuret of potassa throws down a black precipitate. Their composition has been very imperfectly ascertained.

NICO′PHORUS. (From νικη, victory, and φερω, to bear: so called because victors were crowned with it.) A kind of ivy.

NICOTIA′NA. (From Nicott, who first brought it into Europe.) Tobacco.
1. The name of a genus of plants in the Linnæan system. Class, *Pentandria;* Order, *Monogynia.*
2. The former pharmacopœial name of the tobacco. See *Nicotiana tabacum.*

NICOTIANA AMERICANA. American or Virginian tobacco. See *Nicotiana tabacum.*

NICOTIANA MINOR. See *Nicotiana rustica.*

NICOTIANA RUSTICA. The systematic name of the English tobacco. *Nicotiana minor; Priapeia; Hyoscyamus luteus.* This plant is much weaker than the Virginian tobacco, the leaves are chiefly used to smoke vermin, though they promise, from their more gentle operation, to be a safer remedy in some cases than the former.

NICOTIANA TABACUM. The systematic name of the Virginian tobacco-plant. *Petum,* by the Indians; *Ta bacum; Hyoscyamus peruvianus; Picelt. Nicotiana —foliis lanceolato-ovatis sessilibus decurrentibus florentibus acutis,* of Linnæus, is the plant employed medicinally. It is a very active narcotic and sternutatory. A decoction of the leaves is much esteemed in some diseases of the skin, and is by some said to be a specific against the itch. The fumes and the decoction are employed in obstinate constipations of the bowels, and very frequently with success; it is necessary, however, to caution the practitioner against an effect mostly produced by its exhibition, namely, syncope, with cold sweats; and, in some instances, death. Vauquelin has obtained a peculiar principle from this plant, in which its active properties reside. See *Nicotin.*

NICOTIN. A peculiar principle obtained by Vauquelin, from tobacco. It is colourless, and has the peculiar taste and smell of the plant. It dissolves both in water and alkohol: it is volatile and poisonous.

[" Evaporate the expressed juice to one-fourth its bulk; and, when cold, strain it through fine linen; evaporate nearly to dryness; digest the residue in alkohol, filter and evaporate to dryness; dissolve this again in alkohol, and again reduce it to a dry state. Dissolve the residue in water, saturate the acid which it contains with weak solution of potassa, introduce the whole into a retort, and distil to dryness, redissolve, and again dissolve three or four times successively in water, from which solution it may be obtained by very gradual evaporation."—*Webs. Man. of Chem.* A.]

NICTITATIO. Twinkling, or winking of the eyes.

NIDULANS. (From *nidulor,* to place in a nest.) Nidulate: applied to the seeds of some fruits, which are imbedded on their surface; as those of the strawberry.

NIGE′LLA. (*Quasi nigrella;* from *niger,* black: so named from its black seed.)
1. The name of a genus of plants in the Linnæan system. Class, *Polyandria;* Order, *Pentagynia.*
2. The pharmacopœial name of the plant called devil-in-a-bush, or fennel-flower.

NIGELLA OFFICINARUM. See *Agrostemma githago*
NIGELLA SATIVA. The systematic name of the devil in-a-bush. Fennel-flower. *Melanthium; Melaspermum.* It was formerly employed medicinally as an expectorant and deobstruent, but is now fallen into disuse.

NIGELLA′STRUM. (From *nigella,* fennel flower.) See *Agrostemma githago.*

NIGER. Black. Applied to some parts and diseases from their colour; as *Pigmentum nigrum · morbus niger.*

NIGHT. *Nox.* Many diseases and plants have this for their trivial name, because of some peculiar circumstance connected with the period; as night mare nightshade, &c

Night-blindness. See *Nyctalopia.*

Nightmare. See *Oneirodynia gravans.*

NIGHTSHADE. See *Solanum, Phytolacca,* and *Atropa.*

Nightshade, American. See *Phytolacca decandria.*

Nightshade, deadly. See *Atropa belladonna.*

Nightshade, Palestine. See *Solanum sanctum.*

Nightshade, woody. See *Solanum dulcamara.*

NIGRINE. An ore of titanium.

NIGRI'TIES. (From *niger,* black.) A caries is called *nigrities ossium,* a blackness of the bone.

NI'HILUM ALBUM. *Nihil album.* A name formerly given to the flowers, or oxide of zinc.

NI'NZI RADIX. See *Sium ninsi.*

NI'NZIN. See *Sium ninsi.*

NIPPLE. *Papilla.* The small projecting proportion in the middle of the breasts of men and women. It is much larger in the latter, and has several openings in it, the excretory ducts of the lacteal glands.

NIPPLE-WORT. See *Lapsana.*

NISUS FORMATIVUS. (*Nisus, &c.* m.) A creative or formative effort.

NITIDUS. Polished, smooth, shining: applied in botany to stems, &c.; as in the Chærophyllum sylvestre. See *Caulis.*

NITRAS AMMONIÆ. See *Ammoniæ nitras.*

NITRAS ARGENTI. See *Argenti nitras.*

NITRAS POTASSÆ. See *Nitric acid.*

NITRAS POTASSÆ FUSUS. *Sal prunellæ; Nitrum tabulatum.* This salt, besides the nitric acid and potassa, contains a little sulphuric acid. See *Nitric acid.*

NITRAS SODÆ. *Alkali minerale nitratum; Nitrum cubicum.* Its virtues are similar to those of nitrate of potassa, for which it may be safely substituted.

NITRATE. (*Nitras, atis,* f.; from *nitrum,* nitre.) A salt formed by the union of the nitric acid, with salifiable bases; as the nitrate of potassa, soda, silver, &c.

Nitrate of potassa. See *Nitric acid.*

Nitrate of silver. See *Argenti nitras.*

NITRE. Ni'τρον. *Nitrum; Potassæ nitras; Saltpetræ; Alaurat; Algali; Atac; Baurack; Acusto; Halinitrum.* The common name for saltpetre or the nitrate of potassa. A perfect neutral salt, formed by the union of the nitric acid with the vegetable alkali, thence called nitrate of potassa. Its taste is cooling, and it does not alter the colour of the syrup of violets. Nitre exists in large quantities in the earth, and is continually formed in inhabited places; it is found in great quantities upon walls which are sheltered from the rain. It is of great use in the arts; it is the principal ingredient in gunpowder; and, burned with different proportions of tartar, forms the substances called fluxes. It is of considerable importance in medicine, as a febrifuge, diuretic, and antiphlogistic remedy, in doses of from five to twenty grains. See *Nitric acid.*

NITRIC ACID. *Acidum nitricum.* "The two principal constituent parts of our atmosphere, when in certain proportions, are capable, under particular circumstances, of combining chemically into one of the most powerful acids, the nitric. If these gases be mixed in a proper proportion in a glass tube about a line in diameter, over mercury, and a series of electric shocks be passed through them for some hours, they will form nitric acid; or, if a solution of potassa be present with them, nitrate of potassa will be obtained. The constitution of this acid may be further proved, analytically, by driving it through a red-hot porcelain tube, as thus it will be decomposed into oxygen and nitrogen gases. For all practical purposes, however, the nitric acid is obtained from nitrate of potassa, from which it is expelled by sulphuric acid.

Three parts of pure nitrate of potassa, coarsely powdered, are to be put into a glass retort, with two of strong sulphuric acid. This must be cautiously added, taking care to avoid the fumes that arise. Join to the retort a tubulated receiver of large capacity, with an adopter interposed, and lute the junctures with glazier's putty. In the tubulure fix a glass tube, terminating in another large receiver, in which is a small quantity of water; and if you wish to collect the gaseous products, let a bent glass tube from this receiver communicate with a pneumatic trough. Apply heat to the receiver by means of a sand bath. The first product that passes into the receiver is generally red and fuming; but the appearances gradually diminish, till the
104

acid comes over pale, and even colourless, if the materials used were clean. After this it again becomes more and more red and fuming, till the end of the operation; and the whole mingled together will be of a yellow or orange colour.

Empty the receiver, and again replace it. Then introduce by a small funnel, very cautiously, one part of boiling water in a slender stream, and continue the distillation. A small quantity of a weaker acid will thus be obtained, which can be kept apart. The first will have a specific gravity of about 1.500, if the heat have been properly regulated, and if the receiver was refrigerated by cold water or ice. Acid of that density, amounting to two-thirds of the weight of the nitre, may thus be procured. But commonly the hea' is pushed too high, whence more or less of the acid is decomposed, and its proportion of water uniting to the remainder, reduces its strength. It is not profitable to use a smaller proportion of sulphuric acid, when a concentrated nitric is required. But when only a dilute acid, called in commerce *aquafortis,* is required, then less sulphuric acid will suffice, provided a portion of water be added. One hundred parts of good nitre, sixty of strong sulphuric acid, and twenty of water, form economical proportions.

In the large way, and for the purposes of the arts, extremely thick cast iron or earthen retorts are employed, to which an earthen head is adapted, and connected with a range of proper condensers. The strength of the acid too is varied, by putting more or less water in the receivers. The nitric acid thus made generally contains sulphuric acid, and also muriatic, from the impurity of the nitrate employed. If the former, a solution of nitrate of barytes will occasion a white precipitate; if the latter, nitrate of silver will render it milky. The sulphuric acid may be separated by a second distillation from very pure nitre, equal in weight to an eighth of that originally employed; or by precipitating with nitrate of barytes, decanting the clear liquid, and distilling it. The muriatic acid may be separated by proceeding in the same way with nitrate of silver, or with litharge, decanting the clear liquid, and redistilling it, leaving an eighth or tenth part in the retort. The acid for the last process should be condensed as much as possible, and the redistillation conducted very slowly; and if it be stopped when half is come over, beautiful crystals of muriate of lead will be obtained on cooling the remainder, if litharge be used, as Steinacher informs us; who also adds, that the vessel should be made to fit tight by grinding, as any lute is liable to contaminate the product.

As this acid still holds in solution more or less nitrous gas, it is not in fact nitric acid, but a kind of nitrous. It is, therefore, necessary to put it into a retort, to which a receiver is added, the two vessels not being luted, and to apply a very gentle heat for several hours, changing the receiver as soon as it is filled with red vapours. The nitrous gas will thus be expelled, and the nitric acid will remain in the retort as limpid and colourless as water. It should be kept in a bottle and secluded from the light, otherwise it will lose part of its oxygen.

What remains in the retort is a bisulphate of potassa, from which the superfluous acid may be expelled by a pretty strong heat, and the residuum, being dissolved and crystallized, will be sulphate of potassa.

As nitric acid in a fluid state is always mixed with water, different attempts have been made to ascertain its strength, or the quantity of real acid contained in it.

The nitric acid is of considerable use in the arts. It is employed for etching on copper; as a solvent of tin to form with that metal a mordant for some of the finest dyes; in metallurgy and assaying; in various chemical processes, on account of the facility with which it parts with oxygen, and dissolves metals; in medicine as a tonic, and as a substitute for mercurial preparations in syphilis and affections of the liver, as also in form of vapour to destroy contagion. For the purposes of the arts it is commonly used in a diluted state, and contaminated with the sulphuric and muriatic acids, by the name of *aquafortis.* This is generally prepared by mixing common nitre with an equal weight of sulphate of iron, and half its weight of the same sulphate calcined, and distilling the mixture; or by mixing nitre with twice its weight of dry powdered clay, and distilling in a reverberatory furnace. Two kinds are found in the shops, one called *double aqua-fortis*, which is about half the strength of nitric acid ; the other simply *aquafortis*, which is half the strength of the double.

A compound made by mixing two parts of the nitric acid with one of muriatic, known formerly by the name of *aqua regia*, and now by that of *nitro-muriatic acid*, has the property of dissolving gold and platina. On mixing the two acids, heat is given out, an effervescence takes place, and the mixture acquires an orange colour. This is likewise made by adding gradually to an ounce of powdered muriate of ammonia four ounces of double aquafortis, and keeping the mixture in a sand heat till the salt is dissolved ; taking care to avoid the fumes, as the vessel must be left open ; or by distilling nitric acid with an equal weight, or rather more, of common salt.

On this subject we are indebted to Sir H. Davy for some excellent observations, published by him in the first volume of the Journal of Science. If strong *nitrous* acid, saturated with nitrous gas, be mixed with a saturated solution of muriatic acid gas, no other effect is produced than might be expected from the action of nitrous acid of the same strength on an equal quantity of water ; and the mixed acid so formed has no power of action on gold or platina. Again, if muriatic acid gas, and nitrous gas, in equal volumes, be mixed together over mercury, and half a volume of oxygen be added, the immediate condensation will be no more than might be expected from the formation of nitrous acid gas. And when this is decomposed, or absorbed by the mercury, the muriatic acid gas is found unaltered, mixed with a certain portion of nitrous gas.

It appears then that *nitrous* acid, and muriatic acid gas, have no chemical action on each other. If *colourless nitric* acid and muriatic acid of commerce be mixed together, the mixture immediately becomes yellow, and gains the power of dissolving gold and platinum. If it be gently heated, pure chlorine arises from it, and the colour becomes deeper. If the heat be longer continued, chlorine still rises, but mixed with nitrous acid gas. When the process has been very long continued till the colour becomes very deep, no more chlorine can be procured, and it loses its power of acting upon platinum and gold. It is now *nitrous* and muriatic acids. It appears then from these observations, which have been very often repeated, that nitromuriatic acid owes its peculiar properties to a mutual decomposition of the nitric and muriatic acids ; and that water, chlorine, and nitrous acid gas, are the results. Though nitrous gas and chlorine have no action on each other when perfectly dry, yet if water be present, there is an immediate decomposition, and nitrous acid and muriatic acid are formed. 118 parts of strong liquid nitric acid being decomposed in this case, yield 67 of chlorine. *Aqua regia* does not oxidise gold and platina. It merely causes their combination with chlorine.

A bath made of nitro-muriatic acid, diluted so much as to taste no sourer than vinegar, or of such a strength as to prick the skin a little, after being exposed to it for twenty minutes or half an hour, has been introduced by Dr. Scott of Bombay as a remedy in chronic syphilis, a variety of ulcers and diseases of the skin, chronic hepatitis, bilious dispositions, general debility, and languor. He considers every trial as quite inconclusive where a ptyalism, some affection of the gums, or some very evident constitutional effect, has not arisen from it. The internal use of the same acid has been recommended to be conjoined with that of the partial or general bath.

With the different bases the nitric acid forms *nitrates*.

The *nitrate of barytes*, when perfectly pure, is in regular octahedral crystals, though it is sometimes obtained in small shining scales.

The *nitrate of potassa* is the salt well known by the name of *nitre* or *saltpetre*. It is found ready formed in the East Indies, in Spain, in the kingdom of Naples, and elsewhere, in considerable quantities ; but nitrate of lime is still more abundant. Far the greater part of the nitrate made use of is produced by a combination of circumstances which tend to compose and condense nitric acid. This acid appears to be produced in all situations where animal matters are completely decomposed with access of air, and of proper substances with which it can readily combine. Grounds fre-

quently trodden by cattle, and impregnated with their excrements, or the walls of inhabited places, where putrid animal vapours abound, such as slaughter-houses, drains, or the like, afford nitre by long exposure to the air. Artificial nitre beds are made by an attention to the circumstances in which this salt is produced by nature. Dry ditches are dug, and covered with sheds, open at the side, to keep off the rain. These are filled with animal substances, such as dung, or other excrements, with the remains of vegetables, and old mortar, or other loose calcareous earth ; this substance being found to be the best and most convenient receptacle for the acid to combine with. Occasional watering, and turning up from time to time, are necessary to accelerate the process, and increase the surfaces to which the air may apply ; but too much moisture is hurtful. When a certain portion of nitrate is formed, the process appears to go on more quickly ; but a certain quantity stops it altogether ; and after this cessation, the materials will go on to furnish more, if what is formed be extracted by lixiviation. After a succession of many months, more or less, according to the management of the operation, in which the action of a regular current of fresh air is of the greatest importance, nitre is found in the mass. If the beds contained much vegetable matter, a considerable portion of the nitrous salt will be common saltpetre; but if otherwise, the acid will, for the most part, be combined with the calcareous earth. It consists of 6.75 acid + 6 potassa.

To extract the saltpetre from the mass of earthy matter, a number of large casks are prepared, with a cock at the bottom of each, and a quantity of straw within, to prevent its being stopped up. Into these the matter is put, together with wood-ashes, either strewed at top, or added during the filling. Boiling water is then poured on, and suffered to stand for some time ; after which it is drawn off, and another water added in the same manner, as long as any saline matter can be thus extracted. The weak brine is heated, and passed through other tubs, until it becomes of considerable strength. It is then carried to the boiler, and contains nitre and other salts; the chief of which is common culinary salt, and sometimes muriate of magnesia. It is the property of nitre to be much more soluble in hot than cold water ; but common salt is very nearly as soluble in cold as in hot water. Whenever, therefore, the evaporation is carried by boiling to a certain point, much of the common salt will fall to the bottom, for want of water to hold it in solution, though the nitre will remain suspended by virtue of the heat. The common salt thus separated is taken out with a perforated ladle, and a small quantity of the fluid is cooled, from time to time, that its concentration may be known by the nitre which crystallizes in it. When the fluid is sufficiently evaporated, it is taken out and cooled, and a great part of the nitre separates in crystals ; while the remaining common salt continues dissolved, because equally soluble in cold and in hot water. Subsequent evaporation of the residue will separate more nitre in the same manner. By the suggestion of Lavoisier, a much simpler plan was adopted ; reducing the crude nitre to powder, and washing it twice with water.

This nitre, which is called nitre of the first boiling, contains some common salt, from which it may be purified by solution in a small quantity of water, and subsequent evaporation ; for the crystals thus obtained are much less contaminated with common salt than before ; because the proportion of water is so much larger, with respect to the small quantity contained by the nitre, that very little of it will crystallize. For nice purposes, the solution and crystallization of nitre are repeated four times. The crystals of nitre are usually of the form of six-sided flattened prisms, with dihedral summits. Its taste is penetrating ; but the cold produced by placing the salt to dissolve in the mouth, is such as to predominate over the real taste at first. Seven parts of water dissolve two of nitre, at the temperature of sixty degrees; but boiling water dissolves its own weight. 100 parts of alkohol, at a heat of 176°, dissolve only 2.9.

On being exposed to a gentle heat, nitre fuses ; and in this state, being poured into moulds, so as to form little round cakes, or balls, it is called *sal prunella*, or *crystal mineral*. This at least is the way in which this salt is now usually prepared, conformably to the directions of Boerhaave, though in most dispensatories a twenty-fourth part of sulphur was directed to be de-flagrated on the nitre before it was poured out. This salt should not be left on the fire after it has entered into fusion, otherwise it will be converted into a *ni-trate* of potassa. If the heat be increased to redness, the acid itself is decomposed, and a considerable quantity of tolerably pure oxygen gas is evolved, succeeded by nitrogen.

This salt powerfully promotes the combustion of inflammable substances. Two or three parts mixed with one of charcoal, and set on fire, burn rapidly; azote and carbonic acid gas are given out, and a small portion of the latter is retained by the alkaline residuum, which was formerly called *clyssus of nitre*. Three parts of nitre, two of subcarbonate of potassa, and one of sulphur, mixed together in a warm mortar, form the *fulminating powder*; a small quantity of which, laid on a fire shovel, and held over the fire till it begins to melt, explodes with a loud sharp noise. Mixed with sulphur and charcoal, it forms *gunpowder*.

Three parts of nitre, one of sulphur, and one of fine saw-dust, well mixed, constitute what is called the powder of fusion. If a bit of base copper be folded up and covered with this powder in a walnut-shell, and the powder be set on fire with a lighted paper, it will detonate rapidly, and fuse the metal into a globule of sulphuret without burning the shell.

Silex, alumina, and barytes, decompose this salt in a high temperature, by uniting with its base. The alumina will effect this even after it has been made into pottery.

The uses of nitre are various. Beside those already indicated, it enters into the composition of fluxes, and is extensively employed in metallurgy; it serves to promote the combustion of sulphur in fabricating its acid; it is used in the art of dying; it is added to common salt for preserving meat, to which it gives a red hue; it is an ingredient in some frigorific mixtures; and it is prescribed in medicine, as cooling, febrifuge, and diuretic; and some have recommended it mixed with vinegar as a very powerful remedy for the sea scurvy.

Nitrate of soda, formerly called *cubic* or *quadrangular nitre,* approaches in its properties to the nitrate of potassa; but differs from it in being somewhat more soluble in cold water, though less in hot, which takes up little more than its own weight; in being inclined to attract moisture from the atmosphere; and in crystallizing in rhombs, or rhomboidal prisms. It may be prepared by saturating soda with the nitric acid; by precipitating nitric solutions of the metals, or of the earths, except barytes, by soda; by lixiviating and crystallizing the residuum of common salt distilled with three-fourths its weight of nitric acid; or by saturating the mother waters of nitre with soda instead of potassa.

Nitrate of strontian may be obtained in the same manner as that of barytes, with which it agrees in the shape of its crystals, and most of its properties.

Nitrate of lime, the *calcareous nitre* of older writers, abounds in the mortar of old buildings, particularly those that have been much exposed to animal effluvia, or processes in which azote is set free. Hence it abounds in nitre beds, as was observed when treating of the nitrate of potassa. It may also be prepared artificially by pouring dilute nitric acid on carbonate of lime.

The *nitrate of ammonia* possesses the property of exploding, and being totally decomposed, at the temperature of 600°; whence it acquired the name of *nitrum flammans*. The readiest mode of preparing it is by adding carbonate of ammonia to dilute nitric acid till saturation takes place. If this solution be evaporated in a heat between 70° and 100°, and the evaporation not carried too far, it crystallizes in hexahedral prisms, terminating in very acute pyramids. If the heat rise to 212°, it will afford, on cooling, long fibrous silky crystals: if the evaporation be carried so far as for the salt to concrete immediately on a glass rod by cooling, it will form a compact mass. According to Sir H. Davy, these differ but little from each other, except in the water they contain.

When dried as much as possible without decomposition, it consists of 6.75 acid + 2.125 ammonia + 1.125 water.

The chief use of this salt is for affording nitrous oxide on being decomposed by heat.

Nitrate of magnesia, magnesian nitre, crystallizes

in four-sided rhomboidal prisms, with oblique or truncated summits, and sometimes in bundles of small needles. Its taste is bitter, and very similar to that of nitrate of lime, but less pungent. It is fusible, and decomposable by heat, giving out first a little oxygen gas, then nitrous oxide, and lastly nitric acid. It deliquesces slowly. It is soluble in an equal weight of cold water, and in but little more hot, so that it is scarcely crystallizable but by spontaneous evaporation.

The two preceding species are capable of combining into a triple salt, an ammoniaco-magnesian nitrate, either by uniting the two in solution, or by a partial decomposition of either by means of the base of the other. This is slightly inflammable when suddenly heated; and by a lower heat is decomposed, giving out oxygen, azote, more water than it contained, nitrous oxide, and nitric acid. The residuum is pure magnesia.

From the activity of the nitric acid as a solvent of earths in analyzation, the *nitrate of glucine* is better known than any other of the salts of this new earth. Its form is either pulverulent, or a tenacious or ductile mass. Its taste is at first saccharine, and afterward astringent. It grows soft by exposure to heat, soon melts, its acid is decomposed into oxygen and azote, and its base alone is left behind. It is very soluble and very deliquescent.

Nitrate, or rather *supernitrate of alumina,* crystallizes, though with difficulty, in thin, soft, pliable flakes. It is of an austere and acid taste, and reddens blue vegetable colours. It may be formed by dissolving in diluted nitric acid, with the assistance of heat, fresh precipitated alumina, well washed but not dried. It is deliquescent, and soluble in a very small portion of water. Alkohol dissolves its own weight. It is easily decomposed by heat.

Nitrate of zircone crystallizes in small, capillary, silky needles. Its taste is astringent. It is easily decomposed by fire, very soluble in water, and deliquescent. It may be prepared by dissolving zircone in strong nitric acid; but, like the preceding species, the acid is always in excess.

Nitrate of yttria may be prepared in a similar manner. Its taste is sweetish and astringent. It is scarcely to be obtained in crystals; and if it be evaporated by too strong a heat, the salt becomes soft like honey, and on cooling, concretes into a stony mass." *Ure's Chem. Dict.*

NITRIC ACID OXYGENIZED. The apparent oxygenation of nitric acid by Thenard, ought to be regarded merely as the conversion of a portion of its combined water into deutoxide of hydrogen.

Nitric oxide. See *Nitrogen, deutoxide of.*

Nitric oxide of Mercury. See *Hydrargyri nitrico-oxidum.*

NITRICO-OXIDUM HYDRARGYRI. See *Hydrargyri nitrico-oxydum.*

NITROGEN. (From νιτρον, nitre, and γεννάω, to generate: so called because it is the generator of nitre.) Azot; Azote. "An important elementary or undecomposed principle. As it constitutes four-fifths of the volume of atmospheric air, the readiest mode of procuring azote is to abstract its oxygenous associate, by the combustion of phosphorus or hydrogen. It may also be obtained from animal matters, subjected in a glass retort to the action of nitric acid, diluted with 8 or 10 times its weight of water.

Azote possesses all the physical properties of air. It extinguishes flame and animal life. It is absorbable by about 100 volumes of water. Its spec. gravity is 0.9722. 100 cubic inches weigh 29.65 grains. It has neither taste nor smell. It unites with oxygen in four proportions, forming four important compounds. These are,

I. *Protoxide of azote,* called also nitrous oxide, protoxide of nitrogen, and gaseous oxide of azote.

This combination of nitrogen and oxygen was formerly called the dephlogisticated nitrous gas, but now gaseous oxide of nitrogen or nitrous oxide. It was first discovered by Priestley. Its nature and properties have since been investigated (though not very accurately) by a society of Dutch chemists.

Sir Humphrey Davy has examined with uncommon accuracy the formation and properties of all the substances concerned in its production. He has detected the sources of error in the experiments of Priestley, and the Dutch chemists, and to him we are indebted for a thorough knowledge of this gas. We shall, therefore, exhibit the philosophy of this gaseous fluid, as we find it in his researches concerning the nitrous oxide.

Properties. It exists in the form of a permanent gas. A candle burns with a brilliant flame and crackling noise in it; before its extinction the white inner flame becomes surrounded with a blue one. Phosphorus introduced into it, in a state of *actual* inflammation, burns with increased splendour, as in oxygen gas. Sulphur introduced into it when burning with a feeble blue flame is instantly extinguished; but when in a state of *vivid inflammation*, it burns with a rose-coloured flame. Ignited charcoal burns in it more brilliantly than in atmospheric air. Iron wire, with a small piece of wood affixed to it, when inflamed, and introduced into a vessel filled with this gas, burns vehemently, and throws out bright scintillating sparks. No combustible body, however, burns in it, unless it be previously brought to a state of vivid inflammation. Hence sulphur may be melted, and even sublimed in it, phosphorus may be liquefied in it without undergoing combustion. Nitrous oxide is pretty rapidly absorbed by water that has been boiled; a quantity of gas equal to rather more than half the bulk of the water may be thus made to disappear, the water acquires a sweetish taste, but its other properties do not differ perceptibly from common water. The whole of the gas may be expelled again by heat. It does not change blue vegetable colours. It has a distinctly sweet taste, and a faint but agreeable odour. It undergoes no diminution when mingled with oxygen or nitrous gas. Most of the liquid inflammable bodies, such as æther, alkohol, volatile and fat oils, absorb it rapidly and in great quantity. Acids exert but little action on it. The affinity of the neutro-saline solutions for gaseous oxide of nitrogen is very feeble. Green muriate and green sulphate of iron, whether holding nitrous gas in solution, or not, do not act upon it. None of the gases, when mingled with it, suffer any perceptible change at common temperatures; the muriatic and sulphurous acid gases excepted, which undergo a slight expansion. Alkalies freed from carbonic acid, exposed in the dry or solid form, have no action upon it; they may, however, be made to combine with it in the nascent state, and then constitute *saline compounds* of a peculiar nature. These combinations deflagrate when heated with charcoal, and are decomposed by acids; the gaseous oxide of nitrogen being disengaged. It undergoes no change whatever from the simple effect of light. The action of the electric spark, for a long while continued, converts it into a gas, analogous to atmospheric air and nitrous acid; the same is the case when it is made to pass through an ignited earthen tube. It explodes with hydrogen in a variety of proportions, at very high temperatures; for instance, when electric sparks are made to pass through the mixture. Sulphuretted, heavy, and light carburetted hydrogen gases, and gaseous oxide of carbon, likewise burn with it when a strong red heat is applied. 100 parts by weight of nitrous oxide, contain 36.7 of oxygen and 63.3 of nitrogen; 100 cubic inches weigh 50 grains at 55° temperature and 30 inches atmospheric pressure. Animals, when wholly confined in gaseous oxide of nitrogen, give no signs of uneasiness for some moments, but they soon become restless and then die. When gaseous oxide of nitrogen is mingled with atmospheric air, and then received into the lungs, it generates highly pleasurable sensations; the effects it produces on the animal system are eminently distinguished from every other chemical agent. It excites every fibre to action, and rouses the faculties of the mind, inducing a state of great exhilaration, an irresistible propensity to laughter, a rapid flow of vivid ideas, and unusual vigour and fitness for muscular exertions, in some respects resembling those attendant on the pleasantest period of intoxication, without any subsequent languor, depression of the nervous energy, or disagreeable feelings; but more generally followed by vigour, and a pleasurable disposition to exertion, which gradually subsides.

Sir H. Davy first showed, that by breathing a few quarts of it, contained in a silk bag, for two or three minutes, effects analogous to those occasioned by drinking fermented liquors were produced. Individuals, who differ in temperament, are, however, as we might expect, differently affected.

Sir H. Davy describes the effect it had upon him as follows:—'Having previously closed my nostrils, and exhausted my lungs, I breathed four quarts of nitrous

oxide from and into a silk bag. The first feelings were similar to those produced in the last experiment (giddiness); but in less than half a minute, the respiration being continued, they diminished gradually, and were succeeded by a sensation analogous to gentle pressure on all the muscles, attended by a highly pleasurable thrilling, particularly in the chest and the extremities. The objects around me became dazzling, and my hearing more acute. Towards the last inspiration the thrilling increased, the sense of muscular power became greater, and at last an irresistible propensity to action was indulged in. I recollect but indistinctly what followed: I know that my motions were various and violent.

'These effects very soon ceased after respiration. In ten minutes I had recovered my natural state of mind. The thrilling in the extremities continued longer than the other sensations.

'The gas has been breathed by a very great number of persons, and almost every one has observed the same things. On some few, indeed, it has no effect whatever, and on others the effects are always painful.

'Mr. J. W. Tobin, (after the first imperfect trials,) when the air was pure, experienced sometimes sublime emotions with tranquil gestures, sometimes violent muscular action, with sensations indescribably exquisite; no subsequent debility—no exhaustion—his trials have been very numerous. Of late he has only felt sedate pleasure. In Sir H. Davy the effect is not diminished.

'Mr. James Thomson. Involuntary laughter, thrilling in his toes and fingers, exquisite sensations of pleasure. A pain in the back and knees, occasioned by fatigue the day before, recurred a few minutes afterward. A similar observation, we think, we have made on others; and we impute it to the undoubted power of the gas to increase the sensibility of nervous power, beyond any other agent, and probably in a peculiar manner.

'Mr. Thomas Pople. At first unpleasant feelings of tension; afterward agreeable luxurious languor, with suspension of muscular power; lastly, powers increased both of body and mind.

'Mr. Stephen Hammick, surgeon of the Royal Hospital, Plymouth. In a small dose, yawning and languor. It should be observed that the first sensation has often been disagreeable, as giddiness; and a few persons, previously apprehensive, have left off inhaling as soon as they felt this. Two larger doses produced a glow, unrestrainable tendency to muscular action, high spirits, and more vivid ideas. A bag of common air was first given to Mr. Hammick, and he observed that it produced no effect. The same precaution against the delusions of imagination was of course frequently taken.

Mr. Robert Southey could not distinguish between the first effects and an apprehension of which he was unable to divest himself. His first definite sensations were, a fulness and dizziness in the head, such as to induce a fear of falling. This was succeeded by a laugh which was involuntary, but highly pleasurable, accompanied with a peculiar thrilling in the extremities; a sensation perfectly new and delightful. For many hours after this experiment, he imagined that his taste and smell were more acute, and is certain that he felt unusually strong and cheerful. In a second experiment, he felt pleasure still superior, and has once poetically remarked, that he supposes the atmosphere of the highest of all possible heavens to be composed of this gas.

'Robert Kinglake, M.D. Additional freedom and power of respiration, succeeded by an almost delirious, but highly pleasurable sensation in the head, which became universal with increased tone of the muscles. At last, an intoxicating placidity absorbed for five minutes all voluntary power, and left a cheerfulness and alacrity for several hours. A second stronger dose produced a perfect trance for about a minute; then a glow pervaded the system. The permanent effects were an invigorated feeling of vital power, and improved spirits. By both trials, particularly by the former, old rheumatic feelings seemed to be revived for the moment.

'Mr. Wedgewood breathed atmospheric air first, without knowing it was so. He declared it to have no effect, which confirmed him in his disbelief of the power of the gas. After breathing this some time however, he threw the bag from him, kept breathing on laboriously with an open mouth, holding his nose with his left hand, without power to take it away, though aware of the ludicrousness of his situation: all his muscles seemed to be thrown into vibrating motions; he had a violent inclination to make antic gestures, seemed lighter than the atmosphere, and as if about to mount. Before the experiment, he was a good deal fatigued after a long ride, of which he permanently lost all sense. In a second experiment, nearly the same effect, but with less pleasure. In a third, much greater pleasure.

Such are the properties that characterize the nitrous oxide.

The Dutch chemists and some French and German philosophers assert that it cannot be respired; that burning phosphorus, sulphur, and charcoal, are extinguished in it, &c. It is probable they did not examine it in a state of purity, for it is otherwise difficult to account for these and many other erroneous opinions.

Method of obtaining the protoxide of nitrogen.—Gaseous oxide of nitrogen is produced, when substances, having a strong affinity with oxygen, are brought into contact with nitric acid, or with nitrous gas. It may therefore be obtained by various processes, in which nitrous gas or nitric acid is decomposed by substances capable of attracting the greater part of their oxygen. The most commodious and expeditious, as well as the cheapest mode of obtaining it, is by decomposing nitrate of ammonia *at a certain temperature*, in the following manner:—

1. Introduce into a glass retort some pure nitrate of ammonia, and apply the heat of an Argand's lamp; the salt will soon liquefy, and, when it begins to boil, gas will be evolved. Increase the heat gradually till the body and neck of the retort become filled with a semi-transparent milky white vapour. In this state the temperature of the fused nitrate is between 340°

and 480°. After the decomposition has proceeded for a few minutes, so that the gas evolved quickly enlarges the flame of a taper held near the orifice of the retort, it may be collected over water, care being taken during the whole process, never to suffer the temperature of the fused nitrate to rise above 500° Fahr. which may easily be judged of, from the density of the vapours in the retort, and from the quiet ebullition of the fused nitrate; for, if the heat be increased beyond this point, the vapours in the retort acquire a reddish and more transparent appearance; and the fused nitrate begins to rise, and occupy twice the bulk it did before. The nitrous oxide after its generation, is allowed to stand over water, for at least six hours, and is then fit for respiration or other experiments.

Explanation.—Nitrate of ammonia consists of nitric acid and ammonia; nitric acid is composed of nitrous gas and oxygen: and ammonia consists of hydrogen and nitrogen: At a temperature of about 480° the attractions of hydrogen for nitrogen in ammonia, and that of nitrous gas for oxygen in nitric acid, are *diminished*: while, on the contrary, the attractions of the hydrogen of ammonia for the oxygen of the nitric acid, and that of the nitrogen of the ammonia for the nitrous gas of the nitric acid, are *increased*; hence, all the former affinities are broken, and new ones produced, namely, the hydrogen of the ammonia attracts the oxygen of the nitric acid, the result of which is *water*; the nitrogen of the ammonia combines with the liberated nitrous gas, and forms *nitrous oxide*. The water and nitrous oxide produced, probably exist in binary combination in the aëriform state, at the temperature of the decomposition.

Such is the philosophy of the production of protoxide of nitrogen, by decomposing nitrate of ammonia at that temperature, given by Davy.

To illustrate this complicated play of affinity more fully, the following sketch may not be deemed superfluous.

A Diagram exhibiting the production of Gaseous Oxide of Nitrogen, by decomposing Nitrate of Ammonia, at 480° Fahr.

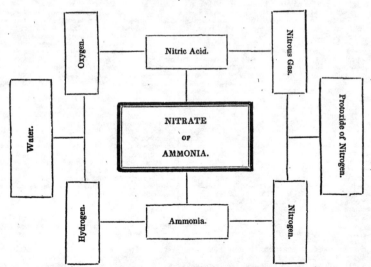

Sir Humphrey Davy has likewise pointed out, that, when the heat employed for decomposing nitrate of ammonia is raised above the before-stated temperature, another play of affinities takes place, the attractions of nitrogen and hydrogen for each other and of oxygen for nitrous gas are still more diminished, while that of nitrogen for nitrous gas is totally destroyed, and that of hydrogen for oxygen increased to a greater extent. A new attraction likewise takes place, namely, that of nitrous gas for nitric acid to form *nitrous acid vapour*,

and a new arrangement of principles is rapidly produced: the nitrogen of the ammonia having no affinity for any of the single principles at this temperature, enters into no binary compound; the oxygen of the nitric acid forms water with the hydrogen, and the nitrous gas combines with the nitric acid to form *nitrous acid vapour.*

All these substances most probably exist in combination, at the temperature of their production: and at a lower temperature assume the form of *nitrous acid nitrous gas, nitrogen,* and *water;* and hence we see the necessity of not heating the nitrate of ammonia above the before-stated temperature.

On account of the rapid absorption of gaseous oxide of nitrogen by water, it is economical to preserve the fluid which has been used to confine this gas, and to make use of it for collecting other quantities of it. In order to hasten its production, the nitrate of ammonia may be previously freed from its water of crystallization by gently fusing it in a glass of Wedgwood's bason for a few minutes, and then keeping it for use in a well-stopped bottle.

2. Nitrous oxide may likewise be obtained by exposing common nitrous gas to alkaline sulphites, particularly to sulphite of potassa containing its full quantity of water of crystallization. The nitrous oxide produced from nitrous gas by sulphite of potassa has all the properties of that generated from the decomposition of nitrate of ammonia.

The conversion of nitrous gas into nitrous oxide, by these bodies, depends on the abstraction of a portion of its oxygen by the greater affinity of the sulphite presented to it. The nitrogen and remaining oxygen assume a more condensed state of existence, and constitute nitrous oxide.

3. Nitrous oxide may also be obtained by mingling together nitrous gas and sulphuretted hydrogen gas. The volume of gases in this case is diminished, sulphur deposited, ammonia, water, and nitrous oxide are formed.

The change of principles which take place in this experiment, depends upon the combination of the hydrogen of the sulphuretted hydrogen gas, with different portions of the oxygen and nitrogen of the nitrous gas, to form water and ammonia, while it deposites sulphur. The remaining oxygen and nitrogen being left in due proportion constitute nitrous oxide.

Remark.—This singular exertion of attraction by a simple body appears highly improbable *a priori;* but the formation of ammonia, and the non-oxygenation of the sulphur, elucidate the fact. In performing this experiment, care should be taken that the gases should be rendered as dry as possible; for the presence of water considerably retards the decomposition.

4. Nitrous oxide may also be produced by preventing alkaline sulphurets to nitrous gas. Davy observed that a solution of sulphuret of strontian, or barytes, answers this purpose best.

This decomposition of nitrous gas is not solely produced by the abstraction of oxygen from the nitrous gas, to form sulphuric acid. It depends equally on the decomposition of the sulphuretted hydrogen dissolved in the solution or liberated from it. In this process, sulphur is deposited and sulphuric acid formed.

5. Nitrous oxide is obtained in many circumstances similar to those in which nitrous gas is produced. Dr. Priestley found that nitrous oxide was evolved, together with nitrous gas, during the solution of iron, tin, and zinc in nitric acid.

It is difficult to ascertain the exact rationale of these processes, for very complicated agencies of affinities take place. Either the nascent hydrogen arising from the decomposition of the water by the metallic substance may combine with portions of the oxygen and nitrogen of the nitrous gas; and thus by forming water and ammonia, convert it into nitrous oxide; or the metallic substance may attract at the same time oxygen from the water and nitrous gas, while the nascent hydrogen of the water seizes upon a portion of the nitrogen of the nitrous gas, to form ammonia. The analogy between this process and the decomposition of nitrous gas by sulphuretted hydrogen, renders the first opinion most probable.

Such are the principal methods of obtaining nitrous oxide. There are no reasons, Davy thinks, for supposing that nitrous oxide is formed in any of the processes of nature, and the nice equilibrium of affinity by which it is constituted forbids us to hope for the power of composing it from its simple principles. We must be content to produce it artificially.

II. *Deutoxide of azote,* termed likewise nitrous gas, or nitric oxide.

The name of nitrous gas is given to an aëriform fluid, consisting of a certain quantity of nitrogen and oxygen, combined with caloric. It is an elastic, colourless fluid, having no sensible taste; it is neither acid nor alkaline; it is exceedingly hurtful to animals, pro-

ducing instant suffocation whenever they attempt to breathe it. The greater number of combustible bodies refuse to burn in it. It is nevertheless capable of supporting the combustion of some of these bodies. Phosphorus burns in nitrous gas when introduced into it in a state of inflammation: pyrophorus takes fire in it spontaneously.

It is not decomposable by water, though 100 cubic inches of this fluid, when freed from air, absorb about five cubic inches of the gas. This solution is void of taste; it does not redden blue vegetable colours; the gas is expelled again when the water is made to boil or suffered to freeze. Nitrous gas has no action on nitrogen gas even when assisted by heat. It is decomposed by several metals at high temperatures.

Its specific gravity, when perfectly pure, is to that of atmospheric air as about 1.04 to 1.

Ardent spirits, saccharine matters, hydro-carbonates, sulphurous acid, and phosphorus, have no action on it at the common temperature. It is not sensibly changed by the action of light. Heat dilates it. It rapidly combines with oxygen gas at common temperatures, and converts it into nitrous acid. Atmospheric air produces the same effect, but with less intensity. It is absorbable with green sulphate, muriate and nitrate of iron, and decomposable by alkaline, terrene, and metallic sulphurets, and other bodies, that have a strong affinity for oxygen; but it is not capable of combining with them chemically, so as to form saline compounds From the greatest number of bodies which absorb it, it may be again expelled by the application of heat.

It communicates to flame a greenish colour before extinguishing it; when mixed with hydrogen gas this acquires the property of burning with a green flame. It is absorbable by nitric acid and renders it fuming.

When exposed to the action of caloric in an ignited porcelain tube, it experiences no alteration, but when electric sparks are made to pass through it, it is decomposed and converted into nitrous acid, and nitrogen gas. Phosphorus does not shine in it. It is composed of about eight parts of oxygen, and seven of nitrogen.

Methods of obtaining deutoxide of nitrogen.—1. Put into a small proof, or retort, some copper wire or pieces of the same metal, and pour on it nitric acid of commerce diluted with water, an effervescence takes place, and nitrous gas will be produced. After having suffered the first portions to escape on account of the atmospheric air contained in the retort, collect the gas in the water-apparatus as usual. In order to obtain the gas in a pure state, it must then be shook for some time in contact with water. The water in this instance suffers no alteration; on the contrary, the acid undergoes a partial decomposition; the metal robs some of the nitric acid of the greatest part of its oxygen, and becomes oxidised; the acid having lost so much of its oxygen, becomes thereby so altered, that at the usual temperature it can exist no longer in the liquid state, but instantly expands and assumes the form of gas; ceasing at the same time to act as an acid, and exhibiting different properties: but the acid remaining undecomposed combines with the oxide of copper, and forms nitrate of copper.

Instead of presenting copper to nitric acid, iron, zinc, mercury, or silver, may be made use of. The metals best suited for the production of nitrous gas are silver, mercury, and copper.

2. Deutoxide of nitrogen may likewise be obtained by synthesis. This method of obtaining it we owe to Dr. Milner of Cambridge.

Into the middle of an earthern tube about 20 inches long and three-fourths of an inch wide, open at both ends, put as much coarsely-powdered manganese as is sufficient nearly to fill it. Let this tube traverse a furnace having two openings opposite to each other. To one end of the tube lute a retort containing water strongly impregnated with ammonia, and to the other adapt a bent glass tube which passes into the pneumatic trough. Let a fire be kindled in the furnace, and when the manganese may be supposed to be red hot, apply a gentle heat to the retort, and drive over it the vapour of the ammonia; the consequence will be that nitrous gas will be delivered at the farther end of the tube, while the ammonia enters the other end; and this effect does not take place without the presence of the alkali.

Explanation.—Ammonia consists of hydrogen and nitrogen; its hydrogen combines with the oxygen which is given out by the ignited manganese, and forms water; its nitrogen unites at the same time to another portion of the oxygen, and constitutes the nitrous gas.

There is a cause of deception in this experiment, against which the operator ought to be on his guard, lest he should conclude no nitrous gas is formed, when, in reality, there is a considerable quantity. The ammonia, notwithstanding every precaution, will frequently pass over undecomposed. If the receiver in the pneumatic trough is filled with water, great part of this will indeed be presently absorbed; but still some portion of it will mix with the nitrous gas formed in the process. Upon admitting the atmospheric air, the nitrous gas will become decomposed, and the red nitrous fumes instantly unite with the alkali. The receiver is presently filled with white clouds of nitrate of ammonia; and in this manner a wrong conclusion may easily be drawn from the want of the orange colour of the nitrous fumes. A considerable quantity of nitrous gas may have been formed, and yet no orange colour appear, owing to this circumstance; and therefore it is easy to understand how a small quantity of nitrous gas may be most effectually disguised by the same cause.

Dr. Milner also obtained nitrous gas, by passing ammoniacal gas over sulphate of iron deprived of its water of crystallization.

III. Nitrous acid. See *Nitric acid.*
IV. Nitric acid. See *Nitrous acid.*

Azote combines with chlorine and iodine, to form two very formidable compounds:—

1. The *chloride of azote* was discovered about the beginning of 1812, by Dulong; but its nature was first investigated and ascertained by Sir H. Davy.

Put into an evaporating porcelain basin a solution of one part of nitrate or muriate of ammonia in 10 of water, heated to about 100°, and invert into it a wide-mouthed bottle, filled with chlorine. As the liquid ascends, by the condensation of the gas, oily-looking drops are seen floating on its surface, which collect together, and fall to the bottom in large globules. This is *chloride of azote.* By putting a thin stratum of common salt into the bottom of the basin, we prevent the decomposition of the chloride of azote, by the ammoniacal salt. It should be formed only in very small quantities. The *chloride of azote,* thus obtained, is an oily-looking liquid, of a yellow colour, and a very pungent intolerable odour, similar to that of chlorocarbonous acid. Its sp. gr. is 1.653. When tepid water is poured into a glass containing it, it expands into a volume of elastic fluid, of an orange colour, which diminishes as it passes through the water.

'I attempted,' says Sir H. Davy, 'to collect the products of the explosion of the new substance, by applying the heat of a spirit-lamp to a globule of it, confined in a curved glass tube over water; a little gas was at first extricated; but long before the water had attained the temperature of ebullition, a violent flash of light was perceived, with a sharp report; the tube and glass were broken into small fragments, and I received a severe wound in the transparent *cornea* of the eye, which has produced a considerable inflammation of the eye, and obliges me to make this communication by an amanuensis. This experiment proves what *extreme* caution is necessary in operating on this substance, for the quantity I used was scarcely as large as a grain of mustard-seed.'—It evaporates pretty rapidly in the air; and *in vacuo* it expands into a vapour, which still possesses the power of exploding by heat. When it is cooled artificially in water, or the ammoniacal solution, to 40° F., the surrounding fluid congeals; but when alone, it may be surrounded with a mixture of ice and muriate of lime, without freezing.

It gradually disappears in water, producing azote; while the water becomes acid, acquiring the taste and smell of a weak solution of nitro-muriatic acid.

With muriatic and nitric acids, it yields azote; and, with dilute sulphuric acid, a mixture of azote and oxygen. In strong solutions of ammonia it detonates; with weak ones, it affords azote.

When it was exposed to pure mercury, out of the contact of water, a white powder (calomel) and azote were the results. 'The action of mercury on the compound,' says Sir H. 'appeared to offer a more correct

and less dangerous mode of attempting its analysis; but on introducing two grains under a glass tube filled with mercury, and inverted, a violent detonation occurred, by which I was slightly wounded in the head and hands, and should have been severely wounded, had not my eyes and face been defended by a plate of glass, attached to a proper cap; a precaution very necessary in all investigations of this body.' In using smaller quantities, and recently distilled mercury, he obtained the results of the experiments, without any violence of action.

A small globule of it, thrown into a glass of olive oil, produced a most violent explosion; and the glass, though strong, was broken into fragments. Similar effects were produced by its action on oil of turpentine and naphtha. When it was thrown into ether or alkohol, there was a very slight action. When a particle of it was touched under water by a particle of phosphorus, a brilliant light was perceived under the water, and permanent gas was disengaged, having the characters of azote.

When quantities larger than a grain of mustard seed were used for the contact with phosphorus, the explosion was always so violent as to break the vessel in which the experiment was made. On tinfoil and zinc it exerted no action; nor on sulphur and resin. But it detonated most violently when thrown into a solution of phosphorus in ether or alkohol.

The mechanical force of this compound in detonation, seems superior to that of any other known, not even excepting the ammoniacal fulminating silver. The velocity of its action appears to be likewise greater.

2. *Iodide of azote.* Azote does not combine directly with iodine. We obtain the combination only by means of ammonia. It was discovered by Courtois, and carefully examined by Colin. When ammoniacal gas is passed over iodine, a viscid shining liquid is immediately formed, of a brownish-black colour, which, in proportion as it is saturated with ammonia, loses its lustre and viscosity. No gas is disengaged during the formation of this liquid, which may be called *iodide of ammonia.* It is not fulminating. When dissolved in water, a part of the ammonia is decomposed; its hydrogen forms hydriodic acid; and its azote combines with a portion of the iodine, and forms the fulminating powder. We may obtain the iodide of azote directly, by putting pulverulent iodine into common water of ammonia. This indeed is the best way of preparing it; for the water is not decomposed, and seems to concur in the production of this iodide, only by determining the formation of hydriodate of ammonia.

The iodide of azote is pulverulent, and of a brownish-black colour. It detonates from the smallest shock, and from heat, with a feeble violet vapour. When properly prepared, it often detonates spontaneously. Hence, after the black powder is formed, and the liquid ammonia decanted off, we must leave the capsule containing it in perfect repose.

When this iodide is put into potassa water, azote is disengaged, and the same products are obtained as when iodine is dissolved in that alkaline lixivium. The hydriodate of ammonia, which has the property of dissolving a great deal of iodine, gradually decomposes the fulminating powder, while azote is set at liberty. Water itself has this property, though in a much lower degree. As the elements of iodide of azote are so feebly united, it ought to be prepared with great precautions, and should not be preserved. In the act of transferring a little of it from a platina capsule to a piece of paper, the whole exploded in my hands, though the friction of the particles on each other was inappreciably small.

The strongest arguments for the compound nature of azote are derived from its slight tendency to combination, and from its being found abundantly in the organs of animals which feed on substances that do not contain it.

Its uses in the economy of the globe are little understood. This is likewise favourable to the idea that the real chemical nature is as yet unknown, and leads to the hope of its being decomposable.

It would appear that the atmospheric azote and oxygen spontaneously combine in other proportions, under certain circumstances, in natural operations. Thus we find, that mild calcareous or alkaline matter favours the formation of nitric acid, in certain regions of the earth; and that they are essential to its production in our artificial arrangements, and forming nitre from decomposing animal and vegetable substances."

NITROGEN, PROTOXIDE OF. See *Nitrogen*.

NITROGEN, DEUTOXIDE OF. See *Nitrogen*.

NITROLEUCIC ACID. (*Acidum nitro-leucicum :* so called from its being obtained by the action of *nitric acid* on *leucine*.) *Leucine* is capable of uniting to nitric acid, and forming a compound, which Braconnot has called the nitro-leucic acid. When we dissolve leucine in nitric acid, and evaporate the solution to a certain point, it passes into a crystalline mass, without any disengagement of nitrous vapour, or of any gaseous matter; if we press this mass between blotting paper, and redissolve it in water, we shall obtain from this by concentration, fine, divergent, and nearly colourless needles. These constitute the new acid. It unites to the bases, forming salts which fuse on red-hot coals. The nitro-leucates of lime and magnesia are unalterable in the air.

NITRO-MURIATIC ACID. *Aqua regia*. When nitric and muriatic acids are mixed, they become yellow, and acquire the power of readily dissolving gold, which neither of the acids possessed separately. This mixture evolves chlorine, a partial decomposition of both acids having taken place; and water, chlorine, and nitrous acid gas are thus produced, that is, the hydrogen of the muriatic acid abstracts oxygen from the nitric to form water. The result must be chlorine and nitrous acid.—*Brande*.

NITRO-SACCHARIC ACID. *Acidum nitro-saccharicum*. Nitro-saccharine acid. When we heat the *sugar of gelatine* with nitric acid, they dissolve without any apparent disengagement of gas, and if we evaporate this solution to a proper degree, it forms, on cooling, a crystalline mass. On pressing this mass between the folds of blotting-paper, and recrystallizing them, we obtain beautiful prisms, colourless, transparent, and slightly striated. These crystals are very different from those which serve to produce them; and constitute, according to Braconnot, a true acid, which results from the combination of the nitric acid itself, with the sweet matter of which the first crystals are formed. Thenard conceives it is the *nitrous* acid which is present.

Nitro-saccharic acid has a taste similar to that of the tartaric; only it is a little sweetish. Exposed to the fire in a capsule, it froths much, and is decomposed with the diffusion of a pungent smell. Thrown on burning coals, it acts like saltpetre. It produces no change in saline solutions. Finally, it combines with the bases, and gives birth to salts which possess peculiar properties. For example, the salt which it forms with lime is not deliquescent, and is very little soluble in strong alkohol. That which it produces with the oxide of lead detonates to a certain degree by the action of heat.—*Ann. de Chimie et de Phys*. xiii 113.

NITRO-SULPHURIC ACID. A compound, consisting of one part nitre dissolved in about ten of sulphuric acid.

NITROUS. *Nitrosus*. Of or belonging to nitre.

NITROUS ACID. *Acidum nitrosum*. Fuming nitrous acid. It appears to form a distinct genus of salts, that may be termed *nitrites*. But these cannot be made by a direct union of their component parts, being obtainable only by exposing a nitrate to a high temperature, which expels a portion of its oxygen in the state of gas, and leaves the remainder in the state of a nitrate, if the heat be not urged so far, or continued so long, as to effect a complete decomposition of the salt. In this way the nitrates of potassa and soda may be obtained, and perhaps those of barytes, strontian, lime, and magnesia. The nitrites are particularly characterized, by being decomposable by all the acids except the carbonic, even by the nitric acid itself, all of which expel them from nitrous acid. We are little acquainted with any one except that of potassa, which attracts moisture from the air, changes blue vegetable colours to green, is somewhat acrid to the taste, and when powdered emits a smell of nitric oxide.

The acid itself is best obtained by exposing nitrate

of lead to heat in a glass retort. Pure *nitrous* acid comes over in the form of an orange-coloured liquid It is so volatile as to boil at the temperature of 82°. Its specific gravity is 1.450. When mixed with water it is decomposed, and nitrous gas is disengaged, occasioning effervescence. It is composed of one volume of oxygen united with two of nitrous gas. It therefore consists ultimately, by weight, of 1.75 nitrogen + 4 oxygen; by measure, of 2 oxygen + 1 nitrogen. The variously coloured acids of nitre are not *nitrous* acids, but nitric acid impregnated with nitrous gas, the deutoxide of nitrogen or azote.

Nitrous oxide. See *Nitrogen*.

NI'TRUM. This name was anciently given to na tron, but in modern times to nitre. See *Nitre*.

NITRUM PURIFICATUM. See *Nitre*.

NITRUM VITRIOLATUM. Sulphuric acid and soda. See *Sodæ sulphas*.

NO'BILIS. (*Quasi noscibilis ;* from *nosco*, to know.) Noble. Some parts of animals, and of plants, are so named by way of eminence ; as a valve of the heart, and the more perfect metals, as gold and silver.

NOCTAMBULATION. *Noctambulatio ;* from *nox*, night, and *ambulo*, to walk.) *Noctisurgium*. Walking in the night, when asleep. See *Oneirodynia activa*.

NOCTISU'RGIUM. See *Noctambulation*.

Nocturnal emission. See *Gonorrhœa dormientium*.

Nodding cnicus. See *Cnicus cernuus*.

NODE. *Nodus*. A hard circumscribed tumour, proceeding from a bone, and caused by a swelling of the periosteum ; they appear on every part of the body, but are more common on such as are thinly covered with muscles, as the os frontis, forepart of the tibia, radius, and ulna. As they increase in size, they become more painful from the distention they occasion in the periosteum. When they continue long, the bone becomes completely carious.

NODOSUS. Knotty: nodose. Applied to the form of the seed-vessel of the *Cucurbita melopepo*.

NODUS. (From *anad*, to tie, Hebrew.) A node or swelling upon a bone. See *Node*.

NO'LI ME TANGERE. A species of herpes affecting the skin and cartilages of the nose, very difficult to cure, because it is exasperated by most applications. The disease generally commences with small, superficial spreading ulcerations of the alæ of the nose, which become more or less concealed beneath fufuraceous scabs. The whole nose is frequently destroyed by the progressive ravages of this peculiar disorder, which sometimes cannot be stopped or retarded by any treatment, external or internal.

NO'MA. (From *νεμω*, to eat.) An ulcer that sometimes attacks the cheek or vulva of young girls. It appears in the form of red and somewhat livid spots , is not attended with pyrexia, pain, or tumour, and in a few days becomes gangrenous.

NON-NATURAL. *Res non-naturales*. Under this term, ancient physicians comprehend air, meat and drink, sleep and watching, motion and rest, the retentions and excretions, and the affections of the mind ; or, in other words, those principal matters which do not enter into the composition of the body, but at the same time are necessary to its existence.

NO'NUS. (*Quasi novenus ;* from *novem*, nine.) The ninth. Sometimes applied to the coracoid muscle of the shoulder.

NO'PAL. *Nopalnochetzth*. The plant that feeds the cochineal insect.

NORLA'NDICÆ BACCÆ. See *Rubus arcticus*. ₁

NOSE. *Nasus*. See *Nares*.

Nose, bleeding of. See *Epistaxis*.

NOSOCO'MIUM. (From *νοσος*, a disease, and *κομεω*, to take care of.) *Nosodochium*. An hospital or infirmary for the sick.

NOSODO'CHIUM. See *Nosocomium*.

NOSOLOGY. (*Nosologia ;* from *νοσος*, a disease, and *λογος*, a discourse.) The doctrine of the names of diseases. Modern physicians understand by nosology, the arrangement of diseases in classes, orders, genera, species, &c. The following are the approved arrangements of the several nosologists. That of Dr. Cullen is generally adopted in this country, and next to it the arrangement of Sauvages.

Synoptical View of the Classes, Orders, and Genera, according to the CULLENIAN System.

CLASS I.—PYREXIÆ.

ORDER I.
FEBRES.
§ 1. *Intermittentes.*
1. Tertiana
2. Quartana
3. Quotidiana.
§ 2. *Continuæ.*
4. Synocha
5. Typhus
6. Synochus.
ORDER II.
PHLEGMASIÆ.
7. Phlogosis
8. Ophthalmia
9. Phrenitis
10. Cynanche
11. Pneumonia
12. Carditis
13. Peritonitis
14. Gastritis
15. Enteritis
16. Hepatitis
17. Splenitis
18. Nephritis
19. Cystitis
20. Hysteritis
21. Rheumatismus
22. Odontalgia
23. Podagra
24. Arthropuosis.
ORDER III.
EXANTHEMATA.
25. Variola
26. Varicella
27. Rubeola
28. Scarlatina
29. Pestis
30. Erysipelas
31. Miliaria
32. Urticaria
33. Pemphigus
34. Aphtha.
ORDER IV.
HÆMORRHAGIÆ
35. Epistaxis
36. Hæmoptysis
37. Hæmorrhois
38. Menorrhagia.
ORDER V.
PROFLUVIA
39. Catarrhus
40. Dysenteria

CLASS II.—NEUROSES.

ORDER I.
COMATA.
41. Appoplexia
42. Paralysis.
ORDER II.
ADYNAMIÆ.
43. Syncope
44. Dyspepsia
45. Hypochondriasis
46. Chlorosis.
ORDER III.
SPASMI.
47. Tetanus
48. Convulsio
49. Chorea
50. Raphania
51. Epilepsia
52. Palpitatio
53. Asthma
54. Dyspnœa
55. Pertussis
56. Pyrosis
57. Colica
58. Cholera
59. Diarrhœa
60. Diabetes
61. Hysteria
62. Hydrophobia.
ORDER IV.
VESANIÆ.
63. Amentia
64. Melancholia
65. Mania
66. Oneirodynia.

CLASS III.—CACHEXIÆ.

ORDER I.
MARCORES.
67. Tabes
68. Atrophia.
ORDER II.
INTUMESCENTIÆ.
§ 1. *Adiposæ.*
69. Polysarcia
§ 2. *Flatuosæ.*
70. Pneumatosis
71. Tympanites
72. Physometra.
§ 3. *Aquosæ.*
73. Anasarca
74. Hydrocephalus
75. Hydrorachitis
76. Hydrothorax
77. Ascites
78. Hydrometra
79. Hydrocele.
§ 4. *Solidæ.*
80. Physconia
81. Rachitis.
ORDER III.
IMPETIGINES.
82. Scrofula
83. Syphilis
84. Scorbutus
85. Elephantiasis
86. Lepra
87. Frambœsia
88. Trichoma
89. Icterus.

CLASS IV.—LOCALES.

ORDER I.
DYSÆSTHESIÆ.
90. Caligo
91. Amaurosis
92. Dysopia
93. Pseudoblepsis
94. Dysecoea
95. Paracusis
96. Anosmia
97. Agheustia
98. Anæsthesia.
ORDER II.
DYSOREXIÆ.
§ 1. *Appetitus erronei.*
99. Bulimia
100. Polydipsia
101. Pica
102. Satyriasis
103. Nymphomania
104. Nostalgia.
§ 2. *Appetitus deficientes.*
105. Anorexia
106. Adipsia
107. Anaphrodisia.
ORDER III.
DYSCINESIÆ
108. Aphonia
109. Mutitas
110. Paraphonia
111. Psellismus
112. Strabismus
113. Dysphagia
114. Contractura.
ORDER IV.
APOCENOSES.
115. Profusio
116. Ephidrosis
117. Epiphora
118. Ptyalismus
119. Enuresis
120. Gonorrhœa.
ORDER V.
EPISCHESES.
121. Obstipatio
122. Ischuria
123. Dysuria
124. Dyspermatismus
125. Amenorrhœa.
ORDER VI.
TUMORES.
126. Aneurisma
127. Varix
128. Ecchymoma
129. Scirrhus
130. Cancer
131. Bubo
132. Sarcoma
133. Verruca
134. Clavus
135. Lupia
136. Ganglion
137. Hydatis
138. Hydarthrus
139. Exostosis.
ORDER VII.
ECTOPIÆ.
140. Hernia
141. Prolapsus
142. Luxatio.
ORDER VIII.
DYALYSES.
143. Vulnus
144. Ulcus
145. Herpes
146. Tinea
147. Psora
148. Fractura
149. Caries

Synoptical View of the System of SAUVAGES.

CLASS I.—VITIA.

ORDER I.
MACULÆ.
Genus 1. Leucoma
2. Vitiligo
3. Ephelis
4. Gutta rosea
5. Nævus
6. Ecchymoma.
ORDER II.
EFFLORESCENTIÆ.
7. Herpes
8. Epinyctis
9. Psydracia
10. Hydroa.
ORDER III.
HYMATA.
11. Erythema
12. Œdema
13. Emphysema
14. Scirrhus
15. Phlegmone
16. Bubo
17. Parotis
18. Furunculus
19. Anthrax
20. Cancer
21. Paronychia
22. Phimosis.
ORDER IV.
EXCRESCENTIÆ.
23. Sarcoma
24. Condyloma
25. Verruca
26. Pterygium
27. Hordeolum
28. Bronchocele
29. Exostosis
30. Gibbositas
31. Lordosis.
ORDER V.
CYSTIDES.
32. Aneurisma
33. Varix
34. Hydatis
35. Marisca
36. Staphyloma
37. Lupia
38. Hydarthrus
39. Apostema
40. Exomphalus
41. Oscheocele.
ORDER VI.
ECTOPIÆ.
42. Exophthalmia
43. Blepharoptosis
44. Hypostaphyle
45. Paraglossa
46. Proptoma
47. Exania
48. Exocyste
49. Hysteroptosis
50. Enterocele
51. Epiplocele
52. Gasterocele
53. Hepatocele
54. Splenocele
55. Hysterocele
56. Cystocele
57. Encephalocele
58. Hysteroloxia
59. Parochidium
60. Exarthrema
61. Diastasis
62. Laxarthrus.
ORDER VII.
PLAGÆ.
63. Vulnus
64. Punctura
65. Excoriatio
66. Contusio
67. Fractura
68. Fissura
69. Ruptura
70. Amputatura
71. Ulcus
72. Exulceratio
73. Sinus
74. Fistula
75. Rhagas
76. Eschara
77. Caries
78. Arthrocace.

NOSOLOGY.

CLASS II.—FEBRES

ORDER I.	82. Typhus	85. Tritæophya	88. Tertiana
CONTINUÆ.	83. Hectica.	86. Tetartophya.	89. Quartana
79. Ephemera	ORDER II.	ORDER III.	90. Erratica.
80. Synocha	REMITTENTES.	INTERMITTENTES.	
81. Synochus	84. Amphimerina	87. Quotidiana	

CLASS III.—PHLEGMASIÆ.

ORDER I.	97. Erysipelas	103. Pleuritis	109. Cephalitis
EXANTHEMATICÆ	98. Scarlatina	104. Gastritis	110. Cynanche
91. Pestis	99. Essera	105. Enteritis	111. Carditis
92. Variola	100. Aphtha.	106. Epiploitis	112. Peripneumonia.
93. Pemphigus	ORDER II.	107. Metritis.	113. Hepatitis
94. Rubeola	MEMBRANACEÆ.	ORDER III.	114. Splenitis
95. Miliaris	101. Phrenitis	PARENCHYMATOSÆ.	115. Nephritis.
96. Purpura	102. Paraphrenesis	108. Cystitis	

CLASS IV.—SPASMI.

ORDER I.	ORDER II.	126. Pandiculatio	ORDER IV.
TONICI PARTIALES.	TONICI GENERALES.	127. Apomyttosis	CLONICI GENERALES
116. Strabismus	122. Tetanus	128. Convulsio	132. Rigor
117. Trismus	123. Catochus.	129. Tremor	133. Eclampsia
118. Obstipitas	ORDER III.	130. Palpitatio	134. Epilepsia
119. Contractura	CLONICI PARTIALES.	131. Claudicatio.	135. Hysteria
120. Crampus	124. Nystagmus		136. Scelotyrbe
121. Priapismus.	125. Carphologia		137. Beriberia.

CLASS V.—ANHELATIONES.

ORDER I.	141. Singultus	144. Dyspnœa	149. Rheuma
SPASMODICÆ.	142. Tussis.	145. Asthma	150. Hydrothorax
138. Ephialtes	ORDER II.	146. Orthopnœa	151. Empyema.
139. Sternutatio	OPPRESSIVÆ.	147. Angina	
140. Oscedo	143. Stertor	148. Pleurodyne	

CLASS VI.—DEBILITATES.

ORDER I.	161. Anæsthesia.	168. Paraphonia	ORDER V
DYSÆSTHESIÆ.	ORDER II.	169. Paralysis	COMATA
152. Cataracta	ANEPITHYMIÆ.	170. Hemiplegia	176. Catalepsis
153. Caligo	162. Anorexia	171. Paraplexia.	177. Ecstasis
154 Amblyopia	163. Adipsia	ORDER IV.	178. Typhomania
155. Amaurosis	164. Anaphrodisia.	LEIPOPSYCHIÆ.	179. Lethargus
156 Anosmia	ORDER III.	172. Asthenia	180. Cataphora
157. Agheustia	DYSCINESIÆ.	173. Leipothymia	181. Carus
158. Dysecœa	165. Mutitas	174. Syncope	182. Apoplexia.
159. Paracusis	166. Aphonia	175. Asphyxia.	
160. Cophosis	167. Psellismus		

CLASS VII.—DOLORES.

ORDER I.	ORDER II.	201. Cardiogmus.	ORDER V.
VAGI.	CAPITIS	ORDER IV.	EXTERNI ET ARTUUM
183. Arthritis	193. Cephalalgia	ABDOMINALES IN-	210. Mastodynia
184. Ostocopus	194. Cephalæa	TERNI.	211. Rachialgia
185. Rheumatismus	195. Hemicrania	202. Cardialgia	212. Lumbago
186. Catarrhus	196. Ophthalmia	203. Gastrodynia	213. Ischias
187. Anxietas	197. Otalgia	204. Colica	214. Proctalgia
188. Lassitudo	198. Odontalgia.	205. Hepatalgia	215. Pudendagra
189. Stupor	ORDER III.	206. Splenalgia	
190. Pruritus	PECTORIS.	207. Nephralgia	
191. Algor	199. Dysphagia	208. Dystocia	
192. Ardor.	200 Pyrosis	209. Hysteralgia.	

CLASS VIII.—VESANIÆ.

ORDER I.	ORDER II.	229. Nymphomania	236. Dæmonomania.
HALLUCINATIONES.	MOROSITATES.	230. Tarantismus	VESANIÆ ANOMALÆ
216 Vertigo	222. Pica	231. Hydrophobia.	237. Amnesia
217. Suffusio	223. Bulimia	ORDER III.	238. Agrypnia.
218. Diplopia	224. Polydipsia	DELIRIA.	
219. Syrigmos	225. Antipathia	232. Paraphrosyne	
220. Hypochondriasis	226. Nostalgia	233. Amentia	
221. Somnambulismus.	227. Panophobia	234. Melancholia	
	228. Satyriasis	235. Mania	

CLASS IX.—FLUXUS.

ORDER I.	247. Hæmorrhois	ORDER III.	267. Leucorrhœa
SANGUIFLUXUS.	248. Dysenteria	SERIFLUXUS.	268. Gonorrhœa
239. Hæmorrhagia	249. Melæna	258. Ephidrosis	269. Dyspermatismus
240. Hæmoptysis	250. Nausea	259. Epiphora	270. Galactirrhœa
241. Stomacace	251. Vomitus	260. Coryza	271. Otorrhœa.
242. Hæmatemesis	252. Ileus	261. Ptyalismus	ORDER IV.
243. Hæmaturia	253. Cholera	262. Anacatharsis	AERIFLUXUS.
244. Menorrhagia	254. Diarrhœa	263. Diabetes	272. Flatulentia
245. Abortus.	255. Cœliaca	264. Enuresis	273. Ædopsophia
ORDER II.	256. Lienteria	265. Dysuria	274. Dysodia
ALVIFLUXUS.	257. Tenesmus	266. Pyuria	
246. Hepatirrhœa			

CLASS X.—CACHEXIÆ.

ORDER I.	276. Phthisis	ORDER II.	280. Pneumatosis
MACIES.	277. Atrophia	INTUMESCENTIÆ.	281. Anasarca
275. Tabes.	278. Aridura.	279. Polysarcia	282. Phlegmatia

P D

283. Physconia
284. Graviditas.

ORDER III.
HYDROPES PARTIALES.
285. Hydrocephalus
286. Physocephalus
287. Hydrorachitis
288. Ascites
289. Hydrometra
290. Physometra

291. Tympanites
292. Meteorismus
293. Ischuria.

ORDER IV.
TUBERA.
294. Rachitis
295. Scrofula
296. Carcinoma
297. Leontiasis
298. Malis
299. Frambœsia.

ORDER V.
IMPETIGINES
300. Syphilis
301. Scorbutus
302. Elephantiasis
303. Lepra
304. Scabies
305. Tinea.

ORDER VI.
ICTERITIÆ
306. Aurigo
307. Melasicterus

308. Phænigmus
309. Chlorosis.

ORDER VII.
CACHEXIÆ ANOMALÆ.
310. Phthiriasis
311. Trichoma
312. Alopecia
313. Elcosis
314. Gangræna
315. Necrosis

Synoptical View of the System of LINNÆUS.
CLASS I.—EXANTHEMATICI.

ORDER I.
CONTAGIOSI.
1. Morta
2. Pestis

3. Variola
4. Rubeola
5. Petechia
6. Syphilis.

ORDER II.
SPORADICI
7. Miliaria
8. Uredo

9. Aphtha.

ORDER III.
SOLITARII
10. Erysipelas

CLASS II.—CRITICI.

ORDER I.
CONTINENTES.
11. Diaria
12. Synocha
13. Synochus
14. Lenta.

ORDER II.
INTERMITTENTES.
15. Quotidiana
16. Tertiana
17. Quartana

18. Duplicana
19. Errana.
ORDER III.
EXACERBANTES.
20. Amphimærina

21. Tritæus
22. Tetartophia
23. Hemitritæa
24. Hectica.

CLASS III.—PHLOGISTICI.

ORDER I.
MEMBRANACEI.
25. Phrenitis
26. Paraphrenesis
27. Pleuritis
28. Gastritis

29. Enteritis
30. Proctitis
31. Cystitis.
ORDER II.
PARENCHYMATICI.
32. Sphacelismus

33. Cynanche
34. Peripneumonia
35. Hepatitis
36. Splenitis
37. Nephritis
38. Hysteritis.

ORDER III.
MUSCULOSI.
39. Phlegmone.

CLASS IV.—DOLOROSI.

ORDER I.
INTRINSECI.
40. Cephalalgia
41. Hemicrania
42. Gravedo
43. Ophthalmia
44. Otalgia
45. Odontalgia

46. Angina
47. Soda
48. Cardialgia
49. Gastrica
50. Colica
51. Hepatica
52. Splenica
53. Pleuritica

54. Pneumonica
55. Hysteralgia
56. Nephritica
57. Dysuria
58. Pudendagra
59. Proctica.

ORDER II.
EXTRINSECI
60. Arthritis
61. Ostocopus
62. Rheumatismus
63. Volatica
64. Pruritus.

CLASS V.—MENTALES.

ORDER I.
IDEALES.
65. Delirium
66. Paraphrosyne
67. Amentia
68. Mania
69. Dæmonia
70. Vesania

71. Melancholia
ORDER II.
IMAGINARII.
72. Syringmos
73. Phantasma
74. Vertigo
75. Panophobia
76. Hypochondriasis

77. Somnambulismus.
ORDER III.
PATHETECI.
78. Citta
79. Bulimia
80. Polydipsia
81. Satyriasis
82. Erotomania

83. Nostalgia
84. Tarantismus
85. Rabies
86. Hydrophobia
87. Cacositia
88. Antipathia
89. Anxietas.

CLASS VI.—QUIETALES.

ORDER I.
DEFECTIVI.
90. Lassitudo
91. Languor
92. Asthenia
93. Lipothymia
94. Syncope
95. Asphyxia.

ORDER II.
SOPOROSI.
96. Somnolentia
97. Typhomania
98. Lethargus
99. Cataphora
100. Carus
101. Apoplexia
102. Paraplegia
103. Hemiplegia

104. Paralysis
105. Stupor
ORDER III.
PRIVATIVI.
106. Morosis
107. Oblivio
108. Amblyopia
109. Cataracta
110. Amaurosis
111. Scotomia

112. Cophosis
113. Anosmia
114. Ageustia
115. Aphonia
116. Anorexia
117. Adipsia
118. Anæsthesia
119. Atecnia
120. Atonia.

CLASS VII.—MOTORII.

ORDER I.
SPASTICI.
121. Spasmus
122. Priapismus
123. Borborygmos
124. Trismos
125. Sardiasis
126. Hysteria

127. Tetanus
128. Catochus
129. Catalepsis
130. Agrypnia.
ORDER II.
AGITATORII.
131. Tremor
132. Palpitatio

133. Orgasmus
134. Subsultus
135. Carpologia
136. Stridor
137. Hippos
138. Psellismus
139. Chorea
140. Beriberi.

ORDER III.
AGITATORII.
141. Rigor
142. Convulsio
143. Epilepsia
144. Hieranosos
145. Raphania

CLASS VIII.—SUPPRESSORII.

ORDER I.
SUFFOCATORII.
146. Raucedo
147. Vociferatio
148. Risus
149. Fletus
150. Suspirium
151. Oscitatio
114

152. Pandiculatio
153. Singultus
154. Sternutatio
155. Tussis
156. Stertor
157. Anhelatio
158. Suffocatio
159. Empyema

160. Dyspnœa
161. Asthma
162. Orthopnœa
163. Ephialtes.
ORDER II.
CONSTRICTORII.
164. Anglutitio
165. Flatulentia

166. Obstipatio
167. Ischuria
168. Dysmenorrhœa
169. Dyslochia
170. Aglactatio
171. Sterilitas.

NOSOLOGY.

CLASS IX.—EVACUATORII.

ORDER I.
CAPITIS.
172 Otorrhœa
173. Epiphora
174. Hæmorrhagia
175. Coryza
176. Stomacace
177. Ptyalismus.
ORDER II.
THORACIS.
178. Screatus
179. Expectoratio

180. Hæmoptysis
181. Vomica.
ORDER III.
ABDOMINIS.
182. Ructus
183. Nausea
184. Vomica
185. Hæmatemesis
186. Iliaca
187. Cholera
188. Diarrhœa
189. Lienteria

190. Cœliaca
191. Cholirica
192. Dysenteria
193. Hæmorrhois
194. Tenesmus
195. Crepitus.
ORDER IV.
GENITALIUM.
196. Enuresis
197. Stranguria
198. Diabetes
199. Hæmaturia

200. Glus
201. Gonorrhœa
202. Leucorrhœa
203. Menorrhagia
204. Parturitio
205. Abortus
206. Mola.
ORDER V
CORPORIS EXTERNI
207. Galactia
208. Sudor.

CLASS X.—DEFORMES.

ORDER I.
EMACIANTES.
209. Phthisis
210. Tabes
211. Atrophia
212. Marasmus
213. Rachitis.

ORDER II.
TUMIDOSI.
214. Polysarcia
215. Leucophlegmatia
216. Anasarca
217. Hydrocephalus
218. Ascites

219. Hyposarca
220. Tympanites
221. Graviditas.
ORDER III.
DECOLORES.
222. Cachexia
223. Chlorosis

224. Scorbutus
225. Icterus
226. Plethora.

CLASS XI.—VITIA.

ORDER I.
HUMORALIA.
227. Aridura
228. Digitium
229. Emphysema
230. Oedema
231. Sugillatio
232. Inflammatio
233. Abscessus
234. Gangrena
235. Sphacelus.
ORDER II.
DIALYTICA.
236. Fractura
237. Luxatura
238. Ruptura
239. Contusura
240. Profusio
241. Vulnus
242. Amputatura
243. Laceratura
244. Punctura
245. Morsura
246. Combustura.
247. Excoriatura
248. Intertrigo
249. Rhagas.
ORDER III.
EXULCERATIONES.
250. Ulcus

251. Cacoethes
252. Noma
253. Carcinoma
254. Ozena
255. Fistula
256. Caries
257. Arthrocace
258. Cocyta
259. Paronychia
260. Pernio
261. Pressura
262. Arctura.
ORDER IV.
SCABIES.
263. Lepra
264. Tinea
265. Achor
266. Psora
267. Lippitudo
268. Serpigo
269. Herpes
270. Varus
271. Bacchia
272. Bubo
273. Anthrax
274. Phlyctæna
275. Pustula
276. Papula
277. Hordeolum
278. Verruca

279. Clavus
280. Myrmecium
281. Eschara.
ORDER V.
TUMORES PROTUBE-RANTES.
282. Aneurisma
283. Varix
284. Scirrhus
285. Struma
286. Atheroma
287. Anchylosis
288. Ganglion
289. Natta
290. Spinola
291. Exostosis.
ORDER VI.
PROCIDENTIÆ.
292. Hernia
293. Prolapsus
294. Condyloma
295. Sarcoma
296. Pterygium
297. Ectropium
298. Phimosis
299. Clitorismus.
ORDER VII.
DEFORMATIONES.
300. Contractura
301. Gibber

302. Lordosis
303. Distortio
304. Tortura
305. Strabismus
306. Lagophthalmia
307. Nyctalopia
308. Presbytia
309. Myopia
310. Labarium
311. Lagostoma
312. Apella
313. Atreta
314. Plica
315. Hirsuties
316. Alopecia
317. Trichiasis.
ORDER VIII
MACULÆ.
318. Cicatrix
319. Nævus
320. Morphæa
321. Vibex
322. Sudamen
323. Melasma
324. Hepatizon
325. Lentigo
326. Ephelis

Synoptical View of the System of VOGEL.

CLASS I.—FEBRES.

ORDER I.
INTERMITTENTES.
1. Quotidiana
2. Tertiana
3. Quartana
4. Quintana
5. Sextana
6. Septana
7. Octana
8. Nonana
9. Decimana
10. Vaga
11. Menstrua
12. Tertiana duplex
13. Quartana duplex
14. Quartana triplex.
ORDER II.
CONTINUÆ.
§ 1. *Simplices.*
15. Quotidiana
16. Synochus
17. Amatoria
18. Phrenitis

19. Epiala
20. Causos
21. Elodes
22. Lethargus
23. Typhomania
24. Leipyria
25. Phricodes
26. Lyngodes
27. Assodes
28. Cholerica
29. Syncopalis
30. Hydrophobia
31. Oscitans
32. Ictericodes
33. Pestilentialis
34. Siriasis.
§ 2. *Compositæ.*
¶ 1. *Exanthematicæ.*
35. Variolosa
36. Morbillosa
37. Miliaris
38. Petechialis
39. Scarlatina

40. Urtica
41. Bullosa
42. Varicella
43. Pemphigodes
44. Aphthosa.
¶ 2. *Inflammatoriæ.*
45. Phrenismus
46. Chemosis
47. Ophthalmites
48. Otites
49. Angina
50. Pleuritis
51. Peripneumonia
52. Mediastina
53. Pericarditis
54. Carditis
55. Paraphrenitis
56. Gastritis
57. Enteritis
58. Hepatitis
59. Splenitis
60. Mesenteritis
61. Omentitis

62. Peritonitis
63. Mycolitis
64. Pancreatica
65. Nephritis
66. Cystitis
67. Hysteritis
68. Erysipelacea
69. Podagrica
70. Panaritia
71. Cyssotis.
¶ 3. *Symptomaticæ*
72. Apoplectica
73. Catarrhalis
74. Rheumatica
75. Hæmorrhoidalis
76. Lactea
77. Vulneraria
78. Suppuratoria
79. Lenta
80. Hectica

CLASS II.—PROFLUVIA.

ORDER I.
HÆMORRHAGIÆ.
81. Hæmorrhagia
82. Epistaxis
83. Hæmoptoe

84. Hæmoptysis
85. Stomacace
86. Odontirrhœa
87. Otorrhœa
88. Ophthalmorrhagia

89. Hæmatemesis
90. Hepatirrhœa
91. Catarrhexis
92. Hæmaturia
93. Cystirrhagia

94. Stymatosis
95. Hæmatopedesis
96. Menorrhagia
97. Abortio.

NOSOLOGY.

ORDER II.
APOCENOSES
98. Catarrhus
99. Epiphora
100. Coryza
101. Otopuosis
102. Otoplatos
103 Ptyalismus

104. Vomica
105. Diarrhœa
106. Puorrhœa
107. Dysenteria
108. Lienteria
109. Cœliaca
110. Cholera
111. Pituitaria

112. Leucorrhois
113. Eneuresis
114. Diuresis
115. Diabetes
116. Puoturia
117. Chylaria
118. Gonorrhœa
119. Leucorrhœa

120. Exoneirosis
121. Hydropedesis
122. Galactia
123. Hypercatharsi
124. Ecphyse
125. Dysodia.

CLASS III.—EPISCHESES.

126. Gravedo
127. Flatulentia

128. Obstipatio
129. Ischuria

130. Amenorrhœa
131. Dyslochia

132. Deuteria
133. Agalaxis.

CLASS IV.—DOLORES.

134. Anxietas
135. Blestrismus
136. Pruritus
137. Catapsyxis
138. Rheumatismus
139. Arthritis
140. Cephalalgia
141. Cephalæa
142. Clavus
143. Hemicrania
144. Carebaria
145. Odontalgia

146. Hæmodia
147. Odaxismus
148. Otalgia
149. Acataposis
150. Cionis
151. Himantesis
152. Cardiogmus
153. Mastodynia
154. Soda
155. Periadynia
156. Pneumatosis
157 Cardialgia

158. Encausis
159. Nausea
160. Colica
161. Eilema
162. Ileus
163. Stranguria
164. Dysuria
165. Lithiasis
166. Tenesmus
167. Clunesia
168. Cedma
169. Hysteralgia

170. Dysmenorrhæa
171. Dystochia
172. Atocia
173. Priapismus
174. Psoriasis
175. Podagra
176. Osteocopus
177. Psophos
178. Volatica
179. Epiphlogisma.

CLASS V.—SPASMI.

180. Tetanus
181. Opisthotonus
182. Episthotonus
183. Catochus
184. Tremor
185. Frigus
186. Horror
187. Rigor
188. Epilepsia
89. Eclampsia
190. Hieranosos

191. Convulsio]
192. Raphania
193. Chorea
194. Crampus
195. Scelotyrbe]
196. Angone
197. Glossocele
198. Glossocoma
199. Hippos
200. Illosis
201. Cinclesis

202. Cataclasis
203. Cillosis
204. Sternutatio
205. Tussis
206. Clamor
207. Trismus
208. Capistrum
209. Sardiasis
210. Gelasmus
211. Incubus
212. Singultus

213. Palpitatio
214. Vomitus
215. Ructus
216. Ruminatio
217. Oesophagtamus
218. Hypochondriasis
219. Hysteria
220. Phlogosis
221. Digitium.

CLASS VI.—ADYNAMIÆ.

222. Lassitudo
223. Asthenia
224. Torpor
225. Adynamia
226. Paralysis
227. Paraplegia
228. Hemiplegia
229. Apoplexia
230. Catalepsis
231. Carus
232. Coma
233. Somnolentia
234. Hypophasis
235. Ptosis
236. Amblyopia
237. Mydriasis

238. Amaurosis
239. Cataracta
240. Synizezis
241. Glaucoma
242. Achlys
243. Nyctalopia
244. Hemeralopia
245. Hemalopia
246. Dysicoia
247. Surditas
248. Anosmia
249. Apogeusis
250. Asaphia
251. Clangor
252. Raucitas
253. Aphonia

254. Leptophonia
255. Oxyphonia
256. Rhenophonia
257. Mutitas
258. Traulotis
259. Psellotis
260. Ichnophonia
261. Battarismus
262. Suspirium
263. Oscitatio
264. Pandiculatio
265. Apnæa
266. Macropnœa
267. Dyspnœa
268. Asthma
269. Orthopnœa

270. Pnigma
271. Renchus
272. Rhochmos
273. Lipothymus
274. Syncope
275. Asphyxia
276. Apepsia
277. Dyspepsia
278. Diapthora
279. Anorexia
280. Anatrope
281. Adipsia
282. Acyisis
283. Agenesia
284. Anodynia.

CLASS VII.—HYPÆRESTHESES.

285. Antipathia
286 Agrypnia
287. Phantasma
288. Caligo
289. Hæmalopia

290. Marmaryge
291. Dysopia
292. Susurrus
293. Vertigo
294. Apogeusia

295. Polydipsia
296. Bulimus
297. Addephagia
298. Cynorexia
299. Allotriophagia

300. Malacia
301. Pica
302. Bombus
303. Celsa.

CLASS VIII.—CACHEXIÆ.

304. Cachexia
305. Chlorosis
306. Icterus
307. Melanchlorus
308. Atrophia
309. Tabes
310. Phthisis

311. Hydrothorax
312. Rachitis
313. Anasarca
314. Ascites
315. Hydrocystis
316. Tympanites
317. Hysterophyse

318. Scorbutus
319. Syphilis
320. Lepra
321. Elephantiasis
322. Elephantia
323. Plica
324. Phthiriasis

325. Physconia
326. Paracyisis
327. Gangræna
328. Sphacelus.

CLASS IX.—PARANOIÆ.

329. Athymia
330. Delirium
331. Mania

332. Melancholia
333. Ecstasis
334. Ecplexis

335. Enthusiasmus
336. Stupiditas
337. Amentia

338. Oblivio
339. Somnium
340. Hypnobatasis

CLASS X.—VITIA.

ORDER I.
INFLAMMATIONES.
341. Ophthalmia
342. Blepharotis
343. Erysipelas
344. Hieropyr
345. Paronychia
346. Onychia

347. Encausis
348. Phimosis
349. Paraphimosis
350. Pernio.
ORDER II.
HUMORES.
351. Phlegmone
352. Furunculus

353. Anthrax
354. Abscissus
355. Onyx
356. Hippopyon
357. Phygethlon
358. Empyema
359. Phyma
360. Ecthymata

361. Urticaria
362. Parulis
363. Epulis
364. Anchylops
365. Paraglossa
366. Chilon
367. Scrofula
368. Bubon

369. Bronchocele	408. Aneurisma	443. Herpes	478. Anapleusis
370. Parotis	409. Cirsocele	444. Scabies	479. Spasma
371. Gongrona	410. Gastrocele	445. Aquula	480. Contusio
372. Sparganosis	411. Hepatocele	446. Hydroa	481. Diabrosis
373. Coilima	412. Splenocele	447. Variola	482. Agomphiasis
374. Scirrhus	413. Hysterocele	448. Varicella	483. Eschara
375. Cancer	414. Hygrocirsocele	449. Purpura	484. Piptonychia
376. Sarcoma	415. Sarcocele	450. Encauma.	485. Cacoethes
377. Polypus	416. Physocele	ORDER V.	486. Therioma
378. Condyloma	417. Exostosis	MACULÆ.	487. Carcinoma
379. Ganglion	418. Hyperostosis	451. Ecchymoma	488. Phagedæna
380. Ranula	419. Pædarthrocace	452. Petechiæ	489. Noma
381. Terminthus	420. Encystis	453. Morbilli	490. Sycosis
382. Oedema	421. Staphyloma	454. Scarlatæ	491. Fistula
383. Encephalocele	422. Staphylosis	455. Lentigo	492. Sinus
384. Hydrocephalum	423. Fungus	456. Urticaria	493. Caries
385. Hydropthalmia	424. Tofus	457. Stigma	494. Achores
386. Spina bifida	425. Flemen.	458. Vibex	495. Crusta lactea
387. Hydromphalus	ORDER III.	459. Vitiligo	496. Favus
388. Hydrocele	EXTUBERANTIÆ.	460. Leuce	497. Tinea
389. Hydrops scroti	426. Verruca	461. Cyasma	498. Argemon
390. Steatites	427. Porrus	462. Lichen	499. Ægilops
391. Pneumatosis	428. Clavus	463. Selina	500. Ozæna
392. Emphysema	429. Callus	464. Nebula.	501. Aphthæ
393. Hysteroptosis	430. Encanthis	ORDER VI.	502. Intertrigo
394. Cystoptosis	431. Pladarotis	DISSOLUTIONES.	503. Rhacosis.
395. Archoptoma	432. Pinnula	465. Vulnus	ORDER VII.
396. Bubonocele	433. Pterygium	466. Ruptura	CONCRETIONES.
397. Oscheocele	434. Hordeolum	467. Rhagas	504. Ancyloblepharon
398. Omphalocele	435. Grando	468. Fractura	505. Zynizesis
399. Merocele	436. Varus	469. Fissura	506. Dacrymoma
400. Enterocele ovularis	437. Gutta rosacea	470. Plicatio	507. Ancyloglossum
401. Ischiatocele	438. Ephelis	471. Thlasis	508. Ancylosis
402. Elytrocele	439. Esoche	472. Luxatio	509. Cicatrix
403. Hypogastrocele	440. Exoche.	473. Subluxatio	510. Dactylion
404. Cystocele	ORDER IV.	474. Diachalasis	
405. Cyrtoma	PUSTULÆ & PAPULÆ.	475. Attritis	
406. Hydrenterocele	441. Epinyctis	476. Porrigo	
407. Varix	442. Phlyctæna	477. Aposyrma	

CLASS XI.—DEFORMITATES.

511. Phoxos	524. Hirsuties	537. Gryposis	550. Saniodes
512. Gibber	525. Canities	538. Nævus	551. Cripsorchis
513. Caput obstipum	526. Distrix	539. Montrositas	552. Hermaphrodites
514. Strabismus	527. Xirasia	540. Polysarcia	553. Dionysiscus
515. Myopiasis	528. Phalacrotis	541. Ichnotis	554. Artetiscus
516. Lagophthalmus	529. Alopecia	542. Rhicnosis	555. Nefrendis
517. Trichiasis	530. Madarosis	543. Varus	556. Spanopogon
518. Ectropium	531. Ptilosis	544. Valgus	557. Hyperartetisci
519. Entropium	532. Rodatio	545. Leiopodes	558. Galiancon
520. Rhœas	533. Phalangosis	546. Apella	559. Galbulus
521. Rhyssemata	534. Coloboma	547. Hypospadiæos	560. Mola.
522. Lagocheilos	535. Cercosis	548. Urorhœas	
523. Malachosteon	536. Cholosis	549. Atreta	

A Synoptical View of the System of SAGAR.

CLASS I.—VITIA.

ORDER I.	18. Emphysema	37. Marisca	58. Bubonocele
MACULÆ.	19. Scirrhus	38. Hydatis	59. Opodeocele
1. Leucoma	20. Inflammatio	39. Staphyloma	60. Ischiocele
2. Vitiligo	21. Bubo	40. Lupia	61. Colpocele
3. Ephelis	22. Parotis	41. Hydarthrus	62. Perinæocele
4. Nævus	23. Furunculus	42. Apostema	63. Peritonæorixis
5. Ecchymoma.	24. Anthrax	43. Exomphalus	64. Encephalocele
ORDER II.	25. Cancer	44. Oscheophyma.	65. Hysteroloxia
EFFLORESCENTIÆ.	26. Paronychia	ORDER VI.	66. Parorchidium
6. Pustula	27. Phimosis.	ECTOPIÆ.	67. Exarthrema
7. Papula	ORDER IV.	45. Exophthalmia	68. Diastasis
8. Phlycthæna	EXCRESCENTIÆ.	46. Blepharoptosis	69. Loxarthrus
9. Bacchia	28. Sarcoma	47. Hypostaphyle	70. Gibbositas
10. Varus	29. Condyloma	48. Paraglossa	71. Lordosis.
11. Herpes	30. Verruca	49. Proptoma	ORDER VII.
12. Epinyctis	31. Pterygium	50. Exania	DEFORMITATES
13. Hemeropathos	32. Hordeolum	51. Exocystis	72. Lagostoma
14. Psydracia	33. Trachelophyma	52. Histeroptosis	73. Apella
15. Hydra.	34. Exostosis.	53. Colpoptosis	74. Polymerisma
ORDER III.	ORDER V.	54. Gastrocele	75. Epidosis
PHYMATA.	CYSTIDES.	55. Omphalocele	76. Anchylomerisma
16. Erythema	35. Aneurysma	56. Hepatocele	77. Hirsuties.
17. Oedema	36. Varix	57. Merocele	

CLASS II.—PLAGÆ.

ORDER I.	81. Morsus	ORDER II.	87. Sutura
SOLUTIONES.	82. Excoriatio	SOLUTIONES.	88. Paracentesis
recentes, cruentæ.	83. Contusio	recentes, cruentæ, artifi-	ORDER III.
78. Vulnus	84. Ruptura.	ciales.	SOLUTIONES.
79. Punctura		85. Operatio	incruentæ.
80. Sclopetoplaga		86. Amputatio	89. Ulcus

117

90. Exulceratio
91. Fistula
92. Sinus

93. Eschara
94. Caries
95. Arthrocace.

ORDER IV.
SOLUTIONES.
anomalæ.
96. Rhagas

97. Ambustio
98. Fractura
99. Fissura.

CLASS III.—CACHEXIÆ.

ORDER I.
MACIES.
100. Tabes
101. Phthisis
102. Atrophia
103. Hæmataporia
104. Aridura.

ORDER II.
INTUMESCENTIÆ.
105. Plethora
106. Polysarcia
107. Pneumatosis
108. Anasarca
109. Phlegmatia
110. Physconia

111. Graviditas.
ORDER III.
HYDROPES *partiales.*
112. Hydrocephalus
113. Physocephalus
114. Hydrorachitis
115. Ascites
116. Hydrometra
117. Physometra
118. Tympanites
119. Meteorismus.

ORDER IV.
TUBERA.
120. Rachitis
121. Scrofula

122. Carcinoma
123. Leontiasis
124. Malis
125. Framboesia.
ORDER V.
IMPETIGINES.
126. Syphilis
127. Scorbutus
128. Elephantiasis
129. Lepra
130. Scabies
131. Tinea.

ORDER VI.
ICTERITIE.
132. Aurigo

133. Melasicterus
134. Phœnigmus
135. Chlorosis.
ORDER VII.
ANOMALÆ
136. Phthiriasis
137. Trichoma
138. Alopecia
139. Elcosis
140. Grangræna
141. Necrosis.

CLASS IV.—DOLORES.

ORDER I.
VAGI.
142. Arthritis
143. Ostocopus
144. Rheumatismus
145. Catarrhus
146. Anxietas
147. Lassitudo
148. Stupor
149. Pruritus
150. Algor

151. Ardor.
ORDER II.
CAPITIS.
152. Cephalalgia
153. Cephalæa
154. Hemicrania
155. Ophthalmia
156. Otalgia
157. Odontalgia.

ORDER III.
PECTORIS.
158. Pyrosis
159. Cardiogmus.
ORDER IV.
ABDOMINIS.
160. Cardialgia
161. Gastrodynia
162. Colica
163. Hepatalgia
164. Splenalgia

165. Nephralgia
166. Hysteralgia.
ORDER V.
EXTERNARUM
167. Mastodynia
168. Rachialgia
169. Lumbago
170. Ischias
171. Proctalgia
172. Pudendagra
173. Digitium.

CLASS V.—FLUXUS.

ORDER I.
SANGUIFLUXUS.
174. Hæmorrhagia
175. Hæmoptysis
176. Stomacace
177. Hæmatemesis
178. Hæmaturia
179. Metrorrhagia
180. Abortus.

ORDER II.
ALVIFLUXUS.
sanguinolenti.
181. Hepatirrhœa

182. Hæmorrhois
183. Dysenteria
184. Melæna.
ORDER III.
ALVIFLUXUS.
non sanguinolenti.
185. Nausea
186. Vomitus
187. Ileus
188. Cholera
189. Diarrhœa
190. Cœliaca
191. Lienteria

192. Tenesmus
193. Proctorrhœa.
ORDER IV.
SERIFLUXUS.
194. Ephidrosis
195. Epiphora
196. Coryza
197. Ptyalismus
198. Anacatharsis
199. Diabetes
200. Enuresis
201. Pyuria
202. Leucorrhœa

203. Lochiorrhœa
204. Gonorrhœa
205. Galactirrhœa
206. Otorrhœa.
ORDER V.
AERIPLUXUS.
207. Flatulentia
208. Ædopsophia
209. Dysodia

CLASS VI.—SUPPRESSIONES.

ORDER I.
EGERENDORUM.
210. Adiapneustia
211. Sterilitas
212. Ischuria
213. Dysuria

214. Aglactatio
215. Dyslochia.

ORDER II.
INGERENDORUM
216. Dysphagia
217. Angina.

ORDER III
IMI VENTRIS.
218. Dysmenorrhœa
219. Dystocia
220. Dyshæmorrhois
221. Obstipatio.

CLASS VII.—SPASMI.

ORDER I.
TONICI PARTIALES.
222. Strabismus
223. Trismus
224. Obstipitas
225. Contractura
226. Crampus
227. Priapismus.

ORDER II.
TONICI GENERALES.
228. Tetanus
229. Catochus.
ORDER III.
CHRONICI PARTIALES.
230. Nystagmus
231. Carphologia

232. Subsultus
233. Pandiculatio
234. Apomistosis
235. Convulsio
236. Tremor
237. Palpitatio
238. Claudicatio.

ORDER IV.
CHRONICI GENERALES.
239. Phricasmus
240. Eclampsia
241. Epilepsia
242. Hysteria
243. Scelotyrbe
244. Beriberia.

CLASS VIII.—ANHELATIONES.

ORDER I.
SPASMODICÆ.
245. Ephialtes
246. Sternutatio
247. Oscedo

248. Singultus
249. Tussis.
ORDER II.
SUPPRESSIVÆ.
250. Stertor

251. Dyspnœa
252. Asthma
253. Orthopnœa
254. Pleurodyne
255. Rheuma

256. Hydrothorax
257. Empyema.

CLASS IX.—DEBILITATES.

ORDER I.
DYSÆSTHESIÆ.
258. Amblyopia
259. Caligo
260. Cataracta
261. Amaurosis
262. Anosmia
263. Agheustia
264. Dysecœa
265. Paracusis
266. Cophosis

267. Anæsthesia.
ORDER II.
ANEPYTHYMIÆ.
268. Anorexia
269. Adipsia
270. Anaphrodisia.
ORDER III.
DYSCINESIÆ.
271. Mutitas
272. Aphonia
273. Psellismus

274. Cacophonia
275. Paralysis
276. Hemiplegia
277. Paraplexia.
ORDER IV.
LEIPOPSYCHIÆ.
278. Asthenia
279. Lipothymia
280. Syncope
281. Asphyxia.

ORDER V.
COMATA.
282. Catalepsis
283. Ectasis
284. Typhomania
285. Lethargus
286. Cataphora
287. Carus
288. Apoplexia.

NOSOLOGY.

CLASS X.—EXANTHEMATA.

Order I. CONTAGIOSA.		Order II. NON-CONTAGIOSA.	
289. Pestis	291. Pemphigus	295. Miliares	297. Essera
290. Variola	292. Purpura	296. Erysipelas	298. Aphtha.
	293. Rubeola		
	294. Scarlatina.		

CLASS XI.—PHLEGMASIÆ.

Order I. MUSCULOSÆ.	Order II. MEMBRANACÆ.	307. Enteritis	311. Peripneumonia
299. Phlegmone	303. Phrenitis	308. Epiploitis	312. Hepatitis
300. Cynanche	304. Diaphragmitis	309. Cystitis.	313. Splenitis
301. Myositis	305. Pleuritis	Order III. PARENCHYMATOSÆ.	314. Nephritis
302 Carditis.	306. Gastritis	310. Cephalitis	315. Metritis.

CLASS XII.—FEBRES.

Order I. CONTINUÆ	319. Typhus	322. Tritæophya	325. Tertiana
316. Judicatoria	320. Hectica.	323. Tetartophya.	326. Quartana
317. Humoraria	Order II. REMITTENTES.	Order III. INTERMITTENTES.	327. Erratica.
318. Frigeraria	321. Amphimerina	324. Quotidiana	

CLASS XIII.—VESANIÆ.

Order I. HALLUCINATIONES.	Order II. MOROSITATES.	340. Satyriasis	346. Amentia
328. Vertigo	334. Pica	341. Nymphomania	347. Melancholia
329. Suffusio	335. Bulimia	342. Tarantismus	348. Dæmonomania
330. Diplopia	336. Polydipsia	343. Hydrophobia	349. Mania.
331. Syrigmos	337. Antipathia	344. Rabies.	Order IV. ANOMALÆ.
332. Hypochondriasis	338. Nostalgia	Order III. DELIRIA.	350. Amnesia
333. Somnambulismus.	339. Panophobia	345. Paraphrosyne	351. Agrypnia

Synoptical View of the System of Dr. MacBride.

CLASS I.—UNIVERSAL DISEASES.

Order I. FEVERS.	12. Rheumatism	29. Eclampsia	40. Melancholia.
1. Continued	13. Ostocopus	30. Hieranosos:	Order IX. CACHEXIES, or *Humoral Diseases.*
2. Intermittent	14. Headache	Order VI. WEAKNESSES AND PRIVATIONS.	41. Corpulency
3. Remittent	15. Toothache		42. Dropsy
4. Eruptive	16. Earache	31. Coma	43. Jaundice
5. Hectic.	17. Pleurodyne	32. Palsy	44. Emphysema
Order II. INFLAMMATIONS.	18. Pain in the stomach	33. Fainting.	45. Tympany
6. External	19. Colic	Order VII. ASTHMATIC DISORDERS.	46. Physconia
7. Internal.	20. Lithiasis		47. Atrophia
Order III. FLUXES.	21. Ischuria	34. Dyspnœa	48. Ostosarcosis
8. Alvine	22. Proctalgia.	35. Orthopnœa	49. Sarcostosis
9. Hæmorrhage	Order V. SPASMODIC DISEASES.	36. Asthma	50. Mortification
10. Humoral discharge.	23. Tetanus	37. Hydrothorax	51. Scurvy
Order IV. PAINFUL DISEASES.	24. Catochus	38. Empyema.	52. Scrofula
11. Gout	25. Locked jaw	Order VIII. MENTAL DISEASES.	53. Cancer
	26. Hydrophobia		54. Lues Venerea.
	27. Convulsion	39. Mania	
	28. Epilepsy		

CLASS II.—LOCAL DISEASES.

Order I. OF THE INTERNAL SENSES.	Order IV. OF THE SECRETIONS AND EXCRETIONS.	95. Hiccup	118. Impetigo
55. Loss of memory	74. Epiphora	96. Cough	119. Leprosy
56. Hypochondriasis	75. Coryza	97. Vomiting	120. Elephantiasis
57. Loss of judgment.	76. Ptyalism	98. Palpitation of the heart	121. Frambœsia
Order II. OF THE EXTERNAL SENSES.	77. Anacatharsis	99. Chorea	122. Herpes
	78. Otorrhœa	100. Trismus	123. Maculæ
58. Blindness	79. Diarrhœa	101. Nystagmus	124. Alopecia
59. Depraved sight	80. Incontinence of urine.	102. Cramp	125. Trichoma
60. Deafness	81. Pyuria	103. Scelotyrbe	126. Scald head
61. Depraved hearing	82. Dysuria	104. Contraction	127. Phthiriasis.
62. Loss of smell	83. Constipation	105. Paralysis	Order VII. DISLOCATIONS.
63. Depraved smell	84. Tenesmus	106. Anchylosis	
64. Loss of taste	85. Dysodia	107. Gibbositas	128. Hernia
65. Depraved taste	86. Flatulence	108. Lordosis	129. Prolapsus
66. Loss of feeling.	87. Ædopsophia.	109. Hydarthrus.	130. Luxation.
Order III. OF THE APPETITES.	Order V. IMPEDING DIFFERENT ACTIONS.	Order VI. OF THE EXTERNAL HABIT.	Order VIII. SOLUTIONS OF CONTINUITY.
67. Anorexia	88. Aphonia	110. Tumour	131. Wound
68. Cynorexia	89. Mutitas	111. Excrescence	132. Ulcer
69. Pica	90. Paraphonia	112. Aneurism	133. Fissure
70. Polydipsia	91. Dysphagia	113. Varix	134. Fistula
71. Satyriasis	92. Wry neck	114. Papulæ	135. Burn, or scald
72. Nymphomania	93. Angone	115. Phlyctœnæ	136. Excoriation
73. Anaphrodisia.	94. Sneezing	116. Pustulæ	137. Fracture
		117. Scabies, or Psora	138. Caries.

CLASS III.—SEXUAL DISEASES.

Order I. GENERAL, *proper to Men.*	Order II. LOCAL, *proper to Men.*	143. Gonorrhœa virulenta	147. Crystalline
139. Febris testicularis	141. Dyspermatismus	144. Priapism	148. Hernia humoralis
140. Tabes dorsalis.	142. Gonorrhœa simplex	145. Phimosis	149. Hydrocele
		146. Paraphimosis	150. Sarcocele

151. Cirsocele.	155. Menorrhagia	161. Mastodynia.	165. Physometra
ORDER III. GENERAL, proper to Women.	156. Hysteralgia	ORDER IV. LOCAL, proper to Women.	166. Prolapsus uteri
	157. Graviditas		167. ———— ——— vaginæ
152. Amenorrhœa	158. Abortus	162. Hydrops ovarii	168. Polypus uteri
153. Chlorosis	159. Dystochia	163. Scirrhus ovarii	
154. Leucorrhœa	160. Febris puerperalis	164. Hydrometra	

CLASS IV.—INFANTILE DISEASES.

ORDER I. GENERAL.	172. Aphthæ	ORDER II. LOCAL.	179. Purpura
169. Colica meconialis	173. Eclampsia	176. Imperforation	180. Crusta lactea.
170. Colica lactentium	174. Atrophia	177. Anchyloglossum	
171. Diarrhœa infantum	175. Rachitis.	178. Aurigo	

Synoptical view of Dr. GOOD'S System.

CLASS I. CŒLIACA. *Diseases of the Digestive Function.*

ORDER 1. ENTERICA. Affecting the alimentary canal.
Genus 1. ODONTIA. Misdentition.
Species 1. O. dentitionis. Teething.
2. O. dolorosa. Toothache.
3. O. stuporis. Tooth-edge.
4. O. deformis. Deformity of the teeth.
5. O. edentula. Toothlessness.
6. O. incrustans. Tartar of the teeth.
7. O. excrescens. Excrescent gums.
Genus 2. PTYALISMUS. Ptyalism.
Species 1. P. acutus. Salivation.
2. P. chronicus. Chronic ptyalism.
3. P. iners. Drivelling.
Genus 3. DYSPHAGIA. Dysphagy.
Species 1. D. constricta. Constrictive dysphagy.
2. D. atonica. Atonic dysphagy.
3. D. globosa. Nervous quinsy.
4. D. uvulosa. Uvula dysphagy.
5. D. linguosa. Lingual dysphagy.
Genus 4. DIPSOSIS. Morbid thirst.
Species 1. D. avens. Immoderate thirst.
2. D. expers. Thirstlessness.
Genus 5. LIMOSIS. Morbid appetite.
Species 1. L. avens. Voracity.
2. L. expers. Long fasting.
3. L. pica. Depraved appetite.
4. L. cardiagica. Heartburn. Waterbrash.
5. L. flatus. Flatulency.
6. L. emesis. Sickness. Vomiting.
7. L. dyspepsia. Indigestion.
Genus 6. COLICA. Colic.
Species 1. C. ileus. Iliac passion.
2. C. rhachialgica. Painter's colic.
3. C. cibaria. Surfeit.
4. C. flatulenta. Wind-colic.
5. C. constipata. Constipated colic.
6. C. constricta. Constrictive colic.
Genus 7. COPOSTATRIS. Costiveness.
Species 1. C. constipata. Constipation.
2. C. obstipata. Obstipation.
Genus 8. DIARRHŒA. Looseness.
Species 1. D. fusa. Feculent looseness.
2. D. biliosa. Bilious looseness.
3. D. mucosa. Mucous looseness.
4. D. chylosa. Chylous looseness.
5. D. lienteria. Lientery.
6. D. serosa. Serous looseness.
7. D. tabulosa. Tabular looseness.
8. D. gypsata. Gypseous looseness.
Genus 9. CHOLERA. Cholera.
Species 1. C. biliosa. Bilious cholera.
2. C. flatulenta. Flatulent cholera.
3. C. spasmodica. Spasmodic cholera.
Genus 10. ENTEROLITHUS. Intestinal concretions.
Species 1. E. bezoardus. Bezoar.
2. E. calculus. Intestinal calculus.
3. E. scybalum. Scybalum.
Genus 11. HELMINTHIA. Worms.
Species 1. H. alvi. Alvine worms.
2. H. podicis. Anal worms.
3. erratica. Erratic worms.
Genus 12. PROCTICA. Proctica.
Species 1. P. simplex. Simple proctica.
2. P. spasmodica. Spasmodic stricture of the rectum.
3. P. callosa. Callous stricture of the rectum.
4. P. tenesmus. Tenesmus.
5. P. marica. Piles.
6. P. exania. Prolapse of the fundament.
ORDER 2. SPLANCHNICA. Affecting the collatitious viscera.

Genus 1. ICTERUS. Yellow jaundice.
Species 1. I. cholœus. Biliary jaundice.
2. cholelithicus. Gallstone jaundice.
3. I. spasmodicus. Spasmodic jaundice
4. I. hepaticus. Hepatic jaundice.
5. I. infantum. Jaundice of Infants.
Genus 2. MELÆNA. Melena.
Species 1. M. cholœa. Black or green jaundice
2. M. cruenta. Black vomit.
Genus 3. CHOLOLITHUS. Gall-stone.
Species 1. C. quiescens. Quiescent gall-stone
2. C. means. Passing of gall-stones
Genus 4. PARABISMA. Visceral turgescence.
Species 1. P. hepaticum. Turgescence of the liver
2. P. splenicum. Turgescence of the spleen.
3. P. pancreaticum. Turgescence of the pancreas.
4. P. mesentericum. Turgescence of the mesentery.
5. P. intestinale. Turgescence of the intestines.
6. P. omentale. Turgescence of the omentum.
7. P. complicatum. Turgescence compounded of various organs.

CLASS II PNEUMATICA. *Diseases of the Respiratory Function.*

ORDER 1. PHONICA. Affecting the vocal avenues
Genus 1. CORYZA. Running at the nose.
Species 1. C. entonica. Entonic coryza.
2. C. atonica. Atonic coryza.
Genus 2. POLYPUS. Polypus.
Species 1. P. elasticus. Compressible polypus.
2. P. coriaceus. Cartilaginous polypus.
Genus 3. RHONCHUS. Rattling in the throat
Species 1. R. stertor. Snoring.
2. R. cerchnus. Wheezing.
Genus 4. APHONIA. Dumbness.
Species 1. A. elinguium. Elingual dumbness
2. A. atonica. Atonic dumbness.
3. A. surdorum. Deaf dumbness.
Genus 5. DYSPHONIA. Dissonant voice.
Species 1. D. susurrans. Whispering voice.
2. D. puberum. Voice of puberty.
3. D. immodulata. Immelodious voice.
Genus 6. PSELLISMUS. Dissonant speech.
Species 1. P. bambalia. Stammering.
2. P. blæsitas. Misenunciation.
ORDER 2. PNEUMONICA. Affecting the lungs, their membranes, or motive power.
Genus 1. BEX. Cough.
Species 1. B. humida. Common or humid cough.
2. B. sicca. Dry cough.
3. B. convulsiva. Hooping-cough.
Genus 2. LARYNGISMUS. Laryngic suffocation.
Species 1. L. stridulus. Stridulus construction of the larynx.
Genus 3. DYSPNŒA. Anhelation.
Species 1. D. chronica. Short-breath.
2. D. exacerbans. Exacerbating anhelation.
Genus 4. ASTHMA. Asthma.
Species 1. A. siccum. Dry or nervous asthma.
2. A. humidum. Humid or common asthma.
Genus 5. EPHIALTES. Incubus.
Species 1. E. vigilantium. Day-mare.
2. E. nocturnus. Night-mare.
Genus 6. STERNALGIA. Suffocative breast-pang.
Species 1. S. ambulantium. Acute breast-pang.
2. S. chronica. Chronic breast-pang.
Genus 7. PLEURALGIA. Pain in the side.
Species 1. P. acuta. Stitch.
2. P. chronica. Chronic pain in the side.
CLASS III. HÆMATICA. *Diseases of the Sanguinous Function.*
ORDER 1. PYRETICA. Fevers

Genus 1. EPHEMERA. Diary fever.
Species 1. E. mitis. Mild diary fever.
2. E. acuta. Acute diary fever.
3. E. sudatoria. Sweating fever.
Genus 2. ANETUS. Intermitting fever. Ague.
Species 1. A. quotidianus Quotidian ague.
2. A. tertianus. Tertian ague.
3. A. quartanus. Quartan ague.
4. A. erraticus. Irregular ague.
5. A. complicatus. Complicated ague.
Genus 3. EPANETUS. Remittent fever.
Species 1. E. mitis. Mild remittent.
2. E. malignus. Malignant remittent.
3. E. hectica. Hectic fever.
Genus 4. ENECIA. Continued fever.
Species 1. E. cauna. Inflammatory fever.
2. E typhus. Typhous fever.
3. E. synochus. Synochal fever.
ORDER 2. PHLOGISTICA. Inflammations.
Genus 1. APOSTEMA. Aposteme.
Species 1. A. commune. Common aposteme.
2. Apsoaticum. Psoas abscess.
3. A. hepaticum. Abscess of the liver.
4. A. empyema. Lodgment of matter in the chest.
5. A vomica. Vomica.
Genus 2. PHLEGMONE. Phlegmon
Species 1. P. communis. Common phlegmon.
2. P. parulis. Gum-boil.
3. P. auris. Imposthume of the ear.
4. P. parotidea. Parotid phlegmon.
5. P. mammæ. Abscess of the breast.
6. P. bubo. Bubo.
7. P. phimotica. Phimotic phlegmon.
Genus 3. PHYMA. Tubercle.
Species 1. P. hordeolum. Sty.
2. P. furunculus. Boil.
3. *P.* sycosis. Ficous phyma.
4. P. anthrax. Carbuncle.
Genus 4. IONTHUS. Whelk.
Species 1. I. varus. Stone pock.
2. I. corymbyfer. Carbunculated face. Rosy drop.
Genus 5. PHLYSIS. Phlysis.
Species 1. P. paronychia. Whitlow.
Genus 6. ERYTHEMA. Inflammatory blush.
Species 1. E. œdematosum. Œdematous inflammation.
2. E. erysipelatosum. Esysipelatous inflammation.
3. E. gangrenosum. Gangrenous inflammation.
4. E. vesiculare. Vesicular inflammation.
5. E. pernio. Chilblain.
6. E. entertrigo. Fret.
Genus 7. EMPRESMA. Visceral inflammation.
Species 1. E. cephalites. Inflammation of the brain.
2. E. otitis. Inflammation of the ear.
3. E. parotitis. Mumps.
4 E. parithmitis. Quincy.
5. E. laryngitis. Inflammation of the larynx
6. E. bronchitis. Croup.
7. E. pneumonitis. Peripneumony.
8. E. pleuritis. Pleurisy
9. E. carditis. Inflammation of the heart.
10. E. peritonitis. Inflammation of the peritoneum.
11. E. gastritis. Inflammation of the stomach.
12. E. enteritis. Inflammation of the bowels.
13. E. hepatitis. Inflammation of the liver.
14. E. splenitis. Inflammation of the spleen.
15. E. nephritis. Inflammation of the kidney.
16. E. cystitis. Inflammation of the bladder.
17. E. hysteritis. Inflammation of the womb.
18. E. orchitis Inflammation of the testicles.
Genus 8. OPHTHALMIA. Ophthalmy.
Species 1. O. taraxis. Lachrymose ophthalmy.
2. O. iridis. Inflammation of the iris.
3. O. purulenta. Purulent ophthalmy.
4. O. glutinosa. Glutinous ophthalmy.
5. O. chronica. Lippitude. Blear-eye.
Genus 9. CATARRHUS. Catarrh.
Species 1. C, communis. Cold in the head or chest.
2. C. epidemicus. Influenza.
Genus 10. DYSENTERIA. dysentery.
Species 1. D. simplex. Simple Dysentery.
2. D. pyretica. Dysenteric fever.

Genus 11. BUCNEMIA. Tumid leg.
Species 1. B. sparganosis. Puerperal tumid leg.
2. B. tropica. Tumid leg of hot climates.
Genus 12. ARTHROSIA. Articular inflammation.
Species 1. A. acuta. Acute rheumatism.
2. A. chronica. Chronic inflammation.
3. A. podagra. Gout.
4. A. hydarthrus. White-swelling.
ORDER 3. EXANTHEMATICA. Eruptive fevers. Ex anthems.
Genus 1. EXANTHESIS. Rash exanthem.
Species 1. E. rosalia. Scarlet fever
2. rubeola. Measles.
3. E. urticaria. Nettle-rash.
Genus 2. EMPHLYSIS. Achorous exanthem.
Species 1. E. miliaria. Miliary fever.
2. E. aphtha. Thrush.
3. E. vaccina. Cow-pox.
4. E. varicella. Water-pox.
5. E. pemphigus Vesicular fever.
6. E. erysipelas. St. Anthony's fire.
Genus 3. EMPYESIS. Pustulous exanthem.
Species 1. E. variola. Smallpox.
Genus 4. ANTHRACIA. Carbuncular exanthem.
Species 1. A. pestis. Plague.
2. A. rubula. Yaws.
ORDER 4. DYSTHETICA. Cachexies.
Genus 1. PLETHORA. Plethora.
Species 1. P. entenica. Sanguineous plethora.
2. P. atonica. Serous plethora.
Genus 2. HÆMORRHAGIA. Hemorrhage.
Species 1. H. entonica. Entonic hæmorrhage.
2. H. atonica. Atonic hæmorrhage.
Genus 3. MARASMUS. Emaciation.
Species 1. M. atrophia. Atrophy.
2. M. climactericus. Decay of nature.
3. M. Tabes. Decline.
4. M. phthisis. Consumption
Genus 4. STRUMA. Scrofula.
Species 1. S. vulgaris. King's evil.
Genus 5. CARCINUS. Cancer.
Species 1. C. vulgaris. Common cancer.
Genus 6. LUES. Venereal disease.
Species 1. L. syphilis. Pox.
2. L. syphilodes. Bastard pox.
Genus 7. ELEPHANTIASIS. Elephant-skin.
Species 1. E. arabica. Arabian elephantiasis. Black leprosy.
2. E. italica. Italian elephantiasis.
3. E. asturiensis. Asturian elephantiasis.
Genus 8. CATACAUSIS. Catacausis.
Species 1. C. ebriosa. Enebriate catacausis.
Genus 9. PORPHYRA. Scurvy.
Species 1. P. simplex. Petechial scurvy.
2. P. hæmorrhagica. Land-scurvy.
3. P. nautica. Sea-scurvy.
Genus 10. EXANGIA. Exangia.
Species 1. E. aneurisma. Aneurism.
2. E. varix. Varix.
3. E. cyania. Blue-skin.
Genus 11. GANGRÆNA. Gangrene.
Species 1. G. sphacelus. Mortification.
2. G. ustilaginea. Mildew-mortification.
3. G. necrosis. Dry-gangrene.
4. G. caries. Caries.
Genus 12. ULCUS. Ulcer.
Species 1. U. incarnans. Simple healing ulcer.
2. U. vitiorum. Depraved ulcer.
3. U. sinuosum. Sinuous ulcer.
4. U. tuberculosum. Warty. Excrescent ulcer.
5. U. cariosum. Carious ulcer.
CLASS IV. NEUROTICA. *Diseases of the Nervous Function.*
ORDER 1. PHRENICA. Affecting the intellect.
Genus 1. ECPHRONIA. Insanity. Craziness.
Species 1. E. melancholia. Melancholy
2. E. mania. Madness.
Genus 2. EMPATHEMA. Ungovernable passion.
Species 1. E. entonicum. Empassioned excitement.
2. E. atonicum. Empassioned depression.
3. E. inane. Hair-brained passion.
Genus 3. ALUSIA. Illusion. Hallucination.
Species 1. A. elatio. Sentimentalism. Mental extravagance.
2. A. hypochondriasis. Hypochondrism. Low spiritedness.

Genus 4. APHLIXIA. Revery.
Species 1. A. socors. Absence of mind.
  2. A. intenda. Abstraction of mind.
  3. A. otiosa. Brown study.
Genus 5. PARONIRIA. Sleep-disturbance.
Species 1. P. ambulans. Sleep-walking.
  2. P. loquens. Sleep-talking.
  3. P. salax. Night pollution.
Genus 6. MORIA. Fatuity.
Species 1. M. imbecillis. Imbecility.
  2. M. demens. Irrationality.
ORDER 2. ÆSTHETICA. Affecting the sensation.
Genus 1. PAROPSIS. Morbid-sight.
Species 1. P. lucifuga. Night-sight.
  2. P. noctifuga. Day-sight.
  3. P. longinqua. Long-sight.
  4. P. propinqua. Short-sight.
  5. P. lateralis. Skew-sight.
  6. P. illusoria. False-sight.
  7. P. caligo. Opaque cornea.
  8. P. glaucosis. Humeral opacity.
  9. P. cataracta. Cataract.
  10. P. synizesis. Closed pupil.
  11. P. amaurosis. Drop serene.
  12. P. staphyloma. Protuberant eye.
  13. P. stabismus. Squinting.
Genus 2. PARACUSIS. Morbid hearing.
Species 1. P. acris. Acute hearing.
  2. P. obtusa. Hardness of hearing.
  3. P. perversa. Perverse hearing.
  4. P. duplicata. Double hearing.
  5. P. illusoria. Imaginary sounds.
  6. P. surditas. Deafness.
Genus 3. PAROSMIS. Morbid smell.
Species 1. P. acris. Acute smell.
  2. P. obtusa. Obtuse smell.
  3. P. expers. Want of smell.
Genus 4. PARAGEUSIS. Morbid taste.
Species 1. P. acute. Acute taste.
  2. P. obtusa. Obtuse taste.
  3. P. expers. Want of taste.
Genus 5. PARAPSIS. Morbid touch.
Species 1. P. acris. Acute sense of touch or general feeling.
  2. P. expers. Insensibility of touch or general feeling.
  3. P. illusoria. Illusory sense of touch or general feeling.
Genus 6. NEURALGIA. Nerve-ache.
Species 1. N. faciei. Nerve-ache of the face.
  2. N. pedis. Nerve-ache of the foot.
  3. N. mammæ. Nerve-ache of the breast.
ORDER 3. CINETICA. Affecting the muscles.
Genus 1. ENTASIA. Constrictive spasm.
Species 1. E priapismus. Priapism
  2. E. loxia. Wry neck.
  3. E. articularis. Muscular stiff-joint.
  4. E. systremma. Cramp.
  5. E. trismus. Hooked-jaw.
  6. E. tetanus. Tetanus.
  7. E. lyssa. Rabies. Canine madness.
  8. E. acrostimus. Suppressed pulse.
Genus 2. CLONICUS. Clonic spasm.
Species 1. C. singultus. Hiccough.
  2. C. sternutatio. Sneezing.
  3. Palpitatio. Palpitation.
  4. C. nectitatio. Wrinkling of the eyelids.
  5. C. subsultus. Twitching of the tendons.
  6. C. pandiculatio. Stretching.
Genus 3. SYNCLONUS. Synclonic spasm
Species 1. S. tremor. Trembling.
  2. S. chorea. St. Vitus's dance.
  3. S. ballismus. Shaking palsy.
  4. S. raphania. Raphania.
  5. S. beriberia. Barbiers.
ORDER 4. SYSTATICA. Affecting several, or all the sensorial powers, simultaneously.
Genus 1. AGRYPNIA. Sleeplessness.
Species 1. A. excitata. Irritative wakefulness.
  2. A. pertesa. Chronic wakefulness.
Genus 2. DYSPHORIA. Restlessness.
Species 1. D. simplex. Fidgets.
  2. D. anxietas. Anxiety.
Genus 3. ANTIPATHIA. Antipathy
Species 1. A. sensilis. Sensile antipathy.
  2. A. insensilis. Insensile antipathy.
Genus 4. CEPHALÆA. Headache

Species 1. C. gravans. Stupid headache.
  2. C. intensa. Chronic headache.
  3. C. hemicrania. Megrim.
  4. C. pulsatilis. Throbbing headache.
  5. C. nauseosa. Sick headache.
Genus 5. DINUS. Dizziness.
Species 1. D. vertigo. Vertigo.
Genus 6. SYNCOPE. Syncope.
Species 1. S. simplex. Swooning.
  2. S. recurrens. Fainting fit.
Genus 7. SYSPASIA. Comatose spasm.
Species 1. S. convulsio. Convulsion.
  2. S. hysteria. Hysterics.
  3. S. epilepsia. Epilepsy.
Genus 8. CARUS. Torpor.
Species 1. C. asphyxia. Asphyxy. Suspended animation.
  2. C. ecstasis. Ecstacy.
  3. C. catalepsia. Catalepsy.
  4. C. lethargus. Lethargy.
  5. C. apoplexia. Apoplexy.
  6. C. paralysis. Palsy.
CLASS V. GENETICA.—*Diseases of the Sexual Function.*
ORDER 1. CENOTICA. Affecting the fluids.
Genus 1. PARAMENIA. Mismenstruation.
Species 1. P. obstructionis. Obstructed menstruation.
  2. P. difficilis. Laborious menstruation.
  3. P. superflua. Excessive menstruation.
  4. P. erroris. Vicarious menstruation.
  5. P. cessationis. Irregular cessation of the menses.
Genus 2. LECORRHÆA. Whites.
Species 1. L. communis. Common whites.
  2. L. nabothi. Labour-show.
  3. L. senescentium. Whites of advaned life.
Genus 3. BLENORRHŒE. Gonorrhœa.
Species 1. B. simplex. Simple urethral running.
  2. B. luodes. Clap.
  3. B. chronica. Gleet.
Genus 4. SPERMORRHŒA. Seminal flux.
Species 1. S. entonica. Entonic seminal flux.
  2. S. atonica. Atonic seminal flux.
Genus 5. GALACTIA. Mislactation.
Species 1. G. præmatura. Premature milkflow.
  2. G. defectiva. Deficient milkflow.
  3. G. depravata. Depraved milkflow.
  4. G. erratica. Erratic milkflow.
  5. G. virorum. Milkflow in males.
ORDER 2. ORGASTICA. Affecting the orgasm.
Genus 1. CHLOROSIS. Green-sickness.
Species 1. C. entonica. Entonic green-sickness.
  2. C. atonica. Atonic green-sickness.
Genus 2. PROCOTIA. Genital precocity.
Species 1. P. masculina. Male precocity.
  2. P. feminina. Female precocity
Genus 3. LAGNESIS. Lust.
Species 1. L. salacitas. Salacity.
  2. L. furor. Lascivious madness.
Genus 4. AGENESIA. Male sterility.
Species 1. A. impotens. Male impotency.
  2. A. dyspermia. Seminal misemission.
  3. A. incongrua. Copulative incongruity.
Genus 5. AMPHORIA. Female sterility. Barrenness.
Species 1. A. impotens. Barrenness of impotency.
  2. A. paramenica. Barrenness of mismenstruation.
  3. A. impercita. Barrenness of irrespondence.
  4. A. incongrua. Barrenness of incongruity.
Genus 6. ÆDOPTOSIS. Genital prolapse.
Species 1. Æ. uteri. Falling down of the womb.
  2. Æ. vaginæ. Prolapse of the vagina.
  3. Æ. vesicæ. Prolapse of the bladder
  4. Æ. complicata. Complicated genita. prolapse.
  5. Æ. polyposa. Genital excrescence.
ORDER 3. CARPOTICA. Affecting the impregnation.
Genus 1. PARACYESIS. Morbid pregnancy.
Species 1. P. irritativa. Constitutional derangement of pregnancy.
  2. P. uterina. Local derangement of pregnancy.
  3. P. abortus. Abortion.
Genus 2. PARODYNIA. Morbid labour.
Species 1. P. atonica. Atonic labour.
  2. P. implastica. Unpliant labour.
  3. P. sympathetica. Complicated labour.

Species 4. P. perversa. Preternatura presentation.
5. P. amorphica. Impracticable labour.
6. P. pluralis. Multiplicate labour.
7. P. secundaria. Sequential labour.
Genus 3. **Eccyesis.** Extra-uterine fœtation.
Species 1. E. ovaria. Ovarian exfœtation.
2. E. tubalis. Tubal exfœtation.
3. E. abdominalis. Abdominal exfœtation.
Genus 4. **Pseudocyesis.** Spurious pregnancy.
Species 1. P. molaris. Mole.
2. P. inanis. False conception.

CLASS VI. ECCRITICA.—*Diseases of the Excernent Functions.*

Order 1. Mesotica. Affecting the parenchyma.
Genus 1. **Polysarchia.** Corpulency
Species 1. P. adiposa. Obesity.
Genus 2. **Emphyma.** Tumour.
Species 1 E. sarcoma. Sarcomatous tumour.
2. E. encystis. Encysted tumour.
3. E. exostosis. Bony tumour.
Genus 3. **Parostia.** Mis-ossification.
Species 1. P. fragilis. Fragility of the bones.
2. P. flexilis. Flexility of the bones.
Genus 4. **Cyrtosis.** Contortion of the bones.
Species 1. C. rhachia. Rickets.
2. C. cretinismus. Cretinismus.
Genus 5. **Osthexia.** Osthexy.
Species 1. O. infarciens. Parenchymatous orthexy.
2. O. implexa. Vascular osthexy.
Order 2. Catotica. Affecting internal surfaces.
Genus 1. **Hydrops.** Dropsy.
Species 1. H. cellularis. Cellular dropsy.
2. H. capitis. Dropsy of the head.
3. H. spinæ. Dropsy of the spine.
4. H. thoracis. Dropsy of the chest.
5. H. abdominis. Dropsy of the belly.
6. H. ovarii. Dropsy of the ovaries.
7. H. tubalis. Dropsy of the Fallopian tubes.
8. H. uteri. Dropsy of the womb.
9. H. scroti. Dropsy of the scrotum.
Genus 2. **Emphysema.** Inflation, wind dropsy.
Species 1. E. cellulare. Cellular inflation.
2. E. abdominis. Tympany.
Genus 3. **Paruria.** Mismicturition.
Species 1. P. inops. Destitution of urine.
2. P. retentionis. Stoppage of urine.
3. P. stillatitia. Strangury.
4. P. mellita. Saccharine urine. Diabetes.
5. P. incontinens. Incontinence of urine.
6. P. incocta. Unassimulated urine.
7. P. erratica. Erratic urine.
Genus 4. **Lithia.** Urinary calculus.
Species 1. L. renalis. Renal alculus.
2. L. vesicalis. Stone in the bladder.
Order 3. Acrotica. Affecting the external surface.
Genus 1. **Ephidrosis.** Morbid sweat.
Species 1. E. profusa. Profuse sweat.
2. E. cruenta. Bloody sweat.
3. E. partialis. Partial sweat.
4. E. discolor. Coloured sweat.
5. E. olens. Scented sweat.
6. E. arenosa. Sandy sweat.
Genus 2. **Exanthesis.** Cutaneous-blush.
Species 1. E. rescola. Rose-rash.
Genus 3. **Exormia.** Papulous skin.
Species 1. E. strophulus. Gum-rash.
2. E. lichen. Lichenous-rash.
3. E. prurigo. Pruriginous-rash.
4. E. milium. Millet-rash.
Genus 4. **Lepidosis.** Scale-skin.
Species 1. L. pityriasis. Dandrift.
2. L. lepriasis. Leprosy.
3. L. psoriasis. Dry-scall.
4. L. icthyiasis. Fish-skin.
Genus 5. **Ecphlysis.** Blains.
Species 1. E. pompholyx Water-blebs.
2. E. herpes. Tetter.
3. E. rhypea. Sordid blain.
4. E. eczema. Heat eruption.
Genus 6. **Ecpyesis.** Humid scall.
Species 1. E. impetigo. Running scall.
2. E. porrigo. Scabby scall.
3. E. ecthyma. Papulous scall.
4. E. scabies. Itch.
Genus 7. **Malis.** Cutaneous vermination
Species 1. M. pediculi. Lousiness.
2. M. pulicis Flea-bites.

Species 3. M. acari. Tick-bite.
4. M. filatiæ. Guinea-worm.
5. M. œstri. Gadfly-bite.
6. M. gordii. Hair-worm.
Genus 8. **Ecphyma.** Cutaneous excrescence.
Species 1. E. caruncula. Caruncle.
2. E. verruca. Wart.
3. E. clavus. Corn.
4. E. callus. Callus.
Genus 9. **Trichosis.** Morbid hair.
Species 1. T. setosa. Bristly hair.
2. T. plica. Platted hair.
3. T. hirsuties. Extraneous hair.
4. T. distrix. Forky hair.
5. T. poliosis. Gray hairs.
6. T. arthrix. Baldness.
7. T. area. Areated hair.
8. T. decolor. Miscoloured hair.
Genus 10. **Epichrosis.** Macular skin.
Species 1. E. leucasmus. Veal-skin.
2. E. spilus. Mole.
3. E. lenticula. Freckles.
4. E. ephelis. Sun-burn.
5. E. aurigo. Orange-skin.
6. E. pœcilia. Pyeballed-skin.
7. E. alphosis. Albino-skin.

NOSTA'LGIA. (From *νοϛεω*, to return, and *αλγος*, pain.) A vehement desire for revisiting one's country. A genus of disease in the class *Locales,* and order *Dysorexiæ,* of Cullen, known by impatience when absent from one's native home, and a vehement desire to return, attended with gloom and melancholy, loss of appetite, and want of sleep.

NOSTRUM. This word means *our own,* and is very significantly applied to all quack medicines, the composition of which is kept a secret from the public, and known only to the inventor.

Notched leaf. See *Erosus.*
NO'THUS. (Νοθος, spurious.) Spurious. 1. Those ribs which are not attached to the sternum are called *costæ nothæ,* the spurious ribs.

2. Diseases so called which only resemble others which they really are not: as *peripneumonia notha,* &c.
NOTIÆ'US. (From *νωτον,* the back.) An epithet of the spinal marrow.
NOTIO'DES. (From *νοτις,* moisture.) Applied to a fever, attended with a vitiation of the fluids, or a colliquative wasting.
NOVACULITE. See *Whetslate.*
NUBE'CULA. (Dim. of *nubes,* a cloud.) A little cloud. 1. A cloud in the urine.

2. A white speck in the eye.
NUCAMENTUM. See *Amentum.*
NUCES GALLÆ. Common galls.
NUCES PURGANTES. See *Ricinus.*
NUCESTA. See *Myristica moschata.*
NU'CHA. *Nucha capitis.* The hind part or nape of the neck. The part is so called where the spinal marrow begins.
NUCI'STA. The nutmeg.
NUCK, **Anthony,** a distinguished Dutch physician and anatomist, flourished at the Hague, and subsequently at Leyden, in the latter part of the 17th century. He filled the office of professor of anatomy and surgery in the latter university, and was also president of the college of surgeons. He pursued his dissections with great ardour, cultivating both human and comparative anatomy at every opportunity. He contributed some improvements also to the practice of surgery. He died about the year 1692.
NU'CLEUS. (*E nuce,* from the nut.) 1. A kernel or fruit enclosed in a hard shell.

2. When the centre of a tumour or morbid concretion, as a stone of the bladder, has an obvious difference from the surrounding parts, that is called the nucleus: thus a cherry-stone and other things have been found in calculi of the bladder, forming the nucleus of that concretion.
NU'CULÆ SAPONA'RIÆ. See *Sapindus saponaria.*
NUDUS. Naked. Applied to flowers, leaves, stems, receptacles, seeds, &c. of plants. A flower is said to be naked when the calyx is wanting, as in the tulip, and white lily; and a leaf when it is destitute of all kinds of clothing or hairiness, as in the genus *orchis :* the stem is naked that bears no leaves, scales, or any other vesture, as *Cuscuta europea:* the receptacle of the *Leontodon taraxacum* and *Lactuca,* the seeds of the gymnospermal plants, &c.

NUMMULA'RIA. (From *nummus*, money: so called because its leaves are round, and of the size of the old silver twopence.) See *Lysimachia nummularia.*

NUT. See *Nux.*

Nut, Barbadoes. See *Jatropha curcas.*

Nut, cocoa. See *Cocos nucifera.*

Nut, Pistachia. See *Pistacia vera.*

Nut, purging. See *Jatropha curcas.*

NUTMEG. See *Myristica moschata.*

NUTRITION. *Nutritio.* Nutrition may be considered the completion of the assimilating functions. The food changed by a series of decompositions animalized and rendered similar to the being which it is designed to nourish, applies itself to those organs, the loss of which it is to supply; and this identification of nutritive matter to our organs constitutes nutrition.

The living body is continually losing its constituent parts.

"From the state of the embryo to the most advanced old age, the weight and volume of the body are almost continually changing; the different organs and tissues present infinite variations in their consistence, colour, elasticity, and sometimes their chemical composition. The volume of the organs augments when they are often in action; on the contrary, their size diminishes when they remain long at rest. By the influence of one or other of these causes, their chemical and physical properties present remarkable variations. Many diseases often produce in a very short time, remarkable changes in the exterior conformation, and in the structure of a great number of organs.

If madder is mixed with the food of an animal, in fifteen or twenty days the bones present a red tint, which disappears when the use of it is left off.

There exists, then, in the organs, an insensible motion of the particles which produce all these modifications. It is this that is called *nutrition,* or *nutritive action.*

This phenomenon, which the observing spirit of the ancients had not permitted to escape, was to them the object of many ingenious suppositions that are still admitted. For example, it is said that, by means of the nutritive action, the whole body is renewed, so that, at a certain period, it does not possess a single particle of the matter that composed it formerly. Limits have even been assigned to this total renewal: some have fixed the period of three years; others think it not complete till seven: but there is nothing to give probability to these conjectures; on the contrary, certain well-proved facts seem to render them of no avail.

It is well known that soldiers, sailors, and several savage people colour their skins with substances which they introduce into the tissue of this membrane itself: the figures thus traced preserve their form and colour during their lives, should no particular circumstances occur. How can this phenomenon agree with the renewal of the skin according to these authors? The recent use of nitrate of silver internally, in the cure of epilepsy, furnishes a new proof of this kind. After some months' use of this substance, some sick persons have had their skin coloured of a grayish blue, probably by a deposition of the salt in the tissue of this membrane, where it is immediately in contact with the air. Several individuals have been in this state for some years without the tint becoming weaker; while in others it has diminished by degrees, and disappeared in two or three years.

In resting on the suppositions which we have spoken, it is admitted, in the metaphorical language now used in physiology, that the atoms of the organs can only serve for a certain period in their composition; that in time they *wear,* and become at last improper to enter into their composition; and that they are then absorbed and replaced by new atoms proceeding from the food.

It is added, that the animal matters of which our excretions are composed are the *detritus* of the organs, and that they are principally composed of atoms that can no longer serve in their composition, &c. &c.

Instead of discussing these hypotheses, we shall mention a few facts from which we have some idea of the nutritive movement.

A. In respect to the rapidity with which the organs change their physical and chemical properties by sickness or age, it appears that nutrition is more or less rapid according to the tissues. The glands, the muscles, the skin, &c., change their volume, colour, consistence, with great quickness the tendons, the fibrous

membranes, the bones, the cartilages, appear to have a much slower nutrition, for their physical properties change but slowly by the effect of age and disease.

B. If we consider the quantity of food consumed proportionably to the weight of the body, the nutritive movement seems more rapid in infancy and youth, than in the adult and in old age; it is accelerated by the repeated action of the organs, and retarded by repose. Indeed, children and young people consume more food than adults and old people: these last can preserve all their faculties by the use of a very small quantity of food. All the exercises of the body, hard labour, require necessarily a greater quantity, or more nutritive food; on the contrary, perfect repose permits of longer abstinence.

C. The blood appears to contain most of the principles necessary to the nutrition of the organs; the fibrine, the albumen, the fat, the salts, &c., that enter into the composition of the tissues, are found in the blood. They appear to be deposited in their parenchyma at the instant when the blood traverses them; the manner in which this deposite takes place is entirely unknown. There is an evident relation between the activity of the nutrition of an organ and the quantity of blood it receives. The tissues that have a rapid nutrition have larger arteries; when the action of an organ has determined an acceleration of its nutrition, the arteries increase in size.

Many proximate principles that enter into the composition of the organs are not found in the blood: as osmazome, the cerebral matter, gelatine, &c. They are, therefore, formed from other principles in the parenchyma of the organs, in some chemical but unknown manner

D. Since chemical analysis has made known the nature of the different tissues of the animal economy, they have been all found to contain a considerable portion of azote. Our food being also partly composed of this simple body, the azote of our organs likewise probably comes from them; but several eminent authors think that it is derived from respiration; others believe that it is formed by the influence of life solely. Both parties insist particularly upon the example of the herbivorous animals, which are supported exclusively upon non-azotized matter; upon the history of certain people that live entirely upon rice and maize; upon that of negroes who can live a long time without eating any thing but sugar; lastly, upon what is related of *caravans,* which, in traversing the deserts, have for a long time had only gum in place of every sort of food. Were it indeed proved by these facts, that men can live a long time without azotized food, it would be necessary to acknowledge that azote has an origin different from the food; but the facts cited by no means prove this. In fact, almost all the vegetables upon which man and the animals feed contain more or less azote; for example, the impure sugar that the negroes eat presents a considerable portion of it; and with regard to the people, as they say, who feed upon rice or maize, it is well known that they eat milk or cheese: now *casein* is the most azotized of all the nutritive proximate principles.

E. A considerable number of tissues in the economy appear to have no nutrition, properly so called: as the epidermis, the nails, the hair, the teeth, the colouring matter of the skin, and, perhaps, the cartilages.

These different parts are really secreted, by particular organs, as the teeth and the hair; or by parts which have other functions at the same time, as the nails and epidermis. The most of the parts formed in this mode wear by the friction of exterior bodies, and are constantly renewed if they are entirely carried away, they are capable of reproduction. A very singular fact is, that they continue to grow several days after death.—*Magendie's Physiology.*

NUTRI'TUM UNGUENTUM. A composition of litharge, vinegar, and oil.

NUX. (*Nux, cis.* f.) A nut, or fruit, which has a hard shell.

Botanists consider this as distinct from the drupa, and define it a pericarp, the seed being contained in a hard bony shell.

From the number of seeds it contains, it is called,

1. *Monosperm,* having one; as in *Corylus avellana.*

2. *Disperm,* with two; as in *Halesia.*

From its loculaments:

1. *Unilocular, bilocular, trilocular*, with one, two, or three; as in *Corylus, Lygeum*, and *Elais*.

From its figure:

1. *Alate*, winged; as in *Pinus thuja*.
2. *Angulate*; as in *Cypressus*.
3. *Ovate*; as in *Corylus* and *Carpinus*.
4. *Quadrangular*; as in *Halesia*.
5. *Tetragone*; as in *Peladium* and *Mesua*.
6. *Reniform*; as in *Anacardium*.
7. *Spinous*; as in *Trapa natans*.

NUX AQUATICA. See *Trapa natans*.
NUX AROMATICA. The nutmeg.
NUX BARBADENSIS. See *Jatropha curcas*.
NUX BASILICA. The walnut.
NUX BEN. See *Guilandina moringa*.
NUX CATHARTICA. The garden spurge.
NUX CATHARTICA AMERICANA. See *Jatropha curcas*.
NUX INDICA. The cocoa-nut.
NUX JUGLANS. See *Juglans*.
NUX MEDICA. The maldivian nut.
NUX METELLA. The nux vomica.
NUX MOSCHATA. See *Myrystica moschata*.
NUX MYRISTICA. See *Myristica moschata*.
NUX PERSICA. The walnut.
NUX PISTACIA. See *Pistacia vera*.
NUX PURGANS. See *Jatropha curcas*.
NUX SERAPIONIS. St. Ignatius's bean.
NUX VOMICA. See *Strychnos*.

NYCTALO'PIA. (From νυξ, the night, and ωψ, an eye.) *Imbecillitas oculorum*, of Celsus. A defect in vision, by which the patient sees little or nothing in the day, but in the evening and night sees tolerably well. The proximate cause is various:

1. From a periodical amaurosis, or gutta serena, when the blind paroxysm begins in the morning and terminates in the evening.

2. From too great a sensibility of the retina, which cannot bear the meridian light. See *Photophobia*.

3. From an opaque spot in the middle of the crystalline lens. When the light of the sun in the meridian contracts the pupil, there is blindness: about evening, or in more obscure places, the pupil dilates, hence the rays of light pass through the limbus of the crystalline lens.

4. From a disuse of light; thus persons who are educated in obscure prisons see nothing immediately in open meridian light; but by degrees their eyes are accustomed to distinguish objects in daylight.

5. From an immoveable mydriasis; for in this instance the pupil admits too great a quantity of light, which the immobile pupil cannot moderate; hence the patient, in a strong light, sees little or nothing.

6. From too great a contraction of the pupil. This admits not a sufficiency of lucid rays, in bright light, but towards night the pupil dilates more, and the patient sees better.

7. *Nyctalopia endemica*. A whole people have been nyctalopes, as the Æthiopians, Africans, Americans, and Asiatics. A great flow of tears are excreted all the day from their eyes; at night they see objects.

8. From a commotion of the eye; from which a man in the night saw all objects distinctly.

NYCTO'BASIS. (From νυξ, the night, and βαινω, to go.) Walking in the sleep.

NY'MPHA. (From νυμφα, a water-nymph: so called because it stands in the water-course.) *Alæ internæ minores clitoridis; Colliculum; Collicula; Myrtocheilides; Labia minora*. The membranous fold, situated within the labia majora, on each side of the entrance of the vagina uteri.

NYMPHÆ'A. (From νυμφα, a water-nymph; because it grows in watery places.) The name of a genus of plants in the Linnæan system. Class, *Polyandria*; Order, *Monogynia*. The water-lily.

NYMPHÆA ALBA. *Leuconymphæa. Nenuphar. Micro-leuconymphæa*. The systematic name of the white water-lily. This beautiful plant was formerly employed medicinally as a demulcent, and slightly anodyne remedy. It is now laid aside.

NYMPHÆA GLANDIFERA. See *Nymphæa nelumbo*.

NYMPHÆA LOTUS. The Egyptian lotus. An aquatic plant, a native of both Indies. The root is conical, firm, about the size of a middling pear, covered with a blackish bark, and set round with fibres. It has a sweetish taste, and, when boiled or roasted, becomes as yellow within as the yelk of an egg. The plant grows in abundance on the banks of the Nile, and is there much sought after by the poor, who, in a short time, collect enough to supply their families with food for several days.

NYMPHÆA LUTEA. *Nymphæa major lutea*, of Caspar Bauhin. The systematic name of the yellow water-lily. This beautiful plant was employed formerly with the same intention as the white water-lily and, like it, is now fallen into disuse. Lindestolpe informs us, that, in some parts of Sweden, the roots, which are the strongest part, were, in times of scarcity, used as food, and did not prove unwholesome.

NYMPHÆA NELUMBO. *Faba ægyptiaca; Cyamus ægyptiacus; Nymphæa indica; Nymphæa glandifera*. The pontic, or Egyptian bean. This plant grows on marshy grounds in Egypt, and some of the neighbouring countries. The fruit is eaten either raw or boiled, and is a tonic and astringent.

NYMPHOI'DES. (From νυμφαια, the water-lily, and ειδος, likeness.) Resembling the water-lily; as *Menyanthes nymphoides*.

NYMPHOMA'NIA. (From νυμφα, nympha, and μανια, madness.) *Furor uterinus*. Called by the Arabians, *Acrai; Brachuna; Arascon; Arsatum; Œstromania*. A genus of disease in the class *Locales*, and order *Dysorexiæ*, of Cullen, characterized by excessive and violent desire for coition in women. The effects, as described by Juvenal, in his sixth satire, are most humiliating to human nature. It acknowledges the same causes as satyriasis; but as females, more especially in warm climates, have a more irritable fibre, they are apt to suffer more severely than the males.

It is a species of madness, or a high degree of hysterics. Its immediate cause is a preternatural irritability of the uterus and pudenda of women, or an unusual acrimony of the fluids in these parts. Its presence is known by the wanton behaviour of the patient; she speaks and acts with unrestrained obscenity, and, as the disorder increases, she scolds, cries, and laughs, by turns. While reason is retained, she is silent, and seems melancholy, but her eyes discover an unusual wantonness. The symptoms are better or worse, until the greatest degree of the disorder approaches, and then, by every word and action, her condition is too manifest.

NYMPHOTOMIA. (From νυμφα, the nympha, and τεμνω, to cut.) The operation of removing the nympha when too large.

NYSTA'GMUS. (From νυςαω, to sleep.) A twinkling of the eyes, such as happens when a person is very sleepy. Authors also define nystagmus to be an involuntary agitation of the oculary bulb. It is known by the instability or involuntary and constant motions of the globe of the eye, from one canthus to another, or in some other directions. Sometimes it is accompanied with a hippus, or an alternate and repeated dilatation and constriction of the pupil. The species are, 1. Nystagmus, from fear. This agitation is observed under the operation for the cataract; and it is checked by persuasion, and waiting a short space of time. 2. Nystagmus, from sand or small gravel falling in the eye. 3. Nystagmus, from a catarrh, which is accompanied with much inflammation. 4. Nystagmus, from saburra in the primæ viæ, as is observed in infants afflicted with worms, and is known by the signs of saburra. 5. Nystagmus symptomaticus, which happens in hysteric, epileptic, and sometimes in pregnant persons, and is a common symptom accompanying St. Vitus's dance.

O

OAK. See *Quercus*.

Oak, Jerusalem. See *Chenopodium botrys*.

Oak, sea. See *Fucus vesiculosus*.

Oak, willow-leaved. See *Quercus phellos*.

[*Oaks, American.* See *Quercus.* A.]

OAT. See *Avena*.

OBELÆ′A. (From οβελος, a dart, or a spit.) *Obelæa sagittalis,* an epithet for the sagittal suture of the skull.

OBELISCOTHE′CA. (From οβελισκος, an obelisk, and θηκα, a bag: so called from the shape of its seed-bags.) The dwarf sunflower. *Cystus helianthemum.*

OBESITY. See *Polysarcia.*

OBLESION. (From *ob,* against, and *lædo,* to hurt.) An injury done to any part.

OBLI′QUUS. Oblique. 1. In anatomy. A term applied to parts from their direction.

2. In botany, it means the same as *radix obliquus,* but sometimes it means twisted. *Folium obliquum,* for example, is a leaf, one part of which is vertical, the other horizontal ; as in *Fritillaria obliqua.*

OBLIQUUS ASCENDENS ABDOMINIS. See *Obliquus internus abdominis.*

OBLIQUUS ASCENDENS INTERNUS. See *obliquus internus abdominis.*

OBLIQUUS AURIS. See *Laxator tympani.*

OBLIQUUS CAPITIS INFERIOR. See *Obliquus inferior capitis.*

OBLIQUUS CAPITIS SUPERIOR. See *Obliquus superior capitis.*

OBLIQUUS DESCENDENS ABDOMINIS. See *Obliquus externus abdominis.*

OBLIQUUS DESCENDENS EXTERNUS. See *Obliquus externis abdominis.*

OBLIQUUS EXTERNUS. See *Obliquus externus abdominis.*

OBLIQUUS EXTERNUS ABDOMINIS. A muscle of the abdomen: so named by Morgagni, Albinus, and Winslow. It is the *Obliquus descendens* of Vesalius and Douglas, and the *Obliquus major* of Haller, and some others. By Dumas it is named *Ilio-pubicosto-abdominal.* It is a broad, thin muscle, fleshy posteriorly, and tendinous in the middle and lower part, and is situated immediately under the integuments, covering all the other muscles of the lower belly. It arises from the lower edges of the eight, and sometimes, though rarely, of the nine inferior ribs, not far from their cartilages, by as many distinct fleshy portions, which indigitate with corresponding parts of the serratus major anticus, and the latissimus dorsi. From these several origins, the fibres of the muscle descend obliquely forwards, and soon degenerate into a broad and thin aponeurosis, which terminates in the linea alba. About an inch and a half above the pubes, the fibres of this aponeurosis separate from each other, so as to form an aperture, which extends obliquely inwards and forwards, more than an inch in length, and is wider above than below, being nearly of an oval figure. This is what is sometimes, though erroneously, called the *ring* of the abdominal muscles, *annulus abdominis,* for it belongs only to the external oblique, there being no such opening either in the obliquus internus, or in the transversalis, as some writers, and particularly Douglas and Cheselden, would give us to understand. This opening, or ring, serves for the passage of the spermatic vessels in men, and of the round ligament of the uterus in women, and is of a larger size in the former than in the latter. The two tendinous portions, which, by their separation, form this aperture, are called the *columns* of the ring. The anterior, superior, and inner column, which is the broadest and thickest of the two, passes over the symphysis pubis, and is fixed to the opposite os pubis; so that the anterior column of the right obliquus externus intersects that of the left, and is, as it were, interwoven with it, by which means their insertion is strengthened, and their attachment made firmer. The posterior, inferior, and exterior column, approaches the anterior one as it descends, and is fixed behind and below it to the os pubis of the same side. The fibres of that part of the

obliquus externus, which arises from the two inferior ribs, descend almost perpendicularly, and are inserted, tendinous and fleshy, into the outer edge of the anterior half of the spine of the ilium. From the anterior superior spinous process of that bone, the external oblique is stretched tendinous to the os pubis, forming what is called *Poupart's* and sometimes *Fallopius's* ligament, Fallopius having first described it. Winslow, and many others, name it the *inguinal* ligament. But, after all, it has no claim to this name, it being nothing more than the tendon of the muscle, which is turned or folded inwards at its interior edge. It passes over the blood-vessels of the lower extremity, and is thickest near the pelvis; and in women, from the greater size of the pelvis, it is longer and looser than in men. Hence we find that women are most liable to crural herniæ; whereas men, from the greater size of the ring of the external oblique, are most subject to the inguinal. From this ligament, and from that part of the tendon which forms the ring, we observe a detachment of tendinous fibres, which are lost in the *fascia lata* of the thigh. This may, in some measure, account for the pain which, in cases of strangulated herniæ, is felt when the patient stands upright, and which is constantly relieved upon bending the thigh upwards. This muscle serves to draw down the ribs in expiration; to bend the trunk forwards when both muscles act, or to bend it obliquely in one side, and, perhaps, to turn it slightly upon its axis, when either acts singly; it also raises the pelvis obliquely when the ribs are fixed; it supports and compresses the abdominal viscera, assists in the evacuation of the urine and fæces, and is likewise useful in parturition.

OBLIQUUS INFERIOR. See *Obliquus inferior capitis,* and *Obliquus inferior oculi.*

OBLIQUUS INFERIOR CAPITIS. This muscle of the head, the *obliquus inferior sive major,* of Winslow, and the *Spini axoido-tracheli-altoidien,* of Dumas, is larger than the obliquus superior capitis. It is very obliquely situated between the two first vetebræ of the neck. It arises tendinous and fleshy from the middle and outer side of the spinous process of the second vertebra of the neck, and is inserted tendinous and fleshy into the lower and posterior part of the transverse process of the first vertebra. Its use is to turn the first vertebra upon the second, as upon a pivot, and to draw the face towards the shoulder.

OBLIQUUS INFERIOR OCULI. *Obliquus minor oculi,* of Winslow, and *Maxillo, scleroticien,* of Dumas. An oblique muscle of the eye, that draws the globe of the eye forwards, inwards, and downwards. It arises by a narrow beginning from the outer edge of the orbitar process of the superior maxillary bone, near its junction with the lachrymal bone, and running obliquely outwards, is inserted into the sclerotic membrane of the eye.

OBLIQUUS INFERIOR SIVE MAJOR. See *Obliquus inferior capitis.*

OBLIQUUS INTERNUS. See *Obliquus internus abdominis.*

OBLIQUUS INTERNUS ABDOMINIS. *Musculus acclivis.* A muscle of the abdomen. The *Obliquus ascendens,* of Vesalius, Douglas, and Cowper; the *Obliquus minor,* of Haller; the *Obliquus internus,* of Winslow ; the *Obliquus ascendens internus,* of Innes; and the *Iliolumbo-costi abdominal,* of Dumas. It is situated immediately under the external oblique, and is broad and thin like that muscle, but somewhat less considerable in its extent. It arises from the spinous processes of the three inferior lumbar vertebræ, and from the posterior and middle part of the os sacrum, by a thin tendinous expansion, which is common to it and to the serratus posticus inferior; by short tendinous fibres, from the whole spine of the ilium, between its posterior tuberosity and its anterior and superior spinous process; and from two-thirds of the posterior surface of what is called Fallopius's ligament, at the middle of which we find the round ligament of the uterus in women, and the spermatic vessels in men, passing under the thir edge of this muscle; and in the latter, it likewise sends off some fibres, which descend upon the spermatic chord, as far as the tunica vaginalis of the testis, and constitute what is called the *cremaster* muscle, which surrounds, suspends, and compresses the testicle. From these origins, the fibres of the internal oblique run in different directions; those of the posterior portion ascend obliquely forwards, the middle ones become less and less oblique, and at length run in a horizontal direction, and those of the anterior portion extend obliquely downwards. The first of these are inserted, by very short tendinous fibres, into the cartilages of the fifth, fourth, and third of the false ribs; the fibres of the second, or middle portion, form a broad tendon, which, after being inserted into the lower edge of the cartilage of the second false rib, extends towards the linea alba, and separates into two layers; the anterior layer, which is the thickest of the two, joins the tendon of the obliquus externus, and runs over the two upper thirds of the rectus muscle, to be inserted into the linea alba; the posterior layer runs under the rectus, adheres to the anterior surface of the tendon of the transversalis, and is inserted into the cartilages of the first of the false, and the last of the true ribs, and likewise into the linea alba. By this structure we may perceive that the greater part of the rectus is enclosed, as it were, in a sheath. The fibres of the anterior portion of the internal oblique, or those which arise from the spine of the ilium and the ligamentum Fallopii, likewise form a broad tendon, which, instead of separating into two layers, like that of the other part of the muscle, runs over the lower part of the rectus, and adhering to the under surface of the tendon of the external oblique, is inserted into the forepart of the pubes. This muscle serves to assist the obliquus externus; but it seems to be more evidently calculated than that muscle is to draw the ribs downwards and backwards. It likewise serves to separate the false ribs from the true ribs, and from each other.

OBLIQUUS MAJOR ABDOMINIS. See *Obliquus externus abdominis.*

OBLIQUUS MAJOR CAPITIS. See *Obliquus inferior capitis.*

OBLIQUUS MAJOR OCULI. See *Obliquus superior oculi.*

OBLIQUUS MINOR ABDOMINIS. See *Obliquus internus abdominis.*

OBLIQUUS MINOR CAPITIS. See *Obliquus superior capitis.*

OBLIQUUS MINOR OCULI. See *Obliquus inferior oculi.*

OBLIQUUS SUPERIOR CAPITIS. Riolanus, who was the first that gave particular names to the oblique muscles of the head, called this muscle *obliquus minor,* to distinguish it from the inferior, which, on account of its being much larger, he named *obliquus major.* Spigelius afterward distinguished the two, from their situation with respect to each other, into *superior* and *inferior;* and in this he is followed by Cowper and Douglas. Winslow retains both names. Dumas calls it *Trachelo-altoido-occipital.* That used by Albinus is here adopted. This little muscle, which is nearly of the same shape as the *recti capitis,* is situated laterally between the occiput and the first vertebra of the neck, and is covered by the complexus and the upper part of the splenius. It arises, by a short thick tendon, from the upper and posterior part of the transverse process of the first vertebra of the neck, and, ascending obliquely inwards and backwards, becomes broader, and is inserted, by a broad flat tendon, and some few fleshy fibres, into the os occipitis, behind the back part of the mastoid process, under the insertion of the complexus and splenius, and a little above that of the rectus major. The use of this muscle is to draw the head backwards, and perhaps to assist in its rotatory motion.

OBLIQUUS SUPERIOR OCULI. *Trochlearis; Longissimus oculi. Obliquus major,* of Winslow; and *Optico-trochlei-scleroticien,* of Dumas. An oblique muscle of the eye, that rolls the globe of the eye, and turns the pupil downwards and outwards. It arises like the straight muscles of the eye from the edge of the foramen opticum at the bottom of the orbit, between the rectus superior and rectus internus; from thence runs straight along the papyraceous portion of the ethmoid bone to the upper part of the orbit, where a cartilaginous trochlea is fixed to the inside of the internal angular process of the os frontis, through which its tendon passes, and runs a little downwards and out-

wards, enclosed in a loose membranaceous sheath, to be inserted into the sclerotic membrane.

OBLIQUUS SUPERIOR SIVE MINOR. See *Obliquus superior capitis.*

OBLIQUUS SUPERIOR SIVE TROCHLEARIS. See *Obliquus superior oculi.*

OBLONGUS. In botany applied to leaves, petals, seeds, &c. which are three or four times longer than broad. This term is used with great latitude, and serves chiefly in a specific character to contrast a leaf, which has a variable, or not very decided form, with others that are precisely round, ovate, linear, &c.

The *petals* of the genus Citrus and Hedera, and those of the Narcissus moschatus, are *oblong,* and the *seeds* of the Boerhaavia diffusa.

OBOVATUS. Obovate. Used in botany to designate leaves, &c. which are ovate with a broader end uppermost: as those of the primrose and daisy. Linnæus at first used the words *obversi ovatum.*

OBSIDIAN. A mineral, of which there are two kinds, the translucent and transparent.

1. The *translucent obsidian.* This is of a velvet black colour, and occurs in beds in porphyry and various secondary trap rocks in Iceland and Tokay.

2. The transparent is of a duck-blue colour, imbedded in pearl-stone porphyry in Siberia and Mexico.

OBSIDIA'NUM. (So called from its resemblance to a kind of stone, which one Obsidius discovered in Ethiopia, of a very black colour, though sometimes pellucid, and of a muddy water.) 1. A species of glass. See *Obsidian.*

2. Pliny says that *obsidianum* was a sort of colour with which vessels were glazed. Hence the name is applied, by Libavius, to glass of antimony.

OBSTETRIC. (*Obstetricus:* from *obstetrix,* a nurse.) Belonging to midwifery.

OBSTIPA'TIO. (From *obstipo,* to stop up.) Costiveness. A genus of disease in the class *Locales,* and order *Epischeses* of Cullen, comprehending three species:

1. *Obstipatio debilium,* in weak and commonly dyspeptic persons.

2. *Obstipatio rigidorum,* in persons of rigid fibres, and a melancholic temperament.

3. *Obstipatio obstructorum.* from obstructions. See *Colica.*

OBSTRUE'NOA. (From *obstruo,* to shut up.) Whatever closes the orifices of the ducts or vessels.

OBSTUPEFACIE'NTIA. (From *obstupefacio,* to stupefy.) Narcotics.

OBTUNDE'NTIA. (From *obtundo,* to make blunt.) Substances which sheath or blunt irritation, and are much the same as demulcents. They consist chiefly of bland, oily, or mucilaginous matters, which form a covering on inflamed and irritable surfaces, particularly those of the stomach, lungs, and anus.

OBTURA'TOR. A stopper up, or that which covers any thing.

OBTURATOR EXTERNUS. *Extra-pelvio-pubi-trochanterien,* of Dumas. This is a small flat muscle, situated obliquely at the upper and anterior part of the thigh, between the pectinalis and the forepart of the foramen thyroideum, and covered by the abductor brevis femoris. It arises tendinous and fleshy from all the inner half of the circumference of the foramen thyroideum, and likewise from part of the obturator ligament. Its radiated fibres collect and form a strong roundish tendon, which runs outwards, and, after adhering to the capsular ligament of the joint, is inserted into a cavity at the inner and back part of the root of the great trochanter. The chief uses of this muscle are to turn the thigh obliquely outwards, to assist in bending the thigh, and in drawing it inwards. It likewise prevents the capsular ligament from being pinched in the motions of the joint.

OBTURATOR INTERNUS. *Marsupialis, seu obturator internus,* of Douglas. *Marsupialis seu bursalis,* of Cowper; and *Intrapelvio-trochanterien,* of Dumas. A considerable muscle, a great part of which is situated within the pelvis. It arises, by very short tendinous fibres, from somewhat more than the upper half of the internal circumference of the foramen thyroideum of the os innominatum. It is composed of several distinct fasciculi, which terminate in a roundish tendon that passes out of the pelvis, through the niche that is between the spine and the tuberosity of the ischium, and, after running between the two portions of the gemini, which enclose it as in a sheath, is inserted

127

into the cavity at the root of the great trochanter, after adhering to the adjacent part of the capsular ligament of the joint. This muscle rolls the os femoris obliquely outwards, by pulling it towards the ischiatic niche, upon the cartilaginous surface of which its tendon, which is surrounded by a membraneous sheath, moves as upon a pulley.

OBTURATOR NERVE. A nerve of the thigh, that is lost upon the muscles situated on the inside of the thigh.

OBTUSUS. Blunt. Applied to a leaf which terminates in a segment of a circle; as that of the *Linum catharticum*. This formed leaf has a small point *obtusum cum acumine*, in the *Statyce limonium*. The petals of the *Tropæolum majus* are obtuse.

OCCIPITAL. *Occipitalis.* Belonging to the occiput or back part of the head.

OCCIPITAL BONE. *Os occipitis; Os memoriæ; Os nervosum; Os basilare.* This bone, which forms the posterior and inferior part of the skull, is of an irregular figure, convex on the outside and concave internally. Its external surface, which is very irregular, serves for the attachment of several muscles. It affords several inequalities, which sometimes form two semicircular hollows separated by a scabrous ridge. The inferior portion of the bone is stretched forwards in form of a wedge, and hence is called the *cuneiform* process, or basilary process. At the base of this process, situated obliquely on each side of the foramen magnum, are two flat, oblong protuberances, named *condyles.* They are covered with cartilage, and serve for the articulation of the head with the first vertebra of the neck. In the inferior portion of this bone, at the basis of the cranium, and immediately behind the cuneiform process, we observe a considerable hole, through which the medulla oblongata passes into the spine. The nervi accessorii, the vertebral arteries, and sometimes the vertebral veins likewise, pass through it. Man being designed for an erect posture, this foramen magnum is found nearly in the middle of the basis of the human cranium, and at a pretty equal distance from the posterior part of the occiput, and the anterior part of the lower jaw; whereas in quadrupeds it is nearer the back part of the occiput. Besides this hole, there are four other smaller foramina, viz. two before, and two behind the condyles. The former serve for the transmission of the ninth pair of nerves, and the two latter for the veins which pass from the external parts of the head to the lateral sinuses. On looking over the internal surface of the os occipitis, we perceive the appearance of a cross, formed by a very prominent ridge, which rises upwards from near the foramen magnum, and by two transverse sinuosities, one on each side of the ridge. This cross occasions the formation of four fossæ, two above and two below the sinuosities. In the latter are placed the lobes of the cerebellum, and in the former the posterior lobes of the brain. The two sinuosities serve to receive the lateral sinuses. In the upper part of this bone is seen a continuation of the sinuosity of the longitudinal sinus; and at the basis of the cranium we observe the inner surface of the cuneiform process made concave, for the reception of the medulla oblongata. The occipital bone is thicker and stronger than any of the other bones of the head, except the petrous part of the ossa temporum; but it is of unequal thickness. At its lateral and inferior parts, where it is thinnest, it is covered by a great number of muscles. The reason for so much thickness and strength in this bone, seems to be, that it covers the cerebellum, in which the least wound is of the utmost consequence; and that it is, by its situation, more liable to be fractured by falls than any other bone of the cranium. For if we fall forwards, the hands are naturally put out to prevent the forehead's touching the ground; and if on one side, the shoulders in a great measure protect the sides of the head; but if a person fall backwards, the hind part of the head consequently strikes against the earth, and that too with considerable violence. Nature therefore has wisely constructed this bone so as to be capable of the greatest strength at its upper part, where it is the most exposed to injury. The os occipitis is joined, by means of the cuneiform process, to the sphenoid bone, with which it often ossifies, and makes but one bone in those who are advanced in life. It is connected to the parietal bones by the lambdoidal suture, and to the temporal bones by the additamentum of the temporal

suture. The head is likewise united to the trunk by means of this bone. The two condyles of the occipital bone are received into the superior oblique processes of the atlas, or first vertebra of the neck, and it is by means of this articulation that a certain degree of motion of the head backwards and forwards is performed. But it allows only very little motion to either side; and still less of a circular motion, which the head obtains principally by the circumvolution of the atlas on the second vertebra, as is described more particularly in the account of the vertebræ. In the fœtus, the os occipitis is divided by an unossified cartilaginous substance, into four parts. One of these, which is the longest, constitutes all that portion of the bone which is above the foramen magnum; two others, which are much smaller, compose the inside of the foramen magnum, and include the condyloid processes; and the fourth is the cuneiform process. This last is sometimes not completely united with the rest, so as to form one bone, before the sixth or seventh year.

OCCIPITA'LIS. See *Occipito-frontalis* and *Occipital.*

OCCIPITO. Names compounded of this word belong to the occiput.

OCCIPITO-FRONTALIS. *Digastricus cranii; Epicranius,* of Albinus. *Frontalis et occipitalis,* of Winslow and Cowper; and *Occipito-frontal,* of Dumas. A single, broad, digastric muscle, that covers the cranium, pulls the skin of the head backwards, raises the eyebrows upwards, and at the same time, draws up and wrinkles the skin of the forehead. It arises from the posterior part of the occiput, goes over the upper part of the os parietale and os frontis, and is lost in the eyebrows.

O'CCIPUT. The hinder part of the head. See *Caput.*

OCCLUSUS. Shut up. Applied to the florets of the fig, which are shut up in the fleshy receptacle that forms the fruit.

OCCULT. *Occultus.* Hidden. A term that has been much used by writers that had not clear ideas of what they undertook to explain; and which served therefore only for a cover to their ignorance: hence, occult cause, occult quality, occult disease.

OCHE'MA. (From οχεω, to carry.) A vehicle, or thin fluid.

OCHETEU'MA. (From οχετος, a duct.) The nostril.

U'CHETUS. (From οχεω, to convey.) A canal or duct. The urinary or abdominal passages.

O'CHEUS. (From οχεω, to carry.) The bag of the scrotum.

O'CHRA. (From ωχρος, pale: so named because it is often of a pale colour.)

1. Ochre. An argillaceous earth impregnated with iron of a red or yellow colour. The Armenian bole, and other earths, are often adulterated with ochre.

2. The forepart of the tibia.

OCHROITS. See *Cerite.*

O'CHRUS. (From ωχρος, pale: so called from the pale muddy colour in its flowers.) A leguminous plant, or kind of pulse.

OCHTHO'DES. (From οχθος, importing the tumid lips of ulcers, callous, tumid.) An epithet for ulcers, whose lips are callous and tumid, and consequently difficult to heal.

OCIMA'STRUM. (Diminutive of *ocimum,* basil.) Wild white campion, or basil.

OCREA. A term used by Rottball, to the membrane that enfolds the flower-stalks in *Cyperus,* and which Sir J. Smith thinks is a species of bractea.

OCTA'NA. (From *octo,* eight.) An erratic intermitting fever, which returns every eighth day.

OCTANDRIA. (From οκτω, eight, and ανηρ, a husband.) The name of a class of plants in the sexual system of Linnæus, consisting of those which have hermaphrodite flowers, furnished with eight stamina.

OCTA'VUS HUMERI. The *Teres minor.*

OCTA'VUS HUMERI PLACENTINI. The *Teres minor.*

OCULA'RES COMMUNES. A name for the nerves called *Motores oculorum.*

OCULA'RIA. (From *oculus,* the eye: so called from its uses in disorders of the eye.) See *Euphrasia.*

O'CULUS. The eye. See *Eye.*

OCULUS BOVINUS. See *Hydrophthalmia.*

OCULUS BOVIS. See *Chrysanthemum leucanthemum.*

Oculus bubulus. See *Hydrophthalmia*

Oculus christi. Austrian flea-bane: a species of *Inula*, sometimes used as an adstringent by continental physicians.

Oculus elephantinus. A name given to *Hydrophthalmia*.

Oculus genu. The knee-pan.

Oculus lachrymans. The *Epiphora*.

Oculus mundi. A species of *Opal*, generally of a yellowish colour. By lying in water it becomes of an amber colour, and also transparent.

Oculi adductor. See *Rectus internus oculi*.

Oculi attollens. See *Rectus superior oculi.*

Oculi cancrorum. See *Cancer*.

Oculi depressor. See *Rectus inferior oculi.*

Oculi elevator. See *Rectus superior oculi.*

Oculi levator. See *Rectus superior oculi.*

Oculi obliquus inferior. See *Obliquus inferior oculi.*

Oculi obliquus major. See *Obliquus superior oculi.*

Oculi obliquus minor. See *Obliquus inferior oculi.*

O'CYMUM. (From ωκυς, swift: so called from its quick growth.) *Ocymum*. The name of a genus of plants in the Linnæan system. Class, *Didynamia*; Order, *Gymnospermia*.

Ocymum basilicum. The systematic name of the common or citron basil. *Basilicum. Ocimum—foliis ovatis glabris; calycibus ciliatis*, of Linnæus. This plant is supposed to possess nervine qualities, but is seldom employed but as a condiment to season high dishes, to which it imparts a grateful odour and taste.

Ocymum caryophyllatum. *Ocimum minimum* of Caspar Bauhin. Small or bush basil. This plant is mildly balsamic. Infusions are drank as tea, in catarrhous and uterine disorders, and the dried leaves are made into cephalic, and sternutatory powders. They are, when fresh, very juicy, of a weak aromatic and very mucilaginous taste, and of a strong and agreeable smell improved by drying.

Odaxi'smos. (From οδους, a tooth.) A biting sensation, pain, or itching in the gums.

ODONTA'GO'GOS. (From οδους, a tooth, and αγω, to draw.) The name of an instrument to draw teeth, one of which, made of lead, Forrestus relates to have been hung up in the temple of Apollo, denoting, that such an operation ought not to be made, but when the tooth was loose enough to draw with so slight a force as could be applied with that.

ODONTA'GRA. (From οδους, a tooth, and αγρα, a seizure.) 1. The toothache.

2. The gout in the teeth.

3. A tooth-drawer.

ODONTA'LGIA. (From οδους, a tooth, and αλγος, pain.) *Odontia; Odaxismus.* The toothache. This well-known disease makes its attack by a most violent pain in the teeth, most frequently in the molares, more rarely in the incisorii, reaching sometimes up to the eyes, and sometimes backwards into the cavity of the ear. At the same time, there is a manifest determination to the head, and a remarkable tension and inflation of the vessels takes place, not only in the parts next to that where the pain is seated, but over the whole head.

The toothache is sometimes merely a rheumatic affection, arising from cold, but more frequently from a carious tooth. It is also a symptom of pregnancy, and takes place in some nervous disorders. It may attack persons at any period of life, though it is most frequent in the young and plethoric. From the variety of causes which may produce this affection, it has been named by authors odontalgia cariosa, scorbutica, catarrhalis, arthritica, gravidarum hysterica, stomachica, and rheumatica.

O'DONTALGIC. (*Odontalgicus;* from οδονταλγια, the toothache.) Medicines which relieve the toothache.

Many empirical remedies have been proposed for the cure of the toothache, but have not in any degree answered the purpose. When the affection is purely rheumatic, blistering behind the ear will almost always remove it: but when it proceeds from a carious tooth, the pain is much more obstinate. In this case it has been recommended to touch the pained part with a hot iron, or with oil of vitriol, in order to destroy the aching nerve; to hold spirits in the mouth; to put a drop of

oil of cloves into the hollow of the tooth, or a pill made of camphor, opium, and oleum caryophylli. Others recommend gum mastich, dissolved in oleum terebinthinæ, applied to the tooth upon a little cotton. The great Boerhaave is said to have applied camphor, opium, oleum caryophylli, and alkohol, upon cotton. The caustic oil which may be collected from writing paper, rolled up tight, and set fire to at the end, will sometimes destroy the exposed nervous substance of a hollow tooth. The application of radix pyrethri, by its power of stimulating the salivary glands, either in substance or in tincture, has also been attended with good effects. But one of the most useful applications of this kind, is strong nitrous acid, diluted with three or four times its weight of spirit of wine, and introduced into the hollow of the tooth, either by means of a hair pencil or a little cotton. When the constitution has had some share in the disease, the Peruvian bark has been recommended, and perhaps with much justice, on account of its tonic and antiseptic powers. When the pain is not fixed to one tooth, leeches applied to the gum are of great service. But very often all the foregoing remedies will fail, and the only infallible cure is to draw the tooth.

ODONTIA. The name of a genus of diseases in Good's Nosology. Class *Cœliaca;* Order, *Enterica.* Pain, or derangement of the teeth or their involucres. It has seven species, viz. *Odontia dentitionis; dolorosa; stupores; deformis; edentula; incrustans; excrescens.*

ODONTIASIS. (From οδοντιαω, to put forth the teeth.) Dentition, or cutting teeth. See *Dentition* and *Teeth.*

Odo'ntica. (From οδους, a tooth.) Remedies for pains in the teeth.

ODONTIRRHŒ'A. (From οδους, a tooth, and ρεω, to flow.) Bleeding from the socket of the jaw, after drawing a tooth.

ODO'NTIS. (From οδους, a tooth: so called because its decoction was supposed useful in relieving the toothache.) A species of lychnis.

ODONTI'TIS. Inflammation of a tooth. See *Odontalgia.*

ODONTOGLY'PHUM. (From οδους, a tooth, and γλυφω, to scrape.) An instrument for scaling and scraping the teeth.

ODONTOID. (*Odontoides;* from οδους, a tooth and ειδος, form; because it is shaped like a tooth.) Tooth-like. See *Dentatus.*

ODONTOLI'THOS. (From οδους, a tooth, and λιθος, a stone.) The tartar, or stony crust upon the teeth.

ODONTOPHY'IA. (From οδους, a tooth, and φυω, to grow.) Dentition, or cutting teeth.

Odontotri'mma. (From οδους, a tooth, and τριβω, to wear away.) A dentifrice, or medicine, to clean the teeth.

ODORIFEROUS. (From the smell which the secretion from them has.) Some glands are so called.

Odoriferous glands. *Glandulæ odoriferæ.* These glands are situated around the corona glandis of the male, and under the skin of the labia majora and nymphæ of females. They secrete a sebaceous matter, which emits a peculiar odour.

ODOUR. Smell. This, which is the emanation of an odoriferous body, is generally ascribed to a portion of the body itself, converted into vapour: but from some experiments lately instituted it would seem probable, that in many cases the odour is owing not to the substance itself, but to a gas or vapour resulting from its combination with an appropriate vehicle, capable of diffusion in space.

Œ'A. (Οιη: from οιω, to bear; so named from its fruitfulness.) The service tree, Cratægus termi nalis.

ŒCONOMY. (*Œconomia:* from οικος, a house, and νομος, a law.) *Œconomia animalis.* The conduct of nature in preserving bodies and following her usual order; hence animal œconomy and vegetable œconomy, &c.

ŒDE'MA. (From οιδεω, to swell.) A synonyme of anasarca. See *Anasarca.*

ŒDEMATO'DES. (From οιδεω, to swell, and ειδος, resemblance.) Like to an œdema.

Œdemosa'rca. (From οιδημα, a swelling, and σαρξ, flesh.) A tumour mentioned by Severinus, of a middle nature, between an *œdema* and *sarcoma.*

ŒNA'NTHE. (From οινος, wine, and ανθος, a flower: so called because its flowers smell like the vine.)

1. The botanical name of a genus of the umbelliferous plants. Class, *Pentandria ;* Order, *Digynia.*

2. The pharmacopœial name of the hemlock dropwort. See *Œnanthe crocata.*

ŒNANTHE CROCATA. The hemlock dropwort. *Œnanthe—chærophylli foliis* of Linnæus. An active poison that has too often proved fatal, by being eaten in mistake instead of water-parsnip. The juice, nevertheless, cautiously exhibited, promises to be an efficacious remedy in inveterate scorbutic eruptions. The root of this plant is not unpleasant to the taste, and esteemed to be most delecterious of all the vegetables which this country produces. Mr. Howel, Surgeon at Haverfordwest, relates, that "eleven French prisoners had the liberty of walking in and about the town of Pembroke. Three of them being in the fields a little before noon, dug up a large quantity of this plant, which they took to be wild celery, to eat with their bread and butter for dinner. After washing it, they all three ate, or rather tasted of the roots. As they were entering the town, without any previous notice of sickness at the stomach, or disorder in the head, one of them was seized with convulsions. The other two ran home, and sent a surgeon to him. The surgeon endeavoured first to bleed, and then to vomit him ; but those endeavours were fruitless, and he died presently. Ignorant of the cause of their comrade's death, and of their own danger, they gave of these roots to the other eight prisoners, who ate of them with their dinner. A few minutes afterward the remaining two who gathered the plants were seized in the same manner as the first, of which one died ; the other was bled, and a vomit, with great difficulty, forced down, on account of his jaws being, as it were, locked together. This operated, and he recovered, but was some time affected with dizziness in his head, though not sick, or the least disordered in the stomach. The other eight being bled and vomited immediately, were soon well." At Clonmell, in Ireland, eight boys mistaking this plant for water-parsnip, ate plentifully of its roots. About four or five hours after the eldest boy became suddenly convulsed, and died: and before the next morning four of the other boys died in a similar manner. Of the other three, one was maniacal several hours, another lost his hair and nails, but the third escaped unhurt. Stalpaart Vander Wiel mentions two cases of the fatal effects of this root; these, however, were attended with great heat in the throat and stomach, sickness, vertigo, and purging; they both died in the course of two or three hours after eating the root. Allen, in his Synopsis Medicinæ, also relates, that four children suffered greatly by eating this poison. In these cases great agony was experienced before the convulsion supervened: vomitings likewise came on, which were encouraged by large draughts of oil and warm water, to which their recovery is ascribed. The late Sir William Watson, who refers to the instances here cited, also says, that a Dutchman was poisoned by the leaves of the plant boiled in pottage. It appears, from various authorities, that most brute animals are not less affected by this poison than man: and Lightfoot informs us, that a spoonful of the juice of this plant given to a dog, rendered him sick and stupid: but a goat was observed to eat the plant with impunity. The great virulence of this plant has not, however, prevented it from being taken medicinally. In a letter from Dr. Poulteney to Sir William Watson, we are told that a severe and inveterate cutaneous disorder was cured by the juice of the root, though not without exciting the most alarming symptoms. Taken in the dose of a spoonful, in two hours afterward, the head was affected in a very extraordinary manner, followed with violent sickness and vomiting, cold sweats, and rigors; but this did not deter the patient from continuing the medicine, in somewhat less doses, till it effected a cure.

ŒNA'REA. (Οιναρεη: from οιναρα, the cuttings of vines.) The ashes prepared of the twigs, &c. of vines.

ŒNELÆ'UM. (From οινος, wine, and ελαιον, oil.) A mixture of oil and wine.

ŒNO'GALA. (From οινος, wine, and γαλα, milk.) A sort of potion made of wine and milk. According to some, it is wine as warm as new milk

ŒNO GARUM. From οινος, wine, and γαρον, garum. A mixture of wine and garum.

ŒNO'MELI. (From οινος, wine, and μελι, honey.) Mead, or wine, made of honey, or sweetened with honey.

ŒNO'PLI. (From οινος, wine.) The great jubebtree. The juice of the fruit is like that of the grape.

ŒNOSTA'GMA. (From οινος, wine, and ςαζω, to distil.) Spirit of wine.

ŒNO'THERA. (From οινος, wine: so called because its dried roots smell like wine.) A species of lysimachia.

ŒNOTHIONIC ACID. (*Œnothionicus ;* from οινος, wine.) An acid produced during the distillation of sulphuric æther, and found in the residue according to Sertuerner.

ŒNUS. (From οινος, wine.) Wine.

ŒNUS ANTHINOS. Flowery wine. Galen says it is *Œnos anthosmias,* or wine impregnated with flowers, in which sense it is an epithet for the *Cyceon.*

ŒNUS ANTHOSMIAS. (From ανθος, a flower, and οσμη, a smell.) Sweet-scented wine.

ŒNUS APEZESMENUS. A wine heated to a great degree, and prescribed with other things, as garlic, salt, milk, and vinegar.

ŒNUS APODÆDUS. Wine in which the dais, or tæda, hath been boiled.

ŒNUS DEUTERUS. Wines of the second pressing.

ŒNUS DIACHEOMENUS. Wine diffused in larger vessels, cooled and strained from the lees, to render it thinner and weaker ; wines thus drawn off are called *saccus,* and *saccata,* from the bag through which they are strained.

ŒNUS GALACTODES. Wine with milk, or wine made as warm as new milk.

ŒNUS MALACUS. *Œnus malthacus.* Soft wine. Sometimes it means weak and thin, opposed to strong wine ; or mild in opposition to austere.

ŒNUS MELICHROOS. Wine in which is honey.

ŒNUS ŒNODES. Strong wine.

ŒNUS STRAPHIDIOS LEUCOS. White wine made from raisins.

ŒNUS TETHALASMENOS. Wine mixed with sea-water.

ŒSOPHAGÆ'US. (From οισοφαγος, the gullet.) The muscle forming the sphincter œsophagi.

ŒSOPHAGI'SMUS. (From οισοφαγος, the gullet.) Difficult swallowing, from spasm.

ŒSO'PHAGUS. (*Œsophagus,* i. m. ; from φιω, to carry, and φαγω, to eat: because it carries the food into the stomach.) The membranous and muscular tube that descends in the neck, from the pharynx to the stomach. It is composed of three tunics, or membranes, viz. a common, muscular, and mucous. Its arteries are branches of the œsophageal, which arises from the aorta. The veins empty themselves into the vena azygos. Its nerves are from the eighth pair and great intercostal; and it is every where under the internal or mucous membrane supplied with glands that separate the mucus of the œsophagus, in order that the masticated bole may readily pass down into the stomach.

ŒSTROMA'NIA. (From οιςρος, the pudenda of a woman, and μαινομαι, to rage.) A furor uterinus. See *Nymphomania.*

Œ'STRUM. (From *œstrus,* a gad-bee: because by its bite, or sting, it agitates cattle.) *Œstrum venereum.* The orgasm, or pleasant sensation, experienced during coition.

ŒSTRUM VENEREUM. 1. The clitoris is so called, as being the seat of the sensation.

2. The sensation is also so called.

Œ'SYPE. (From οις, a sheep, and ρυπος, sordes.) *Œsypos ; Œsypum; Œsypus.* It frequently is met with in the ancient Pharmacy, for a certain oily substance, boiled out of particular parts of the fleeces of wool, as what grows on the flank, neck, and parts most used to sweat.

O'FFA ALBA. (From *phath,* a fragment, Hebrew Van Helmont thus calls the white coagulation which arises from a mixture of a rectified spirit of wine, and of urine ; but the spirit of urine must be distilled from well-fermented urine ; and that must be well dephlegmated, else it will not answer.

OFFICINAL. (*Officinalis ;* from *officina,* a shop.) Any medicine, directed by the colleges of physicians to be kept in the shops, is so termed.

OFFUSCA'TIO. The same as *Amaurosis*.

OIL. (*Oleum*; from *olea*, the olive: this name being at first confined to the oil expressed from the olive.) Oil is defined, by modern chemists, to be a proper juice of a fat or unctuous nature, either solid or fluid, indissoluble in water, combustible with flame, and volatile in different degrees. Oils are never formed but by organic bodies; and all the substances in the mineral kingdom, which present oily characters, have originated from the action of vegetable or animal life. They are distinguished into fat, and essential oils; under the former head are comprehended oil of olives, almonds, rape, ben, linseed, hemp, cocoa, &c. Essential oils differ from fat oils by the following characters: their smell is strong and aromatic; their volatility is such that they rise with the heat of boiling water, and their taste is very acrid; they are likewise much more combustible than fat oils; they are obtained by pressure, distillation, &c. from strong-smelling plants, as that of peppermint, aniseed, caraway, &c. The use of fat oils in the arts, and in medicine, is very considerable; they are medicinally prescribed as relaxing, softening, and laxative remedies; they enter into many medical compounds, such as balsams, unguents, plasters, &c. and they are often used as food on account of the mucilage they contain. See *Olea*. Essential oils are employed as cordial, stimulant, and antispasmodic remedies.

[" *Oil, animal.* The proximate principles of the animal creation consist, like those of vegetables, of a few elementary substances, which, by combination in various proportions, give rise to their numerous varieties. Carbon, hydrogen, oxygen, and nitrogen, are the principal ultimate elements of animal matter; and phosphorus and sulphur are also often contained in it. The presence of nitrogen constitutes the most striking peculiarity of animal, compared with vegetable bodies; but as some vegetables contain nitrogen, so there are certain animal principles, into the composition of which it does not enter.

The presence of nitrogen stamps a peculiarity upon the products obtained by the destructive distillation of animal matter, and which are characterized by the presence of ammonia, formed by the union of hydrogen with the nitrogen. It is sometimes so abundantly generated as to be the leading product; thus, when horns, hoofs, or bones, are distilled *per se*, a quantity of solid carbonate of ammonia, and of the same substance combined with empyreumatic oil, and dissolved in water, are obtained; hence the pharmaceutical preparations called *spirit* and *salt of hartshorn*, and Dipel's *animal oil*. Occasionally the acetic, benzoic, and some other acids, are formed by the operation of heat on animal bodies, and these are found united to the ammonia; cyanogen and hydrocyanic acid frequently occur."—Webs. *Man. Chem.*—A.]

Oil, ætherial. See *Oleum æthereum.*
Oil, almond. See *Amygdalus.*
Oil of allspice. See *Oleum pimentæ.*
Oil of amber. See *Oleum succini.*
Oil of caraway. See *Oleum carui.*
Oil, castor. See *Ricinus communis.*
Oil of chamomile. See *Oleum anthemidis.*
Oil of juniper. See *Oleum juniperi.*
Oil of lavender. See *Oleum lavendulæ.*
Oil of linseed. See *Oleum lini.*
Oil of mace. See *Oleum macis.*
Oil, olive. See *Olea europæa.*
Oil of origanum. See *Oleum origani.*
Oil, palm. See *Cocos butyracea.*
Oil of pennyroyal. See *Oleum pulegii.*
Oil of peppermint. See *Oleum menthæ piperitæ.*
Oil, rock. See *Petroleum.*
Oil of spearmint. See *Oleum menthæ viridis.*
Oil, sulphurated. See *Oleum sulphuratum.*
Oil of turpentine. See *Oleum terebinthinæ rectificatum.*
Oil of vitriol. See *Sulphuric acid.*
OINTMENT. See *Unguentum.*
OISANITE. Pyramidal ore of titanium.
OLDENLANDIA. (In honour of H. B. Oldenland, a Dane, who made a visit to the Cape of Good Hope, about the year 1695, for the purpose of collecting plants, where he soon after died. Linnæus described many plants from his Herbarium.) The name of a genus of plants. Class *Pentandria*; Order, *Digynia*.
OLDENLANDIA UMBELLATA. The roots of this plant

which grows wild on the coast of Coromandel, and is also cultivated there, are used by dyers, and calico printers, for the same purpose as madder with us, giving the beautiful red so much admired in the Madras cottons. .

O'LEA. The name of a genus of plants in the Linnæan system. Class, *Monandria*; Order, *Monogynia*.

OLEA EUROPÆA. The systematic name of the plant from which the olive oil is obtained. *Oliva; Olea sativa. Olea—foliis lanceolatis integerrimis racemis axillaribus coarctatis*, of Linnæus. The olive-tree in all ages has been greatly celebrated, and held in peculiar estimation, as the bounteous gift of heaven; it was formerly exhibited in the religious ceremonies of the Jews, and is still continued as emblematic of peace and plenty. The varieties of this tree are numerous, distinguished not only by the form of the leaves, but also by the shape, size, and colour of the fruit; as the large Spanish olive, the small oblong Provence olive, &c. &c. These, when pickled, are well known to us by the names of Spanish and French olives, which are extremely grateful to many stomachs, and said to excite appetite and promote digestion; they are prepared from the green unripe fruit, which is repeatedly steeped in water, to which some quicklime or alkaline salt is added, in order to shorten the operation: after this, they are washed and preserved in a pickle of common salt and water, to which an aromatic is sometimes added. The principal consumption, however, of this fruit is in the preparation of the common salad oil, or *oleum olivæ* of the pharmacopœias, which is obtained by grinding and pressing them when thoroughly ripe: the finer and purer oil issues first by gentle pressure, and the inferior sorts on heating what is left, and pressing it more strongly. The best olive oil is of a bright pale amber colour, bland to the taste, and without any smell: it becomes rancid by age, and sooner if kept in a warm situation. With regard to its utility, oil, in some shape, forms a considerable part of our food, both animal and vegetable, and affords much nourishment. With some, however, oily substances do not unite with the contents of the stomach, and are frequently brought up by eructation; this happens more especially to those whose stomachs abound with acid.—Oil, considered as a medicine, is supposed to correct acrimony, and to lubricate and relax the fibres; and, therefore, has been recommended internally to obviate the effects of various stimuli, which produce irritation, and consequent inflammation: on this ground it has been generally prescribed in coughs, catarrhal affections, and erosions. The oil of olives is successfully used in Switzerland against the *tænia osculis superficialibus*, and it is in very high estimation in this and other countries against nephritic pains, spasms, colic, constipation of the bowels, &c. Externally it has been found a useful application to bites and stings of various poisonous animals, as the mad dog, several serpents, &c. also to burns, tumours, and other affections, both by itself, or mixed in liniments or poultices. Oil rubbed over the body is said to be of great service in dropsies, particularly ascites. Olive oil enters several officinal compositions, and when united with water, by the intervention of alkali, is usually given in coughs and hoarsenesses.

OLEA'MEN. (From *oleum*, oil.) A thin liniment composed of oils.

OLEA'NDER. (From *olea*, the olive-tree, which it resembles.) The rose-bay.

OLEA'STER. (Diminutive of *olea*, the olive-tree.) The wild olive.

OLE'CRANON. (From ωλενη, the ulna, and κρανον, the head. The elbow, or process of the ulna, upon which a person leans. See *Ulna.*

OLEFIANT GAS. See *Carburetted hydrogen gas.*

OLEIC ACID. "When potassa and hog's lard are saponified, the margarate of the alkali separates in the form of a pearly looking solid, while the fluid fat remains in solution, combined with the potassa. When the alkali is separated by tartaric acid, the oily principle of fat is obtained, which Chevreuil purifies by saponifying it again and again, recovering it two or three times; by which means the whole of the margarine is separated. As this oil has the property of saturating bases and forming neutral compounds, he has called it oleic acid."

O'LENE. (Ωλενη.) The cubit, or ulna

OLEOSA'CCHARUM. (From *oleum*, oil, and *sac-*

charum, sugar. An essential oil ground up with ugar.

OLERACEUS. (From *oleo*, to grow.) *Holeraceus.* Partaking of the nature of pot-herbs.

OLERACEÆ. (From *olus*, a pot-herb.) The name of an order of plants in Linnæus's Fragments of a Natural Method, consisting of such as have incomplete inelegant flowers, heaped together in the calyces; as beta, chenopodium, spinacia, &c.

O'LEUM. See *Oil*.

OLEUM ABIETINUM. The resinous juice which exudes spontaneously from the silver and red firs. It is supposed to be superior to that obtained by wounding the tree.

OLEUM ÆTHEREUM. Æthereal oil. *Oleum vini.* After the distillation of sulphuric æther, carry on the distillation with a less degree of heat until a black froth begins to rise; then immediately remove the retort from the fire. Add sufficient water to the liquor in the retort, that the oily part may float upon the surface. Separate this, and add to it as much lime-water as may be necessary to neutralize the adherent acid, and shake them together. Lastly, collect the æthereal oil which separates. This oil is used as an ingredient in the compound spirit of æther. It is of a yellow colour, less volatile than æther, soluble in alkohol, and insoluble in water.

OLEUM AMYGDALÆ. See *Amygdalus communis.*

OLEUM AMYGDALARUM. See *Amygdalus communis.*

OLEUM ANIMALE. *Oleum animale Dippelii.* An empyreumatic oil obtained by distillation from bones and animal substances. It is sometimes exhibited as an antispasmodic and diaphoretic, in the dose of from ten to forty drops.

OLEUM ANIMALE DIPPELII. See *Oleum animale.*

OLEUM ANISI. Formerly *Oleum essentiale anisi; Oleum e seminibus anisi.* Oil of anise. The essential oil of aniseed possesses all the virtues attributed to the anisum, and is often given as a stimulant and carminative, in the dose of from five to eight drops mixed with an appropriate vehicle. See *Pimpinella anisum.*

OLEUM ANTHEMIDIS. Oil of chamomile, formerly called oleum e floribus chamæmeli. See *Anthemis nobilis.*

OLEUM CAMPHORATUM. See *Linimentum camphoræ.*

OLEUM CARPATHICUM. A fine essential oil, distilled from the fresh cones of the tree which affords the common turpentine. See *Pinus sylvestris.*

OLEUM CARUI. Formerly called *Oleum essentiale carui; Oleum essentiale e seminibus carui.* The oil of caraways is an admirable carminative, diluted with rectified spirit into an essence, and then mixed with any proper fluid. See *Carum.*

OLEUM CARYOPHYLLI AROMATICI. A stimulant and aromatic preparation of the clove. See *Eugenia caryophyllata.*

OLEUM CEDRINUM. *Essentia ae cedro.* The oil of the peel of citrons, obtained, without distillation, in Italy.

OLEUM CINNAMOMI. A warm, stimulant, and delicious stomachic. Given in the dose of from one to three drops, rubbed down with some yelk of egg, in a little wine, it allays violent emotions of the stomach from morbid irritability, and is particularly serviceable in debility of the primæ viæ, after cholera.

OLEUM CORNU CERVI. This is applied externally as a stimulant to paralytic affections of the limbs.

OLEUM GABIANUM. See *Petroleum rubrum.*

OLEUM JUNIPERI. Formerly called *Oleum essentiale juniperi baccæ; Oleum essentiale e baccis juniperi.* Oil of juniper. Oil of juniper-berries possesses stimulant, carminative, and stomachic virtues, in the dose of from two to four drops, and in a larger dose proves highly diuretic. It is often administered in the cure of dropsical complaints, when the indication is to provoke the urinary discharge. See *Juniperus communis.*

OLEUM LAVENDULÆ. Formerly called *Oleum essentiale lavendulæ; Oleum essentiale e floribus lavendulæ.* Oil of lavender. Though mostly used as a perfume, this essential oil may be exhibited internally, in the dose of from one to three drops, as a stimulant in nervous headaches, hysteria, and debility of the stomach. See *Lavenda spica.*

OLEUM LAURI. *Oleum laurinum.* An anodyne and antispasmodic application, generally rubbed on sprains and bruises unattended with inflammation.

OLEUM LIMONIS. The essential oil of lemons pos-

sesses stimulant and stomachic powers, but is principally used externally, mixed with ointments, as a perfume.

OLEUM LINI. Linseed oil is emollient and demulcent, in the dose of from half an ounce to an ounce. It is frequently given in the form of clyster in colics and obstipation. Cold-drawn linseed-oil, with lime-water and extract of lead, forms, in many instances, the best application for burns and scalds. See *Linum usitatissimum.*

OLEUM LUCII PISCIS. See *Esox lucius.*

OLEUM MACIS. *Oleum myristicæ expressum.* Oil of mace. A fragrant sebaceous substance, expressed in the East Indies from the nutmeg. There are two kinds. The best is brought in stone jars, is somewhat soft, of a yellow colour, and resembles in smell the nutmeg. The other is brought from Holland, in flat square cakes. The weak smell and faint colour warrants our supposing it to be the former kind sophisticated. Their use is chiefly external, in form of plaster, unguent, or liniment. See *Myristica moschata.*

OLEUM MALABATHRI. An oil similar in flavour to that of cloves, brought from the East Indies, where it is said to be drawn from the leaves of the cassia-tree.

OLEUM MENTHÆ PIPERITÆ. Formerly called *Oleum essentiale menthæ piperitidis.* Oil of peppermint. Oil of peppermint possesses all the active principle of the plant. It is mostly used to make the simple water. Mixed with rectified spirit it forms an essence, which is put into a variety of compounds, as sugar drops and troches, which are exhibited as stimulants, carminatives, and stomachics. See *Mentha piperita.*

OLEUM MENTHÆ VIRIDIS. Formerly called *Oleum essentiale menthæ sativæ.* Oil of spearmint. This essential oil is mostly in use for making the simple water, but may be exhibited in the dose of from two to five drops as a carminative, stomachic, and stimulant. See *Mentha viridis.*

OLEUM MYRISTICÆ. The essential oil of nutmeg is an excellent stimulant and aromatic, and may be exhibited in every case where such remedies are indicated, with advantage. See *Myristica moschata.*

OLEUM MYRISTICÆ EXPRESSUM. This is commonly called oil of mace. See *Oleum macis.*

OLEUM NEROLI. *Essentia neroli.* The essential oil of the flowers of the Seville orange-tree. It is brought to us from Italy and France.

OLEUM OLIVÆ. See *Olea europea.*

OLEUM ORIGANI. Formerly called *Oleum essentiale origani.* Oil of origanum. A very acrid and stimulating essential oil. It is employed for alleviating the pain arising from caries of the teeth, and for making the simple water of marjoram. See *Origanum vulgare.*

OLEUM PALMÆ. See *Cocos butyracea.*

OLEUM PETRÆ. See *Petroleum.*

OLEUM PIMENTÆ. Oil of allspice. A stimulant and aromatic oil. See *Myrtus pimenta.*

OLEUM PULEGII. Formerly called *Oleum essentiale pulegii.* Oil of penny-royal. A stimulant and antispasmodic oil, which may be exhibited in hysterical and nervous affections. See *Mentha pulegium.*

OLEUM RICINI. See *Ricinus communis.*

OLEUM ROSMARINI. Formerly called *Oleum essentiale rosis marini.* Oil of rosemary. The essential oil of rosemary is an excellent stimulant, and may be given with great advantage in nervous, and spasmodic affections of the stomach. See *Rosmarinus officinalis.*

OLEUM SABINÆ. A stimulating emmenagogue: it is best administered with myrrh, in the form of bolus. See *Juniperis communis.*

OLEUM SASSAFRAS. An agreeable stimulating carminative and sudorific.

OLEUM SINAPEOS. This is an emollient oil, the acrid principle of the mustard remaining in the seed. See *Sinapis alba.*

OLEUM SUCCINI. *Oleum succini rectificatum.* Put amber in an alembic, and with the heat of a sand-bath, gradually increased, distil over an acid liquor, an oil, and a salt contaminated with oil. Then redistil the oil a second and a third time. Oil of amber is mostly used externally, as a stimulating application to paralytic limbs, or those affected with cramp and rheumatism. Hooping-cough, and other convulsive diseases, are said to be relieved also by rubbing the spine with this oil. See *Succinum.*

OLEUM SULPHURATUM. Formerly called *Balsamum sulphuris simplex.* Sulphurated oil. Take of washed su.phur, two ounces; olive oil, a pint. Having heated the oil in a very large iron pot, and the sulphur gradually, stir the mixture after each addition, until they have united. This, which was formerly called simple balsam of sulphur, is an acrid stimulating preparation, and much praised by some in the cure of coughs and other phthisical complaints.

OLEUM SYRIÆ. A fragrant essential oil, obtained by distillation from the balm of Gilead plant. See *Dracocephalum moldavica.*

OLEUM TEMPLINUM. *Oleum templinum verum.* A terebinthinate oil obtained from the fresh cones of the *Pinus abies* of Linnæus.

OLEUM TEREBINTHINÆ RECTIFICATUM. Take of oil of turpentine, a pint; water, four pints. Distil over the oil. Stimulant, diuretic, and sudorific virtues are attributed to this preparation, in the dose of from ten drops to twenty, which are given in rheumatic pains of the chronic kind, especially sciatica. Its chief use internally, however, is as an anthelmintic and styptic. Uterine, pulmonic, gastric, intestinal, and other hæmorrhages, when passive, are more effectually relieved by its exhibition than by any other medicine. Externally it is applied, mixed with ointments and other applications, to bruises, sprains, rheumatic pains, indolent ulcers, burns, and scalds.

OLEUM TERRÆ. See *Petroleum.*

OLEUM VINI. Stimulant and anodyne, in the dose of from one to four drops.

OLEUM VITRIOLI. See *Sulphuric acid.*

OLFACTORY. (*Olfactorius;* from *olfactus,* the sense of smelling.) Belonging to the organ or sense of smelling.

OLFACTORY NERVE. The first pair of nerves are so termed, because they are the organs of smelling. They arise from the corpora striata, perforate the ethmoid bone, and are distributed very numerously on the pituitary membrane of the nose.

OLI'BANUM. (From *lebona,* Chaldean.) See *Juniperus lycia.*

OLIGOTRO'PHIA. (From ολιγος, small, and τρεφω, to nourish.) Deficient nourishment.

OLISTHE'MA. (From ολισθαινω, to fall out.) A luxation.

OLI'VA. See *Olea europea.*

OLIVA'RIS. (From *oliva,* the olive.) *Oliviformis.* Resembling the olive: applied to two eminences on the lower part of the medulla oblongata, called *corpora olivaria.*

OLIVE. See *Olea europea.*

Olive, spurge. See *Daphne mezereum.*

Olive-tree. See *Olea europea.*

OLIVE'NITE. An ore of copper.

OLI'VILE. The name given by Pelletier to the substance which remains after gently evaporating the alkoholic solution of the gum which exudes from the olive-tree. It is a white, brilliant, starchy powder.

OLI'VINE. A subspecies of prismatic chrysolite. Its colour is olive-green. It occurs in basalt, greenstone, porphyry, and lava, and generally accompanied with augite. It is found in Scotland, Ireland, France, Bohemia, &c.

OLLA'RIS LAPIS. Pot-stone.

OLOPHLY'CTIS. (From ολος, whole, and φλυκτις, a pustule.) A small hot eruption covering the whole body.

OLUSA'TRUM. (*Id est olus atrum,* the black herb, from its black leaves.) See *Smyrnium olusatrum.*

OMA. This Greek final usually imports external protuberance; as in *sarcoma, staphyloma, carcinoma,* &c.

OMA'GRA. (From ωμος, the shoulder, and αγρα, a seizure.) The gout in the shoulder.

OMENTI'TIS. (*Omentitis;* from *omentum,* the caul.) Inflammation of the omentum, a species of peritonitis.

OME'NTUM. (From *omen,* a guess: so called because the soothsayers prophesied from an inspection of this part.) *Epiploon.* The caul. An adipose membranous viscus of the abdomen, that is attached to the stomach, and lies on the anterior surface of the intestines. It is thin and easily torn, being formed of a duplicature of the peritoneum, with more or less of fat interposed. It is distinguished into the great omentum and the little omentum.

1. The *omentum majus,* which is also termed *omentum gastrocolicum,* arises from the whole of the great curvature of the stomach, and even as far as the spleen, from whence it descends loosely behind the abdominal parietes, and over the intestines to the navel, and sometimes into the pelvis. Having descended thus far, its inferior margin turns inwards and ascends again, and is fastened to the colon and the spleen, where its vessels enter.

2. The *omentum minus,* or *omentum hepatico-gastricum,* arises posteriorly from the transverse fissure of the liver. It is composed of a duplicature of peritoneum, passes over the duodenum and small lobe of the liver: it also passes by the lobulus spigelii and pancreas, proceeds into the colon and small curvature of the stomach, and is implanted ligamentous into the œsophagus. It is in this omentum that Winslow discovered a natural opening, which goes by his name. If air be blown in at this *foramen of Winslow,* which is always found behind the lobulus spigelii, between the right side of the liver and hepatic vessels, the duodenum, the cavity of the omentum, and all its sacs, may be distended.

The omentum is always double, and between its lamellæ, closely connected by very tender cellular substance, the vessels are distributed and the fat collected. Where the top of the right kidney, and the lobulus spigelii of the liver, with the subjacent large vessels, form an angle with the duodenum, there the external membrane of the colon, which comes from the peritoneum joining with the membrane of the duodenum, which also rises immediately from the peritoneum lying upon the kidney, enters the back into the transverse fissure of the liver for a considerable space, is continuous with its external coat, contains the gall-bladder, supports the hepatic vessels, and is very yellow and slippery. Behind this membranous production, between the right lobe of the liver, hepatic vessels, vena portarum, biliary ducts, aorta, and adjacent duodenum, there is the natural opening just mentioned, by which air may be blown extensively into all the cavity of the omentum. From thence, in a course continuous with this mem brane from the pyloris and the smaller curvature of the stomach, the external membrane of the liver joins in such a manner with that of the stomach, that the thin membrane of the liver is continued out of the fossa of the venal duct, across the little lobe into the stomach stretched before the lobe and before the pancreas. This little omentum, or *omentum hepatico-gastricum,* when inflated, resembles a cone, and, gradually becoming harder and emaciated, it changes into a true ligament, by which the œsophagus is connected to the diaphragm. But the larger omentum, the *omentum gastrocolicum,* is of a much greater extent. It begins at the first accession of the right gastro-epiploic artery to the stomach, being continued there from the upper plate of the transverse mesocolon, and then from the whole great curve of the stomach, as far as the spleen, and also from the right convex end of the stomach towards the spleen, until it also terminates in a ligament that ties the upper and back part of the spleen to the stomach. This is the anterior lamina. Being continued downwards, sometimes to the navel, sometimes to the pelvis, it hangs before the intestines, and behind the muscles of the abdomen, until its lower edge, being reflected upon itself, ascends, leaving an intermediate vacuity between it and the anterior lamina, and is continued to a very great extent, into the external membrane of the transverse colon, and, lastly, into the sinus of the spleen, by which the large blood-vessels are received, and it ends finally on the œsophagus, under the diaphragm. Behind the stomach, and before the pancreas, its cavity is continuous with that of the smaller omentum. To this the *omentum-colicum* is connected, which arises farther to the right than the first origin of the omentum gastrocolicum from the mesocolon, with the cavity of which it is continuous, but produced solely from the colon and its external membrane, which departs double from the intestine. It is prolonged, and terminates by a conical extremity, sometimes of longer, sometimes of shorter extent, above the intestinum cæcum; for all the blood which returns from the omentum and mesocolon goes into the vena portarum, and by that into the liver itself. The omentum gastrocolicum is furnished with blood from each of the gastro-epiploic arteries, by many descending articulated branches, of which the most lateral are the longest, and the lowest anastomose by minute twigs with those of the colon. It also has branches from the splenic, duodenal, and adipose arte

133

ries. The omentum colicum has its arteries from the colon, as also the smaller appendices, and also from the duodenal and right epiploic. The arteries of the small omentum come from the hepatics, and from the right and left coronaries. The omentum being fat and indolent, has very small nerves. They arise from the nerves of the eighth pair, both in the greater and less curvatures of the stomach. The arteries of the mesentery are in general the same with those which go to the intestine, and of which the smaller branches remain in the glands and fat of the mesentery. Various small accessory arteries go to both mesocolons, from the intercostals, spermatics, lumbars, and caspular to the transverse portion from the splenic artery, and pancreato-duodenalis, and to the left mesocolon, from the branches of the aorta going to the lumbar glands. The veins of the omentum in general accompany the arteries, and unite into similar trunks; those of the left part of the gastrocolic omentum into the splenic, and also those of the hepatico-gastric, which likewise sends its blood to the trunk of the vena portarum: those from the larger and right part of the gastro-colic omentum, from the omentum colicum, and from the appendices epiploicæ into the mesenteric trunk. All the veins of the mesentery meet together, and end in the vena portarum, being collected first into two large branches, of which the one, the mesenteric, receives the gastro-epiploic vein, the colicæ mediæ, the iliocolica, and all those of the small intestines, as far as the duodenum: the other, which going transversely, inserts itself into the former, above the origin of the duodenum, carries back the blood of the left gastric veins, and those of the rectum, except the lowermost, which belongs partly to those of the bladder and partly to the hypogastric branches of the pelvis. The vein which is called hæmorrhoidalis interna is sometimes inserted rather into the splenic than into the mesenteric vein. Has the omentum also lymphatic vessels? Certainly there are conglobate glands, both in the little omentum and in the gastrocolicum; and ancient anatomists have observed pellucid vessels in the omentum; and a modern has described them for lacteals of the stomach.

OMENTUM COLICUM. See *Omentum.*

OMENTUM GASTRO-COLICUM. See *Omentum.*

OMENTUM HEPATICO-GASTRICUM. See *Omentum.*

OMO. (From ωμος, the shoulder.) Names compounded with this word belong to muscles which are attached to the scapula.

OMOCO'TYLE. (From ωμος, the shoulder, and κοτυλη, a cavity.) The cavity in the extremity of the neck of the scapula, in which the head of the humerus is articulated.

OMO-HYOIDEUS. A muscle situated between the os hyoides and shoulder, that pulls the os hyoides obliquely downwards. *Coraco hyoideus* of Albinus and Douglas. *Scapulo hyodien* of Dumas. It arises broad, thin, and fleshy, from the superior costa of the scapula, near the semilunar notch, and from the ligament that runs across it; thence ascending obliquely, it becomes tendinous below the sternocleido-mastoideus, and, growing fleshy again, is inserted into the base of the os hyoides.

OMOPLA'TA. (From ωμος, the shoulder, and πλατυς, broad.) The bladebone. See *Scapula.*

OMOPLATO-HYOIDEUS. The same as *Omo-hyoideus.*

OMO'TOCOS. (From ωμος, crude, and τικτω, to bring forth.) A miscarriage.

OMO'TRIBES. (From ωμος, crude, and τριβω, to bruise.) Oil expressed from unripe olives.

OMPHA'CINUM. (From ομφακιον, the juice of unripe grapes.) Oil expressed from unripe olives.

OMPHA'CION. (From ομφακος, an unripe grape.) *Omphacium.* The juice of unripe grapes; and by some applied to that of wild apples, or crabs, commonly called *Verjuice.*

OMPHACITE. A variety of augite of a pale leek-green colour. It occurs in primitive rocks, with precious garnet, in Carinthia.

OMPHACI'TIS. (From ομφακος, an unripe grape.) A small kind of gall-nut, which resembles an unripe grape.

OMPHACO'MELI. (From ομφακος, an unripe grape, and μελι, honey.) An oxymel made of the juice of unripe grapes and honey.

OMPHALOCA'RPUS. (From ομφαλος, the navel, and καρπος, fruit: so called because its fruit resembles a navel.) Cleavers. The *Galium aperine* of Linnæus.

134

OMPHALOCE'LE. (From ομφαλος, the navel, and κηλη, a tumour.) An umbilical hernia. See *Hernia.*

OMPHALO'DES. (From ομφαλος, a navel, and ειδος, resemblance: so named because the calyx is excavated in the middle like the human navel.) A plant resembling the navel, which the leaf of the cotyledon and hydrocotyle does.

OMPHALOMA'NTIA. (From ομφαλος, the navel, and μυντεαω, to prophesy.) The foolish vaticination of midwives, who pretend to foretell the number of the future offspring from the number of knots in the navel.

OMPHALOS. (From ομφιελισκω, to roll up.) The navel. See *Umbilicus.*

OMPHALOTO'MIA. (From ομφαλος, the navel, and τεμνω, to cut.) The division or separation of the navel-string.

ONA'GRA. (From οναγρος, the wild ass.) 1. An American plant: so called because it is said to tame wild beasts.

2. A name for the rheumatism in the elbow.

ONEIRODY'NIA. (From ονειρον, a dream, and οδυνη, anxiety.) Disturbed imagination during sleep. A genus of disease in the class *Neuroses;* and order *Vesaniæ,* of Cullen, containing two species.

1. *Oneirodynia activa,* walking in the sleep.

2. *Oneirodynia gravans,* the incubus, or nightmare. The nervous or indisposed persons are oppressed during sleep with a heavy pressing sensation on the chest, by which respiration is impeded, or the circulation of blood intercepted, to such a degree, as to threaten suffocation. Frightful ideas are recollected on waking, which occupied the dreaming mind. Frequent attempts are made to *cry out,* but often without effect, and the horrors and agitations felt by the patient, are inexpressibly frightful. The sensations generally originate in a large quantity of wind, or indigestible matter in the stomach of *supper-eaters,* which, pressing the stomach against the diaphragm, impede respiration, or render it short and convulsed. Inflated intestines may likewise produce similar effects, or mental perturbations.

There is another species of nightmare mentioned by authors, which has a more dangerous tendency; and this arises from an impeded circulation of blood in the lungs, when lying down, or two great relaxation of the heart and its impelling powers. Epilepsy, apoplexy, or sudden death, are sometimes among the consequences of this species of disturbed sleep. Diseased states of the large vessels, aneurisms, water in the pleura, pericardium, or lungs, empyema, &c. are among the most dangerous causes.

ONEIRO'GMOS. (From ονειρωτ]ω, to dream.) Venereal dreams.

ONEIRO'GONOS. (From ονειρος, a dream, and γονη, the seed.) So the Greeks call an occasional emission of the semen in sleep, when it only happens rarely

ONION. See *Allium cepa.*

Onion sea. See *Scilla.*

ONI'SCUS. (From ονος, an ass: so called because like the ass it requires much beating before it is useful.) 1. The stockfish.

2. The slow-worm.

3. The name of a genus of insects of the order *Aptera* ONISCUS ASELLUS. The systematic name of the woodlouse. *Millepedes; Millepeda.* These insects, though they obtain a place in the pharmacopœias, are very seldom used medicinally in this country; they appear to act as stimulants and slight diuretics, and for this purpose they ought to be administered in a much greater dose than is usually prescribed. The expressed juice of forty or fifty living millepedes, given in a mild drink, has been said to cure very obstinate jaundices.

ONI'TIS. (From ονος, an ass, because asses covet it.) The *Origanum vulgare,* or wild marjoram.

ONOBRY'CHIS. (From ονος, an ass, and βρυχω, to bray: so called, according to Blanchard, because the smell or taste makes asses bray.) See *Hedysarum onobrychis.*

ONO'NIS. (From ονος, an ass: because it interrupts asses when at plough.) 1. The name of a genus of plants in the Linnæan system. Class, *Diadelphia;* Order, *Decandria.*

2. The pharmacopœial name of the rest-harrow See *Ononis spinosa.*

ONONIS ARVENSIS. See *Ononis spinosa.*

ONONIS SPINOSA. The systematic name of the rest-harrow. *Resta bovis; Arresta bovis; Remora aratri.* The roots of this plant have a faint unpleasant smell, and a sweetish, bitterish, somewhat nauseous taste. Their active matter is confined to the cortical part, which has been sometimes given in powder, or other forms, as an aperient and diuretic.

ONOPO'RDIUM. (Ονοπορδον; from ονος, an ass, and περδω, to break wind: so named from its being much coveted by asses, and from the noise it makes upon pressure.) 1. The name of a genus of plants in the Linnæan system. Class, *Syngenesia;* Order, *Polygamia æqualis.*

2. The pharmacopœial name of the cotton-thistle. See *Onopordium acanthium.*

ONOPORDIUM ACANTHIUM. The systematic name of he cotton-thistle. *Carduus tomentosus.* The plant distinguished by this name is thus described by Linnæus, *Onnpordium—calycibus squamosis squamis patentibus; foliis ovato-oblongis, sinuatis.* Its expressed juice has been recommended as a cure for cancer, either applied by moistening lint with it, or mixing some simple farinaceous substance, so as to form a poultice, which should be in contact with the disease, and renewed twice a day.

ONO'SMA. (From οσμη, a sweet smell or savour.) The name of a genus of plants. Class, *Pentandria;* Order, *Monogynia.*

ONOSMA ECHIOIDES. The systematic name of the plant, the root of which is called *Anchusa lutea* in some pharmacopœias. It is supposed to possess emmenagogue virtues.

ONY'CHIA. (From ονυξ, the nail.) A whitlow at the side of the finger nail.

O'NYX. Ονυξ. In surgery. *Unguis.* An abscess, or collection of pus between the lamellæ of the cornea; so called from its resemblance to the stone called onyx. The diagnostic signs are, a white spot or speck, prominent, soft, and fluctuating. The species are:

1. *Onyx superficialis,* arising from inflammation, not dangerous, for it vanishes when the inflammation is resolved by the use of astringent collyria.

2. *Onyx profundus,* or a deep abscess, which is deeper seated between the lamellæ of the cornea, sometimes breaking internally, and forming an hypopium: when it opens externally, it leaves a fistula upon the cornea; whenever the pus is exsiccated, there remains a leucoma.

In mineralogy, Calcedony, in which there is an alternation of white, black, and dark brown layers.

OOEI'DES. (From ωον, an egg, and ειδος, a likeness.) An epithet for the aqueous humour of the eye.

OPACITY. *Opacitas.* The faculty of obstructing the passage of light.

OPAL. Of this silicious stone there are seven kinds, according to Professor Jameson.

1. *Precious opal.* Of a milk-white colour, inclining to blue. It occurs in small veins in clay-porphyry, in Hungary.

2. *Common opal,* of a milk-white colour, found in Cornwall.

3. *Fire opal;* the colour of a hyacinth-red, found only in Mexico.

4. *Mother of pearl opal,* or *cacholong,* a variety of calcedony.

5. *Semi opal,* of a white, brown, or gray colour, found in Greenland, Iceland, and Scotland.

6. *Jasper opal,* or *ferruginous opal.* This is of a scarlet, or gray colour, and comes from Tokay, in Hungary.

7. *Wood opal,* of various colours, and found in alluvial land at Zatravia, in Hungary.

OPERCULUM. (*Operculum, i. n.*; a cover or lid.) The lid or cover of the fringe, called peristomum, of mosses. It is either *convex, accuminate, flat,* or *permanent,* never leaving the fringe: as in Phascum.

OPHI'ASIS. (From οφις, a serpent; so called from the serpentine direction in which the disease travels round the head.) A species of baldness which commences at the occiput, and winds to each ear, and sometimes to the forehead.

OPHIOGLOSSOI'DES. (From οφωγλοσσον, ophioglossum, and ειδος, a likeness.) A fungus resembling the Ophioglossum, or adder's tongue.

OPHIOGLO'SSUM. (From οφις, a serpent, and γλωσσα, a tongue; so called from the resemblance of its fruit.) The name of a genus of plants. Class, *Cryptogamia;* Order, *Filices.* Adder's tongue.

OPHIORRHI'ZA (From οφις, a serpent, and ριζα a root; because the plant, says Hermann, is regarded in Ceylon, as a grand specific for the bite of the naja or riband snake.) The name of a genus of plants. Class, *Pentandria;* Order, *Monogynia.*

OPHIORRHIZA MUNGOS. The systematic name of the plant, the root of which is called *Radix serpentum* in the pharmacopœias. *Mungos radix.* This bitter root is much esteemed in Java, Sumatra, &c. as preventing the effects which usually follow the bite of the *naja,* a venomous serpent, with which view it is eaten by them It is also said to be exhibited medicinally in the cure of intestinal worms.

OPHIOSCO'RODON. (From οφις, a serpent, and σκοροδον, garlic; so named because it is spotted like a serpent.) Broad-leaved garlic.

OPHIOSTA'PHYLUM. (From οφις, a serpent, and ςαφυλη, a berry; so called because serpents feed upon its berries.) White bryony. See *Bryonia alba.*

OPHIO'XYLUM. (From οφις, and ξυλον; because its root spreads in a zigzag manner like the twisting of a serpent.) The name of a genus of plants. Class, *Pentandria;* Order, *Monogynia.* Serpentine-wood plant.

OPHIOXYLUM SERPENTINUM. The systematic name of the tree, the wood of which is termed lignum serpentum. The nature of this root does not appear to be yet ascertained. It is very bitter. In the cure of the bite of venomous serpents and malignant diseases, it is said to be efficacious.

["OPHITES, or *Green Porphyry.* This is a green stone, which to the naked eye appears homogeneous, and varies in colour from blackish green to pistachio green. It contains greenish white crystals of feldspar, which, on the polished surface, often appear in parallelograms, and are sometimes cruciform. Its texture is very compact, and its fracture often splintery. In many cases its fine green colour is undoubtedly produced by epidote. This belongs to the *green porphyry* of the ancients."—*Cleav Min.* A.]

O'PHRYS. Οφρυς. 1. The lowest part of the forehead, where the eyebrows grow.

2. An herb, so called because its juice was used to make the hair of the eyebrows black.

OPHTHA'LMIA. (From οφθαλμος, the eye. *Ophthalmitis.* An inflammation of the membranes of the eye, or of the whole bulb of the eye. The symptoms which characterize this disease are a preternatural redness of the tunica conjunctiva, owing to a turgescence of its blood-vessels; pain and heat over the whole surface of the eye, often attended with a sensation of some extraneous body between the eye and eyelid, and a plentiful effusion of tears. All these symptoms are commonly increased by motion of the eye, or its coverings, and likewise by exposure to light. We judge of the depth of the inflammation by the degree of pain produced by light thrown upon the eye. When the pain produced by light is considerable, we have much reason to imagine that the parts at the bottom of the eye, and especially the retina, are chiefly affected; and, *vice versa,* when the pain is not much increased by this exposure, we conclude with great probability that the inflammation is confined perhaps entirely to the external covering of the eye. In superficial affections of this kind too, the symptoms are in general local; but, whenever the inflammation is deep-seated, it is attended with severe shooting pains through the head, and fever to a greater or less degree commonly takes place. During the whole course of the disease there is for the most part a very plentiful flow of tears, which frequently become so hot and acrid as to excoriate the neighbouring parts; but it often happens after the disease has been of some duration, that together with the tears a considerable quantity of a yellow purulent like matter is discharged, and when the inflammation has either spread to the eyelids, or has been seated there from the beginning, as soon as the tarsi become affected, a discharge takes place of a viscid glutinous kind of matter, which greatly adds to the patient's distress, as it tends to increase the inflammation, by cementing the eyelids so firmly together as to render it extremely difficult to separate them.

Ophthalmia is divided into external, when the inflammation is superficial, and internal, when the inflammation is deep-seated, and the globe of the eye is much affected.

In severe ophthalmia two distinct stages are commonly observable the first is attended with a great deal of heat and pain in the eye and considerable febrile disorder; the second is comparatively a chronic affection without pain and fever. The eye is merely weakened, moister than in the healthy state, and more or less red.

Ophthalmia may be induced by a variety of exciting causes, such as operate in producing inflammation in other situations. A severe cold in which the eyes are affected at the same time with the pituitary cavities, fauces, and trachea: change of weather; sudden transition from heat to cold; the prevalence of cold winds; residence in damp or sandy countries, in the hot season; exposure of the eyes to the vivid rays of the sun; are causes usually enumerated; and considering these t does not seem extraordinary that ophthalmia should often make its appearance as an epidemic, and afflict persons of every age and sex. Besides these exciting causes, writers also generally mention the suppression of some habitual discharge, as of the menses, bleedings from the nose, from hæmorrhoids, &c. Besides which, inflammation of the eyes may be occasioned by the venereal and scrofulous virus.

OPHTHA'LMIC. *Ophthalmicus.* Belonging to the eye.

OPHTHALMIC GANGLION. *Ganglion ophthalmicum.* Lenticular ganglion. This ganglion is formed in the orbit, by the union of a branch of the third or fourth pair with the first branch of the fifth pair of nerves.

OPHTHALMIC NERVE. *Nervus ophthalmicus.* Orbital nerve. The first branch of the ganglion or expansion of the fifth pair of nerves. It is from this nerve that a branch is given off, to form, with a branch of the sixth, the great intercostal nerve.

OPHTHALMICI EXTERNI. See *Motores oculorum.*

OPHTHALMODY'NIA. (From οφθαλμος, an eye, and οδυνη, pain.) A vehement pain in the eye, without, or with very little redness. The sensation of pain is various, as itching, burning, or as if gravel were between the globe of the eye and lids. The species are:

1. *Ophthalmodynia rheumatica,* which is a pain in the muscular expansions of the globe of the eye, without redness in the albuginea. The rheumatic inflammation is serous, and rarely produces redness.

2. *Ophthalmodynia periodica,* is a periodical pain in the eye, without redness.

3. *Ophthalmodynia spasmodica,* is a pressing pain in the bulb of the eye, arising from spasmodic contractions of the muscles of the eye, in nervous, hysteric, and hypochondriac persons. It is observed to terminate by a flow of tears.

4. *Ophthalmodynia from an internal inflammation* of the eye. In this disorder, there is a pain and sensation as if the globe was pressed out of the orbit.

5. *Ophthalmodynia hydrophthalmica.* After a great pain in the inferior part of the os frontis, the sight is obscured, the pupil is dilated, and the bulb of the eye appears larger, pressing on the lid. This species is likewise perceived from an incipient hydropthalmia of the vitreous humour.

6. *Ophthalmodynia arenosa,* is an itching and sensation of pain in the eye, as if sand or gravel were lodged between the globe and lid.

7. *Ophthalmodynia symptomatica,* which is a symptom of some other eye-disease, and is to be cured by removing the exciting cause.

8. *Ophthalmodynia cancrosa,* which arises from cancerous acrimony deposited in the eye, and is rarely curable.

OPHTHALMOPO'NIA. (From οφθαλμος, the eye, and πονεω, to labour.) An intense pain in the eye, whence the light is intolerable.

OPHTHALMOPTO'SIS. (From οφθαλμος, an eye, and πτωσις, a fall.) A falling down of the globe of the eye on the cheek, canthus, or upwards, the globe itself being scarce altered in magnitude. The cause is a relaxation of the muscles, and ligamentous expansions of the globe of the eye. The species are:

1. *Ophthalmoptosis violenta,* which is generated by a violent contusion or strong stroke, as happens sometimes in boxing. The eye falls out of the socket on the cheek or canthus of the eye, and from the elongation and extension of the optic nerve occasions immediate blindness.

2. *Ophthalmoptosis,* from a tumour within the orbit. An exostosis, toph, abscess, encysted tumours, as atheroma, hygroma; or scirrhus, forming within the orbit, or induration of the orbital adeps, may throw

the bulb of the eye out of the socket upwards, downwards, or towards either canthus.

3. *Ophthalmoptosis paralytica,* or the paralytic ophthalmoptosis, which arises from a palsy of the recti muscles, whence a stronger power in the oblique muscles of the bulb.

4. *Ophthalmoptosis staphylomatica,* when the staphyloma depresses the inferior eyelid, and extends on the cheek.

OPIATE. (*Opiatum;* from the effects being like that of opium.) A medicine that procures sleep, &c. See *Anodyne.*

O'PION. Οπιον. Opium.

OPI'SMUS. (From οπιον, opium.) An opiate confection.

OPISTHENAR. (From οπισθεν, backwards, and θεδαρ, the palm.) The back part of the hand.

OPISTHOCRA'NIUM. (From οπισθεν, backward, and κρανιον, the head.) The occiput, or hinder part of the head.

OPISTHOCYPHO'SIS. (From οπισθεν, backward, and κυφωσις, a gibbosity.) A curved spine.

OPISTHO'TONOS. (From οπισθεν, backward, and τεινω, to draw.) A fixed spasm of several muscles, so as to keep the body in a fixed position, and bent backwards. Cullen considers it as a variety of tetanus. See *Tetanus.*

O'PIUM. (Probably from οπος, juice; or from οπι, Arabian.) The inspissated juice of the poppy. See *Papaver somniferum.*

OPOBA'LSAMUM. (From οπος, juice, and βαλσαμον, balsam.) See *Amyris gileadensis.*

OPOCA'LPASON. (From οπος, juice, and καλπασον, a tree of that name.) *Opocarpason.* A kind of bdellium which resembles myrrh, but is poisonous.

OPODELDOC. A term of no meaning, frequently mentioned by Paracelsus. Formerly it signified a plaster for all external injuries, but now is confined to a camphorated soap liniment.

OPODEOCE'LE. A rupture through the foramen ischii, or into the labia pudendi.

OPO'PANAX. (*Opopanax, acis.* f.; from οπος, juice, and παναξ, the panacea.) See *Pastinaca opopanax.*

OPO'PIA. (From οπτομαι, to see.) The bones of the eyes.

OPO'RICE. (From οπωρα, autumnal fruits.) A conserve made of ripe fruits.

OPPILA'TIO. (From *oppilo,* to shut up.) *Oppilation* is a close kind of obstruction; for, according to Rhodius, it signifies, not only to shut out, but also to fill.

OPPILATI'VA. (From *oppilo,* to shut up.) Medicines or substances which shut up the pores of the skin.

OPPO'NENS. Opposing. A name given to some muscles from their office.

OPPONENS POLLICIS. See *Flexor ossis metacarpi pollicis.*

OPPOSITIFOLIUS. Applied to a flower-stalk, when opposite to a leaf; the Geranium molle, and Sium angustifolium, afford examples of the *Pedunculus oppositifolius.*

OPPOSITUS. Opposite to each other; as the leaves of *Saxifraga oppositifolia,* and *Ballote nigra.*

OPPRE'SSION. *Oppressio.* The catalepsy, or any pressure upon the brain. See *Compression.*

OPSI'GONOS. (From οψι, late, and γινομαι, to be born.) A dens sapientiæ, or late cut tooth.

OPTIC. (*Opticus;* from οπτομαι, to see.) Relating to the eye.

OPTIC NERVE. *Nervus opticus.* The second pair of nerves of the brain. They arise from the thalami nervorum opticorum, perforate the bulb of the eye, and in it form the retina.

OPU'NTIA. (*Ab Opunte,* from the city *Opus,* near which it flourished.) See *Cactus.*

ORACHE. See *Atriplex hortensis,* and *Chenopodium.*

ORANGE. See *Citrus aurantium.*

Orange, Seville. See *Citrus aurantium.*

Orange, shaddock. See *Shaddock.*

ORBICULA'RE OS. *Os pisiforme.* The name of a bone of the carpus. Also a very small round bone, not larger than a pin-head, that belongs to the internal ear.

ORBICULA'RIS. (From *orbiculus,* a little ring: so called from its shape.) This name is given to some muscles which surround the part like a ring.

ORBICULARIS ORIS. *Sphincter labiorum,* of Douglas:

semi-orbicularis, of Winslow ; *constrictor oris* of Cowper; and *labial*, of Dumas. A muscle of the mouth, formed in a great measure by those of the lips; the fibres of the superior descending, those of the inferior ascending and decussating each other about the corner of the mouth, they run along the lip to join those of the opposite side, so that the fleshy fibres appear to surround the mouth like a sphincter. Its use is to shut the mouth, by contracting and drawing both lips together, and to counteract all the muscles that assist in opening it.

ORBICULARIS PALPEBRARUM. A muscle common to both the eyelids. *Orbicularis palpebrarum ciliaris*, of authors ; and *maxillo palpebral*, of Dumas. It arises by a number of fleshy fibres from the outer edge of the orbitar process of the superior maxillary bone, and from a tendon near the inner angle of the eye ; these fibres run a little downwards and outwards, over the upper part of the cheek, below the orbit, covering the under eyelid, and surround the external angle, being closely connected only to the skin and fat; they then run over the superciliary ridge of the os frontis, towards the inner canthus, where they mix with the fibres of the occipito-frontalis and corrugator supercilii : then covering the upper eyelid, they descend to the inner angle opposite to their inferior origin, and firmly adhere to the internal angular process of the os frontis, and to the short round tendon which serves to fix the palpebræ and muscular fibres arising from it. It is inserted into the nasal process of the superior maxillary bone, by a short round tendon, covering the anterior and upper part of the lachrymal sac, which tendon can be easily felt at the inner canthus of the eye. The use of this muscle is to shut the eye, by drawing both lids together, the fibres contracting from the outer angle towards the inner, press the eyeball, squeeze the lachrymal gland, and convey the tears towards the puncta lachrymalia.

ORBICULARIS PALPEBRARUM CILIARIS. See *Orbicularis palpebrarum*.

ORBICULATUS. Orbiculate. Applied to a leaf that is circular or orbicular, the length and breadth being equal, and the circumference an even circular line. Precise examples of this are scarcely to be found. Some species of pepper approach it, and the leaf of the Hedysarum styracifolium is perfectly orbicular, except a notch at the base.

ORBIT. *Orbitum*. The two cavities under the forehead, in which the eyes are situated, are termed orbits. The angles of the orbits are called *canthi*. Each orbit is composed of seven bones, viz. the frontal, maxillary, jugal, lachrymal, ethmoid, palatine, and sphenoid. The use of this bony socket is to maintain and defend the organ of sight, and its adjacent parts.

O'RCHEA. Galen says it is the *scrotum*.

ORCHIDEÆ. (From *orchis*, a plant so called.) The name of an order in Linnæus's Fragments of a Natural Method, consisting of those which have fleshy roots and orchideal corolls.

ORCHIDEUS. Orchideal: resembling the orchis.

ORCHIS. (Ορχις, a testicle ; from ορεγομαι, to desire.) 1. A testicle.

2. The name of a genus of plants in the Linnæan system. Class, *Gynandria*; Order, *Diandria*.

ORCHIS BIFOLIA. The systematic name of the butterfly orchis, the root of which is used indifferently with that of the male orchis. See *Orchis mascula*.

ORCHIS MASCULA. The systematic name of the male orchis. Dog's stones. Male orchis. *Satyrion*. *Orchis—bulbis indivisis, nectarii labio quadrilobo crenulato, cornu obtuso petalis dorsalibus reflexus* of Linnæus. The root has a place in the Materia Medica of the Edinburgh pharmacopœia, on account of the glutinous slimy juice which it contains. The root of the *orchis bifolia* is also collected. Satyrion root has a sweetish taste, a faint and somewhat unpleasant smell. Its mucilaginous or gelatinous quality has recommended it as a demulcent. Salep, which is imported here from the East, is a preparation of an analogous root which is considered as an article of diet, is accounted extremely nutritious, as containing a great quantity of farinaceous matter in a small bulk. The supposed aphrodisiac qualities of this root, which have been noticed ever since the days of Dioscorides, seems, says Dr. Woodville, to be founded on the fanciful doctrine of signatures; thus, *orchis*, i. e. ορχις, *testiculus habet radices, instar testiculorum*.

ORCHIS MORIO. The systematic name of the orchis, from the root of which the salep is made. Salep is a farinaceous powder imported from Turkey. It may be obtained from several other species of the same genus of plants. It is an insipid substance, of which a small quantity, by proper management, converts a large portion of water into a jelly, the nutritive powers of which have been greatly overrated. Salep forms a considerable part of the diet of the inhabitants of Turkey, Persia, and Syria. The method of preparing salep is as follows :—The new root is to be washed in water, and the fine brown skin which covers it is to be separated by means of a small brush, or by dipping the root in warm water, and rubbing it with a coarse linen cloth. The roots thus cleaned are to be spread on a tin plate, and placed in an oven, heated to the usual degree, where they are to remain six or ten minutes. In this time they will have lost their milky whiteness, and acquired a transparency like horn, without any diminution of bulk. Being arrived at this state, they are to be removed in order to dry and harden in the air, which will require several days to effect; or they may be dried in a few hours, by using a very gentle heat. Salep, thus prepared, contains a great quantity of vegetable aliment; as a wholesome nourishment it is much superior to rice; and has the singular property of concealing the taste of salt water. Hence, to prevent the dreadful calamity of famine at sea, it has been proposed that the powder of it should constitute part of the provisions of every ship's company. With regard to its medicinal properties, it may be observed, that its restorative, mucilaginous, and demulcent qualities, render it of considerable use in various diseases, when employed as aliment, particularly in sea-scurvy, diarrhœa, dysentery, symptomatic fever, arising from the absorption of pus, and the stone or gravel.

ORCHITIS. (From ορχις, a testicle.) *Hernia humoralis*. Swelled testicle. A very common symptom attending a gonorrhœa is a swelling of the testicle, which is only sympathetic, and not venereal, because the same symptoms follow every kind of irritation on the urethra, whether produced by strictures, injections, or bougies. Such symptoms are not similar to the actions arising from the application of venereal matter, for suppuration seldom occurs, and, when it does, the matter is not venereal. The swelling and inflammation appear suddenly, and as suddenly disappear, or go from one testicle to the other. The epididymis remains swelled, however, even for a considerable time afterward.

The first appearance of swelling is generally a soft pulpy fulness of the body of the testicle, which is tender to the touch; this increases to a hard swelling accompanied with considerable pain. The epididymis, towards the lower end of the testicle, is generally the hardest part. The hardness and swelling, however, often pervade the whole of the epididymis. The spermatic cord, and especially the vas deferens, are often thickened, and sore to the touch. The spermatic veins sometimes become varicose. A pain in the loins, and sense of weakness there, and in the pelvis, are other casual symptoms. Colicky pains; uneasiness in the stomach and bowels; flatulency; sickness, and even vomiting; are not unfrequent. The whole testicle is swelled, and not merely the epididymis, as has been asserted.

The inflammation of the part most probably arises from its sympathizing with the urethra. The swelling of the testicle coming on, either removes the pain in making water, and suspends the discharge, which does not return till such swelling begins to subside, or else the irritation in the urethra, first ceasing, produces a swelling of the testicle, which continues till the pain and discharge return; thus rendering it doubtful which is the cause and which the effect. Occasionally, however, the discharge has become more violent, though the testicle has swelled; and such swelling has even been known to occur after the discharge has ceased; yet the latter has returned with violence, and remained as long as the hernia humoralis.

Hernia humoralis, with stoppage of the discharge, is apt to be attended with strangury. A very singular thing is, that the inflammation more frequently comes on when the irritation in the urethra is going off, than when at its height.

The enlargement of the testicle, from cancer and

scrofula, are generally slow in their progress : that of a hernia humoralis very quick.

O'RCHOS. (From ορχος, a plantation or orchard : so called from the regularity with which the hairs are inserted.) The extremities of the eyelids, where the eyelashes grow.

ORCHO'TOMY. (*Orchotcmia*; from ορχις, a testicle, and τεμνω, to cut.) Castration. The operation of extracting a testicle.

ORDER. A term applied by naturalists and nosologists to designate a division that embraces a number of genera which have some circumstances common to them all. See *Genus, Plants, sexual system of*, and *Nosology*.

Orders, natural, of plants. See *Natural*.

ORE. The mineral substance from which metals are extracted.

OREOSELI'NUM. (From ορος, a mountain, and σελινον, parsley : so named because it grows wild upon mountains.) Mountain parsley. See *Athamanta*.

ORE'STION. (From ορος, a mountain.) In Dioscorides it is the *Helenium*, or a kind of elecampane, growing upon mountains.

OREXIA. (From ορεγομαι, to desire.) *Orexis*. A desire or appetite.

ORE'XIS. Seo *Orexia*.

ORGAN. Οογανον. *Organum*. A part of the body capable of the performance of some perfect act or operation. They are distinguished by physiologists by their functions, as organs of sense, organs of motion, organs of sensation, digestive organs, &c.

ORGANIC. Of or belonging to an organ. In the present day this term is in general use to distinguish a disease of structure from a functional disease ; thus, when the liver is converted into a hard tuberculated or other structure, it is called an *organic* disease ; but when it merely furnishes a bad bile, the disease is said to be *functional*.

["ORGANIC RELICS. These fossil relics are of two kinds, *Petrifactions* and *Conservatives*. -

Petrifactions, or *Substitutions*, are those relics, which are entirely made up of mineral substances, which have gradually run into the places occupied by organized bodies as those bodies decayed, and assumed their forms.

Conservatives, or *Preservatives*, are those relics, or parts thereof, which still consist of the very same substances, which originally composed the living organized being.

An organic relic may partake of both kinds. The shell of an oyster, being chiefly carbonate of lime, may still remain, which would be a *conservative*. While the enclosed animal matter will be entirely decayed, and mineral matter occupy its place and imitate its form, which would be a *petrifaction*.

Organic relics are *named* by annexing the termination *lithos* (a stone) to the scientific name of the living organized being. As ichthyolithos is composed of ιχθυς (a fish) and λιθος (a stone). That is, a fish becoming stone. In English, *lithos* is changed to *lite*, as *ichthyolite*. Sometimes the letter *l* is left out, as lacerta (lizard) would make *lacertit*, (a petrified lizard). This abridged method has now come into general use." —*Eat. Geol.* A.]

ORGASM. See *Orgasmus*.

ORGASMUS. (From οργαω, " appeto impatienter ; proprie de anemantibus dicitur, quæ turgent libidine." *Scapula*.) Salacity.

ORGASTICA. The name of an order of the class *Genetica*, in Good's Nosology. Diseases affecting the orgasm. Its genera are, *chlorosis, præotia, lagnesis, agenesia, aphorca, œdoptosis*.

ORIBASIUS, an eminent physician of the 4th century, was born at Pergamus, or, according to others, at Sardes, where he resided for some time. He is mentioned as one of the most learned and accomplished men of his age, and the most skilful in his profession ; and he not only obtained great public reputation, but also the friendship of the Emperor Julian, who appointed him quæstor of Constantinople. But after the death of that prince he suffered a severe reverse ; he was stripped of his property, and sent into banishment among the Barbarians. He sustained his misfortunes, however, with great fortitude ; and the dignity of his character, with his professional skill and kindness, gained him the veneration of these rude people, among whom he was adored as a tutelary god. At length he

was recalled to the imperial court, and regained the public favour. He was chiefly a compiler ; but some valuable practical remarks first occur in his writings. He made, at the request of Julian, extensive " Collec tions" from Galen, and other preceding authors, in about seventy books, of which only seventeen now remain ; and afterward made a " Synopsis of this vast work for the use of his son, in nine books : there are also extant four books, in medicines and diseases, entitled " Euporistorum Libri." He praises highly local evacuations of blood, especially by scarifications, which had been little noticed before : and he affirms, that he was himself cured of the plague by it, having lost in this way two pounds of blood from the thighs on the second day of the disease. He first described a singular species of insanity, under the name of *lycanthropia*, in which the patient wanders about by night among the tombs, as if changed into a wolf : though such a disease is noticed in the New Testament.

ORICHALCUM. The brass of the ancients.

ORI'CIA. (From *Oricus*, a city of Epirus, near which it grows.) A species of fir or turpentine-tree, from Oricus.

ORIENTALIA FOLIA. The leaves of senna were so called.

ORI'GANUM. (From ορος, a mountain, and γανοω, to rejoice : so called because it grows upon the side of mountains.)

1. The name of a genus of plants in the Linnæan system. Class, *Didynamia*; Order, *Gymnospermia*.

2. The pharmacopœial name of the wild marjoram. See *Origanum vulgare*.

ORIGANUM CRETICUM. See *Origanum dictamnus*

ORIGANUM DICTAMNUS. The systematic name of the dittany of Crete. *Dictamnus creticus; Origanum creticum; Onitis*. The leaves of this plant, *Origanum—foliis inferioribus tomentosis, spicis nutantibus* of Linnæus, are now rarely used ; they have been recommended as emmenagogue and alexipharmic.

ORIGANUM MARJORANA. The systematic name of sweet marjoram. *Marjorana*. This plant, *Origanum—foliis ovatis obtusis, spicis subrotundis compactis pubescentibus* of Linnæus, has been long cultivated in our gardens, and is in frequent use for culinary purposes. The leaves and tops have a pleasant smell, and a moderately warm, aromatic, bitterish taste. They yield their virtues to aqueous and spirituous liquors, by infusion, and to water in distillation, affording a considerable quantity of essential oil. The medicinal qualities of the plant are similar to those of the wild plant (see *Origanum vulgare*) ; but being much more fragrant, it is thought to be more cephalic, and better adapted to those complaints known by the name of nervous ; and may therefore be employed with the same intentions as lavender. It was directed in the *pulvis sternutatorius*, by both pharmacopœias, with a view to the agreeable odour which it communicates to the asarabacca, rather than to its errhine power, which is very inconsiderable ; but it is now wholly omitted in the Pharm. Lond. In its recent state, it is said to have been successfully applied to scirrhous tumours of the breast.

ORIGANUM SYRIACUM. The Syrian herb mastich. See *Teucrium marum*.

ORIGANUM VULGARE. The systematic name of the wild marjoram. *Marjorana; Mancurana; Origanum heracleoticum; Onitis; Zazarhendi herba. Origanum—spicis subrotundis paniculatis conglomeratis, bractis calyce longioribus ovatis* of Linnæus. This plant grows wild in many parts of Britain. It has an agreeable aromatic smell, approaching to that of marjoram, and a pungent taste, much resembling thyme, to which it is likewise thought to be more allied in its medicinal qualities, and therefore deemed to be em menagogue, tonic, stomachic, &c. The dried leaves, used instead of tea, are said to be exceedingly grateful. They are employed in medicated baths and fomentations.

ORIS CONSTRICTOR. See *Orbicularis oris*.

ORLEANA TERRA. (*Orleana*, so named from the place where it grows.) See *Bixa orleana*.

ORMSKIRK. The name of a place in which Hill lived, who invented a medicine for the cure of hydrophobia, and died without making known its composition. The analysis of Drs. Black and Hepburn demonstrates it to be half an ounce of powder of chalk ; three drachms of Armenian bole ; ten grains of alum; one drachm of powder of elecampane root; six drops of oil of anise. This dose is to be taken every morning for six times in a glass of water, with a small proportion of fresh milk.

ORNITHO'GALUM. (From ορνις, a bird, and γαλα, milk: so called from the colour of its flowers, which are like the milk found in eggs.) The name of a genus of plants in the Linnæan system. Class, *Hexandria;* Order, *Monogynia.*

ORNITHOGALUM MARITIMUM, a kind of wild onion. See *Scilla.*

ORNITHOGLOSSUM. (From ορνις, a bird, and γλωσσα, a tongue: so called from its shape.) Bird's tongue. The seeds of the ash-tree are sometimes so called.

ORNITHOLOGY. (*Ornithologia;* from ορνις, a bird, and λογος, a discourse.) That part of natural history which treats of birds.

ORNITHOPO'DIUM. (From ορνις, a bird, and πους, a foot: so called from the likeness of its pods to a bird's claw.) Bird's foot; scorpion wort. The *Ornithropus perpusillus,* and *Scorpioides,* of Linnæus, are so called.

O'RNUS. (From *orn,* Heb.) The ash-tree which affords manna.

OROBA'NCHE. (From οροβος, the wild pea, and αγχω, to suffocate: so called because it twines round the orobus and destroys it.) The name of a genus of plants in the Linnæan system. Class, *Gynandria* and *Didynamia;* Order, *Angiospermia.*

OROBRY'CHIS. (From οροβος, the wood-pea, and βρυχω, to eat.) The same as orobance.

O'ROBUS. (From ερεπ]ω, to eat.) 1. The name of a genus of plants in the Linnæan system. Class, *Diadelphia;* Order, *Decandria.*

2. The pharmacopœial name of the ervum. See *Ervum.*

OROBUS TUBEROSUS. The heath-pea. The root of this plant is said to be nutritious. The Scotch islanders hold them in great esteem, and chew them like tobacco.

OROSELI'NUM. See *Athamanta.*

ORPIMENT. *Orpimentum.* A sulphuret of arsenic. Native orpiment is found in yellow, brilliant, and, as it were, talky masses, often mixed with realgar, and sometimes of a greenish colour. See *Arsenic.*

ORPINE. See *Sedum telephium.*

ORRHOPY'GIUM. (From ορος, the extremity, and πυγη, the buttocks.) The extremity of the spine, which is terminated by the os coccygis.

O'RRHOS. (From ρεω, to flow.) 1. Serum, whey.

2. The raphe of the scrotum.

3. The extremity of the sacrum.

ORRIS. See *Iris.*

Orris, Florentine. See *Iris florentina.*

Orseille. See *Lichen rocella.*

ORTHITE. A mineral; so named because it always occurs in straight layers, generally in felspar. It resembles gadolinite. It is found in the mine of Fimbo in Sweden.

ORTHOCO'LON. (From ορθος, straight, and κωλον, a limb.) It is a species of stiff joint, when it cannot be bended, but remains straight.

ORTHOPNŒ'A. ·(From ορθος, erect, and πνοη, breathing.) A very quick and laborious breathing, during which the person is obliged to be in an erect posture.

ORVA'LE. (*Orvale,* French.) A species of clary or horminum.

ORVIETA'NUM, a medicine that resists poisons; from a mountebank of Orvieta, in Italy, who first made himself famous by taking such things upon the stage, after doses of pretended poisons; though some say its inventor was one Orvietanus, and that it is named after him.

ORY'ZA. (From *orez,* Arabian.) 1. The name of a genus of plants in the Linnæan system. Class, *Triandria.* Order, *Digynia.* The rice plant.

2. The pharmacopœial name for rice. See *Oryza sativa.*

ORYZA SATIVA. The systematic name of the plant which affords the rice, which is the principal food of the inhabitants in all parts of the East, where it is boiled, and eaten either alone or with their meat. Large quantities of it are annually sent into Europe, and it meets with a general esteem for family purposes. The people of Java have a method of making puddings of rice,

which seems to be unknown here; but it is not difficult to put in practice if it should merit attention. They take a conical earthen pot, which is open at the large end, and perforated all over. This they fill about half full with rice, and putting it into a large earthen pot of the same shape, filled with boiling water, the rice in the first pot soon swells, and stops the perforations, so as to keep out the water. By this method the rice is brought to a firm consistence, and forms a pudding, which is generally eaten with butter, oil, sugar, vinegar, and spices. The Indians eat stewed rice with good success against the bloody flux; and in most inflammatory disorders they cure themselves with only a decoction of it. The spirituous liquor called arrack is made from this grain. Rice grows naturally in moist places, and will not come to perfection, when cultivated, unless the ground be sometimes overflowed or plentifully watered. The grain is of a gray colour when first reaped; but the growers have a method of whitening it before it is sent to market. The manner of performing this, and beating it out in Egypt, is thus described by Hasselquist: They have hollow iron cylindrical pestles, about an inch diameter, lifted by a wheel worked with oxen. A person sits between the pestles, and, as they rise, pushes forward the rice, while another winnows and supplies fresh parcels. Thus they continue working until it is entirely free from chaff. Having in this manner cleaned it, they add one-thirtieth part of salt, and rub them both together, by which the grain acquires a whiteness; then it is passed through a sieve, to separate the salt again from it. In the island of Ceylon they have a much more expeditious method of getting out the rice; for, in the field where it is reaped, they dig a round hole, with a level bottom, about a foot deep, and eight yards diameter, and fill it with bundles of corn. Having laid it properly, the women drive about half a dozen oxen continually round the pit; and thus they will tread out forty or fifty bushels a day. This is a very ancient method of treading out corn, and is still practised in Africa upon other sorts of grain.

OS. 1. (*Os, ossis.* n.) A bone. See *Bone.*

2. (*Os, oris.* n.) The mouth.

Os EXTERNUM. The entrance into the vagina is so named in opposition to the mouth of the womb, which is called the *os internum.*

Os INTERNUM. The orifice or mouth of the uterus.

Os LEONIS. The *Antirrhinum linaria.*

Os SPONGIOSUM. The spongy bones are two in number, and are called *ossa spongiosa inferiora.* The ethmoid bone has two turbinated portions, which are sometimes called the superior spongy bones. These bones, which, from their shape, are sometimes called *ossa turbinata,* have, by some anatomists, been described as belonging to the ethmoid bone; and by others, as portions of the ossa palati. In young subjects, however, they are evidently distinct bones. They consist of a spongy lamella in each nostril. The convex surface of this lamina is turned towards the septum narium, and its concave part towards the maxillary bone, covering the opening of the lachrymal duct into the nose. From their upper edge arise two processes: the posterior of these, which is the broadest, hangs as it were upon the edge of the antrum highmorianum; the anterior one joins the os unguis, and forms a part of the lachrymal duct. These bones are complete in the fœtus. They are lined with the pituitary membrane; and, besides their connexion with the ethmoid bone, are joined to the ossa maxillaria superiora, ossa palati, and ossa unguis. Besides these ossa spongiosa inferiora, there are sometimes two others, situated lower down, one in each nostril. These are very properly considered as a production of the sides of the maxillary sinus turned downwards. In many subjects, likewise, we find other smaller bones standing out into the nostrils, which, from their shape, might also deserve the name of *turbinata,* but they are uncertain in their size, situation, and number.

Os TINCÆ. See *Tincæ os.*

[OSBORN, JOHN C. M.D. the eldest son of Dr. John Osborn, was born at Middletown, Connecticut, September, 1766. He received his classical education at Middletown, under the Rev. Enoch Huntington, an eminent scholar; and his medical education exclusively under his father. He was not distinguished by any academic honour till he became eminent in his profession in North Carolina, to which state he re moved in 1787. Here he was well known as a successful practitioner, and was repeatedly placed at the head of the Medical Society of the district. He came to the city of New-York in 1807, and was shortly after introduced to a large scene of practice. He was created Professor of the Institutes of Medicine, in the Medical Faculty of Columbia College, and upon the union of that Faculty with the College of Physicians and Surgeons, he was appointed Professor of Obstetrics and the Diseases of Women and Children. He died of a pulmonary disorder in the island of St. Croix, upon the day of his landing, March 5th, 1819.

With his professional erudition, Dr. Osborn united great literary acquirements, and his knowledge of books was varied and extensive. These acquisitions he often displayed in his course of public instruction. His view of the Materia Medica as a science was equalled by few, and his knowledge of the actual medical qualities of the native productions of our soil, was a subject which he delighted to investigate, and in his practice, and by his instructions, he earnestly enjoined an acquaintance with these important remedial agents.

Dr. Osborn was a man of much more science and eminence in his profession than either his father or grandfather, and possessed a very fine taste for poetry, belles lettres, and painting. While he was quite a young man, Mr. Barlow submitted to him and his friend, the late Richard Alsop, Esq. the manuscript of the Vision of Columbus, for their correction and revision, previous to its publication. His taste in painting was highly cultivated, and he might have attained to great eminence as an artist."—*Thach. Med. Biog.* A.]

OSCE'DO. A yawning.

OSCHEOCE'LE. (From *οσχεον*, the scrotum, and *κηλη*, a tumour.) 1. Any tumour of the scrotum.

2. A scrotal hernia.

O'SCHEON. *Οσχεον*. The scrotum. Galen gives the name to the *os uteri.*

OSCHEO'PHYMA. (From *οσχεον*, the scrotum, and *φυμα*, a tumour.) A swelling of the scrotum.

OSCILLATION. Vibration. See *Irritability.*

O'SCITANS. (From *oscito*, to gape.) Yawning. Gaping.

OSCITA'TIO. (From *oscito*, to gape.) Yawning. Gaping.

OSCULATO'RIUS. (From *osculo*, to kiss : so called because the action of kissing is performed by it.) The sphincter muscle of the lips.

O'SCULUM. (Diminutive of *os*, a mouth.) A little mouth.

OSMAZOME. If cold water, which has been digested for a few hours on slices of raw muscular fibre, with occasional pressure, be evaporated, filtered, and then treated with pure alkohol, a peculiar animal principle will be dissolved, to the exclusion of the salts. By dissipating the alkohol with a gentle heat, the osmazome is obtained. It has a brownish-yellow colour, and the taste and smell of soup. Its aqueous solution affords precipitates, with infusion of nut-galls, nitrate of mercury, and nitrate and acetate of lead.

OSMIUM. A new metal lately discovered by Tennant among platina, and so called by him from the pungent and peculiar smell of its oxide.

OSMUND. See *Osmunda regalis.*

OSMU'NDA. (From *Osmund*, who first used it.) The name of a genus of plants. Class, *Cryptogamia*; Order, *Filices.*

OSMUNDA REGALIS. *Filix florida.* The systematic name of the osmund-royal. Its root possesses astringent and emmenagogue virtues.

O'SPHYS. *Οσφυς.* The loins.

OSSA SPONGEOSA. See *Os spongiosum.*

OSSI'CULUM. A little bone.

OSSICULA AUDITUS. The small bones of the internal ear are four in number, viz. the malleus, incus, stapes, and os orbiculare; and are situated in the cavity of the tympanum. See *Malleus, Incus, Stapes,* and *Orbiculare os.*

OSSIFICATION. (*Ossificatio*; from *os*, a bone, and *facio*, to make.) See *Osteogeny.*

OSSI'FRAGA. (From *os*, a bone, and *frango*, to break.) A petrified root, called the bone-binder, from its supposed virtues in uniting fractured bones.

OSSI'FRAGUS. See *Osteocolla.*

OSSI'VORUS. (From *os*, a bone, and *voro*, to devour.) Applied to a species of tumour or ulcer which destroys the bone.

140

OSTA'GRA. (From *οστεον*, a bone, and *αγρα*, a laying hold of.) A forceps to take out bones with.

OSTEI'TES. (From *οςεον*, a bone.) The bone-binder See *Osteocolla.*

OSTEOCO'LLA. (From *οςεον*, a bone, and *κολλαω* to glue.) *Ossifraga; Holosteus; Osteites; Amos teus; Osteolithos; Stelochites.* Glue-bone, stone, or bone-binder. A particular carbonate of lime found in some parts of Germany, particularly in the Marché of Brandenburg, and in other countries. It is met with in loose sandy grounds, spreading from near the surface to a considerable depth, into a number of ramifications like the roots of a tree. It is of a whitish colour, soft while under the earth, friable when dry, rough on the surface, for the most part either hollow within, or filled with a solid wood, or with a powdery white matter. It was formerly celebrated for promoting the coalition of fractured bones, and the formation of callus, which virtues are not attributed to it in the present day.

OSTEO'COPUS. (From *οςεον*, a bone, and *κοπος*, uneasiness.) A very violent fixed pain in any part of the bone.

OSTEOGE'NICA. (From *οςεον*, a bone, and *γενναω*, to beget.) Medicines which promote the generation of a callus.

OSTEOGENY. (*Osteogenia*; from *οςεον*, a bone, and *γενεια*, generation.) The growth of bones. Bones are either formed between membranes, or in the substance of cartilage; and the bony deposition is effected by a determined action of arteries. The secretion of bone takes place in cartilage in the long bones, as those of the arm, leg, &c.; and between two layers of membrane, as in the bones of the skull, where true cartilage is never seen. Often the bony matter is formed in distinct bags, and there it grows into form, as in the teeth; for each tooth is formed in its little bag, which, by injection, can be filled and covered with vessels. An artery of the body can assume this action, and deposite bone, which is formed also where it should not be, in the tendons and in the joints, in the great arteries and in the valves, in the flesh of the heart itself, or even in the soft and pulpy substance of the brain.

Most of the bones in the fœtus are merely cartilage before the time of birth. This cartilage is never hardened into bone, but from the first it is an organized mass. It has its vessels, which are at first transparent, but which soon dilate; and whenever the red colour of the blood begins to appear in them, ossification very quickly succeeds, the arteries being so far enlarged as to carry the coarser parts of the blood. The first mark of ossification is an artery which is seen running into the centre of the jelly which is formed. Other arteries soon appear, and a net-work of vessels is formed, and then a centre of ossification begins, stretching its rays according to the length of the bone, and then the cartilage begins to grow opaque, yellow, brittle: it will no longer bend, and a bony centre may easily be discovered. Other points of ossification are successively formed, preceded by the appearance of arteries. The ossification follows the vessels, and buries and hides those vessels by which it is formed. The vessels advance towards the end of the bone, the whole body of the bone becomes opaque, and there is left a small vascular circle only at either end. The heads are separated from the body of the bone by a thin cartilage, and the vessels of the centre, extending still towards the extremities of the bone, perforate the cartilage, pass into the head of the bone, and then its ossification also begins, and a small nucleus of ossification is formed in its centre. Thus the heads and the body are at first distinct bones, formed apart, joined by a cartilage, and not united till the age of fifteen or twenty years. Then the deposition of bone begins; and while the bone is laid by the arteries, the cartilage is conveyed away by the absorbing vessels; and while they convey away the superfluous cartilage, they model the bone into its due form, shape out its cavities, cancelli and holes, remove the thinner parts of the remaining cartilage, and harden it into due consistence. The earth which constitutes the hardness of bone, and all its useful properties, is inorganized, and lies in the interstices of bone, where it is made up of gelatinous matter to give it consistence and strength, furnished with absorbents to keep it in health, and carry off its wasted parts; and pervaded by blood-vessels to supply it with new matter. During all the process of ossification, the absorbents proportion their action to the stimulus which is applied to them: they carry away the serous fluid, when jelly is to take its place; they remove the jelly as the bone is laid; they continue removing the bony particles also, which (as in a circle) the arteries continually renew. This renovation and change of parts goes on even in the hardest bones, so that after a bone is perfectly formed, its older particles are continually being removed, and new ones are deposited in their place. The bony particles are so deposited in the flat bones of the skull as to present a radiated structure, and the vacancies between the fibres which occasion this appearance, are found by injection to be chiefly passages for blood-vessels. As the fœtus increases in size, the osseous fibres increase in number, till a lamina is produced; and as the bone continues to grow, more laminæ are added, till the more solid part of a bone is formed. The ossification which begins in cartilage is considerably later than that which has its origin between membranes. The generality of bones are incomplete until the age of puberty, or between the fifteenth and twentieth years, and in some few instances not until a later period. The small bones of the ear, however, are completely formed at birth.

OSTEOGRAPHY. (*Osteographia;* from ος ̔εον, a bone, and γραφω, to describe.) The description of the bones. See *Bone.*

OSTEOLI'THOS. (From ος ̔εον, a bone, and λιθος, a stone.) See *Osteocolla.*

OSTEOLOGY. (*Osteologia;* from ος ̔εον, a bone, and λογος, a discourse.) The doctrine of the bones. See *Bone.*

OSTEOPŒDION. (From ος ̔εον, a bone, and παις, παιδος, an infant.) *Lithopœdion.* A term given to the mass of an extra-uterine fœtus, which had become osseous, or of an almost stony consistence.

OSTHEXIA. (From ος ̔ωδης, osseous or bony, and εξις, habit.) The name in Good's Nosology of a genus of diseases. Class, *Eccritica;* Order, *Mesotica.* Osthexy or ossific diathesis. It has two species, *Osthexia infarciens; implexa.*

OSTIA'RIUS. (From *ostium,* a door.) The pylorus has been so called.

OSTI'OLA. (Diminutive of *ostium,* a door.) The valves or gates of the heart.

OSTIUM. A door or opening. Applied to small foramina or openings.

O'STREA. (From ος ̔ρακον, a shell.) The oyster. The shell of this fish is occasionally used medicinally; its virtues are similar to those of the carbonate of lime. See *Creta.*

OSTRU'THIUM. See *Imperatoria.*

OSY'RIS. (Οσυρις of Dioscorides, which he describes as a small shrub with numerous, dark, tough branches; and Professor Martyn conjectures its derivation from οζος, a branch. Some take the *antirrhinum linaria* for the true *Osyris.*) The name of a genus of plants in the Linnæan system. Class, *Diœcia;* Order, *Triandria.*

OSYRIS ALBA. *Cassia poetica lobelli; Cassia latinorum; Cassia lignea monspeliensium; Cassia monspeliensium.* Poet's cassia or gardrobe; Poet's rosemary. The whole shrub is astringent. It grows in the southern parts of Europe.

OTA'LGIA. (From ους, the ear, and αλγος, pain,) The earache.

OTENCHY'TES. (From ωτος, the genitive of ους, an ear, and εγχευω, to pour in.) A syringe for the ears.

OTHO'NNA. (From οθονη, lint: so called from the softness of its leaves.) A species of celandine.

O'TICA. (From ους, the ear.) Medicines against diseases of the ear.

OTI'TES. (From ους, the ear.) An epithet of the little finger, because it is commonly made use of in scratching the ear.

OTI'TIS. (From ους, the ear.) Inflammation of the internal ear. It is known by pyrexia, and an excruciating and throbbing pain in the internal ear, that is sometimes attended with delirium.

OTOPLA'TOS. (From ους, the ear.) A stinking ulcer behind the ear.

OTOPYO'SIS. (From ους, the ear, and πυον, pus.) A purulent discharge from the ear.

OTORRHÆ'A. (From ους, the ear, and ρεω, to flow.) A discharge from the ear.

OVA'LE FORAMEN. See *Foramen ovale.*

OVALIS. Oval. Some parts of animals and ve-

getables receive this name from being of this shape as foramen ovale, centrum ovale, folium ovale, receptaculum ovale.

OVARIAN. Ovarial. Belonging to the ovarium.

OVA'RIUM. (Diminutive of *ovum,* an egg.) The ovaria are two flat oval bodies, about one inch in length, and rather more than half in breadth and thickness, suspended in the broad ligaments, about the distance of one inch from the uterus behind, and a little below the Fallopian tubes. To the ovaria, according to the idea of their structure entertained by different anatomists, various uses have been assigned, or the purpose they answer has been differently explained. Some have supposed that their texture was glandular, and that they secreted a fluid equivalent to, and similar to the male semen; but others, who have examined them with more care, assert, that they are ovaria in the literal acceptation of the term, and include a number of vesicles, or ova, to the amount of twenty-two of different sizes, joined to the internal surface of the ovaria by cellular threads or pedicles; and that they contain a fluid which has the appearance of thin lymph. These vesicles are, in fact, to be seen in the healthy ovaria of every young woman. They differ very much in their number in different ovaria, but are very seldom so numerous as has just been stated. All have agreed that the ovaria prepare whatever the female supplies towards the formation of the fœtus; and this is proved by the operation of spaying, which consists in the extirpation of the ovaria, after which the animal not only loses the power of conceiving, but desire is for ever extinguished. The outer coat of the ovaria, together with that of the uterus, is given by the peritoneum; and whenever an ovum is passed into the Fallopian tube, a fissure is observed at the part through which it is supposed to have been transferred. These fissures healing, leave small longitudinal cicatrices on the surface, which are said to enable us to determine, whenever the ovarium is examined, the number of times a woman has conceived. The corpora lutea are oblong glandular bodies of a yellowish colour, found in the ovaria of all animals when pregnant, and, according to some, when they are salacious. They are said to be calyces, from which the impregnated ovum has dropped; and their number is always in proportion to the number of conceptions found in the uterus. They are largest and most conspicuous in the early state of pregnancy, and remain for some time after delivery, when they gradually fade and wither till they disappear. The corpora lutea are very vascular, except at their centre, which is whitish; and in the middle of the white part is a small cavity, from which the impregnated ovum is thought to have immediately proceeded. The ovaria are the seat of a particular kind of dropsy, which most commonly happens to women at the time of the final cessation of the menses, though not unfrequently at a more early period of life. It is of the encysted kind, the fluid being sometimes limpid and thin, and at others discoloured and gelatinous. In some cases it has been found contained in one cyst, often in several; and in others the whole tumefaction has been composed of hydatids not larger than grapes. The ovaria are also subject, especially a short time after delivery, to inflammation, terminating in suppuration, and to scirrhous and cancerous diseases, with considerable enlargement. In the former state, they generally adhere to some adjoining part, as the uterus, rectum, bladder, or external integuments, and the matter is discharged from the vagina by stool, by urine, or by an external abscess of the integuments of the abdomen.

OVATUS. Ovate. Leaves, petals, seeds, &c. are so called when of the shape of an egg cut lengthwise, the base being rounded, and broader than the extremity, a very common form of leaves; as in Vinca major, and Urtica pilulifera, and the *petals* of the Allium flavum, and Narcissus psuedo-narcissus; the *receptacle* of the Omphalea, and seeds of the Quercus.

OVIDUCT. (*Oviductus;* from *ovum,* an egg, and *ductus,* a canal.) The duct or canal through which the ovum, or egg, passes. In the human species, the Fallopian tube is so called, which runs from the ovary to the bottom of the womb.

OVIPAROUS. (From *ovum,* an egg, and *pario,* to bring forth.) Animals which exclude their young in the egg, which are afterward hatched.

OVO'RUM TESTÆ. Egg-shells. A testaceous absorbent.

OVULUM. A little egg. See *Ovum.*

O'VUM. 1. An egg. See *Egg.*

2. The vesicles in the ovarium of females are called the ova, or ovula. When fecundation takes place in one or more of these, they pass, after a short time, along the Fallopian tube into the uterus.

"*Developement of the ovum in the uterus.*—The ovum, in the first moments of its abode in the uterus, is free and unattached; its volume is nearly that which it had in quitting the ovarium; but, in the course of the second month, its dimensions increase, it becomes covered with filaments of about a line in length, which ramify in the manner of blood-vessels, and are implanted into the *decidua.* In the third month, they are seen only on one side of the ovum, the others have nearly disappeared; but those which remain have acquired a greater extent, thickness, and consistence, and are more deeply implanted into the deciduous membrane; taken together they form the *placenta.* The ovum, in the rest of its surface, presents only a soft flocculent layer called *decidua reflexa.* The ovum continues to increase until the end of pregnancy, in which its volume is nearly equal to that of the uterus; but its structure suffers important changes which we will examine.

At first its two membranes have yielded to its enlargement, while becoming thicker or more resisting: the exterior is called *chorion;* the other *amnion.* The liquid contained by the latter augments in proportion to the volume of the ovum. In the second month of pregnancy, there exists also a certain quantity of liquid between the chorion and amnion, but it disappears during the third month.

Up to the end of the third week, the ovum presents nothing indicative of the presence of the germ; the contained liquid is transparent, and partly coagulable as before. At this period there is seen, on the side where the ovum adheres to the uterus, something slightly opaque, gelatinous, all the parts of which appear homogeneous; in a short time, certain points become opaque, two distinct vesicles are formed, nearly equal in volume, and united by a pedicle, one of which adheres to the amnion by a small filament. Almost at the same time a red spot is seen in the midst of this last, from which yellowish filaments are seen to take their rise: this is the heart, and the principal sanguiferous vessels. At the beginning of the second month, the head is very visible, the eyes form two black points, very large in proportion to the volume of the head; small openings indicate the place of the ears and nostrils; the mouth, at first very large, is contracted afterward by the developement of the lips, which happens about the sixtieth day, with that of the ears, nose, extremities, &c.

The developement of all the principal organs happens successively until about the middle of the fourth month; then the state of the *embryo* ceases, and that of the *fœtus* begins, which is continued till the termination of pregnancy. All the parts increase with more or less rapidity during this time, and draw towards the form which they must present after birth. Before the sixth month, the lungs are very small, the heart large, but its four cavities are confounded, or at least difficult to distinguish; the liver is large, and occupies a great part of the abdomen; the gall-bladder is not full of bile, but of a colourless fluid not bitter; the small intestine, in its lower part, contains a yellowish matter, in small quantity, called *meconium;* the testicles are placed upon the sides of the superior lumbar vertebræ; the ovaria occupy the same position. At the end of the seventh month, the lungs assume a reddish tint which they had not before; the cavities of the heart become distinct; the liver preserves its large dimensions, but removes a little from the umbilicus; the bile shows itself in the gall-bladder; the meconium is more abundant, and descends lower in the great intestine; the ovaria tend to the pelvis, the testicles are directed to the inguinal rings. At this period the fœtus is capable of life, that is, it could live and breathe if expelled from the uterus. Every thing becomes more perfect in the eighth and ninth months. We cannot here follow the interesting details of this increase of the organs; they belong to anatomy: we shall consider the physiological phenomena that relate to them.

Functions of the ovum, and of the fœtus.—The ovum begins to grow as soon as it arrives in the cavity of the uterus; its surface is covered with asperities that are

142

quickly transformed into sanguiferous vessels: there is then life in the ovum. But we have no idea of this mode of existence; probably the surface of the ovum absorbs the fluids with which it is in contact, and these, after having undergone a particular elaboration by the membranes, are afterward poured into the cavity of the amnion.

What was the germ before its appearance? Did it exist, or was it formed at that instant? Does the little almost opaque mass that composes it contain the rudiments of all the organs of the fœtus and the adult, or are these created the instant they begin to show themselves? What can be the nature of a nutrition so complicated, so important, performed without vessels, nerves, or apparent circulation? How does the heart move before the appearance of the nervous system? Whence comes the yellow blood that it contains at first? &c. &c. No reply can be given to any of these questions in the present state of science.

We know very little of what happens in the embryo, whose organs are only yet rudely delineated; nevertheless, there is a kind of circulation recognised. The heart sends blood into the large vessels, and into the rudimentary placenta; probably blood returns to the heart by veins, &c.—But when the new being has reached the fœtal state, as most of the organs are very apparent, then it is possible to recognise some of the functions peculiar to that state.

The circulation is the best known of the functions of the fœtus: it is more complicated than that of the adult, and is performed in a manner quite different. In the first place, it cannot be divided into venous and arterial; for the fœtal blood has sensibly every where the same appearance, that is, a brownish red tint: in other respects it is much the same as the blood of the adult; it coagulates, separates into clot, and serum, &c I do not know why some learned chemists have believed that it does not contain fibrin.

The placenta is the most singular and one of the most important organs of the circulation of the fœtus: it succeeds to those filaments which cover the ovum during the first months of pregnancy. Very small at first, it soon acquires a considerable size. It adheres by its exterior surface, to the uterus, presents irregular furrows, which indicate its division into several lobes or *cotyledons,* the number and form of which are not determined. Its fœtal surface is covered by the chorion and amnion, except at its centre, into which the umbilical cord is inserted. Its parenchyma is formed of sanguiferous vessels, divided and subdivided. They belong to the divisions of the umbilical arteries, and to the radicles of the vein of the same name. The vessels of one lobe do not communicate with those of the adjoining lobes; but those of the same *cotyledon* anastomose frequently, for nothing is more easy than to make injections pass from one to another.

The *umbilical cord* extends from near the centre of the placenta to the umbilicus of the child; its length is often near two feet; it is formed by the two umbilical arteries and the vein, connected by a very close cellular tissue, and is covered by the two membranes of the ovum.

In the first months of pregnancy, a vesicle, which receives small vessels, being a prolongation of the mesenteric artery and the meseraic vein, is found in the body of the cord, between the chorion and the amnion, near the umbilicus. This vesicle is not analagous to the *allantoid;* it represents the membranes of the yelk of birds and reptiles, and the umbilical vesicle of the *mammalia.* It contains a yellowish fluid which seems to be absorbed by the veins of its parietes.

The umbilical vein, arising from the placenta, and then arriving at the umbilicus, enters the abdomen, and reaches the inferior surface of the liver; there it divides into two large branches, one of which is distributed to the liver, along with the *venâ porta,* while the other soon terminates in the *vena cava* under the name of *ductus venosus.* This vein has two valves, one at the place of its bifurcation, and the other at the junction with the *vena cava.*

The heart and the large vessels of the fœtus capable of life, are very different from what they become after birth; the valve of the vena cava is large; the partition of the auricles presents a large opening provided with a semilunar valve, called *foramen ovale.* The pulmonary artery, after having sent two small branches to the lungs, terminates almost immediately in the aorta, in the concave aspect of the arch; it is called in this place *ductus arteriosus.*

The last character proper to the circulating organs of the fœtus, is the existence of the *umbilical arteries,* which arise from the internal iliacs, are directed over the sides of the bladder, attach themselves to the *ura-chus,* pass out of the abdomen by the umbilicus, and go to the placenta, where they are distributed as has been mentioned above.

According to this disposition of the circulating apparatus of the fœtus, it is evident that the motion of the blood ought to be different in it from that in the adult. If we suppose that the blood sets out from the placenta, it evidently passes through the umbilical vein as far as the liver; there, one part of the blood passes into the liver, and the other into the vena cava: these two directions carry it to the heart by the interior vena cava; being arrived at this organ, it penetrates into the right auricle, and into the left by the *foramen ovale,* at the instant in which the auricles are dilated. At this instant, the blood of the inferior vena cava is inevitably mixed with that of the superior. How, indeed, could two liquids of the same nature, or nearly so, remain isolated in a cavity in which they arrive at the same time, and which contracts to expel them. I am not ignorant that Sebatier, in his excellent *Treatise on the Circulation of the Fœtus,* has maintained the contrary, but his arguments do not change my opinion in this respect. However it may be, the contraction of the auricle succeeds their dilatation; the blood is thrown into the two ventricles the instant they dilate; these, in their turn, contract, and drive out the blood, the left into the aorta, and the right into the pulmonary artery; but as this artery terminates in the aorta, it is clear that all the blood of the two ventricles passes into the aorta, except a very small portion that goes to the ungs. Under the influence of these two agents of impulsion, the blood is made to flow through all the divisions of the aorta, and returns to the heart by the venæ cavæ. Lastly, it is carried to the placenta by the umbilical arteries, and returns to the fœtus by the vein of the chord.

It is easy to conceive the use of the foramen ovale, and the ductus arteriosus: the left auricle, receiving little or no blood from the lungs, could not furnish any to the left ventricle if it did not receive it from the opening in the partition of the auricles. On the other hand, the lungs have no functions to fulfil, if all the blood of the pulmonary artery were distributed in them, the impulsive force of the right ventricle would have been vainly consumed; while, by means of the ductus arteriosus, the force of both ventricles is employed to move the blood of the aorta; without the joint action of both ventricles, probably the blood could not have reached the placenta, and returned again to the heart. The motions of the heart are very rapid in the fœtus; they generally exceed 120 in a minute: the circulation possesses necessarily a proportionate rapidity.

A delicate question now presents itself for examination. What are the relations of the circulation of the mother with that of the fœtus?—In order to arrive at some precise notion on this point, the mode of junction of the uterus and placenta must first be examined.

Anatomists differ in this respect. It was long believed that the uterine arteries anastomosed directly with the radicles of the umbilical vein, and that the last divisions of the arteries of the placenta opened into the veins of the uterus; but the acknowledged impossibility of making matters injected into the uterine veins pass into the umbilical veins, and reciprocally to cause liquid matters injected into the umbilical arteries to reach the veins of the uterus, caused this idea to be renounced. It is at present generally admitted, that the vessels of the placenta and those of the uterus do not anastomose.

Notwithstanding the high authority of Boerhaave, it cannot be admitted that the fœtus continually swallows the waters of the amnion, and digests it for its nourishment. Its stomach, indeed, contains a viscid matter in considerable quantity: but it has no resemblance to the *liquor amnii;* it is very acid and gelatinous; towards the pylorus, it is somewhat gray, and opaque; it appears to be converted into chyme in the stomach, in order to pass into the small intestine, where, after having been acted upon by the bile, and perhaps by the pancreatic juice, it furnishes a peculiar chyle. The remainder descends afterward into the lar e intestine,

where it forms the meconium, which is evidently the result of digestion during gestation. Whence does the digested matter come? It is probably secreted by the stomach itself, or descends from the œsophagus; there is nothing, however, to prevent the fœtus from swallowing in certain cases, a few mouthfuls of the liquor amnii; and this seems to be proved by certain hairs, like those of the skin, being found in the meconium It is important to remark, that the meconium is a substance containing very little azote. Nothing is yet known regarding the use of this digestion of the fœtus; it is probably not essential to its growth, since infants have been born without a stomach, or any thing similar. Some persons say they have seen chyle in the thoracic duct of the former.

Exhalations seem to take place in the fœtus; for al its surfaces are lubricated nearly in the same manner as afterward: fat is in abundance; the humours of the eye exist: cutaneous transpiration very probably takes place also, and mixes continually with the liquor amnii. With regard to this last liquor, it is difficult to say whence it derives its origin; no sanguineous vessels appear to be directed to the amnion, and it is nevertheless probable that this membrane is its secreting organ.

The cutaneous and mucous follicles are developed, and seem to possess an energetic action, especially from the seventh month; the skin is then covered by a pretty thick layer of fatty matter, secreted by the follicles: several authors have improperly considered it as a deposite of the liquor amnii. The mucus is also abundant in the last two months of gestation.

All the glands employed in digestion have a considerable volume, and seem to possess some activity; the action of the others is little known. It is not known, for example, whether the kidneys form urine, or whether this fluid is injected by the urethra into the cavity of the amnion. The testicles and mammæ seem to form a fluid that resembles neither milk nor semen, and which is found in the *vesiculæ seminales* and lactiferous canals.

What can be said about the nutrition of the fœtus? Physiological works contain only vague conjectures on this point; it appears certain that the placenta draws from the mother the materials necessary for the developement of the organs, but what these materials are, or how they are directed, we do not know."—*Magendie's Physiology.*

OVUM PHILOSOPHICUM. *Ovum chymicum.* A glass body, round like an egg.

OVUM RUFFUM. An obsolete alchemistic term used in the transmutation of metals.

Ox-eye-daisy. See *Chrysanthemum leucanthemum*

Ox's tongue. See *Picris echioides.*

OXALATE. *Oxalas.* A salt formed by the combination of the oxalic acid with a salifiable basis; thus, *oxalate of ammonia.*

OXALIC ACID. *Acidum oxalicum.* "This acid, which abounds in wood sorrel, and which, combined with a small portion of potassa, as it exists in that plant, has been sold under the name of *salt of lemons,* to be used as a substitute for the juice of that fruit, particularly for discharging ink-spots and iron moulds, was long supposed to be analagous to that of tartar. In the year 1776, however, Bergman discovered that a powerful acid might be extracted from sugar by means of the nitric; and a few years afterward Scheele found this to be identical with the acid existing naturally in sorrel. Hence the acid began to be distinguished by the name of *saccharine,* but has since been known in the new nomenclature by that of oxalic.

It may be obtained, readily and economically, from sugar in the following way: to six ounces of nitric acid in a stoppered retort, to which a large receiver is luted, add, by degrees, one ounce of lump sugar coarsely powdered. A gentle heat may be applied during the solution, and nitric oxide will be evolved in abundance. When the whole of the sugar is dissolved, distil off a part of the acid, till what remains in the retort has a syrupy consistence, and this will form regular crystals, amounting to 58 parts from 100 of sugar. These crystals must be dissolved in water, recrystallized, and dried on blotting paper.

Oxalic acid crystallizes in quadrilateral prisms, the sides of which are alternately broad and narrow, and summits dihedral; or, if crystallized rapidly, in small irregular needles. They are efflorescent in dry air, but attract a little humidity if it be damp; are soluble in one part of hot and two of cold water; and are decomposable by a red heat, leaving a small quantity of coaly residuum. 100 parts of alkohol take up near 56 at a boiling heat, but not above 40 cold. Their acidity is so great, that when dissolved in 3600 times their weight of water, the solution reddens litmus paper, and is perceptibly acid to the taste.

The oxalic acid is a good test for detecting lime, which it separates from all the other acids, unless they are present in excess. It has likewise a greater affinity for lime than for any other of the bases, and forms with it a pulverulent, insoluble salt, not decomposable except by fire, and turning syrup of violets green.

Oxalic acid acts as a violent poison when swallowed in the quantity of 2 or 3 drachms; and several fatal accidents have lately occurred in London, in consequence of its being improperly sold instead of Epsom salts. Its vulgar name of salts, under which the acid is bought for the purpose of whitening boot-tops, occasion these lamentable mistakes. But the powerfully acid taste of the latter substance, joined to its prismatic or needle-formed crystallization, are sufficient to distinguish it from every thing else. The immediate rejection from the stomach of this acid by an emetic, aided by copious draughts of warm water containing bicarbonate of potassa, or soda, chalk, or carbonate of magnesia, are the proper remedies.

With *barytes* it forms an insoluble salt; but this salt will dissolve in water acidulated with oxalic acid, and afford angular crystals. If, however, we attempt to dissolve these crystals in boiling water, the excess of acid will unite with the water, and leave the oxalate, which will be precipitated.

The *oxalate of strontian* too is a nearly insoluble compound.

Oxalate of magnesia too is insoluble, unless the acid be in excess.

The *oxalate of potassa* exists in two states, that of a neutral salt, and that of an acidule. The latter is generally obtained from the juice of the leaves of the *oxalis acetosella*, wood-sorrel, or *rumex acetosa*, common sorrel. The expressed juice, being diluted with water, should be set by for a few days, till the feculent parts have subsided, and the supernatant fluid is become clear; or it may be clarified, when expressed, with the whites of eggs. It is then to be strained off, evaporated to a pellicle, and set in a cool place to crystallize. The first product of crystals being taken out, the liquor may be further evaporated, and crystallized; and the same process repeated till no more can be obtained. In this way Schlereth informs us about nine drachms of crystals may be obtained from two pounds of juice, which are generally afforded by ten pounds of wood-sorrel. Savary, however, says, that ten parts of wood-sorrel in full vegetation yield five parts of juice, which give little more than a two-hundredth of tolerably pure salt. He boiled down the juice, however, in the first instance, without clarifying it; and was obliged repeatedly to dissolve and recrystallize the salt to obtain it white.

This salt is in small, white, needley, or lamellar crystals, not alterable in the air. It unites with barytes, magnesia, soda, ammonia, and most of the metallic oxides, into triple salts. Yet its solution precipitates the nitric solutions of mercury and silver in the state of insoluble oxalates of these metals, the nitric acid in this case combining with the potassa. It attacks iron, lead, tin, zinc, and antimony.

This salt, besides its use in taking out ink-spots, and as a test of lime, forms with sugar and water a pleasant, cooling beverage; and, according to Berthollet, it possesses considerable powers as an antiseptic.

The neutral oxalate of potassa is very soluble, and assumes a gelatinous form, but may be brought to crystallize in hexahedral prisms with dihedral summits, by adding more potassa to the liquor than is sufficient to saturate the acid.

Oxalate of soda likewise exists in two different states, those of an acidulous and a neutral salt, which in their properties are analogous to those of potassa.

The *acidulous oxalate of ammonia* is crystallizable, not very soluble, and capable, like the preceding acidules, of combining with other bases, so as to form triple salts. But if the acid be saturated with ammonia, we obtain a neutral oxalate, which on evaporation yields very fine crystals in tetrahedral prisms with dihedral summits, one of the planes of which cuts off

144

three sides of the prism. This salt is decomposable by fire, which raises from it carbonate of ammonia, and leaves only some slight traces of a coaly residuum. Lime, barytes, and strontian unite with its acid, and the ammonia flies off in the form of gas

The oxalic acid readily dissolves *alumina*, and the solution gives, on evaporation, a yellowish transparent mass, sweet and a little astringent to the taste, deliquescent, and reddening tincture of litmus, but not syrup of violets. This salt swells up in the fire, loses its acid, and leaves the alumina a little coloured."

OX'ALIS. (From οξυς, sharp: so called from the sharpness of its juice.) The name of a genus of plants in the Linnæan system. Class, *Decandria*; Order *Pentagynia*. Wood-sorrel.

OXALIS ACETOSELLA. The systematic name of the wood-sorrel. *Lujula*; *Alleluja*. *Oxalis—foliis ternatis, scapo unifloro, flore albo, capsulis pentagonis elasticis, radice squamoso-articulata*, of Linnæus. This plant grows wild in the woods, and flowers in April and May. The leaves are shaped like a heart, standing three together on one stalk. The acetosella is totally inodorous, but has a grateful acid taste, on which account it is used in salads. Its taste is more agreeable than the common sorrel, and approaches nearly to that of the juice of lemons, or the acid of tartar, with which it corresponds in a great measure in its medical effects, being esteemed refrigerant, antiscorbutic, and diuretic. It is recommended by Bergius, in inflammatory, bilious, and putrid fevers. The principal use, however, of the acetosella, is to allay inordinate heat, and to quench thirst; for this purpose, a pleasant whey may be formed by boiling the plant in milk, which under certain circumstances may be preferable to the conserve directed by the London College, though an extremely grateful and useful medicine. Many have employed the root of Lujula, probably on account of its beautiful red colour rather than for its superior efficacy. A salt is prepared from this plant, known by the name of essential salt of lemons, which is an acidulous oxalate of potassa, and commonly used for taking ink-stains out of linen. What is sold under the name of essential salt of lemons in this country, is said by some to consist of cream of tartar, with the addition of a small quantity of sulphuric acid. The leaves of wood-sorrel when employed externally in the form of poultices, are powerful suppurants, particularly in indolent scrofulous humours.

OXA'LME. (From οξυς, sharp, and αλς, salt.) A mixture of vinegar and salt.

Oxid. See *Oxide*.

OXIDATION. The process of converting metals and other substances into oxides, by combining with them a certain portion of oxygen. It differs from acidification in the addition of oxygen not being sufficient to form an acid with the substance oxided.

OXIDE. (*Oxydum, i*, n.; formed of *oxygen*, with the terminal *ide*. See *Ide*.) Oxyd. Oxid. Oxyde. A substance combined with oxygen without being in the state of an acid. Many substances are susceptible of several stages of oxidizement, on which account chemists have employed various terms to express the characteristic distinctions of the several oxides. The specific name is often derived from some external character, chiefly the colour; thus we have the black and red oxides of iron, and of mercury: the white oxide of zinc: but in most instances the denominations proposed by Dr. Thompson are adopted. When there are several oxides of the same substance, he proposes the terms *protoxyde, deutoxyde, tritoxyde*, signifying the first, second, and third stage of oxidizement. Or if two oxides only are known, he proposes the appellation of *protoxyde* for that at the minimum, and of *peroxyde* for that at the maximum of oxidation. The compounds of oxides and water in which the water exists in a condensed state, are termed *hydrates*, or *hydroxures*.

Oxide of carbon, gaseous. See *Carbon, gaseous oxide of*.

Oxide, nitric. See *Nitrogen*.

Oxide, nitrous. See *Nitrogen*.

OXYCA'NTHA. (From οξυς, sharp, and ακανθα, a thorn: so called from the acidity of its fruit.) The barberry.

OXYCANTHA GALENI. See *Berberis*.

OXYCE'DRUS. (From οξυ, acutely, and κεδρος, a cedar: so called from the sharp termination of its leaves.) 1. A kind of cedar

2. Spanish juniper, a species of *juniperus*.

OXYCO'CCOS. (From οξυς, acid, and κοκκος a berry: so named from its acidity.) See *Vaccinium oxycoccos*.

OXY'CRATUM. (From οξυς, acid, and κεραννυμι, to mix.) Oxycrates. Vinegar mixed with such a portion of water as is required, and rendered still milder by the addition of a little honey.

OXYCRO'CEUM EMPLASTRUM. (From οξυς, acid, and κρκος, crocus, saffron.) A plaster in which there is much saffron, but no vinegar necessary, unless in dissolving some gums.

Oxyd. See *Oxide.*

Oxyde. See *Oxide.*

OXYDE'RCICA. (From οξυς, acute, and δερκω, to see.) Medicines which sharpen the sight.

OXYDULE. Synonymous with protoxide.

O'XYDUM. (So called from oxygen, which enters into its composition.) See *Oxide.*

OXYDUM ANTIMONII. See *Antimonii oxydum.*

OXYDUM ARSENICI ALBUM. See *Arsenic.*

OXYDUM CÚPRI VIRIDE ACETATUM. See *Verdigris.*

OXYDUM FERRI LUTEUM. See *Ferri subcarbonas.*

OXYDUM FERRI NIGRUM. Black oxide of iron. The scales which fall from iron, when heated, consist of iron combined with oxygen. These have been employed medicinally, producing the general effects of chalybeates, but not very powerfully.

OXYDUM FERRI RUBRUM. Red oxide of iron. In this the metal is more highly oxidized than in the black. It may be formed by long continued exposure to heat and air. Its properties in medicine are similar to other preparations of iron. It is frequently given internally.

OXYDUM HYDRARGYRI CINEREUM. See *Hydrargyri oxydum cinereum.*

OXYDUM HYDRARGYRI NIGRUM. See *Hydrargyri oxydum cinereum.*

OXYDUM HYDRARGYRI RUBRUM. See *Hydrargyri oxydum rubrum.*

OXYDUM PLUMBI ALBUM. See *Plumbi subcarbonas.*

OXYDUM PLUMBI RUBRUM. See *Lead.*

OXYDUM PLUMBI SEMIVITREUM. See *Lythargyrus.*

OXYDUM STIBII ALBUM. See *Antimonii oxydum.*

OXYDUM STIBII SEMIVITREUM. A vitreous oxide of antimony. It was formerly called *Vitrum antimonii* and consists of an oxide of antimony with a little sulphur; it is employed to make antimonial wine.

OXYDUM STIBII SULPHURATUM. This is an oxide of antimony with sulphur, and was formerly called *Hepar antimonii; Crocus metallorum; Crocus antimonii.* It was formerly exhibited in the cure of fevers and atonic diseases of the lungs. Its principal use now is in preparing other medicines.

OXYDUM ZINCI. See *Zinci oxydum.*

OXYDUM ZINCI SUBLIMATUM. See *Zinci oxydum.*

OXYGARUM. (From οξυς, acid, and γαρον, garum.) A composition of garum and vinegar.

OXYGEN. (*Oxygenium;* from οξυς, acid, and γενναω, to generate; because it is the generator of acidity.) This substance, although existing sometimes in a solid and sometimes in an aëriform state, is never distinctly perceptible to the human senses, but in combination.

We know it only in its combination, by its effects. Nature never presents it solitary: chemists do not know how to insulate it. It is a principle which was long unknown. It is absorbable by combustible bodies, and converts them into oxides or acids. It is an indispensable condition of combustion, uniting itself always to bodies which burn, augmenting their weight, and changing their properties. It may be disengaged in the state of oxygen gas, from burned bodies, by a joint accumulation of caloric and light. It is highly necessary for the respiration of animals. It exists universally dispersed through nature, and is a constituent part of atmospheric air, of water, of acids, and of all bodies of the animal and vegetable kingdoms.

One of the most remarkable combinations into which it is capable of entering, is that which it forms with light and caloric. The nature of that mysterious union has not been ascertained, but it is certain that, in that state, it constitutes the gaseous fluid called OXYGEN GAS.

Properties of oxygen gas.—Oxygen gas is an elastic invisible fluid, like common air, capable of indefinite expansion and compression. It has neither taste nor odour, nor does it show any traces of an acid. Its spe-

cific gravity, as determined by Kirwan, is 0.00135, that of water being 1.0000; it is, therefore, 740 times lighter than the same bulk of water. Its weight is to atmospheric air as 1103 to 1000. One hundred and sixteen cubic inches of oxygen gas weigh 39.38 grains. It is not absorbed by water, but entirely absorbable by combustible bodies, which, at the same time, disengage its caloric and light, producing in consequence a strong heat and flame. It rekindles almost extinct combustible bodies. It is indispensable to respiration, and is the cause of animal heat. It hastens germination. It combines with every combustible body, with all the metals and with the greater number of vegetable and animal substances. It is considered as the cause of acidity; and from this last property is derived the name *oxygen*, a word denoting the origin of acidity.

The act of its combining with bodies is called *oxidisement*, or *oxygenation;* and the bodies with which it is combined are called *oxides*, or *acids.*

Oxygen gas is the chief basis of the pneumatic doctrine of chemistry.

Methods of obtaining oxygen gas.—We are at present acquainted with a great number of bodies from which we may, by art, produce oxygen gas. It is most amply obtained from the oxides of manganese, lead, or mercury; from nitrate of potassa; from the green leaves of vegetables, and from oxychlorate of potassa or soda. Besides these, there are a great many other substances from which oxygen gas may be procured.

1. In order to procure oxygen gas in a state of great purity, pure oxychlorate of potassa or soda must be made use of. With this view, put some of the salt into a small earthen or glass retort, the neck of which is placed under the shelf of the pneumatic trough, filled with water; and heat the retort by means of a lamp. The salt will begin to melt, and oxygen gas will be obtained in abundance, and of great purity, which may be collected and preserved over water.

Explanation.—Oxychlorate of potassa consists of oxygen, chlorine, and potassa. At an elevated temperature, a decomposition takes place, the oxygen unites to the caloric, and forms oxygen gas. The oxychlorate becomes therefore converted into simple chlorate of potassa.

2. Oxygen gas may likewise be obtained from the green leaves of vegetables.

For this purpose fill a bell-glass with water, introduce fresh gathered green leaves under it, and place the bell, or receiver, inverted in a vessel containing the same fluid; expose the apparatus to the rays of the sun, and very pure oxygen gas will be liberated.

The emission of oxygen gas is proportioned to the vigour of the plant and the vivacity of the light; the quantity differs in different plants, and under different circumstances.

Explanation.—It is an established fact, that plants decompose carbonic acid, and probably water, which serve for their nourishment; they absorb the hydrogen and carbon of these fluids, disengaging a part of the oxygen in a state of purity. Light, however, favours this decomposition greatly; in proportion as the oxygen becomes disengaged, the hydrogen becomes fixed in the vegetable, and combines partly with the carbon and partly with the oxygen, to form the oil, &c. of the vegetable.

3. Nitrate of potassa is another substance frequently made use of for obtaining oxygen gas, in the following manner:

Take any quantity of this salt, introduce it into a coated earthen or glass retort, and fit to it a tube, which must be plunged into the pneumatic trough, under the receiver filled with water. When the apparatus has been properly adjusted, heat the retort gradually, till it becomes red-hot; the oxygen gas will then be disengaged rapidly.

Explanation.—Nitrate of potassa consists of nitric acid and potassa. Nitric acid consists again of oxygen and nitrogen. On exposing the salt to ignition, a partial decomposition of the acid takes place; the greatest part of the oxygen of the nitric acid unites to caloric, and appears under the form of oxygen gas. The other part remains attached to the potassa in the state of nitrous acid. The residue in the retort is, therefore, nitrate of potassa, if the process has been carried only to a certain extent.

Remark.—If too much heat be applied, particularly towards the end of the process, a total decomposition ot the nitric acid takes place: the oxygen gas, in that case, will therefore be mingled with nitrogen gas. The weight of the two gases, when collected, will be found to correspond very exactly with the weight of the acid which had been decomposed. The residue then left in the retort is potassa.

4. Black oxide of manganese, however, is generally made use of for obtaining oxygen gas, on account of its cheapness. This native oxide is reduced to a coarse powder; a stone, or rather an iron retort, is then charged with it and heated. As soon as the retort becomes ignited, oxygen gas is obtained plentifully.

Explanation.—Black oxide of manganese is the metal called manganese fully saturated with oxygen, together with many earthy impurities; on applying heat, part of the solid oxygen quits the metal and unites to caloric, in order to form oxygen gas; the remainder of the oxygen remains united to the metal with a forcible affinity: the metal, therefore, approaches to the metallic state, or is found in the state of a gray oxide of manganese.

One pound of the best manganese yields upwards of 1400 cubic inches of oxygen gas, nearly pure. If sulphuric acid be previously added to the manganese, the gas is produced by a less heat, and in a larger quantity; a glass retort may then be used, and the heat of a lamp is sufficient.

5. Red oxide of mercury yields oxygen gas in a manner similar to that of manganese.

Explanation.—This oxide consists likewise of solid oxygen and mercury, the combination of which takes place on exposing mercury to a heat of about 610° Fahr. At this degree it attracts oxygen, and becomes converted into an oxide; but if the temperature be increased, the attraction of oxygen is changed. The oxygen then attracts caloric stronger than it did the mercury; it therefore abandons it, and forms oxygen gas. The mercury then reappears in its metallic state.

6. Red oxide of lead yields oxygen gas on the same principle.

Oxygenated muriatic acid. See *Chlorine*.

OXYGENATION. *Oxygenatio.* This word is often used instead of oxidation, and frequently confounded with it: but it differs in being of more general import, as every union with oxygen, whatever the product may be, is an oxygenation; but oxidation takes place only when an oxide is formed.

Oxygenized muriatic acid. See *Muriatic acid oxygenized.*

Oxygenized nitric acid. See *Nitric acid oxygenized.*

OXYGLY'CUM. (From οξυς, acid, and γλυκυς, sweet.) Honey mixed with vinegar.

OXYIODE. A term applied by Sir H. Davy to the triple compounds of oxygen, iodine, and the metallic bases. Lussac calls them *iodates.*

OXYLA'PATHUM. (From οξυς, acid, and λαπαθον, the dock: so named from its acidity.) See *Rumex acutus.*

O'XYMEL. (*Oxymel, llis.* n.; from οξυς, acid, and μελι, honey.) *Apomeli. Adipson.* Honey and vinegar boiled to a syrup. *Mel acetatum.* Now called *Oxymel simplex.* Take of clarified honey, two pounds; acetic acid a pint. Boil them down to a proper consistence, in a glass vessel, over a slow fire. This preparation of honey and vinegar possesses aperient and expectorating virtues; and is given, with these intentions, in the cure of humoral asthma, and other diseases of the chest, in doses of one or two drachms. It is also employed in the form of gargle, when diluted with water.

OXYMEL ÆRUGINIS. See *Linimentum æruginis.*

OXYMEL COLCHICI. Oxymel of meadow saffron is an acrid medicine, but is nevertheless employed, for its diuretic virtues, in dropsies.

OXYMEL SCILLÆ. Take of clarified honey, three pounds; vinegar of squills, two pints. Boil them in a glass vessel, with a slow fire, to the proper thickness. Aperient, expectorant and detergent virtues, are attri-

buted to the honey of squills. It is given in doses of two or three drachms, along with some aromatic water, as that of cinnamon, to prevent the great nausea which it would otherwise be apt to excite. In large doses it proves emetic.

OXYMU'RIAS HYDRARGYRI. See *Hydrargyri oxymurias.*

OXYMURIATIC ACID. See *Chlorine.*

OXYMYRRHI'NE. (From οξυς, acute. and μυρρινη, the myrtle: so called from its resemblance to myrtle, and its pointed leaves.) *Oxymyrsine.* See. *Myrtus communis.*

OXYMYRSINE. See *Oxymyrrhine.*

OXYODIC ACID. See *Iodic acid.*

OXYNI'TRUM. (From οξυς, acid, and νιτρον, nitre.) A composition chiefly of vinegar and nitre.

OXYO'PIA. (From οξυς, acute, and ωψ, the eye.) The faculty of seeing more acutely than usual. Thus there have been instances known of persons who could see the stars in the daytime. The proximate cause is a preternatural sensibility of the retina. It has been known to precede the gutta serena; and it has been asserted that prisoners, who have been long detained in darkness, have learned to read and write in darkened places.

OXYPHLEGMA'SIA. (From οξυς, acute, and φλεγω, to burn.) An acute inflammation.

OXYPHŒ'NICON. (From οξυς, acid, and φοινιξ, the tamarind; a native of Phœnicia.) See *Tamarindus.*

OXYPHO'NIA. (From οξυς, sharp, and φωνη, the voice.) An acuteness of voice. See *Paraphonia.*

OXYPRUSSIC ACID. See *Chlorocyanic acid.*

OXYRE'GMA. (From οξυς, acid, and ερευγω, to break wind.) An acid eructation.

OXYRRHO'DINON. (From οξυς, acid, and ροδινον, oil of roses.) A composition of the oil of roses and vinegar.

OXYSACCHA'RUM. (From οξυς, acid, and σακχαρον, sugar.) A composition of vinegar and sugar.

OXYSAL DIAPHORETICUM. A preparation of Angelo Sala. It is a fixed salt, loaded with more acid than is necessary to saturate it.

OXY'TOCA. (From οξυς, quick; and τικτω, to bring forth.) Medicines which promote delivery.

OXYTRIPHY'LLUM. (From οξυς, acid, and τριφυλλον, trefoil; so named from its acidity.) See *Oxalis acetosella.*

OYSTER. See *Ostrea.*

Oyster-shell. See *Ostrea.*

OZÆ'NA. (From οζη, a stench.) An ulcer situated in the nose, discharging a fœtid purulent matter, and sometimes accompanied with caries of the bones. Some authors have signified by the term, an ill-conditioned ulcer in the antrum. The first meaning is the original one. The disease is described as coming on with a trifling tumefaction and redness about the ala nasi, accompanied with a discharge of mucus, with which the nostril becomes obstructed. The matter gradually assumes the appearance of pus, is most copious in the morning, and is sometimes attended with sneezing, and a little bleeding. The ulceration occasionally extends round the ali nasis to the cheek, but seldom far from the nose, the ala of which also it rarely destroys. The ozæna is often connected with scrofulous and venereal complaints. In the latter cases, portions of the ossa spongiosa often come away. After the complete cure of all venereal complaints, an exfoliating dead piece of bone will often keep up symptoms similar to those of the ozæna, until it is detached. Mr. Pearson remarks, that the ozæna frequently occurs as a symptom of the cachexia syphiloidea. It may perforate the septum nasi, destroy the ossa spongiosa, and even the ossa nasi. Such mischief is now more frequently the effect of the cachexia syphiloidea, than of lues venerea. The ozæna must not be confounded with abscesses in the upper jawbone.

O'ZYMUM. (From οζω, to smell: so called from its fragrance.) See *Ocymum.*

148

P

P. A contraction of *pugillus,* a pupil, or eighth part of a handful, and sometimes a contraction of *pars* or *partes,* a part or parts.

P. Æ. A contraction of *partes æqualis.*

P. P. A contraction of *pulvis patrum,* Jesuit's powder; the *Cinchona lancif. lia.*

PAAW, PETER, was born at Amsterdam, in 1564. After studying four years at Leyden, he went to Paris, and other celebrated schools, for improvement; and took his degree at Rostock. Thence he repaired to Padua, and attended the dissections of Fabricius ab Aquapendente; and, possessing a good memory, as well as great assiduity, he evinced such respectable acquirements, that he was appointed to a medical professorship on his return to Leyden in 1589. His whole ambition was centred in supporting the dignity and utility of this office; and he obtained general esteem. Anatomy and botany were his favourite pursuits; and Leyden owes to him the establishment of its botanic garden. He died in 1617. Besides some commentaries on parts of Hippocrates and other ancient authors, he left a treatise on the Plague, and several other works, chiefly anatomical.

PA'BULUM. (From *pasco,* to feed.) Food, aliment.

PABULUM VITÆ. The food of life. Such are the different kinds of aliment. The animal heat and spirits are also so called.

PACCHIONI, ANTONIO, was born at Reggio, in 1664. After studying there for some time he went to complete himself at Rome under the celebrated Malpighi; who subsequently introduced him into practice at Tivoli, where he resided six years with considerable reputation. He then returned to Rome, and assisted Lancisi in his explanation of the plates of Eustachius. He devoted also great attention to dissection, particularly of the membranes of the brain. In his first work, he assigned to the dura mater a contractile power, whereby it acted upon the brain; this notion obtained temporary celebrity, but it was confuted by Baglivi, and other anatomists. He afterward announced the discovery of glands near the longitudinal sinus, from which he alleged lymphatics pass to the pia mater; this involved him in farther controversies. He was a member of several learned academies, and died in 1726. Among his posthumous works is one on the mischief of epispastics in many diseases.

Pacchionian glands. See *Glandulæ Pacchioniæ.*

PACHY'NTICA. (From παχυνω, to incrassate.) Medicines which incrassate or thicken the fluids.

PA'CHYS. Παχυς, thick. The name of a disorder described by Hippocrates, but not known by us.

PA'DUS. A name borrowed from Theophrastus, who gives no other account of his *παδος,* than that it greatly delights in a shady situation, like the yew. The term is now applied to the bird-cherry. See *Prunus padus.*

["PAGODITE (or Bildstein of Werner). Nothing is known of the natural situation or associations of this mineral. It is brought from China, and always under some artificial form; and hence it is sometimes called Figure or Sculpture stone, or Bildstein. These figures are supposed often to represent the idols or pagodas of the Chinese. The Bildstein is susceptible of a polish." —*Cleav. Min.* A.]

PÆDANCHO'NE. (From παις, a child, and αγχω, to strangulate.) A species of quinsy common among children.

PÆDARTHRO'CACE. (From παις, a boy, αρθρον, a joint, and κακον, an evil.) The joint evil. A scrofulous affection producing an ulceration of the bones which come ajoint.

PÆNEA. See *Penæa.*

PÆO'NIA. (From *Pæon,* who first applied it to medicinal purposes.) Pæony.

1. The name of a genus of plants in the Linnæan system. Class, *Polyandria;* Order, *Digynia.*

2. The pharmacopœial name of the common pæony. See *Pæonia officinalis.*

PÆONIA OFFICINALIS. The systematic name of the common pæony; male and female pæony. This plant,

Pæonia.—foliis oblongis, of Linnæus, has long been considered as a powerful medicine; and, till lately, had a place in the catalogue of the Materia Medica; in which the two common varieties of this plant are indiscriminately directed for use: and, on the authority of G. Bauhin, improperly distinguished into male and female pæony.

The roots and seeds of pæony have, when fresh, a faint, unpleasant smell, somewhat of the narcotic kind, and a mucilaginous subacid taste, with a slight degree of bitterness and astringency. In drying, they lose their smell and part of their taste. Extracts made from them by water are almost insipid, as well as inodorous; but extracts made by rectified spirits are manifestly bitterish, and considerably adstringent. The flowers have rather more smell than any of the other parts of the plant, and a rough sweetish taste, which they impart, together with their colour, both to water and spirit.

The roots, flowers, and seeds of pæony have been esteemed in the character of an anodyne and corroborant, but more especially the roots; which, since the days of Galen, have been very commonly employed as a remedy for the epilepsy. For this purpose, it was usual to cut the root into thin slices, which were to be attached to a string, and suspended about the neck as an amulet; if this failed of success, the patient was to have recourse to the internal use of this root, which Willis directs to be given in the form of a powder, and in the quantity of a drachm, two or three times a day, by which, as we are informed, both infants and adults were cured of this disease. Other authors recommended the expressed juice to be given in wine, and sweetened with sugar, as the most effectual way of administering this plant. Many writers, however, especially in modern times, from repeated trials of the pæony in epileptic cases, have found it of no use whatever; though Professor Home, who gave the radix pæoniæ to two epileptics at the Edinburgh infirmary, declares that one received a temporary advantage from its use. Of the good effects of this plant, in other disorders, we find no instances recorded.

PAIGIL. See *Primula veris.*

PAIN. Αλγη. Οδυνη. *Dolor.* Any unpleasant sensation, or irritation.

Painter's colic. See *Colica pictonum.*

PAKFONG. The white copper of the Chinese, said to be an alloy of copper, nikel, and zinc.

PALATE. See *Palatum.*

PALATI CIRCUMFLEXUS. See *Circumflexus palati.*

PALATI LEVATOR. See *Levator palati.*

PALATI os. The palate bone. The palate is formed by two bones of very irregular figure. They are placed between the ossa maxillaria superiora and the os sphenoides at the back part of the roof of the mouth, and extend from thence to the bottom of the orbit. Each of these bones may be divided into four parts, viz. the inferior, or square portion, the pterygoid process, the nasal lamella, and orbitar process. The first of these, or the square part of the bone, helps to form the palate of the mouth. The upper part of its internal edge rises into a spine, which makes part of the septum narium. The *pterygoid* process, which is smaller above than below, is so named from its being united with the pterygoid process of the sphenoid bone, with which it helps to form the pterygoid fossæ. It is separated from the square part of the bone, and from the nasal lamella, by an oblique fossa, which, applied to such another in the os maxillare, forms a passage for a branch of the fifth pair of nerves. The *nasal* lamella is nothing more than a very thin bony plate, which arises from the upper side of the external edge of the square part of the bone. Its inner surface is concave, and furnished with a ridge, which supports the back part of the os spongiosum inferius. Externally it is convex, and firmly united to the maxillary bone. The *orbitar* process is more irregular than any other part of the bone. It has a smooth surface, when it helps to form the orbit; and, when viewed in its place, we see it contiguous to that part of the orbit which is formed by the os maxillare, and appearing as a small triangle at the inner extremity of the orbitar process of this last-mentioned bone. This fourth part of the os palati likewise helps to form the zygomatic fossa on each side, and there its surface is concave. Between this orbitar process and the sphenoid bone, a hole is formed, through which an artery, vein, and nerve are transmitted to the nostrils. The ossa palati are complete in the fœtus. They are joined to the ossa maxillaria superiora, os sphenoides, os ethmoides, ossa spongiosa inferiora, and vomer.

PALATI TENSOR. See *Circumflexus*.

PALATO. Names compounded of this word belong to muscles which are attached to the palate.

PALATO-PHARYNGEUS. (So called from its origin in the palate and insertion in the pharynx.) A muscle situated at the side of the entry of the fauces. *Thyro-staphilinus* of Douglas. *Thyro-pharyngo-staphilinus*, of Winslow; and *palato-pharyngien*, of Dumas. It arises by a broad beginning from the middle of the velum pendulum palati at the root of the uvula posteriorly, and from the tendinous expansion of the circumflexus palati. The fibres are collected within the posterior arch behind the tonsils, and run backwards to the top and lateral part of the pharynx, where the fibres are scattered and mixed with those of the stylopharyngeus. It is inserted into the edge of the upper and back part of the thyroid cartilage. Its use is to draw the uvula and velum pendulum palati downwards and backwards, and at the same time to pull the thyroid cartilage and pharynx upwards, and shorten it; with the *constrictor superior pharyngis* and tongue, it assists in shutting the passage into the nostrils; and in swallowing, it thrusts the food from the fauces into the pharynx.

PALATO-SALPINGEUS. (From *palatum*, the palate, and σαλπιγξ, a trumpet; so called from its origin in the palate, and its trumpet-like shape.) See *Circumflexus*.

PALATO-STAPHILINUS. See *Azygos uvulæ*.

PALATUM. (*Palatum, i. n.*; from *palo*, to hedge in; because it is staked in, as it were, by the teeth.) 1. The palate or roof of the mouth.

2. An eminence of the inferior lip of the corolla of personate flowers which closes them; as in *Antirrhinum*. See *Corolla*.

PALATUM MOLLE. The soft palate. This lies behind the bony palate; and from the middle of it the uvula hangs down.

PALEA. (*Palae, æ. f.*; chaff.) Chaff, or short, linear, obtuse dry scales.

PALEA DE MECHA. A name given by some to the *Juncus odoratus*.

PALEACEUS (From *palea*, chaff.) Chaffy, or covered with chaff. Applied by botanists to the receptacles of plants; as those of the *Xeranthemum. Zinnia, Anthemis*, &c. See *Receptaculum*.

PALIMPI'SSA. (From παλιν, repetition, and πισσα, pitch.) Dioscorides says, that dry pitch is thus named, because it is prepared of pitch twice boiled.

PALINDRO'MIA. (Παλιν, again, and δρομος, a course.) This term is used by Hippocrates for any regurgitation of humours to the more noble parts: and sometimes for the return of a distemper.

PALIU'RUS. (From παλλω, to move, and ουρον, urine; so called from its diuretic qualities.) The *Rhamnus paliurus*.

PALLADIUM. A new metal, first found by Dr. Wollaston, associated with platina, among the grains of which he supposes its ores to exist, or an alloy of it with iridium and osmium; scarcely distinguishable from the crude platina, though it is harder and heavier.

PALLAS, PETER SIMON, was born at Berlin, where his father was professor of Surgery, in 1741. He applied early and assiduously to his studies, particularly to dissection, insomuch that he was enabled, at the age of 17, to read a public course on anatomy. He then went to Halle, and in 1759 to Gottingen, where a severe illness for some time interrupted his pursuits; but he afterward made numerous experiments on poisons, and dissections of animals; and composed a very ingenious treatise on those which are found within others, particularly the worms occurring in the human body. In the following year, he took his degree at Leyden, then travelled through Holland and England, directing his attention almost entirely to natural history. In 1762, his father recalled him to Berlin; but allowed him soon after to settle at the Hague, where he could better prosecute his favourite studies; the fruit of

which shortly appeared in a valuable treatise on zoophytes, and some other publications : and he was admitted into the Royal Society of London, and the Academy Naturæ Curiosorum, to which he had sent interesting papers. About this period he meditated a voyage to the Cape of Good Hope, and other Dutch settlements; but his father again recalled him in 1766. However, in the following year, he was induced by Catharine II. to become professor of natural history at St. Petersburgh. Thence, in 1768, he set out, with some other philosophers, on a scientific tour, as far as Siberia, which occupied six years. Of this he afterward published a most interesting account in five quarto volumes comprehending every thing memorable in the several provinces which he had visited. This was followed by a particular history of the Mongul tribes, who had, at different periods, overrun the greater part of Asia, and whom he clearly proved to be a distinct race from the Tartars. In 1777 he read before the academy a dissertation on the formation of mountains, and the changes which this globe has undergone, particularly in the Russian empire. He also published, from time to time, numerous works relative to zoology, botany, agriculture, and geography. About the year 1784, he received signal proofs of the empress's favour : who not only considerably increased his salary, and conferred upon him the order of St. Vladimir, but learning that he wished to dispose of his collection of natural history, gave him a greater price than he had valued it at, and allowed him the use of it during his life. In 1794, he travelled to the Crimea, of which he published an account on his return : and his health now beginning to decline, the empress presented him an estate in that province, with a liberal sum for his establishment. Unfortunately, however, the situation was particularly unhealthy, and proved very injurious to his family. At length he determined to visit his brother, and his native city, where he died shortly after, in 1811.

PALLIATIVE. (*Palliativus*; from *pallio*, to dissemble.) A medicine given only with an intent to palliate or relieve pains in a fatal disease.

Palm oil. See *Cocos butyracea*.

PALMA CHRISTI. See *Ricinus*.

PAL'MA. (From παλλω, to move.) 1. The palm of the hand. 2. A palm-tree. See *Palmæ*.

PALMÆ. (From *palma*, the hand; so called because the leaves are extended from the top like the finger upon the hand.) Palms. One of the natural families of plants which have trunks similar to trees, but come under the term stipes, the tops being frondescent, that is, sending off leaves. Palms are the most lofty, and in some instances, the most long-lived of plants, and have therefore justly acquired the name of trees. Yet Sir James Smith observes, paradoxical as it may seem, they are rather perennial herbaceous plants, having nothing in common with the growth of trees in general. Palms are formed of successive circular crowns of leaves, which spring directly from the root. These leaves and their footstalks are furnished with bundles of large sap-vessels, and returning-vessels, like the leaves of trees, when one circle of them has performed its office, another is formed within it, which, being confined below, necessarily rises a little above the former. Thus, successive circles grow one above the other; by which the vertical increase of the plant is almost without end. Each circle of leaves is independent of its predecessor, and has its own cluster of vessels; so that there can be no aggregation of woody circles.

PALMARIS. (*Palmaris*; from *palma*, the hand.) Belonging to the hand.

PALMARIS BREVIS. *Palmaris brevis vel caro quadrata*, of Douglas; and *Palmare cutané*, of Dumas. A small, thin, cutaneous flexor muscle of the hand, situated between the wrist and the little finger. Fallopius tells us that it was discovered by Cananus. Winslow names it *palmaris cutaneus*. It arises from a small part of the internal annular ligament, and inner edge of the aponeurosis palmaris, and is inserted by small bundles of fleshy fibres into the os pisiforme, and into the skin and fat that cover the abductor minimi digiti. This muscle seems to assist in contracting the palm of the hand.

PALMARIS CUTANEUS. See *Palmaris brevis*.

PALMARIS LONGUS. A flexor muscle of the arm

situated on the fore-arm, immediately under the integuments. *Ulnaris gracilis*, of Winslow; and *Epitrochlo carpi palmaire*, of Dumas. It arises tendinous from the inner condyle of the os humeri, but soon becomes fleshy, and after continuing so about three inches, terminates in a long slender tendon, which, near the wrist, separates into two portions, one of which is inserted into the internal annular ligament, and the other loses itself in a tendinous membrane, that is nearly of a triangular shape, and extends over the palm of the hand, from the carpal ligaments to the roots of the fingers, and is called *aponeurosis palmaris*. Some of the fibres of this expansion adhere strongly to the metacarpal bones, and separate the muscles and tendons of each finger. Several anatomical writers have considered this aponeurosis as a production of the tendon of this muscle, but seemingly without reason, because we now and then find the latter wholly inserted into the carpal ligament, in which case it is perfectly distinct from the aponeurosis in question; and, in some subjects, the palmaris longus is wanting, but the aponeurosis is always to be found. Rhodius, indeed, says that the latter is now and then deficient: but there is good reason to think that he was mistaken. This muscle bends the hand, and may assist in its pronation: it likewise serves to stretch the aponeurosis palmaris.

PALMATUS. Palmate. Applied to leaves, cut, as it were, into several oblong, nearly equal segments, about half-way, or rather more, towards the base, leaving an entire space like the palm of the hand; as in *Passiflora cœrulea*.

PA'LMOS. (From παλλω, to beat.) A palpitation of the heart.

PA'LMULA. (Diminutive of *palma*, the hand: so called from its shape.) 1. A date.

2. The broad and flat end of a rib.

PA'LPEBRA. (*A palpitando*, from their frequent motion.) The eyelid, distinguished into upper and under; at each end they unite and form the canthi.

Palpebræ superioris, levator. See *Levator palpebræ superioris.*

Palpebrarum aperiens rectus. See *Levator palpebræ superioris.*

PALPITA'TIO. 1. A palpitation or convulsive motion of a part.

2. Palpitation of the heart. A genus of diseases in the class *Neuroses*, and order *Spasmi*, of Cullen.

PALSY. See *Paralysis.*

PALUDA'PIUM. (From *Palus* a lake, and *apium*, smallage: so named because it grows in and about rivulets.) A species of smallage.

PA'LUS SANCTUS. A name of guaiacum.

PAMPHI'LIUM. (From πας, all, and φιλος, grateful: so called from its extensive usefulness.) A plaster described by Galen.

PAMPINIFORM. (*Pampiniformis*; from *pampinus*, a tendril, and *forma*, a likeness.) Resembling a tendril; applied to the spermatic chord and the thoracic duct.

PANA'CEA. (From παν, the neuter of πας, all, and ακεομαι, to cure.) An epithet given by the ancients to those remedies which they conceived would cure every disease. Unfortunately for men of the present day there are no such remedies.

PANACEA DUCIS HOLSATIÆ. The sulphate of potassa.

PANACEA DUPLICATA. Sulphate of potassa.

PANACEA VEGETABILIS. Saffron.

PANADA. (Diminutive of *pane*, bread, Ital.) *Panata; Panatella.* Bread boiled in water to the consistence of pap. Dry biscuits soaked are the best for this purpose.

PANALE'THES. (From παν, all, and αληθης, true.) A name of a cephalic plaster, from its universal efficacy.

PA'NARIS. (Corrupted from *paronychia*.) See *Paronychia.*

PANARI'TIA. (Corrupted from *paronychia*.) See *Paronychia.*

PA'NAX. (A name borrowed from the old Greek botanists, whose παναξ, or πανακης, was so denominated from παν, all, and ακος, medicine, because of its abundant virtues. The name being unoccupied, Linnæus adopted it for the Chinese ginseng, that famous restorative and panacea, the reputed virtues of which yield in no respect to the ancient panax.) 1. The name of a genus of plants in the Linnæan system. Class, *Polygamia*; Order, *Diœcia.*

2. A name of the Hercules' all-heal. See *Laserpitium chironium.*

PANAX QUINQUEFOLIUM. The systematic name of the plant which affords the ginseng root. *Ginseng; Panax—foliis ternis quinatis* of Linnæus. The root is imported into this country scarcely the thickness of the little finger, about three or four inches long, frequently forked, transversely wrinkled, of a horny texture, and both internally and externally of a yellowish white colour. To the taste it discovers a mucilaginous sweetness, approaching to that of liquorice, accompanied with some degree of bitterness, and a slight aromatic warmth. The Chinese ascribe extraordinary virtues to the root of ginseng, and have no confidence in any medicine unless in combination with it. In Europe, however, it is very seldom employed.

PANCHRE'STOS. (From παν, all, and χρησος, useful: so named from its general usefulness.) *Panchreston.* 1. An epithet of a collyrium described by Galen.

2. It has the same signification as *Panacea.*

PANCHYMAGO'GA. (From παν, all, χυμος, *succus*, humour, and αγω, *duco*, to lead or draw.) This term is ascribed to such medicines as are supposed to purge all humours equally alike; but this is a conceit now not minded.

PANCE'NUS. (From πας, all, and κοινος, common.) Epidemic. Applied to popular diseases, which attack all descriptions of persons.

PANCRA'TIUM. (From πας, all, and κρατεω, to conquer: so called from its virtues in overcoming all obstructions.) See *Scilla.*

PA'NCREAS. (From πας, all, and κρεας, flesh: so called from its fleshy consistence.) A glandular viscus of the abdomen, of a long figure, compared to a dog's tongue, situated in the epigastric region under the stomach. It is composed of innumerable small glands, the excretory ducts of which unite and form one duct, called the pancreatic duct, which perforates the duodenum with the ductus communis choledochus, and conveys a fluid, in its nature similar to saliva, into the intestines. The pancreatic artery is a branch of the splenic. The veins evacuate themselves into the splenic vein. Its nerves are from the par vagum and great intercostal. The use of the pancreas is to secrete the pancreatic juice, which is to be mixed with the chyle in the duodenum. The quantity of the fluid secreted is uncertain; but it must be very considerable, if we compare it with the weight of the saliva, the pancreas being three times larger, and seated in a warmer place. It is expelled by the force of the circulating blood, and the pressure of the incumbent viscera in the full abdomen. Its great utility appears from its constancy, being found in almost all animals; nor is this refuted by the few experiments in which a part of it was cut out from a robust animal, without occasioning death; because the whole pancreas cannot be removed without the duodenum: for even a part of the lungs may be cut out without producing death, but they are not, therefore, useless. It seems principally to dilute the viscid cystic bile, to mitigate its acrimony, and to mix it with the food. Hence, it is poured into a place remote from the duct from the liver, as often as there is no gall-bladder. Like the rest of the intestinal humours it dilutes and resolves the mass of aliments, and performs every other office of the saliva.

PANCREATIC. (*Pancreaticus*; from *pancreas*, the name of a viscus.) Of or belonging to the pancreas.

Pancreatic duct. See *Ductus pancreaticus.*

Pancreatic juice. See *Pancreas.*

PANCRE'NE. (From πας, all, and κρηνη, a fountain.) A name of the pancreas from its great secretion.

PANDALI'TIUM. A whitlow.

PANDEMIC. (*Pandemicus*; from παν, all, and δημος, the people.) A disease is so termed which attacks all or a great many persons in the same place and at the same time. A pandemic disease is one which is very general.

PANDICULA'TIO. (From *pandiculo*, to gape and stretch.) Pandiculation, or a restless stretching or gaping, such as accompanies the cold fit of an ague.

PANDURIFORMIS. Fiddle-shaped; applied to a leaf, which is oblong, broad at the two extremities, and contracted in the middle, as in the fiddle dock, *Rumex pulcher.*

PANICULA A panicle. A species of compound

inflorescence which bears the flowers in a sort of loose, subdivided, bunch or cluster, without any order, appearing like a branched spike. The flowers of the *Æsculus hippo-castanum*, *Rhus cotinus*, *Gypsophylla paniculata*, and *Syringa vulgaris*, are good examples of a panicle; but this species of inflorescence occurs most in grasses, as in *Poa aquatica*.

1. When the stalks are distant, lax, or spreading, it is called *Panicula patula;* as in *Campanula patula*.

2. *Panicula coartata*, is a dense or crowded one, observed in *Campanula rapunculus*.

3. *P. dichotoma*, forked; as in *Linum flavum*.

4. *P. brachiata*, crossing each other in pairs; as in *Salvia paniculata*.

5. *P. divaricata*, a more spreading one than the patulous; as in the *Pnenanthes muralis*.

PA'NICUM. (*A paniculis*, from its many panicles; the spike consisting of innumerable thick seeds, disposed in many panicles.) The name of a genus of plants in the Linnæan system. Class, *Triandria;* Order, *Digynia*.

PANICUM ITALICUM. The systematic name of the plant which affords the Indian millet-seed, which is much esteemed in Italy, being a constant ingredient in soups, and made into a variety of forms for the table.

PANICUM MILIACEUM. The systematic name of the plant which affords the millet-seed. They are esteemed as a nutritious article of diet, and are often made into puddings in this country.

PA'NIS. Bread. See *Bread*.

PANIS CUCULI. See *Oxalis acetosella*.

PANIS FORCINUS. A species of cyclamen.

PANNI'CULUS. (From *pannus*, cloth.) 1. A piece of fine cloth.

2. The cellular and carnous membranes are so called from their resemblance to a piece of fine cloth.

PANNO'NICA. (From *pannus*, a rag: so called because its stalk is divided into many uneven points, like the end of a piece of rag.) Hawk-weed, or *Hypochæris*.

PA'NNUS. (From πενω, to labour.)

1. A piece of cloth.

2. A tent for a wound.

3. A speck in the eye, resembling a bit of rag.

4. An irregular mark upon the skin.

PANO'CTIA. A bubo in the groin.

PANOPHO'BIA. (From *παν*, all, and *φοβος*, fear.) *Pantophobia*. That kind of melancholy which is principally characterized by groundless fears.

PANSY. See *Viola tricolor*.

PANTAGO'GA. (From *πας*, all, and *αγω*, to drive out.) Medicines which expel all morbid humours.

PANTO'LMIUS. (From *πας*, all, and *τολμαω*, to dare: so named from its general uses.) A medicine described by Ægineta.

PANTOPHO'BIA. See *Panophobia*.

PA'NUS. (From πενω, to work.) 1. A weaver's roll.

2. A soft tumour, like a weaver's roll.

PAPA'VER. (*Papaver*, *eris.* n.; from *pappa*, pap: so called because nurses used to mix this plant in children's food to relieve the colic and make them sleep.) 1. The name of a genus of plants in the Linnæan system. Class, *Polyandria;* Order, *Monogynia*. The poppy.

2. The pharmacopœial name of the white poppy. See *Papaver somniferum*.

PAPAVER ERRATICUM. See *Papaver rhœas*.

PAPAVER NIGRUM. The black poppy. This is merely a variety of the white poppy, producing black seeds. See *Papaver somniferum*.

PAPAVER RHŒAS. The systematic and pharmacopœial name of the red corn poppy. *Papaver erraticum*. *Papaver—capsulis glabris globosis, caule-piloso multifloro;—foliis pennatifidis incisis* of Linnæus. The heads of this species, like those of the somniferum, contain a milky juice of a narcotic quality; from which an extract is prepared, that has been successfully employed as a sedative. The flowers have somewhat of the smell of opium, and a mucilaginous taste, accompanied with a slight degree of bitterness. A syrup of these flowers is directed in the London Pharmacopœia, which has been thought useful as an anodyne and pectoral, and is prescribed in coughs and catarrhal affections. See *Syrupus rhœados*.

PAPAVER SOMNIFERUM. The systematic name of

150

the white poppy, from which opium is obtained. Linnæus describes the plant:—*Papaver—calycibus, cap sulisque glabris, foliis amplexicaulibus incisis*. This drug is also called *opium thebaicum*, from being anciently prepared chiefly at Thebes: *Opion* and *manus Dei*, from its extensive medical virtues, &c. The Arabians called it *affion* and *afium*. It is the concreted milky juice of the capsule or head of the poppy. It is brought from Turkey, Egypt, the East Indies, and other parts of Asia, where poppies are cultivated for this use in fields, as corn among us. The manner in which it is collected has been described long ago by Kæmpfer, and others; but the most circumstantial detail of the culture of the poppy, and the method of procuring the opium, is that given by Kerr, as practised in the province of Bahar. He says, "The field being well prepared by the plough and harrow, and reduced to an exact level superficies, it is then divided into quadrangular areas of seven feet long, and five feet in breadth, leaving two feet of interval, which is raised five or six inches, and excavated into an aqueduct for conveying water to every area, for which purpose they have a well in every cultivated field. The seeds are sown in October or November. The plants are allowed to grow six or eight inches distant from each other, and are plentifully supplied with water; when the young plants are six or eight inches high, they are watered more sparingly. But the cultivator spreads all over the areas a nutriment compost of ashes, human excrements, cow dung, and a large portion of nitrous earths, scraped from the highways and old mud walls. When the plants are nigh flowering, they are watered profusely, to increase the juice. When the capsules are half grown, no more water is given, and they begin to collect the opium. At sunset they make two longitudinal double incisions upon each half-ripe capsule, passing from below upwards, and taking care not to penetrate the internal cavity of the capsule. The incisions are repeated every evening until each capsule has received six or eight wounds; then are they allowed to ripen their seeds. The ripe capsules afford little or no juice. If the wound was made in the heat of the day, a cicatrix would be too soon formed. The night dews, by their moisture, favour the exstillation of the juice. Early in the morning, old women, boys, and girls, collect the juice by scraping it off the wounds with a small iron scoop, and deposite the whole in an earthen pot, where it is worked by the hand in the open sunshine, until it becomes of a considerable spissitude. It is then formed into cakes of a globular shape, and about four pounds in weight, and laid into little earthen basins to be further exsiccated. These cakes are covered over with the poppy or tobacco leaves, and dried until they are fit for sale. Opium is frequently adulterated with cow dung, the extract of the poppy plant procured by boiling, and various other substances which they keep in secrecy." This process, however, is now but rarely practised, the consumption of this drug being too great to be supplied by that method of collection.

The best sort of the *officinal opium* is the expressed juice of the heads, or of the heads and the upper part of the stalks inspissated by a gentle heat. This was formerly called *meconium*, in distinction from the true opium, which issues spontaneously.

The inferior sorts (for there are considerable differences in the quality of this drug,) are said to be prepared by boiling the plant in water, and evaporating the strained decoction; but as no kind of our opium will totally dissolve in water, the juice is most probably extracted by expression. Newman was informed by some Turks at Genoa and Leghorn, that in some places the heads, stalks, and leaves are committed to the press together, and that this juice inspissated affords a very good opium.

On this head Dr. Lewis remarks, that the point has not yet been fully determined. It is commonly supposed, that whatever preparations the Turks may make from the poppy for their own use, the opium brought to us is really the milky juice collected from incisions made in the heads, as described by Kæmpfer. It is certain that an extract made by boiling the heads, or the heads and stalks in water, is much weaker than opium; but it appears also, that the pure milky tears are considerably stronger.

The principles separable from opium are, a resin, gum, besides a minute portion of saline matter, and water and earth, which are intimately combined together, insomuch that all the three dissolve almost equally in water and in spirit.

Four ounces of opium, treated with alkohol, yielded three ounces and four scruples of resinous extract; five drachms and a scruple of insoluble impurities remaining. On taking four ounces more, and applying water at first, Newman obtained two ounces five drachms and one scruple of gummy extract; the insoluble part amounting here to seven drachms and a scruple. In distillation, alkohol brought over little or nothing; but the distilled water was considerably impregnated with the peculiar ill smell of opium.

From this analysis may be estimated the effects of different solvents upon it. Alkohol and proof spirit dissolving its resin, afford tinctures possessing all its virtues. Water dissolves its gummy part, which is much less active; but a part of the resin is at the same time taken up by the medium of the gum. Wines also afford solutions possessing the virtues of opium. Vinegar dissolves its active matter, but greatly impairs its power.

A new vegetable alkali, to which the name of *morphia* is given, has also been extracted from opium. It is in this alkali that the narcotic principle resides. It was first obtained pure by Sertürner, in the year 1817. Two somewhat different processes for procuring it have been given by Robiquet and Choulant. According to the former, a concentrated infusion of opium is to be boiled with a small quantity of common magnesia for a quarter of an hour. A considerable quantity of a grayish deposite falls. This is to be washed on a filter with cold water; and, when dry, acted on by weak alkohol for some time, at a temperature beneath ebullition. In this way, very little morphia, but a great quantity of colouring matter, is separated. The matter is then to be drained on a filter, washed with a little cold alkohol, and afterward boiled with a large quantity of highly rectified alkohol. This liquid being filtered while hot, on cooling, it deposites the morphia in crystals, and very little coloured. The solution in alkohol, and crystallization being repeated two or three times, colourless morphia is obtained.

The theory of this process is the following: Opium contains a meconiate of morphia. The magnesia combines with the meconic acid, and the morphia is displaced.

Choulant directs us to concentrate a dilute watery infusion of opium, and leave it at rest till it spontaneously let fall its sulphate of lime in minute crystals. Evaporate to dryness; dissolve in a little water, and throw down any remaining lime and sulphuric acid, by the cautious addition, first of oxalate of ammonia, and then of muriate of barytes. Dilute the liquid with a large body of water, and add caustic ammonia to it as long as any precipitate falls. Dissolve this in vinegar, and throw it down again with ammonia. Digest on the precipitate about twice its weight of sulphuric æther, and throw the whole upon a filter. The dry powder is to be digested three times in caustic ammonia, and as often in cold alkohol. The remaining powder being dissolved in twelve ounces of boiling alkohol, and the filtered hot solution being set aside for 18 hours, deposites colourless transparent crystals, consisting of double pyramids. By concentrating the supernatant alkoholic solution, more crystals may be obtained.

Dr. Thomson directs us to pour caustic ammonia into a strong infusion of opium, and to separate the brownish-white precipitate by the filter; to evaporate the infusion to about one-sixth of its volume, and mix the concentrated liquid with more ammonia. A new deposite of impure morphia is obtained. Let the whole of the deposites be collected on the filter, and washed with cold water. When well drained, pour a little alkohol on it, and let the alkoholic liquid pass through the filter. It will carry off a good deal of the colouring matter, and very little of the morphia. 'Dissolve the impure morphia thus obtained, in acetic acid, and mix the solution which has a very deep brown colour, with a sufficient quantity of ivory-black. This mixture is to be frequently agitated for 24 hours, and then thrown on the filter. The liquid passes through quite colourless. If ammonia be now dropped into it, pure morphia falls in the state of a white powder. If we dissolve this precipitate in alkohol, and evaporate that liquid slowly we obtain the morphia in pretty regular

crysta . It is perfectly white, has a pearly lustre, is destitute of smell, but has an intensely bitter taste; and the shape of the crystals in all my trials was a four-sided rectangular prism.'—*Annals of Phil.*, June, 1820. On the above process, it should be observed, that the acetic solution must contain a good deal of phosphate of lime, derived from the ivory-black; and that therefore those who have used that precipitate for morphia in medicine, have been disappointed. The subsequent solution in alkohol, however, and crystallization, render it pure.

Choulant says, it crystallizes in double four-sided pyramids, whose bases are squares or rectangles; sometimes in prisms with trapezoidal bases.

It dissolves in 82 times its weight of boiling water; and the solution on cooling deposites regular, colourless, transparent crystals. It is soluble in 36 times its weight of boiling alkohol, and in 42 times its weight of cold alkohol, of 0.92. It dissolves in eight times its weight of sulphuric æther. All these solutions change the infusion of brazil-wood to violet, and the tincture of rhubarb to brown. The saturated alkoholic and æthereous solutions, when rubbed on the skin, leave a red mark.

Sulphate of morphia crystallizes in prisms, which dissolve in twice their weight of distilled water.

Nitrate of morphia yields needle-form crystals in stars, which are soluble in 1½ times their weight of distilled water.

Muriate of morphia is in feather-shaped crystals and needles. It is soluble in 10½ times its weight of distilled water.

The acetate crystallizes in needles, the tartrate in prisms, and the carbonate in short prisms.

Morphia acts with great energy on the animal economy. A grain and a half taken at three different times, produced such violent symptoms upon three young men of 17 years of age, that Sertürner was alarmed lest the consequences should have proved fatal.

Morphia, according to its discoverer, melts in a gentle heat; and in that state has very much the appearance of melted sulphur. On cooling, it again crystallizes. It burns easily; and, when heated in close vessels, leaves a solid resinous black matter, having a peculiar smell.

The use of this celebrated medicine, though not unknown to Hippocrates, can be clearly traced to Diagoras, who was nearly his cotemporary; and its importance has ever since been gradually advanced by succeeding physicians of different nations. Its extensive practical utility, however, has not been long well understood; and in this country perhaps may be dated from the time of Sydenham. Opium is the chief narcotic now employed; it acts directly upon the nervous power, diminishing the sensibility, irritability, and mobility of the system; and, according to Cullen, in a certain manner suspending the motion of the nervous fluid to and from the brain, and thereby inducing sleep, one of its principal effects. From this sedative power of opium, by which it allays pain, inordinate action, and restlessness, it naturally follows that it may be employed with advantage in a great variety of diseases. Indeed, there is scarcely any disorder in which, under some circumstances, its use is not found proper; and though in many cases it fails of producing sleep, yet, if taken in a full dose, it occasions a pleasant tranquillity of mind, and a drowsiness which approaches to sleep, and which always refreshes the patient. Besides the sedative power of opium, it is known to act more or less as a stimulant, exciting the motion of the blood. By a certain conjoined effort of this sedative and stimulant effect, opium has been thought to produce intoxication, a quality for which it is much used in eastern countries.

The principal indications which opium is capable of fulfilling are, supporting the actions of the system, allaying pain and irritation, relieving spasmodic action, inducing sleep, and checking morbidly increased secretions. It is differently administered, as it is designed to fulfil one or other of these indications.

Where opium is given as a stimulus, it ought to be administered in small doses, frequently repeated, and slowly increased, as by this mode the excitement it produces is best kept up. But where the design is to mitigate pain or irritation, or the symptoms arising from these, it ought to be given in a full dose, and at distant intervals, by which the state of diminished power and sensibility is most completely induced.

One other general rule, with respect to the administration of opium, is, that it ought not to be given in any pure inflammatory affection, at least until evacuations have been used, or unless means are employed to determine it to the surface, and produce a diaphoresis.

In continued fevers, not of the pure inflammatory kind, opium is administered sometimes as a general stimulus, and at other times to allay irritation. The great practical rule in such cases is, that it ought to be given in such quantities only, that the pulse becomes slower and fuller from its operation. Its exhibition is improper where local inflammation, especially of the brain, or of its membranes, exists.

An intermittent fever, an opiate renders the paroxysms milder, and facilitates the cure. Dr. Cullen recommends the union of opium with bark, which enables the stomach to bear the latter in larger doses, and adds considerably to its efficacy.

In the profluvia and cholera, opium is employed to lessen the discharge, and is frequently the principal remedy in effecting the cure. In passive hæmorrhagy, it is useful by its stimulant power. In retrocedent gout it is used as a powerful stimulant.

In convulsive and spasmodic diseases it is advantageously administered, with the view of relieving symptoms, or even of effecting a cure; and in several of them it requires to be given to a very great extent.

In lues venerea it promotes the action of mercury, and relieves the irritation arising either from that remedy, or the disease.

In the year 1779, opium was introduced into practice as a specific against the lues venerea. It was employed in several of the military hospitals, where it acquired the reputation of a most efficacious remedy ; and Dr. Michaelis, physician of the Hessian forces, published an account of a great number of successful experiments made with it, in the first volume of the Medical Communications, in the year 1784. Opium was afterward given as an anti-venereal remedy in some foreign hospitals. Many trials were also made of its virtues in several of the London hospitals, and in the Royal Infirmary at Edinburgh. Very favourable reports of its efficacy in removing venereal complaints were published by different practitioners; but, at the same time, so many deductions were to be made, and so many exceptions were to be admitted, that it required little sagacity to discover, that most of the advocates for this medicine reposed but a slender and fluctuating confidence in its anti-venereal powers. Mr. Pearson made several experiments on the virtues of opium in lues venerea, at the Lock Hospital, in the years 1784 and 1785 ; and published a narrative of its effects, in the second volume of the Medical Communications. "The result of my experiments," says he, "was very unfavourable to the credit of this new remedy ; and I believe that no surgeon in this country relies on opium as a specific against the venereal virus. I have been long accustomed to administer opium with great freedom during the mercurial course; and the experience of nearly twenty years has taught me, that, when it is combined with mercury, the proper efficacy of the latter is not in any measure increased ; that it would not be safe to rely upon a smaller quantity of the mineral specific, nor to contract the mercurial course within a shorter limit than where no opium has been employed. This representation will not, I presume, admit of controversy; yet we frequently hear people expressing themselves upon this head, as if opium manifested some peculiar qualities in venereal complaints, of a distinct nature from its well-known narcotic properties, and thus afforded an important aid to mercury in the removal of lues venerea." Perhaps it may not be useful to disentangle this subject from the perplexity in which such indefinite language necessarily involves it. Opium, when given in conjunction with mercury, by diminishing the sensibility of the stomach and bowels, prevents many of those inconveniences which this mineral is apt to excite in the primæ viæ; and thus its admission into the general system is facilitated. Mercury will likewise often produce a morbid irritability, accompanied with restlessness and insomnolescence; and it sometimes renders venereal sores painful, and disposed to spread. These accidental evils, not necessarily connected with the

152

venereal disease, may be commonly alleviated, and often entirely removed, by a judicious administration of opium; and the patient will consequently be enabled to persist in using the mineral specific. It, however, must be perfectly obvious, that opium, in conferring this sort of relief, communicates no additional virtues to mercury ; and that, in reality, it assists the constitution of the patient, not the operation of the medicine with which it is combined. The salutary effects of mercury as an antidote may be diminished or lost by the supervention of vomiting, dysentery, &c. Opium will often correct these morbid appearances, and so will spices, wine, and appropriate diet, &c. ; yet it would be a strange use of words to urge, wherever these articles of food were beneficial to a venereal patient, that they concurred in augmenting the medicinal virtues of mercury. It may be supposed that the majority of medical men would understand by the terms, "to assist a medicine in curing a contagious disease," that the drug conjoined with the specific actually increased its medicinal efficacy; whereas, in the instances before us, it is the human body only which has been aided to resist the operation of certain noxious powers, which would render a perseverance in the antidote prejudicial or impossible. The soothing qualities of this admirable medicine can scarcely be estimated too highly. Yet we must be ware of ascribing effects to them which have no existence; since a confidence in the anti-venereal virtue of opium would be a source of greater mischief than its most valuable properties would be able to compensate.

Opium is employed with laxatives in colic, and often prevents ileus and inflammation, by relieving the spasm.

It is given also to promote healthy suppuration, and is a principal remedy in arresting the progress of gangrene.

The sudorific property of opium is justly considered of considerable power, more especially in combination with ipecacuan or antimony. The compound powder of ipecacuan, consisting of one part of ipecacuan, one part of opium, and eight of sulphate of potassa, is a very powerful sudorific, given in a dose from 15 to 25 grains. The combination of opium with antimony is generally made by adding 30 to 40 drops of antimonial wine to 25 or 30 drops of tincture of opium, and forming them into a draught.

Opium, taken into the stomach in immoderate doses, proves a narcotic poison, producing vertigo, tremors, convulsions, delirium, stupor, stertor, and, finally, fatal apoplexy.

Where opium has been taken so as to produce these dangerous consequences, the contents of the stomach are first to be evacuated by a powerful emetic, as a solution of the sulphate of zinc. Large draughts of vinegar, or any of the native vegetable acids, are then to be swallowed. Moderate doses of brandy, or a strong infusion of coffee, have also been found useful.

Respecting the external application of opium, authors seem not sufficiently agreed. Some allege, that when applied to the skin it allays pain and spasm, procures sleep, and produces all the salutary or dangerous effects which result from its internal use ; while others say, that thus applied it has little or no effect whatever. It has also been asserted, that when mixed with caustic it diminishes the pain which would otherwise ensue ; and if this be true, it is probably by decreasing the sensibility of the part. Injected by the rectum, it has all the effect of opium taken into the stomach; but to answer this purpose, double the quantity is to be employed. Applied to the naked nerves of animals, it produces immediate torpor and loss of power in all the muscles with which the nerves communicate.

The requisite dose of opium varies in different persons and in different states of the same person. A quarter of a grain will in one adult produce effects which ten times the quantity will not do in another and a dose that might prove fatal in cholera or colic, would not be perceptible in many cases of tetanus, or mania. The lowest fatal dose to those unaccustomed to take it, seems to be about four grains; but a dangerous dose is so apt to produce vomiting, that it has seldom time to occasion death. When given in too small a dose, it often produces disturbed sleep, and other disagreeable consequences; and in some cases it seems impossible to be made to agree in any dose or *form.* Often, on the other hand, from a small dose sound sleep and alleviation of pain will be produced; while a larger one occasions vertigo and delirium. Some prefer the repetition of small doses; others the giving a full dose at once; its operation is supposed to last about eight hours; this, however, must depend upon circumstances. The usual dose is one grain. The officinal preparations of this drug are numerous. The following are among the principal: *Opium purificatum, pilula saponis cum opio, pulvis cornu usti cum opio, tinctura opii, tinctura camphoræ composita,* and *confectio opii:* it is also an ingredient in the *pulvis ipecacuanhæ compositus, electuarium japonicum pulvis cretæ compositus cum opio,* &c. The capsules of the poppy are also directed for medicinal use in the form of fomentation; and in the *syrupus papaveris,* a useful anodyne, which often succeeds in procuring sleep where opium fails; it is, however, more especially adapted to children. The seeds of this species of poppy contain a bland oil, and in many places are eaten as food; as a medicine, they have been usually given in the form of emulsion in catarrhs, stranguries, &c.

PAP'AW. The fruit of a species of *carica.* See *Carica papaya.*

PAPILIONACEUS. Papilionaceous. A term applied to the corolla of plants when they are irregular and spreading, and thus resemble somewhat the butterfly. The various petals which compose such a flower are distinguished by appropriate names: *vexillum,* the standard, the large one at the back; *alæ,* the two side petals; and *carina,* the heel, consisting of two petals united or separate, embracing the internal organs.

PAPIL'LA. (From *pappus,* down. See *Ulla.*)
1. The nipple of the breast. See *Nipple.*
2. The fine terminations of nerves, &c. as the nervous papillæ of the tongue, skin, &c.

PAPILLÆ MEDULLARES. Small eminences on the medulla oblongata.

PAPILLA'RIS HERBA. See *Lapsana.*

PAPILLOSUS. Papillose. Applied to stalks connected with soft tubercles; as the ice plant, *Mesembryanthemum crystallinum.*

PAPPOSUS. Pappose: furnished with a pappus or seed-down; as the seeds of the *Leontodon taraxacum.*

PAPPUS. 1. The hair on the middle of the chin. See *Capillus.*
2. The *seed-down.* This is restrained by Gærtner to the chaffy, feathery, or bristly crown of many seeds that have no pericarpium, and which originates in a partial calyx crowning the summits of each of these seeds, and remaining after the flower is fallen; as in the seeds of dandelion, goats-beard.

The same term is used by the generality of botanists for the feathery crown of seeds furnished with a capsule, as well as for a similar appendage to the base or sides of any seeds, neither of which can originate from a calyx. For the former of these, Gærtner adopts the term *coma;* for the latter, *pubes;* which last also serves for any downiness or wool about the *testa* of a seed; as in the cotton plant, and *Blandfordia nobilis.*

The varieties of the pappus are,
1. *P. fessilis,* on the apex of the seed, without any footstalk; as in *Asclepias syriaca, Nerium oleander,* and *Epilobium.*
2. *P. stipitatus,* elevated on a footstalk; as in *Leontodon taraxacum.*
3. *P. plumosus,* when the radii of the footstalked pappus are hairy laterally; as in *Tragopogon pratense.*

The *lana pappiformis* of authors is not a pappus, but hairs which only surround the seed; as in *Eryophorum.*

PAP'ULA. (*Papula, æ. f.;* diminutive of *pœppa,* a dug or nipple. See *Ulla.*) A very small and acuminated elevation of the cuticle, with an inflamed base, not containing a fluid, nor tending to suppuration. The duration of papulæ is uncertain, but they terminate for the most part in scurf.

PARABYSMA. (*Parabysma, atis. n.;* from *παραβυω,* congestion, infarction, coacervation.) Dr. Good has applied this term to a genus of diseases, (comprehended by Cullen and others under that of physcoma,) Class, *Cœliaca;* Order, *Splanchnica.* Visceral turgescence. It has seven species. *Parabysma hepati-*

cum; splenicum; pancreaticum; mesentericum; in testinale; omentale; complicatum

PA'R. (*Par, aris.* n; a pair.) A pair.

PAR CUCULLARE. So Casserius calls the *Crico aorytænoid muscle.*

PAR VAGUM. The eighth pair of nerves. They arise from the corpora olivaria of the medulla oblongata, and proceed into the neck, thorax, and abdomen. In the neck the par vagum gives off two branches, the lingual and superior laryngeal; and, in the thorax, four branches, the recurrent laryngeal, the cardiac, the pulmonary, and the œsophageal plexuses. At length the trunks of the nervi vagi, adjacent to the mediastinum, run into the stomach, and there form the stomachic plexus, which branches to the abdominal plexuses.

PARACELSUS, a native of Switzerland, born about the year 1493. His father is said to have been a practitioner in medicine, and inspired him with a taste for chemistry. He very early commenced a sort of rambling life, assuming the pompous names of *Phillipus, Aureolus, Theophrastus, Paracelsus, Bombastus de Hohenheim;* and after visiting the schools of France, Italy, and Germany, he sought for information during several years among quacks of every description, pretending that he had found the principles of the medical art altogether erroneous. He appears to have possessed the talent of imposing upon mankind in an eminent degree; for even the learned Erasmus is said to have consulted him. It cannot be a matter of surprise, that, by the bold use of active medicines, especially mercury, antimony, and opium, he should have effected some remarkable cures: these cases were displayed with the usual exaggeration, while those, in which he failed, or did mischief, passed unnoticed. His reputation, however, became so great, that the magistrates of Basle engaged him, at a large salary, to fill the chair of medicine in their university Accordingly, in 1527, he began delivering lectures, sometimes in barbarous Latin, oftener in German; but, though he gained at first some enthusiastic adherents, the ridiculous vanity which he displayed, despising every other authority in medicine, whether ancient or modern, soon created such disgust, that he was left without an audience. A quarrel with the magistrates, on account of a decision against his demand of fees, which was deemed exorbitant, decided him in the following year to leave the place. He subsequently resided in Alsace, and other parts of Germany, leading a life of extreme intemperance, in the lowest company; yet occasional instances of extraordinary success in his practice still preserved him some reputation, notwithstanding numerous failures. But the most striking proof of the folly of his pretensions was given in his own person; for, after announcing that he was in possession of an elixir which would prolong human life to an indefinite period, he died at Saltzburg, in 1541, of a fever. It must be acknowledged, however, that Paracelsus was of material service to medicine, by showing that many active medicines might be safely employed; and particularly as having been one of the first to exhibit mercury in the cure of syphilis, which had been in vain attempted by the Galenical remedies then in use. He published little during his life, but a great number of posthumous treatises appeared under his name, which are too replete with absurdities to deserve enumeration.

PARACENTE'SIS. (From *παρακεντεω,* to pierce through.) The operation of tapping to evacuate the water in ascites, dropsy of the ovarium, &c.

PARACMA'STICOS. (From *παρακμαζω,* to decline.) *Paracme.* The declension of any distemper; also according to Galen, that part of life where a person is said to grow old, and which he reckons from 35 to 49, when he is said to be old.

PARA'COE. (From *παρα,* diminutive, and *ακουω,* to hear.) Dulness of hearing.

PARACOLLE'TICA. (From *παρακολλαομαι,* to glue together.) Agglutinants, or substances which unite parts preternaturally separated.

PARA'COPE. (From *παρακοπτω,* to be delirious) In Hippocrates, it is a slight delirium.

PARACRUSIS. (From *παρακρουω,* to deprecate.) A slight disarrangement of the faculties, where the patient is inattentive to what is said to him.

PARACU'SIS. (From *παρα,* wrong, and *ακουω,* to hear.) Depraved hearing. Deafness. A genus of disease in the class *Locales*, and order *Dysæsthesiæ*, of Cullen. It is occasioned by any thing that proves injurious to the ear, as loud noises from the firing of cannon, violent colds, particularly affecting the head, inflammation or ulceration of the membrane, hard wax, or other substances interrupting sounds, too great a dryness, or too much moisture in the parts; or by atony, debility, or paralysis of the auditory nerves. In some instances it ensues in consequence of preceding diseases, such as fever, syphilis, &c. and in others it depends upon an original defect in the structure or formation of the ear. In that last instance, the person is usually not only deaf, but likewise dumb. There are two species.

1. *Paracusis imperfecta; Surditas.* When existing sounds are not heard as usual.

2. *Paracusis imaginaria*, called also *Sussurus ; Syrigmus ; Syringmos; Tinnitus aurium.* When imaginary sounds are heard, not from without, but excited within the ear.

PARACYESIS. (From παρα, male; and κυησις, *graviditas.*) The name of a genus of diseases in Good's Nosology; Class, *Genetica ;* Order, *Carpotica.* Morbid pregnancy. It has three species, viz. *Paracyesis irritativa, uterina, abortus.*

PARACYNA'NCHE. (From παρα, κυων, a dog, and αλχω, to strangle.) A species of quinsy. See *Cynanche.*

PARADI'SUS. (Hebrew.) A pungent seed resembling the cardamom, named from its virtues. See *Amomum.*

PARADISI GRANA. See *Amomum.*

PARAGEUSIS. (From παρα, male, γευω, *gustum præbeo.*) The name of a genus of diseases in Good's Nosology: Class, *Neurotica ;* Order, *Æsthetica.* Morbid taste. It comprehends three species, viz. *Parageusis acuta, obtusa, expers.*

PARAGLO'SSA. (From παρα, and γλωσσα, the tongue.) A prolapsus of the tongue, a swelled tongue.

PARAGO'GE. (From παραγω, to adduce.) This term signifies that fitness of the bones to one another, which is discernible in their articulation; and bones which are thereby easier of reduction, when dislocated, are by Hippocrates called παραγωγοτερα.

PARALA'MPSIS. (From παραλαμπω, to shine a little.) Some writers use this word to express a cicatrix in the transparent part of the cornea of the eye.

PARALLE'GMA. (From παραλλαττω, to change. *Parallaxis.* The transmutation of a solid part from its proper place, as where one part of a broken bone lies over another.

PARALLA'XIS. See *Parallagma.*

PARALLE'LA. (From παραλληλος, parallel.) A sort of scurf or leprosy, affecting only the palms of the hands, and running down them in parallel lines.

PARALO'GIA. (From παραλεγω, to talk absurdly.) A delirium in which the patient talks wildly.

PARALO'PHIA. (From παρα, near, and λοφια, the first vertebra of the back.) The lower and lateral part of the neck near the vertebræ, according to some anatomical writers, as Keil, &c.

PARA'LYSIS. (From παραλυω, to loose, or weaken.) *Catalysis; Attonitus morbus; Tremor.* The palsy. A genus of disease in the Class *Neuroses,* and Order *Comata,* of Cullen, known by a loss or diminution of the power of voluntary motion, affecting certain parts of the body, often accompanied with drowsiness. In some instances, the disease is confined to a particular part; but it more usually happens that one entire side of the body from the head downwards is affected. The species are:

1. *Paralysis partialis,* partial, or palsy of some particular muscle.

2. *Paralysis hemiplegica,* palsy of one side longitudinally.

3. *Paralysis paraplegica,* palsy of one half of the body, taken transversely, as both legs and thighs.

4. *Paralysis venenata,* from the sedative effects of poisons. Paralysis is also symptomatic of several diseases, as worms, scrofula, syphilis, &c.

It may arise in consequence of an attack of apoplexy. It may likewise be occasioned by any thing that prevents the flow of the nervous power from the brain into the organs of motion; hence tumours, overdistention, and effusion, often give rise to it. It may also be occasioned by translations of morbid matter to the head, by the suppression of usual evacuations, and

by the pressure made on the nerves by luxations, fractures, wounds, or other external injuries. The long-continued application of sedatives will likewise produce palsy, as we find those, whose occupations subject them to the constant handling of white lead, and those who are much exposed to the poisonous fumes of metals or minerals, are very apt to be attacked with it. Whatever tends to relax and enervate the system, may likewise prove an occasional cause of this disease.

Palsy usually comes on with a sudden and immediate loss of the motion and sensibility of the parts; but, in a few instances, it is preceded by a numbness, coldness, and paleness, and sometimes by slight convulsive twitches. When the head is much affected, the eye and mouth are drawn on one side, the memory and judgment are much impaired, and the speech is indistinct and incoherent. If the disease affects the extremities, and has been of long duration, it not only produces a loss of motion and sensibility, but likewise a considerable flaccidity and wasting away in the muscles of the parts affected.

When palsy attacks any vital part, such as the brain, heart, or lungs, it soon terminates fatally. When it arises as a consequence of apoplexy, it generally proves very difficult to cure. Paralytic affections of the lower extremities ensuing from any injury done to the spinal marrow, by blows and other accidents, usually prove incurable. Palsy, although a dangerous disease in every instance, particularly at an advanced period of life, is sometimes removed by the occurrence of a diarrhœa or fever.

The morbid appearances to be observed on dissections in palsy are pretty similar to those which are to be met with in apoplexy; hence collections of blood, and of serous fluids, are often found effused on the brain, but more frequently the latter; and in some instances the substance of this organ seems to have suffered an alteration. In palsy, as well as in apoplexy the collection of extravasated fluid is generally on the opposite side of the brain to that which is affected.

The general indications are, to remove, as far as possible, any compressing cause, and to rouse gradually the torpid portion of the nervous system. It will sometimes be proper, where the attack is sudden, the disease originating in the head, with great determination of blood to that part, particularly in a plethoric habit, to open the temporal artery, or jugular vein, or apply cupping glasses to the neck, and exhibit active purges, with the other means pointed out under apoplexy. But where the patient is advanced in life, of a debilitated constitution, and not too full of blood, the object should rather be to procure regular and healthy discharges from the bowels, obviate irritation in the brain by blisters in the neighbourhood, and procure a steady determination to the skin by gently stimulant diaphoretics, as ammonia, guaiacum, &c. in moderate doses regularly persevered in. Emetics have been sometimes very useful under these circumstances, but would be dangerous where congestion in the brain existed. Certain narcotic substances have been found occasionally successful, as aconite, arnica, toxicodendron, nux vomica, and opium; but the tendency of the latter to produce fulness of the vessels of the head must greatly limit its use. Various local means of increasing the circulation, and nervous energy in the affected parts, are resorted to in this complaint, often with decided benefit. In all cases it is proper to keep up sufficient warmth in the limb, or the disease may be rendered incurable. But in addition to this, in tedious cases, fomentations, the vapour bath, friction, electricity, and a variety of stimulant, rubefacient, or even vesicatory, embrocations, liniments, and plasters, may assist materially in the recovery of the patient. In the use of some of these it should be a rule to begin near the boundary of the disease, and carry them onward, as the amendment proceeds, not only as they will be more likely to answer a good purpose, but also because there would be some risk in stimulating too powerfully an extreme part. A suitable diet, according to the habit of the patient, warm clothing, the prudent use of the bath, and other means calculated to strengthen the system, must not be neglected.

PARALYSIS HERBA. (From παραλυω, to weaken: so called from its use in paralytic disorders.) The cowslip and primrose are sometimes so termed. See *Primula veris,* and *Primula vulgaris.*

PARAMENIA. (From παρα, wrong, and μην, the

menses.) The name of a genus of diseases in Good's Nosology. Class, *Genetica;* Order, *Cenotica.* Mismenstruation. It has five species, viz. *Paramenia obstructionis, difficilis, superfluus, erroris, cessationis.*

PARAME'RIA. (From παρα, near, and μηρος, the .high.) The inward parts of the thigh.

PARA'MESUS. (From παρα, near, and μεσος, the middle.) The ring-finger, or that which is between the middle and the little fingers.

PARAMO'RPHLÆ. (From παρα, wrong, and μορφη, form.) The name of a class of diseases of the nutritive powers in Dr. Young's Nosology. Diseases of Structure.

PARANEURISMI. (From παρα, wrong, and νευρον, a nerve. The name given by Dr. Young to a class of diseases. Nervous disease.

["PARANTHINE of Haüy, or *Scapolite* of Jameson. This rare mineral, sometimes massive, usually appears in long prismatic crystals, having four or eight sides. The latter form, which may be called a four-sided .prism, truncated on its lateral edges, is sometimes terminated by four-sided summits, whose faces are inclined to the alternate lateral planes, on which they stand, at angles of 120°. The primitive form is a four-sided prism, which is very easily divisible, parallel to the diagonals of its bases, which are squares. The crystals, usually long, sometimes cylindrical or acicular, are often in groupes, composed of parallel, diverging, or intermingled prisms.

The longitudinal fracture is foliated; indeed, some crystals might be mistaken for little plates of mica, arranged in the direction of its axis. The cross fracture is often uneven.

The Scapolite presents a considerable diversity of colour, lustre, and hardness, which appears to arise in part from a partial decomposition, perhaps the loss of the water of crystallization."—*Cleav. Min.* A.]

PARANŒ'A. (From παρα, diminutive, and νοεω, to understand.) *Paranoia.* Alienation of mind; defect of judgment.

PARAPE'CHYUM. (From παρα, near, and πηχυς, the cubit.) That part of the arm from the elbow to the wrist.

PARAPHIMO'SIS. (From παρα, about, and φιμοω, to bridle.) A disorder wherein the prepuce, being retracted towards the root of the penis, cannot be returned again over the glans, but makes a sort of ligature behind the corona. It is easily known; the glans is uncovered, the skin tumefied on the corona, and above it forms a circular collar or stricture, which, from the skin being unequally extended, becomes indented, and makes several rings round the part. This disease may proceed from two causes; as first from the imprudence of young people, and sometimes also of grown persons, who having the end of their prepuce too straight, cannot uncover their glans without pain, and when they have done it, neglect returning it so soon as they ought; and thus the contracted part of the prepuce forms a constriction behind the glans. Soon after, the glans and penis swell, and the prepuce being consequently very much distended, is affected in the same manner; an inflammation seizes upon both, and swellings quickly appear upon the stricture formed by the prepuce, so that the whole may be liable to a gangrene, if not speedily relieved. The second thing that may produce a paraphimosis; is a venereal virus. In adults, whose glans is uncovered, there frequently arise venereal chancres in the prepuce after impure coition, which before they digest, are generally attended with inflammation, more or less considerable. This inflammation is alone sufficient to render the prepuce too straight for the size of the penis, in consequence of which a swelling or inosculation may ensue like that before mentioned; and this is what is termed a paraphimosis.

PARAPHO'NIA. (From παρα, wrong, and φωνη, sound.) Alteration of the voice. A genus of disease in the Class *Locales,* and Order *Dyscinesiæ,* of Cullen, comprehending six species, viz.

1. *Paraphonia puberum.* About the age of puberty the change of voice from an acute and soft to a grave and harsh tone.

2. *Paraphonia rauca.* The voice hoarse and rough from dryness of flaccid tumour of the fauces.

3. *Paraphonia resonans.* Rough voice from obstruction of the nares, with hissing sound in the nose.

4. *Paraphonia palatina.* From the uvula wanting, or divided, and commonly attended with hare-lip, the voice rough, obscure, and disagreeable.

5. *Paraphonia clangens.* An acute, shrill, and weak toned voice.

6. *Paraphonia comatosa.* A sound emitted at inspiration from relaxation of the velum palati, and of the glottis.

PARA'PHORA. (From παραφερω, to transfer.) A slight kind of delirium, or light-headedness in a fever. Some use this word for a delirium in general.

PARAPHRENE'SIS. A delirium; also a paraphrenitis.

PARAPHRENI'TIS. (From παρα, *male,* not rightly and *phrenitis,* inflammation of the brain ; so called because its symptoms resemble those of the phrenitis, or inflammation of the brain, which it is not.) *Paraphrenesis; Diaphragmatitis.* An inflammation of the diaphragm. A genus of disease in the Class *Pyrexiæ,* and Order *Phlegmasiæ,* of Cullen, known by delirium, with difficulty of breathing, and pain in the region of the diaphragm, and which requires the same treatment as inflammation of the lungs.

PARAPHRO'SYNE. (From παραφρονεω, to be estranged in mind.) The same as *Mania.*

PARAPHYMO'SIS. See *Paraphimosis.*

PARAPLE'GIA. (From παραπλησσω, to strike inharmoniously.) Palsy of one half of the body taken transversely. A species of paralysis. See *Paralysis.*

PARAPOPLE'XIA. (From παρα; diminutive, and αποπληξια, an apoplexy.) A slight apoplexy.

PARAPSIS. (From παρα, and απτομαι, *perperam tango.*) The name of a genus of diseases in Good's Nosology, Class *Neurotica;* Order *Æsthetica.* Morbid touch. It embraces three species, *Parapsis acris, expers, illusoria.*

PARARTHRE'MA. (From παρα, and αρθρον, a joint.) A slight luxation. A tumour from protrusion, as in hernia.

PARARTHRE'MATA. (The plural of *pararthrema.*) See *Pararthrema.*

PARARY'THMOS. (From παρα, and ρυθμος, number.) A pulse not suitable to the age of the person

PARASCEPA'STRA. (From παρα, and σκεπαζω, to cover.) A cap or bandage to go round the whole head.

PARA'SCHIDE. (From παρα, and σχιζω, to cleave.) A fragment or fissure in a broken bone.

PARASITÆ. The name of an order of plants in Linnæus's Fragments of a Natural Method.

PARASITIC. (*Parasiticus;* from παρασιτος a parasite or hanger on.) An animal is so termed that receives its nourishment in the bodies of others; as worms, polypes, hydatids, &c.

A plant is so called which sends its roots into other plants, from which it draws its nourishment; as the Epidendrum vanilla. See *Arrhizus.*

PARASITICUS. Parasitical.

PARASITUS. (Παρασιτος, a parasite.) A parasite: applied to animals and vegetables which draw their nourishment from others of the same kingdom, living within the interior of animals, or having their roots fixed in the barks of vegetables.

PARA'SPHAGIS. (From παρα, near, and σφαγη, the throat.) The part of the neck contiguous to the clavicles.

PARA'STATA. (From παριστημι, to stand near.) It signifies any thing situated near another.

PARA'STATA. (From παριστημι, to stand near.) The *Epididymis* of Hippocrates. Herophilus and Galen called these the *Varicosæ, Parastatæ,* to distinguish them from the *Glandulæ Parastatæ,* now called *Prostatæ.* Rufus Ephesius called the tubæ Fallopianæ by the name of *Parastatæ Varicosæ.*

PARASTRE'MMA. (From παρα στρεφω, to distort, or pervert.) A perversion, or convulsive distortion of the mouth, or any part of the face.

PARASYNA'NCHE. See *Paracynanche.*

PARA'THENAR. (From παρα, near, and θεναρ, the sole of the foot.) A muscle situated near the sole of the foot.

PARATHENAR MINOR. See *Flexor brevis minimi digiti pedis.*

PARANTHINE. See *Scapolite.*

PARDA'LIUM. (From παρδος, the panther.) An ointment smelling like the panther.

PARE', AMBROSE, a French surgeon, was born at Lavel, in 1509. He commenced the study of the surgical profession early in life, and practised it with great zeal both in hospitals and in the army. His reputation at length rose very high, and he was appointed surgeon in ordinary to Henry II. in 1552 ; which office he held also under the three succeeding kings. Charles IX. derived material assistance from his professional skill, and gave a signal proof of his gratitude ; for Paré, being a Huguenot, would have been included in the horrible massacre of St. Bartholomew's, had not the king sent for him on the preceding night, and ordered him not to leave the royal chamber. After having been long esteemed as the first surgeon of his time, and beloved for his private virtues, he died in the year 1590. He was the author of some works, which were universally read, and translated into most of the languages of Europe, containing a body of surgical science. He was a man of original mind, and a real improver of his art, especially in the treatment of gunshot wounds ; adopting a lenient method, instead of the irritating and cauterizing applications previously in use. He was also a bold and successful operator ; and displayed on many occasions all the resources of an enlightened surgeon. He appears, however, to have borrowed freely from the Italian writers and practitioners, especially in anatomy. There is also an affectation of reference to the works of the ancients in his writings, for he was by no means well versed in these, and indeed obliged to request another to translate into French some of the books of Galen, which he wished to consult.

PAREC'CRISES. (From παρα, wrong, and εκκρινω, to secern or secrete.) The name of a class of diseases in Dr. Young's Nosology.—Diseases of secretion.

PAREGORIC. (*Paregoricus* ; from παραγορεω, to mitigate, to assuage.) That which allays pain.

Paregoric elixir. See *Tinctura camphoræ composita.*

PAREI'A. Παρεια. That part of the face which is between the eyes and chin.

PAREI'RA BRAVA. See *Cissampelos.*

PARENCE'PHALIS. (From παρα, near, and εγκεφαλος, the brain.) See *Cerebellum.*

PARE'NCHYMA. (From παρεγχνω, to strain through ; because the ancients believed the blood was strained through it.) 1. The spongy and cellular substance or tissue, that connects parts together. It is applied to the connecting medium of the substance of the viscera.

2. The green juicy layer of barks which lies immediately under the epidermis of trees.

PA'RESIS. (From παριημι, to relax.) An imperfect palsy.

PARGASITE. Common actynolite.

PARHAEMA'SIÆ. (From παρα, wrong, and αιμα, blood.) The name of a class of diseases in Dr. Young's Nosology. Sanguine diseases.

PARIE'RA BRAVA. (A Spanish word.) See *Cissampelos.*

PARIETALE OS. (*Parietalis* ; from *paries*, a wall : because they defend the brain like walls.) *Ossa verticis. Ossa sincipitis. Ossa verticalia vel bregmatis.* The parietal bones are two arched and somewhat quadrangular bones, situated one on each side of the superior part of the cranium. Each of these bones forms an irregular square. They are thicker above than below ; but are somewhat thinner, and at the same time more equal and smooth than the other bones of the cranium. The only foramen we observe in them, is a small one towards the upper and posterior part of each. It has been named the parietal foramen, and serves for the transmission of a small vein to the longitudinal sinus. In many subjects this foramen is wanting. On the inner surface of these bones are the marks of the vessels of the dura mater, and of the convoluted surface of the brain. On the inside of their upper edge we may likewise observe a considerable furrow, which corresponds with the longitudinal sinus of the dura mater ; and lower down, towards their posterior and inferior angle, is a smaller one for part of the lateral sinuses. These bones are joined to each other by the sagittal suture ; to the os sphenoides, and ossa temporum, by the squamous suture ; to the os occipitis by the lambdoidal suture ; and to the os frontis by the coronal suture. Their connexion with this latter bone is well worthy our attention. We shall find, that in the middle of the suture, where the os frontis from its size and flatness is the most in danger of being injured, it rests upon the arch formed by the parietal bones ; whereas, at the sides, the parietal bones are found resting upon the os frontis, because this same arch is there in the greatest danger from

156

pressure. In new-born infants, the ossa parietalia are separated from the middle of the divided os frontis by a portion of the cranium, then unossified. When the finger is applied to this part, the motion of the brain, and the pulsation of the arteries of the dura mater, may be easily distinguished. In general, the whole of this part is completely ossified before we are seven years of age.

PARIETA'RIA. (From *paries*, a wall ; because it grows upon old walls, among rubbish.) 1. The name of a genus of plants in the Linnæan system. Class, *Polygamia* ; Order, *Monœcia.*

2. The pharmacopœial name of the wall pellitory. See *Parietaria officinalis.*

PARIETARIA OFFICINALIS. The systematic name of the wall pellitory. *Parietaria ; foliis lanceolato-ovatis, pedunculis dichotomis, calycibus diphyllis,* of Linnæus. This plant has no smell, and its taste is simply herbaceous. In the practice of the present day, it is wholly laid aside, although it was formerly in high estimation as a diuretic.

PA'RIS. (So called in reference to the youth of that name, who adjudged the golden apple to Venus, this herb bearing but one seed.) 1. The name of a genus of plants in the Linnæan system. Class, *Octandria* ; Order, *Tetragynia.*

2. The pharmacopœial name of the herb Paris. See *Paris quadrifolia.*

PARIS QUADRIFOLIA. The systematic name of the herb Paris, or true love. The colour and smell of this plant indicate its possessing narcotic powers. The leaves and berries are said to be efficacious in the cure of hooping-cough, and to act like opium. Great caution is requisite in their exhibition, as convulsions and death are caused by an overdose. The root possesses emetic qualities.

PARI'STHMIA. (From παρα, and ισθμιον, the part of the throat where the tonsils are. A part of the throat near the tonsils, or disorders of the tonsils.

PARISTHMIO'TOMUS. (From παρισθμια, the tonsils, and τεμνω, to cut.) An instrument with which the tonsils were formerly scarified.

PARISTHMITIS. Inflammation of parts about the fauces.

PARODO'NTIS. (From παρα, near, and οδους, a tooth.) A painful tubercle upon the gums.

PARODYNIA. (From παρα, *male,* and ωδιν, or ωδις ινος, *dolor parturientis.*) The name of a genus of disease in Good's Nosology. Class, *Genetica* ; Order, *Carpotica.* Morbid labour. It embraces seven species, viz. *Parodynia atonica ; implastica ; sympathetica ; perversa ; amorphica ; pleuralis ; secundaria.*

PARONIRIA. (From παρα, and ονειρον, a dream, i. e. depraved, disturbed, or morbid dreaming.) The name of a genus of diseases in Good's Nosology. Class, *Neurotica* ; Order, *Phrenica.* Sleep, disturbance. It has three species, viz. *Paroniria ambulans ; loquens,* and *salax.*

PARONY'CHIA. (From παρα, about, and ονυξ, the nail.) *Panaris ; Panaritium.* A whitlow, or whitloe. Any collection of pus formed in the fingers is termed by authors, panaris, or whitloe, and is an abscess of the same nature with those arising in other parts of the body. These abscesses are situated more or less deep, which has induced the writers upon the subject to divide them into several species : accordingly they have ranged them under four heads, agreeably to the places where they are formed. The first kind of panaris is formed under the cuticle, on one side of the nail, and sometimes all round it. The second is seated in the fat lying under the skin, between that and the sheath which involves the flexor tendons. The third is described by authors to be formed within the sheath ; and they still add a fourth species, arising between the periosteum and the bone.

PARO'PLÆ. (From παρα, near, and ωψ, the eye.) The external angles of the eyes.

PAROPSIS. (From παρα, *male,* and οψις, *visus* sight.) The name of a genus of diseases in Good' Nosology. Class, *Neurotica* ; Order, *Phrenica.* Morbid sight. It has thirteen species ; viz. *Paropsis lucifuga ; noctifuga ; longingua ; propingua ; lateralis ; illusoria ; caligo ; glaucosis ; catarracti ; synizesis ; amaurosis ; staphyloma ;* and *strabismus.*

PAROPTE'SIS. (From παρα, and οπ]αω, to roast.) A provocation of sweat, by making a patient approach the fire, or by placing him in a bagnio.

PARORA'SIS. (From παρα, diminutive, and οραω, to see.) An imbecility of sight.

PARORCHI'DIUM. (From παρα, and ορχις, a testicle.) A tumour in the groin, occasioned by the testicle, which is passing into the scrotum.

PAROSMIS. (From παρα, *male*, bad; and οζω, *olfacio*, to smell.) The name of a genus of diseases in Good's Nosology. Class, *Neurotica;* Order, *Œsthetica;* Morbid smell. It has three species; viz. *Parosmis acris, obtusa,* and *expers.*

PAROSTIA. (From παρα, and οστεον, a bone.) The name of a genus of diseases in Good's Nosology. Class, *Eccritica;* Order, *Mesotica.* Misossification. Its species are two, viz. *Parostia fragilis,* and *flexus.*

PAROTID GLAND. (*Parotideus;* from παρα, about, and ους, the ear.) *Glandula parotidea; Parotis.* A large conglomerate and salival gland, situated under the ear, between the mamillary process of the temple bone and the angle of the lower jaw. The excretory duct of this gland opens in the mouth, and is called, from its discoverer, the *Stenonian* duct.

PAROTIDE'A. (From παρωτις, the parotid gland.) The trivial name of a species of quinsy, in which the parotid gland, neck, and throat, are considerably affected. See *Cynanche parotidea.*

PARO'TIS. (From παρα, near, and ους, the ear.) See *Parotid gland.*

PAROTITIS. Inflammation of the parotid gland. See *Cynanche parotidea.*

PAROXYSM. (*Paroxysmus;* from παροξυνω, to aggravate.) 1. An obvious increase of the symptoms of a disease which lasts a certain time and then declines.

2. A periodical attack or fit of a disease.

Parsley, black mountain. See *Athamanta oreoselinum.*

PARSLEY. See *Apium petroselinum.*

Parsley, Macedonian. See *Bubon macedonicum.*

PARSNIP. See *Pastinaca sativa.*

Parsnip, water. See *Sium modiflorum.*

PARTHENIA'STRUM. (Diminutive of *parthonium,* tansy.) A species of *parthenium.*

PA'RTHENIS. The same as parthenium.

PARTHE'NIUM. (From παρθενος, a virgin: so called because of its uses in diseases of young women.) See *Matricaria parthenium.*

PARTHENIUM MAS. See *Tanacetum.*

PARTITUS. A botanical term: partite, cut, as it were, almost to the base, and according to the number of incisions; *bipartite* when two, *tripartite* when three, *quadripartite* when four, *quinquepartite* when five, &c.

[PARTRIDGE BERRY. See *Gaultheria.* A.]

PARTURITION. *Parturitio;* from *pario.* The expulsion of the foetus from the uterus.

After seven months of pregnancy, the foetus has all the conditions for breathing, and exercising its digestion; it may then be separated from its mother, and change its mode of existence; childbirth rarely, however, happens at this period: most frequently the foetus remains two months longer in the uterus, and it does not pass out of this organ till after the revolution of nine months.

Examples are related of children being born after ten full months of gestation, but these cases are very doubtful, for it is very difficult to know exactly the period of conception. The legislation, in France, however, has fixed the principle, that childbirth may take place the 299th day of pregnancy.

Nothing is more curious than the mechanism by which the foetus is expelled; every thing happens with wonderful precision; all seems to have been foreseen, and calculated to favour its passage through the pelvis, and the genital parts.

The physical causes that determine the exit of the foetus are the contraction of the uterus, and that of the abdominal muscles; by their force the liquor amnii flows out, the head of the foetus is engaged in the pelvis, it goes through it, and soon passes out by the valve, the folds of which disappear; these different phenomena take place in succession, and continue a certain time: they are accompanied with pains more or less severe, with swelling and softening of the soft parts of the pelvis, and external genital parts, and with an abundant mucous secretion in the cavity of the vagina. All these circumstances, each in its own way, favour the passage of the foetus.

To facilitate the study of this complicated action, it must be divided into several periods.

The first period of childbirth.—It is constituted by the precursory signs Two or three days before childbirth, a flow of mucus takes place from the vagina, the external genital parts swell, and become softer; it is the same with the ligaments that unite the bones of the pelvis; the *cervix uteri* flattens, its opening is enlarged, its edges become thinner; slight pains, known under the name of *flying pains,* are felt in the loins and abdomen.

Second period.—Pains of a peculiar kind come on: they begin in the lumbar region, and seem to be propagated towards the *cervix uteri,* or the *rectum;* they are renewed only after considerable intervals, as a quarter, or half an hour. Each of them is accompanied with an evident contraction of the body of the uterus, with tension of its neck, and dilatation of the opening; the finger directed into the vagina discovers that the envelopes of the foetus are pushed outward, and that there is a considerable tumour which is called *the waters:* the pains very soon become stronger, and the contractions of the uterus more powerful; the membranes break, and a part of the liquid escapes; the uterus contracts on itself, and is applied to the surface of the foetus.

Third period.—The pains and contractions of the uterus increase considerably; they are instinctively accompanied by the contraction of the abdominal muscles. The woman who is aware of their effect is inclined to favour them, in making all the muscular efforts of which she is capable: her pulse then becomes stronger and more frequent; her face is animated, her eyes shine, her whole body is in extreme agitation, perspiration flows in abundance. The head is then engaged in the pelvis; the occiput, placed at first above the left acetabulum, is directed inward and downward, and comes below and behind the arch of the pubis.

Fourth period.—After some instants of repose, the pains and expulsive contractions resume all their activity; the head presents itself at the vulva, makes an effort to pass, and succeeds when there happens to be a contra on sufficiently strong to produce this effect. The head being once disengaged, the remaining parts of the body easily follow on account of their smaller volume. The section of the umbilical cord is then made, and a ligature is put round it at a short distance from the umbilicus.

Fifth period.—If the accoucheur has not proceeded immediately to the extraction of the placenta after the birth of the child, slight pains are felt in a short time, the uterus contracts freely, but with force enough to throw off the placenta, and the membranes of the ovum: this expulsion bears the name of *delivery* During the twelve or fifteen days that follow childbirth, the uterus contracts by degrees upon itself, the woman suffers abundant perspirations, her mammae are extended by the milk that they secrete; a flow of matter, which takes place from the vagina, called *lochia,* first sanguiferous, then whitish, indicates that the organs of the woman resume, by degrees, the disposition that they had before conception."—*Magendie.*

PARU'LIS. (From παρα, near, and ουλον, the gum.) An inflammation, boil, or abscess in the gums.

PARURIA. (From παρω, *perperam,* and ουρεω, to make water.) The name of a genus of diseases in Good's Nosology. Class, *Eccritica;* Order, *Catotica.* Mismicturition. It embraces seven species, viz. *Paruria inops; retentionis; stillatitia; mellita; incontinens; incocta,* and *erratica.*

PARY'GRON. (From παρα, and υγρος, humid.) A liquid or moist preparation for allaying a topical inflammation.

PASI'PHILUS. (From πας, all, and φιλος, grateful, from its general usefulness.) A name given to a plaster.

PA'SMA. (From πασσω, to sprinkle over.) See *Catapasma.*

PA'SSA. (From *pando,* to spread.)
1. A grape or raisin.
2. In Paracelsus it is a whitloe.

PASSA MINOR. See *Uva passa minor.*

PASSAVA'NTICUS. (From πας, all, and αναινω, to dry up.) An epithet given by Schroder to a powder, which dries up, and evacuates morbid humours.

PASSIFLO'RA. (Altered by Linnæus, from *flos*

passionis of preceding botanists: a term applied to the beautiful genus in question, because the instruments of Christ's passion were thought to be represented in the parts of the fructification.) The name of a genus of plants in the Linnæan system. Class, *Gyandria;* Order, *Pentandria.*

PASSIFLORA LAURIFOLIA. Bay-leaved passion-flower. A native of Surinam. The fruit of this tree grows to the size of a small lemon, which it greatly resembles. It has a delicious smell and flavour, and is excellent for quenching thirst, abating heat of the stomach, increasing the appetite, recruiting the spirits, and allaying the heat in fevers.

PASSIFLORA MALIFORMIS. Apple-shaped granadilla. The fruit of this species of passion-flower is esteemed a delicacy in the West Indies, where it is served up at table in desserts. They are not unwholesome.

PASSION. (*Passio, onis.* f.; from *patior,* to suffer.) By passion, is generally understood an instinctive feeling become extreme and exclusive. A man of strong passion neither hears, sees, nor exists, but through the feeling which agitates him; and as the violence of his feeling is such that it is extremely painful, it has been called *passion* or *suffering.* The passions have the same end as instinct; like them, they incline animals to act according to the general laws of animated nature.

We see in man passions which he has in common with the animals, and which consist of animal wants, become excessive; but he has others which are displayed only in the social state. These are *social* wants grown to excess.

The *animal passions* have a twofold design, the preservation of the individual, and of the species.

To the preservation of the individual belong fear, anger, sorrow, hatred, excessive hunger, &c. To the preservation of the species, excessive venereal desires, jealousy; the fury which is felt when the young ones are in danger, &c.

Nature has made this sort of passions very powerful, and which are equally so in a state of civilization.

The passions which belong to the social state are only the social wants carried to an excess. Ambition is the inordinate love of power; avarice, th love of riches, become excessive; hatred and revenge, that natural and impetuous desire to injure whoever hurts us; the passion of gaming, and almost all the vices, which are also passions, are violent inclinations to increase the feeling of existence; violent love is an elevation of the venereal desires, &c.

Some of the passions are allayed, or extinguished by gratification; others become more irritated by it. The first sort are therefore often the cause of happiness, as is seen in philanthropy and love; while the latter sort necessarily causes misery. Misers, ambitious and envious people, are examples of the last.

If our necessities develope the intellect, the passions are the principle or the cause of every thing *great* which man performs, whether good or bad. Great poets, heroes, great criminals, and conquerors, are men of strong passions."

Passion, cœliac. See *Diarrhœa cœliaca.*
Passion, hysteric. See *Hysteria.*
Passion, iliac. See *Iliac Passion.*

PASSU'LA. A small raisin.

PASSULÆ MAJORES. See *Uva passa major.*

PASSULA'TUM. (From *passula,* a fig, or raisin.) This is a term given by Dispensatory writers to some medicines where raisins are the chief ingredient; as the electuarium passulatum, &c.

PA SSUM. (From *passa,* a grape, or raisin.) Raisin wine.

PA'STA. A round cake or lozenge.

PASTA REGIA. (From ϖασσω, to sprinkle.) A lozenge, or small cake, sprinkled over with some dry powdered substance.

PASTI'LLUM. (Diminutive of *pasta,* a lozenge.) *Pastillus.* A troch or pastil. A little lump of paste, or ball, made to take like a lozenge.

PASTINA'CA. (*A pastu;* from its usefulness as a food.) 1. The name of a genus of plants in the Linnæan system. Class, *Pentandria;* Order, *Digynia.* Parsnip.

2. The pharmacopœial name of the parsnip. See *Pastinaca sativa.*

PASTINACA OPOPANAX. The systematic name of the plant which yields opopanax. The plant from whence

this gum resin is procured is known by the names of *opoponacum; panax heracleum; panax costinum; panax pastinacea; kyna.* Hercules' all heal; and opopanax-wort. *Pastinaca—foliis pinnatis, foliolis basi antica excisis,* of Linnæus. Opopanax is the gummiresinous juice, obtained by means of incisions made at the bottom of the stalk of the plant, from which it gradually exudes, and by undergoing spontaneous concretion, assumes the appearance under which we have it imported from Turkey and the East Indies, viz. sometimes in little drops or tears, more commonly in irregular lumps, of a reddish yellow colour on the out side, with specks of white; internally of a paler colour, and frequently variegated with large white pieces. Opopanax has a strong, disagreeable smell, and a bitter, acrid, somewhat nauseous taste. It is only employed in the present practice as an antispasmodic, in combination with other medicines, although it was formerly in high estimation as an attenuant, deobstruent, and aperient. Its antispasmodic virtues are less powerful than galbanum, and more so than ammoniacum. It has no place in the Edinburgh Pharmacopœia, but is directed by the London College.

PASTINACA SATIVA. The systematic name of the parsnip. The cultivated or garden parsnip is the *Pastinaca :—foliolis simpliciter pinnatis,* of Linnæus. *Elaphoboscum,* of the ancients. Its roots are sweet and nutritious, and in high esteem as an article of food. They possess an aromatic flavour, more especially those of the wild plant, and are exhibited in calculous complaints for their diuretic and sheathing qualities.

PATE'LLA. (Diminutive of *patina,* a dish: so named from its shape.) *Rotula.* The knee-pan. A small flat bone, which, in some measure, resembles the common figure of the heart, with its point downwards, and is placed at the forepart of the joint of the knee. It is thicker in its middle part than at its edge. Anteriorly it is a little convex, and rough for the insertion of muscles and ligaments: posteriorly it is smooth, covered with cartilage, and divided by a middle longitudinal ridge, into two slightly concave surfaces, of which the external one is the largest and deepest. They are both exactly adapted to the pulley of the os femoris. The edges of this posterior surface are rough and prominent where the capsular ligament is attached, and below is a roughness at the point of the bone, where the upper extremity of a strong tendinous ligament is fixed, which joins this bone to the tuberosity at the upper end of the tibia. This ligament is of considerable thickness, about an inch in breadth, and upwards of two inches in length. The patella is composed internally of a cellular substance, covered by a thin bony plate; but its cells are so extremely minute, that the strength of the bone is, upon the whole, very considerable. In new-born children it is entirely cartilaginous. The use of this bone seems to be, to defend the articulation of the joint of the knee from external injury. It likewise tends to increase the power of the muscles which act in the extension of the leg, by re moving their direction farther from the centre of motion, in the manner of a pulley. When we consider the manner in which it is connected with the tibia, we find that it may very properly be considered as an appendix to the latter, which it follows in all its motions, so as to be to the tibia what the olecranon is to the ulna; with this difference, however, that the patella is moveable, whereas the olecranon is a fixed process. Without this mobility, the rotatory motion of the leg would have been prevented.

PATENS. Spreading. Applied to leaves, metals, &c.; as the stem of the *Atriplex portulacoides.*

PATHE'TICI. (*Patheticus;* from ϖαθος, an affection; because they direct the eyes to express the passions of the mind.) *Nervi pathetici; Trochleatores* The fourth pair of nerves. They arise from the crura of the cerebellum laterally, and are distributed in the musculus obliquus superior, *seu* trochlearis.

PATHOGNOMONIC. (*Pathognomonicus;* from ϖαθος, a disease, and γινωσκω, to know.) A term given to those symptoms which are peculiar to a disease. They are also termed proper or characteristic symptoms.

PATHOLOGY. (*Pathologia;* from ϖαθος, a disease, and λογος, a discourse.) The doctrine of diseases. It comprehends *nosology, ætiology, symptomatology, semeiotics,* and *therapeia.*

PATIE'NTIA. (From *patior,* to bear, or suffer.)

The name of the herb monk's rhubarb, from its gentle purging qualities. See *Rumex patientia.*

PATIENCE. See *Rumex patientia.*

PA'TOR NARIUM. (From *pateo,* to be opened.) The sinus, cavity, or chasm of the nose.

PA'TRUM CORTEX. (So called from the Jesuits, termed fathers in the church of Rome, who first spread its use in Europe.) See *Cinchona.*

PATU'RSA. The venereal disease.

Paul's betony. See *Veronica.*

PAULI'NA CONFECTIO. (From ϖανω, to rest.) A warm opiate, similar to the *Confectio opii;* so called by Aristarchus, which is the same with the *Confectio archigenis.*

PAULITE. See *Hypersthene.*

PAU'LUS. See *Ægineta.*

PAVA'NA. See *Croton tiglium.*

PA VOR. (From *paveo,* to fear: so called from the dread there is of approaching or touching a person affected with it.) The itch.

PEA. The *pisum sativum* of Linnæus. A species of pulse of great variety, and much in use as a nourishing article of diet.

PEA-STONE. A variety of limestone.

PEACH. See *Amygdalus persica.*

PEAGLE. See *Primula veris.*

PEAR. See *Pyrus communis.* Of pears there are many varieties, affording a wholesome nourishment.

PEARL. See *Margarita.*

PEARL-ASH. An impure potassa obtained by lixiviation from the ashes of plants. See *Potassa.*

Pearl barley. See *Hordeum.*

PEARL SINTER. Fiorite. A variety of silicious sinter, of a white and gray colour, and found on volcanic tuff on the Vicentine.

PEARLSTONE. A sub-species of indivisible quartz of Jameson and Mohs. It is generally of a gray colour, and occurs in great beds in clay porphyry, near Tokay in Hungary, and in Ireland.

PECHBLENDE. An ore of uranium.

PECHE'DION. Πηχεδιον. The perinæum.

PECHU'RIM CORTEX. A highly aromatic bark, the produce of a species of *Laurus.* It is extremely fragrant, like unto that of cinnamon, which it greatly resembles in its properties. In Lisbon it is much esteemed in the cure of dysenteries, and for allaying obstinate vomitings.

PECHU'RIM FABA. See *Faba pechurim.*

PECHU'RIS. See *Faba pechurim.*

PECHYA'GRA. (From πηχυς, the cubit, and αγρα, a seizure.) The gout in the elbow.

PE'CHYS. Πηχυς. The cubit, or elbow.

PECHYTY'RBE. An epithet for the scurvy.

PECQUET, JOHN, was a native of Dieppe, and graduated at Montpelier. He pursued the study of anatomy with great ardour and ingenuity, which he evinced by the discovery of the thoracic duct, and the receptaculum chyli, while yet a student, in 1647. He then settled to practise in his native town; but soon after repaired to Paris, with a view of demonstrating completely the important vessels which he had discovered; and he succeeded in tracing the progress of the chyle into the left subclavian vein. He published an account of this discovery, with a Dissertation on the Circulation of the Blood, and Motion of the Chyle, in 1651; and his fame, in consequence, speedily extended throughout Europe, though some denied the truth, others the originality, of it. Besides his anatomical skill, he was a man of considerable acquirements, and became a Member of the Royal Academy of Sciences. He is said, however, to have shortened his life by an unfortunate attachment to spirituous liquors, and died in 1674.

Pecquet's duct. See *Thoracic duct.*

PE'CTEN. The pubes, or share-bone.

[" *Pectic acid.* M. H. Braconnot has given the name of *pectic acid* to a principle found by him in several plants which have the property of being coagulated by alkohol, metallic solutions, the acids, &c. It appears to be the same substance discovered by Prof. Torrey, of New-York, in the Tuckahoe, *Sclerotium giganteum,* a fungus common in the sandy barrens of the southern states, and to which he gave the name of *Sclerotin.* It is readily soluble in a solution of caustic potassa, and this solution is gelatinized by almost every known body."—*Webs. Man. Chem.* A.]

PECTINA'LIS. (So named from its arising at the pecten, or pubes.) *Pectinæus,* of authors, and *Pubio*

femoral, of Dumas. A small flat muscle, situated obliquely between the pubes and the little trochanter, at the upper and anterior part of the thigh. It arises broad and fleshy from all the anterior edge of the os pectinis, or pubis, as it is more commonly called, as far as its spine, and descending obliquely backwards and outwards, is inserted by a short and broad tendon, into the upper and anterior part of the linea aspera of the os femoris, a little below the lesser trochanter. This muscle serves to bend the thigh, by drawing it upwards and inwards, and likewise assists in rolling it outwards.

PECTINATUS. (From *pecten,* a comb.) Pectinate.

1 A term applied to a pennatifid leaf, the segments of which are remarkably narrow and parallel, like the teeth of a comb; as the lower leaves of the *Hottonia palustris,* and *Meriophyllum verticillatum.*

2. The fasciculated muscular fibres of the right us ricle of the heart are called musculi pectinati.

PECTINÆUS. See *Pectinalis.*

PECTORAL. (*Pectoralis;* from *pectus,* the breast.) Of or belonging to, or that which relieves disorders of the chest.

PECTORA'LIS. *Musculus pectoralis.* See *Pectoralis major.*

PECTORALIS MA'JOR. A broad, thick, fleshy, and radiated muscle, situated immediately under the integuments, and covering almost the whole anterior part of the breast. *Pectoralis,* of authors; and *sterno-costo-clavio-humeral,* of Dumas. Winslow calls it *pectoralis major,* to distinguish it from the serratus anticus, which he has named *pectoralis minor.* It arises from the cartilaginous extremities of the fifth and sixth ribs, from the last of which its tendinous fibres descend over the upper part of the obliquus externus and rectus abdominis, helping to form a part of the sheath in which the latter is included. It likewise springs from almost the whole length of the sternum by short tendinous fibres, which evidently decussate those on the other side; and tendinous and fleshy from more than a third of the anterior part of the clavicle. From these origins the fibres run in a folding manner towards the axilla, and are inserted by a broad tendon into the os humeri, above the insertion of the deltoid muscle, and at the outer side of the groove which lodges the tendon of the long head of the biceps. Some of its fibres likewise extend into that groove; and, from the lower part of this tendon, which is spread near two inches along the os humeri, we find it sending off other fibres, which help to form the fascia that covers the muscles of the arm. It often happens that that part of the pectoralis which arises from the clavicle, is separated from the inferior portion, so as to appear like a distinct muscle. This has induced Winslow to divide it into parts, one of which he calls the *clavicular,* and the other the *thoracic* portion. Sometimes these two portions are inserted by separate tendons, which cross one another at the upper and inner part of the os humeri, the tendon of the thoracic portion being inserted at the outer edge of the bicipital groove, immediately behind the other. This muscle, and the latissimus dorsi, form the cavity of the axilla, or arm-pit. The use of the pectoralis is to move the arm forwards, or to raise it obliquely towards the sternum. It likewise occasionally assists in moving the trunk upon the arm, thus, when we exert any efforts with the hand, as in raising ourselves from off an arm-chair, or in sealing a letter, the contraction of this muscle is particularly observable. To these uses Haller adds that of assisting in respiration, by raising the sternum and ribs. He tells us he well remembers, that when this muscle was affected by rheumatism, his breathing was incommoded; and that, when troubled with difficulty of respiration, he had often found himself greatly relieved by raising and drawing back his shoulders, keeping his arms at the same time firmly fixed. Winslow, however, has denied this use, and Albinus has omitted it, probably because it does not take place in a natural state.

PECTORALIS MINOR. *Serratus anticus* of Albinus. A fleshy and pretty considerable muscle, situated at the anterior and lateral part of the thorax, immediately under the pectoralis major. Douglas and Cowper call this muscle *Serratus minor anticus;* and Winslow gives it the name of *Pectoralis minor;* and Dumas calls it *Costo coracoideus.* It arises from the upper edges of the third, fourth, and fifth ribs, near where they join with their cartilages by an equal number of tendinous and fleshy digitations, which have been compared to the teeth of a saw, whence this and some other muscles, from their having a similar origin, or insertion, have gotten the name of *serrati*. From these origins it becomes thicker and narrower as it ascends, and is inserted by a flat tendon into the upper part of the coracoid process of the scapula. The principal use of this muscle is to draw the scapula forwards and downwards; and when that is fixed, it may likewise serve to elevate the ribs.

PECTORIS OS. See *Sternum.*

PE'CTUS. (*Pectus, oris.* n.) The breast. See *Thorax.*

PECTU'SCULUM. (Diminutive of *pectus,* the breast: so named from its shape.) The metatarsus.

PEDATUS. (From *pes,* a foot.) Pedate. A term applied to a particular kind of leaf, which is ternate with its lateral leaflets compounded in their forepart; as in *Helleborus niger* and *fœtidus,* and *Arum dracunculus.*

PEDE'THMUS. (From πηδαω, to leap.) The motion of the arteries from the impulse of the blood. The pulse.

PEDIA'SMUS. (From πεδιον, a field.) An epithet of a species of wild myrrh.

PEDICELLATUS. (From *pedicellus,* a partial flower-stalk.) Having a small stalk: applied to a nectary which rests on a stalk: as in *Aconitum napellus.*

PEDICELLUS. A partial flower-stalk. See *Pedunculus.*

PEDICULA'RIA. (From *pediculus,* a louse; so called from its use in destroying lice.) See *Delphinium staphisagria.*

PEDICULA'TIO. *Morbus pedicularis.* Φθειριασις. That disease of the body in which lice are continually bred on the skin.

PEDI'CULUS. (Diminutive of *pes,* a foot: so named from its many small feet.)

1. A louse. The name of a genus of insects, of the order *Aptera.* Two species are found on the human body, the *Pediculus humanus,* the common louse; and *the P. pubis,* or crab-louse.

2. A pedicle or footstalk of a flower, or leaf. See *Pedunculus.*

PEDICUS. See *Extensor brevis digitorum pedis.*

PEDILU'VIUM. (From *pes* the foot, and *lavo,* to wash.) A bath for the feet.

PE'DION. (From πους, the foot.) The sole of the foot.

PE'DORA. (From *pes,* a foot.) The sordes of the eyes, ears, and feet.

PEDUNCULUS. A peduncle, or a flower-stalk, or that which springs from the stem, and bears the flowers and fruit, and not the leaves.

Pedicellus is a partial flower-stalk; the ultimate subdivision of a general one, as in the cowslip.

The pedunculus is,

1. *Caulinus,* cauline, when it grows immediately out of the main stem, especially of a tree; as in *Averrhoa bilimbi.*

2. *Rameus,* growing out of the main branch; as in *Eugenia mulaccensis.*

3. *Axillaris,* growing either from the bosom of a leaf, that is, between it and the stem, as in *Anchusa sempervirens;* or between a branch and a stem, as in *Ruppia maritima.*

4. *Oppositifolius,* opposite to a leaf; as in *Geranium pyrenacum.*

5. *Internodis,* proceeding from the intermediate part of a branch between two leaves; as in *Ehretia internodis.*

6. *Gemmaceus,* growing out of a leaf bud; as in *Berberis vulgaris.*

7. *Terminalis,* when it terminates a stem or branch; as in *Centaurea scabiosa.*

8. *Lateralis,* when situated on the side of a stem or branch; as in *Erica vagans.*

9. *Solitarius,* either single on a plant; as in *Rubus chamæmorus;* or only one in the same place, as in *Antirrhinum spurium.*

10. *Pedunculi aggregati,* clustered flower-stalks, when several grow together; as in *Verbascum nigrum.*

11. *Sparsi,* dispersed irregularly over the plant or branches; as in *Ranunculus sceleratus.*

12. *Uniflori, biflori, triflori, &c.* bearing one, two, three, or more flowers.

13. *Multiflori,* many-flowered; as *Daphne laureola.* When there is no flower-stalk, the flowers are said to

be *sessiles;* as in *Centaurea calc rapa,* and the dock ders.

PEGANELÆ'UM. (From ωηγανον, rue, and ελαιον oil.) Oil of rue.

PEGANE'RUM. (From πηγανον, rue.) A plaster composed of rue.

PE'GANUM. (From πηγνυω, to compress: so called, because, by its dryness, it condenses the seed.) Rue. See *Ruta.*

PE'GE. (Πηγη, a fountain.) The internal angles of the eyes are called *pega.*

PELADA. A species of baldness, a shedding of the hair from a venereal cause.

PELA'GRA. *Elephantiasis italica.* This disease does not appear to have been noticed by any of our nosologists, except Dr. Good. Indeed, few accounts of it have hitherto been published, although the peculiar symptoms with which it is attended, and the fatal consequences which generally ensue from it, render it equally curious and important. In certain districts, as Milan and Padua, in Italy, where it is peculiarly prevalent, it is computed to attack five inhabitants out of every hundred. The following account of this singular disease is extracted from Dr. Jansen's treatise on the subject, who had seen the disease at Milan:

About the month of March or April, when the season invites the farmers to cultivate their fields, it often happens that a shining red spot suddenly arises on the back of the hand, resembling the common erysipelas, but without much itching or pain, or indeed any other particular inconvenience. Both men and women, girls and boys, are equally subject to it. Sometimes this spot affects both hands, without appearing on any other part of the body. Not uncommonly it arises also on the shins, sometimes on the neck, and now and then, though very rarely, on the face. It is sometimes also seen on the breasts of women, where they are not covered by the clothes, but such parts of the body as are not exposed to the air, are very seldom affected; nor has it ever been observed to attack the palm of the hand, or the sole of the foot. This red spot elevates the skin a little, producing numerous small tubercles of different colours; the skin becomes dry and cracks, and the epidermis sometimes assumes a fibrous appearance. At length it falls off in white furfuraceous scales; but the shining redness underneath still continues, and, in some instances, remains through the following winter. In the mean time, excepting this mere local affection, the health is not the least impaired, the patient performs all his rural labours as before, enjoys a good appetite, eats heartily, and digests well. The bowels are generally relaxed at the very commencement of the disease, and continue so throughout its whole course. All the other excretions are as usual; and, in females, the menses return at their accustomed periods, and in their proper quantity. But what is most surprising is, that in the month of September, when the heat of the summer is over, in some cases sooner, in others later, the disorder generally altogether disappears, and the skin resumes its natural healthy appearance. This change has been known to take place as early as the latter end of May or June, when the disease has only been in its earliest stage. The patients, however, are not now to be considered as well; the disease hides itself, but is not eradicated: for no sooner does the following spring return, but it quickly reappears, and generally is accompanied with severer symptoms. The spot grows larger, the skin becomes more unequal and hard, with deeper cracks. The patient now begins to feel uneasiness in the head, becomes fearful, dull, less capable of labour and much wearied with his usual exertions. He is exceedingly affected with the changes of the atmosphere, and impatient both of cold and heat. Nevertheless he generally gets through his ordinary labour, with less vigour and cheerfulness indeed than formerly, but still without being obliged to take to his bed; and as he has no fever, his appetite continues good, and the chylopoietic viscera perform their proper functions. When the pelagra has even arrived at this stage, the returning winter, nevertheless, commonly restores the patient to apparent health; but the more severe the symptoms have been, and the deeper root the disease has taken, the more certainly does the return of spring produce it with additional violence. Sometimes the disease in the skin disappears, but the other symptoms remain notwithstanding. The powers both of the mind and body now become daily more enfeebled; peevishness watchings, vertigo, and, at length, complete melancholy, supervene. Nor is there a more distressing kind of melancholy any where to be seen, than takes place in this disease. "On entering the hospital at Legnano," says Dr. Jansen, "I was astonished at the mournful spectacle I beheld, especially in the women's ward. There they all sat, indolent, languid, with downcast looks, their eyes expressing distress, weeping without cause, and scarcely returning an answer when spoken to; so that a person would suppose himself to be among fools and mad people: and, indeed, with very good reason; for gradually this melancholy increases, and at length ends in real mania.

"Many, as I had an opportunity of observing in this hospital, were covered with a peculiar and characteristic sweat, having a very offensive smell, which I know not how better to express than by comparing it to the smell of mouldy bread. A person accustomed to see the disease would at once recognise it by this single symptom. Many complained of a burning pain at night in the soles of the feet, which often deprived them of sleep. Some with double vision: others with fatuity; others with visceral obstructions; others with additional symptoms. Nevertheless, fever still keeps off, the appetite is unimpaired, and the secretions are regularly carried on. But the disease goes on increasing, the nerves are more debilitated, the legs and thighs lose the power of motion, stupor or delirium comes on, and the melancholy terminates in confirmed mania. In the hospital at Legnano, I saw both men and women in this maniacal state. Some lay quiet; others were raving, and obliged to be tied down to the bed, to prevent them from doing mischief to themselves and others. In almost all these the pulse was small, slow, and without any character of fever. One woman appeared to have a slight degree of furor uterinus; for, at the sight of men she became merry, smiled, offered kisses, and by her gestures desired them to come towards her. Some were occupied in constant prayers; some pleased themselves with laughter, and others with other things. But it was remarkable, that all who were in this stage of the disease, had a strong propensity to drown themselves. They now begin to grow emaciated, and the delirium is often followed by a species of tabes. A colliquative diarrhœa comes on, which no remedy can stop, as also has been observed in nostalgia. Sometimes, in the pelagra, the diarrhœa comes on before the delirium, and the delirium and stupor mutually interchange with each other. The appetite often suddenly failed, so that the sick will sometimes go for near a week without tasting food. Not uncommonly it returns as suddenly, so that they eagerly devoured whatever was offered them, and this even at times when they are horribly convulsed. The convulsions with which they are attacked, are most shocking to see, and are of almost every kind, catalepsy excepted, which has been described by writers. I saw one girl in bed, who was violently distorted by opisthotonos every time she attempted to rise. Some are seized with emprosthotonos; and others with other species of tetanus. At length, syncope and death close the tragedy, often without any symptom of fever occurring through the whole course of the disease." The first stage of the pelagra, in which the local affection only takes place, Dr. Jansen observes, continues in some instances for a great length of time; persons being occasionally met with in whom it has lasted six or eight, or even fifteen years, disappearing regularly every winter, and returning again in the spring. This occasions some of the inhabitants to pay little attention to it; although, in other cases, it reaches its greatest height after the second or third attack. It appears that this disease is not infectious, and that the causes producing it are yet unascertained. It has been supposed, by some, to arise from the heat of the sun's rays; and hence it is now and then called *mal de sole ;* but this does not produce any similar disease in other parts of the world, where it is in an equal or even much greater degree than at Milan; no disease in any respect resembling it, having hitherto been noticed in such regions, except the lepra asturiensis described by Thiery, and after him by Sauvages. In this, a tremour of the head and trunk of the body takes place, which does not happen in the pelagra. This, however, is the principal difference in the two diseases.

PELA´NUM. (From *πηλος,* mud: so called from its muddy consistence.) A collyrium.

PELECA´NUS. (From *πελεκαω,* to perforate.) 1. The bird called the pelican.
2. An instrument to draw teeth: so named from its curvature at the end resembling the beak of a pelican.
PELECI´NUM. (From *πελεκυς,* a hatchet: so called because its seeds are shaped like a two-edged hatchet.) The hatchet-vetch.
PELIOM. A blue-coloured mineral, very similar to iolite, found in Bodenmais, in Bohemia.
PELIO´MA. (From *πελος,* black.) An extravasation of blood of a livid colour.
PELLICULA. A pellicle or slender skin. In medicine, it is applied to such an appearance of the surface of urine, and to very delicate membraneous productions. In botany, to the delicate skin which covers some seeds; as the almond, &c.
PELLITORY. See *Parietaria.*
Pellitory, bastard. See *Achillea ptarmica.*
Pellitory of Spain. See *Anthemis pyrethrum.*
PE´LMA. (From *πελω,* to move forwards.) The sole of the foot, or a sock adapted to the sole of the foot.
PELTA. (*Pelta,* a shield or buckler.) A variety of the calyculus, called the shield, which is the fruit, of an oblong, flat, and obtuse form, observed in the lichen tribe.
PELTA´LIS CARTILAGO. (From *pelta,* a buckler: so called from its shape.) The scutiform cartilage of the larynx.
PELTA´TUS. (From *pelta,* a shield.) Peltate: applied to leaves which have the stalk inserted into their middle, like the arm of a man holding a shield; as in *Tropæolum majus,* and *Hydrocotule vulgaris.*
PELVIC. (*Pelvicus ;* from *pelvis,* the lower part of the trunk of the body.) Pertaining to the pelvis.
PELVIC LIGAMENTS. The articulation of the os sacrum with the last lumbar vertebra, and with the ossa innominata, is strengthened by means of a strong transverse ligament, which passes from the extremity and lower edge of the last lumbar vertebra, to the posterior and internal surface of the spine of the ilium. Other ligaments are extended posteriorly from the os sacrum to the ossa ilia on each side, and, from the direction of their fibres, may be called the lateral ligaments. Besides these, there are many shorter ligamentous fibres, which are seen stretched from the whole circumference of the articulating surfaces of these two bones. But the most remarkable ligaments of the pelvis are the two *sacro-ischiatic* ligaments, which are placed towards the posterior and inferior part of the pelvis. One of these may be called the greater, and the other the lesser sacro-ischiatic ligament. The first of these is attached to the posterior edge of the os sacrum, to the tuberosity of the ilium, and to the first of the three divisions of the os coccygis. Its other extremity is inserted into the inner surface of the tuberosity of the ischium. At its upper part it is of considerable breadth, after which it becomes narrower, but expands again before its insertion into the ischium, and extending along the tuberosity of that bone to the lower branch of the os pubis where it terminates in a point, forms a kind of falx, one end of which is loose, while the other is fixed to the bone. The lesser sac-ischiatic ligament is somewhat thicker than the former, and is placed obliquely before it. It extends from the transverse processes of the os sacrum, and the tuberosity of the spine of the ilium, on each side, to the spine of the ischium. These two ligaments not only serve to strengthen the articulation of the ossa innominata with the os sacrum, but to support the weight of the viscera contained in the pelvis, the back and lower part of which is closed by these ligaments. The posterior and external surface of the greater ligament likewise serves for the attachment of some portions of the gluteus maximus and gemini muscles. The symphysis pubis is strengthened internally by a transverse ligament, some of the fibres of which are extended to the obturator ligament.
PE´LVIS. (From *πελυς,* a basin; because it is shaped like a basin used in former times.) The cavity below the belly. It contains the rectum and urinary bladder, the internal organs of generation, and has its muscles and bones.
PELVIS, BONES OF. The pelvis consists, in the child, of many pieces, but in the adult, it is formed of four bones, of the os sacrum behind, the ossa innominata on either side, and the os coccygis below. See *Sacrum, Innominatum os,* and *Coccygis os.* It is wide and expanded at its upper part, and contracted at its inferior

aperture The uppe ,... the pelvis, properly so called, is bounded by an oval ring, which parts the cavity of the pelvis from the cavity of the abdomen. This circle is denominated the brim of the pelvis; it is formed by a continued and prominent line along the upper part of the sacrum, the middle of the ilium, and the upper part, or crest, of the os pubis. The circle of the brim supports the impregnated womb; keeps it up against the pressure of labour-pains; and sometimes this line has been " as sharp as a paper-folder, and has cut across the segment of the womb;" and so by separating the womb from the vagina, has rendered delivery impossible; and the child escaping into the abdomen the woman has died. The lower part of the pelvis is denominated the outlet. It is composed by the arch of the ossa pubis, and by the sciatic ligaments; it is wide and dilateable, to permit the delivery of the child; but being sometimes too wide, it permits the child's head to press so suddenly, and with such violence upon the soft parts, that the perineum is torn.

The marks of the female skeleton have been sought for in the skull, as in the continuation of sagittal suture; but the truest marks are those which relate to that great function by which chiefly the sexes are distinguished; for while the male pelvis is large and strong, with a small cavity, narrow openings, and bones of greater strength, the female pelvis is very shallow and wide, with a large cavity and slender bones, and every peculiarity which may conduce to the easy passage of the child.

The office of the pelvis is to give a steady bearing to the trunk, and to connect it with the lower extremities, by a sure and firm joining, to form the centre of all the great motions of the body, to contain the internal organs of generation, the urinary bladder, the rectum, and occasionally part of the small intestines, and to give support to the gravid uterus.

PELVIS AURIUM. The cochlea of the ear.

PELVIS CEREBRI. The infundibulum.

PEMPHIGO'DES. (From πεμφιξ, a blast of wind.) A fever distinguished by flatulencies and inflations, in which a sort of aerial vapour was said to pass through the skin.

PE'MPHIGUS. (From πεμφιξ, a bubble, or vesicle.) *Febris bullosa; Exanthemata serosa; Morta; Pemphigus helveticus; Pemphigus major; Pemphigus minor.* The vesicular fever. A fever attended by successive eruptions of vesicles about the size of almonds, which are filled with a yellowish serum, and in three or four days subside. The fever may be either synoch or typhus. It is a genus of disease in the class *Pyrexia,* and order *Exanthemata,* of Cullen. The latest writers on this disease contend, that it is sometimes acute and sometimes a chronic affection; that the former is constantly attended with fever, the latter is constantly without; that in neither case is it an acrimonious or contagious matter thrown out by the constitution, but pure serum, secreted by the cutaneous exhalent arteries. So rare was the disease when Dr. Cullen wrote, that he never saw it but once, in a case which was shown to him by Dr. Home. Dr. David Stuart, then physician to the hospital of Aberdeen, published an account of it in the Edinburgh Medical Commentaries. The patient was a private soldier of the 73d regiment, aged 18, formerly a pedler, and naturally of a healthy constitution. About twenty days before, he had been seized with the measles, when in the country; and in marching to town on the second day of their eruption, he was exposed to cold; upon which they suddenly disappeared. On his arrival at Aberdeen, he was quartered in a damp under-ground apartment. He then complained of sickness at stomach, great oppression about the præcordia, headache, lassitude, and weariness on the least exertion, with stiffness and rigidity of his knees and other joints. He had been purged, but with little benefit. About ten days before, he observed on the inside of his thighs, a number of very small, distinct red spots, a little elevated above the surface of the skin, and much resembling the first appearance of the small-pox. This eruption gradually spread itself over his whole body, and the pustules continued every day to increase in size.

Upon being received into the hospital, he complained of headache, sickness at stomach, oppression about the præcordia, thirst, sore throat, with difficulty of swallowing; his tongue was foul, his skin felt hot and feverish, pulse from 110 to 120 rather depressed, belly costive

eyes dull and languid, but without delirium. The whole surface of the skin was interspersed with vesicles, or phlyctænæ, of the size of an ordinary walnut; many of them were larger, especially on the arms and breast. In the interstices, between the vesicles, the appearance of the skin was natural, nor was there any redness round their base; the distance from one to another was from half an inch to a handbreath, or more. In some places two or three were joined together, like the pustules in the confluent small-pox. A few vesticles had burst of themselves, and formed a whitish scab or crust. These were mostly on the neck and face; others showed a tolerable laudable pus. However, by far the greatest number were perfectly entire, turgid, and of a bluish colour. Upon opening them, it was evident that the cuticle elevated above the cutis, and distended with a thin, yellowish, semi-pellucid serum, formed this appearance. Nor was the surface of the cutis ulcerated, or livid; but of a red florid colour, as when the cuticle is separated by a blister, or superficial burning. No other person laboured under a similar disease, either in the part of the country from which he came, or where he resided, in Aberdeen.

Since the publication of this case of pemphigus, by Dr. Stuart, observations on this disease have been published by Dr. Dickson, of Dublin, by Mr. Gaitskell and Mr. Upton, in the Mem. of the Medical Society of London. Some subsequent observations on pemphigus were published in the London Med. Journal, by Mr. Thomas Christie. From a case which Mr. Christie describes, he is disposed to agree with Dr. Dickson, in thinking, that sometimes, at least, pemphigus is not contagious. He remarks, however, that the pemphigus described by some foreign writers was extremely infectious; circumstances which, he thinks, may lead to a division of the disease into two species, the pemphigus simplex, and complicatus, both of which, but especially the last, seem to vary much with respect to mildness and malignity.

PEMPHIGUS MAJOR. A title under which pemphigus is spoken of by Sauvages, who defines it an eruption of phlyctænæ, about the size of a hazel-nut, filled with a thin yellow serum. See *Pemphigus.*

PEMPHIGUS MINOR. In this species the vesicles are no larger than garden peas.

PE'MPHIS. A species of *Lythrum.*

PEMPHIX. A vesicle, or bubble. See *Pemphigus.*

PEMPTÆ'US. (From πεμπτος, the fifth.) An ague, the paroxysm of which returns every fifth day.

PENÆ'A. (A name given by Linnæus in memory of the learned Peter Pena, a native of France, and an excellent scientific botanist.) 1. A genus of plants in the Class *Tetrandria;* Order *Monogynia.*

2. The name of a species of polygala.

PENÆA MUCRONATA. The systematic name of the plant which is said to afford the sarcocolla. This is brought from Persia and Arabia in small grains of a pale yellow colour, having also sometimes mixed with them a few of a deep red colour. Its taste is bitter, but followed with some degree of sweetness. It has been chiefly used for external purposes, and, as its name imports, has been thought to agglutinate wounds and ulcers; but this opinion now no longer exists.

PENDULUS. Pendulous. Hanging. Applied to roots, leaves, flowers, seeds, &c. as the root of the *Spiræa filipendula,* and *Pæonia officinalis,* which consits of knobs connected by filaments; and the seeds of the *Magnolia grandiflora,* which are suspended by their filaments.

PENETRA'NTIA. (From *penetro,* to pierce through.) Medicines which pass through the pores and stimulate.

PENICILLIFO'RMIS. (From *penicillus,* a pencil-brush, and *forma,* likeness.) Peniciliform. 1. Applied to the stigma of milium paspalium.

2. The extremities of the arteries which secrete the bile, are so called.

PENICI'LLUS. (Dim. of *peniculum,* a brush.) *Penicillum.* 1. A tent, or pledget.

2. The secreting extremities of the vena portæ are called *penicilli.* See *Liver.*

PENI'DIUM. A kind of clarified sugar with a mixture of starch, made up into small rolls. The confectioners call it barley-sugar.

PE'NIS. (*A pendendo,* from its hanging down.) *Membrum virile.* The cylindrical part that hangs down under the mons veneris, before the scrotum of males.

t is divided by anatomists into the root, body, and head, called the *glans penis*. It is composed of common integuments, two corpora cavernosa, and one corpus spongiosum, which surrounds a canal, the *urethra*, that proceeds from the bladder to the apex of the penis, where it opens by the *meatus urinarius*. See *Urethra*. The fold of the skin that covers the glans penis is termed the prepuce. The arteries of the penis are from the hypogastric and ischiatic. The vein of the penis, *vena magna ipsius penis*, empties itself into the hypogastric vein. The absorbents of this organ are very numerous, and run under the common integuments to the inguinal glands: absorbents also are found in great plenty in the urethra. The glands of the penis are, Cowper's glands, the prostate, muciparous, and odoriferous glands. The nerves of the penis are branches of the sacral and ischiatic.

PENIS CEREBRI. The pineal gland.

PENIS ERECTOR. See *Erector penis*.

PENIS MULIEBRIS. See *Clitoris*.

PENNYROYAL. See *Mentha pulegium*.

Pennyroyal, hart's. See *Mentha cervina*.

PENTADA'CTYLON. (From πεντε, five, and δακτυλος, a finger: so called because it has five leaves upon each stalk, like the fingers upon the hand.) 1. The herb cinquefoil.

2. A name for the ricinus, the leaf of which resembles a hand.

PENTAGONUS. (From πεντε, five, and γωνια, an angle.) Five-sided: applied to leaves synonymously with quinqueangular, as in *Geranium peltatum*.

PENTAMY'RUM. (From πεντε, five, and μυρον, ointment.) An ointment composed of five ingredients.

PENTA'NDRIA. (From πεντε, five, and ανηρ, a husband.) The name of a class of plants in the sexual system of Linnæus, embracing those which have hermaphrodite flowers and five stamens.

PENTANEU'RON. (From πεντε, five, and νευρον, a string: so called because it has five-ribbed leaves.) *Pentapleurum.* Ribwort. See *Plantago lanceolata*.

PENTAPHA'RMACON. (From πεντε, five, and φαρμακον, *remedium*, remedy.) Any medicine consisting of five ingredients.

PENTAPHYLLOI'DES. (From πενταφυλλον, cinquefoil, and ειδος, likeness: so called from its resemblance to cinquefoil.) See *Fragaria sterilis*.

PENTAPHY'LLUM. (From πεντε, five, and φυλλον, a leaf: so named because it has five leaves on each stalk.) See *Potentilla reptans*.

PENTAPHYLLUS. (From πεντε, five, and φυλλον, a leaf.) Pentaphyllous, or five-leaved: applied to leaves, calyces, &c. as the flower-cup of the *Ranunculus bulbosus*.

PENTAPLEU'RUM. See *Pentaneuron*.

PENTA'TOMUM. (From πεντε, five, and τεμνω, to cut: so called because its leaves are divided into five segments.) Cinquefoil. The *Potentilla reptans*.

PENTO'ROBUS. (From πεντε, five, and οροβος, the wood-pea: so called because it has five seeds resembling the wood-pea.) The herb peony. See *Pæonia officinalis*.

PEONY. See *Pæonia*.

PEPA'NSIS. (From πεπαινω, to concoct.) *Pepasmus.* The maturation or concoction of humours.

PEPA'SMUS. The same as pepansis.

PEPA'STICA. (From πεπαινω, to concoct.) Digestive medicines.

PEPERINE. A fatty resinous matter, obtained by Pelletier from black pepper, by digesting it in alkohol, and evaporating the solution.

PE'PITA NUX. St. Ignatius's bean.

PE'PLION. (From πεπλος, the herb devil's-milk.) *Peplos ; Peplus.* The *Euphorbia peplus*.

PEPO. (From πεπτο, to ripen.)

I. In botanical definitions, a fleshy succulent pericarpium, or seed-vessel, the seeds of which are inserted into the sides of the fruit.

From its figure, the pepo is called,
1. *Globosus ;* as in Cucumis colocynthus.
2. *Oblongus ;* as Cucumis sativ is.
3. *Lagenæformis ;* as Cucurbit i lagenaria.
4. *Curvatus ;* as Cucumis flexuosus.
5. *Nodosus ;* as Cucumis melopepo.
6. *Fusiformis ;* as Cucumis chale.
7. *Echinatus ;* as Cucumis anguria.
8. *Verrucosus ;* as Cucurbita verrucosa.
9. *Scaber ;* as Cucumis sativus.

II. See *Cucurbita*.

PEPPER. See *Piper nigrum*.

Pepper, black. See *Piper nigrum*.

Pepper, Guinea. See *Capsicum annuum*.

Pepper, Jamaica. See *Myrtus pimenta*.

Pepper, long. See *Piper longum*.

Pepper, poorman's. See *Polygonum hydropiper*.

Pepper, wall. See *Sedum acre*.

Pepper, water See *Polygonum hydropiper*.

PEPPERMINT See *Mentha piperita*.

PEPPERWORT. See *Lepidium iberus*.

PE'PTIC. (*Pepticus ;* from πεπτω, to ripen.) That which promotes digestion, or is digestive.

PERACUTE. Very sharp. Diseases are thus called when very severe, or aggravated beyond mea sure; as subacute is applied to such as are not very acute, or so severe as they generally are.

PERCHLORIC ACID. *Acidum perchloricum.* Oxychloric acid. If about 3 parts of sulphuric acid be poured on one of chlorate of potassa in a retort, and after the first violent action is over, heat be gradually applied, to separate the deutoxide of chlorine, a saline mass will remain, consisting of bisulphate of potassa and perchlorate of potassa. By one or two crystallizations, the latter salt may be separated from the former. It is a neutral salt, with a taste somewhat similar to the common muriate of potassa. It is very sparingly soluble in cold water, since at 60°, only 1-55th is dissolved; but in boiling water it is more soluble. Its crystals are elongated octahedrons. It detonates feebly when triturated with sulphur in a mortar. At the heat of 412°, it is resolved into oxygen and muriate of potassa, in the proportion of 46 of the former to 54 of the latter. Sulphuric acid, at 280°, disengages the perchloric acid. For these facts science is indebted to Count Von Stadion. It seems to consist of 7 primes of oxygen, combined with one of chlorine, or 7.0 + 4.5. These curious discoveries have been lately verified by Sir H. Davy. The other perchlorates are not known.

Mr. Wheeler describes an ingenious method which he employed to procure chloric acid from the chlorate of potassa. He mixed a warm solution of this salt with one of fluosilicic acid. He kept the mixture moderately hot for a few minutes, and to ensure the perfect decomposition of the salt, added a slight excess of the acid. Aqueous solution of ammonia will show, by the separation of silica, whether any of the fluosilicic acid be left after the decomposition of the chlorate. Thus we can effect its complete decomposition The mixture becomes turbid, and fluosilicate of po tassa is precipitated abundantly in the form of a gelatinous mass. The supernatant liquid will then contain nothing but chloric acid, contaminated with a small quantity of fluosilicic. This may be removed by the cautious addition of a small quantity of solution of chlorate. Or, after filtration, the whole acid may be neutralized by carbonate of barytes, and the chlorate of that earth, being obtained in crystals, is employed to procure the acid, as directed by Gay Lussac.

PERCIVAL, THOMAS, was born at Warrington, in 1740. He studied for three years with great assiduity, at Edinburgh: then came to London, and was chosen a Fellow of the Royal Society; after which he visited different places on the Continent, and took his degree at Leyden. In 1767, he settled at Manchester, and continued there till the period of his death, in 1804, in the unremitting exercise of his medical duties. Dr. Percival possessed, in an eminent degree, those moral and intellectual endowments, which are calculated to form a distinguished physician. He has been well characterized as an author without vanity, a philosopher without pride, a scholar without pedantry, and a Christian without guile. His earlier inquiries were directed to medical, chemical, and philosophical subjects, which he pursued with great judgment, combining the cautious but assiduous use of experiment with scientific observation, and much literary research. His papers were published collectively, under the title of "Essays, Medical and Experimental," in three volumes; which have passed through many editions, and obtained him considerable reputation. His subsequent publications were of a moral nature, and originally conceived for the improvement of his children. But his last work, entitled "Medical Ethics," which appeared in 1803, is adapted for the use of the profession, and will form a lasting monument of his integrity and wisdom. He contributed also numerous papers on various subjects to the Memoirs of the Literary and Philosophical Society of Manchester, which he had been mainly instrumental in establishing, and which did not cease to manifest a grateful sense of his merits, by the continued appointment of him to the presidency.

PERCOLATION. (*Percolatio*, strained through; from *per*, through, and *colo*, to strain.) It is generally applied to animal secretion, from the office of the glands being thought to resemble that of a strainer in transmitting the liquors that pass through them.

PERDE'TUM. In Paracelsus it is the root of skirret, or *Sium sisarum.*

PERDI'CIUM. (From περδιξ, a partridge: so called because partridges were said to feed upon it.) The *Parietaria officinalis*, or pellitory of the wall.

PERENNIAL. See *Perennis.*

PERENNIS. Perennial; lasting for years: applied to plants in opposition to those which live only one or two years; thus the elm, oak, fir, &c. are perennial.

Perennial worm-grass. See *Spigelia.*

PERETE'RION. (From περαω, to dig through.) The perforating part of the trepan.

PERFOLIA'TA. (From *per*, and *folium*: so called because the leaves surround the stem, like those of a cabbage.) See *Bupleurum perfoliatum.*

PERFOLIATUS. (From *per*, through, and *folium*, a leaf.) Perfoliate: applied to leaves when the stem runs through them, as in *Bupleurum rotundifolium*, and *Chlora perfoliata.*

PE'RFORANS. See *Flexor profundus forans.*

PERFORANS, SEU FLEXOR PROFUNDUS. See *Flexor longus digitorum pedis profundus perforans.*

PERFORANS, SEU FLEXOR TERTII INTERNODII DIGITORUM PEDIS. See *Flexor longus digitorum pedis profundus perforans.*

PERFORANS, VULGO PROFUNDUS. See *Flexor profundus perforans.*

PERFORATA. (From *perforo*, to pierce through: so called because its leaves are full of holes.) See *Hypericum.*

PERFORA'TUS. See *Flexor brevis digitorum pedis*, and *Flexor sublimis perforatus.*

PERFORATUS, SEU FLEXOR SECUNDI INTERNODII DIGITORUM PEDIS. See *Flexor brevis digitorum pedis perforatus sublimis.*

PERIA'MMA. (From περιαπτο, to hang round.) An amulet, or charm, which was hung round the neck to prevent infection.

PERIA'NTHIUM. (From περι, and ανθος, a flower.) The calyx properly and commonly so called, when it is contiguous to and makes a part of the flower, as the five green leaves which encompass a rose, including their urn-shaped base; the tubular part comprehending the scales in the pinks, or the globular scaly cup in Centaurea. The tulip is a naked flower, having no calyx at all. The perianth is of infinite variety of forms.

From its number of leaves, it is,

1. *Monophyllous*, formed of one only; as in Datura stramonium.
2. *Diphyllous*; as in Papaver rhœas.
3. *Triphyllous*; as in Canna indica.
4. *Tetraphyllous*; as in Lunaria annua.
5. *Pentaphyllous*; as in Ranunculus.

From the division of its edge,

1. *Undivided*; without any irregularity; as in the female of the Quercus robur.
2. *Partite*, or divided almost to the base; hence *bipartite* or *bilabeate*, in Salvia officinalis; *tripartite*, in Stratiotes aloides; *quadripartite*, in Œnothera biennis: *quinquepartite*, in Nerium oleander; *duodecempartite*, in Sempervivum tectorum.
3. *Cloven*, cut as it were to the middle only; hence, *bifid*, in Adoxa moschatellina; *trifid*, in Asarum canadense; *quinquefid*, in Œsculus hippocastanum.
4. *Dentate*, in Marrubium vulgare; *quinquedentate*, in Cucumis and Cucurbita, the female flowers.
5. *Serrate*, in Centaurea cyanus.

From its *figure*,

1. *Tubulosum*; as in Datura stramonium.
2. *Patens*, with spreading leaflets; as in Borago officinalis.
3. *Reflexum*, its laciniated portions turned backward; as in Œnothera biennis.
4. *Inflatum*, pouched and hollow; as in Cucubalus behen, and Physalis alkekengi in fruit.

From its colour

Coloratum, when of any other than green; a i is Gomphrena globosa.

From the disposition of the germen,

1. *Superum*, when the perianth and corols are above. Hence the remains are visible on the fruit, as in roses, pears, &c.
2. *Inferum*, when below the germen; as in the poppy and water-lily.

From the number on each flower,

1. *Simplex*, when one; as in Nicotiana tabacum.
2. *Duplex*, double; as in Malva, Althæa, Hibiscus, &c.
3. *Calyculatum*, or *acutum*, having a lesser one, or scales down to the base; as in Dianthus caryophyllus
Nullum, when wanting; as in tulips.

From its situation with respect to the fructification,

1. *Perianthum floris*, when belonging to the male.
2. *P. fructus*, when with the pistils.
3. *P. fructificationis*, containing both stamina and pistils in the flower.

From its duration,

1. *Caducum*, falling off early; as in Papaver
2. *Deciduus*, very late; as in Tilia Europœa.
3. *Peristens*; as in Hyosciamus.
4. *Marescens*, withered, but yet conspicuous on the fruit; as in Pyrus, Mespilus, &c.

PERIBLE'PSIS. (From περιβλεπω, to stare about.) That kind of wild look which is observed in delirious persons.

PERI'BOLE. (From περιβαλλω, to surround.) A word used frequently by Hippocrates in different senses. Sometimes it signifies the dress of a person; at others a translation of the morbific humours from the centre to the surface of the body.

PERIBRO'SIS. An ulceration or erosion, at the corners or uniting parts of the eyelids. This disorder most frequently affects the internal commissure of the eyelids. The species are, 1. *Peribrosis*, from the acrimony of the tears, as may be observed in the epiphora.

2. *Peribrosis*, from an ægylops, which sometimes extends to the commissure of the eyelids.

PERICARDI'TIS. (From περικαρδιον, the pericardium.) Inflammation of the pericardium. See *Carditis.*

PERICA'RDIUM. (From περι, about, and καρδια, the heart.) The membranous bag that surrounds the heart. Its use is to secrete and contain the vapour of the pericardium, which lubricates the heart, and thus preserves it from concreting with the pericardium.

PERICA'RPIA. (From περι, about, and *carpus*, the wrist.) Medicines that are applied to the wrist.

PERICARPIALIS. Belonging to the pericarpium of plants: thus the spines of the Datura stramonium on the fruit, are called pericarpial.

PERICARPIUM. The seed-vessel or covering of the seed of plants, which is mostly membranous, leathery, woody, pulpy, or succulent. The membranous are,

1. Capsula.	5. Lomentum.
2. Siliqua.	6. Folliculus.
3. Silicula.	7. Samara.
4. Legumen.	

The woody seed-vessels are

8. Strobulus.	9. Nux.

The fleshy ones,

10. Pomum.	12. Drupa.
11. Pepo.	

The succulent,

13. Bacca.

The seed-vessel is extremely various in different plants, and is formed of the germen enlarged. It is not an essential part of a plant, the seeds being frequently naked, and guarded only by the calyx, as is the case with the plants of the order *Gymnospermia*, also in the great class of compound flowers, *Syngenesia.*

The use of the seed-vessel is to protect the seeds till ripe, and then, in some way or other, to promote their dispersion, either scattering them by its elastic power, or serving for the food of animals, in the dung of which the seeds vegetate, or promoting the same end by various other means. The same organ which remains closed so long as it is juicy or moist, splits or flies asunder when dry, thus scattering the seeds in weather most favourable for their success. By an extraordinary provision of nature, however, in some annual species of Mesembryanthemum, natives of sandy deserts in

Africa, the seed-vessel opens only in rainy weather; otherwise the seeds might, in that country, lie long exposed before they met with sufficient moisture to vegetate.

PERICHÆ'TIUM. (From περι, about, and χαιτη, a hair or bristle.) A scaly sheath, investing the fertile flower, and consequently the base of the fruit-stalk, of some mosses. In the genus *Hypnum* it is of great consequence, not only by its presence, constituting a part of the generic character, but by its differences in shape, proportion, and structure, serving frequently to discriminate species. Linnæus appears by his manuscripts, Sir James Smith informs us, to have intended adding this to the different kinds of calyx, though it is not one of the seven enumerated in his printed works.

PERICHO'NDRIUM. (From περι, about, and χονδρος, a cartilage.) The membrane that covers a cartilage.

PERICHRI'SIS. (From περι, about, and χριω, to anoint.) A liniment.

PERICHRI'STA. (From περι, around, and χριω, to anoint.) Any medicines with which the eyelids are anointed, in an ophthalmia.

PERICLA'SIS. (From περι, about, and κλαω, to break.) It is a term used by Galen for such a fracture of the bone as quite divides it, and forces it through the flesh into sight Or a fracture with a great wound, wherein the bone is laid bare.

PERICLY'MENUM. (From περικλυζω, to roll round: so called because it twists itself round whatever is near it.) The honeysuckle or woodbine. See *Lonicera.*

PERICNE'MIA. (From περι, about, and κνημη, the tibia.) The parts about the tibia.

PERICRA'NIUM. (From περι, about, and κρανιον, the cranium.) The membrane that is closely connected to the bones of the head or cranium.

PERIDE'SMICA. (From περι, about, and δεσμος, a ligature.) 1. Parts about a ligament.

2. A suppression of urine, from stricture in the urethra.

PERIDIUM. The name given by Person to the round membranous dry case of the seeds of some of the angiosperm mushrooms.

PERIDOT. See *Chrysolite.*

PERI'DROMOS. (From περι, about, and δρομος, a course.) The extreme circumference of the hairs of the head.

PERIE'RGIA. Περιεργια. Any needless caution or trouble in an operation, as περιεργος is one who despatches it with unnecessary circumstances: both the terms are met with in Hippocrates, and others of the Greek writers.

PERIESTE'COS. (From περιςημι, to surround, or to guard.) An epithet for diseases, signs, or symptoms, importing their being salutary, and that they prognosticate the recovery of the patient.

PERI'GRAPHE. (From περιγραφω, to circumscribe.) 1. An inaccurate description, or delineation.

2. In Vesalius, *perigraphe* signifies certain white lines and impressions, observable in the musculus rectus of the abdomen.

PE'RIN. (From πηρα, a bag.) A testicle. Some explain it the *Perinæum;* others say it is the *Anus.*

PERINÆOCE'LE. (From περιναιον, the perinæum, and κηλη, a rupture.) A rupture in the perinæum.

PERINÆ'UM. (From περινεω, to flow round, because that part is generally moist.) The space between the anus and organs of generation.

PERINÆUS TRANSVERSUS. See *Transversus perinæi.*

PERINYCTIS. (*Perinyctis, idis,* f.; from περι and νυξ, the night. Little swellings like nipples; or, as others relate, pustules, or pimples, which break out in the night.

PERIO'STEUM. (From περι, about, and οςεον, a bone.) The membrane which invests the external surface of all the bones, except the crowns of the teeth. It is of a fibrous texture, and well supplied with arteries, veins, nerves, and absorbents. It is called *pericranium,* on the cranium; *periorbita,* on the orbits; *perichondrium,* when it covers cartilage; and *peridesmium,* when it covers ligament. Its use appears to be to distribute the vessels on the external surfaces of bones.

PERIPHIMO'SIS. See *Phimosis.*

PERIPLEUMO'NIA. See *Pneumonia.*

PERIPNEUMO'NIA. (From περι, and πνευμων,

the lung.) Peripneumony, or inflammation of the lungs. See *Pneumonia.*

PERIPNEUMONIA NOTHA. Bastard or spurious peripneumony. Practitioners, it would appear, do not all affix this name to the same disease; some affirming it to be a rheumatic affection of the respiratory muscles, while others consider it as a mild peripneumony. It is characterized by difficulty of breathing, great oppression at the chest, with obscure pains, coughs, and occasionally an expectoration. Spurious peripneumony is sometimes so slight as to resemble only a violent catarrh; and, after the employment of a few proper remedies, goes off by a free and copious expectoration; but sometimes the symptoms run high, and an effusion of serum into the bronchia takes place, which destroys the patient.

PERIPYD'MA. (From περι, about, and πυον, pus) A collection of matter about any part, as round a tooth, in the gums.

PERIRRHE'XIS. (From περι, about, and ρηγνυμι, to break.) A breaking off, or a separation round about, either of corrupted bones, or of dead flesh.

PERIRRHŒ'A. (From περιρρεω, to flow about.) A reflux of humours in a dropsical case to any of the larger emunctories for its excretion.

PERISCYPHI'SMUS. (From περι, about, and κυφος, gibbous.) An incision made across the forehead, or from one temple to another, over the upper part of the os frontis. It was formerly made to cover a considerable inflammation or defluxion from the eyes.

PERISTALTIC. (*Peristalticus;* from περιςελλω, to contract.) The vermicular motion of the intestines, by which they contract and propel their contents, is called peristaltic. A similar motion takes place in the Fallopian tubes, after conception, by means of which the ovum is translated from the ovarium into the uterus.

PERISTAPHYLI'NUS. (From περι, about, and ςαφυλη, the uvula.) A muscle which is connected with the uvula.

PERISTE'RIUM. (From περιςερος, a pigeon: so called because pigeons covet it.) See *Verbena officinalis.*

PERISTOMA. See *Peristomium.*

PERISTOMIUM. (From περι, around, and ςομα, the mouth or opening of the capsule.) *Peristoma* The fringe-like membranous margin which, in many mosses, borders the orifice of the theca or capsule. It is either simple or double, and consists either of separate teeth, or of a plated or jagged membrane. The external fringe is mostly of the former kind; the inner, when present, of the latter. The number of teeth, remarkably constant in each genus and species, is either four, eight, sixteen, thirty-two, or sixty-four. On these Hedwig and his followers have placed great dependence.

PERISTRO'MA. (From περιςυρεννυω, to strew about.) Properly signifies any covering.

PERISY'STOLE. (From περιςελλω, to compress.) The pause or time between a contraction and dilatation of the heart.

PERITE'RION. (From περι, and τηρεω, to preserve.) The perforating part of the trepan.

PERITONÆORE'XIS. (From περιῖονaιον, the peritonæum, and ρησσω, to break.) A bursting of the peritonæum.

PERITONÆ'UM. (From περιτεινω, to extend round.) A strong simple membrane, by which all the viscera of the abdomen are surrounded. It has an exceedingly smooth, exhaling, and moist internal surface. Outwardly, it is every where surrounded by cellular substance, which, towards the kidneys, is very loose and very fat; but is very short at the lower tendon of the transverse muscles. It begins from the diaphragm, which it completely lines, and at the last fleshy fibres of the ribs, and the external lumbar fibres, it completes the septum, in conjunction with the pleura, with which it is continuous through the various intervals of the diaphragm. Posteriorly, it descends before the kidneys; anteriorly, behind the abdominal muscles. It dips into the pelvis from the bones of the pubes, passes over the bladder, and descends behind; and being again carried backwards at the entrance of the ureters, in two linear folds, it rejoins upon the intestinum rectum that part of itself which invests the loins, and in this situation lies before the rectum. The cellular texture, which covers the peritonæum on the outside, is continued into sheaths in very many places; of which, one receives the testicle on each side, another the iliac vessels of the pelvis, viz. the obturatoria, those of the penis and bladder, and the aorta, and, ascending to the breast, accompanies the œsophagus and vertebræ; by means of which, there is a communication between the whole body and the peritonæum, well known in dropsical people. It has various prolongations for covering the viscera. The shorter productions of this membrane are called ligaments; and are formed by a continuous reduplication of the peritonæum, receding from its inner surface, enclosing cellular substance, and extending to some viscus, where its plates separate, and, having diverged, embrace the viscus; but the intermediate cellular substance always accompanies this membranaceous coat, and joins it with the true substance of the viscus. Of this short kind of production, three belong to the liver, one or two to the spleen, and others to the kidneys, and to the sides of the uterus and vagina. By these means, the tender substance of the viscera is defended from injury by any motion or concussion, and their whole mass is prevented from being misplaced by their own weight, and from injuring themselves, being securely connected with the firm sides of the peritonæum.

PERITONI'TIS. (From ωεριτοναι, the peritonæum.) An inflammation of the peritonæum. A genus of disease in the Class *Pyrexiæ*, and Order *Phlegmasiæ*, of Cullen, known by the presence of pyrexia, with pain in the abdomen, that is increased when in an erect position, but without other proper signs of inflammation of the abdominal viscera. When the inflammation attacks the peritonæum of the viscera, it takes the name of the viscus; thus, *peritonitis, hepatitis, peritonitis intestinalis, peritonitis omentalis*, or *epiploitis*, or *omentitis, peritonitis mesenterii*, &c.

All these Dr. Cullen considers under the general head of peritonitis, as there are no certain signs by which they can be distinguished from each other, and the method of cure must be the same in all. He however distinguishes three species.

1. *Peritonitis propria;* when the peritonæum, strictly so called, is inflamed.

2. *Peritonitis omentalis. Omentitis. Epiploitis*, when the omentum is affected.

3. *Peritonitis mesenterica*, when the mesentery is inflamed.

PERIZO'MA. (From περιζωννυμι, to gird round.) This term strictly signifies a girdle; but by Hildanus, and some other chirurgical writers, it is applied to those instruments for supporting ruptures, which we commonly call trusses. Some also express by it the diaphragm.

PE'RLA. (Ital. and Span. *perl*, Welch, *perlen*, Germ.) See *Margarita*.

Perlate acid. A name given by Bergman to the acidulous phosphate of soda, Haupt having called the phosphate of soda *Sal mirabile perlatum.*

PE'RNIO. A kibe or chilblain. A species of *erythema*, of Cullen. Chilblains are painful inflammatory swellings, of a deep purple or leaden colour, to which the fingers, toes, heels, and other extreme parts of the body are subject, on being exposed to a severe degree of cold. The pain is not constant, but rather pungent and shooting at particular times, and an insupportable itching attends. In some instances the skin remains entire, but in others it breaks and discharges a thin fluid. When the degree of cold has been very great, or the application long continued, the parts affected are apt to mortify and slough off, leaving a foul ill-conditioned ulcer behind. Children and old people are more apt to be troubled with chilblains than those of a middle age; and such as are of a scrofulous habit are remarked to suffer severely from them.

PE'RONE. (From πειρω, to fasten: so called because it fastens together the tibia and the muscles.) The fibula.

PERONE'US. (*Peroneus*, περοναιος; from *perone*, the fibula.) Belonging to the fibula.

PERONEUS ANTICUS. See *Peroneus brevis.*

PERONEUS BREVIS. This muscle is the *peroneus secundus*, seu *anticus*, of Douglas; the *peroneus medius*, seu *anticus* of Winslow; the *peronæus secundus* of Cowper; and *petit-pcroneo sus-metatarsien*, of Dumas. It arises, by an acute, thin, and fleshy origin, from the anterior and outer part of the fibula, its fibres continuing to adhere to the lower half of that bone. Its

round tendon passes through the groove in the malleo lus externus, along with that of the peroneus longus, after which it runs in a separate groove to be inserted into the upper and posterior part of the tubercle at the basis of the metatarsal bone that supports the little toe Its use is to assist the peroneus longus.

PERONEUS LONGUS. This muscle, which is the *peroneus primus*, seu *posticus*, of Douglas; *peroneus maximus*, seu *posterior*, of Winslow; *peronæus primus*, of Cowper; and *tibi peroneo-tarsien*, of Dumas, is situated somewhat anteriorly along the outer side of the leg. It arises tendinous and fleshy from the external lateral part of the head of the tibia, and likewise from the upper anterior surface and outer side of the *perone* or fibula, its fibres continuing to adhere to the outer surface of the latter, to within three or four inches of the malleolus externus. It terminates in a long round tendon, which runs obliquely behind the malleolus internus, where it passes through a cartilaginous groove in common with the peroneus brevis, being bound down by an annular ligament. When it has reached the os calcis. it quits the tendon of the peroneus brevis, and runs obliquely inwards along a groove in the os cuboides, under the muscles on the sole of the foot, to be inserted into the outside of the posterior extremity of the metatarsal bone that supports the great toe. Near the insertion of this muscle we find a small *bursa mucosa.* This muscle draws the foot outwards, and likewise assists in extending it.

PERONEUS MAXIMUS. See *Peroneus longus.*

PERONEUS MEDIUS. See *Peroneus brevis.*

PERONEUS POSTICUS. See *Peroneus longus.*

PERONEUS PRIMUS. See *Peronéus longus.*

PERONEUS SECUNDUS. See *Peroneus brevis.*

PERONEUS TERTIUS. This is the name given by Al binus to a muscle which, by some writers, is called *nonus Vesalii*, or Vesalius's ninth muscle of the foot; but by most considered in the present day as a portion of the extensor longus digitorum pedis. It is situated at the anterior, inferior, and outer part of the leg, along the outer edge of the last described muscle, to which it is intimately united. It arises fleshy from the anterior surface of the lower half of the fibula, and from the adjacent part of the interosseous ligament. Its fibres run obliquely downwards, towards a tendon which passes under the annular ligament, and then running obliquely outwards, it is inserted into the root of the metatarsal bone that supports the little toe. This muscle assists in bending the foot.

PERPENDICULARIS. Applied to parts of plants, as the root of the Daucus carota, which goes straight down into the earth.

PE'RSICA. (From *Persia*, its native soil.) The peach. See *Amygdalus persica.*

PERSICA'RIA. (From *Persica*, the peach-tree: so called because its blossoms are like those of the peach.) See *Polygonum persicaria.*

PERSICARIA MITIS. See *Polygonum persicaria.*

PERSICARIA URENS. See *Polygonum hydropiper.*

PE'RSICUS IGNIS. A carbuncle. Avicenna says, it is that species of carbuncle which is attended with pustules and vesications.

[PERSIMMON. See *Diospyros. A.*]

PERSISTENS. Permanent. Applied to flower-cups remaining a long time after the flower, as that of the Hyosciamus niger.

PERSI'STENS FEBRIS. A regular intermitting fever, the paroxysms of which return at constant and stated hours.

PERSONA'TA. (From *persona*, a mask; because, says Pliny, the ancient actors used to mask themselves with the leaves of this plant.) See *Arctium lappa.*

PERSONATUS. Personate. A term applied to a monopetalous corolla, when irregular, and closed by a kind of palate; as in Antirrhinum.

PERSPIRATION. *Perspiratio.* The vapour that is secreted by the extremities of the cutaneous arteries from the external surface of the body. It is distinguished into *sensible* and *insensible.* The former is separated in the form of an invisible vapour, the latter so as to be visible in the form of very little drops adhering to the epidermis. The *secretory organ* is composed of the extremities of the cutaneous arteries. The *smell* of the perspirable fluid, in a healthy man, is fatuous and animal; its *taste* manifestly salt and ammoniacal. In *consistence* it is vaporous or aqueous; and its *specific gravity* in the latter state is greater than that of water

For the most part it is yellowish, from the passage of the subcutaneous oil, and sebaceous matter of the subcutaneous glands.

Whatever form it takes, the liquid that escapes from the skin is composed, according to Thenard, of a great deal of water, a small quantity of acetic acid, of muriate of soda and potassa, a small quantity of earthy phosphate, an atom of oxide of iron, and a trace of animal matter. Berzelius considers the acid of sweat not the same as acetic acid, but like the lactic acid of Scheele. The skin exhales, besides, an oily matter, and some carbonic acid.

Many experiments have been made to determine the quantity of transpiration which is formed in a given time, and the variations that this quantity undergoes according to circumstances. The first attempts are due to Sanctorius, who, during thirty years, weighed every day, with extreme care, and an indefatigable patience, his food and his drink, his solid and liquid excretions, and even himself. Sanctorius, in spite of his zeal and perseverance, arrived at results that were not very exact. Since his time, several philosophers and physicians have been employed on the same subject with more success; but the most remarkable labour in this way is that of Lavoisier and Seguin. These philosophers were the first who distinguished the loss that takes place by pulmonary transpiration from that of the skin. Seguin shut himself up in a bag of *gummed silk*, tied above his head, and presenting an opening, the edges of which were fixed round his mouth by a mixture of turpentine and pitch. In this manner only, the humour of the pulmonary transpiration passed into the air. In order to know the quantity, it was sufficient to weigh himself, with the bag, at the beginning and end of the experiment, in a very fine balance. By repeating the experiment out of the bag, he determined the whole quantity of humour transpired; so that, by deducting from this the quantity that he knew had passed out from the lungs, he had the quantity of humour exhaled by the skin. Besides, he took into account the food that he had used, his excretions solid and liquid, and generally all the causes that could have any influence upon the transpiration. By following this plan, the results of Lavoisier and Seguin are these :—

1st, The greatest quantity of insensible transpiration (the pulmonary included) is 25.6 grains troy per minute; consequently, 3 ounces, 1 drachm, 36 grains, per hour; and 6 pounds, 4 ounces, 6 drachms, 24 grains, in 24 hours.

2d, The least considerable loss is 8.8 grains per minute; consequently, 2 pounds, 2 ounces, 3 drachms, in 24 hours.

3d, It is during the digestion that the loss of weight occasioned by insensible transpiration is at its minimum.

4th, The transpiration is at its maximum immediately after dinner.

5th, The mean of the insensible transpiration is 14.4 grains per minute; in the mean 14.4 grains, 8.8 depend on cutaneous transpiration, and 5.6 upon the pulmonary.

6th, The cutaneous transpiration alone varies during and after repasts.

7th, Whatever quantity of food is taken, or whatever are the variations of the atmosphere, the same individual, after having augmented in weight by all the food that he has taken, returns, in 24 hours, to the same weight, nearly that he was the day before, provided he is not growing, or has not eaten to excess.

It is much to be wished that this interesting labour had been continued, and that authors had not limited their studies to insensible transpiration, but had extended their observations to the sweat.

Whenever the humour of transpiration is not evaporated, as soon as it is in contact with the air, it appears at the surface of the skin in the form of a layer of quid of variable thickness. Now, this effect may happen because the transpiration is too copious, or because of the diminution of the dissolvent force of the air. We perspire in an air hot and humid, by the influence of the two causes joined; we would perspire with more difficulty in an air of the same heat, but dry. Certain parts of the body transpire more copiously, and sweat with more facility, than others; such are the hands and the feet, the armpits, the groins, the brow, &c. Generally the skin of these parts receives a greater proportional quantity of blood :

and, in some people, the armpit, the sole of the foot, and the intervals between the toes, do not come so easily in contact with the air.

The sweat does not appear to have every where the same composition; every one knows that its odour is variable according to the different parts of the body. It is the same with its acidity, which appears much stronger in the armpits and feet than elsewhere.

The cutaneous transpiration has numerous uses in the animal economy, keeps up the suppleness of the epidermis, and thus favours the exercise of the tact and the touch. It is by evaporation along with that of the lungs, the principal means of cooling, by which the body maintains itself within certain limits of temperature; also its expulsion from the economy appears very important, for every time that it is diminished or suspended, derangements of more or less consequence follow, and many diseases are not arrested until a considerable quantity of sweat is expelled.

Beside water, it cannot be doubted that *carbon* is also emitted from the skin; but in what state, the experiments hitherto made do not enable us to decide. Cruickshanks found, that the air of the glass vessel in which his hand and foot had been confined for an hour, contained carbonic acid gas; for a candle burned dimly in it, and it rendered lime-water turbid. And Jurine found, that air which had remained for some time in contact with the skin, consisted almost entirely of carbonic acid gas. The same conclusion may be drawn from the experiments of Ingenhousz and Milly. Trousset has lately observed, that air was separated copiously from a patient of his, while bathing.

Besides water and carbon, or carbonic acid gas, the skin emits also a particular odorous substance. That every animal has a peculiar smell, is well known : the dog can discover his master, and even trace him to a distance by the scent. A dog, chained up several hours after his master had set out on a journey of some hundred miles, followed his footsteps by the smell. But it is needless to multiply the instances of this fact; they are too well known to every one. Now, this smell must be owing to some peculiar matter which is constantly emitted; and this matter must differ somewhat, either in quantity or some other property, as we see that the dog easily distinguishes the individual by means of it. Cruickshanks has made it probable, that this matter is an oily substance, or at least that there is an oily substance emitted by the skin. He wore repeatedly, night and day, for a month, the same under waistcoat of fleecy hosiery, during the hottest part of the summer. At the end of this time, he always found an oily substance accumulated in considerable masses on the nap of the inner surface of the waistcoat, in the form of black tears. When rubbed on paper, it rendered it transparent, and hardened on it like grease. It burned with a white flame, and left behind it a charry residuum.

Berthollet has observed the perspiration acid; and he has concluded, that the acid which is present is the phosphoric; but this has not been proved. Fourcroy and Vauquelin have ascertained, that the scurf which collects upon the skins of horses, consists chiefly of phosphate of lime, and urea is even sometimes mixed with it.

According to Thenard, however, who has lately endeavoured more particularly to ascertain this point, the acid contained in sweat is the acetous; which, he likewise observes, is the only free acid contained in urine and in milk, this acid existing in both of them when quite fresh. His account of his examination of it is as follows :—

The sweat is more or less copious in different individuals; and its quantity is perceptibly in the inverse ratio of that of the urine. All other circumstances being similar, much more is produced during digestion than during repose. The maximum of its production appears to be twenty-six grains and two-thirds in a minute; the minimum nine grains, troy weight. It is much inferior, however, to the pulmonary transpiration; and there is likewise a great difference between their nature and manner of formation. The one is a product of a particular secretion, similar in some sort to that of the urine; the other, composed of a great deal of water and carbonic acid, is the product of a combustion gradually effected by the atmospheric air.

The sweat, in a healthy state, very sensibly reddens litmus paper or infusion. In certain diseases, and particularly in putrid fevers, it is alkaline; yet its taste is always rather saline, and more similar to that of salt than acid. Though colourless, it stains linen. Its smell is peculiar, and insupportable when it is concentrated, which is the case in particular during distillation. But before he speaks of the trials to which he subjected it, and of which he had occasion for a great quantity, he describes the method he adopted for procuring it, which was similar to that of Cruickshanks.

Human sweat, according to Thenard, is formed of a great deal of water, free acetous acid, muriate of soda, an atom of phosphate of lime and oxide of iron, and an inappreciable quantity of animal matter, which approaches much nearer to gelatin than to any other substance.

Perspiration varies in respect to, 1. The *temperature of the atmosphere.* Thus men have a more copious, viscid, and higher-coloured sweat in summer than in winter, and in warm countries than in colder regions. 2. *Sex.* The sweat of a man is said to smell more acrid than that of a woman. 3. *Age.* The young are more subject to sweat than the aged, who, during the excessive heat of the summer, scarcely sweat at all. 4. *Ingesta.* An alliacious sweat is perceived from eating garlick; a leguminous from pease; an acid from acids; a fœtid from animal food only; and a rancid sweat from fat foods, as is observed in Greenland. A long abstinence from drink causes a more acrid and coloured sweat; and the drinking a great quantity of cold water in summer, a limpid and thin sweat. 5. *Medicines.* The sweat of those who have taken musk, even moderately, and asafœtida, or sulphur, smells of their respective natures. 6. *Region of the body.* The sweat of the head is greasy; on the forehead it is more aqueous; under the axillæ very unguinous; and in the interstices of the toes, it is very fœtid, forming in the most healthy man blackish sordes. 7. *Diseases.* In this respect it varies very much in regard to quantity, smell, and colour; for the sweat of gouty persons is said to turn blue vegetable juices to a red colour. Some men also have a lucid sweat, others a sweat tinging their linen of a cerulean colour.

The uses of the insensible perspiration are, 1. To *liberate* the blood from superfluous animal gas, azote, and water. 2. To eliminate the noxious and heterogeneous excrements; hence the acrid, rancid, leguminous, or putrid perspiration of some men. 3. To *moisten* the external surface of the body, lest the epidermis, cutis, and its nervous papillæ, be dried up by the atmospheric air. 4. To *counterbalance* the suppressed pulmonary transpiration of the lungs; for when it is suppressed, the cutaneous is increased; hence the nature of both appears to be the same.

The use of the sensible perspiration, or sweat, in a healthy man, is scarcely observable, unless from an error of the non-naturals. Its first effect on the body is always prejudicial, by exhausting and drying it, although it is sometimes of advantage. 1. By supplying a watery excretion: thus when the urine is deficient, the sweat is often more abundant. In this manner an aqueous diarrhœa is frequently cured by sweating. 2. By eliminating, at the same time, any morbid matter. Thus various miasmata are critically expelled, in acute and chronic diseases, with the sweat.

PERTU'SSIS. (From *per*, much, and *tussis*, cough.) The hooping-cough. A genus of diseases in the class *Neuroses,* and order *Spasmi,* of Cullen, known by a convulsive strangulating cough, with hooping, returning by fits, that are usually terminated by a vomiting; and by ts being contagious.

Children are most commonly the subjects of this disease, and it seems to depend on a specific contagion, which affects them but once in their life. The disease being once produced, the fits of coughing are often repeated without any evident cause; but, in many cases, the contagion may be considered as only giving the predisposition, and the frequency of the fits may depend upon various exciting causes, such as violent exercise, a full meal, the having taken food of difficult digestion, and irritation of the lungs by dust, smoke, or disagreeable odours. Emotions of the mind may likewise prove an exciting cause.

Its proximate or immediate cause seems to be a viscid matter or phlegm lodged about the bronchia, trachea, and fauces, which sticks so close as to be expectorated with the greatest difficulty. Some have supposed it to be a morbid irritability of the stomach,

with increased action of its mucous glands; but the affection of the stomach which takes place in the disease, is clearly only of a secondary nature, so that this opinion must be erroneous.

The hooping-cough usually comes on with a difficulty of breathing, some degree of thirst, a quick pulse, and other slight febrile symptoms, which are succeeded by a hoarseness, cough, and difficulty of expectoration. These symptoms continue perhaps for a fortnight or more, at the end of which time the disease puts on its peculiar and characteristic form, and is now evident, as the cough becomes convulsive, and is attended with a sound, which has been called a hoop.

When the sonorous inspiration has happened, the coughing is again renewed, and continues in the same manner as before, till either a quantity of mucus is thrown up from the lungs, or the contents of the stomach are evacuated by vomiting. The fit is then terminated, and the patient remains free from any other for some time, and shortly afterward returns to the amusements he was employed in before the fit, expresses a desire for food, and when it is given to him, takes it greedily. In those cases, however, where the attack has been severe, he often seems much fatigued, makes quick inspirations, and falls into a faint.

On the first coming on of the disease, there is little or no expectoration; or if any, it consists only of thin mucus; and as long as this is the case, the fits of coughing are frequent, and of considerable duration; but on the expectoration becoming free and copious, the fits of coughing are less frequent, as well as of shorter duration.

By the violence of coughing, the free transmission of blood through the lungs is somewhat interrupted, as likewise the free return of the blood from the head, which produces that turgescence and suffusion of the face, which commonly attend the attack, and in some instances brings on a hæmorrhage either from the nose or ears.

The disease having arrived at its height, usually continues for some weeks longer, and at length goes off gradually. In some cases it is, however, protracted for several months, or even a year.

Although the hooping-cough often proves tedious, and is liable to return with violence on any fresh exposure to cold, when not entirely removed, it nevertheless is seldom fatal, except to very young children, who are always likely to suffer more from it than those of a more advanced age. The danger seems indeed always to be in proportion to the youth of the person, and the degree of fever, and difficulty of breathing, which accompany the disease, as likewise the state of debility which prevails.

It has been known in some instances to terminate in apoplexy and suffocation. If the fits are put an end to by vomiting, it may be regarded as a favourable symptom, as may likewise the taking place of a moderate and free expectoration, or the ensuing of a slight hæmorrhage from the nose or ears.

Dissections of those who die of the hooping-cough usually show the consequence of the organs of respiration being affected, and particularly those parts which are the seat of catarrh. When the disease has been long protracted, it is apt to degenerate into pulmonary consumption, asthma, or visceral obstructions, in which last case the glands of the mesentery are found in a hard and enlarged state.

In the treatment of this disease it must be borne in mind, that in the early period palliative measures can only be employed; but when it continues merely from habit, a variety of means will often at once put a stop to it. In the first stage in mild cases very little is required, except obviating occasional irritation, keeping the bowels regular, &c. But where it puts on a more serious character, the plan will differ accordingly as it is attended with inflammatory symptoms, or exhibits a purely spasmodic form. In the former case, it may be sometimes proper in plethoric habits to begin by a full bleeding, or leeches to the chest, if the patient be very young, then clear the bowels effectually, apply a blister, and exhibit antimonials, or squill, in nauseating doses, assisted perhaps by opium, to promote diaphoresis and expectoration. An occasional emetic, where the breathing is much oppressed with wheezing, in young children particularly, may afford material relief When the disorder is more of the spasmodic character, some of these means may still be useful, as blisters, and nauseating medicines, so far as the strength will admit; but the remedies of greatest efficacy are the narcotics, as opium, conium, &c. exhibited in adequate doses. In the chronic or habitual stage of the disease, almost any thing, which produces a considerable impression on the constitution, will occasionally succeed: but we chiefly rely on sedative and antispasmodic, or on tonic remedies, accordingly as there are marks of irritability, or of mere debility in the system. Of the former description, opium is perhaps the best, especially in conjunction with squill, given in a full dose at night, and in small quantities swallowed slowly from time to time during the day. Conium, asafœtida, &c. may however occasionally answer better in particular constitutions Among the tonics the cinchona is often highly efficacious, where no appearances of local disease attend ; some of the metallic preparations also, particularly sulphate of zinc, may be much relied upon. Sometimes stimulant applications to the chest, but still more certainly opiate frictions, will be found to cure this disorder. The same is very often accomplished by a change of air, indeed occasionally after the failure of most remedies. The cold bath also, where there is no local disease, may have an excellent effect; assisted by warm clothing, especially wearing some kind of fur over the chest. Fear and other emotions of the mind, strangury induced by the use of the lytta, &c. &c. rank also among the remedies of pertussis.

Peruvian balsam. See *Myroxylon peruiferum.*
Peruvian bark. See *Cinchona.*
PERUVIA′NUS CORTEX. See *Cinchona.*
PERUVIANUS CORTEX FLAVUS. See *Cinchona cordifolia.*
PERUVIANUS CORTEX RUBER. See *Cinchona oblongifolia.*
PERVIGI′LIUM. (From *per*, much, and *vigilo*, to watch.) Watching, or a want of sleep. See *Vigilance.*
PERVI′NCA. (From *pervincio*, to tie together.) So called because its stringy roots were used for binding substances together. See *Vinca minor.*
PES. (*Pes, dis.* m.; a foot.) The foot.
PES ALEXANDRINUS. See *Anthemis pyrethrum.*
PES CAPRÆ. Goat's foot, a species of *Oxalis;* also a species of *Convolvulus.*
PES CATI. See *Gnaphalium dioicum.*
PES COLOMBINUS. See *Geranium rotundifolium.*
PES HIPPOCAMPI. The name of two columns at the end of the fornix of the brain, which diverge posteriorly.
PES LEONIS. See *Alchemilla.*
PES TIGRIDIS. Tiger's foot. A species of *Ipomœa.*
PESSARY. (*Pessarium;* from ωεσσω, to soften.) An instrument that is introduced into the vagina to support the uterus.
PESTILENCE. A plague.
PESTILENTIAL. (*Pestilentialis;* from *pestes*, the plague.) An epidemic, malignant, and contagious disease, approaching to the nature of the plague.
PESTILENTWORT. See *Tussilago petasites.*
PESTILOCHIA. See *Aristolochia virginiana.*
PE′STIS. The plague. A genus of disease in the class *Pyrexiæ*, and order *Exanthemata*, of Cullen, characterized by typhus, which is contagious in the extreme, prostration of strength, buboes, and carbuncles, petechiæ, hæmorrhage, and colliquative diarrhœa.

By some writers the disease has been divided into three species; that attended with buboes ; that attended with carbuncles; and that accompanied with petechiæ. This division appears wholly superfluous. Dr. Russel, in his elaborate treatise on the plague, makes mention of many varieties; but when these have arisen, they seem to have depended in a great measure on the temperament and constitution of the air at the time the disease became epidemical, as likewise on the patient's habit of body at the time of his being attacked with it.

The plague is by most writers considered as the consequence of a pestilential contagion, which is propagated from one person to another by association, or by coming near infected materials.

It has been observed, that it generally appears as early as the fourth or fifth day after infection: but it has not yet been ascertained how long a person who has laboured under the disease is capable of infecting others, nor how long the contagion may lurk in an unfavourable habit without producing the disease, and may yet be communicated, and the disease excited, in habits more susceptible of the infection. It has generally been supposed, however, that a quarantine of 40

days is much longer than is necessary for persons, and probably for goods also. Experience has not yet deter mined how much of this term may be abated. "If ₄ am not much mistaken," observes Dr. Thomas, "the Board of Trade has, however, very lately, under the sanction of the College of Physicians, somewhat abridged it."

It sometimes happens, that after the application of the putrid vapour, the patient experiences only a considerable degree of languor and slight headache for many days previous to a perfect attack of the disease: but it more usually comes to pass, that he is very soon seized with great depression of strength, anxiety, palpitations, syncope, stupor, giddiness, violent headache, and delirium, the pulse becoming at the same time very weak and irregular.

These symptoms are shortly succeeded by nausea, and a vomiting of a dark bilious matter, and in the further progress of the disease, carbuncles make their appearance ; buboes arise in different glands, such as the parotid, maxillary, cervical, axillary, and inguinal ; or petechiæ hæmorrhagies and a colliquative diarrhœa, ensue, which denote a putrid tendency prevailing to a great degree in the mass of the blood.

Such are the characteristic symptoms of this malignant disease, but it seldom happens that they are all to be met with in the same person. Some, in the advanced state of the disease, labour under buboes, others under carbuncles, and others again are covered with petechiæ.

The plague is always to be considered as attended with imminent danger, and when it prevailed in this country about 200 years ago, proved fatal to most of those who were attacked with it. It is probable, however, that many of them died from want of care and proper nourishment, as the infected were forsaken by their nearest friends; because in Turkey and other countries, where attention is paid to the sick, a great many recover.

When the disease is unattended by buboes, it runs its course more rapidly, and is more generally fatal, than when accompanied by such inflammations. The earlier they appear, the milder usually is the disease. When they proceed kindly to suppuration, they always prove critical, and ensure the patient's recovery. A gentle diaphoresis, arising spontaneously, has been known in many instances likewise to prove critical. When carbuncles show a disposition to gangrene, the event will be fatal. Petechiæ, hæmorrhages, and colliquative diarrhœa, denote the same termination.

Dissections of the plague have discovered the gallbladder full of black bile, the liver very considerably enlarged, the heart much increased in size, and the lungs, kidneys, and intestines beset with carbuncles. They have likewise discovered all the other appearances of putrid fever.

PETALUM. A petal. The name of the coloured leaflets of the corolla of a flower. The great variety of form, duration, &c. of the petals, give rise to the following names.

From their duration,
1. *Petalo patentia ;* as in Rosa canina.
2. *Patentissima ;* very spreading.
3. *Erecta ;* as in Allium nigrum.
4. *Conniventia ;* as in Rumex.
5. *Distantia ;* as in Cucubalus bacciferus.
From the figure of the border,
6. *Acuminata ;* as in Saxifraga stellaris.
7. *Setacea ;* as in Tropæolum minus.
8. *Apice cohærentia ;* as in Vitis vinifera.
9. *Apice reflexa ;* as in Anemone pratensis
10. *Aristata ;* as in Galium aristatum.
11. *Bifida ;* as in Silene nocturna.
12. *Bipartita ;* as in Alsine media.
13. *Biloba ;* as in Geranium striatum.
14. *Carinata ;* as in Curum carui.
15. *Concava ;* as in Ruta graveolens.
16. *Cordata ;* as in Sium selinum.
17. *Hirsuta ;* as in Menyanthes trifoliata.
18. *Ciliata ;* as in Asclepias undulata.
19. *Crenata ;* as in Linum usitatissimum
20. *Dentata ;* as in Silene lucitanica.
21. *Serrata ;* as in Dianthus arboreus.
22. *Cuneiforma ;* as in Epidendrum cordatum.
23. *Emarginata ;* as in Allium roseum.
24. *Inflexa ;* as in Pimpinella.
25. *Reflexa ;* as in Pancratium zelanicum.

26. *Involuta;* as in Anethum.
27. *Integra;* as in Nigella arvensis.
28. *Laciniata;* as in Reseda.
29. *Lanceolata;* as in Narcissus minor.
30. *Linearia;* as in Tussilago farfara.
31. *Lineata;* as Scilla lucitanica.
32. *Punctata;* as in Melanthium capense.
33. *Maculata;* as in Digitalis purpurea.
34. *Oblonga;* as in Citrus and Hedera.
35. *Obtusa;* as in Tropæolum majus.
36. *Orata;* as in Allium flavum.
37. *Plana;* as in Pancratium maritimum.
38. *Subrotunda;* as in Rosa centifolia.
39. *Truncata;* as in Hura crepitans.
40. *Coronata;* as in Nerium oleander.

The claw of the petal is very long, in Dianthus and Saponaria; and *connate,* in Malva sylvestris and oxalis.

PETALIFORMIS. Petaliform, like a petal; applied to the stigma of the Iris germanica.

PETALITE. A mineral found in the mine of Uts, in Sweden, interesting from its analysis having led to the knowledge of a new alkali.

PETALO'DES. (From πεταλον, a leaf, or thin scale.) This term is by Hippocrates applied to a urine which hath in it flaky substances resembling leaves.

PETASI'TES. (From πετασος, a hat: so named because its leaves are shaped like a hat.) See *Tussilago petasites.*

PETE'CHIA. (From the Italian *petechio,* a fleabite, because they resemble the bites of fleas.) A red or purple spot, which resembles a flea-bite.

PETIOLATUS. Petiolate: applied to leaves which are formed with a stalk, whether long or short, simple or compound, as most leaves are: as in Verbasum nigrum, &c.

PETIOLUS. (From *pes,* a foot.) A petiole. The footstalk or leafstalk of a plant. The term is applied exclusively to the stalk of the leaf.

It is distinguished into the *apex,* which is inserted into the leaf, and the *base,* which comes from the stem.

From its figure it is called,

1. *Linearis,* equal in breadth throughout; as in Citrus medica.
2. *Alatus;* as in Citrus aurantium.
3. *Appendiculatus,* when furnished with leaflets at its base; as in Dipsacus pilosus.
4. *Teres,* round throughout; as in Pisum sativum.
5. *Semiteres,* round on one side, and flat on the other.
6. *Triquetrus,* three-sided.
7. *Angulatus,* having angles.
8. *Cuniliculatus,* channelled to its very base, where it is sometimes greatly dilated and concave; as in Angelica sylvestris.
9. *Compressus,* compressed towards its base; as in Populus tremula.
10. *Clavatus,* thicker towards the apex; as in Cacalia suaveolens.
11. *Spinescens,* becoming a spine after the fall of the leaf; as in Rhamnus catharticus.

From its insertion the petiolus is called,

12. *Insertus,* as in most trees, and the Pirus communis.
13. *Articulatus;* as in Oxalis acetocella.
14. *Adnatus,* adhering so to the stem, that it cannot be displaced without injuring the bark.
15. *Decurrens,* adhering at its base, and going some little way down the stem; as in Pisum ochrus.
16. *Amplexicaulis,* surrounding the stem at its base; as in Senecio hastatus.
17. *Vaginans,* surrounding the stem with a perfect tube; as in Canna indica.

From its length with respect to the leaf, it is said to be *brevissimus,* when much shorter, and *longissimus,* when longer; as in Anemone hepatica, and Geranium terebinthinatum.

It is distinguished also into *simple,* when not divided; as in most leaves: and *compound,* when divided into lateral branches; as in all compound leaves.

PETIT, JOHN LEWIS, was born at Paris in 1674. From his childhood he displayed a remarkable degree of penetration, which gained him the attachment of M. de Littre, a celebrated anatomist, who resided in his father's house. He took a pleasure, even at the

age of seven, in witnessing the process of dissection and being allowed to attend the demonstrations of that gentleman. he made such progress, that when scarcely twelve years old, the superintendence of the anatomical theatre was confided to him. He afterward studied surgery, and was admitted master at Paris in 1700 He became, as it were, the oracle in his profession in that city, and his fame extended throughout Europe. He was sent for to the kings of Poland and Spain, whom he restored to health: they endeavoured to retain him near their persons by liberal offers, but he preferred his native place. He became a member of the Academy of Sciences; and was appointed Director of the Academy of Surgery, and Censor and Royal Professor at the schools. He was likewise chosen a Fellow of the Royal Society of London. He died in 1750. Many memoirs were communicated by him to the French academies. His only separate publication was a Treatise on the Diseases of the Bones, which passed through several editions, but involved him in much controversy. Some posthumous works, relating to surgical diseases and operations, likewise appeared under his name.

PETRA'PIUM. (From *petra,* a rock, and *apium,* parsley: so called because it grows in stony places.) See *Bubon macedonicum.*

PETRELE'UM. (From πετρα, a rock, and ελαιον, oil.) An oil or liquid bitumen which distils from rocks.

PETRIFACTIONS. Stony matters deposited either in the way of incrustation, or within the cavities of organized substances, are called petrifactions. Calcareous earth being universally diffused and capable of solution in water, either alone, or by the medium of carbonic acid or sulphuric acid, which are likewise very abundant, is deposited whenever the water or the acid becomes dissipated. In this way we have incrustations of limestone or of selenite in the form of stalactites or dropstones from the roofs of caverns, and in various other situations.

The most remarkable observations relative to petrifactions are thus given by Kirwan:—

1. That those of shells are found on, or near, the surface of the earth; those of fish deeper; and those of wood deepest. Shells in specie are found in immense quantities at considerable depths.
2. That those organic substances that resist putrefaction most, are frequently found petrified; such as shells, and the harder species of woods: on the contrary, those that are aptest to putrefy are rarely found petrified; as fish, and the softer parts of animals, &c.
3. That they are most commonly found in strata of marl, chalk, limestone, or clay, seldom in sandstone, still more rarely in gypsum; but never in gneiss, granite, basaltes, or shorle; but they sometimes occur among pyrites, and ores of iron, copper, and silver and almost always consist of that species of earth, stone, or other mineral that surrounds them, sometimes of silex, agate, or carnelion.
4. That they are found in climates where their originals could not have existed.
5. That those found in slate or clay are compressed and flattened.

PETRO'LEUM. (From *petra,* a rock, and *oleum,* oil.) The name of petroleum is given to a liquid bituminous substance which flows between rocks, or in different places at the surface of the earth. See *Bitumen.*

["In the *United States* it is found, sometimes abundantly, in *Kentucky,* the western parts of *Pennsylvania,* and in *New-York,* at Seneca Lake, &c. It usually floats on the surface of springs, which, in many cases, are known to be in the vicinity of coal. It is sometimes called Seneca or Genesee oil."—*Cleav. Min.* A.]

PETROLEUM BARBADENSE. Barbadoes tar. This is chiefly obtained from the island of Barbadoes, and is sometimes employed externally in paralytic diseases See *Bitumen.*

PETROLEUM RUBRUM. *Oleum gabianum.* Red petroleum. A species of rock-oil of a blackish-red colour, of thicker consistence, with a less penetrating and more disagreeable smell than the other kinds of petroleum. It is abundant about the village of Gabian in Languedoc. It is a species of bitumen. See *Bitumen.*

PETROLEUM SULPHURATUM. A stimulating balsamic remedy given in coughs, asthmas, and other affections of the chest.

ETROPHARYNGÆ'US. A muscle which arises in the petrose portion of the temporal bone, and is inserted into the pharynx.

PETRO-SALPINGO STAPHYLINUS. See *Levator palati*.

PETROSELI'NUM. (From πετρα, a rock, and σελινον, parsley.) See *Apium petroselinum*.

PETROSELINUM MACEDONICUM. See *Bubon*.

PETROSELINUM VULGARE. See *Apium petroselinum*.

PETRO'SILEX. Compact felspar. A species of coarse flint, of a deep blue or yellowish green colour. It is interspersed in veins through rocks; and from this circumstance derives its name.

["PETUNTZE. This would probably be arranged under the common variety of felspar, had it not received some additional importance from its use in the manufacture of porcelain. It appears, in fact, to be that variety of felspar, which the Chinese call *Petuntze*.

"It is nearly or quite opaque, and its colour is usually whitish or gray. It has in most cases less lustre than common felspar. Its fracture is lamellar, although its masses often have a coarse granular structure.

"It most frequently occurs in beds, and usually contains a little quartz. Its powder is said to have a slightly saline taste.

"It is employed in the enamel of porcelain ware, and enters, in certain proportions, into the composition of the porcelain itself. Any variety of felspar, which contains very little or no metallic oxide, would, undoubtedly, answer the same purpose."—*Cleav. Min.* A.]

PEUCE'DANUM. (From πευκη, the pine-tree: so called from its leaves resembling those of the pine-tree.) 1. The name of a genus of plants. Class, *Pentandria*; Order, *Digynia*.

2. The pharmacopœial name of the hog's fennel. See *Peucedanum officinale*.

PEUCEDANUM OFFICINALE. The systematic name of the hog's fennel. *Marathrum sylvestre; Marathrophyllum; Pinastellum; Fœniculum porcinum*. The plant which bears these names in the pharmacopœias is the *Peucedanum:—foliis quinquepartitis, filiformibus linearibus*, of Linnæus. The root is the officinal part; it has a strong fœtid smell, somewhat resembling that of sulphureous solutions, and an acrid, unctuous, bitterish taste. Wounded when fresh, in the spring or autumn, particularly in the former season, in which the root is most vigorous, it yields a considerable quantity of yellow juice, which soon dries into a solid gummy resin, which retains the taste and strong smell of the root. This, as well as the root, is recommended as a nervine and anti-hysteric remedy.

PEUCEDANUM SILAUS. The systematic name of the meadow saxifrage. *Saxifraga vulgaris ; Saxifraga anglica ; Hippomarathrum ; Fœniculum erraticum*. English or meadow saxifrage. The roots, leaves, and seeds of this plant have been commended as aperients, diuretics, and carminatives; and appear, from their aromatic smell, and moderately warm, pungent, bitterish taste to have some claim to these virtues. They are rarely used.

PEWTER. A compound metal, the basis of which is tin. The best sort consists of tin alloyed with about a twentieth or less of copper or other metallic bodies, as the experience of the workmen has shown to be the most conducive to the improvement of its hardness and colour, such as lead, zinc, bismuth, and antimony There are three sorts of pewter, distinguished by the names of plate, trifle, and ley-pewter. The first was formerly much used for plates and dishes; of the second are made the pints, quarts, and other measures of beer; and of the ley-pewter, wine measures and large vessels.

The best sort of pewter consists of 17 parts of antimony to 100 parts of tin; but the French add a little copper to this kind of pewter. A very fine silver-looking metal is composed of 100 pounds of tin, eight of antimony, one of bismuth, and four of copper. On the contrary, the ley-pewter, by comparing its specific gravity with those of the mixtures of tin and lead, must contain more than a fifth part of its weight of lead.

PEYE'RI GLANDULÆ. Peyer's glands. The small glands situated under the villous coat of the intestines.

PEZIZA. (Somewhat altered from the Greek πεζικη, which is derived from πεζα, the sole of the foot. Pliny

speaks of the *pezizæ*, as the Greek appellation of such fungi, as grow without any stalk or apparent root.) The name of a genus of plants. Class, *Cryptogamia* ; Order, *Fungi*.

PEZI'ZA AURICULÆ. *Auricula judæ ; Fungus sambucinus ; Agaricus auriculæ forma*. Jew's ears. A membranaceous fungus. *Peziza concava rugosa auriformis*, of Linnæus, which resembles the human ear. Its virtues are adstringent, and when employed (by some its internal use is not thought safe), it is made into a decoction, as a gargle for relaxed sore throats.

PHACIA. (Φακια, a lentil.) A cutaneous spot or blemish, called by the Latins *lentigo* and *lenticula*.

PHÆNO'MENON. (From φαινω, to make appear.) An appearance which is contrary to the usual process of nature.

PHAGEDÆ'NA. (From φαγω, to eat.) A species of ulcer that spreads very rapidly.

PHAGEDÆNIC. (*Phagedænicus* ; from φαγω, to eat.) 1. An ulceration which spreads very rapidly 2. Applications that destroy fungous flesh.

PHALACROTIS. (From φαλακρος, bald.) Baldness

PHA'LACRUM. (From φαλακρος, bald.) A surgical instrument, with a blunt, smooth top; as a probe.

PHALA'NGES. The plural of *Phalanx*.

PHALANGO'SIS. (From φαλαγξ, a row of soldiers.) 1. An affection of the eyelids, where there are two or more rows of hairs upon them.

2. A morbid inversion of the eyelids.

PHA'LANX. (*Phalanx, gis.* f.; from φαλαγξ, a battalion.) The small bones of the fingers and toes, which are distinguished into the first, second, and third phalanx.

PHA'LARIS. (From φαλος, white, shining: so named from its white shining seed, supposed to be the φαλαρος of Dioscorides.) The name of a genus of plants. Class, *Triandria*; Order, *Digynia*. Canary grass.

PHALARIS CANARIENSIS. Canary grass. The seed of this plant is well known to be the common food of canary-birds. In the Canary islands, the inhabitants grind it into meal, and make a coarse sort of bread with it.

PHA'LLUS. (Named after the φαλλος of the Greeks, to which it bears a striking resemblance.) The name of a genus, of the Order *Fungi* ; Class, *Cryptogamia*.

PHALLUS ESCULENTUS. The systematic name of morel fungus. It grows on moist banks and wet pastures, and springs up in May. It is used in the same manner as the truffle, for gravies and stewed dishes, but gives an inferior flavour.

PHALLUS IMPUDICUS. The systematic name of the plant called *Fungus phalloides*, stink-horns. A fungus which is, at a distance, intolerably fœtid, so that it is oftener smelled than seen, being supposed to be some carrion, and therefore avoided; when near it has only the pungency of volatile alkali. It is applied to allay pain in the limbs.

PHANTA'SMA. (From φανταζω, to make appear.) Imagination.

PHA'RICUM. (From *Pharos*, the island from whence it was brought.) A violent kind of poison.

PHARMACEU'TIC. (*Pharmaceuticus* ; from φαρμακευω, to exhibit medicines.) Belonging to pharmacy. See *Pharmacy*.

PHARMACOCHY'MIA. (From φαρμακον, a medicine, and χυμια, chemistry.) Pharmaceutic chemistry, or that part of chemistry which respects the preparation of medicines.

PHARMACOLITE. Native arseniate of lime.

PHARMACOPŒ'IA. (From φαρμακον, a medicine, and ποιεω, to make.) A dispensatory, or book of directions for the composition of medicines approved of by medical practitioners, or published by authority. The following are the most noted, viz.

P. Amstelodamensis.	P. Edinburgensis.
P. Argentoratensis.	P. Hofniensis.
P. Augetoratensis.	P. Londinensis.
P. Bateana.	P. Norimbergensis.
P. Brandenburgensis.	P. Parisiensis.
P. Brandenburgica.	P. Ratisbonensis.
P. Bruxellensis.	P. Regia.

PHARMACOPO'LA. (From φαρμακον, a medicine, and πωλεω, to sell.) An apothecary or vender of medicines.

PHARMACOPO'LIUM. (From φαρμακον, a medicine, and πωλεω, to sell.) A druggist's or apothecary's shop.

PHARMACOPO′SIA. (From φαρμακον, a medicine, and ποσις, a potion.) A liquid medicine.

PHARMACOTHE′CA. (From φαρμακον, a medicine, and τιθημι, to place.) A medicine-chest.

PHARMACY. (*Pharmacia*; from φαρμακον, a medicine.) The art of preparing remedies for the treatment of diseases.

The articles of the Materia Medica, being generally unfit for administration in their original state, are subjected to various operations, mechanical or chemical, by which they become adapted to this purpose. Herein consists the practice of pharmacy, which therefore requires a previous knowledge of the sensible and chemical properties of the substances operated on. The qualities of many bodies are materially changed by heat, especially in conjunction with air and other chemical agents ; the virtues of others reside chiefly in certain parts, which may be separated by the action of various menstrua, particularly with the assistance of heat ; and the joint operation of remedies on the human body is often very different from what would be anticipated, from that which they exert separately ; hence in the preparations and compositions of the Pharmacopœias, we are furnished with many powerful as well as elegant forms of medicine.

[*Pharmacy, College of.* A College of Pharmacy was instituted in the City of New-York, in 1829, by the Druggists and Apothecaries, with the following provisions :

"No person hereafter engaging in such business, shall be admitted as a member, unless he has been regularly educated as a Druggist or Apothecary, or has received a diploma from this college, and is of correct moral deportment.

"It shall be the duty of the board of Trustees, to recommend suitable persons as Lecturers on Materia Medica, Chemistry, and Pharmacy, and on such other branches of science as may be useful in the instruction of Apothecaries, who shall be elected by a majority, at a general meeting of the college.

"The Trustees shall have power to publish in a pamphlet form, from time to time, such original essays or extracts from books of science, as may in their opinion be deemed useful for the advancement of knowledge, connected with the business of Druggists or Apothecaries.—*Extr. from circular.* A.]

PHARYNGE′THRON. Φαρυγγεθρον. The pharynx, or fauces.

PHARYNGE′US. (From φαρυγξ, the pharynx.) Belonging to or affecting the pharynx ; thus cynanche pharyngea, &c.

PHARYNGOSTAPHYLI′NUS. A muscle originating in the pharynx, and terminating in the uvula.

PHARYNGOTO′MIA. (From φαρυγξ, the pharynx, and τεμνω, to cut.) The operation of cutting the pharynx.

PHA′RYNX. (Απο του φερω, because it conveys the food into the stomach.) The muscular bag at the back part of the mouth. It is shaped like a funnel, adheres to the fauces behind the larynx, and terminates in the œsophagus. Its use is to receive the masticated food, and to convey it into the œsophagus.

PHASE′OLUS. (From φασηλος, a little ship, or galliot, which its pods were supposed to resemble.) The name of a genus of plants. Class, *Diadelphia*; Order, *Decandria*.

PHASEOLUS CRETICUS. A decoction of the leaves of this plant, called by the Americans Cajan and Cayan, is said to restrain the bleeding from piles when excessive.—*Ray.*

PHASEOLUS VULGARIS. The systematic name of the kidney-bean. This is often called the *French* bean; when young and well boiled it is easy of digestion, and delicately flavoured. They are less liable to produce flatulency than pease.

PHASGA′NIUM. (From φασγανον, a knife : so called because its leaves are shaped like a knife, or sword.) The herb swordgrass.

PHASIANUS. 1. The name of a genus of birds, of the order *Gallinœ*.

2. The pheasant.

PHASIANUS COLCHICUS. The common pheasant.

PHASIANUS GALLUS. The common or wild cock.

PHAT′NIUM. (From φατνη, a stall.) The socket of a tooth.

PHELLA′NDRIUM. (From φελλος, the cork-tree, and ανδριος, male: so called because it floats upon the water like cork.) The name of a genus of plants. Class, *Pentandria*; Order, *Digynia*.

PHELLANDRIUM AQUATICUM. The systematic name of the water-fennel, or fine-leaved water hemlock. *Fœniculum aquaticum; Cicutaria aquatica.* The plant which bears this name in the pharmacopœias is the *Phellandrium—foliorum ramificationibus divaricatis,* of Linnæus. It possesses vertiginous and poisonous qualities, which are best counteracted by acids, after clearing the primæ viæ. The seeds are recommended by some, in conjunction with Peruvian bark, in the cure of pulmonary phthisis.

PHE′MOS. (From φιμοω, to shut up.) A medicine against a dysentery.

["PHENICIN is produced by stopping the action of the sulphuric acid on indigo before it is converted into cerulin ; diluting, filtering, and washing the mixture with water, when it becomes of a bottle-green colour : muriate of potassa is added to the blue washings which are finally obtained, when the phenicin is precipitated of a fine reddish purple colour. It is soluble in water, and in alkohol, forming blue-coloured solutions, and is easily converted into cerulin by the action of water. From its ultimate analysis, Mr. Crum is disposed to consider phenicin as constituted, of 1 indigo$+$2 water."—*Webs. Man. Chem.* A.]

PHILADE′LPHUS. (From φιλεω, to love, and αδελφος, a brother: so called because, by its roughness, it attaches itself to whatever is near it.) See *Galium aparine.*

PHILANTHRO′PUS. (From φιλεω, to love, and ανθρωπος, a man: so called from its uses.) 1. A medicine which relieves the pain of the stone.

2. The herb goose-grass, because it sticks to the garments of those who touch it. See *Galium aparine.*

PHILO′NIUM. (From *Philo,* its inventor.) A warm opiate.

PHILONIUM LONDINENSE. An old name of the *Confectio opii.*

PHI′LTRUM. (From φιλεω, to love.) 1. A philtre or imaginary medicine, to excite love.

2. The depression on the upper lip, where lovers say lute.

PHILLY′RIA. (Πιλλυρια of Dioscorides, supposed to be so called from *Phillyria,* the mother of Chiron, who first applied it medicinally. The name of a genus of plants, Class, *Diandria*; Order, *Monogynia.* Mock privet.

PHIMO′SIS. (From φιμω, to bind up.) A constriction or straitness of the extremity of the prepuce, which, preventing the glans from being uncovered, is often the occasion of many troublesome complaints. It may arise from different causes, both in children and grown persons. Children have naturally the prepuce very long; and as it exceeds the extremity of the glans, and is not liable to be distended, it is apt to contract its orifice. This often occasions a lodgment of a small quantity of urine between that and the glans, which, if it grows corrosive, may irritate the parts so as to produce an inflammation. In this case, the extremity of the prepuce becomes more contracted, and consequently the urine more confined. Hence the whole inside of the prepuce excoriates and suppurates; the end of it grows thick and swells, and in some months becomes callous. At other times it does not grow thick, but becomes so strait and contracted as hardly to allow the introduction of a probe. The only way to remove this disorder is by an operation. A phimosis may affect grown persons from the same cause as little children ; though there are some grown persons who cannot uncover their glans, or at least not without pain, and yet have not the extremity of the prepuce so contracted as to confine the urine from passing, we notwithstanding find them sometimes troubled with a phimosis, which might be suspected to arise from a venereal taint, but has, in reality, a much more innocent cause. There are, we know, sebaceous glands, situated in the prepuce, round the corona, which secrete an unctuous humour, which sometimes becomes acrimonious, irritates the skin that covers the glans, and the irritation extended to the internal membrane of the prepuce, they both become inflamed, and yield a purulent serum, which cannot be discharged, because the glans is swelled, and the orifice of the prepuce contracted. We find also some grown persons, who, though they never uncovered the glans, have been subject to phimosis from a venereal cause. In some, it is owing to gonorrhœa, where the matter lodged between the prepuce and the glans occasioned the same excoriation as the discharge before mentioned from the sebaceous glands. In others, it proceeds from venereal chancres on the prepuce, the glans, or the frænum; which producing an inflammation either on the prepuce or glans, or both, the extremity of the foreskin contracts, and prevents the discharge of the matter. The parts, in a very little time, are greatly tumefied, and sometimes a gangrene comes on in less than two days.

PHLEBORRHA'GIA. (From φλεψ, a vein, and ρηγνυμι, to break out.) A rupture of a vein.

PHLEBOTOMY. (*Phlebotomia;* φλεψ, a vein, and τεμνω, to cut.) The opening of a vein.

PHLEGM. (*Phlegma, atis.* n.; from φλεγω, to burn or to excite.) In chemistry it means water from distillation, but, in the common acceptation of the word, it is a thick and tenacious mucus secreted in the lungs.

PHLEGMAGO'GA. (From φλεγμα, phlegm, and αγω, to drive out.) Medicines which promote the discharge of phlegm.

PHLEGMA'SIA. (From φλεγω, to burn.) An inflammation.

PHLEGMASIA DOLENS. A very improper name given by Dr. Hull to a disease noticed by some of the French writers, under the name of the *L'enflure des jambes et des cuisses de la femme accouché;* while others have called it *dépôt du lait,* from its supposed cause. By the Germans it is called *Œdema lacteum,* and by the English *the white leg.* This disease principally affects women in the puerperal state; in a few instances it has been observed to attack pregnant women; and, in one or two cases, nurses, on losing their children, have been affected by it. Women of all descriptions are liable to be attacked by it during and soon after childbed; but those, whose limbs have been pained or anasarcous during pregnancy, and who do not suckle their offspring, are more especially subject to it. It has rarely occurred oftener than once in the same female. It supervenes to easy and natural, as well as to difficult and preternatural births. It sometimes makes its appearance in twenty-four or forty-eight hours after delivery, and at other times, not till a month or six weeks after; but, in general, the attack takes place from the tenth to the sixteenth day of the lying-in. It has, in many instances, attacked women who were recovering from puerperal fever; and, in some cases, has supervened or succeeded to thoracic inflammation. It not uncommonly begins with coldness and rigors; these are succeeded by heat, thirst, and other symptoms of pyrexia; and then pain, stiffness, and other symptoms of topical inflammation supervene. Sometimes the local affection is from the first accompanied with, but is not preceded by, febrile symptoms. Upon other occasions, the topical affection is neither preceded by puerperal fever, nor rigors, &c.; but soon after it has taken place, the pulse becomes more frequent, the heat of the body is increased, and the patient is affected with thirst, headache, &c. The pyrexia is very various in degree in different patients, and sometimes assumes an irregular remittent or intermittent type. The complaint generally takes place on one side only at first, and the part where it commences is various; but it most commonly begins in the lumbar, hypogastric, or inguinal region, on one side, or in the hip, or top of the thigh, and corresponding labium pudendi. In this case, the patient first perceives a sense of pain, weight, and stiffness, in some of the above-mentioned parts, which are increased by every attempt to move the pelvis, or lower limb. If the part be carefully examined, it generally is found rather fuller or hotter than natural, and tender to the touch, but not discoloured. The pain increases, always becomes very severe, and, in some cases, is of the most excruciating kind. It extends along the thigh, and when it has subsisted for some time, longer or shorter in different patients, the top of the thigh and the labium pudendi become greatly swelled, and the pain is then sometimes alleviated, but accompanied with a greater sense of distention. The pain next extends down to the knee, and is generally the most severe on the inside and back of the thigh, in the direction of the internal cutaneous and the crural nerves; when it has continued for some time, the whole of the thigh becomes swelled, and the pain is somewhat re-

lieved. The pain then extends down the leg to the foot, and is commonly the most severe in the direction of the posterior tibial nerve; after some time, the part last attacked begins to swell, and the pain abates in violence, but is still very considerable, especially on any attempt to move the limb. The extremity being now swelled throughout its whole extent, appears perfectly or nearly uniform, and it is not perceptibly lessened by an horizontal position, like an œdematose limb. It is of the natural colour, or even whiter, is hotter than natural; excessively tense, and exquisitely tender when touched. When pressed by the finger in different parts, it is found to be elastic, little, if any, impression remaining, and that only for a very short time. If a puncture, or incision, be made into the limb, in some instances, no fluid is discharged; in others, a small quantity only issues out, which coagulates soon after; and in others a large quantity of fluid escapes, which does not coagulate; but the whole of the effused matter cannot be drawn off in this way. The swelling of the limb varies both in degree and in the space of time requisite for its full formation. In most instances, it arrives at double the natural size, and in some cases at a much greater. In lax habits, and in patients whose legs have been very much affected with ana sarca during pregnancy, the swelling takes place more rapidly than in those who are differently circumstanced; it sometimes arrives, in the former class of patients, at its greatest extent in twenty-four hours, or less, from the first attack.

Instead of beginning invariably at the upper part of the limb, and descending to the lower, this complaint has been known to begin in the foot, the middle of the leg, the ham, and the knee. In whichsoever of these parts it happens to begin, it is generally soon diffused over the whole of the limb, and, when this has taken place, the limb presents the same phenomena, exactly, that have been stated above, as observable when the inguen, &c. are first affected.

After some days, generally from two to eight, the febrile symptoms diminish, and the swelling, heat, tension, weight, and tenderness of the lower extremity, begin to abate, first about the upper part of the thigh, or about the knee, and afterward in the leg and foot. Some inequalities are found in the limb, which, at first, feel like indurated glands, but, upon being more nicely examined, their edges are not so well defined as those of conglobate glands; and they appear to be occasioned by the effused matter being of different degrees of consistence in different points. The conglobate glands of the thigh and leg are sometimes felt distinctly, and are tender to the touch, but are seldom materially enlarged: and as the swelling subsides, it has happened, that an enlargement of the lymphatic vessels, in some part of the limb, has been felt, or been supposed to be felt.

The febrile symptoms having gradually disappeared, the pain and tenderness of the limb being much relieved, and the swelling and tension being considerably diminished, the patient is debilitated and much reduced, and the limb feels stiff, heavy, benumbed, and weak. When the finger is pressed strongly against it for some time, in different points, it is found to be less elastic than at first, in some places retaining the impression of the finger for a longer, in other places for a shorter time, or scarcely at all. And, if the limb be suffered to hang down, or if the patient walk much, it is found to be more swelled in the evening, and assumes more of an œdematose appearance. In this state the limb continues for a longer or shorter time, and is commonly at length reduced wholly, or nearly, to the natural size.

Hitherto the disease has been described as affecting only one of the inferior extremities, and as terminating by resolution, or the effusion of a fluid that is removed by the absorbents; but, unfortunately, it sometimes happens, that after it abates in one limb, the other is attacked in a similar way. It also happens, in some cases, that the swelling is not terminated by resolution; for sometimes a *suppuration* takes place in one or both legs, and ulcers are formed which are difficult to heal. In a few cases, a gangrene has supervened. In some instances, the patient has been destroyed by the violence of the disease, before either suppuration or gangrene have happened.

The *predisposing causes* of this disease, when it occurs during the pregnant or puerperal state, or in a short time afterward, appear to be, 1st, *The increased irritability and disposition to inflammation which prevail during pregnancy, and in a still higher degree for some time after parturition.* 2dly, *The over-distended, or relaxed state of the blood-vessels of the inferior part of the trunk and of the lower extremities, produced during the latter months of utero-gestation.*

Among the *exciting causes* of this disease may be enumerated, 1st, *Contusions,* or violent exertions of the lower portions of the abdominal and other muscles inserted in the pelvis, or thighs, or of the muscles of the inferior extremities, and contusions of the cellular texture connected with these muscles, during a tedious labour. 2dly, *The application of cold and moisture,* which are known to act very powerfully upon every system in changing the natural distribution of the circulating fluids, and, consequently, in a system predisposed by parturition, may assist in producing the disease, by occasioning the fluids to be impelled, in unusual quantity, into the weakened vessels of the lumbar, hypogastric, and inguinal regions, and of the inferior extremities. 3dly, *Suppression,* or diminution of the lochia, and of the secretion or milk, which, by inducing a plethoric state of the sanguiferous system, may occasion an inflammatory diathesis, may favour congestion, and the determination of an unusual quantity of blood to the vessels of the parts just mentioned, and thus contribute to the production of an inflammation of these parts. 4thly, *Food taken in too large quantity, and of a too stimulating quality,* especially when the patient does not give suck. This cause both favours the production of plethora, and stimulates the heart and arteries to more frequent and violent action; the effects of which may be expected to be particularly felt in the lumbar, hypogastric, or inguinal regions, and in the lower extremities, from the state of their blood-vessels. 5thly, *Standing, or walking too much,* before the arteries and veins of the lower half of the body have recovered sufficiently from the effects of the distention which existed during the latter months of pregnancy. This must necessarily occasion too great a determination of blood to these parts, and consequently too great a congestion in them; whence they will be more stimulated than the upper parts of the body, and inflammation will sometimes be excited in them.

From an attentive consideration of the whole of the phenomena observable in this disease, and of its remote causes and cure, no doubt remains, Dr. Hull thinks, that *the proximate cause consists in an inflammatory affection, producing suddenly a considerable effusion of serum and coagulating lymph from the exhalants into the cellular membrane of the lymph.*

PHLEGMA'SIÆ. The plural of *phlegmasia.* Inflammations. The name of the second order in the class *Pyrexiæ,* of Cullen's Nosological arrangement, characterized by pyrexia, with topical pain and inflammation; the blood, after venesection, exhibiting a buffy coat.

PHLEGMATORRHA'GIA. (From φλεγμα, mucus, and ρηγνυμι, to break out.) A discharge of thin mucous phlegm from the nose, through cold.

PHLE'GMON. (*Phlegmon, onis.* m.; from φλεγω, to burn.) *Phlegmone.* An inflammation of a bright red colour, with a throbbing and pointed tumour, tending to suppuration.

PHLOGISTON. (From φλογιζω, to burn.) The supposed general inflammable principle of Stahl, who imagined it was pure fire, or the matter of fire fixed in combustible bodies, in order to distinguish it from fire in action, or in a state of liberty.

Phlogisticated air. See *Nitrogen.*

Phlogisticated alkali. See *Alkali phlogisticated.*

Phlogisticated gas. See *Nitrogen.*

PHLOGO'SIS. (From φλογοω, to inflame.) Inflammation. See *Inflammation.*

PHLOGOTICA. (*Phlogoticus;* from φλεγω, to burn.) The name of the second order of the class *Hæmatica,* in Good's Nosology. Inflammation. Its genera are *Apostema; Phlegmone; Phyma; Ionthus; Phlysis; Erythema; Empresma; Ophthalmia; Catarrhus; Dysenteria; Bucnemia; Arthrosia.*

PHLYCTÆ'NA. (Φλυκταινα, small bladders.) *Phlyctis; Phlysis.* A small pellucid vesicle, that contains a serous fluid

PHLYSIS. (From φλυζω, to burn.) The name of a genus of diseases in Good's Nosology. Class, *Hæmatica;* Order, *Phlogotica.* It has only one species, *Phlysis paronychia.* Whitlow.

174

PHLYZA'CIUM. (From φλυζω, to be hot.) A pustule on the skin, excited by fire or heat. See *Pustule.*

PHŒNIGMUS. (From φοινιξ, red.) 1. A redness of the skin, such as is produced by stimulating substances.

2. That which reddens the skin when applied to it.

PHŒ'NIX. (Φοινιξ, of the ancient Greeks, the date palm tree; from which, as a *primitive* word, *Phœnicia,* the land of palm-trees, seems to have derived its name, as likewise *the red colour* phœniceus.) The name of a genus of plants. Class, *Diœcia;* Order, *Triandria.* The date palm-tree.

PHŒNIX DACTYLIFERA. The systematic name of the date-tree. *Phœnix- frondibus pinnatis; foliolis ensiformibus complicatis,* of Linnæus. The fruit is called dactylus or date. Dates are oblong. Before they are ripe, they are rather rough and astringent; but when perfectly matured, they are much of the nature of the fig. See *Ficus carica.* Senegal dates are much esteemed, they having a more sugary, agreeable flavour than those of Ægypt and other places. Dates are aperient.

PHONICA. (*Phonicus;* from φωνη, the voice.) The name of the first order of the class *Pneumatica,* in Good's Nosology. Diseases affecting the vocal avenues. It has six genera, viz. *Coryza; Polypus; Rhonchus; Aphonia; Dysphonia; Psellismus.*

PHOSGENE GAS. (*Phosgene:* so called by its discoverer, Doctor John Davy, from its mode of production.) Chloro-carbonaceous acid, a combination of carbonic oxide and chlorine, made by exposing a mixture of equal volumes of chlorine, and carbonic oxide, to the action of light. It has a peculiar pungent odour, is soluble in water, and is resolved into carbonic and muriatic acid gas.

PHOSPHATE. (*Phosphas;* from *phosphorus.*) A salt formed by the union of phosphoric acid with salifiable bases; thus, *phosphate of ammonia, phosphate of lime,* &c.

PHOSPHATIC ACID. *Acidum phosphaticum.* "This acid is obtained by the slow combustion of cylinders of phosphorus in the air. For which purpose, it is necessary that the air be renewed to support the combustion; that it be humid, otherwise the dry coat of phosphatic acid would screen the phosphorus from farther action of the oxygen, and that the different cylinders of phosphorus be insulated, to prevent the heat from becoming too high, which would melt or inflame them, so as to produce phosphoric acid. The acid, as it is formed, must be collected in a vessel, so as to lose as little of it as possible. All these conditions may be thus fulfilled: We take a parcel of glass tubes, which are drawn out to a point at one end; we introduce into each a cylinder of phosphorus a little shorter than the tube; we dispose of these tubes alongside of one another to the amount of 30 or 40, in a glass funnel, the beak of which passes into a bottle placed on a plate, covered with water. We then cover the bottle and its funnel with a large bell-glass, having a small hole in its top, and another in its side.

A film of phosphorus first evaporates, then combines with the oxygen and the water of the air, giving birth to phosphatic acid, which collects in small drops at the end of the glass tubes, and falls through the funnel into the bottle. A little phosphatic acid is also found on the sides of the bell-glass, and in the water of the plate. The process is a very slow one.

The phosphatic acid thus collected is very dilute. We reduce it to a viscid consistence, by heating it gently; and better still, by putting it, at the ordinary temperature, into a capsule over another capsule full of concentrated sulphuric acid, under the receiver of an air-pump, from which we exhaust the air.

The acid thus formed is a viscid liquid, without colour, having a faint smell of phosphorus, a strong taste, reddening strongly the tincture of litmus, and denser than water in a proportion not well determined. Every thing leads to the belief that this acid would be solid, could we deprive it of water. When it is heated in a retort, phosphuretted hydrogen gas is evolved, and phosphoric acid remains. The oxygen and hydrogen of the water concur to this transformation. Phosphatic acid has no action, either on oxygen gas, or on the atmospheric air at ordinary temperatures. In combining with water, a slight degree of heat is occasioned. The phosphatic acid in its action on the salifia ole bases is transformed into phosphorous and phosphoric acids, whence proceed phosphites and phosphates."

PHOSPHITE. *Phosphis* A salt formed by the combination of phosphorous acid with salifiable bases; thus, *ammoniacal phosphite*, &c.

Phosphorated hydrogen. See *Phosphorus.*

PHOSPHORESCENCE. The luminous appearance which is given off by phosphorescent bodies.

PHOSPHORIC ACID. *Acidum phosphoricum.* "The base of this acid, or the acid itself, abounds in the mineral, vegetable, and animal kingdoms. In the mineral kingdom it is found in combination with lead, in the green lead ore; with iron, in the bog ores, which afford cold short iron, and more especially with calcareous earth in several kinds of stone. Whole mountains in the province of Estremadura in Spain are composed of this combination of phosphoric acid and lime. Bowles affirms, that the stone is whitish and tasteless, and affords a blue flame without smell when thrown upon burning coals. Prout describes it as a dense stone, not hard enough to strike fire with steel; and says that it is found in strata, which always lie horizontally upon quartz, and which are intersected with veins of quartz. When this stone is scattered upon burning coals, it does not decrepitate, but burns with a beautiful green light, which lasts a considerable time. It melts into a white enamel by the blow-pipe; is soluble with heat, and some effervescence in the nitric acid, and forms sulphate of lime with the sulphuric acid, while the phosphoric acid is set at liberty in the fluid.

The vegetable kingdom abounds with phosphorus, or its acid. It is principally found in plants that grow in marshy places, in turf, and several species of the white woods. Various seeds, potatoes, agaric, soot, and charcoal, afford phosphoric acid, by abstracting the nitric acid from them, and lixiviating the residue. The lixivium contains the phosphoric acid, which may either be saturated with lime by the addition of lime-water, in which case it forms a solid compound; or it may be tried by examination of its leading properties by other chemical methods.

In the animal kingdom it is found in almost every part of the bodies of animals which are not considerably volatile. There is not, in all probability, any part of these organized beings which is free from it. It has been obtained from blood, flesh, both of land and water animals; from cheese; and it exists in large quantities in bones, combined with calcareous earth. Urine contains it, not only in a disengaged state, but also combined with ammonia, soda, and lime. It was by the evaporation and distillation of this excrementitious fluid with charcoal that phosphorus was first made; the charcoal decomposing the disengaged acid and the ammoniacal salt. But it is more cheaply obtained by the process of Scheele, from bones, by the application of an acid to their earthy residue after calcination.

In this process the sulphuric acid appears to be the most convenient, because it forms a nearly insoluble compound with the lime of the bones. Bones of beef, mutton, or veal, being calcined to whiteness in an open fire, lose almost half of their weight. This must be pounded, and sifted; or the trouble may be spared by buying the powder that is sold to make cupels for the assayers, and is, in fact, the powder of burned bones ready sifted. To every two pounds of the powder there may be added about two pounds of concentrated sulphuric acid. Four or five pounds of water must be afterward added to assist the action of the acid; and during the whole process the operator must remember to place himself and his vessels so that the fumes may be blown from him. The whole may be then left on a gentle sand bath for twelve hours or more, taking care to supply the loss of water which happens by evaporation. The next day a large quantity of water must be added, the whole strained through a sieve, and the residual matter, which is sulphate of lime, must be edulcorated by repeated affusions of hot water, till it passes tasteless. The waters contain phosphoric acid nearly free from lime; and by evaporation, first in glazed earthen, and then in glass vessels, or rather in vessels of platina or silver, for the hot acid acts upon glass, afford the acid in a concentrated state, which, by the force of strong heat in a crucible, may be made to acquire the form of a transparent consistent glass, though it is usually of a milky, opaque appearance.

For making phosphorus, it is not necessary o evaporate the water further than to bring it to the consistence of syrup; and the small portion of lime it contains is not an impediment worth the trouble of removing, as it affects the produce very little. But when the acid is required in a purer state, it is proper to add a quantity of carbonate of ammonia, which, by double elective attraction, precipitates the lime that was held in solution by the phosphoric acid. The fluid, being then evaporated, affords a crystallized ammoniacal salt, which may be melted in a silver vessel, as the acid acts upon glass or earthen vessels. The ammonia is driven off by the heat, and the acid acquires the form of a compact glass, as transparent as rock crystal, acid to the taste, soluble in water, and deliquescent in the air.

This acid is commonly pure, but nevertheless may contain a small quantity of soda, originally existing in the bones, and not capable of being taken away by this process, ingenious as it is. The only unequivocal method of obtaining a pure acid appears to consist in first converting it into phosphorus by distillation of the materials with charcoal, and then converting it again into acid by rapid combustion, at a high temperature, either in oxygen or atmospheric air, or some other equivalent process.

Phosphorus may also be converted into the acid state by treating it with nitric acid. In this operation, a tubulated retort with a ground stopper, must be half filled with nitric acid, and a gentle heat applied. A small piece of phosphorus being then introduced through the tube, will be dissolved with effervescence, produced by the escape of a large quantity of nitric oxide. The addition of phosphorus must be continued until the last piece remains undissolved. The fire being then raised to drive over the remainder of the nitric acid, the phosphoric acid will be found in the retort, partly in the concrete and partly in the liquid form.

Sulphuric acid produces nearly the same effect as the nitric; a large quantity of sulphurous acid flying off. But as it requires a stronger heat to drive off the last portions of this acid, it is not so well adapted to the purpose. The liquid chlorine likewise acidifies it.

When phosphorus is burned by a strong heat, sufficient to cause it to flame rapidly, it is almost perfectly converted into dry acid, some of which is thrown up by the force of the combustion, and the rest remains upon the supporter.

This substance has also been acidified by the direct application of oxygen gas passed through hot water in which the phosphorus was liquefied or fused.

The general characters of phosphoric acid are: 1. It is soluble in water in all proportions, producing a specific gravity, which increases as the quantity of acid is greater, but does not exceed 2.687, which is that of the glacial acid. 2. It produces heat when mixed with water, though not very considerable. 3. It has no smell when pure, and its taste is sour, but not corrosive. 4. When perfectly dry, it sublimes in close vessels; but loses this property by the addition of water; in which circumstance it greatly differs from the boracic acid, which is fixed when dry, but rises by the help of water. 5. When considerably diluted with water, and evaporated, the aqueous vapour carries up a small portion of the acid. 6. With charcoal or inflammable matter, in a strong heat, it loses its oxygen, and becomes converted into phosphorus.

Phosphoric acid is difficult of crystallizing.

Though the phosphoric acid is scarcely corrosive, yet, when concentrated, it acts upon oils, which it dis colours, and at length blackens, producing heat, and a strong smell like that of ether and oil of turpentine; but does not form a true acid soap. It has most effect on essential oils, less on drying oils, and least of all on fat oils. Spirit of wine and phosphoric acid have a weak action on each other. Some heat is excited by this mixture, and the product which comes over in distillation of the mixture is strongly acid, of a pungent arsenical smell, inflammable with smoke, miscible in all proportions with water, precipitating silver and mercury from their solutions, but not gold; and although not an ether, yet it seems to be an approximation to that kind of combination.

Phosphoric acid, united with *barytes*, produces an insoluble salt, in the form of a heavy white powder, fusible at a high temperature into a gray enamel. The best mode of preparing it is by adding an alkaline phosphate to the nitrate or muriate of barytes.

The *phosphate of strontian* differs from the preceding in being soluble in an excess of its acid.

Phosphate of lime is very abundant in the native state.

The phosphate of lime is very difficult to fuse, but in a glasshouse furnace it softens, and acquires the semi-transparency and grain of porcelain. It is insoluble in water, but when well calcined, forms a kind of paste with it, as in making cupels. Besides this use of it, it is employed for polishing gems and metals, for absorbing grease from cloth, linen, or paper, and for preparing phosphorus. In medicine it has been strongly recommended against the rickets by Dr. Bonhomme of Avignon, either alone or combined with phosphate of soda. The *burnt hartshorn* of the shops is a phosphate of lime.

An *acidulous phosphate of lime* is found in human urine, and may be crystallized in small silky filaments, or shining scales, which unite together into something like the consistence of honey, and have a perceptibly acid taste. It may be prepared by partially decomposing the calcareous phosphate of bones by the sulphuric, nitric, or muriatic acid, or by dissolving that phosphate in phosphoric acid. It is soluble in water, and crystallizable. Exposed to the action of heat, it softens, liquefies, swells up, becomes dry, and may be fused into a transparent glass, which is insipid, insoluble, and unalterable in the air In these characters it differs from the glacial acid of phosphorus. It is partly decomposable by charcoal, so as to afford phosphorus.

The *phosphate of potassa* is very deliquescent, and not crystallizable, but condensing into a kind of jelly. Like the preceding species, it first undergoes the aqueous fusion, swells, dries, and may be fused into a glass; but this glass deliquesces. It has a sweetish saline taste.

The *phosphate of soda* was first discovered combined with ammonia in urine, by Schockwitz, and was called *fusible* or *microcosmic salt.* Margraff obtained it alone by lixiviating the residuum left after preparing phosphorus from this triple salt and charcoal. Haupt, who first discriminated the two, gave the phosphate of soda the name of *sal mirabile perlatum.* Rouelle very properly announced it to be a compound of soda and phosphoric acid. Bergman considered it, or rather the acidulous phosphate, as a peculiar acid, and gave it the name of *perlate acid.* Guyton-Morveau did the same, but distinguished it by the name of *ouretic:* at length Klaproth ascertained its real nature to be as Rouelle had affirmed.

This phosphate is now commonly prepared by adding to the acidulous phosphate of lime as much carbonate of soda in solution as will fully saturate the acid. The carbonate of lime which precipitates, being separated by filtration, the liquid is duly evaporated so as to crystallize the phosphate of soda; but if there be not a slight excess of alkali, the crystals will not be large and regular. Funcke, of Linz, recommends, as a more economical and expeditious mode, to saturate the excess of lime in calcined bones by dilute sulphuric acid, and dissolve the phosphate of lime that remains in nitric acid. To this solution he adds an equal quantity of sulphate of soda, and recovers the nitric acid by distillation. He then separates the phosphate of soda from sulphate of lime by elutriation and crystallization, as usual. The crystals are rhomboidal prisms of different shapes; efflorescent; soluble in 3 parts of cold, and 1½ of hot water. They are capable of being fused into an opaque white glass, which may be again dissolved and crystallized. It may be converted into an acidulous phosphate by an addition of acid, or by either of the strong acids, which partially, but not wholly, decompose it. As its taste is simply saline, without any thing disagreeable, it is much used as a purgative, chiefly in broth, in which it is not distinguishable from common salt. For this elegant addition to our pharmaceutical preparations, we are indebted to Dr. Pearson. In assays with the blow-pipe it is of great utility; and it has been used instead of borax for soldering.

The *phosphate of ammonia* crystallizes in prisms with four regular sides, terminating in pyramids, and sometimes in bundles of small needles. Its taste is cool, saline, pungent, and urinous. On the fire it comports itself like the preceding species, except that the whole of its base may be driven off by a continuance of the

176

heat, leaving only the acid behind. It is but little more soluble in hot water than in cold, which takes up a fourth of its weight. It is pretty abundant in human urine, particularly after it has become putrid. It is an excellent flux both for assays and the blow-pipe, and in the fabrication of coloured glass and artificial gems.

Phosphate of magnesia crystallizes in irregular hexahedral prisms, obliquely truncated; but is commonly pulverulent, as it effloresces very quickly. It requires fifty parts of water to dissolve it. Its taste is cool and sweetish. This salt too is found in urine.

An *ammoniaco-magnesian phosphate* has been discovered in an intestinal calculus of a horse by Four croy, and since by Bartholdi, and likewise by the former, in some human urinary calculi.

The *phosphate of glucine* has been examined by Vauquelin, who informs us, that it is a white powder, or mucilaginous mass, without any perceptible taste; fusible but not decomposable by heat; unalterable in the air, and insoluble unless in an excess of its acid.

It has been observed, that the phosphoric acid, aided by heat, acts upon silex; and we may add, that it enters into many artificial gems in the state of a silicious phosphate."—*Ure's Chemical Dictionary.*

PHOSPHORITE. A subspecies of apatite. 1. *Common phosphorite.* This is of a yellowish white colour, when rubbed in an iron mortar, or thrown on red-hot coals. It emits a green-coloured phosphoric light. It is found in Estremadura, in Spain.

2. *Earthy phosphorite.* Of a grayish white colour, and consists of dull dusty particles, which phosphoresce on glowing coals. It is found in Hungary.

PHOSPHOROUS ACID. *Acidum phosphorosum.* "This acid was discovered in 1812 by Sir H. Davy. When phosphorus and corrosive sublimate act on each other at an elevated temperature, a liquid called protochloride of phosphorus is formed. Water added to this, resolves it into muriatic and phosphorous acids. A moderate heat suffices to expel the former, and the latter remains associated with water. It has a very sour taste, reddens vegetable blues, and neutralizes bases. When heated strongly in open vessels, it inflames. Phosphuretted hydrogen flies off, and phosphoric acid remains. Ten parts of it heated in close vessels give off one-half of bihydroguret of phosphorus, and leave 8½ of phosphoric acid. Hence the liquid acid consists of 80.7 acid + 19.3 water. Its prime equivalent is 2.5."

PHOSPHORUS. (From φως, light, and φερω, to carry.) *Autophosphorus.* A simple substance which has never been found pure in nature. It is always met with united to oxygen, or in the state of phosphoric acid. In that state it exists very plentifully, and is united to different animal, vegetable, and mineral substances.

"If phosphoric acid be mixed with 1-5th of its weight of powdered charcoal, and the mixture distilled at a moderate red heat, in a coated earthen retort, whose beak is partially immersed in a basin of water, drops of a waxy-looking substance will pass over, and, falling into the water, will concrete into the solid called phosphorus. It must be purified, by straining it through a piece of chamois leather, under warm water. It is yellow and semitransparent. It is as soft as wax, but fully more cohesive and ductile. Its sp. gr. is 1.77. It melts at 99° F. and boils at 550°.

In the atmosphere, at common temperatures, it emits a white smoke, which, in the dark, appears luminous. This smoke is acidulous, and results from the slow oxygenation of the phosphorus. In air perfectly dry, however, phosphorus does not smoke, because the acid which is formed is solid, and, closely incasing the combustible, screens it from the atmospherical oxygen.

When phosphorus is heated in the air to about 148°, it *takes fire,* and burns with a splendid white light, and a copious dense smoke. If the combustion take place within a large glass receiver, the smoke becomes condensed into snowy looking particles, which fall in a successive shower, coating the bottom plate with a spongy efflorescence of *phosphoric acid.* This acid snow soon liquefies by the absorption of aqueous vapour from the air.

When phosphorus is inflamed in oxygen, the light and heat are incomparably more intense; the former dazzling the eye, and the latter cracking the glass vessel. Solid phosphoric acid results; consisting of 1.5 phosphorus + 2.0 oxygen.

When phosphorus is heated in highly rarefied air, three products are formed from it: one is phosphoric acid; one is a volatile white powder; and the third is a red solid of comparative fixity, requiring a heat above that of boiling water for its fusion. The volatile substance is soluble in water, imparting acid properties to it. It seems to be phosphorous acid. The red substance is probably an oxide of phosphorus, since, for its conversion into phosphoric acid it requires less oxygen than phosphorus does. See *Phosphoric, Phosphorous*, and *Hypophosphorous Acids*.

Phosphorus and chlorine combine with great facility, when brought in contact with each other at common temperatures.

1. When chlorine is introduced into a retort exhausted of air, and containing phosphorus, the phosphorus takes fire, and burns with a pale flame, throwing off sparks; while a white substance rises and condenses on the sides of the vessel.

If the chlorine be in considerable quantity, as much as 12 cubic inches to a grain of phosphorus, the latter will entirely disappear, and nothing but the white powder will be formed, into which about 9 cubic inches of the chlorine will be condensed. No new gaseous matter is produced.

The powder is a compound of phosphorus and chlorine, first described as a peculiar body by Sir H. Davy in 1810; and various analytical and synthetical experiments which he made with it, prove that it consists of about 1 phosphorus, and 6.8 chlorine in weight. It is the *bichloride* of phosphorus.

Its properties are very peculiar. It is snow-white, extremely volatile, rising in a gaseous form at a temperature much below that of boiling water. Under pneumatic pressure it may be fused, and then it crystallizes in transparent prisms.

It acts violently on water, decomposing it, whence result the phosphoric and muriatic acids; the former from the combination of the phosphorus with the oxygen, and the latter from that of the chlorine with the hydrogen of the water. It produces flame when exposed to a lighted taper. If it be transmitted through an ignited glass tube, along with oxygen, it is decomposed, and phosphoric acid and chlorine are obtained. The superior fixity of the acid above the chloride, seems to give that ascendancy of attraction to the oxygen here, which the chlorine possesses in most other cases. Dry litmus paper exposed to its vapour in a vessel exhausted of air, is reddened. When introduced into a vessel containing ammonia, a combination takes place, accompanied with much heat, and there results a compound, insoluble in water, undecomposable by acid or alkaline solutions, and possessing characters analogous to earths.

2. The *protochloride* of phosphorus was first obtained in a pure state by Sir H. Davy, in the year 1809. If phosphorus be sublimed through corrosive sublimate, in powder in a glass tube, a limpid fluid comes over as clear as water, and having a specific gravity of 1.45. It emits acid fumes when exposed to the air, by decomposing the aqueous vapour. If paper, imbued with it, be exposed to the air, it becomes acid without inflammation. It does not redden dry litmus paper plunged into it. Its vapour burns in the flame of a candle. When mixed with water, and heated, muriatic acid flies off, and phosphorous acid remains. If it be introduced into a vessel containing chlorine, it is converted into the bichloride; and if made to act upon ammonia, phosphorus is produced, and the same earthy-like compound results as that formed by the bichloride and ammonia.

The compounds of iodine and phosphorus have been examined by Sir H. Davy and Gay Lussac.

Phosphorus unites to iodine with the disengagement of heat, but no light. One part of phosphorus and eight of iodine form a compound of a red orange-brown colour, fusible at about 212°, and volatile at a higher temperature.

One part of phosphorus and 16 of iodine produce a crystalline matter of a grayish-black colour, fusible at 84°.

One part of phosphorus, and 24 of iodine, produce a black substance partially fusible at 115°.

Phosphuretted hydrogen. Of this compound there are two varieties; one consisting of a prime of each constituent, and therefore to be called phosphuretted hydrogen; another, in which the relation of phospho-

rus is one half less, to be called therefore subphosphuretted hydrogen.

1. *Phosphuretted hydrogen.* Into a small retort filled with milk of lime, or potassa water, let some fragments of phosphorus be introduced, and let the heat of an Argand flame be applied to the bottom of the retort, while its beak is immersed in the water of a pneumatic trough. Bubbles of gas will come over which explode spontaneously with contact of air. It may also be procured by the action of dilute muriatic acid on phosphuret of lime. In order to obtain the gas pure, however, we must receive it over mercury. Its smell is very disagreeable. Its sp. grav. is 0.9022. 100 cubic inches weigh 27.5 gr. In oxygen, it inflames with a brilliant white light. In common air, when the gaseous bubble bursts the film of water, and explodes, there rises up a ring of white smoke, luminous in the dark. Water absorbs about 1-40th of its bulk of this gas, and acquires a yellow colour, a bitter taste, and the characteristic smell of the gas. When brought in contact with chlorine it detonates with a brilliant green light; but the products have never been particularly examined.

2. *Subphosphuretted hydrogen.* It was discovered by Sir H. Davy in 1812. When the crystalline hydrate of phosphorous acid is heated in a retort out of the contact of air, solid phosphoric acid is formed, and a large quantity of subphosphuretted hydrogen is evolved. Its smell is fœtid, but not so disagreeably so as that of the preceding gas. It does not spontaneously explode like it with oxygen; but at a temperature of 300° a violent detonation takes place. In chlorine it explodes with a white flame. Water absorbs one-eighth of its volume of this gas.

It is probable that phosphuretted hydrogen gas sometimes contains the subphosphuret and common hydrogen mixed with it.

'There is not, perhaps,' says Sir H. Davy, 'in the whole series of chemical phenomena, a more beautiful illustration of the theory of definite proportions, than that offered in the decomposition of hydrophosphorous acid into phosphoric acid, and hydrophosphoric gas.

'Four proportions of the acid contain four proportions of phosphorus and four of oxygen; two proportions of water contain four proportions of hydrogen and two of oxygen (all by volume.) The six proportions of oxygen unite to three proportions of phosphorus to form three of phosphoric acid, and the four proportions of hydrogen combine with one of phosphorus to form one proportion of hydrophosphoric gas (that is, subphosphuretted hydrogen); and there are no other products.'—*Elements*, p. 297.

Phosphorus and sulphur are capable of combining. They may be united by melting them together in a tube exhausted of air, or under water. In this last case, they must be used in small quantities; as, at the moment of their action, water is decomposed, sometimes with explosions. They unite in many proportions. The most fusible compound is that of one and a half of sulphur to two of phosphorus. This remains liquid at 40° Fahrenheit. When solid, its colour is yellowish-white. It is more combustible than phosphorus, and distils undecompounded at a strong heat. Had it consisted of 2 sulphur—3 phosphorus, we should have had a definite compound of 1 prime of the first—2 of the second constituent. This proportion forms the best composition for phosphoric fire-matches or bottles. A particle of it attached to a brimstone match, inflames when gently rubbed against a surface of cork or wood. An oxide made by heating phosphorus in a narrow-mouthed phial with an ignited wire, answers the same purpose. The phial must be kept closely corked, otherwise phosphorous acid is speedily formed.

Phosphorus is soluble in oils, and communicates to them the property of appearing luminous in the dark. Alkohol and ether also dissolve it, but more sparingly."

The earliest account we have concerning the medicinal use of phosphorus, is in the seventh volume of Haller's Collection of Theses, relating to the history and cure of diseases. The original dissertation is entitled, *De Phosphori Loco Medicamenti adsumpti vir tute medica, aliquot casibus singularibus confirmata, Auctore J. Gabi Mentz.* There are three cases of singular cures performed by means of phosphorus, narrated in this thesis; the history of these cases and cures was sent to Dr. Gabi Mentz, by his father.

The first instance is of a man who laboured under a putrid fever.

The second, is that of a man who laboured under a bilious fever.

The third case is entitled a malignant catarrhal fever, with petechiæ.

The dangerous consequences which are likely to follow the injudicious administration of phosphorus cannot be impressed on the mind more strongly than by reading the cases and experiments which are mentioned by Weickard, in the fourth part of his miscellaneous writings, (Vermischte Medicineche Schrifften, von M. A. Weickard.)

PHOSPHURET. (*Phosphuretum,* from *phosphorus.*) A combination of phosphorus, with a combustible or metallic oxide.

Phosphuretted hydrogen. See *Phosphorus.*

PHOSPHURE'TUM. See *Phosphuret.*

PHOTICITE. A mixture of the silicate and carbosilicate of manganese.

PHOTOPHO'BIA. (From φως, light, and φοβεω, to dread.) Such an intolerance of light, that the eye, or rather the retina, can scarcely bear its irritating rays. Such patients generally wink, or close their eyes in light, which they cannot bear without exquisite pain, or confused vision. The proximate cause is too great a sensibility in the retina. The species are,

1. *Photophobia inflammatoria,* or dread of light from an inflammatory cause, which is a particular symptom of the internal ophthalmia.

2. *Photophobia,* from the disuse of light, which happens to persons long confined in dark places or prisons ; on the coming out of which into light the pupil contracts, and the persons cannot bear light. The depression of the cataract occasions this symptom, which appears as though fire and lightning entered the eye, not being able to bear the strong rays of light.

3. *Photophobia nervea,* or a nervous photophobia, which arises from an increased sensibility of the nervous expansion and optic nerve. It is a symptom of the hydrophobia, and many disorders, both acute and nervous.

4. *Photophobia,* from too great light, as looking at the sun, or at the strong light of modern lamps.

PHOTO'PSIA. (From φως, light, and οψις, vision.) Lucid vision. An affection of the eye in which the patient perceives luminous rays, ignited lines, or coruscations.

PHRA'GMUS. (From φρασσω, to enclose, or fence: so called from their being set round like a fence of stakes.) The rows of teeth.

PHRE'NES. (*Phren,* from φρην, the mind; because the ancients imagined it was the seat of the mind.) The diaphragm.

PHRENE'SIS. See *Phrenitis.*

PHRENIC. (*Phrenicus ;* from φρενες, the diaphragm.) Belonging to the diaphragm.

PHRENIC ARTERY. The arteries going to the diaphragm.

PHRENIC NERVE. Diaphragmatic nerve. It arises from a union of the branches of the third, fourth, and fifth cervical pairs, on each side, passes between the clavicle and subclavian artery, and descends from thence by the pericardium to the diaphragm.

PHRENIC VEIN. The veins coming from the diaphragm.

PHRENICA. (*Phrenicus ;* from φρην, the mind, or intellect.) The name of the first order of diseases of the class *Neurotica,* in Good's Nosology. Diseases affecting the intellect. Its genera are, *Ecphoronia ; Empathema ; Alusia ; Aphlexia ; Paroniria ; Moria.*

PHRENI'TIS. (*Phrenitis, idis.* f. Φρενιτις ; from φρην, the mind.) *Phreneeis ; Phrenetiasis ; Phrenismus ; Cephalitis ; Sphacelismus ; Cephalalgia inflammatoria.* By the Arabians, *karabitus.* Phrenzy or inflammation of the brain. A genus of disease in the Class *Pyrexia,* and Order *Phlegmasiæ,* of Cullen ; characterized by strong fever, violent headache, redness of the face and eyes, impatience of light and noise, watchfulness, and furious delirium. It is symptomatic of several diseases, as worms, hydrophobia, &c. Phrenitis often makes its attacks with a sense of fulness in the head, flushing of the countenance, and redness of the eyes, the pulse being full, but in other respects natural. As these symptoms increase, the patient becomes restless, his sleep is disturbed, or wholly forsakes him. It sometimes comes on, as in the epidemic,

of which Saalman gives an account, with pain, or a peculiar sense of uneasiness of the head, back, loins, and joints; in some cases, with tremor of the limbs, and intolerable pains of the hands, feet, and legs. It now and then attacks with stupor and rigidity of the whole body, sometimes with anxiety and a sense of tension referred to the breast, often accompanied with palpitation of the heart. Sometimes nausea and a painful sense of weight in the stomach, are among the earliest symptoms. In other cases, the patient is attacked with vomiting, or complains of the heart-burn, and griping pains in the bowels. When the intimate connexion which subsists between the brain and every part of the system is considered, the variety of the symptoms attending the commencement of phrenitis is not so surprising, nor that the stomach in particular should suffer, which so remarkably sympathizes with the brain. These symptoms assist in forming the diagnosis between phrenitis and synocha. The pain of the head soon becomes more considerable, and sometimes very acute. "If the meninges," says Dr. Fordyce, "are affected, the pain is acute; if the substance only, obtuse, and sometimes but just sensible." And Dr. Cullen remarks, " I am here, as in other analogous cases, of opinion, that the symptoms above mentioned of an acute inflammation, always mark inflammations of membraneous parts, and that an inflammation of parenchyma, or substance of viscera, exhibits, at least commonly, a more chronic inflammation."

The seat of the pain is various: sometimes it seems to occupy the whole head; sometimes, although more circumscribed, it is deep-seated, and ill-defined. In other cases, it is felt principally in the forehead or occiput. The redness of the face and eyes generally increases with the pain, and there is often a sense of heat and throbbing in the head, the countenance acquiring a peculiar fierceness. These symptoms, for the most part, do not last long before the patient begins to talk incoherently, and to show other marks of delirium. Sometimes, however, Saalman observes, delirium did not come on till the fifth, sixth, or seventh day. The delirium gradually increases, till it often arrives at a state of phrenzy. The face becomes turgid, the eyes stare, and seem as if bursting from their sockets, tears, and sometimes even blood, flowing from them: the patient, in many cases, resembling a furious maniac, from whom it is often impossible to distinguish him, except by the shorter duration of his complaint. The delirium assists in distinguishing phrenitis and synocha, as it is not a common symptom in the latter. When delirium does attend synocha, however, it is of the same kind as in phrenitis.

We should, *a priori,* expect in phrenitis considerable derangement in the different organs of sense, which so immediately depend on the state of the brain. The eyes are incapable of bearing the light, and false vision, particularly that termed *muscæ volitantes,* and flashes of light seeming to dart before the eyes, are frequent symptoms. The hearing is often so acute, that the least noise is intolerable: sometimes, on the other hand, the patient becomes deaf; and the deafness, Saalman observes, and morbid acuteness of hearing, sometimes alternate. Affections of the smell, taste, and touch, are less observable.

As the organs of sense are not frequently deranged in synocha, the foregoing symptoms farther assist the diagnosis between this complaint and phrenitis.

The pulse is not always so much disturbed at an earlier period, as we should expect from the violence of the other symptoms, compared with what we observe in idiopathic fevers. When this circumstance is distinctly marked, it forms, perhaps, the best diagnosis between phrenitis and synocha, and gives to phrenitis more of the appearance of mania. In many cases, however, the fever runs as high as the delirium; then the case often almost exactly resembles a case of violent synocha, from which it is the more difficult to distinguish it if the pulse be full and strong. In general, however, the hardness is more remarkable than in synocha, and in many cases the pulse is small and hard, which may be regarded as one of the best diagnostics between the two complaints, the pulse in synocha being always strong and full. In phrenitis it is sometimes, though rarely, intermitting. The respiration is generally deep and slow, sometimes difficult, now and then interrupted with hiccough, seldom hurried and frequent; a very unfavourable symptom. In many of the cases mentioned by Saalman, pneumonia supervened.

The deglutition is often difficult, sometimes convulsive. The stomach is frequently oppressed with bile, which is an unfavourable symptom; and complete jaundice, the skin and urine being tinged yellow, some-'imes supervenes. Worms in the stomach and bowels are also frequent attendants on phrenitis, and there is reason to believe, may have a share in producing it. The hydrocephalus internus, which is more allied to phrenitis than dropsy of the brain, properly so called, seems often, in part at least, to arise from derangement of the primæ viæ, particularly from worms. We cannot otherwise account for the frequent occurrence of these complaints.

Instead of a superabundance of bile in the primæ viæ, there is sometimes a deficiency, which seems to afford even a worse prognosis. The alvine fæces being of a white colour, and a black cloud in the urine, are regarded by Lobb as fatal symptoms. The black cloud in the urine is owing to an admixture of blood; when unmixed with blood, it is generally pale.

There is often a remarkable tendency to the worst species of hæmorrhagies, towards the fatal termination of phrenitis. Hæmorrhagy from the eyes has already been mentioned. Hæmorrhagy from the intestines also, tinging the stools with a black colour, is not uncommon. These hæmorrhagies are never favourable; but the hæmorrhagies characteristic of synocha, particularly that from the nose, sometimes occur at an earlier period, and, if copious, generally bring relief. More frequently, however, blood drops slowly from the nose, demonstrating the violence of the disease, without relieving it. In other cases, there is a discharge of thin mucus from the nose.

Tremours of the joints, convulsions of the muscles of the face, grinding of the teeth, the face from being florid suddenly becoming pale, involuntary tears, a discharge of mucus from the nose, the urine being of a dark red or yellow colour, or black, or covered with a pellicle, the fæces being either bilious or white, and very fœtid, profuse sweat of the head, neck, and shoulders, paralysis of the tongue, general convulsions, much derangement of the internal functions, and the symptoms of other visceral inflammations, particularly of the pneumonia, supervening, are enumerated by Saalman as affording the most unfavourable prognosis. The delirium changing to coma, the pulse at the same time becoming weak, and the deglutition difficult, was generally the forerunner of death. When, on the contrary, there is a copious hæmorrhagy from the hæmorrhoidal vessels, from the lungs, mouth, or even from the urinary passages, when the delirium is relieved by sleep, and the patient remembers his dreams, when the sweats are free and general, the deafness is diminished or removed, and the febrile symptoms become milder, there are hopes of recovery.

In almost all diseases, if we except those which kill suddenly, as the fatal termination approaches, nearly the same train of symptoms supervenes, viz. those denoting extreme debility of all the functions. Saalman remarks, that the blood did not always show the buffy coat.

Phrenitis, like most other complaints, has sometimes assumed an intermitting form, the fits coming on daily, sometimes every second day. When phrenitis terminates favourably, the typhus, which succeeds the increased excitement, is generally less in proportion to that excitement, than in idiopathic fevers; a circumstance which assists in distinguishing phrenitis from synocha.

The imperfect diagnosis between these complaints is further assisted by the effects of the remedies employed. For in phrenitis, in removing the delirium and other local symptoms, the febrile symptoms in general soon abate. Whereas in synocha, although the delirium and headache be removed, yet the pulse continues frequent, and other marks of indisposition remain for a much longer time.

It will be of use to present, at one view, the circumstances which form the diagnosis between phrenitis and synocha.

Synocha generally makes its attack in the same manner, its symptoms are few and little varied. The symptoms at the commencement of phrenitis are often more complicated, and differ considerably in different cases. Derangement of the internal functions is com-

paratively rare in synocha. In phrenitis it almost constantly attends, and often appears very early. The same observation applies to the derangement of the organs of sense. In synocha, the pulse from the commencement is frequent and strong. In phrenitis, symptoms denoting the local affection often become considerable before the pulse is much disturbed. In phrenitis, we have seen that the pulse sometimes very suddenly loses its strength, the worst species of hæmorrhagies, and other symptoms denoting extreme debility, showing themselves; and such symptoms are generally the forerunners of death: but that when the termination is favourable, the degree of typhus which succeeds it is less in proportion to the preceding excitement than in synocha. Lastly, if we succeed in removing the delirium and other symptoms affecting the head, the state of the fever is found to partake of this favourable change more immediately and completely than in synocha, where, although we succeed in relieving the headache or delirium, the fever often suffers little abatement.

With regard to the duration of phrenitis, Eller observes, that when it proves fatal, the patient generally dies within six or seven days. In many fatal cases, however, it is protracted for a longer time, especially where the remissions have been considerable. Upon the whole, however, the longer it is protracted, providing the symptoms do not become worse, the better is the prognosis.

On the first attack of the disease we must begin by bleeding the patient as largely as his strength will permit: it may be productive of more relief to the head, where the patient cannot spare much blood, if the temporal artery, or the jugular vein be opened; and in the progress of the complaint occasional cupping or leeches may materially assist the other means employed. Active cathartics should be given directly after taking blood, calomel with jalap, followed by some saline compound in the infusion of senna, until the bowels are copiously evacuated. The head should be shaved, and kept constantly cool by some evaporating lotion. Antimonial and mercurial preparations may then be given to promote the several discharges, and diminish arterial action: to which purpose digitalis also may powerfully concur. Blisters to the back of the neck, behind the ears, or to the temples, each perhaps successively, when the violence of the disorder is lessened by proper evacuations, may contribute very much to obviate internal mischief. The head should be kept raised, to counteract the accumulation of blood there; and the antiphlogistic regimen must be observed in the fullest extent. Stimulating the extremities by the pediluvium, sinapisms, &c. may be of some use in the decline of the complaint, where an irritable state of the brain appears.

PHRENETI'ASIS. See *Phrenitis.*

PHRENSY. See *Phrenitis.*

PHTHEIRI'ASIS. (From φθειρ, a louse.) See *Phthiriasis.*

PHTHEI'RIUM. See *Phtheiroctonum.*

PHTHEIRO'CTONUM. (From φθειρ, a louse, and κτεινω, to kill; because it destroys lice.) *Phtheirium.* The herb Staves-acre. See *Delphinium staphisagria.*

PHTHIRI'ASIS. (From φθειρ, a louse.) *Morbus pediculosus; pediculatio; phtheiriasis.* A disease in which several parts of the body generate lice, which often puncture the skin, and produce little sordid ulcers.

PHTHISIS. (From φθιω, to consume.) *Tabes pulmonalis.* Pulmonary consumption. A disease represented by Dr. Cullen as a sequel of hæmoptysis: it is known by emaciation, debility, cough, hectic fever, and purulent expectoration.

Species: 1. *Phthisis incipiens,* incipient, without an expectoration of pus.

2. *Phthisis humida,* with an expectoration of pus.

3. *Phthisis scrophulosa,* from scrofulous tubercles in the lungs, &c.

4. *Phthisis hæmoptoica,* from hæmoptysis.

5. *Phthisis exanthematica,* from exanthemata.

6. *Phthisis chlorotica,* from chlorosis.

7. *Phthisis syphilitica,* from a venereal ulcer in the lungs.

The causes which predispose to this disease are very numerous. The following are, however, the most general: hereditary disposition; particular formation of the body, obvious by a long neck prominent shoulders, and narrow chest; scrofulous diathesis, indicated by a fine clear skin, fair hair, delicate rosy complexion, large veins, thick upper lip, a weak voice, and great sensibility; certain diseases, such as syphilis, scrofula, the small pox, and measles; particular employments, exposing artificers to dust, such as needle-pointers, stone-cutters, millers, &c. or to the fumes of metals or minerals under a confined and unwholesome air; violent passions, exertions, or affections of the mind, as grief, disappointment, anxiety, or close application to study, without using proper exercise; frequent and excessive debaucheries, late watching, and drinking freely of strong liquors: great evacuations, as diarrhœa, diabetes, excessive venery, fluor albus, immoderate discharge of the menstrual flux, and the continuing to suckle too long under a debilitated state; and, lastly, the application of cold, either by too sudden a change of apparel, keeping on wet clothes, lying in damp beds, or exposing the body too suddenly to cool air, when heated by exercise; in short, by any thing that gives a considerable check to the perspiration. The more immediate or occasional causes of phthisis are, hæmoptysis, pneumonic inflammation proceeding to suppuration, catarrh, asthma, and tubercles, the last of which is by far the most general. The incipient symptoms usually vary with the cause of the disease; but when it arises from tubercles, it is usually thus marked: it begins with a short dry cough, that at length becomes habitual, but from which nothing is spit up for some time, except a frothy mucus that seems to proceed from the fauces. The breathing is at the same time somewhat impeded, and upon the least bodily motion is much hurried: a sense of straitness, with oppression at the chest, is experienced: the body becomes gradually leaner, and great languor, with indolence, dejection of spirits, and loss of appetite, prevail. In this state the patient frequently continues a considerable length of time, during which he is, however, more readily affected than usual by slight colds, and upon one or other of these occasions the cough becomes more troublesome and severe, particularly by night, and it is at length attended with an expectoration, which towards morning is more free and copious. By degrees the matter which is expectorated becomes more viscid and opaque, and now assumes a greenish colour and purulent appearance, being on many occasions streaked with blood. In some cases, a more severe degree of hæmoptysis attends, and the patient spits up a considerable quantity of florid, frothy blood. The breathing at length becomes more difficult, and the emaciation and weakness go on increasing. With these, the person begins to be sensible of pain in some part of the thorax, which, however, is usually felt at first under the sternum, particularly on coughing. At a more advanced period of the disease, a pain is sometimes felt on one side, and at times prevails in so high a degree, as to prevent the person from lying easily on that side; but it more frequently happens, that it is felt only on making a full inspiration, or coughing. Even where no pain is felt, it often happens that those who labour under phthisis cannot lie easily on one or other of their sides, without a fit of coughing being excited, or the difficulty of breathing being much increased. At the first commencement of the disease, the pulse is often natural, or perhaps is soft, small, and a little quicker than usual; but when the symptoms which have been enumerated have subsisted for any length of time, it then becomes full, hard, and frequent. At the same time the face flushes, particularly after eating; the palms of the hands, and soles of the feet, are affected with burning heat; the respiration is difficult and laborious; evening exacerbations become obvious, and, by degrees, the fever assumes the hectic form. This species of fever is evidently of the remittent kind, and has exacerbations twice every day. The first occurs usually about noon, and a slight remission ensues about five in the afternoon. This last is, however, soon succeeded by another exacerbation, which increases gradually until after midnight; but, about two o'clock in the morning, a remission takes place, and this becomes more apparent as the morning advances. During the exacerbations the patient is very sensible to any coolness of the air, and often complains of a sense of cold when his skin is, at the same time, preternaturally warm. Of these exacerbations, that of the evening is by far the most considerable. From the first appearance of the

180

hectic symptoms, the urine is high coloured, and deposites a copious branny red sediment. The appetite, however, is not greatly impaired, the tongue appears clean, the mouth is usually moist, and the thirst is inconsiderable. As the disease advances, the fauces put on rather an inflamed appearance, and are beset with aphthæ, and the red vessels of the tunica adnata become of a pearly white. During the exacerbations, a florid circumscribed redness appears on each cheek; but at other times the face is pale, and the countenance somewhat dejected. At the commencement of hectic fever, the belly is usually costive; but in the more advanced stages of it, a diarrhœa often comes on, and this continues to recur frequently during the remainder of the disease; colliquative sweats likewise break out, and these alternate with each other, and induce vast debility. In the last stage of the disease the emaciation is so great, that the patient has the appearance of a walking skeleton; his countenance is altered, his cheeks are prominent, his eyes look hollow and languid, his hair falls off, his nails are of a livid colour, and much incurvated, and his feet are affected with œdematous swellings. To the end of the disease the senses remain entire, and the mind is confident and full of hope. It is, indeed, a happy circumstance attendant on phthisis, that those who labour under it are seldom apprehensive or aware of any danger; and it is no uncommon occurrence to meet with persons labouring under its most advanced stage, flattering themselves with a speedy recovery, and forming distant projects under that vain hope. Some days before death the extremities become cold. In some cases a delirium precedes that event, and continues until life is extinguished.

As an expectoration of mucus from the lungs may possibly be mistaken for purulent matter, and may thereby give us reason to suspect that the patient labours under a confirmed phthisis, it may not be amiss to point out a sure criterion, by which we shall always be able to distinguish the one from the other. The medical world are indebted to the late Mr. Charles Darwin for the discovery, who has directed the experiment to be made in the following manner:

Let the expectorated matter be dissolved in vitriolic acid, and in caustic lixivium, and add pure water to both solutions. If there is a fair precipitation in each, it is a certain sign of the presence of pus; but if there is not a precipitate in either, it is certainly mucus.

Sir Everard Home, in his dissertation on the properties of pus, informs us of a curious, but not a decisive mode of distinguishing accurately between pus and animal mucus. The property he observes, which characterizes pus, and distinguishes it from most other substances, is, its being composed of globules, which are visible when viewed through a microscope; whereas animal mucus, and all chemical combinations of animal substances, appear in the microscope to be made up of flakes. This property was first noticed by the late Mr. John Hunter.

Pulmonary consumption is in every case to be considered as attended with much danger; but it is more so when it proceeds from tubercles, than when it arises in consequence either of hæmoptysis, or pneumonic suppuration. In the last instance, the risk will be greater where the abscess breaks inwardly, and gives rise to empyema, than when its contents are discharged by the mouth. Even cases of this nature have, however, been known to terminate in immediate death. The impending danger is generally to be judged of, however, by the hectic symptoms; but more particularly by the fœtor of the expectoration, the degree of emaciation and debility, the colliquative sweats, and the diarrhœa. The disease has, in many cases, been found to be considerably retarded in its progress by pregnancy; and in a few has been alleviated by an attack of mania.

The morbid appearance most frequently to be met with, on the dissection of those who die of phthisis, is the existence of tubercles in the cellular substance of the lungs. These are small tumours which have the appearance of indurated glands, are of different sizes, and are often found in clusters. Their firmness is usually in proportion to their size, and when laid open in this state they are of a white colour, and of a consistence nearly approaching to cartilage. Although indolent at first, they at length become inflamed, and lastly form 'rile abscesses or vomicæ, which breaking, and pouring their contents into the bronchia, give rise to a purulent expectoration, and thus lay the foundation of phthisis. Such tubercles or vomicæ are most usually situated at the upper and back part of the lungs; but in some instances they occupy the outer part, and then adhesions to the pleura are often formed.

When the disease is partial, only about a fourth of the upper and posterior part of the lungs is usually found diseased; but, in some cases, life has been protracted till not one-twentieth part of them appeared, on dissection, fit for performing their function. A singular observation, confirmed by the morbid collections of anatomists, is, that the left lobe is much oftener affected than the right. The indications are,

1. To moderate inflammatory action.
2. To support the strength, and promote the healing of ulcers in the lungs.
3. To palliate urgent symptoms.

The first object may require occasional small bleedings, where the strength will permit, in the early period of the disease; but in the scrofulous this measure is scarcely admissible. Local pain will more frequently lead to the use of cupping, with or without the scarificator, leeches, blisters, and other modes of deriving the nervous energy, as well as blood, from the seat of the disease. The bowels must be kept soluble by gentle laxatives, as cassia, manna, sulphate of magnesia, &c.: and diaphoresis promoted by saline medicines, or the pulvis ipecacuanhæ compositus. The occasional use of an emetic may benefit the patient by promoting the function of the skin, and expectoration, especially where there is a wheezing respiration. The inhalation of steam, impregnated, perhaps, with hemlock, or ether, may be useful as soothing the lungs, and facilitating expectoration. Certain sedative remedies, particularly digitalis, and hemlock, have been much employed in this disease; and in so far as they moderate the circulation, and relieve pain, they are clearly beneficial: but too much reliance must not be placed upon them. Certain sedatives have been also proposed to be respired by the patient, as hydrogen, &c.; but their utility is very questionable. Among the tonic medicines, the mineral acids are, perhaps, the most generally useful; however, myrrh and chalybeates, in moderate doses, often answer a good purpose. But a great deal will depend on a due regulation of the diet, which should be of a nutritious kind, but not heating, or difficult of digestion: milk, especially that of the ass; farinaceous vegetables; acescent fruits; the different kinds of shell-fish; the lichen islandicus, boiled with milk, &c., are of this description. Some mode of gestation, regularly employed, particularly sailing; warm clothing; removal to a warm climate, or to a pure and mild air in this, may materially concur in arresting the progress of the disease, in its incipient stage. With regard to urgent symptoms, requiring palliation, the cough may be allayed by demulcents, but especially mild opiates swallowed slowly; colliquative sweats, by acids, particularly the mineral: diarrhœa, by chalk and other astringents, but most effectually by small doses of opium.

PHTHISIS PUPILLÆ. An amaurosis.

PHTHO'RIA. (From φθορα, an abortion.) Medicines which promote abortion.

PHU. (φου, or φευ; from phua, Arabian.) The name of a plant. See *Valeriana phu.*

PHYGE'THLON. (From φυω, to grow.) A red and painful tubercle in the arm-pits, neck, and groins.

PHYLACTE'RIUM. (From φυλασσω, to preserve.) An amulet or preservative against infection.

PHYLLA'NTHUS. (From φυλλον, a leaf, and ανθος, a flower; because the flowers in one of the original species, now a *Hylophytta*, grow out of the leaves.) The name of a genus of plants. Class, *Monœcia;* Order, *Monadelphia.*

PHYLLANTHUS EMBLICA. The systematic name of the Indian tree from which the emblic myrobalan is obtained.

PHYLLI'TIS. (From φυλλον, a leaf: so called because the leaves only appear. See *Asplenium scolopendrium.*

PHYMA. (From φυω, to produce.) A tubercle on any external part of the body.

PHY'SALIS. (From φυσαω, to inflate: so called

because its seed is contained in a kind of bladder.) The name of a genus of plants. Class, *Pentandria;* Order, *Monogynia.*

PHYSALIS ALKEKENGI. The systematic name of the winter cherry. *Alkekengi; Halicacabum.* This plant, *Physalis—foliis geminis integris acutis caule herbaceo, inferné subramosa,* of Linnæus, is cultivated in our gardens. The berries are recommended as a diuretic, from six to twelve for a dose, in dropsical and calculous diseases.

PHYSALITE. Prophysalite. A sub-species of primitive topaz of Jameson. A greenish white mineral found in granite in Finbo, in Sweden.

PHYSCO'NIA. (From φυσκων, a big-bellied fellow.) *Hyposarca; Hypersarchidios.* Enlargement of the abdomen. A genus of disease in the class *Cachexiæ,* and order *Intumescentiæ,* of Cullen; known by a tumour occupying chiefly one part of the abdomen, increasing slowly, and neither sonorous nor fluctuating. Species: 1. *Hepatica.* 2. *Splenica.* 3. *Renalis.* 4. *Uterina.* 5. *Ab ovario.* 6. *Mesenterica.* 7. *Omentalis.* 8. *Visceralis.*

PHYSE'MA. (From φυσαω, to inflate.) *Physesis* A windy tumour.

PHYSE'TER. (*Physeter,* from φυσαω, to inflate: so named from its action of blowing and discharging water from its nostrils.) The name of a genus of whale-fish in the Linnæan system.

PHYSETER MACROCEPHALUS. The spermaceti whale Spermaceti, now called in the pharmacopœia *Cetaceum,* is an oily, concrete, crystalline, semi-transparent matter, obtained from the cavity of the cranium of several species of whales, but principally from the *Physeter macrocephalus,* or spermaceti whale. It was formerly very highly esteemed, and many virtues were attributed to it; but it is now chiefly employed in affections of the lungs, primæ viæ, kidneys, &c. as a softening remedy mixed with mucilages. It is also employed by surgeons as an emollient in form of cerates, ointments, &c See also *Ambergris,* and *Balæna macrocephala.*

PHYSIOGNOMY. (*Physiognomia;* from φυσις, nature, and γινωσκω, to know.) The art of knowing the disposition of a person from the countenance.

PHYSIOLOGY. (*Physiologia;* from φυσις, nature, and λογος, a discourse.) That science which has for its object the knowledge of the phenomena proper to living bodies. It is divided into Vegetable Physiology, which is employed in the consideration of vegetables; into Animal or Comparative Physiology, which treats of animals; and into Human Physiology, of which the special object is man.

PHYSIS. Nature.

PHYSOCE'LE. (From φυσα, wind, and κηλη, a tumour.) A species of hernia, the contents of which are distended with wind.

PHYSOCE'PHALUS. (From φυσα, wind, and κεφαλη, the head.) Emphysema of the head. See *Pneumatosis.*

PHYSOME'TRA. (From φυσαω, to inflate, and μητρα, the womb.) *Hysterophyse.* A windy swelling of the uterus. A tympany of the womb. A genus of disease in the class *Cachexiæ,* and order *Intumescentiæ,* of Cullen; characterized by a permanent elastic swelling of the hypogastrium, from flatulent distention of the womb. It is a rare disease, and seldom admits of a cure.

PHYTEU'MA. (*Phyteuma, atis.* n.; from φυτευω, to generate: so called from its great increase and growth.) The name of a genus of plants. Class, *Pentandria;* Order, *Monogynia.*

PHYTEUMA ORBICULARE. *Rapunculus corniculatus.* Horned rampions. By some supposed efficacious in the cure of syphilis.

PHYTOLA'CCA. (*Phytolacca;* from φυτον, a plant, and λακκα, gum lac: so called because it is of the colour of lacca.) The name of a genus of plants. Class, *Decandria;* Order, *Decagynia.*

PHYTOLACCA DECANDRIA. The systematic name of the Pork-physic; Pork-weed; Poke-weed; Red-weed of Virginia; Red night-shade; American night shade. *Solanum racemosum americanum; Solanum magnum virginianum rubrum.* In Virginia and other parts of America, the inhabitants boil the leaves, and eat them in the manner of spinach. They are said to have an anodyne quality, and the juice of the root is violently cathartic. The Portuguese had formerly a trick of mixing the juice of the berries with their red wines, in order to give them a deeper colour: but it was found to debase the flavour. This was represented to his Portuguese majesty, who ordered all the stems to be cut down yearly before they produced flowers, thereby to prevent any further adulteration. This plant has been used as a cure for cancers, but to no purpose.

PHYTOLOGY. (*Phytologia.* From φυτον, an herb, and λογος, a discourse.) That part of the science of natural history, which treats on plants.

PHYTOMINERA'LIS. (From φυτον, a plant, and *mineralis*, a mineral.) A substance of a vegetable and mineral nature; as amber.

PI'A MATER. (*Pia mater,* the natural mother; so called because it embraces the brain, as a good mother folds her child.) *Localis membrana; Meninx tenuis.* A thin membrane, almost wholly vascular, that is firmly accreted to the convolutions of the cerebrum, cerebellum, medulla oblongata, and medulla spinalis. Its use appears to be, to distribute the vessels to, and contain the substance of, the cerebrum.

PI'CA. (*Pica,* the magpie: so named because it is said the magpie is subject to this affection.) *Picatio; Malacia; Allotriophagia; Citta; Cissa.* Longing. Depraved appetite, with strong desire for unnatural food. It is very common to pregnant women and chlorotic girls, and by some it is said to occur in men who labour under suppressed hæmorrhoids.

PI'CEA. (Πιτυς, pitch.) The common or red fir or pitch-tree is so termed. The cones, branches, and every part of the tree, affords the common resin called frankincense. See *Pinus abies.*

PICHU'RIM. See *Pechurim.*

PICNITE. Pyenite. See *Schorlite.*

PI'CRIS. (From πικρος, bitter.) The name of a genus of plants. Class, *Syngenesia;* Order, *Polygamia æquales.*

PICRIS ECHO'IDES. The name of the common ox-tongue. The leaves are frequently used as a pot-herb by the country people, who esteem it good to relax the bowels.

PICROMEL. (From πικρος, bitter, and μεγι, honey : so called from its taste.) The characteristic principle of bile. If sulphuric acid, diluted with five parts of water, be mixed with fresh bile, a yellow precipitate will fall. Heat the mixture, then leave it in repose, and decant off the clear part. What remains was formerly called resin of bile; but it is a greenish compound of sulphuric acid and picromel. Edulcorate it with water, and digest with carbonate of barytes. The picromel now liberated will dissolve in the water. On evaporating the solution, it is obtained in a solid state. Or by dissolving the green sulphate in alkohol, and digesting the solution over carbonate of potassa till it cease to redden litmus paper, we obtain the picromel combined with alkohol.

It resembles inspissated bile. Its colour is greenish-yellow; its taste is intensely bitter at first, with a succeeding impression of sweetness. It is not affected by infusion of galls; but the salts of iron and subacetate of lead precipitate it from its aqueous solution. It affords no ammonia by its destructive distillation. Hence the absence of azote is inferred, and the peculiarity of picromel.

PICROTOXIA. Picrotoxine. The poisonous principle of the cocculus indicus. See *Menispermum cocculus,* and *Cocculus indicus.*

PICTO'NIUS. (From the Pictones, who were subject to this disease.) Applied to a species of colic. It should be rather called colica pictorum, the painter's colic, because, from their use of lead, they are much afflicted with it.

PIE'STRUM. (From πιεζω, to press.) An instrument to compress the head of a dead fœtus, for its more easy extraction from the womb.

Pig-nut. The bulbous root of the *Bunium bulbocastanum,* of Linnæus: so called because pigs are very fond of them, and will dig with their snouts to some depth for them. See *Bunium bulbocastanum.*

PIGME'NTUM. (From *pingo,* to paint.) Pigment. This name is given by anatomists to a mucous substance found in the eye, which is of two kinds. *The pigment of the iris* is that which covers the anterior and posterior surface of the iris, and gives the beautiful variety of colour in the eyes. *The pigment of the choroid membrane* is a black or brownish mucus, which covers the anterior surface of the choroid membrane, contiguous to the retina and the anterior surface of the ciliary processes.

PI'LA HYSTRICIS. The bezoar hystricis.

PILA MARINA. A species of alcyonium found on sea-coasts among wrack. It is said to kill worms, and, when calcined, to be useful in scrofula.

PILE. See *Hæmorrhois.*

PILE-WORT. See *Ranunculus ficaria.*

PILEUS. (*Pileus,* a hat.) That part of a gymnos perm fungus or mushroom, which forms the upper round part or head; as in Boletus, and Agaricus.

PI'LI CONGENITI. The hair of the head, eyebrows, and eyelids, are so termed, because they grow *in utero.*

PI'LI POSTGENITI. The hair which grows from the surface of the body after birth is so termed, in contradiction to that which appears before birth; as the hair of the head, eyebrows, and eyelids.

PILOSE'LLA. (From *pilus,* hair: because its leaves are hairy.) See *Hieracium pilocella.*

Pill, aloëtic, with myrrh. See *Pilulæ aloës cum myrrha.*

Pill, compound aloëtic. See *Pilulæ aloës compositæ.*

Pill, compound calomel. See *Pilulæ hydrargyri submuriatis compositæ.*

Pili, compound galbanum. See *Pilulæ galbani compositæ.*

Pill, compound gamboge. See *Pilulæ cambogiæ compositæ.*

Pill, compound squill. See *Pilulæ scillæ compositæ.*

Pill of iron with myrrh. See *Pilulæ ferri compositæ.*

Pill, mercurial. See *Pilulæ hydrargyri.*

Pill, soap, with opium. See *Pilulæ saponis cum opio.*

PILOSUS. Hairy. Applied to the stems, leaves, and receptacles of plants, as that of the *Cerastium alpinum;* and to the nectary of the *Parnassus palustris,* which is in form of five hairy fascules at the base of the stamina. The receptacle of the *Carthamus tinctorius.*

PI'LULA. (*Pilula, æ,* f.; diminutive of *pila.*) A pill. A small round form of medicine, the size of a pea. The consistence of pills is best preserved by keeping the mass in bladders, and occasionally moistening it. In the direction of masses to be thus divided, the proper consistence is to be looked for at first, as well as its preservation afterward; for if the mass then become hard and dry, it is unfit for that division for which it was originally intended; and this is in many instances such an objection to the form, that it is doubtful whether, for the purposes of the pharmacopœia, the greater number of articles had not better be kept in powder, and their application to the formation of pills, left to extemporaneous direction.

PILULÆ ALOES COMPOSITÆ. Compound aloëtic pills. Take of extract of spike-aloe, powdered, an ounce; extract of gentian, half an ounce; oil of caraway, forty minims; simple syrup, as much as is sufficient. Beat them together, until they form a uniform mass. From fifteen to twenty-five grains prove moderately purgative and stomachic.

PILULÆ ALOES CUM MYRRHA. Aloëtic pills with myrrh. Take of extract of spike aloe, two ounces; saffron, myrrh, of each an ounce; simple syrup, as much as is sufficient. Powder the aloes and myrrh separately; then beat them all together until they form a uniform mass. From ten grains to a scruple of this pill, substituted for the *pilula Rufi,* prove stomachic and laxative, and are calculated for delicate females, especially where there is uterine obstruction.

PILULÆ AMMONIARETI CUPRI. An excellent tonic and diuretic pill, which may be given with advantage in dropsical diseases, where tonics and diuretics are indicated.

PILULÆ CAMBOGIÆ COMPOSITÆ. Compound gamboge pills. Take of gamboge powdered, extract of spike-aloe, powdered, compound cinnamon powder, of each a drachm; soap, two drachms. Mix the powders together; then having added the soap, beat the whole together until they are thoroughly incorporated. These pills are now first introduced into the London pharmacopœia, as forming a more active purgative pill than the pil. aloës cum myrrha, and in this way supplying an article very commonly necessary in practice. The dose is from ten grains to a scruple.

PILULÆ FERRI COMPOSITÆ. Compound iron pills. Pills of iron and myrrh. Take of myrrh, powdered, two drachms; subcarbonate of soda, sulphate of iron, sugar, of each, a drachm. Rub the myrrh with the subcarbonate of soda; add the sulphate of iron, and rub them again; then beat the whole together until they are thoroughly incorporated. These pills answer the same purpose as the mistura ferri composita. The dose is from ten grains to one scruple.

PILULÆ GALBANI COMPOSITÆ. Compound galbanum pills. Formerly called *pilulæ gummosæ*. Take of galbanum gum resin, an ounce; myrrh, sagapenum, of each an ounce and half; asafœtida gum resin, half an ounce; simple syrup, as much as is sufficient. Beat them together until they form a uniform mass. A stimulating antispasmodic and emmenagogue. From half a scruple to half a drachm may be given three times a day in nervous disorders of the stomach and intestines, in hysterical affections and hypochondriasis.

PILULÆ HYDRARGYRI. Mercurial pills. Often from its colour called the blue pill. Take of purified mercury, two drachms; confection of red roses, three drachms; liquorice-root, powdered, a drachm. Rub the mercury with the confection, until the globules disappear; then add the liquorice-root, and beat the whole together, until they are thoroughly incorporated. An alterative and anti-venereal pill, which mostly acts upon the bowels if given in sufficient quantity to attempt the removal of the venereal disease, and therefore requires the addition of opium. The dose is from five grains to a scruple. Three grains of the mass contain one of mercury. Joined with the squill pill, it forms an excellent expectorant and alterative, calculated to assist the removal of dropsical diseases of the chest, and asthmas attended with visceral obstruction.

PILULÆ HYDRARGYRI SUBMURIATIS COMPOSITÆ. Compound pills of submuriate of mercury. Take of submuriate of mercury, precipitated sulphuret of antimony, of each a drachm; guaiacum resin, powdered, two drachms. Rub the submuriate of mercury, first with the precipitated sulphuret of antimony, then with the guiacum resin, and add as much acacia mucilage as may be requisite to give the mass a proper consistence. This is intended as a substitute for the famed Plummer's pill. It is exhibited as a alternative in a variety of diseases, especially cutaneous eruptions, pains of the venereal or rheumatic kind, cancerous and schirrous affections, and chronic ophthalmia. The dose is from five to seven grains. In about five grains of the mass there is one grain of the submuriate of mercury.

PILULÆ SAPONIS CUM OPIO. Pills of soap and opium. Formerly called pilulæ saponaceæ. Take of hard opium powdered, half an ounce; hard soap, two ounces. Beat them together until they are thoroughly incorporated. The dose is from three to ten grains. Five grains of the mass contain one of opium.

PILULÆ SCILLÆ COMPOSITÆ. Compound squill pills. Take of squill root, fresh dried and powdered, a drachm; ginger-root, powdered, hard soap, of each three drachms: ammoniacum, powdered, two drachms. Mix the powders together; then beat them with the soap, adding as much simple syrup as may be sufficient to give a proper consistence. An attenuant, expectorant, and diuretic pill, mostly administered in the cure of asthma and dropsy. The dose is from ten grains to a scruple.

PI'LOS. (Πιλος, wool carded.)
1. In anatomy the short hair which is found all over the body. See *Capillus.*
2. In botany, a hair: which, according to Linnæus, is an excretory duct of a bristle-like form. They are fine, slender, cylindrical, flexible bodies, found on the surfaces of the herbaceous parts of plants. Some of them are the excretory ducts of glands, but many of them are not: and it is not easy to conceive any satisfactory opinion of their use to the plant.

When placed under the microscope they appear to be membraneous tubes, articulated in the majority of instances, often punctured; and in some plants, as the Borago laxiflora, covered with warts. They are either *simple* or undivided, *compound* or branched.

1. *Pili simplices*, the most common form of a simple hair is that of a jointed thread, generally too flexible to support itself, and thus most commonly found bent and waved. According to its degree of firmness, its quantity, and the mode of its application to the surfaces of stems and leaves, it constitutes the characteristic of surfaces: thus, the surface is termed *pilosus*, or hairy, when the hairs are few and scattered, but conspicuous,

as in Hieracium pilocella;—*lanatus*, woolly, when they are complicated, but nevertheless the single hairs are distinguishable, as in Verbascum;—*tomentosus*, shaggy, when they are so thickly matted that the individual hairs cannot be distinguished, and when the position of the hair is nearly parallel with the disk, being at the same time straight, or very slightly curved, and thick although unmatted: it constitutes the *silky* surface, as is seen on the leaves of Potentilla anserina, and Achemilla alpina. In some instances the simple hair is firm enough to support itself erect; in which case it is usually awl-shaped, and the articulations are shorter towards the base, as in Bryonia alba. It does not always, however, terminate in a point, but sometimes in a small knob, as in the newly-evolved succulent shoots of ligneous plants, Belladonna, &c. In some instances also, as on the under disk of the leaves of the Symphitum officinale, the simple hair is hooked towards apex; which occasions the velvety feeling when the finger is passed over the surface of those leaves, the convex part of the curve of the hair being that only which comes in contact with the finger. Another variety of the simple hair is that which has given rise to the term *glanduloso-ciliata:* it is a slender hollow thread, supporting a small, cup-shaped, glandular body, and is rather to be regarded as a stipate gland. ·

2. *Pili compositi* are either, *plumosus*, feathery, which is a simple hair with other hairs attached to it laterally, as in Hieracium undulatum; or it is *ramosus*, branched, that is, lateral hairs are given off from common stalks, as on the petiole of the gooseberry leaf, or it consists of an erect firm stem, from the summit of which smaller hairs diverge in every direction, as in Marrubium peregrinum; or it is *stellatus*, star-like, being composed of a number of simple diverging, awl-shaped hairs, springing from a common centre, which is a small knob sunk in the cutis, as on the leaves of marsh-mallow. Some authors have applied the term *ramenta* to small, flat, or stroplike hairs which are found on the leaves of some of the genus Begonia.—*Thomson.* See *Pubescence.*

PIMELITE. A variety of steatite found at Kosemutz, in Silesia.

PIME'NTA. (From *Pimienta*, the Spanish fir) Pepper. See *Myrtus pimenta.*

PIME'NTO. See *Myrtus pimenta.*

PIMPERNEL. See *Anagallis arvensis.*

Pimpernel, water. See *Veronica beccabunga.*

PIMPINE'LLA. (*Quasi bipinella*, or *bipenula;* from the double pennate order of its leaves.) 1. The name of a genus of plants in the Linnæan system. Class, *Pentandria;* Order, *Digynia.* Pimpinella.

2. The pharmacopœial name of the *Pimpinella alba* and *magna.*

PIMPINELLA ALBA. A variety of the *pimpinella magna,* the root of which is indifferently used with that of the greater pimpinell. The pimpinella saxifraga was also so called.

PIMPINELLA ANISUM. The systematic name of the anise plant. *Anisum; Anisum vulgare. Pimpinella —foliis radicalibus trifidis incisis,* of Linnæus. A native of Egypt. Anise seeds have an aromatic smell, and a pleasant, warm, and sweetish taste. An essential oil and distilled water are prepared from them, which are employed in flatulencies and gripes, to which children are more especially subject; also in weakness of the stomach, diarrhœas, and loss of tone in the primæ viæ. ·

PIMPINELLA ITALICA. The root which bears this name in some pharmacopœias is now fallen into disuse. See *Sanguisorba officinalis.*

PIMPINELLA MAGNA. The systematic name of the greater pimpinella. *Pimpinella nigra.* The root of this plant has been lately extolled in the cure of erysipelatous ulcerations, tinea, capitis, rheumatism, and other diseases.

PIMPINELLA NIGRA. See *Pimpinella magna.*

PIMPINELLA NOSTRAS. See *Pimpinella.*

PIMPINELLA SAXIFRAGA. The systematic name of the Burnet saxifrage. *Tragoselinum.* Several species of pimpinella were formerly used officinally; but the roots which obtain a place in the Materia Medica of the Edinburgh Pharmacopœia, are those of this species of saxifrage, the *Pimpinella—foliis pinnatis, foliolis radicalibus subrotundis, ummis linearibus,* of Linnæus. They have an unpleasant smell; and a hot, pungent, bitterish taste; they are recommended by several writers as a stomachic: in the way of gargle, they have been employed for dissolving viscid mucus, and to stimulate the tongue when that organ becomes paralytic.

PINASTE'LLUM. (From *pinus*, the pine-tree; so called because its leaves resemble those of the pine-tree.) Hog's fennel. See *Peucedanum silans*.

PI'NEA. See *Pinus pinea*.

PINEAL. (*Pinealis*; from *pinea*, a pine-apple, from its supposed resemblance to that fruit.) Formed like the fruit of the pine.

PINEAL GLAND. *Glandula pinealis; Conarium*. A small heart-like substance, about the size of a pea, situated immediately over the corpora quadrigemina, and hanging from the *thalami nervorum opticorum* by two crura or peduncles. Its use is not known. It was formerly supposed to be the seat of the soul.

PINE-APPLE. See *Bromelia ananus*.

Pine-thistle. See *Atractylis gummifera*.

PI'NEUS PURGANS. See *Jatropha curcas*.

PINGUE'DO. (From *pinguis*, fat.) Fat. See *Fat*.

PINGUI'CULA. (From *pinguis*, fat: so called because its leaves are fat to the touch.) The name of a genus of plants. Class, *Diandria*; Order, *Monogynia*.

PINGUICULA VULGARIS. *Sanicula montana; Sanicula eboracensis; Viola palustris: Liparis; Cucullata; Dodecatheon; Plinii*. Butterwort. Yorkshire sanicle. The remarkable unctuosity of this plant has caused it to be applied to chaps, and as a pomatum to the hair. Decoctions of the leaves in broths are used by the common people in Wales as a cathartic.

PINHO'NES INDICI. See *Jatropha curcas*.

PINITE. Micarelle of Kirwan. A blackish green mineral, consisting of silica, alumina, and oxide of iron, found in the granite of St. Michael's Mount, Cornwall, and in porphyry in Scotland.

PINK, INDIAN. See *Spigelia*.

PINNA. (Πιννα, a wing.) 1. The name of the lateral and inferior part of the nose, and the broad part of the ear

2. The leaflet of a pinnate leaf. See *Leaf*.

PINNA'CULUM. (Dim. of *pinna*, a wing.) A pinnacle. A name of the uvula from its shape.

PINNATIFIDUS. Pinnatifid: applied to leaves which are cut transversely into several oblong parallel segments; as in Ipomosis, and Myriophyllum verticillatum.

PINNATUS. Applied to a leaf which has several leaflets proceeding laterally from one stalk, and imitates a pinnatifid leaf. Of this there are several kinds.

1. *Folium pinnatum cum impari*, with an odd or terminal leaflet; as in roses.

2. *F. p. cirrosum*, with a tendril, when furnished with a tendril instead of the odd leaflet; as in the pea and vetch tribe.

3. *F. abruptè pinnatum*, abruptly, without either a terminal leaflet or a tendril; as in the genus Mimosa.

4. *F. oppositè pinnatum*, oppositely, when the leaflets are opposite or in pairs; as in saintfoin, roses, and sium angustifolium.

5. *F. alternatim pinnatum*, alternately, when they are alternate; as in Viscia dumetorum.

6. *F. interruptè pinnatum*, interruptedly, when the principal leaflets are ranged alternately with an intermediate series of smaller ones; as in Spiræa filipendula and fumaria.

7. *F. articulatè pinnatum*, jointedly, with apparent joints in the common foot-stalk; as in Weinmannia pinnata.

8 *F. decursivè pinnatum*, decurrently, when the leaflets are decurrent; as in Eryngium campestre.

9 *F. lyrato pinnatum*, in a lyrate manner, having the terminal leaflet largest, and the rest gradually smaller as they approach the base; as in Erysimum præcox: and with intermediate smaller leaflets; as in Geum rivale, and the common turnip.

10. *F. verticillato pinnatum*, in a whirled manner, the leaflets cut into five divaricated segments, embracing the foot-stalk; as in Sium verticillatum.

PINNULA. The leaflet of bi and tripinnate leaves.

PI'NUS. The name of a genus of plants in the Linnæan system. Class, *Monœcia*; Order, *Monadelphia*. The pine-tree.

PINUS ABIES. *Elate; Thelaia*. The Norway

spruce fir, which affords the Burgundy pitch and common frankincense.

1. *Pix arida*. Formerly called *Pix burgundica*, from the place it was made at. The prepared resin of *Pinus abies—foliis solitariis, subtetragonis acutius culis distichis, ramis infra nudis conis cylindraceis*, of Linnæus. It is of a solid consistence, yet somewhat soft, of a reddish brown colour, and not disagreeable smell. It is used externally as a stimulant in form of plaster in catarrh, pertussis, and dyspnœa.

2. *Abietis resina; Thus*. Common frankincense. This is a spontaneous exudation, and is brought in small masses, or tears, chiefly from Germany, but partly and purest from France. It is applicable to the same purposes as Burgundy pitch, but little used at present.

PINUS BALSAMEA. The systematic name of the tree which affords the Canada balsam. *Abies canadensis* The Canada balsam is one of the purest turpentines, procured from the *Pinus balsamea* of Linnæus, and imported from Canada. For its properties, see *Turpentine*.

PINUS CEDRUS. The wood of this species, cedar wood, is very odorous, more fragrant than that of the fir, and it possesses similar virtues.

PINUS CEMBRA. This affords the Carpathian balsam. *Oleum germanis; Carpathicum*. This balsam is obtained both by wounding the young branches of the *Pinus—foliis quinus, levibus* of Linnæus, and by boiling them. It is mostly diluted with turpentine, and comes to us in a very liquid and pellucid state, rather white.

PINUS LARIX. The systematic name of the tree which gives us the agaric and Venice turpentine. The larch-tree. The Venice turpentine issues spontaneously through the bark of the *Pinus—foliis fasciculatis mollibus obtusiusculis bracteis extra squamas strobilorum extantibus*. Hort. Kew. It is usually thinner than any of the other sorts; of a clear whitish or pale yellowish colour; a hot, pungent, bitterish, disagreeable taste; and a strong smell, without any thing of the aromatic flavour of the Chian kind. For its virtues, see *Turpentine*. See also *Boletus laricis*.

PINUS PICEA. The systematic name of the silver fir.

PINUS PINEA. The systematic name of the stone pine-tree. The young and fresh fruit of this plant is eaten in some countries in the same manner as almonds are here, either alone or with sugar. They are nutritive, aperient, and diuretic.

PINUS SYLVESTRIS. The systematic name of the Scotch fir. *Pinus—foliis geminis rigidis, conis, ovato-conicis longitudine foliorum subgeminis basi rotundatis* of Linnæus, which affords the following officinals.

1. *Common turpentine* is the juice which flows out on the tree being wounded in hot weather. See *Turpentine*.

2. From this the oil is obtained by distillation, mostly with water, in which case yellow resin is left; but if without addition, the residuum is common resin, or colophony. The oil is ordered to be purified in the pharmacopœia. See *Oleum terebinthinæ rectificatum*.

3. When the coal begins to check the exudation of the juice, part of this concretes in the wounds; which is collected, and termed *galipot* in Provence, *barras* in Guienne, sometimes also *white resin*, when thoroughly hardened by long exposure to the air. See *Resina flava*, and *alba*.

4. The *Pix liquida*, or tar, is produced by cutting the wood into pieces, which are enclosed in a large oven constructed for the purpose. It is well known for its economical uses. Tar-water, or water impregnated with the more soluble parts of tar, was some time ago a very fashionable remedy in a variety of complaints, but is in the present practice fallen into disuse.

5. Common pitch is tar inspissated; it is now termed in the pharmacopœia, *Resina nigra*.

PI'PER. (Πεπερι; from πεπτω, to concoct; because by its heat it assists digestion.) Pepper. The name of a genus of plants in the Linnæan system. Class, *Diandria*; Order, *Trigynia*.

PIPER ALBUM. See *Piper nigrum*.

PIPER BRASILIANUM. See *Capsicum annuum*.

PIPER CALECUTICUM. See *Capsicum annuum*.

PIPER CARYOPHYLLATUM. See *Myrtus pimenta*.

PIPER CAUDATUM. See *Piper cubeba*.

PIPER CUBEBA. The plant, the berries of which are called cubebs. *Piper caudatum; Cumamus. Piper—foliis oblique ovatis, seu oblongus venosis acutis, spica solitaria pedunculata oppositifolia, fructibus pedicel-

latis, of Linnæus. The dried berries are of an ash-brown colour, generally wrinkled, and resembling pepper, but furnished each with a slender stalk. They are a warm spice, of a pleasant smell, and moderately pungent taste, imported from Java: and may be exhibited in all cases where warm spicy medicines are indicated, but they are inferior to pepper. Of late they have been successfully given internally in the cure of venereal gonorrhœa.

PIPER DECORTICATUM. White pepper.

PIPER FAVASCI. The clove-berry tree.

PIPER GUINEENSE. See *Capsicum annuum.*

PIPER HISPANICUM. See *Capsicum annuum.*

PIPER INDICUM. See *Capsicum annuum.*

PIPER JAMAICENSE. See *Myrtus pimenta.*

PIPER LONGUM. *Macropiper; Acapatli; Catu-tripali: Pimpilim.* Long pepper. *Piper—foliis cordatis petiolatis sessilibusque*, of Linnæus. The berries or grains of this plant are gathered while green, and dried in the heat of the sun, when they change to a blackish or dark-gray colour. They possess precisely the same qualities as the Cayenne pepper, only in a weaker degree.

PIPER LUSITANICUM. See *Capsicum annuum.*

PIPER MURALE. See *Sedum acre.*

PIPER NIGRUM. *Melanopiper; Molagocodi; Lada; Piper aromaticum.* Black pepper. This species of pepper is obtained in the East Indies, from the *Piper —foliis ovatis septem-nerviis glabris, petiolis simplietssimis*, of Linnæus. Its virtues are similar to those of the other peppers. The black and white pepper are both obtained from the same tree, the difference depending on their preparation and degrees of maturity. Pelletier has extracted a new vegetable principle from black pepper, in which the active part of the grain resides, to which the name of *piperine* is given. To obtain it, black pepper was digested repeatedly in alkohol, and the solution evaporated until a fatty resinous matter was left. This, on being washed in warm water, became of a good green colour. It had a hot and burning taste; dissolved readily in alkohol, less so in æther. Concentrated sulphuric acid gave it a fine scarlet colour. The alkoholic solution after some days deposited crystals, which were purified by repeated crystallization in alkohol and æther. They then formed colourless four-sided prisms, with single inclined terminations. They have scarcely any taste. Boiling water dissolves a small portion; but not cold water. They are soluble in acetic acid, from which combination feather-formed crystals are obtained. This substance fuses at 212° F. The fatty matter left after extracting the piperine, is solid at a temperature near 32°, but liquefies at a slight heat. It has an extremely bitter and acrid taste, is very slightly volatile, tending rather to decompose than to rise in vapour. It may be considered as composed of two oils, one volatile and balsamic; the other more fixed, and containing the acrimony of the pepper.

PIPERINE. The active principle of pepper. See *Piper nigrum.*

PIPERI'TIS. (From *piper*, pepper: so called because its leaves and roots are biting like pepper to the taste.) The herb dittany or lepidium and peppermint.

PIPERITUS. (From *piper*, pepper.) Peppered.

PIPERITÆ. The name of an order of plants in Linnæus's Fragments of a Natural Method, consisting of the Piper, and such as, like it, have flowers in a thick spike.

PIRAMIDALIA CORPORA. See *Corpus pyramidale.*

PIRAMIDA'LIS. (So called from its form.) Of a pyramidal figure.

Piss-a-bed. See *Leontodon taraxacum.*

PISIFORM. (*Pisiformis;* from *pisum*, a pea, and *forma*, likeness.) Pea-like.

PISIFO'RME OS. The fourth bone of the first row of the carpus.

["PISOLITE. This variety of carbonate of lime occurs in globular or spheroidal concretions, usually about the size of a *pea*, though sometimes larger. These concretions are composed of distinct, concentric layers, and almost invariably contain a grain of sand, or some other foreign substance, as a *nucleus.* The pisolite is nearly or quite opaque, and has a dull fracture. Its colour is usually white, often dull or with a shade of yellow, &c.

"These concretions, sometimes detached and scattered are more frequently united by a calcareous cement. Thus united, they form masses of various sizes, and also continuous beds, which are sometimes covered with alluvial deposites.

"The pisolite has been found chiefly near the warm springs of Carlsbad in Bohemia, and the baths of St. Philip in Tuscany.

"The structure of the pisolite, and the situation in which it is found, seem to indicate the mode of formation. The particles of sand, or nuclei of these concretions, were probably raised and suspended by an agitated or rotary motion of certain springs or streams, strongly impregnated with calcareous particles. These particles were then deposited around the floating nuclei, which, being thus incrusted with a series of layers, became sufficiently heavy to fall through the fluid."—*Cleav. Min.* A.]

PISMIRE. See *Formica rufa.*

PISSASPHA'LTUS. (From πισσα, pitch, and ασφαλτος, bitumen.) The thicker kind of rock-oil.

PISTA'CIA. (Πιςακια, supposed to be a Syrian word.) The name of a genus of plants in the Linnæan system. Class, *Diœcia;* Order, *Pentandria.*

PISTACIA LENTISCUS. The systematic name of the tree which affords the mastich. *Mastiche; Mastix. Pistacia—foliis abruptè pinnatis, foliolis lanceolatis*, of Linnæus. A native of the south of Europe. In the island of Chio, the officinal mastich is obtained most abundantly; and, according to Tournefort, by making transverse incisions in the bark of the tree, from whence the mastich exudes in drops, which are suffered to run down to the ground, when, after sufficient time is allowed for their concretion, they are collected for use. Mastich is brought to us in small, yellowish, transparent, brittle tears, or grains; it has a light agreeable smell, especially when rubbed or heated; on being chewed, it first crumbles, soon after sticks together, and becomes soft and white, like wax, without impressing any considerable taste. No volatile oil is obtained from this substance when distilled with water. Pure alkohol and oil of turpentine dissolve it; water scarcely acts upon it; though by mastication it becomes soft and tough, like wax. When chewed a little while, however, it is white, opaque, and brittle, so as not to be softened again by chewing. The part insoluble in alkohol much resembles in its properties caoutchouc. It is considered to be a mild corroborant and astringent; and as possessing a balsamic power, it has been recommended in hæmoptysis, proceeding from ulceration, leucorrhœa, debility of the stomach, and in diarrhœas and internal ulcerations. Chewing this drug has likewise been said to have been of use in pains of the teeth and gums, and in some catarrhal complaints; it is, however, in the present day, seldom used either externally or internally. The wood abounds with the resinous principle, and a tincture may be obtained from it, which is esteemed in some countries in the cure of hæmorrhages, dysenteries, and gout.

PISTACIA NUX. See *Pistacia vera.*

PISTACIA TEREBINTHUS. The systematic name of the tree which gives out the Cyprus turpentine. *Terebinthina de Chio.* Chio or Chian turpentine. This substance is classed among the resins. It is procured by wounding the bark of the trunk of the tree. The best Chio turpentine is about the consistence of honey, very tenacious, clear, and almost transparent; of a white colour, inclining to yellow, and a fragrant smell, moderately warm to the taste, but free from acrimony and bitterness. Its medicinal qualities are similar to those of the other turpentines. See *Turpentines.*

PISTACIA VERA. The systematic name of a large tree, which affords the pistachio-nut. *Pistacia vera—foliis impari pinnatis—foliolis subovatis recurvis*, of Linnæus. An oblong pointed nut, about the size and shape of a filbert, including a kernel of a pale greenish colour, covered with a yellow or greenish skin. Pistachio-nuts have a sweetish unctuous taste, resembling that of sweet almonds, and, like the latter, afford an oil, and may be formed into an emulsion.

Pistachio-nut. See *Pistacia vera.*

PISTACITE. See *Epidote.*

PISTILLUM. (*Pistillum*, a pestle, from its likeness.) A pistil or pointal: the female genital organ of a flower, which, being no less essential than the male, stands within them in the centre of the flower. Linnæus conceived the pistil originated from the pith, and the stamens from the wood, and hence constructed an ingenious hypothesis relative to the propagation of vegetables, which is not destitute of observations and analogies to support it, but not countenanced by the anatomy and physiology of the parts.

A pistil consists of three parts.

1. The *germen*, or rudiment of the young fruit and seed, which of course is essential.

2. The *stylus*, or style, various in length and thickness, sometimes wanting, and, when present, serving merely to elevate the third part.

3. The *stigma*, which is indispensable. The *Nicotiana tabacum* has these organs well displayed.

PISTOLO'CHIA. (From πιςος, faithful, and λοχεια, parturition: so called because it was thought to promote delivery.) Birthwort. See *Aristolochia.*

PISUM. (An ancient name, the origin of which is lost in its antiquity.) The name of a genus of plants. Class, *Diadelphia;* Order, *Decandria.* The pea.

PISUM SATIVUM. The common pea. A very nutritious, but somewhat flatulent article of food.

PITCAIRN, ARCHIBALD, was born at Edinburgh, in 1652. He applied to the study of divinity, and afterward of the law, in that university, with such intensity, that he was threatened with symptoms of consumption, for the removal of which he went to Montpelier, where his attention was diverted to medicine; on his return, he applied himself zealously to the mathematics, which appearing to him capable of elucidating medical subjects, he was determined in consequence to adopt this profession. After attending diligently to the various branches at Edinburgh, he went to complete his medical studies at Paris, and then returned to settle in his native place, where he quickly obtained a large practice and extensive reputation. In 1688 he published a little tract to establish Harvey's claim to the Discovery of the Circulation. About four years after he was invited to become professor of physic at Leyden, which he accepted accordingly; and he ranked among his pupils the celebrated Boerhaave. However, his mathematical illustrations of medicine not being favourably received, he relinquished the appointment in about a year. He returned then to practise at Edinburgh, where his life terminated in 1713. He published while at Leyden, and subsequently, several dissertations to prove the utility of mathematics in medical discussion; which were more than once reprinted. After his death, his lectures were made public, under the title of " Elementa Medicinæ Physico-Mathematica."

PITCH. *Pix.* See *Resina.*

Pitch, *Burgundy.* See *Pinus abies.*

Pitch, *Jews'.* See *Bitumen judaicum.*

Pitch-tree. See *Pinus abies.*

PITCHSTONE. A subspecies of indivisible quartz of a green colour, and vitreo-resinous lustre found in Scotland and Ireland.

PITTA'CIUM. (From πιττα, pitch.) A pitch plaster.

PITTIZITE. Pitchy iron ore.

PITTO'TA. (From πιττα, pitch.) Medicines in which pitch is the principal ingredient.

PITUI'TA. Phlegm, that is, viscid and glutinous mucus.

PITUITARY. Of or belonging to phlegm.

PITUITARY GLAND. *Glandula pituitaria.* A gland situated within the cranium, between a duplicature of the dura mater, in the sella turcica of the sphenoid bone.

PITUITARY MEMBRANE. *Membrana pituitaria.* Schneiderian membrane. The mucous membrane that lines the nostrils and sinuses, communicating with the nose, is so called, because it secretes the mucus of those parts, to which the ancients assigned the name of *pituita.*

PITYRI'ASIS. (From πιτυρον, bran: so named from its branny-like appearance.) A genus in the second order, or scaly diseases, of Dr. Willan's cutaneous diseases. The pityriasis consists of irregular patches of small thin scales, which repeatedly form and separate, but never collect into crusts, nor are attended with redness or inflammation, as in the lepra and scaly tetter. Dr. Willan distinguishes pityriasis from the porrigo of the Latins, which has a more extensive signification, and comprehends a disease of the scalp, terminating in ulceration; whereas the former is, by the best Greek authors, represented as always dry and scaly. Thus, according to Alexander and Paulus, pityriasis is characterized by " the separation of slight furfuraceous substances from the surface of the head, or other parts of the body, without ulceration." Their
186

account of this appearance is conformable to experience; and the two varieties of it which they have pointed out may be denominated, *Pityriasis capitis,* and *Pityriasis versicolor.*

1. *Pityriasis capitis,* when it affects very young infants, is termed by nurses the dandriff. It appears at the upper edge of the forehead and temples, as a slight whitish scurf set in the form of a horse-shoe; on other parts of the head there are large scales, at a distance from each other, flat, and semipellucid. Sometimes, however, they nearly cover the whole of the hairy scalp, being close together, and imbricated. A similar appearance may take place in adults; but it is usually the effect of lepra, scaly tetter, or some general disease of the skin.

Elderly persons have the pityriasis capitis in nearly the same form as infants; the only difference is, that this complaint in old people occasions larger exfoliations of the cuticle.

2. The *pityriasis versicolor* chiefly affects the arms, breast, and abdomen. It is diffused very irregularly; and being of a different colour from the usual skin colour, it exhibits a singular chequered appearance. These irregular patches, which are at first small, and of a brown or yellow hue, appear at the scrobiculus cordis, about the mammæ, clavicles, &c. Enlarging gradually, they assume a tesselated form; in other cases they are branched, so as to resemble the foliaceous lichens growing on the bark of trees; and sometimes when the discoloration is not continuous, they suggest the idea of a map being distributed on the skin like islands, continents, peninsulas, &c. All the discoloured parts are slightly rough, with minute scales, which soon fall off, but are constantly replaced by others. This scurf, or scaliness, is most conspicuous on the sides and epigastric region. The cuticular lines are somewhat deeper in the patches than on the contiguous parts; but there is no elevated border, or distinguishing boundary between the discoloured part of the skin, and that which retains its natural colour The discoloration rarely extends over the whole body. It is strongest and fullest round the umbilicus, on the breasts, and sides; it seldom appears in the skin over the sternum, or along the spine of the back. Interstices of proper skin colour are more numerous, and largest at the lower part of the abdomen and back, where the scales are often small, distinct, and a little depressed. The face, nates, and lower extremities are least affected; the patches are found upon the arms, but mostly on the inside, where they are distinct and of different sizes. The pityriasis versicolor is not a cuticular disease; for when the cuticle is abraded from any of the patches, the sallow colour remains as before in the skin or rete mucosum. This singular appearance is not attended with any internal disorder, nor with any troublesome symptom, except a slight itching or irritation felt on getting into bed, and after strong exercise, or drinking warm liquors. There is in some cases a slight exanthema, partially distributed among the discoloured patches; and sometimes an appearance like the lichen pilaris; but eruptions of this kind are not permanent, neither do they produce any change in the original form of the complaint. The duration of the pityriasis versicolor is always considerable. Dr. Willan has observed its continuance in some persons for four, five, or six years. It is not limited to any age or sex. Its causes are not pointed out with certainty. Several patients have referred it to fruit taken in too great quantities; some have thought it was produced by eating mushrooms; others by exposure to sudden alterations of cold and heat. In some individuals, who had an irritable skin, and occasionally used violent exercise, the complaint has been produced, or at least much aggravated, by wearing flannel next to the skin. It is likewise often observed in persons who had resided for a length of time in a tropical climate.

PIX. (*Pix, picis,* f.; from πισσα.) Pitch. See *Resina.*

PIX ARIDA. See *Pinus abies.*

PIX BURGUNDICA. See *Pinus abies.*

PIX LIQUIDA. Tar or liquid pitch. See *Pinus sylvestris.*

PLACE'BO. I will please: an epithet given to any medicine adapted more to please than benefit the patient.

PLACE'NTA. (From πλακους, a cake, so called

from its resemblance to a cake.) The afterbirth. The membranes of the ovum have usually been mentioned as two, the amnion and the chorion; and the latter has again been divided into the true and the false. The third membrane (which, from its appearance, has likewise been called the villous or spongy, and from the consideration of it as the inner lamina of the uterus, cast off like the exuviæ of some animals, the decidua,) has been described by Harvey, not as one of the membranes of the ovum, but as a production of the uterus. The following is the order of the membranes of the ovum, at the full period of gestation: 1st, There is the outer or connecting, which is flocculent, spongy, and extremely vascular, completely investing the whole ovum, and lining the uterus. 2dly, The middle membrane, which is nearly pellucid, with a very few small blood-vessels scattered over it, and which forms a covering to the placenta and funis, but does not pass between the placenta and uterus. 3dly, The inner membrane, which is transparent, of a firmer texture than the others, and lines the whole ovum, making, like the middle membrane, a covering for the placenta and funis with the two last. The ovum is clothed when it passes from the ovarium into the uterus, where the first is provided for its reception.

These membranes, in the advanced state of pregnancy, cohere slightly to each other, though, in some ova, there is a considerable quantity of fluid collected between them, which, being discharged when one of the outer membranes is broken, forms one of the circumstances which have been distinguished by the name of by or false waters.

Between the middle and inner membrane, upon or near the funis, there is a small, flat, and oblong body, which, in the early part of pregnancy, seems to be a vesicle containing milky lymph, which afterward becomes of a firm, and apparently fatty texture. This is called the *vesicula umbilicalis* ; but its use is not known.

The placenta is a circular, flat, vascular, and apparently fleshy substance, different in its diameter in different subjects, but usually extending about six inches, or upwards, over about one-fourth part of the outside of the ovum in pregnant women. It is more than one inch in thickness in the middle, and becomes gradually thinner towards the circumference from which the membranes are continued. The placenta is the principal medium by which the communication between the parent and child is preserved; but, though all have allowed the importance of the office which it performs, there has been a variety of opinions on the nature of that office, and of the manner in which it is executed.

The surface of the placenta, which is attached to the uterus by the intervention of the connecting membrane, is lobulated and convex; but the other, which is covered with the amnion and chorion, is concave and smooth, except the little eminence made by the blood-vessels. It is seldom found attached to the same part of the uterus in two successive births; and, though it most frequently adheres to the anterior part, it is occasionally fixed to any other, even to the os uteri, in which state it becomes a cause of a dangerous hæmorrhage at the time of parturition. The placenta is composed of arteries and veins, with a mixture of pulpy or cellular substance. Of these vessels there are two orders, very curiously interwoven with each other. The first is a continuation of those from the funis, which ramify on the internal surface of the placenta, the arteries running over the veins, which is a circumstance peculiar to the placenta ; and then, sinking into its substance, anastomose and divide into innumerable small branches. The second order proceeds from the uterus; and these ramify in a similar manner with those from the funis, as appears when a placenta is injected from those of the parent. The veins, in their ramifications, accompany the arteries as in other parts. There have been many different opinions with respect to the manner in which the blood circulates between the parent and child, during its continuance in the uterus. For a long time it was believed that the intercourse between them was uninterrupted, and that the blood propelled by the powers of the parent pervaded, by a continuance of the same force, the vascular system of the fœtus ; but repeated attempts having been made, without success, to inject the whole placenta, funis and fœtus, from the vessels of the parent, or any part of the uterus, from the vessels of the funis it is

now generally allowed, that the two systems of vessels in the placenta, one of which may be called maternal, the other fœtal, are distinct. It is also admitted, that the blood of the fœtus is, with regard to its formation, increase, and circulation, unconnected with, and totally independent of the parent; except that the matter by which the blood of the fœtus is formed must be derived from the parent. It is thought that which has probably undergone some preparatory changes in its passage through the uterus, is conducted by the uterine or maternal arteries of the placenta to some cells or small cavities, in which it is deposited: and that some part of it, or something secreted from it, is absorbed by the fœtal veins of the placenta, and by them conveyed to the fœtus for its nutriment. When the blood which circulates in the fœtus requires any alteration in its qualities, or when it has gone through the course of the circulation, it is carried by the arteries of the funis to the placenta, in the cells of which it is deposited, and then absorbed by the maternal veins of the placenta, and conducted to the uterus, whence it may enter the common circulation of the parent. Thus it appears, according to the opinion of Harvey, that the placenta performs the office of a gland, conveying air, or secreting the nutritious juices from the blood brought from the parent by the arteries of the uterus, and carried to the fœtus by the veins of the funis, in a manner probably not unlike to that in which milk is secreted and absorbed from the breasts. The veins in the placenta are mentioned as the absorbents, because no lymphatic vessels have yet been found in the placenta or funis; nor are there any nerves in these parts; so that the only communication hitherto discovered between the parent and child, is by the sanguineous system. The proofs of the manner in which the blood circulates between the parent and child are chiefly drawn from observations made upon the funis. When it was supposed that the child was supplied with blood in a direct stream from the parent, it was asserted that, on the division of the funis, if that part next to the placenta was not secured by a ligature, the parent would be brought into extreme danger by the hæmorrhage which must necessarily follow. But this opinion, which laid the foundation of several peculiarities in the management of the funis and placenta, is proved not to be true: for, if the funis be compressed immediately after the birth of the child, and while the circulation in it is going on, the arteries between the part compressed and the child throb violently, but those between the compression and the placenta have no pulsation; but the vein between the part compressed and the placenta swells, and that part next to the fœtus becomes flaccid; but if, under the same circumstances, the funis be divided, and that part next the child be not secured, the child would be in danger of losing its life by the hæmorrhage; yet the mother would suffer no inconvenience if the other part was neglected. It is, moreover, proved, that a woman may die of an hæmorrhage occasioned by a separation of the placenta, and the child be nevertheless born, after her death, in perfect health. But if the placenta be injured, without separation, either by the rupture of the vessels which pass upon its inner surface, or in any other way, the child being deprived of its proper blood, would perish, yet the parent might escape without injury.

The receptacle of the fructification of plants has been called placenta. See *Receptaculum*

PLACE'NTULA. (Diminutive of *placenta*.) A small placenta.

PLADARO'TIS. (From πλαδαρος, moist, flaccid.) A fungous and flaccid tumour within the eyelid.

Plaited leaf. See *Plicatus.*

PLANTA'GO. (From *planta*, the sole of the feet: so called from the shape of its leaves, or because its leaves lie upon the ground and are trodden upon.) 1. The name of a genus of plants in the Linnæan system. Class, *Tetrandria*; Order, *Monogynia*. The plantain.

2. The pharmacopœial name of the *Plantago major.*

PLANTAGO CORONOPUS. The systematic name of the buck's-horn plantain. *Coronopodium; Cornu cervinum; Stella terræ*. Its medicinal virtues are the same as those of the other plantains.

PLANTAGO LATIFOLIA. See *Plantago major.*

PLANTAGO MAJOR. The systematic name of the broad-leaved plantain. *Centinervia; Heptapleurum*

Polyneuron ; Plantago latifolia. Plantago—foliis ovatis glabris, scapo tereti, spica flosculis imbricatis, of Linnæus. This plant was retained until very lately in the Materia Medica of the Edinburgh College, in which the leaves are mentioned as the pharmaceutical part of the plant; they have a weak herbaceous smell, an austere, bitterish, subsaline taste ; and their qualities are said to be refrigerant, attenuating, substyptic, and diuretic.

PLANTAGO PSYLLIUM. The systematic name of the branching plantain. *Psyllium; Pulicaris herba; Crystallion,* and *Cynomoia,* of Oribasius. Flea-wort. The seeds of this plant, *Plantago—caule ramoso herbaceo, foliis subdentatis, recurvatis ; capitulis aphyllis,* of Linnæus, have a nauseous mucilaginous taste, and no remarkable smell. The decoction of the seeds is recommended in hoarseness and asperity of the fauces.

PLANTAIN. See *Plantago.*

PLANTAIN-TREE. See *Musa paradisiaca.*

PLANTA'RIS. (From *planta,* the sole of the foot.) *Tibialis gracilis,* vulgo *plantaris,* of Winslow. *Extensor tarsi minor,* vulgo *plantaris,* of Douglas. A muscle of the foot, situated on the leg, that assists the soleus, and pulls the capsular ligament of the knee from between the bones. It is sometimes, though seldom, found wanting on both sides. This long and slender muscle, which is situated under the gastrocnemius externus, arises, by a thin fleshy origin, from the upper and back part of the outer condyle of the os femoris. It adheres to the capsular ligament of the 'oint ; and after running obliquely downwards and outwards, for the space of three or four inches, along the second origin of the gastrocnemius internus, and under the gastrocnemius externus, terminates in a long, thin, and slender tendon, which adheres to the inside of the tendo Achillis, and is inserted into the inside of the posterior part of the os calcis. This tendon sometimes sends off an aponeurosis that loses itself in the capsular ligament, but it does not at all contribute to form the aponeurosis that is spread over the sole of the foot, as was formerly supposed, and as its name would seem to imply. Its use is to assist the gastrocnemii in extending the foot. It likewise serves to prevent the capsular ligament of the knee from being pinched.

PLANTS, SEXUAL SYSTEM OF. The sexual system of plants was invented by the immortal Linnæus, professor of physic and botany at Upsal, in Sweden. It is founded on the parts of fructification, viz. the stamens and pistils; these having been observed with more accuracy since the discovery of the uses for which nature has assigned them, a new set of principles has been derived from them, by means of which the distribution of plants has been brought to a greater precision, and rendered more conformable to true philosophy, in this system, than in any one of those which preceded it. The author does not pretend to call it a natural system, he gives it as artificial only, and modestly owns his inability to detect the order pursued by nature in her vegetable productions; but of this he seems confident, that no natural order can ever be framed without taking in the materials out of which he has raised his own ; and urges the necessity of admitting artificial systems for convenience, till one truly natural shall appear. Linnæus has given us his *Fragmenta methodi naturalis,* in which he has made a distribution of plants under various orders, putting together in each such as appear to have a natural affinity to each other ; this, after a long and fruitless search after the natural method, he gives as the result of his own speculation, for the assistance of such as may engage in the same pursuit.

Not able to form a system after the natural method, Linnæus was more fully convinced of the absolute necessity of adopting an artificial one. For the student to enter into the advantages this system maintain over all others, it is necessary that he be instructed in the science of botany, which will amply repay him for his inquiry. The following is a short outline of the sexual system.

The parts of fructification of a plant are,

1. The *calyx,* called also the empalement, or flower-cup. See *Calyx,* and *Anthodium.*

2. The *corolla,* or foliation, which is the gaudy part of the flower, called vulgarly the leaves of the flower. See *Corolla.*

3. The *stamens,* or threads, called also the chives ; these are considered as the male parts of the flower. See *Stamen.*

4. The *pistil,* or pointal, which is the female part. See *Pistillum.*

5. The *seed-vessel.* See *Pericarpium.*

6. The *seed.* See *Semen.*

7. The *receptacle,* or base, on which these parts are seated. See *Receptaculum.*

The first four, are properly parts of the flower, and the last three parts of the fruit. It is from the number proportion, position, and other circumstances attending these parts of the fructification, that the classes and orders, and the genera they contain, are to be characterized, according to the sexual system.

Such flowers as want the stamens, and have the pistil, are termed *female.*

Those flowers which have the stamens, and want the pistils, are called *male.*

Flowers which have both stamens and pistils are said to be *hermaphrodite.*

Neuter flowers are such as have neither stamens nor pistils.

Hermaphrodite flowers are sometimes distinguished into *male hermaphrodites* and *female hermaphrodites.* This distinction takes place when, although the flower contains the parts belonging to each sex, one of them proves abortive or ineffectual ; if the defect be in the stamina, it is a female hermaphrodite, if in the pistil, a male one.

Plants, in regard to sex, take also their denominations in the following manner:

1. *Hermaphrodite plants* are such as bear flowers *upon the same root* that are all hermaphrodite.

2. *Androgynous plants* are such as, *upon the same root,* bear both male and female flowers, distinct from each other, that is, in separate flowers.

3. *Male plants,* such as bear male flowers only upon the same root.

4. *Female plants,* such as bear female flowers only upon the same root.

5. *Polygamous plants,* such as, either on the same or on different roots, bear hermaphrodite flowers, and flowers of either or both sexes.

The first general division of the whole body of vegetables is, in the sexual system, into twenty-four *classes ;* these again are subdivided into *orders ;* the orders into *genera ;* the genera into *species ;* and the species into *varieties,* where they are worthy of note.

A Table of the Classes and Orders.

CLASSES.	ORDERS.					
1. Monandria.	Monogynia.	Digynia.				
2. Diandria.	Monogynia.	Digynia.	Trigynia.			
3. Triandria.	Monogynia.	Digynia.	Trigynia.			
4. Tetrandria.	Monogynia.	Digynia.	Tetragynia.			
5. Pentandria.	Monogynia.	Digynia.	Trigynia.	Tetragynia.	Pentagynia.	Polygynia.
6. Hexandria.	Monogynia.	Digynia.	Trigynia.	Tetragynia.	Polygynia.	
7. Heptandria.	Monogynia.	Digynia.	Tetragynia.	Heptagynia.		
8. Octandria.	Monogynia.	Digynia.	Trigynia.	Tetragynia.		
9. Enneandria.	Monogynia.	Trigynia.	Hexagynia.			
10. Decandria.	Monogynia.	Digynia.	Trigynia.	Pentagynia.	Decagynia.	
11. Dodecandria.	Monogynia.	Digynia.	Trigynia.	Pentagynia.	Dodecagynia.	
12. Icosandria.	Monogynia.	Digynia.	Trigynia.	Pentagynia.	Polygynia.	
13. Polyandria.	Monogynia.	Digynia.	Trigynia.	Tetragynia.	Pentagynia.	Hexagynia. Polygynia
14. Didynamia.	Gymnospermia.	Angiospermia.				
15. Tetradynamia.	Siliculosa.	Siliquosa.				
16. Monadelphia.	Pentandria.	Decandria.	Enneandria.	Dodecandria.	Polyandria.	

Classes.	Orders
17 Diadelphia.	Pentandria. Hexandria.
18. Polyadelphia.	Pentandria. Icosandria. Polyandria.
19. Syngenesia.	Polygamia æqualis. Polygamia superflua. Polygamia frustranea. Polygamia necessaria. Polygamia segregata. Monogamia.
20. Gynandria.	Diandria. Triandria. Tetrandria. Pentandria. Hexandria. Decandria. Dodecandria. Polyandria.
21. Monœcia.	Monandria. Diandria. Triandria. Tetrandria. Pentandria. Hexandria. Heptandria. Polyandria. Monadelphia. Syngenesia. Gynandria.
22. Diœcia.	Monandria. Diandria. Triandria. Tetrandria. Pentandria. Hexandria. Octandria. Enneandria. Decandria. Dodecandria. Polyandria. Monadelphia. Syngenesia. Gynandria.
23. Polygamia.	Monœcia. Diœcia. Triœcia.
24. Cryptogamia.	Filices. Musci. Algæ. Fungi.
Appendix.	Palmæ.

PLA'NUM OS. (*Planus*, soft, smooth; applied to a bone whose surface is smooth or flat.) The pappyraceous or orbital portion of the ethmoid bone was formerly so called.

PLANUS. Flat. Applied to the receptacle of the fruit of plants; as that of the Helianthus annuus.

PLASMA. A mineral of grass or leek-green colour. It occurs in beds associated with common calcedony, and found also among the ruins at Rome.

PLASTER. See *Emplastrum*.

Plaster, ammoniacum. See *Emplastrum ammoniaci.*

Plaster, ammoniacum, with mercury. See *Emplastrum ammoniaci cum hydrargyro.*

Plaster, blistering fly. See *Emplastrum cantharidis.*

Plaster, compound galbanum. See *Emplastrum galbani compositum.*

Plaster, compound pitch. See *Emplastrum picis compositum.*

Plaster, cumin. See *Emplastrum cumini.*

Plaster, lead. See *Emplastrum plumbi.*

Plaster, mercurial. See *Emplastrum hydrargyri.*

Plaster of opium. See *Emplastrum opii.*

Plaster of Paris. See *Gypsum.*

Plaster, resin. See *Emplastrum resinæ.*

Plaster, soap. See *Emplastrum saponis.*

Plaster, wax. See *Emplastrum ceræ.*

PLA'TA. (From πλατυς, broad.) The shoulder-blade.

PLATER, FELIX, was borne at Basle, in 1536, his father being principal of the College there. He went to complete his medical studies at Montpelier, where he distinguished himself at an early age, and obtained his doctor's degree at twenty. He then settled in his native place, and four years after was appointed to the chair of medicine, and became the confidential physician of the princes and nobles of the Upper Rhine. He possessed an extensive knowledge of the branches of science connected with medicine, and contributed much to the reputation of the University, where he continued a teacher upwards of fifty years. He died in 1614, extremely regretted by his countrymen. The following are his principal works: " De Corporis Humani Structura et Usu," in three books; "De Febribus;" "Praxeos Medicæ, tomi tres;" "Observationum Medicinalium, libri tres."

PLATIA'SMUS. (From πλατυς, broad.) A defect in the speech in consequence of too broad a mouth.

PLA'TINUM. (The name platina was given to this metal by the Spaniards, from the word *plata*, which signifies silver in their language, by way of comparison with that metal, whose colour it imitates: or from the river *Plata*, near which it is found.) *Platina.* A metal which exists in nature, only in a metallic state. Its ore has recently been found to contain, likewise, four new metals, *palladium, iridium, osmium,* and *rhodium,* besides iron and chrome. The largest mass of which we have heard, is one of the size of a pigeon's egg, in possession of the Royal Society of Bergara. It is found in the parishes of Novita and Citaria, north from Choco in Peru, and near Carthagena in South America. In was unknown in Europe before the year 1748. Don Antonio Ulloa then gave the first information concerning its existence, in the narrative of his voyage with the French academicians to Peru.

"The crude platina is to be dissolved in nitro-muriatic acid, precipitated by muriate of ammonia, and exposed to a very violent heat. Then the acid and alkali are expelled, and the metal reduced in an agglutinated state, which is rendered more compact by pressure while red-hot.

Pure or refined platina is by much the heaviest body in nature. Its sp. gr. is 21.5. It is very malleable, though considerably harder than either gold or silver; and it hardens much under the hammer. Its colour on the touchstone is not distinguishable from that of silver. Pure platina requires a very strong heat to melt it; but when urged by a white heat, its parts will adhere together by hammering. This property, which is distinguished by the name of welding, is peculiar to platina and iron, which resemble each other likewise in their infusibility.

Platina is not altered by exposure to air; neither is it acted upon by the most concentrated simple acids, even when boiling, or distilled from it.

The aqua regia best adapted to the solution of platina, is composed of one part of the nitric and three of the muriatic acid. The solution does not take place with rapidity. A small quantity of nitric oxide is disengaged, the colour of the fluid becoming first yellow, and afterward of a deep reddish-brown, which, upon dilution with water, is found to be an immense yellow. This solution is very corrosive, and tinges animal matters of a blackish-brown colour, it affords crystals by evaporation.

Muriate of tin is so delicate a test of platina, that a single drop of the recent solution of tin in muriatic acid gives a bright red colour to a solution of muriate of platina, scarcely distinguishable from water.

If the muriatic solution of platina be agitated with ether, the ether will become impregnated with the metal. The ethereal solution is of a fine pale yellow, does not stain the skin, and is precipitable by ammonia

If the nitro-muriatic solution of platina be precipitated by lime, and the precipitate digested in sulphuric acid, a sulphate of platinum will be formed. A subnitrate may be formed in the same manner. According to Chenevix, the insoluble sulphate contains 54.5 oxide of platinum, and 45.5 acid and water; the insoluble muriate, 70 of oxide; and the subnitrate, 89 of oxide; but the purity of the oxide of platinum in these is uncertain.

Platinum does not combine with sulphur directly, but is soluble by the alkaline sulphurets, and precipitated from its nitro-muriatic solution by sulphuretted hydrogen.

Pelletier united it with phosphorus, by projecting small bits of phosphorus on the metal heated to redness in a crucible; or exposing to a strong heat four parts each of platinum and concrete phosphoric acid with one of charcoal powder. The phosphuret of platinum is of a silvery-white, very brittle, and hard enough to strike fire with steel.

Platinum unites with most other metals. Added in the proportion of one-twelfth to gold, it forms a yellowish white metal, highly ductile, and tolerably elastic.

Platinum renders silver more hard, but its colour more dull.

Copper is much improved by alloying with platinum.

Alloys of platinum with tin and lead are very apt to tarnish.

From its hardness, infusibility, and difficulty of being acted upon by most agents, platinum is of great value for making various chemical vessels. These have, it is true, the inconvenience of being liable to erosion from the caustic alkalies and some of the neutral salts.

Platinum is now hammered in Paris into leaves of extreme thinness. By enclosing a wire of it in a little tube of silver, and drawing this through a steel plate in the usual way, Dr. Wollaston has succeeded in producing platinum wire not exceeding 1-3000th of an inch in diameter.

189

There are two *oxides* of platinum.

1. When 100 parts of the protochloride, or muriate of platinum are calcined, they leave 73.3 of metal; 26.7 of chlorine escape. Hence the prime equivalent of the metal would seem to be 12.3. When the above protochloride is treated with caustic potassa, it is resolved into a black oxide of platinum and chloride of potassium. This oxide should consist of 12.3 metal $+$ 1 oxygen.

2. The peroxide appears to contain three prime proportions. Berzelius obtained it by treating the muriate of platinum with sulphuric acid, at a distilling heat, and decomposing the sulphate by aqueous potassa. The precipitated oxide is a yellowish-brown powder, easily reducible by a red heat to the metallic state.

According to E. Davy, there are two *phosphurets* and three *sulphurets* of platinum.

The salts of platinum have the following general characters:—

1. Their solution in water is yellowish-brown.

2. Potassa and ammonia determine the formation of small orange-coloured crystals.

3. Sulphuretted hydrogen throws down the metal in a black powder.

Ferroprussiate of potassa and infusion of galls occasion no precipitate."

PLATYCO′RIA. (From πλατυς, broad, and κορη, the pupil of the eye.) An enlarged pupil.

PLATYOPHTHA′LMUM. (From πλατυς, broad, and οφθαλμος, the eye: so called because it is used by women to enlarge the appearance of the eye.) Antimony.

PLATYPHY′LLUM. (From πλατυς, broad, and φυλλον, a leaf.) Broad-leaved.

PLATY′SMA-MYOIDES. (From πλατυς, broad, μυς, a muscle, and ειδος, resemblance.) *Musculus cutaneus,* of Winslow. *Quadratus genæ vel latissimus colli,* of Douglas. *Latissimus colli,* of Albinus. *Quadratus genæ, seu tetragonus,* of Winslow; and *thoraco maxilli facial,* of Dumas. A thin muscle on the side of the neck, immediately under the skin, that assists in drawing the skin of the cheek downwards; and when the mouth is shut, it draws all that part of the skin to which it is connected below the lower jaw, upwards.

PLE′CTANÆ. (From πλεκτω, to fold.) The horns of the uterus.

PLE′CTRUM. (From πληττω, to strike: so named from their resemblance to a drum-stick.) The styloid process of the temporal bone, and the uvula.

PLEMPIUS, VOPISCUS FORTUNATUS, was born at Amsterdam in 1601. He commenced his medical studies at Leyden, then travelled for improvement to Italy, and took his degree at Bologna. He settled as a physician in his native city, and acquired a high reputation there; whence he was invited to a professorship at Louvain, whither he repaired in 1633. He adopted, on this occasion, the Catholic religion, and took a new degree, in conformity with the rules of the university. He was soon after nominated principal of the college of Breugel. His death happened in 1671. He increased the reputation of Louvain by the extent of his attainments, and distinguished himself in all the public questions that came under discussion. He was author of many works in Latin and Dutch; in one of which, entitled "Fundamenta, seu Institutiones Medicinæ," he gave a satisfactory proof of his candour, by strenuously advocating the circulation of the blood, of which he had previously expressed doubts.

PLEONASTE. See *Celanite.*

PLERO′SIS. See *Plethora.*

PLE′SMONE. See *Plethora.*

PLETHO′RA. (From πληθω, to fill.) *Plesmone. Plerosis.* 1. An excessive fulness of vessels, or a redundance of blood.

2. A fulness of habit or body.

PLEUMO′NIA. See *Pneumonia.*

PLEU′RA. Πλευρα. A membrane which lines the internal surface of the thorax, and covers its viscera. It forms a great process, the mediastinum, which divides the thorax into two cavities. Its use is to render the surface of the thorax moist by the vapour it exhales. The cavity of the thorax is every where lined by this smooth and glistening membrane, which is in reality two distinct portions or bags, which, by being applied to each other laterally, form the septum

190

called mediastinum: thus divides the cavity into two parts, and is attached posteriorly to the vertebræ of the back; and anteriorly to the sternum. But the two laminæ, of which this septum is formed, do not every where adhere to each other; for at the lower part of the thorax they are separated, to afford a lodgment to the heart; and at the upper part of the cavity they receive between them the thymus gland. The pleura is plentifully supplied with arteries and veins from the internal mammary, and the intercostals. Its nerves, which are very inconsiderable, are derived chiefly from the dorsal and intercostal nerves. The surface of the pleura, like that of the peritonæum and other membranes lining cavities, is constantly bedewed with a serous moisture, which prevents adhesions of the viscera. The mediastinum, by dividing the breast into two cavities, obviates many inconveniences to which we should otherwise be liable. It prevents the two lobes of the lungs from compressing each other when we lie on one side, and consequently contributes to the freedom of respiration, which is disturbed by the least pressure on the lungs. If the point of a sword penetrates between the ribs into the cavity of the thorax, the lungs on that side cease to perform their office, because the air being admitted through the wound, prevents the dilatation of that lobe, while the other lobe, which is separated from it by the mediastinum, remains unhurt, and continues to perform its functions as usual.

PLEURALGIA. (From πλευρα, and ἀλγος, pain.) Pain in the pleura, or side.

["PLEURISY ROOT. This species of root is found from Maine to Georgia, and is readily distinguished from other roots, by its bright orange-coloured flowers. The root when dry is brittle, and easily reduced to powder. Its taste is moderately bitter, and its chief soluble proportions are extractive matter and fœcula. It acts medicinally as a mild diaphoretic, expectorant, and subtonic. It has been much used, in the United States in catarrh, bronchitis, the secondary stages of pneumonia, and in phthisis as a palliative. From some associations of this kind, it is known in many places as *pleurisy root.* It has the property of producing diaphoresis with less previous heat and excitement than attends the use of most vegetable sudorifics. Twenty or thirty grains can be given three times a day, or a gill of the infusion, prepared like that of serpentaria."—*Big. Mat. Med.* A.]

PLEURI′TIS. (*Pleuritis, idis.* f.; from πλευρα, the pleura.) Pleurisy, or inflammation of the pleura. A species of pneumonia, of Cullen. See *Pneumonia.* In some instances the inflammation is partial, or affects one place in particular, which is commonly on the right side; but, in general, a morbid affection is communicated throughout its whole extent. The disease is occasioned by exposure to cold, and by all the causes which usually give rise to all inflammatory complaints; and it attacks chiefly those of a vigorous constitution and plethoric habit. In consequence of the previous inflammation, it is apt, at its departure, to leave behind a thickening of the pleura, or adhesions to the ribs and intercostal muscles, which either lay the foundation of future pneumonic complaints, or render the patient more susceptible of the changes in the state of the atmosphere than before.

It comes on with an acute pain in the side, which is much increased by making a full inspiration, and is accompanied by flushing in the face, increased heat over the whole body, rigors, difficulty of lying on the side affected, together with a cough and nausea, and the pulse is hard, strong, and frequent, and vibrates under the finger when pressed upon, not unlike the tense string of a musical instrument. If blood is drawn, and allowed to stand for a short time, it will exhibit a thick, sizy, or buffy coat on its surface. If the disease be neglected at its onset, and the inflammation proceeds with great violence and rapidity, the lungs themselves become affected, the passage of the blood through them is stopped, and the patient is suffocated; or, from the combination of the two affections, the inflammation proceeds on to suppuration, and an abscess is formed. The prognostic in pleurisy must be drawn from the severity of the symptoms. If the fever and inflammation have run high, and the pain should cease suddenly, with a change of countenance, and a sinking of the pulse, great danger may be apprehended; but if the heat and other febrile symptoms abate gradually, if respiration is performed with greater ease and less pain, and a free and copious expectoration ensues, a speedy recovery may be expected.

The appearances on dissection are much the same as those mentioned under the head of pneumonia, viz. an inflamed state of the pleura, connected with the lungs, having its surface covered with red vessels, and a layer of coagulated lymph lying upon it, adhesions, too, of the substance of the lungs to the pleura. Besides these, the lungs themselves are often found in an inflamed state, with an extravasation either of blood or coagulated lymph in their substance. Tubercles and abscesses are likewise frequently met with. See *Pneumonia*.

PLEUROCOLLE′SIS. (From πλευρα, the pleura, and κολλαω, to adhere.) An adhesion of the pleura to the lungs, or some neighbouring part.

PLEURODY′NIA. (From πλευρα, and οδυνη, pain.) A pain in the side, from a rheumatic affection of the pleura.

PLEURO-PNEUMO′NIA. (From πλευρα, and πνευμονια, an inflammation of the lungs.) An inflammation of the lungs and pleura.

PLEURORTHOPNÆ′A. (From πλευρα, the pleura, ορθος, upright, and πνεω, to breathe.) A pleurisy in which the patient cannot breathe without keeping his body upright.

PLEUROSTHO′TONOS. (From πλευρον, the side, and τεινω, to stretch.) A spasmodic disease, in which the body is bent to one side.

PLE′XUS. (From *plecto*, to plait or knit.) A net-work of vessels. The union of two or more nerves is also called a plexus.

PLEXUS CARDIACUS. The cardiac plexus of nerves is the union of the eighth pair of nerves and great sympathetic.

PLEXUS CHOROIDES. The choroid plexus is a net-work of vessels situated in the lateral ventricle of the brain.

PLEXUS PAMPINIFORMIS. The plexus of vessels about the spermatic chord.

PLEXUS PULMONICUS. The pulmonic plexus is formed by the union of the eighth pair of nerves with the great sympathetic.

PLEXUS RETICULARIS. A net-work of vessels under the fornix of the brain.

PLI′CA. (From *plico*, to entangle. This disease is commonly distinguished by the adjective *Polonica*, it being almost peculiar to the inhabitants of Poland.) *Helotis; Kolto; Rhopalosis; Plica polonica. Trichoma.* Plaited hair. A disease of the hairs, in which they become long and coarse, and matted and glued into inextricable tangles. It is peculiar to Poland, Lithuania, and Tartary, and generally appears during the autumnal season.

PLICA′RIA. (From *plico*, to entangle: so called because its leaves are entangled together in one mass.) Wolf's-claw, or club moss. See *Lycopodium*.

PLICATUS. Plaited, folded. A term applied to leaves, when the disk, especially towards the margin, is acutely folded up and down; as in *Malva crispa.*

PLI′NTHIUS. Πλινθιος. The fourfold bandage.

PLUM. *Pruna.* Three sorts of plums are ranked among the articles of the materia medica; they are all met with in the gardens of this country, but the shops are supplied with them moderately dried, from abroad.

1. The *pruna brignolensia;* the Brignole plum, or prunello, brought from Brignole, in Provence; it is of a reddish yellow colour, and has a very grateful, sweet, subacid taste. 2. The *pruna gallica;* the common or French prune. 3. The *pruna damascena,* or damson. All these fruits possess the same general qualities with the other summer fruits. The prunelloes, in which the sweetness has a greater mixture of acidity than in the other sorts, are used as mild refrigerants in fevers and other hot indispositions. The French prunes and damsons are the most emollient and laxative; they are often taken by themselves, to gently move the belly, where there is a tendency to inflammations. Decoctions of them afford a useful basis for laxative or purgative mixtures, and the pulp, in substance, for electuaries.

Plum, Malabar. See *Eugenia jambos.*

PLUMBA′GO. (From *plumbum*, lead: so called because it is covered with lead-coloured spots.) 1. The name of a genus of plants. Class, *Pentandria;* Order, *Monogynia.*

2. Lead-wort. See *Polygonum persicaria.*
3. Black lead. An ore of a shining blue-black colour, a greasy feel, and unberculated when fractured. See *Graphite.*

PLUMBAGO EUROPÆA. The systematic name of the tooth-wort. *Dentaria; Dentillaria.* This plant is to be distinguished from the pellitory of Spain, which is also called dentaria. It is the *Plumbago—foliis amplexicaulibus, lanceolatis scabris,* of Linnæus. The root was formerly esteemed, prepared in a variety of ways, as a cure for the toothache, arising from caries.

PLUMBI ACETAS. *Cerussa acetata. Plumbi superacetas. Saccharum saturni,* or sugar of lead, from its sweet taste. It possesses sedative and astringent qualities in a very high degree, and is perhaps the most powerful internal medicine in profuse hæmorrhages, especially combined with opium; but its use is not entirely without hazard, as it has sometimes produced violent colic and palsy; wherefore it is better not to continue it unnecessarily. The dose may be from one to three grains. It has been also recommended to check the expectoration, and colliquative discharges in phthisis, but will probably be only of temporary service. Externally it is used for the same purposes as the liquor plumbi subacetatis.

PLUMBI ACETATIS LIQUOR. Solution of acetate of lead, formerly called *aqua lithargyri acetati.* Goulard's extract. Take of semi-vitrified oxide of lead, two pounds; acetic acid, a gallon. Mix, and boil down to six pints, constantly stirring; then set it by, that the feculencies may subside, and strain. It is principally employed in a diluted state, by surgeons, as a resolvent against inflammatory affections.

PLUMBI ACETATIS LIQUOR DILUTUS. Diluted solution of acetate of lead. *Aqua lithargyri acetati composita.* Take of solution of sub-acetate of lead, a fluid drachm; distilled water, a pint; weak spirit, a fluid drachm. Mix. The virtues of this water, the *aqua vegeto-mineralis* of former pharmacopœias, applied externally, are resolvent, refrigerant, and sedative.

PLUMBI CARBONAS. See *Plumbi subcarbonas.*
PLUMBI OXYDUM SEMIVITREUM. See *Lithargyrus.*
PLUMBI SUBCARBONAS. *Carbonas plumbi.* Subcarbonate of lead commonly called cerusse, or white lead This article is made in the large way in white lead manufactories, by exposing thin sheets of lead to the vapour of vinegar. The lead is curled up and put into pots of earthenware, in which the vinegar is, in such a way as to rest just above the vinegar. Hundreds of these are arranged together, and surrounded with dung, the heat from which volatilizes the acetic acid, which is decomposed by the lead, and an imperfect carbonate of lead is formed, which is of a white colour. This preparation is seldom used in medicine or surgery but for the purpose of making other preparations, as the superacetate. It is sometimes employed medicinally in form of powder and ointment, to children whose skin is fretted. It should, however, be cautiously used, as there is great reason to believe that complaints of the bowels of children originate from its absorption. See *Pulvis cerussæ compositus*

PLU′MBUM. See *Lead.*
PLUMBUM CANDIDUM. See *Tin.*
PLUMBUM CINEREUM. Bismuth.
PLUMBUM NIGRUM. Black-lead.
PLUMBUM RUBEUM. The philosopher's stone.
PLUMBUM USTUM. Burnt lead.
PLUMME′RI PILULÆ. Plummer's pills. A composition of calomel, antimony, and guaiacum. See *Pilulæ hydrargyri submuriatis compositæ.*

PLUMULA. (A diminutive of *pluma*, a feather.) A little feather. The expanding embryo or germ of a plant within the seed, resembling a little feather. It soon becomes a tuft of young leaves, with which the young stem, if there be any, ascends. See *Corculum* and *Cotyledon.*

PLUNKET'S CANCER REMEDY. Take crow's foot, which grows in low grounds, one handful; dog's fennel, three sprigs, both well pounded; crude brimstone in powder, three middling thimblefuls; white arsenic the same quantity; incorporated all in a mortar, and made into small balls the size of a nutmeg, and dried in the sun. These balls must be powdered and mixed with the yelk of an egg, and laid over the sore or cancer on a piece of pig's bladder, or stripping of a calf when dropped, which must be cut to the size of the sore, and smeared with the yelk of an egg. This must be applied cautiously to the lips or nose lest any part of it get down; nor is it to be laid on too broad on the face, or too near the heart, nor to exceed the breadth of half-a-crown; but elsewhere as far as the sore goes. The plaster must not be stirred until it drops off of itself, which will be in a week. Clean bandages are often to be put on.

PNEUMATIC. (*Pneumaticus;* from πνευμα, wind, relating to air.) Of or belonging to air or gas.

PNEUMATIC APPARATUS. See *Apparatus, pneumatic.*

PNEUMATICÆ. (From πνευμων, the lung.) The name given by Dr. Good, to the second class of diseases in his Nosology. Diseases of the respiratory function. It has two orders, *Phonica* and *Pneumonica.*

PNEUMATOCE'LE. (From πνευμα, wind, and κηλη, a tumour.) Any species of hernia, that is distended with flatus.

PNEUMATO'MPHALUS. (From πνευμα, wind, and ομφαλος, the navel.) A flatulent, umbilical hernia.

PNEUMATO'SIS. (From πνευματοω, to inflate.) *Emphysema.* Windy swelling. A genus of disease in the Class *Cachexiæ,* and Order *Intumescentiæ,* of Cullen, known by a collection of air in the cellular texture under the skin, rendering it tense, elastic, and crepitating. Air in the cellular membrane is confined to one place; but in a few cases, it spreads universally over the whole body, and occasions a considerable degree of swelling. It sometimes arises spontaneously, which is, however, a very rare occurrence, or comes on immediately after delivery, without any evident cause; but it is most generally induced by some wound or injury done to the thorax, and which affects the lungs; in which case the air passes from these, through the wound, into the surrounding cellular membrane, and from thence spreads over the whole body.

Pneumatosis is attended with an evident crackling noise, and elasticity upon pressure; and sometimes with much difficulty of breathing, oppression, and anxiety.

We are to consider it as a disease by no means unattended with danger; but more probably from the causes which give rise to it, than any hazard from the complaint itself.

The species of pneumatosis are:

1. *Pneumatosis spontanea,* without any manifest cause.

2. *Pneumatosis traumatica,* from a wound.

3. *Pneumatosis venenata,* from poisons.

4. *Pneumatosis hysterica,* with hysteria.

PNEUMO'NIA. (From πνευμων, a lung.) *Pneumonitis; Peripneumonia; Peripneumonia vera.* Inflammation of the lungs. A genus of disease in the Class *Pyrexia,* and Order *Phlegmasiæ,* of Cullen; characterized by pyrexia, difficult respiration, cough, and a sense of weight and pain in the thorax. The species of pneumonia, according to the above nosologist, are,

1. *Peripneumonia.* The pulse not always hard, but sometimes soft: an obtuse pain in the breast: the respiration always difficult; sometimes the patient cannot breathe, unless in an upright posture; the face swelled, and of a livid colour; the cough for the most part with expectoration, frequently bloody.

2. *Pleuritis.* The pulse hard: a pungent pain in one side; aggravated during the time of inspiration; an uneasiness when lying on one side; a very painful cough, dry in the beginning of the disease, afterward with expectoration, and frequently bloody. See *Pleuritis.*

With respect to pneumonia, the most general cause of this inflammation is the application of cold to the body, which gives a check to the perspiration, and determines a great flow of blood to the lungs. It attacks principally those of a robust constitution and plethoric habit, and occurs most frequently in the winter season and spring of the year: but it may arise in either of the other seasons, when there are sudden vicissitudes from heat to cold.

Other causes, such as violent exertions in singing, speaking, or playing on wind instruments, by producing an increased action of the lungs, have been known to occasion peripneumony. Those who have laboured under a former attack of this complaint, are much predisposed to returns of it.

192

The true peripneumony comes on with an obtuse pain in the chest or side, great difficulty of breathing, (particularly in a recumbent position, or when lying on the side affected,) together with a cough, dryness of the skin, heat, anxiety, and thirst. At the first commencement of the disease the pulse is usually full, strong, hard, and frequent; but in a more advanced stage it is commonly weak, soft, and often irregular. In the beginning, the cough is frequently dry and without expectoration; but in some cases it is moist, even from the first, and the matter spit up is various both in colour and in consistence, and is often streaked with blood.

If relief is not afforded in time, and the inflammation proceeds with such violence as to endanger suffocation, the vessels of the neck will become turgid and swelled; the face will alter to a purple colour; an effusion of blood will take place into the cellular substance of the lungs, so as to impede the circulation through that organ, and the patient will soon be deprived of life.

If these violent symptoms do not arise, and the pro per means for carrying off the inflammation have either been neglected, or have proved ineffectual, although adopted at an early period of the disease, a suppuration may ensue, which event is to be known by frequent slight quiverings, and an abatement of the pain and sense of fulness in the part, and by the patient being able to lie on the side which was affected, without experiencing great uneasiness.

When peripneumony proves fatal, it is generally by an effusion of blood taking place in the cellular texture of the lungs, so as to occasion suffocation, which usually happens between the third and seventh days; but it may likewise prove fatal, by terminating either in suppuration or gangrene.

When it goes off by resolution, some very evident evacuation always attends it; such as a great flow of urine, with a copious sediment, diarrhœa, a sweat diffused over the whole body, or a hæmorrhage from the nose; but the evacuation which most frequently terminates the complaint, and which does it with the greatest effect, is a free and copious expectoration of thick white or yellow matter, slightly streaked with blood; and by this the disease is carried off generally in the course of ten or twelve days.

Our opinion as to the event is to be drawn from the symptoms which are present. A high degree of fever attended with delirium, great difficulty of breathing acute pain, and dry cough, denote great danger; on the contrary, an abatement of the febrile symptoms, and of the difficulty of breathing and pain, taking place on the coming on of a free expectoration, or the happening of any other critical evacuation, promises fair for the recovery of the patient. A termination of the inflammation in suppuration is always to be considered as dangerous.

On dissection, the lungs usually appear inflamed; and there is often found an extravasation, either of blood, or of coagulable lymph, in their cellular substance. The same appearances likewise present themselves in the cavity of the thorax, and within the pericardium. The pleura, connected with the lungs, is also in an inflated state, having its surface every where crowded with red vessels. Besides these, abscesses are frequently found in the substance of the lungs, as likewise tubercles and adhesions to the ribs are formed. A quantity of purulent matter is often discovered also in the bronchia. In the early period of this disease we may hope, by active measures, to bring about immediate resolution; but when it is more advanced, we must look for a discharge by expectoration, as the means of restoring the part to a healthy state. We should begin by large and free bleeding, not deterred by the obscure pulse sometimes found in peripneumony, carrying this evacuation to faintness, or to the manifest relief of the breathing. In the subsequent use of this measure, we must be guided by the violence of the disease on the one hand, and the strength of the patient on the other; the scrofulous, in particular, cannot bear it to any extent; and it is more especially in the early part of the complaint, that it produces a full and decisive effect. Under doubtful circumstances it will be better to take blood locally, particularly when there are pleuritic symptoms; with which blisters may co-operate. The bowels must be well evacuated in the first instance, and subsequently kept regular: and antimonials may be given with great advantage com bined often with mercurials to promote the discharges, especially from the skin and lungs. Digitalis is proper also, as lessening the activity of the circulation. The antiphlogistic regimen is to be observed, except that the patient will not bear too free exposure to cold. To quiet the cough, demulcents may be of some use or cooling sialagogues: but where the urgency of the symptoms is lessened by copious depletion, opiates are more to be relied upon ; a little syrup of poppy, for instance, swallowed slowly from time to time ; or a full dose of opium may be given at night to procure sleep, joined with calomel and antimony, that it may not heat the system, but, on the contrary, assist them in promoting the secretions. Inhaling steam will occasionally assist in bringing about expectoration ; or, where there is a wheezing respiration, squill in nauseating or sometimes even emetic, doses may relieve the patient from the viscid matter collected in the air passages. When the expectoration is copious in the decline of the complaint, tonic medicines, particularly myrrh, with a more nutritious diet, become necessary to support the strength: and the same means will be proper, if it should go on to suppuration. Where adhesions have occurred, or other organic change, though the symptoms may appear trifling, much caution is required to prevent the patient falling into *Phthisis ;* on which subject see the management of that disease : and should serous effusion happen, see *Hydrothorax.*

PNEUMONICA. (From πνευμων, the lung.) The name of the second order of diseases in the Class *Pneumatica* of Good's Nosology. Diseases affecting the lungs, their membranes, or motive power. It has six genera, viz. *Bex; Dyspnœa; Asthma; Ephialtes; Sternalgia; Pleuralgia.*

PNEUMOPLEURI'TIS. (From πνευμων, the lungs, and πλευριτις, an inflammation of the pleura.) An inflammation of the lungs and pleura.

PNIGA'LIUM. (From πνιγω, to suffocate.) The nightmare. A disorder in which the patient appears to be suffocated.

PNIX. (From πνιγω, to suffocate.) A sense of suffocation.

POD. See *Siliqua.*

PODA'GRA. (From πους, the foot, and αγρα, a taking, or seizure.) *Febris podagrica. Arthritis ; Dolor podagricus ;* The gout. A genus of disease in the Class *Pyrexiæ,* and Order *Phlegmasiæ,* of Cullen ; known by irregular, pain in the joints, chiefly of the great toe, or at any rate of the hands and feet, returning at intervals: previous to the attack, the functions of the stomach are commonly disturbed. The species are,

1. *Podagra regularis. Arthritis podagra; Arthritis rachialgica ; Arthritis æstiva,* of Sauvages. The regular gout.

2. *Podagra atonica. Arthritis melancholica; hiemalis ; chlorotica ;* and *asthmatica,* of Sauvages. The atonic gout.

3. *Podagra retrograda.* The retrocedent.

4. *Podagra aberrans.* Misplaced or wandering gout.

The gout is a very painful disease, preceded usually by flatulency; and indigestion, and accompanied by fever pains in the joints of the hands and feet, particularly in that of the great toe, and which returns by paroxysms, occurring chiefly in the spring and beginning of winter. The only disorder for which the regular gout can possibly be mistaken, is the rheumatism ; and cases may occur wherein there may be some difficulty in making a just discrimination : but the most certain way of distinguishing them will be, to give due consideration to the predisposition in the habit, the symptoms which have preceded, the parts affected, the recurrences of the disease, and its connexion with other parts of the system. Its attacks are much confined to the male sex, particularly those of a corpulent habit, and robust body ; but every now and then we meet with instances of it in robust females. Those who are employed in constant bodily labour, or who live much upon vegetable food, as likewise those who make no use of wine, or other fermented liquors, are seldom afflicted with the gout. The disease seldom appears at an earlier period of life than from five-and-thirty to forty ; and, when it does, it may be presumed to arise from an hereditary disposition. Indolence, inactivity, and too free a use of tartareous wines, fermented liquors, and animal food, are the principal

U u

causes which give rise to the gout, but t may likewise be brought on by great sensuality and excess in venery, intense and close application to study, long want of rest, grief, or uneasiness of mind, exposure to cold, too free a use of acidulated liquors, a sudden change from a full to a spare diet, the suppression of any accustomed discharge, or by excessive evacuations ; and that it sometimes proceeds from an hereditary disposition, is beyond all doubt, as females who have been remarked for their great abstemiousness, and youths of a tender age, have been attacked with it.

1. *Podagra regularis.* A paroxysm of regular gout sometimes comes on suddenly, without any previous warning; at other times it is preceded by an unusual coldness of the feet and legs, a suppression of perspiration in them, and numbness, or a sense of prickling along the whole of the lower extremities : and with these symptoms the appetite is diminished, the stomach is troubled with flatulency and indigestion, a degree of torpor and languor is felt over the whole body, great lassitude and fatigue are experienced after the least exercise, the body is costive, and the urine pallid. On the night of the attack, the patient perhaps goes to bed in tolerable health, and after a few hours is awakened by the severity of the pain, most commonly in the first joint of the great toe; sometimes, however, it attacks other parts of the foot, the heel, calf of the leg, or perhaps the whole of the foot. The pain resembles that of a dislocated bone, and is attended with the sensation as if cold water was poured upon the part; and this pain, becoming more violent, is succeeded by rigors and other febrile symptoms, together with a severe throbbing and inflammation in the part. Sometimes both feet become swelled and inflamed, so that neither of them can be put to the ground; nor can the patient endure the least motion without suffering excruciating pain. Towards morning, he falls asleep, and a gentle sweat breaks out, and terminates the paroxysm, a number of which constitutes what is called a fit of the gout. The duration of the fit will be longer or shorter, according to the disposition of the body to the disease, the season of the year, and the age and strength of the patient. When a paroxysm has thus taken place, although there is an alleviation of pain at the expiration of some hours, still the patient is not entirely relieved from it ; and, for some evenings successively, he has a return both of pain and fever, which continue, with more or less violence, until morning. The paroxysms, however, prove usually more mild every day, till at length the disease goes off either by perspiration, urine, or some other evacuation ; the parts which have been affected becoming itchy, the cuticle falling off in scales from them, and some slight degree of lameness remaining. At first, an attack of gout occurs, perhaps, only once in two or three years; it then probably comes on every year, and at length it becomes more frequent, and is more severe, and of longer duration, each succeeding fit. In the progress of the disease, various parts of the body are affected, and translations take place from one joint, or limb, to another; and, after frequent attacks, the joints lose their strength and flexibility, and become so stiff as to be deprived of all motion. Concretions, of a chalky appearance, are likewise formed upon the outside of the joints, and nephritic affections of the kidneys arise from a deposite of the same kind of matter in them, which, although fluid at first, becomes gradually dry and firm. This matter is partly soluble in acids, but without effervescence ; and Dr. Wollaston discovered it not to be carbonate of lime, but a compound of the uric or lithic acid and soda.

2. *Podagra atonica.* Atonic gout. It sometimes happens that, although a gouty diathesis prevails in the system, yet, from certain causes, no inflammatory affection of the joints is produced ; in which case, the stomach becomes particularly affected, and the patient is troubled with flatulency, indigestion, loss of appetite, eructations, nausea, vomiting, and severe pains; and these affections are often accompanied with much dejection of spirits, and other hypochondriacal symptoms. In some cases, the head is affected with pain and giddiness, and now and then with a tendency to apoplexy ; and in other cases, the viscera of the thorax suffer from the disease, and palpitations, faintings, and asthma arise. This is what is called atonic gout.

3. *Podagra retrograda.* Retrocedent gout. It sometimes happens, that, after the inflammation has occu-

plied a joint, instead of its continuing the usual time, and so going off gradually, it ceases suddenly, and is translated to some internal part. The term retrocedent gout is applied to occurrences of this nature. When it falls on the stomach, it occasions nausea, vomiting, anxiety, or great pain; when on the heart, it brings on syncope; when on the lungs, it produces an affection resembling asthma: and, when it occupies the head, it is apt to give rise to apoplexy, or palsy.

4. *Podagra aberrans*, or misplaced gout, is when the gouty diathesis, instead of producing the inflammatory affection of the joints, occasions an inflammatory affection of some internal parts, and which appears from the same symptoms that attend the inflammation of those parts from other causes. All occurrences of this nature, as well as of the two former, are to be regarded as attacks of irregular gout, and are to be guarded against as much as possible.

In the regular gout, generally, little medical interference is necessary. The antiphlogistic regimen should be observed, in proportion to the strength of the patient, the bowels kept regular, and the part of a moderate temperature, by covering it with flannel, &c.; it may be useful too to promote a gentle diaphoresis. In young and robust constitutions, where there is no hereditary tendency to the disease, and the inflammation and fever run high, more active evacuations may sometimes be required; and, on the contrary, in persons advanced in life, who have suffered much from the disease, and been accustomed to a generous diet, this must be in some degree allowed, even during the paroxysm, to obviate a metastasis; recommending fish in preference to other animal food, and madeira as the least acescent wine. The application of cold to the part is a dangerous practice; and it is better to abstain from any local measures, lest the favourable progress of the disease should be interrupted. When the paroxysm is terminated, any remaining stiffness of the joint will probably be gradually removed by friction, &c. With respect to the means of obviating future attacks, the chief dependence is to be placed on abstemiousness, with regular moderate exercise. Proper medicines may be occasionally prescribed to remove any dyspeptic symptoms, keep the bowels regular, the skin perspirable, &c. If the disease appear to hang about the patient in the atonic form, a more nutritious diet, with tonic or even stimulant medicines, may be required to re-establish the health, which will probably not be accomplished without a paroxysm intervening. The Bath waters have often been found useful under these circumstances. In the retrocedent gout, the object is to bring back the inflammation to the joint as soon as possible: for which purpose a sinapism, or other stimulant application, should be put upon the part; while ammonia, aromatics, either warm wine, or brandy and water, &c., are administered internally, in proportion to the urgency of the symptoms; but in general the best form of medicine is the combination of opium with some of the stimulants just mentioned, unless where congestion appears in the head. Sometimes blisters or rubefacients may be properly applied over the internal part affected, where this is of importance to life, or even the local abstraction of blood becomes necessary. This, however, holds more especially where the attack is inflammatory, constituting the misplaced gout, and a more antiphlogistic plan must then be pursued: but evacuations cannot be borne to the same extent as in the idiopathic phlegmasiæ.

PODAGRA′RIA. (From *podagra*, the gout: so called because it was thought to expel the gout.) See *Ægopodium podagraria*.

PODECIUM. (From πες, a foot.) The name given by Acharius to the peculiar foot-stalk of the tubercles in the cup lichens.

PODONI′PTRUM. (From ϖους, a foot, and νιπ7ω, to wash.) A bath for the feet.

PODOPHY′LLUM. (From ϖους, a foot, and φυλλον, a leaf; so named from its shape.) A species of wolf's bane.

["PODOPHYLLUM PELTATUM. Stem erect, two leaved; leaves peltate. Inhabits woods, flowers in May, is perennial. Stem one foot high; leaves lobed; flowers, solitary, white; fruit ovate.—*Torrey's Compendium*.

"The *podophyllum peltatum* is an American plant, growing in low shady situations, from New-England

194

to Georgia. The plant has only two leaves, with a flower in the fork, followed by a yellow acid fruit.

"The root is creeping and jointed, and, when dry, it is brittle and easily reduced to powder. Its taste is unpleasant, and, when chewed for some time, becomes intensely bitter. Water and alkonol extract its bitterness. It contains resin, fœcula, bitter extractive, and a portion of gummy substance.

"Podophyllum is one of the most certain and efficacious of the cathartic vegetables, which have been examined in this country. It very nearly resembles jalap in its operation, but is somewhat slower, and continues its effects for a longer time. In irritable stomachs it sometimes occasions nausea, but not more than other medicines of its class. In small doses, it proves a gradual and easy laxative; in large ones, a powerful and long continued purge. It has been particularly recommended in dropsy, to which disease it seems well adapted, by the large evacuations it occasions.

"It is best given in powder. Ten grains taken at night, produce a free operation on the following morning, and twenty grains purge with activity. If calomel be combined with it, it operates sooner and with less griping."—*Big. Mat. Med.* A.]

PODOTHE′CA. (From ϖους, a foot, and τιθημι, to put.) A shoe or stocking. An anatomical preparation, consisting of a kind of shoe of the scarf-skin, with the nails adhering to it, taken from a dead subject.

POECILIA, (Ποικιλια, from ποικιλος, *versicolor*.) The specific name of a species of *Epichrosis* in Good's Nosology, to designate the pye-bald skin, or that affection found among negroes, in which it is marbled generally with alternate spots, or patches of black and white.

Pointed leaf. See *Acuminatus*.

POISON. *Venenum.* That substance which, when applied externally, or taken into the human body, uniformly effects such a derangement in the animal economy as to produce disease, may be defined a poison. It is extremely difficult, however, to give a definition of a poison; and the above is subject to great inaccuracy. Poisons are divided, with respect to the kingdom to which they belong, into animal, vegetable, mineral, and halituous, or aërial.

Poisons, in general, are only deleterious in certain doses; for the most active, in small doses, form the most valuable medicines. There are nevertheless, certain poisons, which are really such in the smallest quantity, and which are never administered medicinally; as the poison of hydrophobia or the plague There are likewise substances which are innocent when taken into the stomach, but which prove deleterious when taken into the lungs, or when applied to an abraded surface; thus carbonic acid is continually swallowed with fermented liquors, and thus the poison of the viper may be taken with impunity; while in spiring carbonic acid kills, and the poison of the viper, inserted into the flesh, often proves fatal.

Several substances also act as poisonous when applied either externally or internally; as arsenic.

When a substance produces disease, not only in mankind, but in all animals, it is distinguished by the term *common poison;* as arsenic, sublimate, &c.; while that which is poisonous to man only, or to animals, and often to one genus merely, is said to be a *relative poison;* thus aloes are poisonous to dogs and wolves: the Phellandrium aquaticum kills horses, while oxen devour it greedily, and with impunity. It appears, then, that substances act as poisonous only in regard to their *dose, the part of the body they are applied to,* and the *subject.*

Poisons enter the body in the following ways:

1. Through the œsophagus alone, or with the food.
2. Through the anus by clysters.
3. Through the nostrils.
4. Through the lungs with the air.
5. Through the absorbents of the skin either whole, ulcerated, cut, or torn.

Poisons have been arranged in six classes:

I.—*Corrosive* or *escharotic poisons.*

They are so named because they usually irritate, inflame, and corrode the animal texture with which they come into contact. Their action is in general more violent and formidable than that of the other poisons. The following list from Orfila contains the principal bodies of this class:—

1 *Mercurial preparations;* corrosive sublimate

red oxide of mercury; turbeth mineral, or yellow subsulphate of mercury; pernitrate of mercury; mercurial vapours.

2. *Arsenical preparations;* such as white oxide of arsenic, and its combination with the bases, called arseniates, arsenic acid, and the arseniates; yellow and red sulphuret of arsenic; black oxide of arsenic, or fly-powder.

3. *Antimonial preparations;* such as tartar emetic, or cream tartrate of antimony; oxide of antimony; kermes mineral; muriate of antimony; and antimonial wine.

4. *Cupreous preparations;* such as verdigris; acetate of copper; the cupreous sulphate, nitrate, and muriate; ammoniacal copper; oxide of copper; cupreous soaps, or grease tainted with oxide of copper; and cupreous wines or vinegars.

5. *Muriate of tin.*

6. *Oxide and sulphate of zinc.*

7. *Nitrate of silver.*

8. *Muriate of gold.*

9. *Pearl-white,* or *the oxide of bismuth,* and the subnitrate of this metal.

10. *Concentrated acids;* sulphuric, nitric, phosphoric, muriatic, hydriodic, acetic, &c.

11. *Corrosive alkalies,* pure or subcarbonated potassa, soda, and ammonia.

12. The *caustic earths,* lime and barytes.

13. *Muriate and carbonate of barytes.*

14. *Glass and enamel powder.*

15. *Cantharides.*

II.—*Astringent poisons.*

1. *Preparations of lead,* such as the acetate, carbonate, wines sweetened with lead, water impregnated with its oxide, food cooked in vessels containing lead, syrups clarified with subacetate of lead, plumbean vapours.

III.—*Acrid poisons.*

1. The *gases;* chlorine, muriatic acid, sulphurous acid, nitrous gas, and nitro-muriatic vapours.

2. *Jatropha manihot,* the fresh root, and its juice, from which cassava is made.

3. *The Indian ricinus,* or Molucca wood.

4. *Scammony.*

5. *Gamboge.*

6. Seeds of *Palma Christi.*

7. *Elaterium.*

8. *Colocynth.*

9. *White hellebore root.*

10. *Black hellebore root.*

11. Seeds of *Stavesacre.*

12. The wood and fruit of the *Ahovai* of Brazil.

13. *Rhododendron chrysanthum.*

14. Bulbs of *Colchicum,* gathered in summer and autumn.

15. The milky juice of the *Convolvulus arvensis.*

16. *Asclepias.*

17. *Œnanthe fistulosa* and *crocata.*

18. Some species of *clematis.*

19. *Anemone pulsatilla.*

20. Root of *Wolf's-bane.*

21. Fresh roots of *Arum maculatum.*

22. Berries and bark of *Daphne mezereum.*

23. The plant and emanations of the *Rhus toxicodendron.*

24. *Euphorbia officinalis.*

25. Several species of *Ranunculus,* particularly the *aquatilis.*

26. *Nitre,* in a large dose.

27. Some muscles and other shell-fish.

IV.—*Narcotic and stupifying poisons.*

1. The *gases;* hydrogen, azote, and oxide of azote.

2. Poppy and opium.

3. The roots of the *Solanum somniferum;* berries and leaves of the *Solanum nigrum;* those of the *Morel* with yellow fruit.

4. The roots and leaves of the *Atropa mandragora.*

5. *Datura stramonium.*

6. *Hyociamus,* or henbane.

7. *Lactuca virosa.*

8. *Paris quadrifolia,* or herb Paris.

9. *Laurocerasus,* or bay laurel and prussic acid.

10. Berries of the *yew-tree.*

11. *Ervum ervilia;* the seeds.

12. The seeds of *Lathyrus cicera.*

13. Distilled water of *bitter almonds.*

14. The effluvia of many of the above plants.

V.—*Narcotico-acrid poisons.*

1. *Carbonic acid;* the gas of charcoal stoves and fermenting liquors.

2. The *manchineel.*

3. *Faba Sancti Ignatii.*

4. The exhalations and juice of the *poison tree* of Macassar, or *Upas-Antiar.*

5. The *Ticunas.*

6. Certain species of *Strychnos.*

7. The whole plant, *Lauro-cerasus.*

8. *Belladonna,* or deadly nightshade.

9. *Tobacco.*

10. Roots of *white bryony.*

11. Roots of the *Cherophyllum sylvestre.*

12. *Conium maculatum,* or spotted hemlock.

13. *Æthusa cynapium.*

14. *Cicuta virosa.*

15. *Anagallis arvensis.*

16. *Mercurialis perennis.*

17. *Digitalis purpurea.*

18. The distilled waters and oils of some of the above plants.

19. The *odorant principle* of some of them.

20. *Woorara* of Guiana.

21. *Camphor.*

22. *Cocculus indicus.*

23. Several *mushrooms.*

24. *Secale cornutum.*

25. *Lolium temulentum.*

26. *Sium latifolium.*

27. *Coriaria myrtifolia.*

VI.—*Septic* or *putrescent poisons*

1. Sulphuretted hydrogen.

2. Putrid effluvia of animal bodies.

3. Contagious effluvia, or fomites and miasmata.

4. Venomous animals; the viper, rattlesnake, scorpion, mad dog, &c.

Antidote for vegetable poisons. Drapiez has ascertained, by numerous experiments, that the fruit of the *Feuillea cordifolia* is a powerful antidote against the vegetable poisons. He poisoned dogs with the rhus toxicodendron, hemlock, and nux vomica; and all those which were left to the effects of the poison died, but those to which the above fruit was administered recovered completely, after a short illness. To see whether the antidote would act in the same way, applied externally to wounds, into which vegetable poisons had been introduced, he took two arrows, which had been dipped into the juice of the *manchenille,* and slightly wounded with them two cats; to one of these wounds he applied a poultice, composed of the fruit of the *feuillea cordifolia,* while the other was left without any application. The former suffered no inconvenience, except from the pain of the wound, which speedily healed; while the other, in a short time, fell into convulsions, and died. This fruit loses these valuable virtues, if kept two years after it is gathered.

Dr. Chisholm states, that the juice of the sugar cane is the best antidote for arsenic.

Dr. Lyman Spalding, of New-York, announces in a small pamphlet, that, for above these fifty years, the *Scutellaria lateriflora* has proved to be an infallible means for the prevention and cure of the hydrophobia, after the bite of rabid animals. It is better applied as a dry powder than fresh. According to the testimonies of several American physicians, this plant, not yet received as a remedy into any European *Materia Medica,* afforded perfect relief in above a thousand cases, as well in the human species as in the brute creation (dogs, swine, and oxen).

[From a personal acquaintance with Dr. Spalding we are enabled to state, that his pamphlet of cases of hydrophobia, said to have been cured by the scutellaria, has led both the French and English physicians into a mistake, in relation to the curative virtues of this plant. There are few physicians in the United States who place any reliance upon it. At the time of the publication of Dr. Spalding's pamphlet, there was great excitement about rabid dogs, and much newspaper discussion on the virtues of *Scutellaria lateriflora,* as a remedy in the cure of hydrophobia. The subject being very popular, Dr. Spalding, by means of the newspapers, collected all the cases of alleged cure, and published them in a pamphlet, without vouching for their authenticity, or knowing whether they could be relied on as correct. Having led physicians into a belief that these were all well authen ticated cases, the Doctor afterward corrected the mistake, by publishing a proper explanation. The writer hereof was invited by the attending physician, to see a patient in the last stage of hydrophobia, who had taken the scutellaria in great quantity, from the time he was bitten until the fatal symptoms occurred. A.]

Method of detecting poisons.

"When sudden death is suspected to have been occasioned by the administration of poison, either wilfully or by accident, the testimony of the physician is occasionally required to confirm or invalidate this suspicion. He may also be sometimes called upon to ascertain the cause of the noxious effects arising from the presence of poisonous substances in articles of diet; and it may, therefore, serve an important purpose to point out concisely the simplest and most practicable modes of obtaining, by experiment, the necessary information.

The only poisons, however, that can be clearly and decisively detected, by chemical means, are those of the mineral kingdom. Arsenic and corrosive sublimate are most likely to be exhibited with the view of producing death; and lead and copper may be introduced undesignedly, in several ways, into our food and drink. The continued and unsuspected operation of the last two may often produce effects less sudden and violent, but not less baneful to health and life than the more active poisons; and their operation generally involves, in the pernicious consequences, a greater number of sufferers.

Method of discovering arsenic.—When the cause f sudden death is believed, from the symptoms preceding it, to be the administration of arsenic, the contents of the stomach must be attentively examined. To effect this, let a ligature be made at each orifice, the stomach removed entirely from the body, and its whole contents washed out into an earthen or glass vessel. The arsenic, on account of its greater specific gravity, will settle to the bottom, and may be obtained separate, after washing off the other substances by repeated effusions of cold water. These washings should not be thrown away, till the presence of arsenic has been clearly ascertained. It may be expected at the bottom of the vessel in the form of a white powder, which must be carefully collected, dried on a filter, and submitted to experiment.

A. Boil a small portion of the powder with a few ounces of distilled water, in a clean Florence flask, and filter the solution.

B. To this solution add a portion of water, saturated with sulphuretted hydrogen gas. If arsenic be present, a golden yellow sediment will fall down, which will appear sooner, if a few drops of acetic acid be added.

C. A similar effect is produced by the addition of sulphuret of ammonia, or hydrosulphuret of potassa.

It is necessary, however, to observe, that these tests are decomposed not only by all metallic solutions, but, by the mere addition of any acid. But among these precipitates, Dr. Bostock assures us, the greatest part are so obviously different as not to afford a probability of being mistaken; the only two which bear a close resemblance to it, are the precipitate from tartarized antimony, and that separated by an acid. In the latter, however, the sulphur preserves its peculiar yellow colour, while the arsenic presents a deep shade of orange; but no obvious circumstance of discrimination can be pointed out between the hydrosulphurets of arsenic and of antimony. Hence Dr. Bostock concludes, that sulphuretted hydrogen and its compounds merit our confidence only as collateral tests. They discover arsenic with great delicacy: sixty grains of water, to which one grain only of liquid sulphuret (hydroguretted sulphuret ?) had been added, was almost instantly rendered completely opaque by one-eightieth of a grain of the white oxide of arsenic in solution.

D. To a little of the solution A, add a single drop of a weak solution of subcarbonate of potassa, and afterward a few drops of a solution of sulphate of copper. The presence of arsenic will be manifested by a yellowish-green precipitate. Or boil a portion of the suspected powder with a dilute solution of pure potassa, and with this precipitate the sulphate of copper when a similar appearance will ensue still more rema kably, if arsenic be present. The colour of this precipitate is perfectly characteristic. It is that of the pigment called Scheele's green. To identify the arsenic with

still greater certainty, it may be proper, at the time e making the experiments on a suspected substance, to perform similar ones, as a standard of comparison, on what is actually known to be arsenic. Let the colour, therefore, produced by adding an alkaline solution of the substance under examination, to a solution of sul phate of copper, be compared with that obtained by a similar admixture of a solution of copper with one of real arsenic in alkali.

The proportions in which the different ingredients are employed, Dr. Bostock has found to have considerable influence on the distinct exhibition of the effect. Those which he has observed to answer best, were one of arsenic, three of potassa, (probably the subcarbonate of, or common salt of tartar,) and five of sulphate of copper. For instance, a solution of one grain of arsenic, and three grains of potassa, in two drachms of water, being mingled with another solution of five grains of sulphate of copper in the same quantity of water, the whole was converted into a beautiful grass green, from which a copious precipitate of the same hue slowly subsided, leaving the supernatant liquor transparent and nearly colourless. The same materials, except with the omission of the arsenic, being employed in the same manner, a delicate sky-blue resulted, so different from the former as not to admit of the possibility of mistake. In this way, one-fortieth of a grain of arsenic, diffused through sixty grains of wa ter, afforded, by the addition of sulphate of copper and potassa in proper proportions, a distinct precipitate of Scheele's green. In employing this test, it is necessary to view the fluid by reflected and not by transparent light, and to make the examination by daylight. To render the effect more apparent, a sheet of white paper may be placed behind the glass in which the mixed fluids are contained; or the precipitation may be effected by mixing the fluids on a piece of writing-paper.

E. The sediments, produced by any of the foregoing experiments, may be collected, dried, and laid on red-hot charcoal. A smell of sulphur will first arise, and will be followed by that of garlic.

F. A process for detecting arsenic has been proposed by Hume, of London, in the *Philosophical Magazine*, for May, 1809, vol. xxxiii. The test which he has suggested, is the fused nitrate of silver, or lunar caustic, which he employs in the following manner:—

Into a clean Florence oil-flask, introduce two or three grains of any powder suspected to be arsenic; add not less than eight ounce-measures of either rain or distilled water; and heat this gradually over a lamp, or a clear coal fire, till the solution begins to boil. Then, while it boils, frequently shake the flask, which may be readily done by wrapping a piece of leather round its neck, or putting a glove upon the hand. To the hot solution, add a grain or two of subcarbonate of potassa or soda, agitating the whole to make the mixture uniform.

In the next place, pour into an ounce-phial, or a small wine-glass, about two table spoonfuls of this solution, and present to the mere surface of the fluid a stick of dry nitrate of silver or lunar caustic. If there be any arsenic present, a beautiful yellow precipitate will instantly appear, which will proceed from the point of contact of the nitrate with the fluid; and settle towards the bottom of the vessel as a flocculent and copious precipitate.

The nitrate of silver, Hume finds, also, acts very sensibly upon *arsenate* of potassa, and decidedly distinguishes this salt from the above solution or *arsenite* of potassa: the colour of the precipitate, occasioned by the *arsenate*, being much darker and more inclined to brick-red. In both cases, he is of opinion, that the test of nitrate of silver is greatly superior to that of sulphate of copper; inasmuch as it produces a much more copious precipitate, when equal quantities are submitted to experiment. The tests he recommends to be employed in their dry state, in preference to that of solution; and that the piece of salt he held on the surface only.

A modified application of this test has since been proposed by Dr. Marcet, whose directions are as follow:—Let the fluid, suspected to contain arsenic, be filtered; let the end of a glass rod, wetted with a solution of pure ammonia, be brought into contact with this fluid, and let the end of a clean rod, similarly wetted with solution of nitrate of silver, be immersed in the mixture If the minutest quantity of arsenic be present, a precipitate of a bright-yellow colour, inclining to orange, will appear at the point of contact, and will readily subside at the bottom of the vessel. As this precipitate is soluble in ammonia, the greatest care is necessary not to add an excess of that alkali. The acid of arsenic, with the same test, affords a brick-red precipitate.—Hume, it may be added, now prepares his test by dissolving a few grains, say ten, of lunar caustic in nine or ten times its weight of distilled water; precipitating by liquid ammonia: and adding cautiously, and by a few drops at once, liquid ammonia, till the precipitate is redissolved, and no longer. To obviate the possibility of any excess of ammonia, a small quantity of the precipitate may be left undissolved. To apply this test, nothing more is required than to dip a rod of glass into this liquor, and then touch with it the surface of a solution supposed to contain arsenic, which will be indicated by a yellow precipitate.

Sylvester has objected to this test, that it will not produce the expected appearance, when common salt is present. He has, therefore, proposed the red acetate of iron as a better test of arsenic, with which it forms a bright-yellow deposite; or the acetate of copper, which affords a green precipitate. Of the two, he recommends the latter in preference, but advises that both should be resorted to in doubtful cases. Dr. Marcet, however, has replied, that the objection arising from the presence of common salt is easily obviated; for if a little diluted nitric acid be added to the suspected liquid, and then nitrate of silver very cautiously till the precipitate ceases, the muriate acid will be removed, but the arsenic will remain in solution, and the addition of ammonia will produce the yellow precipitate in its characteristic form. It is scarcely necessary to add, that the quantity of ammonia must be sufficient to saturate any excess of nitric acid, which the fluid may contain.

A more important objection to nitrate of silver as a test of arsenic is, that it affords, with the alkaline phosphates, a precipitate of phosphate of silver, scarcely distinguishable by its colour from the arseniate of that metal. In answer to this, it is alleged by Hume, that the arsenite of silver may be discriminated by a curdy or flocculent figure, resembling that of fresh precipitated muriate of silver, except that its colour is yellow; while the phosphate is smooth and homogeneous. The better to discriminate these two arsenites, he advises two parallel experiments to be made, upon separate pieces of clean writing-paper, spreading on the one a little of the fresh prepared arsenite, and on the other a little of the phosphate. When these are suffered to dry, the phosphate will gradually assume a black colour, or nearly so, while the arsenite will pass from its original vivid yellow to an Indian yellow, or nearly a fawn colour.

Dr. Paris conducts the trial in the following manner: Drop the suspected fluid on a piece of white paper, making with it a broad line; along this line a stick of lunar caustic is to be slowly drawn several times successively, when a streak will appear of the colour resembling that known by the name of *Indian yellow*. This is equally produced by arsenic and by an alkaline phosphate, but the one from arsenic is rough, curdy, and flocculent, like that from a crayon; that from a phosphate is homogeneous and uniform, resembling a water colour laid smoothly on with a brush. But a more important and distinctive peculiarity soon succeeds; for in less than two minutes the phosphoric yellow fades into a *sad green*, and becomes gradually darker, and ultimately quite black, while on the other hand the arsenic yellow continues permanent, or nearly so, for some time, and then becomes brown. In performing this experiment, the sunshine should be avoided, or the change of colour will take place too rapidly. (*Ann. of Phil.* x. 60.) The author of the *London Dispensatory* adds, that the test is improved by brushing the streak lightly over with liquid ammonia immediately after the application of the caustic, when, if arsenic be present, a bright queen's yellow is produced, which remains permanent for nearly an hour; but that when lunar caustic produces a *white* yellow before the ammonia is applied, we may infer the presence of some alkaline phosphate rather than of arsenic.

G. Smithson proposes to fuse any powder suspected to contain arsenic with nitre: this produces arseniate of potassa, of which the solution affords a brick-red precipitate with nitrate of silver. In cases where any sensible portion of the alkali of the nitre has been set free, it must be saturated with acetous acid, and the saline mixture dried and redissolved in water. So small is the quantity of arsenic required for this mode of trial, that a drop of solution of oxide of arsenic in water (which, at 54° of Fahr. may be estimated to contain one-eightieth its weight of the oxide), mixed with a little nitrate of potassa, and fused in a platinum spoon, affords a very sensible quantity of arseniate of silver. (*Ann. of Phil. N. S.* iv. 127.)

H. Dr. Cooper, President of Columbia College, finds a solution of chromate of potassa to be one of the best tests of arsenic. One drop is turned green by the fourth of a grain of arsenic, by two or three drops of Fowler's mineral solution, or any other arsenite of potassa. The arsenious acid takes oxygen from the chromic, which is converted into oxide of chrome To exhibit the effect, take five watch-glasses; put on one, two or three drops of a watery solution of white arsenic; on the second, as much arsenite of potassa; on the third, one-fourth of a grain of white arsenic in substance; on the fourth, two or three drops of a solution of corrosive sublimate; on the fifth, two or three drops of a solution of copper. Add to each three or four drops of a solution of chromate of potassa. In half an hour, a bright, clear, grass-green colour will appear in numbers 1, 2, 3, unchangeable by ammonia; number 4 will instantly exhibit an orange precipitate; and number 5 a green, which a drop of ammonia will instantly change to blue. (*Silliman's American Journal*, iii.)

I. But the most decisive mode of determining the presence of arsenic (which, though not absolutely indispensable, should always be resorted to, when the suspected substance can be obtained in sufficient quantity) is by reducing it to a metallic state: for its characters are then clear and unequivocal. For this purpose, let a portion of the white sediment, collected from the contents of the stomach, be dried and mixed with three times its weight of black flux; or if this cannot be procured, with two parts of very dry carbonate of potassa (the salt of tartar of the shops), and one of powdered charcoal. Dr. Bostock finds, that for this mixture we may advantageously substitute one composed of half a grain of charcoal, and two drops of oil, to a grain of the sediment. Procure a tube eight or nine inches long, and one-fourth or one-sixth of an inch in diameter, of thin glass, sealed hermetically at one end. Then put into the tube the mixture of the powder and its flux, and if any should adhere to the inner surface, let it be wiped off by a feather, so that the inside of all the upper part of the tube may be quite clean and dry. Stop the end of the tube loosely, with a little paper, and heat the sealed end only, on a chafing-dish of red-hot coals, taking care to avoid breathing the fumes. The arsenic, if present, will rise to the upper part of the tube, on the inner surface of which it will form a thin brilliant coating. Break the tube, and scrape off the reduced metal. Lay a little on a heated iron, when, if it be arsenic, a dense smoke will arise, and a strong smell of garlic will be perceived. The arsenic may be further identified, by putting a small quantity between two polished plates of copper, surrounding it by powdered charcoal, to prevent its escape, binding these tightly together by iron wire, and exposing them to a low red heat. If the included substances be arsenic, a white stain will be left on the copper.

K. It may be proper to observe, that neither the stain on copper, nor the odour of garlic, is produced by the white oxide of arsenic, when heated without the addition of some inflammable ingredient. The absence of arsenic must not, therefore, be inferred, if no smell should be occasioned by laying the white powder on a heated iron.

Dr. Black ascertained that all the necessary experiments, for the detection of arsenic, may be made on a single grain of the white oxide: this small quantity having produced, when heated in a tube with its proper flux, as much of the metal as clearly established its presence.

If the quantity of arsenic in the stomach should be so small, which is not very probable, as to occasion death, and yet to remain suspended in the washings, the whole contents, and the water employed to wash them must be filtered, and the clear liquor assayed for arsenic by the tests B, C, D, and E.

In this case, it is necessary to be careful that the colour of the precipitate is not modified by that of the liquid found in the stomach. If this be yellow, the precipitate by sulphate of copper and carbonate of potassa will appear green, even though no arsenic be present; but on leaving it to settle, decanting off the fluid, and replacing it with water, it will evidently be blue without any tinge of green, being no longer seen through a yellow medium.—(*Dr. Paris.*)

The liquid contents of the stomach may also be evaporated to dryness below 250° Fahr. and the dry mass be exposed to heat at the bottom of a Florence flask, to sublime the arsenic. If dissolved in an oily fluid, Dr. Ure proposes to boil the solution with distilled water, and afterward to separate the oil by the capillary action of wick threads. The watery fluid may then be subjected to the usual tests

In an investigation, the event of which is to affect the life of an accused person, it is the duty of every one who may prepare himself to give evidence, not to rest satisfied with the appearances produced by any one test of arsenic; but to render its presence quite unequivocal by the concurring results of several.

Discovery of corrosive sublimate, baryta, &c.—Corrosive sublimate (the bichloride or oxymuriate of mercury,) next to arsenic, is the most virulent of the metallic poisons. It may be collected by treating the contents of the stomach in the manner already described; but as it is more soluble than arsenic, *viz.* in about nineteen times its weight of water, no more water must be employed than is barely sufficient, and the washings must be carefully preserved for examination.

If a powder should be collected by this operation, which proves, on examination, not to be arsenic, it may be known to be corrosive sublimate by the following characters:

A. Expose a small quantity of it, without any admixture, to heat in a coated glass tube, as directed in the treatment of arsenic. Corrosive sublimate will be ascertained by its rising to the top of the tube, lining the inner surface in the form of a shining white crust.

B. Dissolve another portion in distilled water; and it may be proper to observe how much of the salt the water is capable of taking up.

C. To the watery solution add a little lime-water. A precipitate of an orange yellow colour will instantly appear.

D. To another portion of the solution add a single drop of a dilute solution of sub-carbonate of potassa (salt of tartar). A white precipitate will appear; but, on a still further addition of alkali, an orange-coloured sediment will be formed.

E. The carbonate of soda has similar effects.

F. Sulphuretted water throws down a dark-coloured sediment, which, when dried and strongly heated, is wholly volatilized, without any odour of garlic.

For the detection of corrosive sublimate, Sylvester has recommended the application of galvanism, which exhibits the mercury in a metallic state. A piece of zinc wire, or if that cannot be had, of iron wire about three inches long, is to be twice bent at right angles, so as to resemble the Greek letter Π. The two legs of this figure should be distant about the diameter of a common gold wedding-ring from each other, and the two ends of the bent wire must afterward be tied to a ring of this description. Let a plate of glass, not less than three inches square, be laid as nearly horizontal as possible, and on one side drop some sulphuric acid, diluted with about six times its weight of water, till it spreads to the size of a halfpenny. At a little distance from this, towards the other side, next drop some of the solution supposed to contain corrosive sublimate, till the edges of the two liquids join together; and let the wire and ring prepared as above be laid in such a way that the wire may touch the acid, while the gold ring is in contact with the suspected liquid. If the minutest quantity of corrosive sublimate be present, the ring in a few minutes will be covered with mercury on the part which touched the fluid.

Smithson remarks, that all the oxides and saline compounds of mercury, if laid in a drop of marine acid on gold, with a bit of tin, quickly amalgamate the gold. In this way, a very minute quantity of corrosive sublimate, or a drop of its solution may be tried, and no addition of muriatic acid is then required. Quantities of mercury may thus be rendered evident.

which could not be so by any other means. Even the mercury of cinnabar may be exhibited; but it must previously be boiled with a little sulphuric acid in a platinum spoon, to convert it into sulphate. An exceedingly minute quantity of metallic mercury in any powder may be discovered by placing it in nitric acid on gold, drying, and adding muriatic acid and tin.

The only mineral poison of great virulence that has not been mentioned, and which, from its being little known to act as such, it is very improbable we should meet with, is the carbonate of baryta. This, in the country where it is found, is employed as a poison for rats, and there can be no doubt would be equally destructive to human life. It may be discovered by dissolving it in muriatic acid, and by the insolubility of the precipitate which this solution yields on adding sulphuric acid, or sulphate of soda. Soluble barytic salts, if these have been the means of poison, will be contained in the water employed to wash the contents of the stomach, and will be detected, on adding sulphuric acid, by a copious precipitate.

It may be proper to observe, that the failure of attempts to discover poisonous substances in the alimentary canal after death, is by no means a sufficient proof that death has not been occasioned by poison. For it has been clearly established, by experiments made on animals, that a poison may be so completely evacuated, that no traces of it shall be found, and yet that death may ensue from the morbid changes which it has occasioned in the alimentary canal, or in the general system.

Method of detecting copper or lead.—Copper and lead sometimes gain admission into articles of food, in consequence of the employment of kitchen utensils of these materials.

1. If copper be suspected in any liquor, its presence will be ascertained by adding a solution of pure ammonia, which will strike a beautiful blue colour. If the solution be very dilute, it may be concentrated by evaporation; and if the liquor contain a considerable excess of acid, like that used to preserve pickles, as much of the alkali must be added as is more than sufficient to saturate the acid. In this, and all other experiments of the same kind, the fluid should be viewed by reflected, and not by transmitted light.

If into a newly prepared tincture of guaiacum wood we drop a concentrated solution of a salt of copper, the mixture instantly assumes a blue colour. This effect does not take place when the solution is very weak, for example, when there is not above half a grain of the salt to an ounce of water; but then, by the addition of a few drops of prussic acid, the blue colour is instantly developed of great purity and intensity. This colour is not permanent, but soon passes to a green, and at length totally disappears. For want of prussic acid, distilled laurel-water may be employed. The test produces its effect, even when the proportion of the salt of copper to the water does not exceed 1-45000th. In this minute proportion no other test, whether the prussiate of potassa, soda, or ammonia, gives the least indication of copper.—(*Quart. Journ.* x. 182.)

2. Lead is occasionally found, in sufficient quantity to be injurious to health, in water that has passed through leaden pipes, or been kept in leaden vessels, and sometimes even in pump-water, in consequence of that metal having been used in the construction of the pump. Acetate of lead has also been known to be fraudulently added to bad wines, with the view of concealing their defects.

Lead may be discovered by adding, to a portion of the suspected water, about half its bulk of water impregnated with sulphuretted hydrogen gas. If lead be present, it will be manifested by a dark brown or blackish, tinge. This test is so delicate, that water, condensed by the leaden worm of a still-tub, is sensibly affected by it. Lead is also detected by a similar effect ensuing on the addition of sulphuret of ammonia, or potassa.

The adequacy of this method, however, to the discovery of very minute quantities of lead, has been set aside by the experiments of Dr. Lambe, the author of a skilful analysis of the springs of Leamington Priors, near Warwick. By new methods of examination, he has detected the presence of lead in several spring-waters, that manifest no change on the addition of the sulphuretted test; and has found that metal in the precipitate, separated from such waters by the carbonate of potassa or of soda. In operating on these waters, Dr Lambe noticed the following appearances :

a. The test forms sometimes a dark cloud, with the precipitate affected by alkalies, which has been redissolved in nitric acid.

b. Though it forms, in other cases, no cloud, the precipitate itself becomes darkened by the sulphuretted test.

c. The test forms a white cloud, treated with the precipitate as in *a.* These two appearances may be united.

d. The test neither forms a cloud, nor darkens the precipitate.

e. In the cases *b, c, d,* heat the precipitate, in contact with an alkaline carbonate, to redness; dissolve out the carbonate by water; and treat the precipitate as in *a.* The sulphuretted test then forms a dark cloud with the solution of the precipitate. In these experiments, it is essential that the acid, used to redissolve the precipitate, shall not be in excess; and if it should so happen, that excess must be saturated before the test is applied. It is better to use so little acid, that some of the precipitate may remain undissolved.

f. Instead of the process *e,* the precipitate may be exposed, without addition, to a red heat, and then treated as in *a.* In this case, the test will detect the metallic matter; but with less certainty than the foregoing one.

The nitric acid, used in these experiments, should be perfectly pure; and the test should be recently prepared by saturating water with sulphuretted hydrogen gas. A few drops of nitric acid added to a water containing lead, which has been reduced to 1-8th or 1-10th its bulk by evaporation, and then followed by the addition of a few drops of hydriodate of potassa, produces a yellow insoluble precipitate.

Another mode of analysis, employed by Dr. Lambe, consists in precipitating the lead by solution of common salt; but as muriate of lead is partly soluble in water, this test cannot be applied to small portions of suspected water. The precipitate must be, therefore, collected, from two or three gallons, and heated to redness with twice its weight of carbonate of soda. Dissolve out the soda; add nitric acid, saturating any superfluity; and then apply the sulphuretted test. Sulphate of soda would be found more effectual in this process than the muriate, on account of the greater insolubility of sulphate of lead. This property, indeed, renders sulphate of soda an excellent test of the presence of lead, when held in solution by acids, for it throws down that metal, even when present in very small quantity, in the form of a heavy white precipitate, which is not soluble by acetic acid.

The third process, which is the most satisfactory of all, and is very easy, except for the trouble of collecting a large quantity of precipitate, is the actual reduction of the metal, and its exhibition in a separate form. The precipitate may be mixed with its own weight of alkaline carbonate, and exposed either with or without the addition of a small proportion of charcoal, to a heat sufficient to melt the alkali. On breaking the crucible, a small globule of lead will be found reduced at the bottom. The precipitate from about fifty gallons of water yielded Dr. Lambe, in one instance, about two grains of lead.

For discovering the presence of lead in wine, a test invented by Dr. Hahnemann, and known by the title of Hahnemann's wine test, may be employed. This test is prepared by putting together, into a small phial, sixteen grains of sulphuret of lime, prepared in the dry way (by exposing to a red heat, in a covered crucible, equal weights of powdered lime and sulphur, accurately mixed), and twenty grains of bitartrate of potassa (cream of tartar). The phial is to be filled with water, well corked, and occasionally shaken for the space of ten minutes. When the powder has subsided, decant the clear liquor, and preserve it, in a well-stopped bottle, for use. The liquor, when fresh prepared, discovers lead by a dark coloured precipitate. A further proof of the presence of lead in wines is the occurrence of a precipitate on adding a solution of the sulphate of soda.

Sylvester has proposed the gallic acid as an excellent test of the presence of lead.

The quantity of lead, which has been detected in sophisticated wine, may be estimated at forty grains of the metal in every fifty gallons

When a considerable quantity of acetate of lead has been taken into the stomach (as sometimes, owing to its sweet taste, happens to children), after the exhibition of an active emetic, the hydro-sulphuret of potassa or of ammonia may be given ; or probably a solution of sulphate of soda (Glauber's salt) would render it innoxious."—*Henry's Chem.*

Poison-oak. See *Rhus toxicodendron.*

POLEMO'NIUM. (An ancient name derived from πολεμος, war: because, according to Pliny, kings had contended for the honour of its discovery.) 1. The name of a genus of plants in the Linnæan system Class, *Pentandria ;* Order, *Monogynia.*

2. Wild sage, or *Teucrium scorodonia* of Linnæus.

POLEMONIUM CÆRULEUM. The systematic name of the Greek valerian, or Jacob's ladder, the root of which is esteemed by some as a good astringent against diarrhœas and dysentery.

POLEY-MOUNTAIN. See *Teucrium.*

POLIOSIS .(From πολος, *candidus,* white or hoary.) The specific name of a species of *Trichosis* in Good's arrangement, in which the hairs are prematurely gray or hoary.

PO'LIUM. (From πολιος, white: so called from its white capillaments.) Poley. *Teucrium* of Linnæus.

POLIUM CRETICUM. See *Teucrium creticum.*

POLIUM MONTANUM. See *Teucrium capitatum.*

POLLEN. (*Pollen, inis.* n.; fine flour, or dust.) The powder which adheres to the anthers of the flowers of plants, and which is contained in the anther, and is thrown out chiefly in warm, dry weather, when the coat of the latter contracts and bursts. The pollen, though to the naked eye a fine powder, and light enough to be wafted along by the air, is so curiously formed, and so various in different plants, as to be an interesting and popular object for the microscope. Each grain of it is commonly a membranous bag, round or angular, rough or smooth, which remains entire till it meets with any moisture, being contrary in this respect to the nature of the anther ; then it bursts with great force, discharging its subtile and vivifying vapour.

In the *Helianthus annuus,* the pollen is *echinate*

In *Geraniums, perforate.*

The pollen of *Symphatum* is *didymous.*

That of the *Mallow, dentate.*

It is *angulate* in *Viola odorata.*

Reniforme in *Narcissus ;* and

In *Borago, convolute.*

POLLENIN. The pollen of tulips has been ascertained by Professor John to contain a peculiar substance, insoluble in alkohol, æther, water, oil of turpentine, naphtha, carbonated and pure alkalies; extremely combustible, burning with great rapidity and flame; and hence used at the theatres to imitate lightning.

POLLEX. The thumb, or great toe.

POLYADELPHIA. (From πολυς, many, and αδελφια, a brotherhood.) The name of a class of plants in the sexual system of Linnæus, embracing plants with hermaphrodite flowers, in which several stamina are united by their filaments into three or more distinct bundles.

POLYA'NDRIA. (From πολυς, many, and ανηρ, a husband.) The name of a class of plants in the sexual system of Linnæus. It consists of plants with hermaphrodite flowers, furnished with several stamina, that are inserted into the common receptacle of the flower ; by which circumstance this class is distinguished from *Icosandria,* in which the striking character is the situation of the stamina on the calyx or petals.

POLYCHRE'STUS. (From πολυς, much, and χρησος, useful.) Having many virtues, or uses. Applied to many medicines from their extensive usefulness.

POLYCHROITE. The colouring matter of saffron.

POLYDI'PSIA. (From πολυς, much, and διψη, thirst.) Excessive thirst. A genus of disease in the Class *Locales,* and Order *Dysorexiæ,* of Cullen. It is mostly symptomatic of fever, dropsy, excessive discharges, or poisons,

POLY'GALA. (From πολυς, much, and γαλα, milk; so named from the abundance of its milky juice.) 1. The name of a genus of plants in the Linnæan system, Class, *Diadelphia ;* Order, *Octandria.*

2. The pharmacopœial name of the common milk wort. See *Polygala vulgaris.*

POLYGALA AMARA. This is a remarkably bitter plant

and, though not used in this country, promises to be as efficacious as those in greater repute. It has been given freely in phthisis pulmonalis, and, like other remedies, failed in producing a cure; yet, as a palliative, it claims attention. Its virtues are balsamic, demulcent, and corroborant.

POLYGALA SENEGA. The systematic name of the rattlesnake milk-wort. *Seneka. Polygala—floribus imperbibus spicatis, caule erecto herbaceo simplicissimo, foliis ovato lanceolatis,* of Linnæus. The root of this plant was formerly much esteemed as a specific against the poison of the rattlesnake, and as an antiphlogistic in pleurisy, pneumonia, &c.; but it is now very much laid aside. Its dose is from ten to twenty grains; but when employed, it is generally used in the form of decoction, which, when prepared according to the formula of the Edinburgh Pharmacopœia, may be given every second or third hour.

POLYGALA VULGARIS. The systematic name of the common milk-wort. The root of this plant is somewhat similar in taste to that of the seneka, but much weaker. The leaves are very bitter, and a handful of them, infused in wine, is said to be a safe and gentle purge.

POLYGA'MIA. (From πολυς, many, and γαμος, a marriage.) Polygamy. The name of a class of plants in the sexual system of Linnæus, consisting of polygamous plants, or plants having hermaphrodite flowers, and likewise male and female flowers, or both. The orders of this division are according to the beautiful uniformity or plan which runs through this ingenious system, distinguished upon the principles of the Classes *Monœcia, Diœcia,* and *Triœcia.* It has the five following orders:

1. *Polygamia æqualis.* The name of an order of Class *Syngenesia,* of the sexual system of plants. The florets are all perfect or united, that is, each furnished with perfect stamens.

2. *Polygamia frustranea.* Florets of the disk, with stamens and pistil: those of the radius with merely an abortive pistil, or with not even the rudiments of any.

3. *Polygamia necessaria.* Florets of the disk with stamens only, those of the radius with pistils only.

4. *Polygamia segregata.* Several flowers, either simp.e or compound, but with united anthers, and with a proper calyx, included in one common calyx.

5. *Polygamia superflua.* Florets of the disk, with stamens and pistil: those of the radius with pistil only, but each, of both kinds, forming perfect seed.

POLYGONA'TUM. (From πολυς, many, and γονυ, a joint: so named from its numerous joints or knots.) Solomon's seal. See *Convallaria polygonatum.*

POLY'GONUM. (From πολυς, many, and γονυ, a joint: so named from its numerous joints.) The name of a genus of plants in the Linnæan system. Class, *Octandria;* Order, *Trigynia.* Knot-grass.

POLYGONUM AVICULARE. The systematic name of the knot-grass. *Centumnodia; Polygonum latifolium; Polygonum mas; Sanguinaria.* This plant is never used in this country; it is said to be useful in stopping hæmorrhages, diarrhœas, &c.; but little credit is to be given to this account.

POLYGONUM BACCIFERUM. A species of equisetum, or horse-tail.

POLYGONUM BISTORTA. The systematic name of the officinal bistort. *Bistorta. Polygonum—caule simplicissimo monostachio, foliis ovatis in petiolum decurrentibus,* of Linnæus. This plant is a native of Britain. Every part manifests a degree of stypticity to the taste, and the root is esteemed to be one of the most powerful of the vegetable astringents, and frequently made use of as such, in disorders proceeding from a laxity and debility of the solids, for restraining alvine fluxes, after due evacuations, and other preternatural discharges, both serous and sanguineous. It has been sometimes given in intermitting fevers; and sometimes also, in small doses, as a corroborant and antiseptic, in acute malignant and colliquative fevers; in which intentions Peruvian bark has now deservedly superseded both these and all other adstringents. The common dose of bistort root in substance, is fifteen or twenty grains: in urgent cases it is extended to a drachm. Its astringent matter is totally dissolved both by water and rectified spirits.

POLYGONUM DIVARICATUM. The systematic name of the eastern buckwheat plant. The roots, reduced to a coarse meal, are the ordinary food of the Siberians.

POLYGONUM FAGOPYRUM. The systematic name of the buckwheat. The grain of this plant constitutes the principal food of the inhabitants of Russia, Germany, and Switzerland.

POLYGONUM HYDROPIPER. The systematic name of the poor man's pepper. *Hydropiper.* Biting arse-smart; Lake-weed; Water-pepper. This plant is very common in our ditches; the leaves have an acrid, burning taste, and seem to be nearly of the same nature with those of the arum. They have been recommended as possessing antiseptic, aperient, diuretic virtues, and given in scurvies and cachexies, asthmas, hypochondriacal and nephritic complaints, and wandering gout. The first leaves have been applied externally, as a stimulating cataplasm.

POLYGONUM LATIFOLIUM. Common knot-grass. See *Polygonum aviculare.*

POLYGONUM MAS. See *Polygonum aviculare.*

POLYGONUM MINUS. Rupture-wort. See *Herniaria glabra.*

POLYGONUM PERSICARIA. The systematic name of the *Persicaria* of the old pharmacopœias. *Persicaria mitis; Plumbago.* Arse-smart. This plant is said to possess vulnerary and antiseptic properties; with which intentions it is given in wine to restrain the progress of gangrene.

POLYGONUM SELENOIDES. Parsley breakstone.

POLYPO'DIUM. (From πολυς, many, and πους, a foot: so called because it has many roots.) The name of a genus of plants in the Linnæan system. Class, *Cryptogamia;* Order, *Filices.* Fern, or polypody.

POLYPODIUM ACULEATUM. *Filix aculeata.* Spear-pointed fern. Fallen into disuse.

POLYPODIUM FILIX MAS. *Aspidium filix mas,* of Dr. Smith; *Pteris; Blancnon; Orbasii; Lonchitis.* Male polypody, or fern. The root of this plant has been greatly celebrated for its effects upon the *tænia osculis superficialibus,* or broad tape-worm. Madame Noufer acquired great celebrity by employing it as a specific. This secret was thought of such importance by some of the principal physicians at Paris, who were deputed to make a complete trial of its efficacy, that it was purchased by the French king, and afterward published by his order. The method of cure is the following:—After the patient has been prepared by an emollient glyster, and a supper of panada, with butter and salt, he is directed to take in the morning, while in bed, a dose of two or three drachms of the powdered root of the male fern. The powder must be washed down with a draught of water, and, two hours after, a strong cathartic, composed of calomel and scammony, is to be given, proportioned to the strength of the patient. If this does not operate in due time, it is to be followed by a dose of purging salts, and if the worm be not expelled in a few hours, this process is to be repeated at proper intervals. Of the success of this, or a similar mode of treatment, in cases of tænia, there can be no doubt, as many proofs in this country afford sufficient testimony; but whether the fern-root or the strong cathartic is the principal agent in the destruction of the worm, may admit of a question; and the latter opinion, Dr. Woodville believes, is the more generally adopted by physicians. It appears, however from some experiments made in Germany, that the tænia has, in several instances, been expelled by the repeated exhibition of the root, without the assistance of any purgative.

[POLYPODIUM BAROMETZ. See *Agnus tartaricus* A]

PO'LYPUS. (From πολυς, many, and πους, a foot: from its sending off many ramifications, like legs) 1. The name of a genus of zoophytes.

2. A species of *sarcoma* in Cullen's Nosology. A polypus is a tumour, which is generally narrow where it originates, and then becomes wider, somewhat like a pear. It is most commonly met with in the nose, uterus, or vagina; and has received its name from an erroneous idea, that it usually had several roots, or feet, like zoophyte polypi.

Polypi vary from each other according to the different causes that produce them, and the alterations that happen in them. Sometimes a polypus of the nose is owing to a swelling of the pituitary membrane, which swelling may possess a greater or less space of the membrane, as also its cellular substance, and may affect either one or both nostrils. At other times it arises from an ulcer produced by a caries of some of the bones which form the internal surface of the nostrils. Polypuses are sometimes so soft, that upon the least touch they are lacerated, and bleed; at other times they are very compact, and even scirrhous. Some continue small a great while; others increase so fast as, in a short time, to push out at the nostrils, or extend backwards towards the throat. Le Dran mentions, that he has known them fill up the space behind the uvula, and, turning towards the mouth, have protruded the fleshy arch of the palate so far forwards as to make it parallel with the third *dentes molares*. There are others which, though at first free from any malignant disposition, become afterward carcinomatous, and even highly cancerous. Of whatever nature the polypus is, it intercepts the passage of the air through the nostril, and, when large, forces the *septum narium* into the other nostril, so that the patient is unable to breathe, unless through the mouth. A large *polypus* pressing in like manner upon the spongy bones, gradually forces them down upon the maxillary bones, and thus compresses and stops up the orifice of the *ductus lachrymalis;* nor is it impossible for the sides of the *canalis nasalis* to be pressed together. In which case, the tears, having no passage through the nose, the eye is kept constantly watering, and the *sacchus lachrymalis*, not being able to discharge its contents, is sometimes so much dilated as to form what is called a flat *fistula.* The above writer has seen instances of polypuses so much enlarged as to force down the ossa palati.

The polypus of the uterus is of three kinds, in respect to situation. It either grows from the fundus, the inside of the cervix, or from the lower edge of the os uteri. The first case is the most frequent, the last the most uncommon. Polypi of the uterus are always shaped like a pear, and have a thin pedicle. They are almost invariably of that species which is denominated fleshy, hardly ever being scirrhous, cancerous, or ulcerated.

3. The coagulated substance which is found in the cavities of the heart of those who are some time *in articulo mortis*, is improperly called a polypus.

POLYSA'RCIA. (From πολυς, much, and σαρξ, flesh.) *Polysomatia; Obesitas; Corpulenta; Steatites.* Troublesome corpulency, obesity, or fatness. A genus of diseases in the Class *Cachexiæ*, and Order *Intumescentia*, of Cullen.

POLYSOMA'TIA. (From πολυς, much, and σωμα, a body.) See *Polysarcia*.

POLYSPA'STUM. (From πολυς, much, and σπαω, to draw.) A forcible instrument for reducing luxations.

POLYTRI'CHUM. (From πολυς, many, and θριξ, hair: so called from its resemblance to a woman's hair, or because, in ancient times, women used to dye the hair with it, to keep it from shedding.) *Polytrychon.* 1. The name of a genus of plants in the Linnæan system. Class, *Cryptogamia;* Order, *Musci.*

2. The pharmacopœial name of the golden maidenhair. See *Polytricum commune.*

POLYTRICUM COMMUNE. The systematic name of the golden maidenhair. *Adianthum aureum.* It possesses, in an inferior degree, astringent virtues: and was formerly given in diseases of the lungs and calculous complaints.

POMACEÆ. (From *pomum*, an apple.) The name of an order of plants in Linnæus's Fragments of a Natural Method, consisting of those which have a fruit of a pulpy, esculent, apple, berry, or cherry kind.

POMA'CEUM. (From *pomum*, an apple.) Cider, or the fermented juice of apple.

POMEGRANATE. See *Punica granatum.*

POMPHOLYGO'DES. (From πομφολυξ, a bubble, and ειδος, resemblance.) Urine, with bubbles on the surface.

PO'MPHOLYX. (From πομφος, a bladder.) 1. A small vesicle, or bubble.

2. The whitish oxide of zinc, which adheres to the covers of the crucibles in making brass, in the form of small bubbles.

PO'MPHOS. (From πεμφω, to put forth.) *Pomphus.* A bladder, or watery pustule.

POMUM. 1. An apple.

2. In botanical distinctions and language this is a fleshy pericarpium or seed-vessel, containing a capsule within it, with several seeds. Its species are,

1. *Pomum oblongum;* as in Pyrus communis.

2. *P. baccatum;* as in Pyrus baccata.

3. *P. muricatum;* as in Momordica trifoliata.

4. *P. hispidum;* as in Momordica elaterium.

The navel-like remains is part of the calyx.

The pomum is comprehended by Gærtner under the different kinds of bacca, it being sometimes scarcely possible to draw the line between them. See *Pyrus malus*

POMUM ADAMI. *(Pomum*, an apple: so called in consequence of a whimsical supposition, that part of the forbidden apple which Adam ate, stuck in the throat, and thus became the case.) The protuberance in the anterior part of the neck, formed by the forepart of the thyroid gland.

POMUM AMORIS. See *Solanum lycopersicum.*

Ponderous spar. See *Heavy spar* and *Barytes.*

PO'NS. A bridge. A part of the brain is so called from its arched appearance.

PONS VAROLII. *Corpus annulare; Processus annularis; Eminentia annularis.* Varolius's bridge. An eminence of the medulla oblongata, first described by Varolius. It is formed by the two exterior crura of the cerebellum becoming flattened and passing over the crura of the cerebrum.

PO'NTICA VINA. Acid, feculent, and tartarous wines.

PONTICUM MEL. A poisonous honey.

Poor man's pepper. See *Polygonum hydropiper*, and *Lepidium.*

POPLAR. See *Populus.*

PO'PLES. The ham, or joint of the knee.

POPLITE'AL. *(Popliteus;* from *poples*, the ham.) A small triangular muscle lying across the back part of the knee-joint, is so called.

POPLITEAL ARTERY. *Arteria poplitea.* The continuation of the crural artery, through the hollow of the ham.

POPPY. See *Papaver.*

Poppy, red corn. See *Papaver rhœas.*

Poppy, white. See *Papaver somniferum.*

POPULA'GO. (From *populus*, the poplar; because its leaves resemble those of the poplar.) See *Caltha palustris.*

PO'PULUS. (From πολυς, many; because of the multitude of its shoots.) 1. The name of a genus of plants in the Linnæan system. Class, *Diœcia;* Order *Octandria.*

2. The pharmacopœial name of the black poplar See *Populus nigra.*

POPULUS BALSAMIFERA. See *Fagara.*

POPULUS NIGRA. The systematic name of the black poplar. *Ægeiros.* The young buds, *oculi*, or rudiments of the leaves, which appear in the beginning of the spring, were formerly employed in an officinal ointment. At present they are almost entirely disregarded, though they should seem, from their sensible qualities, to be applicable to purposes of some importance. They have a yellow, unctuous, odorous, balsamic juice.

PO'RCUS. A name for the pudendum muliebre.

PORI BILIARII. The biliary pores or ducts, that receive the bile from the penicilli of the liver, and con vey it to the hepatic duct. See *Liver.*

PORIFORMIS. Resembling a pore: applied to a nectary, when of that appearance, as that of the hyacinth, which has three like pores in the germen.

POROCE'LE. (From πωρος, a callus, and κηλη, a tumour.) A hard tumour of any part, but especially of the testicle.

PORO'MPHALUM (From πωρος, a callus, and ουφαλος, the navel.) A hard tumour of the navel.

PORPHYRA. Dr. Good's name for scurvy. See *Scorbutus.*

PORPHYRY. A compound rock, having a basis, in which the other contemporaneous constituent parts are imbedded. The base is sometimes clay-stone, sometimes hornstone, sometimes compact felspar or pitchstone, pearlstone, and obsidian. The imbedded parts are most commonly felspar and quartz, which are usually crystallized more or less perfectly, and hence they appear sometimes granular. According to Werner, there are two distinct porphyry formations; the oldest occurs in gneiss, in beds of great magnitude; and also in mica-slate and clay-slate. Between Blair in Athole and Dalnacardoch, there is a very fine example of a bed of porphyry-slate in mica. The second porphyry formation is much more widely extended. It consists principally of clay porphyry, while the former consists chiefly of hornstone porphyry and felspar porphyry.

t sometimes contains considerable repositories of ore, in veins. Gold, silver, lead, tin, copper, iron, and manganese occur in it; but chiefly in the newer porphyry, as happens with the Hungarian mines. It occurs in Arran, and in Perthshire between Dalnacardoch and Tummel-bridge.

PORRET. See *Allium porrum.*

PORRI'GO. (*A porrigendo;* from its spreading abroad.) A disease very common among children, in which the skin of the hairy part of the head becomes dry and callous, and comes off like bran upon combing the head.

PO'RRUM. See *Allium porrum.*

PO'RTA. (*A portando,* because through it the blood is carried to the liver.) That part of the liver where its vessels enter.

PORTÆ VENA. See *Vena portæ.*

PORTAIGUILLE. The acutenaculum.

PORTIO. A portion or branch: applied to a nerve.

PORTIO DURA. (One branch of the seven pair of nerves is called *portio dura,* the hard portion, either from its being more firm than the other, or because it runs into the hard part of the skull; and the other the *portio mollis,* or soft portion.) Facial nerve. This nerve arises near the pons, from the crus of the brain, enters the petrous portion of the temporal bone, gives off a branch into the tympanum, which is called the chorda tympani, and then proceeds to form the *pes anserinus* on the face, from whence the integuments of the face are supplied with nerves. See *Facial nerve.*

PORTIO MOLLIS. Auditory nerve. Acoustic nerve. This nerve arises from the medulla oblongata and fourth ventricle of the brain, enters the petrous portion of the temporal bone, and is distributed on the internal ear, by innumerable branches, not only to the cochlea, but also to the membrane lining the vestibulum and semicircular canals, and is the immediate organ of hearing.

Portland powder. A celebrated gout remedy. It consists of various bitters; principally of hoarhound, bithwort, the tops and leaves of germander, ground-pine, and centaury, dried, powdered, and sifted. It is now fallen into disuse.

PORTORA'RIUM. (From *porta,* a door; because it is, as it were, the door or entrance of the intestines.) The right orifice of the stomach.

PORTULA'CA. (From *porto,* to carry, and *lac,* milk; because it increases the animal milk.) 1. The name of a genus of plants in the Linnæan system. Class, *Dodecandria;* Order, *Digynia.*

2. The pharmacopœial name of the purslane. See *Portulaca oleracea.*

PORTULACA OLERACEA. The systematic name of the eatable purslane. *Andrachne; Allium gallicum.* The plant which is so called in dietetical and medical writings, abounds with a watery and somewhat acrid juice, and is often put into soups, or pickled with spices. It is said to be antiseptic and aperient.

PO'RUS. A pore or duct. A term used in anatomy, and botany; the pores of the skin; and particularly applied in botany to the small puncture-like openings in the inferior surface of the genus Boletus.

Po'sCA. Vinegar and water mixed.

POSSE'TUM. Posset. Milk curdled with wine, treacle, or any acid.

POSTE'RIOR. Parts are so named from their relative situation.

POSTERIOR ANNULARIS. *Musculus posterior annularis.* An external interosseal muscle of the hand, that extends and draws the ring-finger inwards.

POSTERIOR AURIS. See *Retrahentes auris.*

POSTERIOR INDICIS. *Musculus posterior indicis.* An internal interosseal muscle of the hand, that extends the fore-finger obliquely, and draws it outwards.

POSTERIOR MEDII. An external interosseal muscle of the hand, that extends the middle finger, and draws it outwards.

POTAMOGEI'TON. (From ποταμος, a river, and γειτων, adjacent: so named because it grows about rivers.) The name of a genus of plants in the Linnæan system. Class, *Tetrandria;* Order, *Tetragynia.*

POTASH. See *Potassa.*

POTA'SSA. (*Potassa, æ. f.;* so called from the pots, or vessels, in which it was first made.) Vegetable alkali: so called because it is obtained in an impure state by the incineration of vegetables. Potass; Potash; Kali. An hydrated protoxide of potassium

302

Table of the saline product of one thousand pounds of ashes of the following vegetables:—
Saline products.

Stalks of Turkey wheat or maise,	198 lbs.
Stalks of sun-flower,	349
Vine branches,	162.6
Elm,	166
Box,	78
Sallow,	102
Oak,	111
Aspen,	61
Beech,	219
Fir,	132
Fern cut in August,	116 { or 125 according to Wildenheim.
Wormwood,	748
Fumitory,	360
Heath,	115 Wildenheim.

On these tables Kirwan makes the following remarks:—

1. That in general weeds yield more ashes, and their ashes much more salt, than woods; and that, consequently, as to salts of the vegetable alkali kind, as potassa, pearlash, cashup, &c. neither America, Trieste, nor the northern countries have any advantage over Ireland.

2. That of all weeds fumitory produces more salt, and next to it wormwood. But if we attend only to the quantity of salt in a given weight of ashes, the ashes of wormwood contain most. Trifolium fibrinum also produces more ashes and salt than fern.

The process for obtaining pot and pearlash is given by Kirwan, as follows:—

1. The weeds should be cut just before they seed, then spread, well dried, and gathered clean.

2. They should be burned within doors on a grate, and the ashes laid in a chest as fast as they are produced. If any charcoal be visible, it should be picked out, and thrown back into the fire. If the weeds be moist, much coal will be found. A close smothered fire, which has been recommended by some, is very prejudicial.

3. They should be lixiviated with twelve times their weight of boiling water. A drop of the solution of corrosive sublimate will immediately discover when the water ceases to take up any more alkali. The earthy matter that remains is said to be a good manure for clayey soils.

4. The ley thus formed should be evaporated to dryness in iron pans. Two or three at least of these should be used, and the ley, as fast as it is concreted, passed from the one to the other. Thus, much time is saved, as weak leys evaporate more quickly than the stronger. The salt thus produced is of a dark colour, and contains much extractive matter, and being formed in iron pots is called potassa.

5. This salt should then be carried to a reverberatory furnace, in which the extractive matter is burned off, and much of the water dissipated: hence it generally loses from ten to fifteen per cent. of its weight. Particular care should be taken to prevent its melting, as the extractive matter would not then be perfectly consumed, and the alkali would form such a union with the earthy parts as could not easily be dissolved. Kirwan adds this caution, because Dr. Lewis and Dossie have inadvertently directed the contrary. This salt thus refined is called pearlash, and must be the same as the Dantzic pearlash.

To obtain this alkali pure, Bethollet recommends, to evaporate a solution of potassa, made caustic by boiling with quicklime, till it becomes of a thickish consistence; to add about an equal weight of alkohol, and let the mixture stand some time in a close vessel. Some solid matter partly crystallized will collect at the bottom; above this will be a small quantity of a dark-coloured fluid; and on the top another lighter. The latter, separated by decantation, is to be evaporated quickly in a silver basin in a sand-heat. Glass, or almost any other metal, would be corroded by the potassa. Before the evaporation has been carried far, the solution is to be removed from the fire, and suffered to stand at rest; when it will again separate into two fluids. The lighter being poured off, is again to be evaporated with a quick heat; and on standing a day or two in a close vessel, it will deposite transparent crystals of pure potassa. If the liquor be evaporated to a pellicle, the potassa will concrete without regular crystallization. In both cases a high-coloured liquor is separated, which is to be poured off; and the potassa must be kept carefully secluded from air.

A perfectly pure solution of potassa will remain transparent on the addition of lime-water, show no effervescence with dilute sulphuric acid, and not give any precipitate on blowing air from the lungs through it by means of a tube.

Pure potassa for experimental purposes may most easily be obtained by igniting cream of tartar in a crucible, dissolving the residue in water, filtering, boiling with a quantity of quicklime, and after subsidence, decanting the clear liquid, and evaporating in a loosely covered silver capsule, till it flows like oil, and then pouring it out on a clean iron plate. A solid white cake of pure hydrate of potassa is thus obtained, without the agency of alkohol. It must be immediately broken into fragments, and kept in a well stoppered phial.

As 100 parts of subcarbonate of potassa are equivalent to about 70 of pure concentrated oil of vitriol, if into a measure tube, graduated into 100 equal parts, we introduce the 70 grains of acid, and fill up the remaining space with water, then we have an alkalimeter for estimating the value of commercial pearlashes, which, if pure, will require for 100 grains one hundred divisions of the liquid to neutralize them. If they contain only 60 per cent. of genuine subcarbonate, then 100 grains will require only 60 divisions, and so on. When the alkalimeter indications are required in pure or absolute potassa, such as constitutes the basis of nitre, then we must use 102 grains of pure oil of vitriol, along with the requisite bulk of water to fill up the volume of the graduated tube.

The hydrate of potassa, as obtained by the preceding process, is solid, white, and extremely caustic; in minute quantities, changing the purple of violets and cabbage to a green, reddened litmus to purple, and yellow tumeric to a reddish-brown. It rapidly attracts humidity from the air, passing into the oil of tartar per deliquium of the chemists; a name, however, also given to the deliquesced subcarbonate. Charcoal applied to the hydrate of potassa at a cherry-red heat, gives birth to carburetted hydrogen, and an alkaline subcarbonate; but at a heat bordering on whiteness, carburetted hydrogen, carbonous oxide, and potassium, are formed. Several metals decompose the hydrate of potassa, by the aid of heat; particularly potassium, sodium, and iron. The fused hydrate of potassa consist of 6 deutoxide of potassium + 1.125 water = 7.125, which number represents the compound prime equivalent. It is used in surgery, as the potential cautery for forming eschars; and it was formerly employed in medicine diluted with broths as a lithontriptic. In chemistry, it is very extensively employed, both in manufactures and as a reagent in analysis. It is the basis of all the common soft soaps. The oxides of the following metals are soluble in aqueous potassa;—Lead, tin, nickel, arsenic, cobalt, manganese, zinc, antimony, tellurium, tungsten, molybdenum.

The preparations of this alkali that are used in medicine are :

1. Potassa fusa.
2. Liquor potassæ.
3. Potassa cum calce.
4. Subcarbonas potassæ.
5. Carbonas potassæ.
6. Sulphas potassæ.
7. Super-sulphas potassæ.
8. Tartras potassæ.
9. Acetas potassæ.
10. Citras potassæ.
11. Oxychloras potassæ.
12. Arsenias potassæ.
13. Sulphuretum potassæ.

Potassa, acetate of. See Potassæ acetas.
Potassa, carbonate of. See Potassæ carbonas.
Potassa, fused. See Potassa fusa.
Potassa, solution of. See Potassæ liquor
Potassa, subcarbonate of. See Potassæ subcarbonas.
Potassa, subcarbonate of, solution of. See Potassæ subcarbonatis liquor.
Potassa, sulphate of. See Potassæ sulphas.
Potassa, sulphuret of. See Potassæ sulphuretum.
Potassa, supersulphate of. See Potassæ supersulphas.

Potassa, supertartrate of. See Tartarum.
Potassa, tartrate of. See Potassæ tartras.
Potassa with lime. See Potassa cum calce.
POTASSA CUM CALCE. Potassa with lime. Calx cum kali puro; Causticum commune fortius; Lapis infernalis sive septicus. Take of solution of potassa three pints; fresh lime, a pound. Boil the solution of potassa down to a pint, then add the lime, previously slaked by the addition of water, and mix them together intimately. This is in common use with surgeons, as a caustic, to produce ulcerations, and to open abscesses.
POTASSA FUSA. Fused potassa. Kali purum; alkali vegetabile fixum causticum. Take of solution of potassa a gallon. Evaporate the water, in a clean iron pot, over the fire, until, when the ebullition has ceased, the potassa remains in a state of fusion; pour it upon a clean iron plate, into pieces of convenient form. This preparation of potassa is violently caustic, destroying the living animal fibre with great energy.
POTASSA IMPURA. See Potassa.
POTASSÆ ACETAS. Acetate of potassa. Acetated vegetable alkali. Kali acetatum; Sal diureticus; Terra foliata tartari; Sal sennerti. Take of subcarbonate of potassa a pound. Strong acetic acid, two pints. Distilled water, two pints. Mix the acid with the water, and add it gradually to the subcarbonate of potassa so long as may be necessary for perfect saturation. Let the solution be further reduced to one-half by evaporation, and strain it: then by means of a water-bath evaporate it, so that on being removed from the fire, it shall crystallize. The acetate of potassa is esteemed as a saline diuretic and deobstruent. It is given in the dose of from gr. x. to 3 ss. three times a day in any appropriate vehicle against dropsies, he patic obstructions, and the like.
POTASSÆ ARSENIAS. See Liquor arsenicalis.
POTASSÆ CARBONAS. Carbonate of potassa. This preparation, which has been long known by the name of Kali aëratum, appeared in the last London Pharmacopœia for the first time. It is made thus:—Take of subcarbonate of potassa made from tartar, a pound: subcarbonate of ammonia, three ounces; distilled water, a pint. Having previously dissolved the sub carbonate of potassa in the water, add the subcarbonate of ammonia; then, by means of a sand bath, apply a heat of 180° for three hours, or until the ammonia shall be driven off; lastly, set the solution by, to crystallize. The remaining solution may be evaporated in the same manner, that crystals may again form when it is set by.
This process was invented by Berthollet. The potassa takes the carbonic acid from the ammonia, which is volatile, and passes off in the temperature employed. It is, however, very difficult to detach the ammonia entirely. Potassa is thus saturated with carbonic acid, of which it contains double the quantity that the pure subcarbonate of potassa does; it gives out this proportion on the addition of muriatic acid, and may be converted into the subsalt, by heating it a short time to redness. It is less nauseous to the taste than the subcarbonate; it crystallizes, and does not deliquesce. Water, at the common temperature, dissolves one-fourth its weight, and at 212°, five-sixths; but this latter heat detaches some of the carbonic acid.
The carbonate of potassa is now generally used for the purpose of imparting carbonic acid to the stomach, by giving a scruple in solution with a table-spoonful of lemon juice, in the act of effervescing.
POTASSÆ CHLORAS. Formerly called oxymuriate of potassa.
POTASSÆ LIQUOR. Solution of potassa. Aqua kali puri; Lixivium saponarium. Take of subcarbonate of potassa a pound, lime newly prepared half a pound. Boiling distilled water, a gallon. Dissolve the potassa in two pints of the water; add the remaining water to the lime. Mix the liquors while they are hot, stir them together, then set the mixture by in a covered vessel; and after it has cooled, strain the solution through a cotton bag.
If any diluted acid dropped into the solution occasion the extrication of bubbles of gas, it will be necessary to add more lime, and to strain it again A pint of this solution ought to weigh sixteen ounces.
POTASSÆ NITRAS. See Nitre.
POTASSÆ SUBCARBONAS. Subcarbonate of potassa, formerly called, Kali præparatum; Sal absinthii; Sal tartari; Sal plantarum. Take of impure potassa

powdered, three pounds; boiling water, three pints and a half. Dissolve the potassa in water, and filter; then pour the solution into a clean iron pot, and evaporate the water over a moderate fire, until the liquor thickens; then let the fire be withdrawn and stir the liquor constantly with an iron rod, until the salt concretes into granular crystals.

A purer subcarbonate of potassa may be prepared in the same manner from tartar, which must be first burned until it becomes ash-coloured.

This preparation of potassa is in general use to form the citrate of potassa for the saline draughts. A scruple is generally directed to be saturated with lemon juice. In this process, the salt which is composed of potassa and carbonic acid is decomposed. The citric acid having a greater affinity for the potassa than the carbonic, seizes it and forms the citrate of potassa while the carbonic acid flies off in the form of air. The subcarbonate of potassa possesses antacid virtues, and may be exhibited with advantage in convulsions and other spasms of the intestines arising from acidity, in calculous and gouty complaints, leucorrhœa, scrofula, and aphthous affections. The dose is from ten grains to half a drachm.

POTASSÆ SUBCARBONATUS LIQUOR. Solution of subcarbonate of potassa. *Aqua kali præparati; Lixivium tartari; Oleum tartari per deliquium.* Take of subcarbonate of potassa, a pound; distilled water, twelve fluid-ounces. Dissolve the subcarbonate of potassa in the water, and then strain the solution through paper.

POTASSÆ SULPHAS. Formerly called *Kali vitriolatum; Alkali vegetabile vitriolatum; Sal de duobus; Arcanum duplicatum; Sal polychrestus; Nitrum vitriolatum; Tartarum vitriolatum.* Take of the salt which remains after the distillation of nitric acid, two pounds; boiling water, two gallons. Mix them that the salt may be dissolved; next add as much subcarbonate of potassa as may be requisite for the saturation of the acid; then boil the solution, until a pellicle appears upon the surface, and, after straining, set it by, that crystals may form. Having poured away the water, dry the crystals on bibulous paper. Its virtues are cathartic, diuretic, and deobstruent; with which intentions it is administered in a great variety of diseases, as constipation, suppression of the lochia, fevers, icterus, dropsies, milk tumours, &c. The dose is from one scruple to half an ounce.

POTASSÆ SULPHURETUM. Sulphuret of potassa. *Kali sulphuratum; Hepar sulphuris.* Liver of sulphur. Take of washed sulphur, an ounce; subcarbonate of potassa, two ounces; rub them together, and put them in a covered crucible, which is to be kept on the fire till they unite. In this process the carbonic acid is drawn off, and a compound formed of potassa and sulphur. This preparation has been employed in several cutaneous diseases with advantage, both internally and in the form of bath or ointment. It has also been recommended in diabetes. The dose is from five to twenty grains.

POTASSÆ SUPERARSENIAS. See *Superarsenias potassæ.*

POTASSÆ SUPERSULPHAS. Supersulphate of potassa. Take of the salt which remains after the distillation of nitric acid, two pounds; boiling water four pints. Mix them together, so that the salt may be dissolved, and strain the solution; then boil it to one-half, and set it by, that crystals may form. Having poured away the water, dry these crystals upon bibulous paper.

POTASSÆ SUPERTARTRAS. See *Tartarum.*

POTASSÆ TARTRAS. Tartrate of potassa, formerly called *Kali tartarisatum; Tartarum solubile; Tartarus tartarisatus; Sal vegetabilis; Alkali vegetabile tartarisatum.* Take of subcarbonate of potassa, sixteen ounces; supertartrate of potassa, three pounds; boiling water, a gallon. Dissolve the subcarbonate of potassa in the water; next add the supertartrate of potassa, previously reduced to powder, gradually, until bubbles of gas shall cease to arise. Strain the solution through paper, then boil it until a pellicle appear upon the surface, and set it by, that crystals may form. Having poured away the water, dry the crystals upon bibulous paper. Diuretic, deobstruent, and eccoprotic virtues are attributed to this preparation.

POTASSIUM. The metallic basis of potassa. "If a thin piece of solid hydrate of potassa be placed between two discs of platinum, connected with the ex-

tremities of a Voltaic apparatus of 200 double plates, four inches square, it will soon undergo fusion; oxygen will separate at the positive surface, and small metallic globules will appear at the negative surface. These form the marvellous metal potassium, first revealed to the world by Sir H. Davy, early in October, 1807.

If iron-turnings be heated to whiteness in a curved gun-barrel, and potassa be melted and made slowly to come in contact with the turnings, air being excluded, potassium will be formed, and will collect in the cool part of the tube. This method of procuring it was discovered by Gay Lussac and Thenard, in 1808. It may likewise be produced, by igniting potassa with charcoal, as Curaudau showed the same year.

Potassium is possessed of very extraordinary properties. It is lighter than water; its sp. gr. being 0.865 to water 1.0. At common temperatures it is solid, soft, and easily moulded by the fingers. At 150° F. it fuses, and in a heat a little below redness it rises in vapour. It is perfectly opaque. When newly cut, its colour is splendent white, like that of silver, but it rapidly tarnishes in the air. To preserve it unchanged, we must enclose it in a small phial, with pure naphtha. It conducts electricity like the common metals. When thrown upon water, it acts with great violence, and swims upon the surface, burning with a beautiful light of a red colour, mixed with violet. The water becomes a solution of pure potassa. When moderately heated in the air, it inflames, burns with a red light, and throws off alkaline fumes. Placed in chlorine, it spontaneously burns with great brilliancy.

On all fluid bodies which contain water, or much oxygen or chlorine, it readily acts; and in its general powers of chemical combination, says its illustrious discoverer, potassium may be compared to the alkahest, or universal solvent, imagined by the alchemists.

Potassium combines with oxygen in different proportions. When potassium is gently heated in common air or in oxygen, the result of its combustion is an orange-coloured fusible substance. For every grain of the metal consumed, about 1 7-10 cubic inches of oxygen are condensed. To make the experiment accurately, the metal should be burned in a tray of platina covered with a coating of fused muriate of potassa.

The substance procured by the combustion of potassium at a low temperature, was first observed in October, 1807, by Sir H. Davy, who supposed it to be the protoxide; but Gay Lussac and Thenard, in 1810, showed that it was in reality the deutoxide or peroxide. When it is thrown into water, oxygen is evolved, and a solution of the protoxide results, constituting common aqueous potassa. When it is fused and brought in contact with combustible bodies, they burn vividly, by the excess of its oxygen. If it be heated in carbonic acid, oxygen is disengaged, and common subcarbonate of potassa is formed.

When it is heated very strongly upon platina, oxygen gas is expelled from it, and there remains a difficultly fusible substance of a gray colour, vitreous fracture, soluble in water without effervescence, but with much heat. Aqueous potassa is produced. The above ignited solid is protoxide of potassium, which becomes pure potassa by combination with the equivalent quantity of water. When we produce potassium with ignited iron-turnings and potassa, much hydrogen is disengaged from the water of the hydrate, while the iron becomes oxidized from the residuary oxygen. By heating together pure hydrate of potassa and boracic acid, Sir H. Davy obtained from 17 to 18 of water from 100 parts of the solid alkali.

By acting on potassium with a very small quantity of water, or by heating potassium with fused potassa, the protoxide may also be obtained. The proportion of oxygen in the protoxide is determined by the action of potassium upon water. 8 grains of potassium produce from water about 9½ cubic inches of hydrogen; and from these the metal must have fixed 4¾ cubic inches of oxygen. But as 100 cubic inches of oxygen weigh 33.9 gr. 4¾ will weigh 1.61. Thus, 9.61 gr. of the protoxide will contain 8 of metal; and 100 will contain 83.25 metal + 16.75 oxygen. From these data, the prime of potassium comes out 4.969; and that of the protoxide 5.969. Sir H. Davy adopts the number 75 for potassium, corresponding to 50 on the oxygen scale.

When potassium is heated strongly in a small quan-

204

tity of common air, the oxygen of which is not sufficient for its conversion into potassa, a substance is formed of a grayish colour, which, when thrown into water, effervesces without taking fire. It is doubtful whether it be a mixture of the protoxide and potassium, or a combination of potassium with a smaller proportion of oxygen than exists in the protoxide. In this case it would be a suboxide, consisting of 2 primes of potassium $= 10 + 1$ of oxygen $= 11$.

When thin pieces of potassium are introduced into chlorine, the inflammation is very vivid; and then potassium is made to act on chloride of sulphur, there is an explosion. The attraction of chlorine for potassium is much stronger than the attraction of oxygen for the metal. Both of the oxides of potassium are immediately decomposed by chlorine, with the formation of a fixed chloride, and the extrication of oxygen.

The combination of potassium and chlorine is the substance which has been improperly called muriate of potassa, and which, in common cases, is formed by causing liquid muriatic acid to saturate solution of potassa, and then evaporating the liquid to dryness and igniting the solid residuum. The hydrogen of the acid here unites to the oxygen of the alkali, forming water, which is exhaled; while the remaining chlorine and potassium combine. It consists of 5 potassium $+ 4.5$ chlorine.

Potassium combines with hydrogen to form potassuretted hydrogen, a spontaneously inflammable gas, which comes over occasionally in the production of potassium by the gun-barrel experiment. Gay Lussac and Thenard describe also a solid compound of the same two ingredients, which they call a hydruret of potassium. It is formed by heating the metal a long while in the gas, at a temperature just under ignition. They describe it as a grayish solid, giving out its hydrogen on contact with mercury.

When potassium and sulphur are heated together, they combine with great energy, with disengagement of heat and light even *in vacuo*. The resulting sulphuret of potassium, is of a dark gray colour. It acts with great energy on water, producing sulphuretted hydrogen, and burns brilliantly when heated in the air, becoming sulphate of potassa. It consists of 2 sulphur $+ 5$ potassium, by Sir H. Davy's experiments. Potassium has so strong an attraction for sulphur, that it rapidly separates it from hydrogen. If the potassium be heated in the sulphuretted gas, it takes fire and burns with great brilliancy; sulphuret of potassium is formed, and pure hydrogen is set free.

Potassium and phosphorus enter into union with the evolution of light; but the mutual action is feebler than in the preceding compound. The phosphuret of potassium, in its common form, is a substance of a dark chocolate colour, but when heated with potassium in great excess, it becomes of a deep gray colour, with considerable lustre. Hence it is probable, that phosphorus and potassium are capable of combining in two proportions. The phosphuret of potassium burns with great brilliancy, when exposed to air, and when thrown into water produces an explosion, in consequence of the immediate disengagement of phosphuretted hydrogen.

Charcoal which has been strongly heated in contact with potassium, effervesces in water, rendering it alkaline, though the charcoal may be previously exposed to a temperature at which potassium is volatilized. Hence, there is probably a compound of the two formed by a feeble attraction.

Of all known substances, potassium is that which has the strongest attraction for oxygen; and it produces such a condensation of it, that the oxides of potassium are denser than the metal itself. Potassium has been skilfully used by Sir H. Davy and Gay Lussac and Thenard, for detecting the presence of oxygen in bodies. A number of substances, undecomposable by other chemical agents, are readily decomposed by this substance."—*Ure's Chem. Dict.*

Potassium, oxide of. The potassa of the shops.

POTATO. The word potato is a degeneration of *batatas*, the provincial name of the root in that part of Peru from which it was first obtained. See *Solanum tuberosum*.

Potato, Spanish. See *Convolvulus batatas*.
[*Potato flies.* See *Cantharides vittatæ.* A.]
[*Potato, wild.* See *Convolvulus panduratus.* A.]
POTENTIAL. *Potentialis.* 1. Qualities which

are supposed to exist in the body in *potentia* only; by which they are capable, in some measure, of effecting and impressing on us the ideas of such qualities, though not really inherent in themselves: in this sense we say, potential heat, potential cold, &c.

2. In a medical sense it is opposed to actual: hence we say, an actual and potential caustic. A red-hot iron is actually caustic; whereas *potassa pura*, and *nitras argentia* are potentially so, though cold to the touch.

Potential cautery. See *Potassa fusa*, and *Argenti nitras.*

POTENTI'LLA. (*A potentia*, from its efficacy.) 1. The name of a genus of plants in the Linnæan system. Class, *Icosandria;* Order, *Polygynia.*

2. The pharmacopœial name of the wild tansy. See *Potentilla anserina.*

POTENTILLA ANSERINA. The systematic name of the silver-weed, or wild tansy. *Argentina; Anserina.* The leaves of this plant, *Potentilla—foliis dentatis, serratis, caule repente, pedunculis unifloris,* of Linnæus, possess mildly adstringent and corroborant qualities; but are seldom used, except by the lower orders.

POTENTILLA REPTANS. The systematic name of the common cinquefoil, or five-leaved grass. *Pentaphyllum.* The roots of this plant, *Potentilla—foliis quinatis, caule repente, pedunculis unifloris,* of Linnæus, have a bitterish styptic taste. They were used by the ancients in the cure of intermittents: but the medicinal quality of cinquefoil is confined, in the present day, to stop diarrhœas and other fluxes.

POTE'RIUM. (From ποτηριον, a cup: so named from the shape of its flowers.) The name of a genus of plants in the Linnæan system. Class, *Monœcia;* Order, *Polyandria.*

POTERIUM SANGUISORBA. The systematic name of the Burnet saxifrage, the leaves of which are often put into cool tankards; they have an adstringent quality.

POTSTONE. *Lapis ollaris.* A greenish-gray mineral, found abundantly on the shores of the lake Como, in Lombardy, in thick beds of primitive slate, and fashioned into culinary vessels in Greenland. It is a subspecies of rhomboidal mica of Jameson.

POTT, PERCIVAL, was born in London, in 1713. It was the wish of his friends to bring him up to the church, in which he might have obtained good patronage; but he had an irresistible inclination to the surgical profession. He was accordingly apprenticed to Mr. Nourse, of St. Bartholomew's Hospital, who gave anatomical lectures; for which he was employed in preparing the subjects, and thus laid the best foundation for chirurgical skill. In 1744, he was elected assistant-surgeon; and, five years after, one of the principal surgeons at the hospital. He had the merit of chiefly bringing about a great improvement in his profession, availing himself of the resources of nature under a lenient mode of treatment, and exploding the frequent use of the cautery, and other severe methods formerly resorted to. In 1756, he had the misfortune to receive a compound fracture of the leg; but the confinement occasioned by this accident led him to compose his "Treatise on Ruptures;" which was soon followed by an account of the Hernia Congenita. In 1758, he produced a judicious essay on "Fistula Lachrymalis;" and, two years after, an elaborate dissertation "On Injuries of the Head;" which was soon followed by "Practical Remarks on the Hydrocele," &c. In 1764, he was elected a Fellow of the Royal Society; and about the same period he instituted a course of lectures on surgery. In the following year, his treatise "On Fistula in Ano" appeared, in which he effected a very great improvement; and, in 1768, some remarks "On Fractures and Dislocations" were added to a new edition of his work on Injuries of the Head. Seven years after this, he published "Chirurgical Observations" on Cataract, Polypus of the Nose Cancer of the Scrotum, Ruptures, and Mortification of the lower Extremities: this was soon succeeded by a "Treatise on the Necessity of Amputation in some Cases;" and by "Remarks on the Palsy of the lower Limbs," from Curvature of the Spine. He had now attained the greatest eminence in his profession, but towards the close of the year 1788, a severe atttack of fever, neglected at first, terminated his active and valuable life.

POUCH. 1. *Sacculus.* In anatomy, a morbid dilatation of any part of a canal, as the intestine.

2. In botany, see *Silicula.*

POUPART'S LIGAMENT. *Ligamentum Poupartii.* Fallopian ligament. Inguinal ligament. A strong ligament, or rather a tendinous expansion of the external oblique muscle, going across from the inferior and anterior spinous process of the ilium to the crista of the os pubis. It is under this ligament that the femoral vessels pass; and, when the intestine or omentum passes underneath it, the disease is called a femoral hernia.

Powder, antimonial. See *Antimonialis pulvis.*

Powder of burnt hartshorn with opium. See *Pulvis cornu usti cum opio.*

Powder, compound, of aloes. See *Pulvis aloës compositus.*

Powder, compound, of chalk. See *Pulvis cretæ compositus.*

Powder, compound, of chalk, with opium. See *Pulvis cretæ compositus cum opio.*

Powder, compound, of cinnamon. See *Pulvis cinnamomi compositus.*

Powder, compound, of contrayerva. See *Pulvis contrayervæ compositus.*

Powder, compound, of ipecacuanha. See *Pulvis ipecacuanhæ compositus.*

Powder, compound, of kino. See *Pulvis kino compositus.*

Powder, compound, of scammony. See *Pulvis scammoneæ compositus.*

Powder, compound, of senna. See *Pulvis sennæ compositus.*

Powder, compound, of tragacanth. See *Pulvis tragacanthæ compositus.*

Power, muscular. See *Irritability,* and *Muscular motion.*

Power, tonic. See *Irritability.*

Præcipitate, red. See *Hydrargyri nitrico-oxydum.*

Præcipitate, white. See *Hydrargyrum præcipitatum album.*

PRÆCO'RDIA (*Præcordia, orum.* n.; from *præ,* before, and *cor,* the heart.) The forepart of the region of the thorax.

PRÆFU'RNIUM. (From *præ,* before, and *furnus,* a furnace.) The mouth of a chemical furnace.

PRÆMORSUS. (From *præmordeo,* to bite off.) Bitten off. In botany, this term is differently applied: the *radix præmorsa* is an abrupt root, naturally, it is supposed, inclined to a taper root; but, from some decay or interruption in its descending point, it becomes abrupt, or, as it were, bitten off; as in the *Scabiosa succisa,* and *Hedypnois hirta.*

The old opinion of this formed root is thus described in Gerald's Herbal: " The great part of the root seemeth to be bitten away: old fantasticke charmers report, that the divel did bite it for envie, because it is an herbe that hath so many good vertues, and is so beneficial to mankinde."

The *folium præmorsum* is jagged, pointed, very blunt, with various irregular notches, as in *Epidendrum præmorsum,* &c.

PRÆPARA'NTIA MEDICAMENTA. Medicines which were supposed to prepare the peccant fluids to pass off.

PRÆPARANTIA VASA. The spermatic vessels of the testicles.

PRÆPUCE. See *Præputium.*

PRÆPU'TIUM. (From *præputo,* to cut off before, because some nations used to cut it off in circumcision.) *Epagogion* of Dioscorides. *Posthe.* The prepuce. The membranous or cutaneous fold that covers the glans penis and clitoris.

PRASE. A green leek-coloured mineral, found in the island of Bute, and in Borrodale.

PRA'SIUM. (From πρασια, a square border: so called from its square stalks.) Hoarhound. See *Marrubium vulgare.*

PRA'SUM. (From πραω, to burn; because of its hot taste.) The leek.

PRA'XIS. (From πρασσω, to perform.) The practice of any thing, as of medicine.

PRECIPITA'TION. (*Præcipitatio;* from *præcipito,* to cast down.) When two bodies are united, for instance, an acid and an oxide, and a third body is added, such as an alkali, which has a greater affinity with the acid than the metallic oxide has, the consequence is, that the alkali combines with the acid, and the oxide, thus deserted, appears in a separate state at the bottom of the vessel in which the operation is performed. This decomposition is commonly known by

the name of *precipitation,* and the substance that sinks is named a *precipitate.* The substance, by the addition of which the phenomenon is produced, is denominated the *precipitant.*

PRE'DISPOSING. (*Prædisponens;* from *prædis pono,* to predispose.) *Causa proëgumena.* That which renders the body susceptible of disease. The most frequent predisposing causes of diseases are, the temperament and habit of the body, idiosyncrasy, age, sex, and structure of the part.

PREDISPOSITION. (*Prædispositio.* That constitution, or state of the solids, or fluids, or of both, which disposes the body to the action of disease.

PREGNANCY. *Utero gestation.* The particular manner in which pregnancy takes place has hitherto remained involved in obscurity, notwithstanding the laborious investigation of the most eminent philosophers of all ages. Although in a state which (with a few exceptions) is natural to all women, it is in general the source of many disagreeable sensations, and often the cause of diseases which might be attended with the worst consequences, if not properly treated.

It is now, however, universally acknowledged, that those women who bear children enjoy, usually, more certain health, and are much less liable to dangerous diseases, than those who are unmarried, or who prove barren.

Signs of pregnancy.—The womb has a very extensive influence, by means of its nerves, on many other parts of the body; hence, the changes which are produced on it by impregnation, must be productive of changes on the state of the general system. These constitute the signs of pregnancy.

During the first fourteen or fifteen weeks, the signs of pregnancy are very ambiguous, and cannot be depended on; for, as they proceed from the irritation of the womb on other parts, they may be occasioned by every circumstance which can alter the natural state of that organ.

The first circumstance which renders pregnancy probable, is the suppression of the periodical evacuation, which is generally accompanied with fulness in the breasts, headache, flushings in the face, and heat in the palms of the hands.

These symptoms are commonly the consequences of suppression, and therefore are to be regarded as signs of pregnancy, in so far only as they depend on it.

As, however, the suppression of the periodical evacuation often happens from accidental exposure to cold, or from the change of life in consequence of marriage, it can never be considered as an infallible sign.

The belly, some weeks after pregnancy, becomes flat, from the womb sinking, and hence drawing down the intestines along with it; but this cannot be looked upon as a certain sign of pregnancy, because an enlargement of the womb from any other cause will produce the same effect.

Many women, soon after they are pregnant, become very much altered in their looks, and have peculiar irritable feelings, inducing a disposition of mind which renders their tempers easily ruffled, and inciting an irresistible propensity to actions of which, on other occasions, they would be ashamed.

In such cases, the features acquire a peculiar sharpness, the eyes appear larger, and the mouth wider, than usual; and the woman has a particular appearance, which cannot be described, but with which women are well acquainted.

These breeding symptoms, as they are called, originate from the irritation produced on the womb by impregnation; and, as they may proceed from any other circumstance which can irritate that organ, they cannot be depended on when the woman is not young, or where there is not a continued suppression for at least three periods.

The irritations on the parts contiguous to the womb are equally ambiguous; and therefore the signs of pregnancy, in the first four months, are always to be considered as doubtful, unless every one enumerated be distinctly and equivocally present.

From the fourth month, the signs of pregnancy are less ambiguous, especially after the womb has ascended into the cavity of the belly. In general, about the fourth month, or a short time after, the child becomes so much enlarged, that its motions begin to be felt by the mother; and hence a sign is furnished at that period called *quickening.* Women very improperly consider this sign as the most unequivocal proof of pregnancy; for though, when it occurs about the period described, preceded by the symptoms formerly enumerated, it may be looked upon as a sure indication that the woman is with child, yet, when there is an irregularity, either in the preceding symptoms or in its appearance, the situation of the woman must be doubtful.

This fact will be easily understood; for as the sensation of the motion of the child cannot be explained, or accurately described, women may readily mistake other sensations for that of quickening. Flatus has often been so pent up in the bowels, that the natural pulsation of the great arteries, of which people are conscious only in certain states of the body, has frequently been mistaken for this feeling.

After the fourth month, the womb rises gradually from the cavity of the pelvis, enlarges the belly, and pushes out the navel: hence the protrusion of the navel has been considered one of the most certain signs of pregnancy in the latter months. Every circumstance, however, which increases the bulk of the belly occasions this symptom; and therefore it cannot be trusted to, unless other signs concur.

The progressive increase of the belly, along with suppression, after having been formerly regular, and the consequent symptoms, together with the sensation of quickening at the proper period, afford the only true marks of pregnancy.

These signs, however, are not to be entirely depended on; for the natural desire which every woman has to be a mother, will induce her to conceal, even from herself, every symptom which may render her situation doubtful, and to magnify every circumstance which can tend to prove that she is pregnant.

Besides quickening and increase of bulk of the belly, another symptom appears in the latter months, which, when preceded by the ordinary signs, renders pregnancy certain beyond a doubt. It is the presence of milk in the breasts. When, however, there is any irregularity in the preceding symptoms, this sign is no longer to be considered of any consequence.

As every practitioner must naturally wish to distinguish pregnancy from disease, the disorders which resemble it should be thoroughly understood, and also their diagnostics. It is, however, necessary to remark, that wherever any circumstance occurs which affords the most distant reason to doubt the case, recourse ought to be had to the advice of an experienced practitioner, and every symptom should be unreservedly described to him.

PREHE'NSIO. (From *prehendo*, to surprise: so named from its sudden seizure.) The catalepsy.

PREHNITE. Of prismatic prehnite there are two subspecies, the *foliated*, and the *fibrous*. The first is of an apple-green colour, found in France, the Savoy and Tyrol, and beautiful varieties in the interior of southern Africa. The fibrous is of a siskin green colour, and occurs in Scotland.

PRESBYO'PIA. (From πρεσβυς, old, and ωψ, the eye; because it is frequent with old men.) That defect of the sight by which objects close are seen confusedly, but, at remoter distances, distinctly. As the myopia is common to infants, so the presbyopia is a malady common to the aged. The proximate cause is a tardy adunation of the rays in a focus, so that it falls beyond the retina. The species are,

1. *Presbyopia* from a flatness of the cornea. By so much the cornea is flatter, so much the less and more ardy it refracts the rays into a focus. This evil arises, 1st, From a want of aqueous or vitreous humour, which is common to the aged; or may arise from some disease; 2d, From a cicatrix, which diminishes the convexity of the cornea: 3d, From a natural conformation of the cornea.

2. *Presbyopia* from too flat a crystalline lens. This evil is most common to the aged, or it may happen from a wasting of the crystalline lens.

3. *Presbyopia* from too small a density of the cornea or humours of the eye. By so much more these humours are thin or rarified, so much the less they refract the rays of light. Whosoever is affected from this cause is cured in older age; for age induces a greater density of the cornea and lens. From this it is an observed fact, that the *presbyopes* are often cured spontaneously, and throw away their glasses, which younger persons in this disease are obliged to use.

4. *Presbyopia* from a custom of viewing continually remote objects; hence artificers who are occupied in remote objects are said to contract this malady. The reason of this phenomenon is not very clear.

5. *Presbyopia senilis.* From a multitude of causes aged persons are presbyopes; from a penury of humours, which render the cornea and lens flatter, and the bulb shorter. When in senile age, from dryness, the bulb of the eye becomes flatter and shorter, and the cornea flatter, those who were short-sighted or myopes before, see now without their concave glasses.

6. *Presbyopia*, from too close a proximity of objects. The focus is shorter of distant, but longer of nearer objects.

7. *Presbyopia* from a coarctated pupil.

8. *Presbyopia mercurialis*, which arises from the use of mercurial preparations. The patient feels a pressing pain in the eye, which, from being touched, is increased, and the bulb of the eye appears as if rigid, and with difficulty can be moved. Near objects the patient can scarcely distinguish, and distant only in a confused manner. Many have supposed this disorder an imperfect amaurosis.

PRE'SBYTÆ. See *Presbyopia.*

PRESBY'TIA. (From προεσβυς, old; because it is usual to old people.) See *Presbyopia.*

PRESU'RA. (From πρηθω, to inflame.) Inflammation at the ends of the fingers from cold.

PRIAPEI'A. See *Nicotiana rustica.*

PRIAPI'SCUS. (From πριαπος, the penis.) 1. A tent made in the form of a penis.
2. A bougie.

PRIAPISM. See *Priapismus.*

PRIAPI'SMUS. (From πριαπος, a heathen god, whose penis is always painted erect.) Priapism. A continual erection of the penis.

PRIA'PUS. (Πριαπος, a heathen god, remarkable for the largeness of his genitals.)
1. The penis or membrum virile.
2. A name of the *nepenthes*, or wonderful plant, from the appendages at the end of the leaves resembling an erected penis.

PRICKLE. See *Aculeus.*

Prickly-heat. See *Lichen tropicus.*

["PRICKLY ASH. Xanthoxylum fraxineum. The *Xanthoxylum fraxineum* is a prickly shrub, found in the northern, middle, and western parts of the United States, in woods and moist shady declivities.

"The leaves and rind of the fruit resemble those of the lemon in their taste and smell, and possess a similar volatile oil. The bark possesses a separate acrid principle, which is communicated to water and alkohol, but does not come over in distillation. The acrimony is not perceived when the bark or liquid is first taken into the mouth, but gradually developes itself by a burning sensation on the tongue and fauces.

"Prickly ash has acquired much reputation as a remedy in chronic rheumatism. In that disease it has an operation analogous to that of mezereon and guaiacum, which it resembles in its sensible properties. Taken in full doses, it produces a sense of heat in the stomach, a tendency to perspiration, and a relief to rheumatic pains.

"Twenty grains can be taken three times a day in powder, or an ounce may be boiled in a quart of water, and the decoction taken during twenty-four hours."— *Big. Mat. Med.* A.]

PRI'MÆ VIÆ. The first passages. The stomach and the intestinal tube are so called, because they are the first passages of what is taken into the stomach; the lacteals the *secundæ viæ*, because the nourishment next goes into them; and lastly, the blood vessels, which are supplied by the lacteals, are called *viæ tertiæ.*

PRIMARY. *Primarius.* A term in very general use in medicine and surgery. It is applied to diseases, to their symptoms, causes, &c. and denotes priority in opposition to what follows, which is secondary; thus, when inflammation of the diaphragm produces furious delirium, the primary disease is the paraphrenitis; so when gallstones produce violent pain, vomiting, &c. which are followed by jaundice, white fæces, portercoloured urine, &c; the pain and vomiting are primary symptoms, the jaundice and white stools are secondary, &c.

Primary teeth. See *Teeth.*

Primrose. See *Primula vulgaris.*

207

PRI'MULA. (From *primulus*, the beginning: so called because it flowers in the beginning of the spring.) The name of a genus of plants in the Linnæan system. Class, *Pentandria;* Order; *Monogynia.*

PRIMULA VERIS. (From *primulus*, the beginning; so called because it flowers in the beginning of the spring.) *Verbasculum.* The cowslip, paigil, or peagle. The flowers of this plant have a moderately strong and pleasant smell, and a somewhat roughish bitter taste. Vinous liquors impregnated with their flavour by maceration or fermentation, and strong infusions of them drank as tea, are supposed to be mildly corroborant, antispasmodic, and anodyne. An infusion of three pounds of the fresh flowers in five pints of boiling water is made in the shops into a syrup of a fine yellow colour, and agreeably impregnated with the flavour of the cowslip.

PRIMULA VULGARIS. The primrose. The leaves and root of this common plant possess sternutatory properties.

PRI'NCEPS ALEXIPHARMACORUM. The Angelica was formerly so much esteemed as to obtain this name.

PRINCIPLES. *Principia.* Primary substances. Substances or particles which are composed of two or more elements; thus water, gelatine, sugar, fibrine, &c. are the principles of many bodies: These principles are composed of elementary bodies, as oxygen, hydrogen, azote, &c. which are undecomposable.

PRINGLE, SIR JOHN, was born in Scotland in 1707, Having determined to make medicine his profession, he went to Edinburgh for a year, and then to Leyden, to profit by the instructions of the celebrated Boerhaave, where he took his degree in 1730. Then settling at Edinburgh, he obtained four years after the appointment of professor of moral philosophy jointly with Mr. Scott. In 1742 he was made physician to the Earl of Stair, who then commanded the British army, and soon after physician to the military hospital in Flanders. He acquitted himself with so much credit, that the Duke of Cumberland, who succeeded to the command, appointed him, in 1745, physician-general to the forces, and subsequently to the royal hospitals, in the Low Countries, when he resigned his Scotch professorship. He soon after accompanied the same nobleman in his expedition against the rebels in Scotland: but in 1747, went again to the army abroad, where he continued till the treaty of Aix-la-Chapelle. The Duke of Cumberland then appointed him his physician, and he settled in London; but the war of 1755 called him again to the army, which, however, he finally quitted three years after. He had been elected a fellow of the Royal Society in 1745, and on settling in London, contributed many papers to their Transactions, particularly his Experiments on Septic and Antiseptic Substances, for which he was presented with the Copleian medal. In 1752 his "Observations on the Diseases of the Army" first appeared, and rapidly passed through several editions, and was translated into other languages: the utility of the work, indeed, equalled the reputation it acquired, and which it still preserves, especially from the importance of the prophylactic measures suggested. After quitting the army, he was admitted a licentiate, and his fame as a physician, as well as philosopher, speedily attained a high pitch; he received successively various appointments about the royal family, was elected a fellow of the College, and in 1766 raised to the dignity of a baronet. Among numerous literary honours from various academies of science in Europe, the highest was conferred upon him in 1770, being then elected president of the Royal Society: the duties of which office he zealously fulfilled for eight years, when declining health compelled his resignation. His discourses on the annual presentation of the Copleian medals displayed so much learning and general information, that their publication was requested. In 1780 he went to Edinburgh for the improvement of his health; but the want of his accustomed society, and the sharpness of the air, compelled him to return in the following year; he presented, however, to the College of Physicians there before his departure ten folio volumes, in manuscript, of "Medical and Physical Observations," with the restriction that they should not be published, nor lent out of the library. His death happened soon after his return to London, namely, in the beginning of 1782.

PRIONO'DES. (From πριων, a saw.) Serrated: applied in old writings to the sutures of the skull.

208

PRI'OR. The first; a term applied to some muscl from their order.

PRIOR ANNULARIS *Musculus prior annularis* Fourth *interosseus*, of Winslow. An internal interosseus muscle of the hand. See *Interossei manus.*

PRIOR INDICIS. *Extensor tertii internodii indicis*, of Douglas. *Seu-metacarpo-lateriphalangien*, of Dumas. An internal interosseus muscle of the hand, which draws the fore-finger inwards towards the thumb, and extends it obliquely.

PRIOR MEDII. *Musculus prior medii; Second interosseus*, of Douglas, and *seu-metacarpo-lateri phalangien*, of Dumas. An external interosseous muscle of the hand. See *Interossei manus.*

PRO RE NATA. A term frequently used in extemporaneous prescriptions, and implies occasionally, as the occasion may require; thus, an aperient dose is directed to be taken *pro re nata.*

PROBANG. A flexible piece of whalebone with sponge fixed at the end.

PROBE. (From *probo*, to try; because surgeon's try the depth and extent of wounds, &c. with it.) *Stylus.* A surgical instrument of a long and slender form.

PRO'BOLE. (Προβολη, a prominence; from προβαλ λω, to project.) See *Apophysis.*

PROBO'SCIS. (From προ, before, and βοσκω, to feed.) A snout or trunk, as that of an elephant, by which it feeds itself.

PROCA'RDIUM. (From προ, before, and καρδια, the stomach or heart.) The pit of the stomach.

PROCATARCTIC. (*Procatarcticus;* from προκα ταρχω, to go before.) See *Exciting cause.*

PROCESS. (*Processus;* from *procedo*, to go before.) An eminence of a bone; as the spinous and transverse processes of the vertebræ.

PROCESSUS. See *Process.*

PROCESSUS CÆCI VERMIFORMIS. See *Intestine.*

PROCESSUS CAUDATUS. See *Lobulus caudatus.*

PROCESSUS CILIARIS. See *Ciliar ligament.*

PROCESSUS MAMILLARES. A name formerly applied to the olfactory nerves.

PROCIDE'NTIA. (From *procido*, to fall down.) A falling down of any part; thus, *procidentia ani*, *uteri*, *vaginæ*, &c.

PROCO'NDYLUS. (From προ, before, and κονδυλος the middle joint of the finger.) The first joint of a fin ger next the metacarpus.

PROCTA'LGIA. (From πρωκτος, the fundament, and αλγος, pain.) A violent pain of the anus. It is mostly symptomatic of some disease, as piles, scirrhus, prurigo, cancer, &c.

PROCTI'CA. (From πρωκτος, the fundament) The name of a genus of diseases in Good's Nosology ; Class, *Cœliaca;* Order, *Enterica.* Pain or derangement about the anus, without primary inflammation It has six species, viz. *Proctica simplex, spasmodica, callosa, tenesmus, marisca, exenia.*

PROCTI'TIS. (From πρωκτος, the anus.) *Clunesia; Cyssotis.* Inflammation of the internal or mucous membrane of the lower part of the rectum.

PROCTOLEUCORRHŒ'A. (From πρωκτος, the anus, λευκος, white, and ρεω, to flow.) *Proctorrhœa.* A purging of white mucus.

PROCTORRHŒ'A. (From πρωκτος, the anus, and ρεω, to flow.) See *Proctoleucorrhœa.*

PRODUCTIO. See *Apophysis.*

PRŒOTIA. (From πρωι, premature.) The name of a genus of diseases in Good's Nosology. Class *Genetica;* Order, *Orgastica.* Genital precocity. It has two species, viz. *Prœotia masculina*, and feminina.

PROCUMBENS. Procumbent. Applied to stems as that of *Lysimachia nemorum.*

PROFLUVIUM. (From *profluo*, to run down.) A flux.

PROFLUVIA. Fluxes. The fifth order in the class *Pyrexiæ*, of Cullen's Nosology, characterized by pyrexia, with increased excretions.

PROFLUVII CORTEX. See *Nerium antidysentericum.*

PROFUNDUS. See *Flexor profundus perforans*

PROFU'SIO. A genus of disease in the class *Locales*, and order *Apocenoses*, of Cullen. A passive loss of blood.

PROGLO'SSIS. (From προ, before, and γλωσσα, the tongue.) The tip of the tongue.

PROGNO'SIS. (From προ, before, and γινωσκω to know.) The foretelling the event of diseases from particular symptoms.

PROGNOSTIC (*Prognosticus*; from προγινωσκω, to know beforehand.) Applied to those symptoms which enable the physician to form his judgment or prognosis of the probable cause or event of a disease.

PROJECTURA. See *Apophysis.*

PROLA′PSUS. (From *prolabor*, to slip down.) *Procidentia; Delapsio; Exania; Proptoma; Proptosis.* A protrusion. A genus of disease in the class *Locales*, and order *Ectopiæ*, of Cullen; distinguished by the falling down of a part that is uncovered.

PROLE′PTICUS. (From προλαμβανω, to anticipate.) Applied to those diseases, the paroxysms of which anticipate each other, or return after less and less intervals of intermission.

PROLIFER. (From *proles*, an offspring, and *fero*, to bear.) Prolific, or proliferous: applied to those stems which shoot out new branches from the summit of the former ones, as in the Scotch fir; *Pinus sylvestris.*

PROMALACTE′RIUM. (From προ, before, and μαλασσω, to soften.) The room where the body is softened previous to bathing.

PROMETOPI′DIUM. (From προ, before, and μετωπον, the forehead.) *Prometopis.* The skin upon the forehead.

PROMETO′PIS. See *Prometopidium.*

PRONATION. *Pronatio.* The act of turning the palm of the hand downwards. It is performed by rotating the radius upon the ulna, by means of several muscles which are termed pronators.

PRONA′TOR. A name given to two muscles of the hand, the pronator radii quadratus, and pronator radii teres; the use of which is to perform the opposite action to that of the supinators, viz. pronation.

PRONATOR QUADRATUS. See *Pronator radii quadratus.*

PRONATOR RADII BREVIS. See *Pronator radii quadratus.*

PRONATOR RADII QUADRATUS. *Pronator quadratus*, of Douglas and Albinus; *Pronator quadratus sive transversus*, of Winslow; *Pronator radii brevis seu quadratus*, of Cowper; *Cubito radial*, of Dumas. This, which has gotten its name from its use and its shape, is a small fleshy muscle, situated at the lower and inner part of the forearm, and covered by the tendons of the flexor muscles of the hand. It arises tendinous and fleshy from the lower and inner part of the ulna, and runs nearly in a transverse direction, to be inserted into that part of the radius which is opposite to its origin, its inner fibres adhering to the interosseous ligament. This muscle assists in the pronation of the hand, by turning the radius inwards.

PRONATOR RADII TERES. *Pronator teres*, of Albinus and Douglas; *Pronator teres, sive obliquus*, of Winslow; *Epitrochloradial*, of Dumas. A small muscle situated at the upper and anterior part of the forearm. It is called *teres*, to distinguish it from the pronator quadratus. It arises tendinous and fleshy from the anterior and inferior part of the outer condyle of the os humeri; and tendinous from the coronoid process of the ulna, near the insertion of the brachialis internus. The median nerve passes between these two portions. From these origins the muscle runs obliquely downwards and outwards, and is inserted, tendinous and fleshy, into the anterior and convex edge of the radius, about the middle of that bone. This muscle, as its name indicates, serves to turn the hand inwards.

PRONERVA′TIO. (From *pro*, before, and *nervus*, a string.) A tendon or string, like the end of a muscle.

PROPAGO. A slip, layer, or cutting of the vine.

PROPHYLACTIC. (*Prophylacticus*; from προ, and φυλασσω, to defend.) Any means made use of to preserve health and prevent disease.

PROPRIETA′TIS ELIXIR. See *Tinctura aloes composita.*

PROPTO′MA. (From προπιπ⁀]ω, to fall down.) *Procidentia.* A relaxation, such as that of the scrotum, of the under lip, of the breasts in females, of the præpuce, or of the ears.

PRCPYE′MA. (From ϖρο, before, and πυον, pus.) A premature collection of pus.

PRO′RA. (From πρωρα, the prow of a vessel.) The occiput.

PROSARTHRO′SIS. (From προς, to, and αρθρow, to articulate.) The articulation which has manifest motion

PROSPE GMA. (From προσπηγνυμι, to fix near., A fixing of humours in one spot.

PRO′STASIS. (From προιςημι, to predominate.) An abundance of morbid humours.

PROSTATE. (*Glandula prostata*; from προ, before, and ιστημι, to stand: because it is situated before the urinary bladder.) *Corpus glandulosum; Adenoides.* A very large, heart-like, firm gland, situated between the neck of the urinary bladder and the bulbous part of the urethra. It secretes the lacteal fluid, which is emitted into the urethra by ten or twelve ducts, that open near the verumontanum, during coition. This gland is liable to inflammation and its consequences.

Prostate inferior muscle. See *Transversis perinei alter.*

PROSTRATUS. Prostrate. Applied synonymously with *depressus*, depressed, to a stem which lies naturally remarkably flat, spreading horizontally over the ground; as in *Coldenia procumbens*, and *Coronopus Ruelli*, swine's cress.

PROTO′GALA. (From πρωτος, first, and γαλα, milk.) The first milk after delivery.

PROTOXYDE. See *Oxide.*

PROTUBERANTIA. 1. A protuberance on any part.

2. An apophysis.

PROXIMATE. (*Causa proxima:* so called because when the exciting cause begins to have effect it is the *proximum*, or next thing that happens.) The proximate cause of a disease may be said to be in reality the disease itself. All proximate causes are either diseased actions of simple fibres, or an altered state of the fluids.

PRUI′NA. (*A perurendo, quod fruges peruent.*) The powder-like appearance after the bloom observed on ripe fruit, especially plums.

PRUNA. (*Pruna, æ. f.;* a live coal.) The carbuncle. See *Anthrax.*

PRUNE. See *Plums.*

PRUNE′LLA. (From *pruno*, a burn; because it heals burns.) 1. The name of a genus of plants in the Linnæan system. Class, *Didynamia;* Order, *Gymnospermia.*

2. The pharmacopœial name of the self-heal. See *Prunella vulgaris.*

3. The name used by Paracelsus for sore throat, or cynanche.

PRUNELLA VULGARIS. The systematic name of the self-heal. *Prunella; Consolida minor; Symphitum minus. Prunella—foliis omnibus ovato oblongis, serratis, petiolatis*, of Linnæus; it is recommended as an adstringent in hæmorrhages and fluxes, as also in gargles against aphthæ and inflammation of the fauces.

PRUNUM. (*Prunum, i. n.;* from *prunus.*) A plum or prune. See *Plums.*

Prunelloe. See *Plum.*

PRUNUM GALLICUM. See *Prunus domestica.*

PRUNUM SYLVESTRE. See *Prunus spinosa.*

PRU′NUS. (*Prunus, i. f.*) 1. A plum.

2. The name of a genus of plants in the Linnæan system. Class, *Icosandria;* Order, *Monogynia.*

PRUNUS ARMENIACA. Apricots, which are the fruit of this plant, are, when ripe, easily digested, and are considered as a pleasant and nutritious delicacy.

PRUNUS AVIUM. The systematic name of the black cherry-tree. *Prunus—umbellis sessilibus, foliis ovato-lanceolatis. subtus pubescentibus, conduplicatis*, of Linnæus. The flavour of the ripe fruit is esteemed by many, and if not taken in too large quantities, they are extremely salutary. A gum exudes from the tree, whose properties are similar to those of gum-arabic.

PRUNUS CERASUS. The systematic name of the red cherry-tree. *Prunus—umbellis subpedunculatis, foliis ovato-lanceolatis, glabris conduplicatis*, of Linnæus. The fruit of this tree, *Cerasa rubra, anglica, sativa*, possess a pleasant, acidulated, sweet flavour, and are proper in fevers, scurvy, and bilious obstructions. Red cherries are mostly eaten as a luxury, and are very wholesome, except to those whose bowels are remarkably irritable.

PRUNUS DOMESTICA. The systematic name of the plum or damson-tree. *Prunus—pedunculis subsolitariis, foliis lanceolato ovatis convolutis, ramis muticis; gemmæ floriferæ aphyllæ*, of Linnæus. Prunes are considered as emollient, cooling, and laxative, espe cially the French prunes, which are directed in th decoction of senna, and other purgatives; and the pulp is ordered in the *electuarium é senna*. The *damson* is only a variety, which, when perfectly ripe, affords a wholesome article for pies, tarts, &c. gently opening the body: but when damsons are not perfectly mature, they produce colicky pains, diarrhœa, and convulsions in children. See *Plums*.

PRUNUS LAURO-CERASUS. The systematic name of the poison laurel. *Lauro-cerasus.* Common or cherry laurel. *Prunus—floribus racemosis foliis sempervirentibus dorso biglandulosis*, of Linnæus. The leaves of the lauro-cerasus have a bitter styptic taste, accompanied with a flavour resembling that of bitter-almonds, or other kernels of the drupaceous fruits: the flowers also manifest a similar flavour. The powdered leaves, applied to the nostrils, excite sneezing, though not so strongly as tobacco. The kernel-like flavour which these leaves impart being generally esteemed grateful, has sometimes caused them to be employed for culinary purposes, and especially in custards, puddings, blanc-mange, &c.; and as the proportion of this sapid matter of the leaf to the quantity of the milk is commonly inconsiderable, bad effects have seldom ensued. But, as the poisonous quality of this laurel is now indubitably proved and known to be the prussic acid which can be obtained in a separate form (See *Prussic acid*), the public ought to be cautioned against its internal use.

The following communication to the Royal Society, by Dr. Madden, of Dublin, contains the first and principal proofs of the deleterious effects of this vegetable upon mankind:—"A very extraordinary accident that fell out here some months ago, has discovered to us a most dangerous poison, which was never before known to be so, though it has been in frequent use among us. The thing I mean is a simple water, distilled from the leaves of the lauro-cerasus; the water is at first milky, but the oil which comes over being, in a good measure, separated from the phlegm, by passing it through a flannel bag, it becomes as clear as common water. It has the smell of bitter almonds, or peach kernel, and has been for many years in frequent use among our housewives and cooks, to give that agreeable flavour to their creams and puddings. It has also been much in use among our drinkers of drams; and the proportion they generally use it in has been one part of laurel-water to four of brandy. Nor has this practice, however frequent, ever been attended with any apparent ill consequences, till some time in the month of September, 1728, when it happened that one Martha Boyse, a servant, who lived with a person who sold great quantities of this water, got a bottle of it from her mistress, and gave it to her mother. Ann Boyse made a present of it to Frances Eaton, her sister, who was a shopkeeper in town, and who, she thought, might oblige her customers with it. Accordingly, in a few days, she gave about two ounces to a woman called Mary Whaley, who drank about two-thirds of what was filled out, and went away. Frances Eaton drank the rest. In a quarter of an hour after Mary Whaley had drunk the water, (as I am informed,) she complained of a violent disorder in her stomach, soon after lost her speech, and died in about an hour, without any vomiting or purging, or any convulsion. The shop-keeper, F. Eaton, sent word to her sister, Ann Boyse, of what had happened, who came to her upon the message, and affirmed that it was not possible the cor-dial (as she called it) could have occasioned the death of the woman; and, to convince her of it, she filled out about three ounces and drank it. She continued talking with F. Eaton about two minutes longer, and was so earnest to persuade her of the liquor's being inoffensive, that she drank about two spoonfuls more, but was hardly well seated in her chair when she died without the least groan, or convulsion. Frances Eaton, who, as before observed, had drank somewhat more than a spoonful, found no disorder in her stomach, or elsewhere; but to prevent any ill consequences, she took a vomit immediately, and has been well ever since."—Dr. Madden mentions another case, of a gentleman at Kilkenny, who mistook a bottle of laurel-water for a bottle of ptisan. What quantity he drank is uncertain, but he died in a few minutes, complaining of a violent disorder in the stomach. In addition to this, we may refer to the unfortunate case of Sir Theodosius Boughton, whose death, in 1780, an English jury declared to be occasioned by this poison

In this case, the active principle of the lauro-cerasus was concentrated by repeated distillations, and given to the quantity of one ounce; the suddenly fatal effects of which must be still in the recollection of the public. To brute animals this poison is almost instantaneously mortal, as amply appears by the experiments of Mad den, Mortimer, Nicholls, Fontana, Langrish, Vater, and others. The experiments conducted by these gen-tlemen, show that the laurel-water is destructive to animal life, not only when taken into the stomach, but also on being injected into the intestines, or applied externally to different organs of the body. It is remarked, by Abbé Fontana, that this poison, even "when applied in a very small quantity to the eyes, or to the inner part of the mouth, without touching the œsophagus, or being carried into the stomach, is capa-ble of killing an animal in a few minutes: while, ap-plied in a much greater quantity to wounds, it has so little activity, that the weakest animals, such as pigeons, resist its action."

The poisonous quality of the species of laurel is the prussic acid; and if we judge from its sensible quali-ties, an analogous principle seems to pervade many other vegetable substances, especially the kernels of drupaceous fruits: and in various species of the amyg-dalus, this sapid principle extends to the flowers and leaves. It is of importance to notice, that this is much less powerful in its action upon human subjects than upon dogs, rabbits, pigeons, and reptiles. To poison man, the essential oil of the lauro-cerasus must be separated by distillation, as in the spirituous or common laurel-water; and unless this is strongly imbued with the oil, or given in a large dose, it proves innocent. Dr. Cullen observes, that the sedative power of the lauro-cerasus, acts upon the nervous system in a dif-ferent manner from opium and other narcotic sub-stances, whose primary action is upon the animal func-tions; for the lauro-cerasus does not occasion sleep, nor does it produce local inflammation, but seems to act directly upon the vital powers. Abbé Fontana supposes that this poison destroys animal life, by ex-erting its effects upon the blood; but the experiments and observations from which he draws this opinion are evidently inconclusive. It may also be remarked, that many of the Abbé's experiments contradict each other. Thus, it appears from the citation given above, that the poison of this vegetable, when applied to wounds, does not prove fatal; but future experiments led the Abbé to assert, that the oil of the lauro-cerasus, whether given internally, or applied to the wounds of animals, is one of the most terrible and deadly poisons known. Though this vegetable seems to have escaped the notice of Stoerck, yet it is not without advocates for its medical use. Linnæus informs us, that in Switzerland it is commonly and successfully used in pulmonary complaints. Langrish mentions its efficacy in agues; and as Bergius found bitter almonds to have this effect, we may, by analogy, conclude that this power of the lauro-cerasus is well established. Bay-lies found that it possessed a remarkable power of di-luting the blood, and from experience, recommended it in all cases of disease supposed to proceed from too dense a state of that fluid; adducing particular in-stances of its efficacy in rheumatisms, asthmas, and scirrhous affections. Nor does this author seem to have been much afraid of the deleterious quality of lauro-cerasus, as he directs a pound of its leaves to be macerated in a pint of water, of which he gives from thirty to sixty drops three or four times a-day.

PRUNUS PADUS. The systematic name of the wild cluster, or bird cherry-tree. *Padus.* The bark and berries of this shrub are used medicinally. The former, when taken from the tree, has a fragrant smell, and a bitter, substringent taste, somewhat similar to that of bitter almonds. Made into a decoction, it cures inter-mittents, and it has been recommended in the cure of several forms of syphilis. The latter are said to cure the dysentery.

PRUNUS SPINOSA. The systematic name of the sloe tree. *Prunus sylvestris; Prunus—pedunculis solita riis, foliis lanceolatis, glabris, ramis spinosis,* of Linnæus. It is sometimes employed in gargles, to tumefactions of the tonsils and uvula, and from its astringent taste was formerly much used in hæmor-rhages, &c.

PRURI'GO. (From *prurio*, to itch.) *Pruritus; Scabies; Psora; Darta; Libido; Pavor.* The prurigo is a genus of disease in the order *Papulous eruptions* of Dr. Willan's cutaneous diseases. As it arises from different causes, or at different periods of life, and exhibits some varieties in its form, he describes it under the titles of prurigo mitis, prurigo formicans, and prurigo senilis. In these, the whole surface of the skin is usually affected; but there are likewise many cases of local prurigo, which will be afterward noticed according to their respective situations.

1. The *Prurigo mitis* originates without any previous indisposition, generally in spring, or the beginning of summer. It is characterized by soft and smooth elevations of the cuticle, somewhat larger than the papulæ of the lichen, from which they also differ by retaining the usual colour of the skin; for they seldom appear red, or much inflamed, except from violent friction. They are not, as in the other case, accompanied with tingling, but with a sense of itching almost incessant. This is, however, felt more particularly on undressing, and often prevent rest for some hours after getting into a bed. When the tops of the papulæ are removed by rubbing or scratching, a clear fluid oozes out from them, and gradually concretes into thin black scabs.

This species of prurigo mostly affects young persons; and its cause may, I think, says Dr. Willan, in general be referred to sordes collected on the skin, producing some degree of irritation, and also preventing the free discharge of the cutaneous exhalation; the bad consequences of which must necessarily be felt at that season of the year when perspiration is the most copious. Those who have originally a delicate or irritable skin, must likewise, in the same circumstances, be the greatest sufferers.

The eruption extends to the arms, breast, back, and thighs, and often continues during two or three months of the summer, if not relieved by proper treatment. When persons affected with it neglect washing the skin, or are uncleanly in their apparel, the eruption grows more inveterate, and at length, changing its form, often terminates in the itch. Pustules arise among the papulæ, some filled with lymph, others with pus. The acarus scabiei begins to breed in the furrows of the cuticle, and the disorder becomes contagious.

2. The *Prurigo formicans* is a much more obstinate and troublesome disease than the foregoing. It usually affects persons of adult age, commencing at all seasons of the year indifferently; and its duration is from four months to two or three years, with occasional short intermissions. The papulæ are sometimes larger, sometimes more obscure, than in the preceding species; but are, under every form, attended with an incessant, almost intolerable itching. They are diffused over the whole body, except the face, feet, and palms of the hands; they appear, however, in the greatest number on those parts which, from the mode of dress, are subjected to tight ligatures; as about the neck, loins, and thighs.

The itching is complicated with other sensations, which are variously described by patients. They sometimes feel as if small insects were creeping on the skin; sometimes as if stung all over by ants; sometimes as if hot needles were piercing the skin in divers places. On standing before a fire, or undressing, and more particularly on getting into bed, these sensations become most violent, and usually preclude all rest during the greatest part of the night. The prurigo formicans is by most practitioners deemed contagious, and confounded with the itch. In endeavouring to ascertain the justness of this opinion, Dr. Willan has been led to make the following remarks: 1. The eruption is, for the most part, connected with internal disorder, and arises when no source of infection can be traced. 2. Persons affected may have constant intercourse with several others, and yet never communicate the disease to any of them. 3. Several persons of one family may have the prurigo formicans about the same time; but he thinks this should be referred rather to a common predisposition than to contagion, having observed that individuals of a family are often so affected at certain seasons of the year, even when they reside at a distance from each other.

Although the prurigo formicans is never, like the former species, converted into the itch, yet it does occasionally terminate in a pustular disease, not contagious.

3. *Prurigo senilis.* This affection does not differ

much in its symptoms and external appearances from the prurigo formicans; but has been thought by medical writers to merit a distinct consideration on account of its peculiar inveteracy. The prurigo is perhaps aggravated, or becomes more permanent in old age from the dry, condensed state of the skin and cuticle which often takes place at that period. Those who are affected with it in a high degree have little more comfort to expect during life, being incessantly tormented with a violent and universal itching. The state of the skin in the prurigo senilis, is favourable to the production of an insect, the pediculus humanus, more especially to the variety of it usually termed body-lice.

These insects, it is well known, are bred abundantly among the inhabitants of sordid dwellings, of jails, work-houses, &c. and in such situations prey upon persons of all ages indiscriminately. But in the prurigo senilis they arise, notwithstanding every attention to cleanliness or regimen, and multiply so rapidly that the patient endures extreme distress, from their perpetual irritation. The nits or eggs are deposited on the small hairs of the skin, and the pediculi are only found on the skin, or on the linen, not under the cuticle, as some authors have represented. In connexion with the foregoing series of complaints, Dr. Willan mentions some pruriginous affections which are merely local. He confines his observations to the most troublesome of these, seated in the podex, præputium, urethra, pubes, scrotum, and pudendum muliebre. Itching of the nostrils, eyelids, lips, or of the external ear, being generally symptomatic of other diseases, do not require a particular consideration.

1. *Prurigo podicis.* Ascarides in the rectum excite a frequent itching and irritation about the sphincter ani, which ceases when the cause is removed by proper medicines. A similar complaint often arises, independently of worms, hæmorrhoidal tumours, or other obvious causes, which is mostly found to affect persons engaged in sedentary occupations; and may be referred to a morbid state of secretion in the parts, founded, perhaps, on a diminution of constitutional vigour. The itching is not always accompanied with an appearance of papulæ or tubercles; it is little troublesome during the day-time, but returns every night soon after getting into bed, and precludes rest for several hours. The complaint continues in this form during three or four months, and has then an intermission, till it is produced again by hot weather, fatigue, watching, or some irregularity in diet. The same disease occurs at the decline of life, under a variety of circumstances.

Women, after the cessation of the catamenia, are liable to be affected with this species of prurigo, more especially in summer or autumn. The skin between the nates is rough and papulated, sometimes scaly, and a little humour is discharged by violent friction. Along with this complaint, there is often an eruption of itching papulæ on the neck, breast, and back; a swelling and inflammation of one or both ears, and a discharge of matter from behind them, and from the external meatus auditorius. The prurigo podicis sometimes occurs as a symptom of the lues venerea.

2. The *prurigo præputii* is owing to an altered state of secretion on the glans penis, and inner surface of the præputium. During the heat of summer there is also, in some persons, an unusual discharge of mucus, which becomes acrimonious, and produces a troublesome itching, and often an excoriation of these parts. Washing of them with water, or soap and water, employed from time to time, relieves the complaint, and should indeed be practised as an ordinary point of cleanliness, where no inconvenience is immediately felt. If the fluid be secreted in too large a quantity, that excess may be restrained, by washes made with the liquor plumbi subacetatis, or by applying the unguentum plumbi superacetatis.

3. *Prurigo urethralis.* A very troublesome itching sometimes takes place at the extremity of the urethra in females, without any manifest cause. It occurs as well in young women as in those who are of an advanced age. On examination, no stricture or tumour has been found along the course of the urethra. Probably, however, the itching may be occasioned by a morbid state of the neck of the bladder, being in some instances connected with pain and difficulty of making water.

An itching at the extremity of the urethra in men is produced by calculi, and by some diseases of the blad der. In cases of stricture an itching is also felt, but near the place where the stricture is situated. Another cause of it is small broken hairs, which are sometimes drawn in from the pubes, between the præputium and glans, and which afterward becoming fixed in the entrance of the urethra, occasion an itching, or slight stinging, particularly on motion. J. Pearson, surgeon of the Lock Hospital, has seen five cases of this kind, and gave immediate relief by extracting the small hair from the urethra.

4. *Prurigo pubis.* Itching papulæ often arise on the pubes, and become extremely sore if their tops are removed by scratching. They are occasioned sometimes by neglect of cleanliness, but more commonly by a species of pediculus, which perforates the cuticle, and thus derives its nourishment, remaining fixed in the same situation. These insects are termed by Linnæus, &c. *pediculi pubis ;* they do not, however, affect the pubes only, but often adhere to the eyebrows, eyelids, and axillæ. They are often found, also, on the breast, abdomen, thighs, and legs, in persons of the sanguine temperament, who have those parts covered with strong hairs. It is remarkable that they seldom or never fix upon the hairy scalp. The great irritation produced by them on the skin, solicits constantly scratching, by which they are torn from their attachments: and painful tubercles arise at the places where they had adhered. When the pediculi are diffused over the greater part of the surface of the body, the patient's linen often appears as if sprinkled with drops of blood.

5. *Prurigo scroti.* The scrotum is affected with a troublesome and constant itching from ascarides within the rectum, from friction by violent exercise in hot weather, and very usually from the pediculi pubis. Another and more important form of the complaint appears in old men, sometimes connected with the prurigo podicis, and referrible to a morbid state of the skin, or superficial gland of the part. The scrotum, in this case, assumes a brown colour, often also becoming thick, scaly, and wrinkled. The itching extends to the skin covering the penis, more especially along the course of the urethra; and has little respite, either by day or night.

6. The *Prurigo pudendi muliebris,* is somewhat analogous to the prurigo scroti in men. It is often a symptomatic complaint in the lichen and lepra ; it likewise originates from ascarides irritating the rectum, and is in some cases connected with a discharge of the fluor albus.

A similar affection arises in consequence of a change of state in the genital organs at the time of puberty, attended with a series of most distressing sensations. Dr. Willan confines his attention to one case of the disorder, which may be considered as idiopathic, and which usually affects women soon after the cessation of the catamenia. It chiefly occurs in those who are of the phlegmatic temperament, and inclined to corpulency. Its seat is the labia pudendi, and entrance to the vagina. It is often accompanied with an appearance of tension or fulness of those parts, and sometimes with inflamed itching papulæ on the labia and mons veneris. The distress arising from a strong and almost perpetual itching in the above situation, may be easily imagined. In order to allay it in some degree, the sufferers have frequent recourse to friction, and to cooling applications; whence they are necessitated to forego the enjoyment of society. An excitement of venereal sensations also takes place from the constant direction of the mind to the parts affected, as well as from the means employed to procure alleviation. The complicated distress thus arising, renders existence almost insupportable, and often produces a state of mind bordering on frenzy.

Deep ulcerations of the parts seldom take place in the prurigo pudendi: but the appearance of aphthæ on the labia and nymphæ, is by no means unusual. From intercourse with females under these circumstances, men are liable to be affected with aphthous ulcerations on the glans, and inside of the præputium, which prove troublesome for a length of time, and often excite an alarm, being mistaken for chancres.

Women, after the fourth month of their pregnancy, often suffer greatly from the prurigo pudendi, attended with aphthæ. These, in a few cases, have been succeeded by extensive ulcerations, which destroyed the nymphæ, and produced a fatal hectic : such instances

are, however, extremely rare. The complaint has, in general, some intervals or remissions; and the aphthæ usually disappear soon after delivery, whether at the full time, or by a miscarriage.

PRURI'TUS. (From *prurio,* to itch.) See *Prurigo Prussian alkali.* See *Alkali, phlogisticated. Prussian blue.* See *Blue, Prussian.*

PRUSSIATE. A salt formed by the union of the prussic acid, or colouring matter of Prussian blue, with a salifiable basis : thus, *prussiate of potassa,* &c.

PRUSSIC ACID. *Acidum prussicum. Acidum hydrocyanicum.* Hydrocyanic acid. "The combination of this acid with iron was long known, and used as a pigment by the name of Prussian blue, before its nature was understood. Scheele's method of obtaining it is this :—Mix four ounces of Prussian blue with two of red oxide of mercury prepared by nitric acid, and boil them in twelve ounces by weight of water, till the whole becomes colourless; filter the liquor, and add to it one ounce of clean iron filings, and six or seven drachms of sulphuric acid. Draw off by distillation about a fourth of the liquor, which will be prussic acid ; though, as it is liable to be contaminated[1] with a portion of sulphuric, to render it pure, it may be rectified by redistilling it from carbonate of lime.

This prussic acid has a strong smell of peach-blossoms, or bitter almonds; its taste is at first sweetish, then acrid, hot, and virulent, and excites coughing; it has a strong tendency to assume the form of gas; it has been decomposed in a high temperature, and by the contact of light, into carbonic acid, ammonia, and carburetted hydrogen. It does not completely neutralize alkalies, and is displaced even by the carbonic acid ; it has no action upon metals, but unites with their oxides, and forms salts for the most part insoluble; it likewise unites into triple salts with these oxides and alkalies; the oxygenated muriatic acid decomposes it.

The peculiar smell of the prussic acid could scarcely fail to suggest its affinity with the deleterious principle that rises in the distillation of the leaves of the laurocerasus, bitter kernels of fruits, and some other vegetable productions; and Schrader, of Berlin, has ascertained the fact, that these vegetable substances do contain a principle capable of forming a blue precipitate with iron ; and that with lime they afford a test of the presence of iron equal to the prussiate of that earth. Dr. Bucholz, of Weimar, and Roloff, of Magdeburg, confirm this fact. The prussic acid appears to come over in the distilled oil.

Prussic acid and its combinations have been lately investigated by Gay Lussac and Vauquelin in France, and Porrett in England.

To a quantity of powdered Prussian blue diffused in boiling water, let red oxide of mercury be added in successive portions till the blue colour is destroyed. Filter the liquid, and concentrate by evaporation till a pellicle appears. On cooling, crystals of prussiate, or cyanide of mercury, will be formed. Dry these, and put them into a tubulated glass retort, to the beak of which is adapted a horizontal tube about two feet long, and fully half an inch wide at its middle part. The first third-part of the tube next the retort is filled with small pieces of white marble, the two other thirds with fused muriate of lime. To the end of this tube is adapted a small receiver, which should be artificially refrigerated. Pour on the crystals muriatic acid, in rather less quantity than is sufficient to saturate the oxide of mercury which formed them. Apply a very gentle heat to the retort. Prussic acid, named hydro cyanic by Gay Lussac, will be evolved in vapour, and will condense in the tube. Whatever muriatic acid may pass over with it, will be abstracted by the marble, while the water will be absorbed by the muriate of lime. By means of moderate heat applied to the tube, the prussic acid may be made to pass successively along; and after being left some time in contact with the muriate of lime, it may be finally driven into the receiver. As the carbonic acid evolved from marble by the muriatic is apt to carry off some of the prussic acid, care should be taken to conduct the heat so as to prevent the distillation of this mineral acid.

Prussic acid thus obtained has the following properties :—It is a colourless liquid, possessing a strong odour; and the exhalation, if incautiously snuffed up the nostrils, may produce sickness or fainting. Its taste is cooling at first, then hot, asthenic in a high degree, and a true poison.

This acid, when compared with the other animal products, is distinguished by the great quantity of nitrogen it contains, by its small quantity of hydrogen, and especially by the absence of oxygen.

When this acid is kept in well-closed vessels, even though no air be present, it is sometimes decomposed in less than an hour. It has been occasionally kept 15 days without alteration; but it is seldom that it can be kept longer, without exhibiting signs of decomposition. It begins by assuming a reddish-brown colour, which becomes deeper and deeper; and it gradually deposites a considerable carbonaceous matter, which gives a deep colour to both water and acids, and emits a strong smell of ammonia. If the bottle containing the prussic acid be not hermetically sealed, nothing remains but a dry charry mass, which gives no colour to water. Thus a prussiate of ammonia is formed at the expense of a part of the acid, and an azoturet of carbon. When potassium is heated in prussic acid vapour mixed with hydrogen or nitrogen, there is absorption without inflammation, and the metal is converted into a gray spongy substance, which melts, and assumes a yellow colour.

Supposing the quantity of potassium employed capable of disengaging from water a volume of hydrogen equal to 50 parts, we find after the action of the potassium,

1. That the gaseous mixture has experienced a diminution of volume amounting to 50 parts.

2. On treating this mixture with potassa and analyzing the residue by oxygen, that 50 parts of hydrogen have been produced.

3. And consequently that the potassium has absorbed 100 parts of prussic vapour; for there is a diminution of 50 parts which would obviously have been twice as great had not 50 parts of hydrogen been disengaged. The yellow matter is prussiate of potassa; properly a prusside of potassium, analogous in its formation to the chloride and iodide, when muriatic and hydriodic gases are made to act on potassium.

The base of prussic acid thus divested of its acidifying hydrogen, should be called, agreeably to the same chemical analogy, prussine. Gay Lussac styles it cyanogen, because it is the principle which generates blue; or, literally, the blue-maker.

Like muriatic and hydriodic acids also, it contains half its volume of hydrogen. The only difference is, that the former have in the present state of our knowledge simple radicals, chlorine and iodine, while that of the latter is a compound of one volume vapour of carbon, and half a volume of nitrogen. This radical forms true prussides with metals.

If the term cyanogen be objectionable as allying it to oxygen, instead of chlorine and iodine, the term hydrocyanic acid must be equally so, as implying that it contains water. Thus we say, hydronitric, hydromuriatic, and hydrophosphoric, to denote the aqueous compounds of the nitric, muriatic, and phosphoric acids. As the singular merit of Gay Lussac, however, has commanded a very general compliance among chemists with his nomenclature, we shall use the terms prussic acid and hydrocyanic indifferently, as has long been done with the words nitrogen and azote.

The prusside or cyanide of potassium gives a very alkaline solution in water, even when a great excess of hydrocyanic vapour has been present at its formation. In this respect it differs from the chlorides and iodides of that metal, which are perfectly neutral.

Barytes, potassa, and soda combine with prussine, forming true prussides of these alkaline oxides; analogous to what are vulgarly called oxymuriates of lime, potassa, and soda. The red oxide of mercury acts so powerfully on prussic acid vapour, when assisted by heat, that the compound which ought to result is destroyed by the heat disengaged. The same thing happens when a little of the concentrated acid is poured upon the oxide. A great elevation of temperature takes place, which would occasion a dangerous explosion if the experiment were made upon considerable quantities. When the acid is diluted, the oxide dissolves rapidly, with a considerable heat, and without the disengagement of any gas. The substance formerly called prussiate of mercury is generated, which when moist may, like the muriates, still retain that name; but when dry is a prusside of the metal.

When the cold oxide is placed in contact with the acid, dilated into a gaseous form by hydrogen, its vapour is absorbed in a few minutes. The hydrogen is unchanged. When a considerable quantity of vapour has thus been absorbed, the oxide adheres to the side of the tube, and on applying heat, water is obtained. The hydrogen of the acid has here united with the oxygen of the oxide to form the water, while their two radicals combine. Red oxide of mercury becomes an excellent reagent for detecting prussic acid.

By exposing the dry prusside of mercury to heat in a retort, the radical cyanogen or prussine is obtained.

From the experiments of Magendie it appears that the pure hydrocyanic acid is the most violent of all poisons. When a rod dipped into it is brought in contact with the tongue of an animal, death ensues before the rod can be withdrawn. If a bird be held a moment over the mouth of a phial containing this acid, it dies. In the Annales de Chimie for 1814, we find this notice:—M. B., Professor of Chemistry, left by accident on a table a flask containing alkohol impregnated with prussic acid; the servant, enticed by the agreeable flavour of the liquid, swallowed a small glass of it. In two minutes she dropped down dead, as if struck with apoplexy. The body was not examined.

"Scharinger, a professor at Vienna," says Orfila, "prepared, six or seven months ago, a pure and concentrated prussic acid; he spread a certain quantity of it on his naked arm, and died a little time thereafter."

Dr. Magendie has, however, ventured to introduce its employment into medicine. He found it beneficial against phthisis and chronic catarrhs. His formulæ is the following :—

Mix one part of the pure prussic or hydrocyanic acid of Gay Lussac with 8½ of water by weight. To this mixture he gives the name of medicinal prussic acid.

Of this he takes 1 gros. or	59 grs. Troy
Distilled water, 1 lb. or	7560 grs.
Pure sugar, 1½ oz. or	708¾ grs.

And mixing the ingredients well together, he administers a table-spoonful every morning and evening. A well-written report of the use of the prussic acid in certain diseases, by Dr. Magendie, was communicated by Dr. Granville to Mr. Brande, and is inserted in the fourth volume of the Journal of Science.

For the following ingenious and accurate process for preparing prussic acid for medicinal uses, I am indebted to Dr. Nimmo of Glasgow.

"Take of the ferroprussiate of potassa 100 grains, of the protosulphate of iron 84½ grains, dissolve them separately in four ounces of water, and mingle them. After allowing the precipitate of the protoprussiate of iron to settle, pour off the clear part, and add water to wash the sulphate of potassa completely away. To the protoprussiate of iron, mixed with four ounces of pure water, add 135 grains of the peroxide of mercury, and boil the whole till the oxide is dissolved. With the above proportions of peroxide of mercury, the protoprussiate of iron is completely decomposed. The vessel being kept warm, the oxide of iron will fall to the bottom; the clear part may be poured off to be filtered through paper, taking care to keep the funnel covered, so that crystals may not form in it by refrigeration. The residuum may be treated with more water, and thrown upon the filter, upon which warm water ought to be poured, until all the soluble part is washed away. By evaporation, and subsequent rest in a cool place, 145 grains of crystals of the prusside, or cyanide of mercury will be procured in quadrangular prisms.

"The following process for eliminating the hydrocyanic acid I believe to be new :—Take of the cyanide of mercury in fine powder one ounce, diffuse it in two ounces of water, and to it, by slow degrees, add a solution of hydrosulphuret of barytes, made by decomposing sulphate of barytes with charcoal in the common way. Of the sulphuret of barytes take an ounce, boil it with six ounces of water, and filter it as hot as possible. Add this in small portions to the cyanide of mercury, agitating the whole very well, and allowing sufficient time for the cyanide to dissolve, while the decomposition is going on between it and the hydrosul phuret, as it is added. Continue the addition of the hydrosulphuret so long as a dark precipitate of sulphuret of mercury falls down, and even allowing a small excess. Let the whole be thrown upon a filter, and kept warm till the fluid drops through ; add more water to wash the sulphuret of mercury, until eight ounces of fluid have passed through the filter, and it has become tasteless. To this fluid, which contains the prussiate of barytes, with a small excess of hydrosulphuret of barytes, add sulphuric acid, diluted with an equal weight of water, and allowed to become cold, so long as sulphate of barytes falls down. The excess of sulphuretted hydrogen will be removed by adding a sufficient portion of carbonate of lead, and agitating very well. The whole may now be put upon a filter, which must be closely covered ; the fluid which passes is the hydrocyanic acid of what is called the *medical* standard strength."

Scheele found that prussic acid occasioned precipitates with only the following three metallic solutions : nitrates of silver and mercury, and carbonate of silver. The first is white, the second black, the third green, becoming blue.

The hydrocyanates are all alkaline, even when a great excess of acid is employed in their formation, and they are decomposed by the weakest acids."—*Ure's Chem. Dict.*

PRUSSINE. Prussic gas. Cyanogen. This is obtained by decomposing the prusside or cyanide of mercury by heat.

When the simple mercurial prusside is exposed to heat in a small glass retort, or tube, shut at one extremity, it soon begins to blacken. It appears to melt like an animal matter, and then the prussine is disengaged in abundance. This gas is pure from the beginning of the process to the end, provided always that the heat be not very high ; for if it were not sufficiently intense to melt the glass, a little azote would be evolved. Mercury is volatilized with a considerable quantity of prusside, and there remains a charry matter of the colour of soot, and as light as lampblack. The prusside of silver gives out likewise prussine when heated ; but the mercurial prusside is preferable to every other.

Prussine or cyanogen is a permanently elastic fluid. Its smell, which it is impossible to describe, is very strong and penetrating. Its solution in water has a very sharp taste. The gas burns with a bluish flame mixed with purple. Its sp. gr., compared to that of air, is 1.8064.

Prussine is capable of sustaining a pretty high heat, without being decomposed. Water, agitated with it for some minutes, at the temperature of 68°, absorbed about 4½ times its volume. Pure alkohol absorbs 23 times its volume. Sulphuric æther and oil of turpentine dissolve at least as much as water. Tincture of litmus is reddened by prussine. The carbonic acid proceeds, no doubt, from the decomposition of a small quantity of prussine and water. It deprives the red sulphate of manganese of its colour, a property which prussic acid does not possess.

Phosphorus, sulphur, and iodine may be sublimed by the heat of a spirit-lamp in prussine, without occasioning any change on it. Its mixture with hydrogen was not altered by the same temperature, or by passing electrical sparks through it. Copper and gold do not combine with it ; but iron, when heated almost to whiteness, decomposes it in part.

In the cold, potassium acts but slowly on prussine, because a crust is formed on its surface, which presents an obstacle to the mutual action. On applying the spirit-lamp, the potassium becomes speedily incandescent ; the absorption of the gas begins, the inflamed disc gradually diminishes, and when it disappears entirely, which takes place in a few seconds, the absorption is likewise at an end.

The compound of prussine and potassium is yellowish. It dissolves in water without effervescence, and the solution is strongly alkaline. Its taste is the same as that of hydrocyanate or simple prussiate of potassa, of which it possesses all the properties.

When a pure solution of potassa is introduced into this gas, the absorption is rapid. If the alkali be not too concentrated, and be not quite saturated, it is scarcely tinged of a lemon-yellow colour. But if the prussine be in excess, we obtain a brown solution, apparently carbonaceous. On pouring potassa combined with prussine into a saline solution of a black oxide of iron, and adding an acid, we obtain Prussian blue.

The instant an acid is poured into the solution of

prussine in potassa, a strong effervescence of carbonic acid is produced, and at the same time a strong smell of prussic acid becomes perceptible. Ammonia is likewise formed, which remains combined with the acid employed and which may be rendered very sensible to the smell by the addition of quicklime. Since, therefore, we are obliged to add an acid in order to form Prussian blue, its formation occasions no farther difficulty.

Soda, barytes, and strontites produce the same effect as potassa. We must, therefore, admit that prussine forms particular combinations with the alkalies, which are permanent till some circumstance determines the formation of new products. These combinations are true salts, which may be regarded as analagous to those formed by acids. In fact, prussine possesses acid characters. It contains two elements, azote and carbon, the first of which is strongly acidifying, according to Gay Lussac. Prussine reddens the tincture of litmus, and neutralizes the bases. On the other hand, it acts as a simple body when it combines with hydrogen ; and it is this double function of a simple and compound body, which renders its nomenclature so embarrassing.

Be this as it may, the compounds of prussine and the alkalies, which may be distinguished by the term *prussides*, do not separate in water like the alkaline chlorurets (oxymuriates), which produce chlorates and muriates.

The metallic oxides do not seem capable of producing the same changes on prussine as the alkalies.

Prussine rapidly decomposes the carbonates at a dull red heat, and prussides of the oxides are obtained. When passed through sulphuret of barytes, it combines without disengaging the sulphur, and renders it very fusible and of a brownish-black colour. When put into water, we obtain a colourless solution, but which gives a deep brown (maroon) colour to muriate of iron. What does not dissolve contains a good deal of sulphate, which is doubtless formed during the preparation of the sulphuret of barytes.

On dissolving prussine in the sulphuretted hydrosulphuret of barytes, sulphur is precipitated, which is again dissolved when the liquor is saturated with prussine, and we obtain a solution having a very deep brown maroon colour. This gas does not decompose sulphuret of silver, nor of potassa.

Prussine and sulphuretted hydrogen combine slowly with each other. A yellow substance is obtained in fine needles, which dissolves in water, does not precipitate nitrate of lead, produces no Prussian blue, and is composed of 1 volume prussine (cyanogen), and 1½ volumes of sulphuretted hydrogen.

Ammoniacal gas and prussine begin to act on each other whenever they come in contact ; but some hours are requisite to render the effect complete. We perceive at first a white thick vapour, which soon disappears. The diminution of volume is considerable, and the glass in which the mixture is made becomes opaque, its inside being covered with a solid brown matter. On mixing 90 parts of prussine, and 227 ammonia, they combined nearly in the proportion of 1 to 1½. This compound gives a dark orange-brown colour to water, but dissolves only in a very small proportion. The liquid produces no Prussian blue with the salts of iron.

In the first volume of the Journal of Science and the Arts, Sir H. Davy has stated some interesting particulars relative to prussine. By heating prusside of mercury in muriatic acid gas, he obtained pure liquid prussic acid and corrosive sublimate. By heating iodine, sulphur, and phosphorus, in contac with prusside of mercury, compounds of these bodies with prussine or cyanogen may be formed. That of iodine is a very curious body. It is volatile at a very moderate heat ; and on cooling collects in flocculi, adhering together like oxide of zinc formed by combustion. It has a pungent smell, and very acrid taste.

PSALLOI'DES. (From ψαλλος, a stringed instrument, and ειδος, a likeness : because it appears as if stringed like a dulcimer.) Applied by the ancients to the inner surface of the fornix of the brain.

PSALTE'RIUM. (A harp : because it is marked with lines that give its the appearance of a harp.) *Lyra.* The medullary body that unites the posterior crura of the fornix of the brain.

PSAMMI'SMUS. (From ψαμμος, sand.) An application of hot sand to any part of the body.

PSAMMO'DES. (From ψαμμος, sand.) ' Applied to urine which deposites a sandy sediment.

PSELLI'SMUS. (From ψελλιζω, to have a hesitation of speech.) *Psellotis.* Defect of speech. A genus of disease in the Class *Locales,* and Order *Dyscinesiæ,* of Cullen.

PSELLO'TIS. See *Psellismus.*

PSEUDA'CORUS. (From ψευδης, false, and ακοροv, the acorus plant: because it resembled and was substituted for that plant.) See *Iris Pseudacorus.*

PSEUDO. (Ψευδης, false.) Spurious. This word is fixed to the name of several diseases, because they resemble them, but are not those diseases; as *Pseudopneumonia, Pseudo-phrenitis.* It is also prefixed to many substances which are only fictitious imitations; as *Pseudamomum,* a spurious kind of amomum, &c.

PSEUDOBLE'PSIS. (From ψευδης, false, and δλεψις, sight.) *Phantasma; Suffusio.* Imaginary vision of objects. A genus of disease in the Class *Locales,* and Order *Dysæthesiæ,* of Cullen; characterized by depraved sight, creating objects, or representing them different from what they are. Species:—
1. *Pseudoblepsis imaginaria,* in which objects are perceived that are not present.
2. *Pseudoblepsis mutans,* in which objects that are present appear somewhat changed.

PSEUDOCYESIS. (From ψευδης, false, and κυησις, pregnancy.) The name of a genus of disease in Good's Nosology. Class, *Genetica;* Order, *Carpotica.* False conception. It has two species, viz. *Pseudocyesis molaris,* and *inanis.*

PSEUDOMELANTHIUM. (From ψευδης, false, and *melanthium,* the name of a plant.) See *Agrostemma githago.*

PSEUDOPYRETHRUM. (From ψευδης, false, and *pyrethrum,* the name of a plant: so called, because when the flowers are chewed they impart a warmth somewhat like that of pyrethrum root.) See *Achillæa ptarmica.*

PSI'DIUM. (Altered by Linnæus from ψιδιας of the ancient Greeks.) The name of a genus of plants in the Linnæan system. Class, *Icosandria;* Order, *Menogynia.*

PSIDIUM POMIFERUM. The systematic name of the apple guava. This plant, and the *pyriferum,* bear fruits, the former like apples, the latter like pears. The apple kind is most cultivated in the Indies, on account of the pulp having a fine acid flavour, whereas the pear species is sweet, and therefore not so agreeable in warm climates. Of the inner pulp of either, the inhabitants make jellies; and of the outer rind they make tarts, marmalades, &c. The latter they also stew and eat with milk, and prefer them to any other stewed fruits. They have an astringent quality, which exists also in every part of the tree, and abundantly in the leaf-buds, which are occasionally boiled with barley, and liquorice, as an excellent drink against diarrhœas. A simple decoction of the leaves, used as a bath, is said to cure the itch, and most cutaneous eruptions.

PSIDIUM PYRIFERUM. The systematic name of the pear guava. See *Psidium pomiferum.*

PSILO'THRA. (From ψιλοω, to denudate.) Applications to remove the hair.

PSILO'THRUM. (From ψιλοω, to depilate: so called because it was used to remove the hair.) The white briony.

PSIMMY'THIUM. (From ψιω, to smooth: so called because of its use as a cosmetic.) Cerusse, or white lead.

PSO'Æ. (Ψοαι, the loins.) *Alopeces; Nefrometræ; Neurometeres.* 1. The loins.
2. The name of two pair of muscles in the loins.

PSO'AS. (From ψοαι, the loins.) Belonging to the loins.

PSOAS ABSCESS. See *Lumbar abscess.*

PSOAS MAGNUS. *Psoas, seu lumbaris internus,* of Winslow. *Pre-lumbo-trochantin,* of Dumas. This is a long, thick, and very considerable muscle, situated close to the forepart and sides of the lumbar vertebræ. It arises from the bodies of the last vertebræ of the back, and of all the lumbar vertebræ laterally, as well as from the anterior surfaces of their transverse processes by distinct tendinous and fleshy slips, that are gradually collected into one mass, which becomes thicker as it descends, till it reaches the last of the lumbar vertebræ, where it grows narrower again, and uniting its outer and posterior edge (where it begins to become tendi-

nous) with the iliacus internus, descends along with that muscle under the ligamentum Fallopii, and goes to be inserted tendinous at the bottom of the trochanter minor, of the os femoris, and fleshy into the bone a little below that process. Between the tendon of this muscle and the ischium, we find a considerable bursa mucosa. This muscle, at its origin, has some connexion with the diaphragm, and likewise with the quadratus lumborum. It is one of the most powerful flexors of the thighs forwards, and may likewise assist in turning it outwards. When the inferior extremity is fixed, it may help to bend the body forwards, and in an erect posture it greatly assists in preserving the equilibrium of the trunk upon the upper part of the thigh.

PSOAS PARVUS. *Pre-lumbo-pubien,* of Dumas. This muscle, which was first described by Riolanus, is situated upon the psoas magnus, at the anterior part of the loins. The psoas parvus arises thin and fleshy from the side of the uppermost vertebra of the loins, and sometimes also from the lower edge of the last vertebra of the back, and from the transverse processes of each of these vertebræ: it then extends over part of the psoas magnus, and terminates in a thin, flat tendon, which is inserted into that part of the brim of the pelvis, where the os pubis joins the ilium. From this tendon a great number of fibres are sent off, which form a thin fascia, that covers parts of the psoas magnus and iliacus internus, and gradually loses itself on the fore part of the thigh. In the human body, this muscle is very often wanting; but in a dog, according to Douglas, it is never deficient. Riolanus was of opinion, that it occurs oftener in men than in women. Winslow asserts just the contrary; but the truth seems to be, that it is as often wanting in one sex as in the other. Its use seems to be to assist the psoas magnus in bending the loins forwards; and when we are lying upon our back, it may help to raise the pelvis.

PSOAS SIVE LUMBARIS INTERNUS. See *Psoas magnus.*

PSO'RA. Ψωρα. *Scabies.* The itch. A genus of disease in the Class *Locales,* and Order *Dyalyses,* of Cullen: appearing first on the wrists, and between the fingers, in small pustules with watery heads. It is contagious.

PSORALEA. (From ψωραλεος, scabby; because the calyx, and other parts of the plant, are more or less besprinkled with glandular dots, giving a scurfy rough ness.) The name of a genus of plants. Class, *Diadelphia;* Order, *Decandria.*

PSORALEA PENTAPHYLLA. The systematic name of the Chexicum contrayerva, *Contrayerva nova,* which is by many as much esteemed as the Dorstenia. It was introduced into Europe soon after the true plant, from Guiana as well as Mexico.

PSORI'ASIS. (From ψωρα, the itch.) The disease to which Dr. Willan gives this title is characterized by a rough and scaly state of the cuticle, sometimes continuous, sometimes in separate patches, of various sizes, but of an irregular figure, and for the most part accompanied with rhagades or fissures of the skin. From the lepra it may be distinguished, not only by the distribution of the patches, but also by its cessation and recurrence at certain seasons of the year, and by the disorder of the constitution with which it is usually attended. Dr. Willan gives the following varieties:
1. *Psoriasis guttata.* This complaint appears in small, distinct, but irregular patches of laminated scales, with little or no inflammation round them. The patches very seldom extend to the size of a six pence. They have neither an elevated border, nor the oval or circular form by which all the varieties of lepra are distinguished; but their circumference is sometimes angular, and seems goes into small serpentine processes. The scale formed upon each of them is thin, and may be easily detached, leaving a red, shining base. The patches are often distributed over the greatest part of the body, but more particularly on the back part of the neck, the breasts, arms, loins, thighs, and legs. They appear also upon the face, which rarely happens in lepra. In that situation, they are red and more rough than the adjoining cuticle, but not covered with scales. The psoriasis guttata often appears on children in a sudden eruption, attended with a slight disorder of the constitution, and spreads over the body within two or three days. In adults it commences with a few scaly patches on the extremities, proceeds very gradually, and has a longer duration

than in children. Its first occurrence is usually in the spring season, after violent pains in the head, stomach, and limbs. During the summer it disappears spontaneously, or may be soon removed by proper applications, but it is apt to return again early in the ensuing spring, and continues so to do for several successive years. When the scales have been removed, and the disease is about to go off, the small patches have a shining appearance, and they retain a dark red, intermixed with somewhat of a bluish colour, for many days, or even weeks, before the skin is restored to its usual state. In the venereal disease there is an eruption which very much resembles the psoriasis guttata, he only difference being a slighter degree of scaliness, and a different shade of colour in the patches, approaching to a livid red, or very dark rose colour. The patches vary in their extent, from the section of a pea, to the size of a silver penny, but are not exactly circular. They rise at first very little, if at all, above the cuticle. As soon, however, as the scales appear on them, they become sensibly elevated; and sometimes the edge or circumference of the patch is higher than the little scales in its centre. This eruption is usually seen upon the forehead, breast, between the shoulders, or in the inside of the forearms, in the groins, about the inside of the thighs, and upon the skin covering the lower part of the abdomen. The syphilitic psoriasis guttata is attended with, or soon followed by, an ulceration of the throat. It appears about six or eight weeks after a chancre has been healed by an ineffectual course of mercury. A similar appearance takes place at nearly the same period, in some cases where no local symptoms had been noticed. When a venereal sore is in a discharging state, this eruption, or other secondary symptoms, often appear much later than the period above mentioned. They may also be kept back three months, or even longer, by an inefficient application of mercury. If no medicine be employed, the syphilitic form of the psoriasis guttata will proceed during several months, the number of the spots increasing, and their bulk being somewhat enlarged, but without any other material alteration.

2 The *Psoriasis diffusa* spreads into large patches irregularly circumscribed, reddish, rough, and chappy, with scales interspersed. It commences, in general, with numerous minute asperities, or elevations of the cuticle, more perceptible by the touch than by sight. Upon these, small distinct scales are soon after formed, adhering by a dark central point, while their edges may be seen white and detached. In the course of two or three weeks all the intervening cuticle becomes rough and chappy, appears red, and raised, and wrinkled, the lines of the skin sinking into deep furrows. The scales which form among them are often slight, and repeatedly exfoliate. Sometimes, without any previous eruption of papulæ, a large portion of the skin becomes dry, harsh, cracked, reddish, and scaly, as above described. In other cases, the disorder commences with separate patches of an uncertain form and size, some of them being small, like those in the psoriasis guttata, some much larger. The patches gradually expand till they become confluent, and nearly cover the part or limb affected. Both the psoriasis guttata and diffusa likewise occur as a sequel of the lichen simplex. This transition takes place more certainly after frequent returns of the lichen. The parts most affected by psoriasis diffusa are the cheeks, chin, upper eyelids, and corners of the eyes, the temples, the external ear, the neck, the fleshy parts of the lower extremities, and the forearm, from the elbow to the back of the hand, along the supinator muscle of the radius. The fingers are sometimes nearly surrounded with a loose scaly incrustation; the nails crack and exfoliate superficially. The scaly patches likewise appear, though less frequently, on the forehead and scalp, on the shoulders, back, and loins, on the abdomen, and instep. This disease occasionally extends to all the parts above mentioned at the same time; but, in general, it affects them successively, leaving one place free, and appearing in others; sometimes again returning to its first situation. The psoriasis diffusa is attended with a sensation of heat, and with a very troublesome itching, especially at night. It exhibits small, slight, distinct scales, having less disposition than the lepra to form thick crusts. The chaps or fissures of the skin, which usually make a part of this complaint, are very sore and painful, but seldom discharge any fluid. When the scales

are removed by frequent washing, or by the application of unguents, the surface, though raised and uneven, appears smooth and shining; and the deep furrows of the cuticle are lined by a slight scaliness. Should any portion of the diseased surface be forcibly excoriated, there issues out a thin lymph, mixed with some drops of blood, which slightly stains and stiffens the linen, but soon concretes into a thin dry scab; this is again succeeded by a white scaliness, gradually increasing, and spreading in various directions. As the complaint declines, the roughness, chaps, scales, &c. disappear, and a new cuticle is formed, at first red, dry, and shrivelled, but which, in two or three weeks, acquires the proper texture. The duration of the psoriasis diffusa is from one to four months. If, in some constitutions, it does not then disappear, but becomes, to a certain degree, permanent, there is, at least, an aggravation or extension of it, about the usual periods of its return. In other cases, the disease, at the vernal returns, differs much as to its extent, and also with respect to the violence of the preceding symptoms. The eruption is, indeed, often confined to a single scaly patch, red, itching, and chapped, of a moderate size, but irregularly circumscribed. This solitary patch is sometimes situated on the temple, or upper part of the cheek, frequently on the breast, the calf of the leg, about the wrist, or within and a little below the elbow joint, but especially at the lower part of the thigh, behind. It continues in any of these situations several months, without much observable alteration. The complaint, denominated with us the bakers' itch, is an appearance of psoriasis diffusa on the back of the hand, commencing with one or two small, rough, scaly patches, and finally extending from the knuckles to the wrist. The rhagades, or chaps, and fissures of the skin, are numerous about the knuckles and ball of the thumb, and where the back of the hand joins the wrist. They are often highly inflamed, and painful, but have no discharge of fluid from them. The back of the hand is a little raised or tumefied, and, at an advanced period of the disorder, exhibits a reddish, glossy surface, without crusts or numerous scales. However, the deep furrows of the cuticle are, for the most part, whitened by a slight scaliness. This complaint is not general among bakers; that it is only aggravated by their business, and affects those who are otherwise disposed to it, may be collected from the following circumstances: 1. It disappears about midsummer, and returns in the cold weather at the beginning of the year; 2. Persons constantly engaged in the business, after having been once affected with the eruption, sometimes enjoy a respite from it for two or three years; 3. When the business is discontinued, the complaint does not immediately cease. The grocers' itch has some affinity with the bakers' itch, or tetter; but, being usually a pustular disease at its commencement, it properly belongs to another genus. Washer-women, probably from the irritation of soap, are liable to be affected with a similar scaly disease on the hands, and arms, sometimes on the face and neck, which, in particular constitutions, proves very troublesome, and of long duration.

3. The *Psoriasis gyrata* is distributed in narrow patches or stripes, variously figured; some of them are nearly longitudinal; some circular, or semicircular, with verniform appendages; some are tortuous, or serpentine; others like earth-worms or leeches: the furrows of the cuticle being deeper than usual, make the resemblance more striking, by giving to them an annulated appearance. There is a separation of slight scales from the diseased surface, but no thick incrustations are formed. The uniform disposition of these patches is singular. I have seen a large circular one situated on each breast above the papillæ; and two or three others of a serpentine form, in analogous situations along the sides of the chest. The back is often variegated in like manner, with convoluted tetters, similarly arranged on each side of the spine. They likewise appear, in some cases, on the arms and thighs, intersecting each other in various directions. A slighter kind of this complaint affects delicate young women and children in small scaly circles or rings, little discoloured; they appear on the cheeks, neck, or upper part of the breast, and are mostly confounded with the herpetic, or pustular ringworm. The psoriasis gyrata has its remissions and returns, like the psoriasis diffusa; it also exhibits, in some cases, patches of the latter dis-

order on the face, scalp, or extremities while the trunk of the body is chequered with the singular figures above described.

4. *Psoriasis palmaria.* This very obstinate species of tetter is nearly confined to the palm of the hand. It commences with a small, harsh, or scaly patch, which gradually spreads over the whole palm, and sometimes appears in a slight degree on the inside of the fingers and wrist. The surface feels rough from the detached and raised edges of the scaly laminæ; its colour often changes to brown or black, as if dirty; yet the most diligent washing produces no favourable effect. The cuticular furrows are deep, and cleft at the bottom longitudinally, in various places, so as to bleed on stretching the fingers. A sensation of heat, pain, and stiffness in the motions of the hand, attends this complaint. It is worse in winter or spring, and occasionally disappears in autumn or summer, leaving a soft, dark-red cuticle; but many persons are troubled with it for a series of years, experiencing only very slight remissions. Every return or aggravation of it is preceded by an increase of heat and dryness, with intolerable itching. Shoemakers have the psoriasis pamaria locally, from the irritation of the wax they so constantly employ. In braziers, tinmen, silversmiths, &c. the complaint seems to be produced by handling cold metals. A long predisposition to it from a weak, languid, hectical state of the constitution, may give effect to different occasional causes. Dr. Willan has observed it in women after lying-in; in some persons it is connected or alternates with arthritic complaints. When the palms of the hands are affected as above stated, a similar appearance often takes place on the soles of the feet; but with the exception of rhagades or fissures, which seem less liable to form there, the feet being usually kept warm and covered. Sometimes, also, the psoriasis palmaria is attended with a thickness of the præputium, with scaliness and painful cracks. These symptoms at last produce a phimosis, and render connubial intercourse difficult or impracticable; so great, in some cases, is the obstinacy of them, that remedies are of no avail, and the patient can only be relieved by circumcision. This affection of the præputium is not exactly similar to any venereal appearance; but rhagades or fissures, and indurated patches within the palm of the hand, take place in syphilis, and somewhat resemble the psoriasis palmaria. The venereal patches are, however, distinct, white, and elevated, having nearly the consistence of a soft corn. From the rhagades there is a slight discharge, very offensive to the smell. The soles of the feet are likewise, in this case, affected with the patches, not with rhagades. When the disease yields to the operation of mercury, the indurated portions of cuticle separate, and a smooth new cuticle is found formed underneath. The fingers and toes are not affected with the patches, &c. in venereal cases.

5. *Psoriasis labialis.* The psoriasis sometimes affects the lip without appearing on any other part of the body. Its characteristics are, as usual, scaliness, intermixed with chaps and fissures of the skin. The scales are of a considerable magnitude, so that their edges are often loose, while the central points are attached; a new cuticle gradually forms beneath the scales, but is not durable. In the course of a few hours it becomes dry, shrivelled, and broken; and, while it exfoliates, gives way to another layer of tender cuticle, which soon, in like manner, perishes. These appearances should be distinguished from the light chaps and roughness of the lips produced by very cold or frosty weather, but easily removed. The psoriasis labialis may be a little aggravated by frost or sharp winds, yet it receives no material alleviation from an opposite temperature. It is not, indeed, confined within any certain limit, or period of duration, having, in several instances, been protracted through all the seasons. The under lip is always more affected than the upper; and the disease takes place more especially in those persons whose lips are full and prominent.

6. *Psoriasis scrotalis.* The skin of the scrotum may be affected in the psoriasis diffusa like other parts of the surface of the body; but sometimes a roughness and scaliness of the scrotum appears as an independent complaint, attended with much heat, itching, tension, and redness. The above symptoms are succeeded by a hard, thickened, brittle texture of the skin, and by painful chaps or excoriations, which are not easily to be healed. This complaint is sometimes produced under the same circumstances as the prurigo scroti, and appears to be in some cases a sequel of it. A species of the psoriasis scrotalis likewise occurs in the lues venerea, but merits no particular attention, being always combined with other secondary symptoms of the disease.

7. *Psoriasis infantilis.* Infants between the ages of two months and two years, are occasionally subject to the dry tetter. Irregular scaly patches, of various sizes appear on the cheeks, chin, breast, back, nates, and thighs. They are sometimes red, and a little rough or elevated; sometimes excoriated, then again covered with a thin incrustation; and, lastly, intersected by chaps or fissures. The general appearances nearly coincide with those of the psoriasis diffusa: but there are several peculiarities in the tetters of infants, which require a distinct consideration.

8. The *Psoriasis inveterata* is characterized by an almost universal scaliness, with a harsh, dry, and thickened state of the skin. It commences from a few irregular, though distinct patches on the extremities. Others appear afterward on different parts, and, becoming confluent, spread at length over all the surface of the body, except a part of the face, or sometimes the palms of the hands, and soles of the feet. The skin is red, deeply furrowed, or wrinkled, stiff and rigid, so as somewhat to impede the motion of the muscles, and of the joints. So quick, likewise, is the production and separation of scales, that large quantities of them are found in the bed on which a person affected with the disease has slept. They fall off in the same proportion by day, and being confined within the linen, excite a troublesome and perpetual itching.

PSO'RICA. (From ψωρα, the itch.) Medicines to cure the itch.

PSOROPHTHA'LMIA. (From ψωρα, the itch, and οφθαλμος, an eye.) An inflammation of the eyelids, attended with ulcerations, which itch very much. By psorophthalmy, Mr. Ware means a case in which the inflammation of the eyelids is attended with an ulceration of their edges, upon which a glutinous matter lodges, and becomes hard, so that in sleep, when they have been long in contact, they become so adherent, that they cannot be separated without pain. The proximate cause is an acrimony deposited in the glands of the eyelids. The species of the psorophthalmia are,

1. *Psorophthalmia crustosa,* which forms dry or humid crusts in the margins of the eyelids.

2. *Psorophthalmia herpetica,* in which small papulæ, itching extremely, and terminating in scurf, are observed.

PSYCHAGO'GICA. (From ψυχη, the mind, and αγω, to move.) Medicines which recover in syncope or apoplexy.

PSYCHO'TROPHUM. (From ψυχος, cold: because it grows in cold places. A name altered by Linnæus from the *Psychotrophum* of Browne, which alludes to the shady place of growth of most of the species. Ψυχοτροφον is an ancient name for an herb-loving shade.) The name of a genus of plants in the Linnæan system. Class, *Pentandria;* Order, *Monogynia.*

PSYCHOTRIA EMETICA. See *Callicocca ipecacuanha.*

PSYCHO'TROPHUM. (From ψυχος, cold, and τρεφω to nourish: so called because it grows in places exposed to the cold.) The herb betony. See *Betonica officinalis.*

PSYCHROLU'TRUM. (From ψυχος, cold, and λουω, to wash.) A cold bath.

PSY'CHTICA. (From ψυχω, to refrigerate.) Refrigerating medicines.

PSYDRA'CIA. (From ψυχος, cold.) Red and somewhat elevated spots, which soon form broad and superficial vesicles, such as those produced by the stinging-nettle, the bites of insects, &c. See *Pustule.*

PSYLLI'UM. (From ψυλλος, a flea: so called because it was thought to destroy fleas.) See *Plantago psyllium.*

PTARMICA. (From πταιρω, to sneeze: so called because it irritates the nose, and provokes sneezing) Sneezewort. See *Achillæa ptarmica.*

PTE'RIS. (From πτερον, a wing: so called from the likeness of its leaves to wings.) The name of a genus of plants in the Linnæan system. Class, *Cryptogamia;* Order, *Filices.*

PTERIS AQUILINA. The systematic name of the

common brake, or female fern. *Filix fœmina.* The plant which is thus called, in the pharmacopœias, is not the *Polypodium filix fœmina,* but the *Pteris—frondibus supradecompositis, foliolis pinnatis, pinnis lanceolatis, infimis, pinnatifidis, superioribus minoribus,* of Linnæus. The root is esteemed as an anthelmintic, and is supposed to be as efficacious in destroying the tapeworm as the root of the male fern.

PTEROCA'RPUS. (From *πζερον,* a wing, and *καρπος,* fruit.) The name of a genus of plants in the Linnæan system.

PTEROCARPUS SANTALINUS. The systematic name of the red saunders-tree. *Santalum rubrum.* There is some reason to believe that several red woods, capable of communicating this colour to spirituous liquors, are sold as red saunders; but the true officinal kind appears, on the best authority, to be of this tree, which is extremely hard, of a bright garnet-red colour, and bears a fine polish. It is only the inner substance of the wood that is used as a colouring matter, and the more florid red is mostly esteemed. On being cut, it is said to manifest a fragrant odour, which is more especially observed in old trees. According to Lewis, this wood is of a dull red, almost blackish colour on the outside, and a deep brighter red within; its fibres are now and then curled, as in knots. It has no manifest smell, and little or no taste; even of extracts made from it with water, or with spirit, the taste is not considerable.

To watery liquors, it communicates only a yellowish tinge, but to rectified spirit a fine deep red. A small quantity of an extract, made with this menstruum, tinges a large one of fresh spirit of the same colour; though it does not, like most other resinous bodies, dissolve in expressed oils. Of distilled oils, there are some, as that of lavender, which receive a red tincture from the wood itself, and from its resinous extract, but the greater number do not. Red saunders has been esteemed as a medicine; but its only use attaches to its colouring property. The juice of this tree, like that of some others, affords a species of sanguis draconis.

PTERY'GIUM. (Πζερυξ, a wing.) A membraneous excrescence which grows upon the internal canthus of the eye chiefly, and expands itself over the albuginea and cornea towards the pupil. It appears to be an extension or promulgation of the fibres and vessels of the caruncula lachrymalis, or semi-lunar membrane, appearing like a wing. The species of pterygium are four:

1. *Pterygium tenue,* seu *ungula,* is a pellucid pellicle, thin, of a cineritious colour, and unpainful; growing out from the caruncula lachrymalis, or membrana semilunaris.

2. *Pterygium crassum,* seu *pannus,* differs from the ungula by its thickness, red colour, and fulness of the red vessels on the white of the eye, and it stretches over the cornea like fasciculi of vessels.

3. *Pterygium malignum,* is a pannus of various colours, painful, and arising from a cancerous acrimony.

4. *Pterygium pingue,* seu *pinguicula,* is a molecule like lard or fat, soft, without pain, and of a light yellow colour, which commonly is situated in the external angle of the eye, and rarely extends to the cornea; but often remains through life.

PTERYGO. Names compounded of this word belong to muscles which are connected with the pterygoid process of the sphenoid bone; as *pterygo-pharyngeus,* &c.

PTERYGO-PHARYNGEUS. See *Constrictor pharyngis superior.*

PTERYGO-STAPHILINUS EXTERNUS. See *Levator palati.*

PTERYGOID. (*Pterygoides;* from *πζερυξ,* a wing, and *ειδος,* resemblance.) Resembling the wing of a bird.

PTERYGOID PROCESS. A wing-like process of the sphenoid bone.

PTERYGOIDE'UM OS. See *Ethmoid bone.*

PTERYGOIDEUS EXTERNUS. (*Pterygoideus,* from its belonging to the processus pterygoides.) *Pterygoideus minor,* of Winslow. *Pterygo-colli-maxillaire,* of Dumas. *Musculus alaris externus.* A muscle placed, as it were, horizontally along the basis of the skull, between the pterygoid process and the condyle of the lower jaw. It usually arises by two distinct heads; one of which is thick, tendinous, and fleshy, from the outer wing of the pterygoid process of the os

sphenoides, and from a small part of the os maxillare adjoining to it; the other is thin and fleshy, from a ridge in the temporal process of the sphenoid bone, just behind the slit that transmits the vessels to the eye. Sometimes this latter origin is wanting, and, in that case, part of the temporal muscle arises from this ridge. Now and then it affords a common origin to both these muscles. From these origins the muscle forms a strong, fleshy belly, which descends almost transversely outwards and backwards, and is inserted, tendinous and fleshy, into a depression in the forepart of the condyloid process of the lower jaw, and into the anterior surface of the capsular ligament that surrounds the articulation of that bone. All that part of this muscle, which is not hid by the pterygoideus internus, is covered by a ligamentous expansion, which is broader than that belonging to the pterygoideus internus, and originates from the inner edge of the glenoid cavity of the lower jaw, immediately before the styloid process of the temporal bone, and extends obliquely downwards, forwards, and outwards, to the inner surface of the angle of the jaw. When these muscles act together, they bring the jaw horizontally forwards. When they act singly, the jaw is moved forwards, and to the opposite side. The fibres that are inserted into the capsular ligament, serve likewise to bring the moveable cartilage forwards.

PTERYGOIDEUS INTERNUS. *Pterygoideus major,* of Winslow. *Pterygo-anguli-maxillaire,* of Dumas. This muscle arises tendinous and fleshy from the whole inner surface of the external ala of the pterygoid process, filling all the space between the two wings; and from that process of the os palati that makes part of the pterygoid fossa. From thence, growing larger, it descends obliquely downwards, forwards, and outwards, and is inserted, by tendinous and fleshy fibres, into the inside of the lower jaw, near its angle. This muscle covers a great part of the *pterygoideus externus;* and along its posterior edge we observe a ligamentous band, which extends from the back part of the styloid process to the bottom of the angle of the lower jaw. The use of this muscle is to raise the lower jaw, and to pull it a little to one side.

PTERYGOIDEUS MAJOR. See *Pterygoideus internus.*

PTERYGOIDEUS MINOR. See *Pterygoideus externus.*

PTILO'SIS. (From *πζιλος,* bald.) See *Madarosis.*

PTI'SANA. (From *πτισσω,* to decorticate, bruise, or pound.) *Ptissana.* 1. Barley deprived of its husks, pounded, and made into balls.

2. A drink is so called by the French, made mostly of farinaceous substances; as barley, rice, grits, and the like, boiled with water, and sweetened to the palate.

PTO'SIS. (From *πιπζω,* to fall.) *Blepharoptosis* An inability of raising the upper eyelid. The affection may be owing to several causes, the chief of which are a redundance of the skin on the eyelid; *a* paralytic state of the levator muscle, and a spasm of the orbicularis.

PTOSIS IRIDIS. *Prolapsus iridis.* A prolapsus of the iris through a wound of the cornea. It is known by a blackish tubercle, which projects a little from the cornea in various forms. The species of the ptosis of the iris are,

1. *Ptosis recens,* or a recent ptosis from a side wound of the cornea, as that which happens, though rarely, in or after the extraction of the cataract.

2. *Ptosis inveterata,* in which the incarcerated prolapsed iris is grown or attached to the wound or ulcer, and has become callous or indurated.

PTYALAGO'GUE. (From *πζυαλον,* spittle, and *αγω,* to excite.) Medicines which promote a discharge of the saliva, or cause salivation.

PTYALI'SMOS. See *Ptyalismus.*

PTYALI'SMUS. (From *πζυαλιζω,* to spit.) A ptyalism or salivation, or increased secretion of saliva from the mouth.

PTY'ALUM. (From *πζυω,* to spit up.) The saliva or mucus from the bronchia.

PTYASMAGO'GA. (From *πζυασμα,* sputum, and *αγω,* to expel.) Medicines which promote the secretion of saliva.

PU'BES. 1. The external part of the organs of generation of both sexes, which after puberty is covered with hair.

2 The down or pubescence on leaves, seeds, &c of some plants.

PUBES SEMINIS. See *Pappus.*

PUBESCENCE. *Pubescentia.* Under this term is included all kinds of down, hairs, and bristle-like bodies found on the surface of the leaves, stems, pods, &c. of plants. They differ considerably in form and texture, but consist of small, slender bodies, which are either soft and yielding to the slightest impression, or rigid and comparatively unyielding: the former are, properly speaking, *pili,* or hairs; the latter bristles, *setæ;* and, therefore, under these two heads every kind of pubescence may be arranged. See *Pilus* and *Seta.*

PUBESCENS. Pubescent: applied to the stigma of the genus *Vicia.*

PUBIS OS. A separate bone of the fœtal pelvis. See *Innominatum os.*

PUDE'NDUM. (From *pudor,* shame.) The parts of generation.

PUDENDA'GRA. (From *pudenda,* the private parts, and αγρα, a seizure.) *Cedma.* The venereal disease has been so named by some. A pain in the private parts.

PUDENDUM MULIEBRE. The female parts of generation.

PUDI'CAL. (*Pudicus;* from *pudor,* shame.) Belonging to the *pudenda.*

PUDICAL ARTERY. *Arteria pudica.* Pudendal artery. A branch of the internal iliac distributed on the organs of generation.

PUERI'LIS MORBUS. The epilepsy.

PUERPERAL. *Puerperalis.* Appertaining to child-bearing; as puerperal convulsions, fever, &c.

PUFFBALL. See *Lycoperdon.*

PUGI'LLUS. (From *pugnus,* the fist.) *Dragmis.* A pugil, or handful.

PULE'GIUM. (From *pulex,* a flea; because the smell of its leaves, burned, destroys fleas.) See *Mentha pulegium.*

PULEGIUM CERVINUM. Hart's pennyroyal. The *Mentha cervina,* of Linnæus.

PULICA'RIA. (From *pulex,* a flea: so named because it was thought to destroy fleas if hung in a chamber.) See *Plantago psyllium.*

PU'LMO. (*Pulmo, onis* m. Plin. πνευμων. Attice πλευμων, *unde, per metathesin pulmo.*) The lung. See *Lung.*

PULMONA'RIA. (From *pulmo,* the lung; so called because of its virtues in affections of the lungs.) The name of a genus of plants in the Linnæan system. Class, *Pentandria;* Order, *Monogynia.* Lungwort.

PULMONARIA ARBOREA. See *Lichen pulmonarius.*

PULMONARIA MACULATA. See *Pulmonaria officinalis.*

PULMONARIA OFFICINALIS. The systematic name of the spotted lungwort. *Pulmonaria maculata; Symphitum maculosum.* Jerusalem cowslips; Jerusalem sage. This plant is rarely found to grow wild in England; but is very commonly cultivated in gardens, where its leaves become broader, and approach more to a cordate shape. The leaves, which are the part medicinally used, have no peculiar smell; but, in their recent state, manifest a slightly astringent and mucilaginous taste: hence it seems not wholly without foundation that they have been supposed to be demulcent and pectoral. They have been recommended in hæmoptoes, tickling coughs, and catarrhal defluxions upon the lungs. The name pulmonaria, however, seems to have arisen rather from the speckled appearance of these leaves resembling that of the lungs, than from any intrinsic quality which experience discovered to be useful in pulmonary complaints.

PULMONARY. *Pulmonaris.* Belonging to the lungs.

PULMONARY ARTERY. The pulmonary artery, *arteria pulmonalis,* arises from the right ventricle of the heart, and soon divides into the right and left, which ramify throughout the lungs, and form a beautiful network on the air vesicles, where they terminate in the veins, *venæ pulmonales,* whose branches at length form four trunks, which empty themselves into the left auricle of the heart.

Pulmonary consumption. See *Phthisis.*

PULMONARY VEIN. See *Pulmonary artery.*

PULMO'NICA. (From *pulmo,* the lungs.) Medicines for the lungs.

PULMONI'TIS. (From *pulmo,* the lungs.) An inflammation of the lungs.

PULSATI'LLA NIGRICANS. (From *pulso,* to beat about: so called from its being perpetually agitated by the air.) See *Anemone pratensis.*

PULSE. *Pulsus.* The beating of the heart and arteries. The pulse is generally felt at the wrist, by pressing the radial artery with the fingers. The action depends upon the impulse given to the blood by the heart; hence physicians feel the pulse, to ascertain the quickness or tardiness of the blood's motion, the strength of the heart, &c. See *Circulation.*

PULSILE'GIUM. (From *pulsus,* the pulse, and *lego,* to tell.) An instrument for measuring the pulse

PULVI'NAR. (From *pulvis,* dust or chaff, with which they are filled.) A medicated cushion.

PULVINA'RIUM. See *Pulvinar.*

PU'LVIS. (*Pulvis, veris.* m.) A powder. *Pulvinarium.* This form of medicine is either coarse or very fine, simple or compound. In the compounded powders, the intimate and complete admixture of the several ingredients, and more especially in those to which any of the more active substances, as opium, scammony, &c. are added, cannot be too strongly recommended, and for this purpose it may be proper to pass them, after they are mixed mechanically, through a fine sieve.

PULVIS ALOES COMPOSITUS. Compound powder of aloes. Formerly called *pulvis aloes cum guaiaco.* Take of extract of spiked aloe, an ounce and a half; guaiacum resin, an ounce; compound powder of cinnamon, half an ounce. Powder the extract of aloe and guaiacum resin separately; then mix them with the compound powder of cinnamon. The dose is from gr. x. to Эj. It is a warm, aperient, laxative powder, calculated for the aged, and those affected with dyspeptic gout attended with costiveness and spasmodic complaints of the stomach and bowels.

PULVIS ALOES CUM CANELLA. A cathartic, deobstruent powder, possessing stimulating and aloëtic properties omitted in the last London Pharmacopœia, as rather suited to the purpose of extemporaneous prescription.

PULVIS ALOES CUM FERRO. This possesses aperient and deobstruent virtues; and is mostly given in chlorosis and constipation. In the London Pharmacopœia this prescription is omitted for the same reason as pulvis aloes cum canella.

PULVIS ALOES CUM GUAIACO. See *Pulvis aloes compositus.*

PULVIS ANTIMONIALIS. See *Antimonialis pulvis.*

PULVIS AROMATICUS. See *Pulvis cinnamomi compositus.*

PULVIS CERUSSÆ COMPOSITUS. This is mostly used in the form of collyrium, lotion, or injection, as a mucilaginous sedative.

PULVIS CHELARUM CANCRI COMPOSITUS. An antacid and adstringent powder, mostly given to children with diarrhœa and acidity of the primæ viæ.

PULVIS CINNAMOMI COMPOSITUS. Compound powder of cinnamon. Formerly called *pulvis aromaticus: species aromatica: species diambræ sine odoratis.* Take of common cinnamon bark, two ounces; cardamom-seeds, an ounce and a half; ginger-root, an ounce; long pepper, half an ounce. Rub them together, so as to make a very fine powder. The dose is from five to ten grains. An elegant stimulant, carminative, and stomachic powder.

PULVIS COBBII. *Pulvis tunguinensis.* This once celebrated powder consists of sixteen grains of musk, and forty-eight grains of cinnabar. It is directed to be mixed in a gill of arrack.

PULVIS CONTRAJERVÆ COMPOSITUS. Take of contrajerva root powdered, five ounces; prepared shells, a pound and a half. Mix. A febrifuge diaphoretic, mostly given in the dose of from one to two scruples in slight febrile affections.

PULVIS CORNU USTI CUM OPIO. Powder of burnt hartshorn with opium. *Pulvis opiatus.* Take of hard opium, powdered, a drachm; hartshorn, burned and prepared, an ounce: cochineal, powdered, a drachm. Mix. This preparation affords a convenient mode of exhibiting small quantities of opium, ten grains containing one of the opium. It is absorbent and anodyne.

PULVIS CRETÆ COMPOSITUS. Compound powder of chalk. *Pulvis e bolo compositus spine opio. Species e scordio sine opio. Diascordium,* 1720. Take of prepared chalk, half a pound; cinnamon bark, four ounces: tormentil root, acacia gum, of each three ounces: long pepper, half an ounce. Reduce them separately into a very fine powder and then mix. The dose is from 3 ss. to 3 i. An astringent, carminative, and stomachic powder, exhibited in the cure of diarrhœa, pyrosis, and diseases arising from acidity of the bowels, inducing much pain.

PULVIS CRETÆ COMPOSITUS CUM OPIO. Compound powder of chalk with opium. *Pulvis e bolo compositus cum opio. Species e cordio cum opio.* Take of compound powder of chalk, six ounces and a half. Hard opium, powdered, four scruples. Mix. The dose from one scruple to two. The above powder, with the addition of opium, in the proportion of one grain to two scruples.

PULVIS IPECACUANHÆ COMPOSITUS. Compound powder of ipecacuanha. Take of ipecacuanha root, powdered, hard opium powder, of each a drachm; sulphate of potassa, powdered, an ounce. Mix. A diaphoretic powder, similar to that of Dr. Dover, which gained such repute in the cure of rheumatisms, and other diseases arising from obstructed perspiration and spasm. The dose is from five grains to a scruple.

PULVIS KINO COMPOSITUS. Compound powder of kino. Take of kino 15 drachms; cinnamon bark, half an ounce; hard opium, a drachm. Reduce them separately to a very fine powder; and then mix. The proportion of opium this astringent contains is one part to twenty. The dose is from five grains to a scruple.

PULVIS MYRRHÆ COMPOSITUS. A stimulant, antispasmodic, and emmenagogue powder, mostly exhibited in the dose of from fifteen grains to two scruples, in uterine obstructions and hysterical affections.

PULVIS OPIATUS. See *Pulvis cornu usti cum opio.*

PULVIS SCAMMONEÆ COMPOSITUS. Compound powder of scammony. *Pulvis comitis Warwicensis.* Take of scammony gum resin, hard extract of jalap, of each two ounces; ginger-root, half an ounce. Reduce them separately to a very fine powder, and then mix. From ten to fifteen grains or a scruple are exhibited as a stimulating cathartic.

PULVIS SCAMMONII CUM ALOE A stimulating cathartic, in the dose of from ten to fifteen grains.

PULVIS SCAMMONII CUM CALOMELANE. A vermifugal cathartic, in the dose of from ten to fifteen grains.

PULVIS SENNÆ COMPOSITUS. Compound powder of senna. *Pulvis diasennæ.* Take of senna leaves, supertartrate of potassa, of each two ounces; scammony gum resin, half an ounce; ginger-root, two drachms. Reduce the scammony gum resin separately, the rest together, to a very fine powder; and then mix. The dose is from one scruple to one drachm. A saline stimulating cathartic.

PULVIS TRAGACANTHÆ COMPOSITUS. Compound powder of tragacanth. *Species diatragacanthæ frigida.* Take of tragacanth powdered, acacia gum powdered, starch, of each an ounce and a half, refined sugar three ounces. Powder the starch and sugar together; then add the tragacanth and acacia gum, and mix the whole. Tragacanth is very difficultly reduced to powder. The dose is from ten grains to a drachm. A very useful demulcent powder, which may be given in coughs, diarrhœas, strangury, &c.

[PULVIS PARTURIENS. In a letter from Dr. John Stearns, of Saratoga county, to Dr. S. Akerly, dated Waterford, January 25th, 1807, is the following narration:—

"In compliance with your request, I hereby transmit you a sample of the *pulvis parturiens*, which I have been in the habit of using for several years with the most complete success. It expedites lingering parturition, and saves to the accoucheur a considerable portion of time, without producing any bad effects on the patient. The cases in which I have generally found this powder to be useful, are when the pains are lingering, have wholly subsided, or are in any way incompetent to exclude the fœtus. Previous to its exhibition, it is of the utmost consequence to ascertain the presentation, and whether any preternatural obstruction prevents the delivery: as the violent and almost incessant action which it induces in the uterus precludes the possibility of *turning.* The pains produced by it are peculiarly *forcing*, though not accompanied with that distress and agony of which the patients frequently complain when the action is much less. My method of administering it is either in decoction or

powder. Boil half a drachm of the powder in half a pint of water, and give one-third every twenty minutes, till the pains commence. In powder, I give from five to ten grains; some patients require larger doses, though I have generally found these sufficient.

"If the dose is large, it will produce nausea and vomiting. In most cases, you will be surprised with the suddenness of its operation; it is, therefore, necessary to be completely ready before you give the medicine, as the urgency of the pains will allow you but a short time afterward. Since I have adopted the use of this powder, I have seldom found a case that detained me more than three hours. Other physicians, who have administered it, concur with me in the success of its operation.

"The *modus operandi* I feel incompetent to explain. At the same time that it augments the action of the uterus, it appears to relax the rigidity of the muscular fibres. May it not produce the beneficial effects of bleeding, without inducing that extreme debility which is always consequent upon copious depletion? This appears to be corroborated by its nauseating effects on the stomach, and the known sympathy between this viscus and the uterus.

"It is a vegetable, and appears to be a spurious growth of rye. On examining a granary, where rye is stored, you will be able to procure a sufficient quantity from among that grain. Rye, which grows in low, wet ground, yields it in greatest abundance."—*New-York Med. Repos.*

This substance, which Dr. Stearns called *pulvis parturiens,* (more correctly pulvis ad parturandum) is the ergot, or spurred rye, or the secale cornutum. The above notice, from the Med. Rep., was the first publication in the United States, in relation to the use of spurred rye in cases of parturition. Since then, to the present time (1829), many trials have been made, and many cases reported of its efficacy in difficult labours. Some physicians have condemned its use, as often proving fatal to the life of the child in delivery. Dr. Bigelow, of Boston, however, has introduced it into his Materia Medica, and given the following account of its use.

"Various species of grain and grasses are subject to a morbid excrescence on some part of the ear or spike, to which the French name *ergot* has been applied. Rye is more frequently affected with this appendage than any other grain. Different conjectures have been offered relative to the nature of this excrescence, the most probable of which is that of Decandolle, who considers the ergot to be a parasitic vegetable, of the tribe of *fungi,* and genus *sclerotium.*

"Ergot resembles a grain of rye, elongated to several times the common length, of an irregular form, and a dark colour. It has a light and brittle texture, and an unpleasant taste. According to Vauquelin, it contains a pale-yellow colouring matter; an oily matter; a violet colouring matter; an acid, probably phosphoric ; and a vegeto-animal matter.

"This substance was formerly suspected of producing certain epidemic diseases—the dry gangrene, and raphania, but the suspicion was probably unfounded. In regard to its immediate effect on the system, the reports of medical authors differ widely, some considering it highly deleterious. From my own observations, I have found that it produces nausea and vomiting, in doses of from a scruple to a drachm ; that it seldom operates upon the bowels; and that large doses produce headache and temporary febrile symptoms. It has very little acrimony, and does not prove sternutatory when snuffed up the nostrils.

"Besides these more general effects, ergot has a specific power of stimulating the uterus during the process of parturition, in a manner that is not known to be produced by any other medicinal agent. This effect is wholly unequivocal, and cannot be confounded with the common uterine efforts. It is moreover certain, or at least its failures are not more frequent than those of any of our most common operative drugs. This operation consists in a powerful, incessant, and unremitting contraction of the uterus, not alternating with intervals of ease, as in common labour, but continuing without intermission until the child is expelled. When ergot is prematurely or injudiciously administered, the child does not breathe at birth, is difficult to resuscitate, and is sometimes irrecoverably dead. This effect has been attributed to a poisonous quality in the ergot, but is obviously the consequence, simply, of long-con tinued and unremitting pressure on the child, a fact pointed out in the New-England Journal, as early as 1812.

"A few medical writers, principally in Europe, in consequence, probably, of not being furnished with a genuine article, in an unimpaired state, have doubted the power of ergot to effect or alter the action of the uterus. But I may safely assert, that, after fifteen years, during which this drug has attracted notice among us, there is scarcely an article of the materia medica, upon the character of which the minds of the profession in this country are more fully made up, than upon this. Indeed our medical journals, and books of materia medica, have teemed with evidences of its activity.

"For obvious reasons, ergot should never be given in natural and favourable cases of labour. It is strongly contraindicated, at all times, by earliness of the stage, rigidity of the soft parts, any unfavourable conformation, or any presentation which requires changing. It is admissible in lingering cases of children ascertained to be dead, and in lingering cases of abortion. It is useful in retained placenta; and, from its power of causing contraction of the uterus, it arrests flooding after delivery. In females habitually subject to profuse hæmorrhage at this period, there is perhaps no better preventive than a full dose of ergot, administered just before delivery. Its efficacy has been repeatedly attested.

"Spurred rye has been administered as an emmenagogue with various success. Its action on the impregnated uterus is much less than it displays in labour; yet the result of many trials has been, on the whole, in favour of its emmenagogue power.

"Ergot is commonly given in powder, boiled or infused in hot water. A drachm may be prepared in this way for a puerperal patient, and one quarter of the mixture, while turbid, given every twenty minutes, till its effect becomes perceptible. In amenorrhœa, ten or fifteen grains may be given, three times a day, and increased if nausea does not ensue."—*Bigelow's Materia Medica.* A.]

PUMICE. A mineral of which there are three species, the glossy, common, and porphyritic, found in the Lipari islands and Hungary.

PUMPION. See *Cucurbita.*

PUNCTATUS. Dotted. Applied to petals of the Melanthium capense: receptacle of the Leontodon taraxacum.

PU'NCTUM. A point. The opening or commencement of a duct of the eye has received this name, because its projection gives it the appearance of a spot.

PUNCTUM AUREUM. Formerly, when a hernia of the intestines was reduced by an incision made through the skin and membrana adiposa, quite down to the upper part of the spermatic vessels, a golden wire was fixed and twisted, so as to prevent the descent of any thing down the tunica vaginalis.

PUNCTUM LACHRIMALE. Lachrymal point. Two small orifices, one of which is conspicuous in each eyelid, at the extremity of the tarsus, near the internal canthus, are called puncta lachrymalia.

PU'NICA. The name of a genus of plants in the Linnæan system. Class, *Icosandria;* Order, *Monogynia.*

PUNICA GRANATUM. The systematic name of the pomegranate. *Granatum. Punica—foliis lanceolatis, caule arboreo,* of Linnæus. The rind of the fruit and the flowers called *Balaustine flowers,* are the parts directed for medicinal use. In their smell there is nothing remarkable, but to the taste they are very astringent, and have successfully been employed as such, in diseases both internal and external.

PUPIL. (*Pupilla;* from *pupa,* a babe: because it reflects the diminished image of the person who looks upon it like a puppet.) The round opening in the middle of the iris, in which we see ourselves in the eye of another.

PUPI'LLA. See *Pupil.*

PUPILLA'RIS. Of or belonging to the pupil.

PUPILLARIS MEMBRANA. (From *pupilla,* the pupil.) See *Membrana pupillaris.*

PUPILLÆ VELUM. See *Membrana pupillaris.*

PURGAME'NTUM. A purge.

PURGATIVE. Whatever increases the peristaltic motion of the bowels, so as to considerably increase the alvine evacuations. See *Cathartic.*

Purging flax. See *Linum catharticum*

Purging-nut. See *Jatropha curcas.*

PURIFORM. (*Puriformis;* from *pus,* and *forma* resemblance.) Like unto the secretion called pus.

PURPURA. (Πορφύρα, the name of a shell of a purple colour: hence purpura, a purple colour.) An efflorescence consisting of small, distinct, purple specks and patches, attended with general debility, but not always with fever, which are caused by an extravasation of the vessels under the cuticle. It is divided into the five following species:

1. *Purpura simplex.* This has the appearance of petechiæ, without much disorder of the constitution, except languor, pain in the limbs, and a sallow complexion. The petechiæ are most numerous on the breast, inside of the arms and legs, and are of various sizes, and commonly circular. There is no itching or other sensation attending the petechiæ.

2. *Purpura hæmorrhagica* is considerably more severe; the petechiæ are of larger size, and interspersed with vibices and ecchymoses, resembling the marks left by the strokes of a whip, or by violent bruises. They appear first on the legs, afterward on the thighs, arms, and trunk of the body; the hands being more rarely spotted with them, and the face generally free. They are of a bright red colour when they first appear, but soon become purple or livid; and when about to disappear they change to a brown or yellowish hue; the cuticle over them appears smooth and shining, but is not sensibly elevated; in a few cases, however, it has been seen raised into a sort of vesicle, containing black blood. This more particularly happens in the spots which appear on the tongue, gums, and palate, and inside of the cheeks and lips where the cuticle is extremely thin; the gentlest pressure on the skin, even feeling of the pulse, will often produce a purple blotch, like that which is left after a severe bruise.

The same state of habit, which gives rise to these effusions under the cuticle, produces likewise copious discharges of blood, especially from the internal parts; they are often very profuse, and suddenly prove fatal; but in other cases they are less copious: sometimes returning every day at stated periods, and sometimes less frequent, and at regular intervals; and sometimes there is a slow and almost incessant oozing of blood. The bleeding occurs from the gums, nostrils, throat, inside of the cheeks, tongue, and lips, and sometimes from the lining membrane of the eyelids, the urethra, and external ear; and also from the internal cavities of the lungs, stomach, bowels, uterus, kidneys, and bladder.

This disease is often preceded by great lassitude, faintness, and pains in the limbs; but not unfrequently it appears suddenly in the midst of apparent good health. It is always accompanied with extreme debility and depression of spirits; the pulse is commonly feeble, and sometimes quickened; and heat, flushing, perspiration, and other symptoms of febrile irritation, occasionally attend. When the disease has continued for some time, the patient becomes sallow, and much emaciated; and some degree of œdema appears on the lower extremities, which afterward extends to other parts of the body. This disease is extremely uncertain in its duration; in some instances it has terminated in a few days, while in others it has continued, not only for many months, but even for years.

The causes of this disease are by no means clearly ascertained: it occurs at every period of life, and in both sexes, but especially in women and in boys before the age of puberty, particularly those who are employed in sedentary occupations, and who live in close and crowded situations. It has sometimes occurred as a sequela, of small-pox, and of measles, and sometimes in the third or fourth week of puerperal confinement. It is supposed that some local visceral obstruction is the cause of the disease in different instances, as artificial bleeding, and purging, tend greatly to relieve it. The ancient physicians attributed the hæmorrhagies from the nose, gums, and other parts, to the morbid enlargement of the spleen.

In the slighter degrees of purpura occurring in children who are ill fed and nursed, and who reside in close places, or in women shut up in similar situations, and debilitated by anxiety of mind, want of proper food, and fatigue, the use of tonics, with the mineral acids, and wine, will doubtless be adequate to the cure of the disease, especially where exercise in the open air can be employed at the same time. But when it occurs in adults, especially those who already have the benefit of exercise in the air of the country, and who have suffered no privation with respect to diet, when it is accompanied with a white and loaded tongue, a quick and somewhat small though sharp pulse, occasional chills and heats, and other symptoms of feverishness, however moderate, and if there be at the same time fixed internal pains, a dry cough, and an irregular state of the bowels (symptoms which may be presumed to indicate some local congestion); then the administration of tonic medicines, particularly wine, cinchona, and other warmer tonics will be found inefficacious, if not decidedly injurious. In such cases, free and repeated doses of medicines containing the submuriate of mercury, and regulated by their effects on the symptoms of the complaint, and by the appearance of the excretions, from the intestines, will be found most beneficial.

If the pains are fixed, the marks of febrile irritation considerable, and the spontaneous hæmorrhage not profuse, local or general blood-letting may be employed with great benefit, especially in robust adults. When the urgency of hæmorrhagic tendency has been diminished by these means, the constitution rallies, though not rapidly, with the assistance of the mineral acids, and cinchona or cascarilla, or some preparation of iron, together with moderate exercise and nutritious diet.

3. *Purpura urticans* is distinguished by commencing in the form of rounded and reddish elevations of the cuticle, resembling wheals, which are not accompanied like the wheals of urticaria by any sensation of tingling and itching. These tumours gradually dilate, but within one or two days they subside to a level of the surrounding cuticle, and their hue becomes darker, and at length livid. They are most common on the legs where they appear with petechiæ, but also appear on the arms, thighs, breast, &c.

It usually occurs in summer and autumn, and lasts from three to five weeks. Some œdema of the extremities usually accompanies it, and it is occasionally preceded by a stiffness and weight of the limbs. The same rules of treatment apply to this as to the preceding varieties of the disease.

4. *Purpura senilis* appears principally along the outside of the forearm, in elderly women, in successive dark purple blotches, of an irregular form, and various magnitude; each of these continues from a week to ten days, when the extravasated blood is absorbed.

Tonics or any other expedient do not appear to exert any influence over the eruption.

5. *Purpura contagiosa*, is an eruption of petechia which occasionally accompanies typhoid fevers; where they occur in close situations, they are merely symptomatic, and are very rarely seen.

PURPURA ALBA. *Purpura rubra.* Many writers term the miliary fever, when the pustules are white, purpura alba; and when they are red, purpura rubra.

PURPURA SCORBUTICA. Petechial eruptions in scurvy.

PURPURIC ACID. *Acidum purpuricum:* so called from its fine red colour. The excrements of the serpent, *Boa constrictor*, consist of pure lithic acid. Dr. Prout found that on digesting this substance thus obtained, or from urinary calculi, in dilute nitric acid, an effervescence takes place, and the lithic acid is dissolved, forming a beautiful purple liquid. The excess of nitric acid being neutralized with ammonia, and the whole concentrated by slow evaporation, the colour of the solution becomes of a deeper purple; and dark red granular crystals, sometimes of a greenish hue externally, soon begin to separate in abundance. These crystals are a compound of ammonia with the acid principle in question. The ammonia was displaced by digesting the salt in a solution of caustic potassa, till the red colour entirely disappeared. This alkaline solution was then gradually dropped into dilute sulphuric acid, which, uniting with the potassa, left the acid principle in a state of purity.

This acid principle is likewise produced from lithic acid by chlorine, and also, but with more difficulty, by iodine. Dr. Prout, the discoverer of this new acid, has, at the suggestion of Dr. Wollaston, called it purpuric acid, because its saline compounds have for the most part a red or purple colour.

This acid, as obtained by the preceding process, usually exists in the form of a very fine powder, of a slightly yellowish or cream colour; and when examined

222

with a magnifier, especially under water, appears to possess a pearly lustre. It has no smell, nor taste. Its spec. grav. is considerably above water. It is scarcely soluble in water. One-tenth of a grain, boiled for a considerable time in 1000 grains of water was not entirely dissolved. The water, however, assumed a purple tint, probably, Dr. Prout thinks, from the formation of a little purpurate of ammonia. Purpuric acid is insoluble in alkohol and æther. The mineral acids dissolve it only when they are concentrated.

PURSLANE. See *Portulaca.*

PURULENT. (*Purulens*, from *pus*.) Having the appearance of pus.

PUS. Matter. A whitish, bland, creamlike fluid, heavier than water, found in phlegmonous abscesses, or on the surface of sores. It is distinguished, according to its nature, into laudable or good pus, scrofulous, serous, and ichorous pus, &c.

Pus taken from a healthy ulcer, near the source of circulation, as on the arm or breast, Sir Everard Home observes, readily separates from the surface of the sore, the granulations underneath being small, pointed, and of a florid red colour, and has the following properties: it is nearly of the consistence of cream; is of a white colour; has a mawkish taste; and, when cold, is inodorous; but, when warm, has a peculiar smell. Examined in a microscope, it is found to consist of two parts, of globules, and a transparent colourless fluid; the globules are probably white, at least they appear to have some degree of opacity. Its specific gravity is greater than that of water. It does not readily go into putrefaction. Exposed to heat, it evaporates to dryness; but does not coagulate. It does not unite with water in the heat of the atmosphere, but falls to the bottom; yet, if kept in a considerable degree of heat, it rises and diffuses itself through the water, and remains mixed with it, even after having been allowed to cool, the globules being decomposed.

Pus varies in its appearance, according to the different circumstances which affect the ulcer that forms it; such as, the degree of violence of the inflammation, also its nature, whether healthy or unhealthy; and these depend upon the state of health, and strength of the parts yielding pus. These changes arise more from indolence and irritability, than from any absolute disease; many specific diseases, in healthy constitutions, producing no change in the appearance of the matter from their specific quality. Thus, the matter from a gonorrhœa, from the small-pox pustules, or the chicken-pock, has the same appearance, and seems to be made up of similar parts, consisting of globules floating in a transparent fluid, like common pus; the specific properties of each of these poisons being superadded to those of pus. Matter from a cancer may be considered as an exception; but a cancerous ulcer is never in a healthy state.

In indolent ulcers, whether the indolence arise from the nature of the parts, or the nature of the inflammation, the pus is made of globules and flaky particles, floating in a transparent fluid; and globules and flakes are in different proportions, according to the degree of indolence: this is particularly observable in scrofulous abscesses, preceded by a small degree of inflammation. That this flaky appearance is no part of true pus, is well illustrated by observing, that the proportion it bears to the globules is greater where there is the least inflammation; and in those abscesses that sometimes occur, which have not been preceded by any inflammation at all, the contents are wholly made up of a curdy or flaky substance of different degrees of consistence, which is not considered to be pus, from its not having the properties stated in the definition of that fluid.

The constitution and part must be in health to form good pus; for very slight changes in the general health are capable of producing an alteration in it, and even of preventing its being formed at all, and substituting in its place coagulating lymph.

This happens most readily in ulcers in the lower extremities, owing to their distance from the source of the circulation rendering them weaker. And it is curious to observe the influence that distance alone has upon the appearance of pus.

Pus differs from chyle in its globules being larger, not coagulating by exposure to the air, nor by heat, which those of chyle do.

The pancreatic juice contains globules, but they are much smaller than those of pus.

Milk is composed of globules, nearly of the same size as those of pus, but much more numerous. Milk coagulates by runnet, which pus does not; and contains oil and sugar, which are not to be discovered in pus.

The cases in which pus is formed, are, properly speaking, all reducible to one, which is, the state of parts consequent to inflammation. For as far as we yet know, observes Sir E. Home, pus has in no instance been met with, unless preceded by inflammation; and although, in some cases, a fluid has been formed independent of preceding inflammation, it differs from pus in many of its properties.

In considering the time required for the formation of pus, it is necessary to take notice of the periods which are found, under different circumstances, to intervene between a healthy or natural state of the parts, and the presence of that fluid after the application of some irritating substance to the skin.

In cases of wounds made into muscular parts, where blood-vessels are divided, the first process which takes place is the extravasation of red blood; the second is the exudation of coagulating lymph, which afterward becomes vascular; and the third, the formation of matter, which last does not, in common, take place in less than two days; the precise time will, however, vary exceedingly, according to the nature of the constitution, and the state of the parts at the time.

If an irritating substance is applied to a cuticular surface, upon which it raises a blister, pus will be formed in about twenty-four hours.

PUSTULA. A little pustule. See *Pustule.*

PUSTULA ORIS. See *Aphthæ.*

PUSTULE. (*Pustula,* a little pustule; from *pus,* matter.) *Ecthyma; Eczema.* Dr. Willan defines a pustule to be an elevation of the cuticle, sometimes globate, sometimes conoidal in its form, and containing pus, or a lymph which is in general discoloured. Pustules are various in their size, but the diameter of the largest seldom exceeds two lines. There are many different kinds of pustules, properly distinguished in medical authors by specific appellations; as, 1. *Phlyzacium,* a small pustule containing pus, and raised on a hard, circular inflamed base, of a vivid red colour. It is succeeded by a thick, hard, dark-coloured scab. 2. *Psydracium,* according to Dr. Willan, a minute pustule, irregularly circumscribed, producing but a slight elevation of the cuticle, and terminating in a laminated scab. Many of these pustules usually appear together, and become confluent. When mature, they contain pus; and, after breaking, discharge a thin watery humour.

PUTA'MEN. (From *puto,* to cut.) The bark or paring of any vegetable, as the walnut. See *Juglans regia.*

PUTAMINEÆ. The name of an order in Linnæus's *Fragments of a Natural Method,* embracing those which have an outer shell, or putamen, over a hard fruit; as in Capparis and Merisoma.

PUTREFACTION. (*Putrefactio; from putrefacio,* to become rotten, to dissolve.) Putrid fermentation. Putrefactive fermentation. The spontaneous decomposition of such animal and vegetable matters as exhale a fœtid smell. The solid and the fluid matters are resolved into gaseous compounds and vapours, which escape and unite an earthy residuum. The requisites to this process are, 1. A certain degree of humidity. 2. The access of atmospheric air. 3. A certain degree of heat: hence the abstraction of the air and water, or humidity, by drying, or its fixation by cold, by salt, sugar, spices, &c., will counteract the process of putrefaction, and favour the preservation of food, on which principle some patents have been obtained. See *Fermentation.*

[" PUZZOLANA. This usually occurs in small fragments, or friable masses, which have a dull, earthy aspect and fracture, and seem to have been baked. Its solidity does not exceed that of chalk. It is seldom tumefied; and its pores are neither so large nor numerous as those of scoria. Its colours are gray, or whitish, reddish, or nearly black.

" By exposure to heat, it loses its power of affecting the needle, and melts into a black slag. A variety, examined by Bergman, yielded silex, 55 to 60; alumine, 19 to 20; iron, 15 to 20; lime, 5 to 6. It often contains distinct articles of pumice, quartz, and scoria.

"Some mineralogists suppose the black puzzolana to be altered scoria; the white to be pumice, and has proceeded from argillaceous minerals, baked or calcined in the interior of the volcano.

" But, whatever may have been its origin, it is ex tremely useful in the preparation of a *mortar,* which *hardens* quickly, even *under water.* When thus employed, it is mixed with a small proportion of lime, perhaps one-third. Mr. Kirwan supposes, that the rapid induration of this mortar arises from the very low oxidation of the iron. If the mortar be a long time exposed to the air, previous to its use, it will not harden.

" The best puzzolana is said to occur in old currents of lava; but, when too earthy, it loses its peculiar properties. That which comes from Naples is generally gray."—*Cleav. Min.* A.]

Putrid Fever. See *Typhus gravior.*

PYLORIC. (*Pyloricus; from pylorus.*) Belonging to the pylorus.

PYLORIC ARTERY. *Arteria pylorica.* A branch of the hepatic artery.

PYLO'RUS. (From πυλη, an entrance, and ουρος, a guard; because it guards, as it were, the entrance of the bowels.) *Janitor; Portorarium; Ostiarius.* The inferior aperture of the stomach, which opens into the intestines.

PYOPOE'TIC. (From πυον, pus, and ποιεω, to make.) Suppurative.

PYORRHŒ'A. (From πυον, pus, and ρεω, to flow.) A purulent discharge from the belly.

PYOTU'RIA. (From πυον, pus, and ουρον, urine.' *Pyuria.* A mucous or purulent urine.

PYRAMIDA'LIS. (From πυραμις, a pyramid.) A muscle in the front of the belly. Fallopius, who is considered as the first accurate describer of this muscle, gave it the name of *pyramidalis,* from its shape: hence it is called *pyramidalis Fallopii,* by Douglas. But Vesalius seems to have been acquainted with it, and to have described it as a part of the rectus. It is called *pyramidalis vel succenturiatus,* by Cowper; and *pubio-ombilical,* by Dumas. It is a very small muscle, situated at the bottom of the forepart of the rectus, and is covered by the same aponeurosis that forms the anterior part of the sheath of that muscle. It arises by short, tendinous fibres, from the upper and forepart of the os pubis. From this origin, which is seldom more than an inch in breadth, its fibres ascend somewhat obliquely, to be inserted into the linea alba, and inner edge of the rectus, commonly at about the distance of two inches from the pubes, and frequently at a greater or less distance, but always below the umbilicus. In some subjects, the pyramidalis is wanting on one or both sides; and, when this happens, the internal oblique is usually found to be of greater thickness at its lower part. Now and then, though rarely, there are two at one side, and only one at the other, and Sa batier has even seen two on each side. Fallopius, and many others after him, have considered it as the congener of the internal oblique; but its use seems to be to assist the lower part of the rectus.

PYRAMIDALIS FACIEI. See *Levator labii superioris alæque nasi.*

PYRENEITE. A grayish-black coloured mineral, found in the Pyrenees.

PYRENOI'DES. (From πυρην, a kernel, and ειδος, likeness: so called from its kernel-like shape.) Applied to the odontoid process of the second vertebra.

PYRETE'RIUM. (From πυρ, fire, and τηρεω, to keep.) The fire-hole of a furnace.

PYRE'THRUM. (From πυρ, fire, because of the hot taste of its root.) See *Anthemis pyrethrum.*

PYRETHRUM SYLVESTRE. See *Achillea ptarmica.*

PYRETICA. The name given by Dr. Good to an order of his class *Hæmatica.* Fevers. It has four genera: *Ephemera; Anetus; Epanetus; Enecia.*

PYRETOLOGY. (*Pyretologia; from* πυρετος, fever, and λογος, a discourse.) A discourse, or doc trine on fevers.

PYRE'XIA. (From πυρ, fire.) Fever.

PYREXIÆ. Febrile diseases. The first class of Cullen's Nosology; characterized by frequency of pulse after a cold shivering, with increase of heat, and especially, among other impaired functions, a diminution of strength.

PYREXIAL. (From *pyrexia,* fever.) Appertaining to fever.

PYRIFO'RMIS. (From *pyrus*, a pear, and *forma*, a shape; shaped like a pear.) A small radiated muscle of the pelvis, situated under the glutæus maximus, along the inferior edge of the glutæus maximus. *Pyriformis*, seu *iliacus externus*, of Douglas and Cowper. Spigelius was the first who gave a name to this muscle, which he called *pyriformis*, from its supposed resemblance to a pear. It is the *pyriformis sive pyramidalis* of Winslow; and *sacrotrochanterien* of Dumas. It arises by three, and sometimes four, tendinous and fleshy origins, from the anterior surface of the second, third, and fourth pieces of the os sacrum, so that this part of it is within the pelvis. From these origins, the muscle grows narrower, and passing out of the pelvis, below the niche in the posterior part of the ilium, from which it receives a few fleshy fibres, is inserted by a roundish tendon, of an inch in length, into the upper part of the cavity at the root of the trochanter major. The use of this muscle is to assist in moving the thigh outwards, and moving it a little upwards.

PYRI'TES. (From πυρ, fire: so called because it strikes fire with steel.) Native compounds of metal with sulphur.

PYRITES ARSENICALIS. Sulphuret of iron with arsenic.

PYRMONT. The name of a village in the circle of Westphalia, in Germany, in which is a celebrated mineral spring. Pyrmont water. *Aqua pyrmontana* is of an agreeable, though strongly acidulated taste, and emits a large portion of gas; which affects the persons who attend at the well, as well as those who drink the fluid, with a sensation somewhat resembling that produced by intoxication. A general view of the analysis of this water will show that it stands the first in rank of the highly carbonated chalybeates, and contains such an abundance of carbonic acid, as not only to hold dissolved a number of carbonic salts, but to show all the properties of this acid uncombined, and in its most active form. Pyrmont water is likewise a strong chalybeate, with regard to the proportion of iron; and it is, besides, a very hard water, containing much selenite and earthy carbonates. The diseases to which this mineral water may be advantageously applied, are the same as those for which the Spa, and others of the acidulated chalybeates, are resorted to; that is, in all cases of debility that require an active tonic that is not permanently heating; as various disorders in the alimentary canal, especially bilious vomiting, and diarrhœa, and complaints that originate from obstructed menstruation. At Pyrmont, the company generally drink this water by glassfuls, in a morning, to the quantity of two, three, or more English pints. Its common operation is by urine; but, if taken copiously, it generally proves laxative; and when it has not this effect, and that effect is wanted, they commonly mix, with the first glass drank in the morning, from one to five or six drachms of some purging salts.

PYROACETIC ACID. (*Acidum pycitricum;* so called because it is obtained by the action of fire on the acetic acid.) Pyroacetic spirit. Obtained by the destructive distillation of the acetates, from which a modified vinegar escapes, called pyroacetic or spirit.

PYROCI'TRIC ACID. *Acidum pyrocitricum.* A new acid obtained by distilling citric acid.

"When citric acid is put to distil in a retort, it begins at first by melting; the water of crystallization separates almost entirely from it by a continuance of the fusion; then it assumes a yellowish tint, which gradually deepens. At the same time there is disengaged a white vapour which goes over, to be condensed in the receiver. Towards the end of the calcination a brownish vapour is seen to form, and there remains in the bottom of the retort a light very brilliant charcoal.

The product contained in the receiver consists of two different liquids. One of an amber yellow colour, and an oily aspect, occupies the lower part; another, colourless and liquid like water, of a very decided acid taste, floats above. After separating them from one another, we perceive that the first has a very strong bituminous odour, and an acid and acrid taste; that it reddens powerfully the tincture of litmus, but that it may be deprived almost entirely of that acidity by agitation with water, in which it divides itself into globules, which soon fall to the bottom of the vessel, and are not long in uniting to one mass, in the manner of oils heavier than water.

In this state it possesses some of the properties of

224

these substances; it is soluble in alkohol, æther, and the caustic alkalies. However, it does not long continue thus; it becomes acid, and sometimes even it is observed to deposite at the end of some days, white crystals, which have a very strong acidity; if we then agitate it anew with water, it dissolves in a great measure, and abandons a yellow or brownish pitchy matter, of a very obvious empyreumatic smell, and which has much analogy with the oil obtained in the distillation of other vegetable matters. The same effect takes place when we keep it under water; it diminishes gradually in volume, the water acquires a sour taste, and a thick oil remains at the bottom of the vessel.

This liquid may be regarded as a combination (of little permanence indeed) of the peculiar acid with the oil formed in similar circumstances.

As to the liquid and colourless portion which floated over this oil, it was ascertained to contain no citric acid *carried over*, nor acetic acid; first, because on saturating it with carbonate of lime, a soluble calcareous salt was obtained; and, secondly, because this salt, treated with sulphuric acid, evolved no odour of acetic acid.

From this calcareous salt the lime was separated by oxalic acid; or the salt itself was decomposed with acetate of lead, and the precipitate treated with sulphuretted hydrogen. By these two processes, this new acid was separated in a state of purity.

Properties of the pyrocitric acid.—This acid is white, inodorous, of a strongly acid taste. It is difficult to make it crystallize in a regular manner, but it is usually presented in a white mass, formed by the interlacement of very fine small needles. Projected on a hot body it melts, is converted into white very pungent vapours, and leaves some traces of carbon. When heated in a retort, it affords an oily-looking acid, and yellowish liquid, and is partially decomposed. It is very soluble in water and in alkohol; water at the temperature of 10° C. (50° F.) dissolves one-third of its weight. The watery solution has a strongly acid taste, it does not precipitate lime or barytes water, nor the greater part of metallic solutions, with the exception of acetate of lead and protonitrate of mercury. With the oxides it forms salts possessing properties different from the citrates.

The *pyrocitrate of potassa* crystallizes in small needles, which are white, and unalterable in the air. It dissolves in about 4 parts of water. Its solution gives no precipitate with the nitrate of silver, or of barytes, while that of the citrate of barytes forms precipitates with these salts.

The *pyrocitrate of lime* directly formed, exhibits a white crystalline mass, composed of needles, opposed to each other, in a ramification form. This salt has a sharp taste. It dissolves in 25 parts of water at 50° Fahr.

The solution of the pyrocitric acid saturated with barytes water, lets fall, at the end of some hours, a very white crystalline powder, which is *pyrocitrate of barytes*. This salt is soluble in 150 parts of cold water, and in 50 of boiling water.

The *pyrocitrate of lead* is easily obtained by pouring pyrocitrate of potassa into a solution of acetate of lead. The pyrocitrate of lead presents itself under the form of a white gelatinous semitransparent mass, which becomes dry in the air."

PYROGOM. A variety of diopside.

PYROLA. (From *pyrus*, a pear: so named because its leaves resemble those of a pear-tree.) 1. The name of a genus of plants in the Linnæan system Class, *Decandria*; Order, *Monogynia.*

2. The pharmacopœial name of the wintergreen. See *Pyrola rotundifolia.*

PYROLA ROTUNDIFOLIA. The systematic name of the round-leaved wintergreen. This elegant little plant, common in our woods, is now forgotten in the practice of medicine. It possesses gently astringent qualities, and has a somewhat bitter taste.

["**PYROLA UMBELLATA** The *pyrola umbellata*, or *wintergreen*, is a common plant of the American forest. Its leaves have a taste intermediate between sweet and bitter, which in the stalk and roots, is combined with some pungency. Spirit extracts these properties; likewise water, though less perfectly. This plant has been formerly used in rheumatism. More recently it has been found a very useful palliative in strangury and nephritis, both in this country and in

Europe. In dropsy it has sometimes exhibited striking effects as a diuretic, a pint of the saturated infusion being taken every twenty-four hours. It has the advantage over the more common diuretics, that it does not offend the stomach, but, on the contrary, invigorates that organ, and assists digestion. The bruised leaves, externally applied, act as a rubefacient and a discutient to indolent swellings."—*Bigelow's Materia Medica.* A.]

PYROLIGNEOUS ACID. (*Acidum pyrolignosum;* so called because it is procured by distilling wood.) "In the destructive distillation of any kind of wood, an acid is obtained, which was formerly called *acid spirit of wood,* and since, pyroligneous acid. Fourcroy and Vauquelin showed that the acid was merely the acetic, contaminated with empyreumatic oil and bitumen. See *Acetic acid.*

Under Acetic Acid will be found a full account of the production and purification of pyroligneous acid. Mouge discovered about two years ago, that this acid has the property of preventing the decomposition of animal substances. Mr. William Dinsdale, of Field Cottage, Colchester, three years prior to the date of Mouge's discovery did propose to the Lords Commissioners of the Admiralty, to apply a pyroligneous acid, (prepared out of the contact of iron vessels, which blacken it,) to the purpose of preserving animal food, wherever their ships might go. As this application may in many cases afford valuable anti-scorbutic articles of food, and thence be eminently conducive to the health of seamen, it is to be hoped that their Lordship's will, ere long, carry into effect Mr. Dinsdale's ingenious plan, as far as shall be deemed necessary. It is sufficient to plunge meat for a few moments into this acid, even slightly empyreumatic, to preserve it as long as you please. 'Putrefaction,' it is said, 'not only stops, but retrogrades.' To the empyreumatic oil a part of this effect has been ascribed; and hence has been accounted for, the agency of smoke in the preservation of tongues, hams, herrings, &c. Dr. Jorg of Leipsic has entirely recovered several anatomical preparations from incipient corruption by pouring this acid over them. With the empyreumatic oil or tar he has smeared pieces of flesh already advanced in decay, and notwithstanding that the weather was hot, they soon became dry and sound. To the above statements Mr. Ramsay of Glasgow, an eminent manufacturer of pyroligneous acid, and well known for the purity of his vinegar from wood, has recently added the following facts in the 5th number of the Edinburgh Philosophical Journal. If fish be simply dipped in redistilled pyroligneous acid, of the specific gravity of 1.012, and afterward dried in the shade, they preserve perfectly well. On boiling herrings treated in this manner, they were very agreeable to the taste, and had nothing of the disagreeable empyreuma which those of his earlier experiments had, which were steeped for three hours in the acid. A number of very fine haddocks were cleaned, split, and slightly sprinkled with salt for six hours. After being drained, they were dipped for about three seconds in pyroligneous acid, then hung up in the shade for six days. On being broiled, the fish were of an uncommonly fine flavour, and delicately white. Beef treated in the same way had the same flavour as Hamburgh beef, and kept as well. Mr. Ramsay has since found, that his perfectly purified vinegar, specific gravity 1.034, being applied by a cloth or sponge to the surface of fresh meat, makes it keep sweet and sound for several days longer in summer than it otherwise would. Immersion for a minute in his purified common vinegar, specific gravity 1.009, protects beef and fish from all taint in summer, provided they be hung up and dried in the shade. When, by frequent use, the pyroligneous acid has become impure, it may be clarified by beating up twenty gallons of it with a dozen of eggs in the usual manner, and heating the mixture in an iron boiler. Before boiling, the eggs coagulate, and bring the impurities to the surface of the boiler, which are of course to be carefully skimmed off. The acid must be immediately withdrawn from the boiler, as it acts on iron."

PYROLITHIC ACID. "When uric acid concretions are distilled in a retort, silvery white plate sublime. These are pyrolithate of ammonia. When their solution is poured into that of subacetate of lead, a pyrolithate of lead falls, which, after proper washing, is to be shaken with water, and decomposed by sulphuretted hydrogen gas. The supernatant liquid is now a solution of pyrolithic acid, which yields small acicular crystals by evaporation. By heat, these melt and sublime in white needles. They are soluble in four parts of cold water, and the solution reddens vegetable blues. Boiling alkohol dissolves the acid, but on cooling it deposites it, in small white grains. Nitric acid dissolves without changing it. Hence, pyrolithic is a different acid from the lithic, which, by nitric acid, is convertible into purpurate of ammonia. The pyrolithate of lime crystallizes in stalactites which have a bitter and slightly acrid taste. It consists of 91.4 acid + 8.6 lime. Pyrolithate of barytes is a nearly insoluble powder. The salts of potassa, soda, and ammonia, are soluble, and the former two crystallizable. At a red heat, and by passing it over ignited oxide of copper, it is decomposed, into oxygen 44.32, carbon 28.29, azote 16.84, hydrogen 10."

PYROMALIC ACID. "When malic or sorbic acid for they are the same, is distilled in a retort, an acid sublimate, in white needles, appears in the neck of the retort, and an acid liquid distils into the receiver. This liquid, by evaporation, affords crystals, constituting a peculiar acid to which the above name has been given. They are permanent in the air, melt at 118° Fahr., and on cooling, form a pearl-coloured mass of diverging needles. When thrown on red-hot coals, they completely evaporate in an acrid, cough-exciting smoke. Exposed to a strong heat in a retort, they are partly sublimed in needles, and are partly decomposed. They are very soluble in strong alkohol, and in double their weight of water, at the ordinary temperature. The solution reddens vegetable blues, and yields white flocculent precipitates with acetate of lead and nitrate of mercury; but produces no precipitate with lime-water. By mixing it with barytes water, a white powder falls, which is redissolved by dilution with water, after which, by gentle evaporation, the pyromalate of barytes may be obtained in silvery plates. These consist of 100 acid, and 185.142 barytes, or in prime equivalents, of 5.25 + 9.75."

PYROMETER. (From πυρ, fire, and μετρον, measure.) To measure those higher degrees of heat to which the thermometer cannot be applied, there have been other instruments invented by different philosophers: these are called *pyrometers.* The most celebrated instrument of this kind, and which has been adopted into general use, is that invented by the late ingenious Mr. Wedgwood.

This instrument is also sufficiently simple. It consists of two pieces of brass fixed on a plate, so as to be 6-10ths of an inch asunder at one end, and 3-10ths at the other; a scale is marked upon them, which is divided into 240 equal parts, each 1-10th of an inch; and with this his gauge, are furnished a sufficient number of pieces of baked clay, which must have been pre pared in a red heat, and must be of given dimensions These pieces of clay, thus prepared, are first to be applied cold, to the rule of the gauge, that there may no mistake take place in regard to their dimensions. Then any one of them is to be exposed to the heat which is to be measured, till it shall have been completely penetrated by it. It is then removed and applied to the gauge. The difference between its former and its present dimensions will show how much it has shrunk; and will consequently indicate to what degree the intensity of the heat to which it was exposed amounted.

High temperatures can thus be ascertained with accuracy. Each degree of Wedgwood's pyrometer is equal to 130° of Fahrenheit's.

PYROMUCIC ACID. (*Acidum pyromucicum;* because it was obtained from the distillation of gum.) Pyromucous acid. "This acid, discovered in 1818, by Houton Labillardiere, is one of the products of the distillation of mucic acid. When we wish to procure it, the operation must be performed in a glass retort furnished with a receiver. The acid is formed in the brown liquid, which is produced along with it, and which contains water, acetic acid, and empyreumatic oil; a very small quantity of the pyromucic acid remaining attached to the vault of the retort, under the form of crystals. These crystals being coloured, are added to the brown liquor, which is then diluted with three or four times its quantity of water, in order to throw down a certain portion of oil. The whole is next filtered, and evaporated to a suitable degree. A great deal of acetic acid is volatilized, and then the new acid crystallizes. On decanting the mother waters, and concentrating them farther, they yield crystals anew; but as these are small and yellowish, it is necessary to make them undergo a second distillation to render them susceptible of being perfectly purified by crystallization. 150 parts of mucic acid furnish about 60 of brown liquor, from which we can obtain 8 to 10 of pure pyromucic acid.

This acid is white, inodorous, of a strongly acid taste, and a decided action on litmus. Exposed to heat in a retort it melts at the temperature of 266° F., then volatilizes, and condenses into a liquid, which passes on cooling into a crystalline mass, covered with very fine needles. It leaves very slight traces of residuum in the bottom of the retort.

On burning coals, it instantly diffuses white, pungent vapours. Air has no action on it. Water at 60° dissolves one twenty-eighth of its weight. Boiling water dissolves it much more abundantly; and on cooling abandons a portion of it, in small elongated plates, which cross in every direction."

Pyro-mucous acid. See *Pyromucic acid.*

PYROPE. A subspecies of dodecahedral garnet, of a dark blood-red colour. It comes from Saxony, and is highly esteemed as a gem.

PYROPHORUS. An artificial product, which takes fire or becomes ignited, on exposure to the air. It is prepared from alum by calcination, with the addition of various inflammable bodies.

PYROPHYSALITE. See *Physalite.*

PYRO'SIS. (From πυροω, to burn.) *Pyrosis suecica*, of Sauvages. *Cardialgia sputatoria*, of Linnæus. A disease called in Scotland the water-brash; in England, black-water. A genus of disease in the class *Neuroses*, and order *Spasmi*, of Cullen; known by a burning pain in the stomach, attended with copious eructation, generally of a watery insipid fluid.

PYROSMALITE. A liver-coloured mineral, which comes from Wermeland.

PYROTARTARIC ACID. (*Acidum pyro-tartaricum*; so called because obtained by the destructive distillation of tartaric acid.) " Into a coated glass retort introduce tartar, or rather tartaric acid, till it is half full, and fit to it a tubulated receiver. Apply heat, which is to be gradually raised to redness. Pyrotartaric acid of a brown colour, from impurity, is found in the liquid products. We must filter these through paper previously wetted, to separate the oily matter. Saturate the liquid with carbonate of potassa; evaporate to dryness; redissolve, and filter through clean moistened paper. By repeating this process of evaporation, solution, and filtration, several times, we succeed in separating all the oil. The dry salt is then to be treated in a glass retort, at a moderate heat, with dilute sulphuric acid. There passes over into the receiver, first of all, a liquor containing evidently acetic acid; but towards the end of the distillation, there is condensed in the vault of the retort, a white and foliated sublimate, which is the pyrotartaric acid, perfectly pure.

It has a very sour taste, and reddens powerfully the tincture of turnsole. Heated in an open vessel, the acid rises in a white smoke, without leaving the charcoaly residuum which is left in a retort. It is very soluble in water, from which it is separated in crystals by spontaneous evaporation. The bases combine with it, forming pyrotartarates, of which those of potassa, soda, ammonia, barytes, strontites, and lime, are very soluble. That of potassa is deliquescent, soluble in alkohol, capable of crystallizing in plates, like the acetate of potassa. This pyrotartarate precipitates both acetate of lead and nitrate of mercury, while the acid itself precipitates only the latter. Rose is the discoverer of this acid, which was formerly confounded with the acetic."

Pyro-tartarous acid. See *Pyro-tartaric acid.*

PYROTE'CHNIA. (From πυρ, fire, and τεχνη, an art.) Chemistry, or that art by which the properties of bodies are examined by fire.

PYRO'TICA. (From πυροω, to burn.) Caustics.

PYROXENE. See *Augite.*

PY'RUS. The name of a genus of plants in the Linnæan system. Class, *Icosandria;* Order, *Pentagynia.*

PYRUS COMMUNIS. The pear-tree. The fruit is analagous to that of the apple, but more delicately flavoured. Its juice, when fermented, forms perry.

PYRUS CYDONIA. The systematic name of the quince-tree. The fruit is termed *Cydonium malum*, or quince. The tree which affords this fruit is the *Pyrus—foliis integerrimis, floribus, solitariis*, of Linnæus. Quince seeds are directed by the London College to be made into a decoction, which is recommended in apthous affections, and excoriations of the mouth and fauces.

PYRUS MALUS. The systematic name of the apple-tree. The common crab-tree is the parent of all the vast variety of apples at present cultivated. Apples, in general, when ripe, afford a pleasant and easily digestible fruit for the table; but, when the stomach is weak, they are very apt to remain unaltered for some days, and to produce dyspepsia. Sour fruits are to be considered unwholesome, except when boiled or baked, and rend red soft and mellow with the addition of sugar.

PYU'LCUM. (From πυον, pus, and ελκω, to draw.) An instrument to extract the pus from the cavity of any sinuous ulcer.

PYU'RIA. See *Pyoturia.*

PYXACA'NTHA. (From πυξος, box, and ακανθα, a thorn.) The barberry, or thorny box-tree.

PY'XIS. (*Pyxis, idis.* f.; so called because it was made with the πυξος, or box-tree.) Properly a box; but, from its resemblance, the cavity of the hip-bone, or acetabulum, has been sometimes so called.

Q

Q. P. An abbreviation of *quantum placet*, as much as you please.

Q. S. The contraction for *quantum sufficit*, a sufficient quantity.

Q. V. An abbreviation of *quantum vis*, as much as you will.

QUADRANGULUS. Quadrangular. Often used to express form of muscles, leaves, &. The receptacle of the *Dorstenia houstonii*, and *contrayerva*, is quadrangulara.

QUADRA'TUS. (From *quadra*, square: so called from its figure.) See *Depressor labii inferioris.*

QUADRATUS FEMORIS. *Tuber-ischiotrochanterien*, of Dumas. A muscle of the thigh, situated on the outside of the pelvis. It is a flat, thin, and fleshy muscle, but not of the shape its name would seem to indicate. It is situated immediately betow the gemini. It arises tendinous and fleshy from the external surface and lower edge of the tuberosity of the ischium, and is inserted by short tendinous fibres into a ridge which is seen extending from the bases of the trochanter major to that of the trochanter minor. Its use is to bring the os femoris outwards.

QUADRATUS GENÆ. See *Platysma-myoides.*

QUADRATUS LABII INFERIORIS. See *Depressor labii inferioris.*

QUADRATUS LUMBORUM. *Quadratus, seu lumbaris externus*, of Winslow. *Ilio-lumbicostal*, of Dumas. A muscle situated within the cavity of the abdomen. This is a small, flat, and oblong muscle, that has gotten the name of *quadratus*, from its shape, which is that of an irregular square. It is situated laterally, at the lower part of the spine. It arises tendinous and fleshy from about two inches from the posterior part of the spine of the ilium. From this broad origin it ascends obliquely inwards, and is inserted into the transverse processes of the four superior lumbar vertebræ, into the lower edge of the last rib, and, by a small tendon, that passes up under the diaphragm into the side of the last vetebra of the back. When this muscle acts singly, it draws the loins to one side; when both muscles act, they serve to support the spine, and perhaps to bend it forwards. In laborious respiration, the quadratus lumborum may assist in pulling down the ribs.

QUADRATUS MAXILLÆ INFERIORIS. See *Platysmamyoides.*

QUADRATUS RADII. See *Pronator radii-quadratus.*

QUADRI'GA. (From *quatuor*, four, and *jugum*, a yoke.) A bandage which resembles the trappings of a four-horse cart.

["QUADROXALATE OF POTASSA. This may be composed by several methods. It was formed by Dr. Wollaston by digesting the *bin-oxalate* in nitric or muriatic acid. The alkali is divided into two parts, one of which unites with the mineral acid, and the other half remains in combination with the oxalic acid. It forms beautiful crystals, which may be obtained pure by solution, and a second crystallization.

"If three parts by weight of the quadroxalate be decomposed by burning, and the alkali, which is thus disengaged, be mixed with a solution of one part of the crystallized salt, the latter is exactly neutralized. Hence the quadroxalate contains four times the acid that exists in the oxalate. The analysis of this class of salts, from which Dr. Wollaston drew a striking exemplification of the law of simple multiples discovered by Mr. Dalton, may be recapitulated as follows:

	Atoms of base.		Atoms of acid.	Base.		Acid.		Equiv. num.
The oxalate consists of	1	+	1	48	+	36	=	84
The bin-oxalate......	1	+	2	48	+	72	=	120
The quadroxalate...	1	+	4	48	+	144	=	192

"Estimating, therefore, from the weights of their atoms, 100 of potassa should be united, in the oxalate, with 75 of acid; in the bin-oxalate with 150; and in the quadroxalate with 300."—*Web.'s Manual of Chemistry. A.*]

QUARTA'NA. *Febris quartana.* A fourth-day ague. Of this species of ague, as well as the other kinds, there are several varieties noticed by authors. The most frequent of these are, 1. The double quartan, with two paroxysms, or fits, on the first day, none on the second and third, and two again on the fourth day. 2. The double quartan, with a paroxysm on the first day, another on the second, but none on the third. 3. The triple quartan, with three paroxysms every fourth day. 4. The triple quartans with a slight paroxysm every day, every fourth paroxysm being similar. See also *Febris intermittens.*

QUARTATION. An operation, in assaying, by which the quantity of one thing is made equal to a fourth part of another thing.

QUARTZ. This name is given to a genus of minerals which Jameson divides into two species, *rhomboidal quartz*, and indivisible quartz.

The *rhomboidal* contains fourteen subspecies. 1. Amethyst. 2. Rock crystal. 3. Milk quartz, which is of a rose red, and milk-white colour. It is found in Bavaria. 4. Common quartz of many colours, and is one of the most abundant minerals in nature. 6. Cat's eye. 7. Fibrous quartz of a grayish or yellowish white colour, found on the banks of the Moldau, in Bohemia. 8. Iron flint. 9. Hornstone. 10. Flinty slate. 11. Flint. 12. Calcedony. 13. Heliotrope. 14. Jasper.

The *indivisible* quartz has nine subspecies. 1. Floatstone. 2. Quartz or siliceous sinter, of which there are three kinds, the common, opaline, and pearly. 3. Hyalite. 4. Opal. 5. Mænilite. 6. Obsidian. 7. Pitchstone. 8. Pearlstone. 9. Pumicestone.

[QUARTZ RESINITE COMMUNE. See *Halb-opal. A.*]

QUA'SSIA. (From a slave of the name of *Quassi*, who first used it with uncommon success as a secret remedy in the malignant endemic fevers which frequently prevailed at Surinam.) 1. The name of a genus of plants in the Linnæan system. Class, *Decandria;* Order, *Monogynia.*

2. The pharmacopœial name of the bitter quassia. See *Quassia amara.*

QUASSIA AMARA. The systematic name of the bitter quassia-tree. The root, bark, and wood of this tree, *Quassia—floribus hermaphroditis, foliis impari-pinnatis, foliolis oppositis, sessilibus, petiolo articulato alato, floribus racemosis,* of Linnæus, are all comprehended in the catalogues of the materia medica. The tree is a native of South America, particularly of Surinam, and also of some of the West India islands.

The roots are perfectly ligneous; they may be medically considered in the same light as the wood, which is now most generally employed, and seems to differ

from the bark in being less intensely bitter; the latter is therefore thought to be a more powerful medicine. Quassia has no sensible odour; its taste is that of a pure bitter, more intense and durable than that of almost any other known substance; it imparts its virtues more completely to watery than to spirituous menstrua, and its infusions are not blackened by the addition of sulphate of iron. The watery extract is from a sixth to a ninth of the weight of the wood, the spirituous about a twenty-fourth. Quassia, as before observed, derived its name from a negro named Quassi, who employed it with uncommon success as a secret remedy in the malignant endemic fevers, which frequently prevailed at Surinam. In consequence of a valuable consideration, this secret was disclosed to Daniel Rolander, a Swede, who brought specimens of the quassia wood to Stockholm, in the year 1756; and since then the effects of this drug have been generally tried in Europe, and numerous testimonies of its efficacy published by many respectable authors. Various experiments with quassia have likewise been made, with a view to ascertain its antiseptic powers; from which it appears to have considerable influence in retarding the tendency to putrefaction; and this, Professor Murray thinks, cannot be attributed to its sensible qualities, as it possesses no astringency whatever; nor can it depend upon its bitterness, as gentian is much bitterer, yet less antiseptic. The medicinal virtues ascribed to quassia are those of a tonic, stomachic, antiseptic, and febrifuge. It has been found very effectual in restoring digestion, expelling flatulencies, and removing habitual costiveness, produced from debility of the intestines, and common to a sedentary life. Dr. Lettsom, whose extensive practice gave him an opportunity of trying the effects of quassia in a great number of cases, says, "In debility, succeeding febrile diseases, the Peruvian bark is most generally more tonic and salutary than any other vegetable hitherto known; but in hysterical atony, to which the female sex is so prone, the quassia affords more vigour and relief to the system than the other, especially when united with the vitriolum album, and still more with the aid of some absorbent." In dyspepsia, arising from hard drinking, and also in diarrhœas, the doctor exhibited the quassia with great success. But with respect to the tonic and febrifuge qualities of quassia, he says, "I by no means subscribe to the Linnæan opinion, where the author declares, 'me quidem judice chinchinam longe superat.'" It is very well known, that there are certain peculiarities of the air, and idiosyncrasies of constitution, unfavourable to the exhibition of Peruvian bark, even in the most clear intermissions of fever; and writers have repeatedly noticed it. But this is comparatively rare. About midsummer, 1785, Dr. L. met with several instances of low remittent and nervous fevers, wherein the bark uniformly aggravated the symptoms, though given in intermissions the most favourable to its success, and wherein quassia, or snakeroot, was successfully substituted. In such cases, he mostly observed, that there was great congestion in the hepatic system, and the debility at the same time discouraged copious evacuations. And in many fevers, without evident remissions to warrant the use of the bark, while at the time increasing debility began to threaten the life of the patient, the Doctor found that quassia, or snakeroot, singly or combined, upheld the vital powers, and promoted a critical intermission of fever, by which an opportunity was afforded for the bark to effect a cure. It may be given in infusion, or in pills made from the watery extract; the former is generally preferred, in the proportion of three or four scruples of the wood to twelve ounces of water.

QUASSIA SIMAROUBA. The systematic name of the simarouba quassia. *Simarouba; Simaraba; Euonymus; Quassia—floribus monoicis, foliis abrupte pinnatis, foliolis alternis subpetiolatis petiolo nudo floribus paniculatis,* of Linnæus. The bark of this tree, which is met with in the shops, is obtained from the roots; and, according to Dr. Wright of Jamaica, it is rough, scaly, and warted; the inside, when fresh, is a full yellow, but when dried, paler: it has but little smell; the taste is bitter, but not disagreeable. It is esteemed in the West Indies, in dysenteries and other fluxes, as restoring tone to the intestines, allaying their spasmodic motions, promoting the secretions by urine and perspiration, and removing lowness of spirits attending those diseases. It is said also that it soon

Yy 2

disposes the patient to sleep; takes off the gripes and tenesmus, and changes the stools to their natural colour and consistence.

QUA'TRIO. (From *quatuor*, four: so called because it has four sides.) The astragalus.

Queen of the meadow. See *Spiræa ulmaria*

QUERCERA. See *Epialus*.

[QUERCITRON. See *Quercus tinctoria*. A.]

QUE'RCULA. (*Quercula*; diminutive of *quercus*, the oak: so called because it has leaves like the oak.) An antiquated name of the germander. See *Teucrium chamædrys*.

QUE'RCUS. (From *quero*, to inquire; because divinations were formerly given from oaks by the Druids.) The oak.

1. The name of a genus of plants in the Linnæan system. Class *Monœcia*; Order, *Polyandria*.

2. The pharmacopœial name of the oak. See *Quercus robur*.

QUERCUS CERRIS. The systematic name of the tree which affords the *Nux galla*. *Galla maxima orbiculata*. The gall-nut. By this name is usually denoted any protuberance, tubercle, or tumour, produced by the puncture of insects on plants and trees of different kinds. These galls are of various forms and sizes, and no less different with regard to their internal structure. Some have only one cavity, and others a number of small cells, communicating with each other. Some of them are as hard as the wood of the tree they grow on, while others are soft and spongy; the first being termed gall-nuts, and the latter berry-galls, or apple-galls.

The gall used in medicine is thus produced:—the *cynips quercus folii*, an insect of the fly-kind, deposites its eggs in the leaves and other tender parts of the tree. Around each puncture an excrescence is presently formed, within which the egg is hatched, and the worm passes through all the stages of its metamorphosis, until it becomes a perfect insect, when it eats its way out of its prison. The best oak-galls are heavy, knotted, and of a bluish colour, and are obtained from Aleppo. They are nearly entirely soluble in water, with the assistance of heat. From 500 grains of Aleppo galls, Sir Humphry Davy obtained by infusion 185 grains of solid matter, which on analysis appeared to consist of tannin 130; mucilage, and matter rendered insoluble by evaporation, 12; gallic acid, with a little extractive matter, 31; the remainder, calcareous earth and saline matter, 12. Another sort comes from the south of Europe, of a light brownish or whitish colour, smooth, round, easily broken, less compact, and of a much larger size. The two sorts differ only in size and strength, two of the blue galls being supposed equivalent in this respect to three of the others.

Oak-galls are supposed to be the strongest astringent in the vegetable kingdom. Both water and spirit take up nearly all their virtue, though the spirituous extract is the strongest preparation. The powder is, however, the best form; and the dose is from a few grains to half a drachm.

They are not much used in medicine, though they are said to be beneficial in intermittents. Dr. Cullen has cured agues, by giving half a drachm of the powder of galls every two or three hours during the intermission; and by it alone, or joined with camomile flowers, has prevented the return of the paroxysms. But the Doctor states the amount of his results only to be this: that, "in many cases, the galls cured the intermittents; but that it failed also in many cases in which the Peruvian bark afterward proved successful." A fomentation, made by macerating half an ounce of bruised galls in a quart of boiling water for an hour, has been found useful for the piles, the prolapsus ani, and the fluor albus, applied cold. An injection, simply astringent, is made by diluting this fomentation, and used in gleets and leucorrhœa. The camphorated ointment of galls has been found also serviceable in piles, after the use of leeches; and is made by incorporating half a drachm of camphor with one ounce of hog's lard, and adding two drachms of galls in very fine powder. In fact, galls may be employed for the same purposes as oak-bark, and are used under the same forms.

QUERCUS ESCULUS. The systematic name of the Italian oak, whose acorns are, in times of scarcity, said to afford a meal of which bread is made.

QUERCUS MARINA. See *Fucus vesiculosus*.

QUERCUS PHELLOS. The systematic name of the willow-leaved oak, the acorns of which are much sweeter than chesnuts, and much eaten by the Indians. They afford, by expression, an oil little inferior to oil of almonds.

QUERCUS ROBUR. The oak-tree. *Balanos*. *Quercus —foliis oblongis, glabris sinuatis, lobis rotundis glandibus oblongis*, of Linnæus. This valuable tree is indigenous to Britain. Its adstringent effects were sufficiently known to the ancients, but it is the bark which is now directed for medicinal use by our pharmacopœias. Oak-bark manifests to the taste a strong adstringency, accompanied with a moderate bitterness. Like other adstringents, it has been recommended in agues, and for restraining hæmorrhages, alvine fluxes, and other immoderate evacuations. A decoction of it has likewise been advantageously employed as a gargle, and as a fomentation or lotion in *procidentia recti et uteri*.

The fruit of this tree was the food of the first ages; but when corn was cultivated, acorns were neglected. They are of little use with us, except for fattening hogs and other cattle and poultry. Among the Spaniards, the acorn, or *glans iberica*, is said to have long remained a delicacy, and to have been served up in the form of a dessert. In dearths, acorns have been sometimes dried, ground into meal, and baked as bread. Bartholin relates that they are used in Norway for this purpose. The inhabitants of Chio held out a long siege without any other food; and in a time of scarcity in France, A. D. 1709, they recurred to this food. But they are said to be hard of digestion, and to occasion headaches, flatulency, and colics. In Smoland, however, many instances occur, in which they have supplied a salutary and nutritious food. With this view they are previously boiled in water and separated from their husks, and then dried and ground; and the powder is mixed with about one-half, or one-third of corn flour. A decoction of acorns is reputed good against dysenteries and colics: and a pessary of them is said to be useful in immoderate fluxes of the menses. Some have recommended the powder of acorns in intermittent fever; and in Brunswick, they mix it with warm ale, and administer it for producing a sweat in cases of erysipelas. Acorns roasted and bruised have restrained a violent diarrhœa. For other medical uses to which they have been applied, see Murray's Appar Medic. vol. i. page 100.

From some late reports of the Academy of Sciences, at Petersburgh, we learn that acorns are the best substitute to coffee that has been hitherto known. To communicate to them the oily properties of coffee, the following process is recommended. When the acorns have been toasted brown, add fresh butter in small pieces to them, while hot in the ladle, and stir them with care, cover the ladle and shake it, that the whole may be well mixed. The acorns of the Holm oak are formed at Venice into cups about one inch and a half in diameter, and somewhat less in depth. They are used for dressing leather, and instead of galls for dying woollen cloth black.

QUERCUS SUBER. The systematic name of the cork tree. *Suber*. The fruit of this tree is much more nutritious than our acorns, and is sweet and often eaten when roasted in some parts of Spain. The bark, called cork, when burned, is applied as an astringent application to bleeding piles, and to allay the pain usually attendant on hæmorrhoids, when mixed with an ointment. Pessaries and other chirurgical instruments are also made of this useful bark.

["QUERCUS ALBA. White oak. Most, and perhaps all the species of oak, have a high degree of astringency, depending upon tannin, which they possess in great quantities, and on account of which they are extensively used in the preparation of leather. The white oak is one of the American species, which is most esteemed for this property. The bark of the young branches is probably more astringent than that of the trunk, on account of the mass of dead cortical layers, which constitutes a part of the thickness of the latter. Oak-bark has been given in some instances as a substitute for cinchona, to which, however, it is greatly inferior. Its chief use is an external astringent and antiseptic. A strong decoction is employed with advantage as a gargle in cynanche, and as a lotion in gangrenous ulcers and offensive discharges of different kinds."—*Big. Mat. Med.* A.]

["Quercus tinctoria. Black oak. This is also native species, the bark of which affords the extract known to dyers, by the name of *quercitron*. Its properties are similar to those of the preceding. Both are very common trees, and are properly substituted for the *quercus robur*, of European Dispensatories, which is not found here.'—*Big. Mat. Med.* A.]

[Querci americanæ. American oaks. These have been described and delineated by Andrew Michaux, in his history of the oaks of America. He describes *twenty-nine* species and varieties of oaks growing spontaneously in North America. He arranges them in the following manner, viz.

"*Methodical disposition of American oaks.*
SECTION I.
Quercus, foliis adultæ plantæ muticis; fructu pedunculato; fructificatione annua:—Specie ôta biennil.
DIVISION 1.
Foliis—lobatis.
Species 1. Quercus obtusiloba, upland white oak, iron oak.
. 2. Q. macrocarpa, over cup, white oak.
.. 3. Q. lyrata, water white oak.
.. 4. Q. alba—variety, *pennatifida,* } white oaks.
              repanda, }
DIVISION 2.
Foliis—dentatis.
Species 5. Q. Prinus—var. *palustris*—swamp chesnut oak.
              monticola—mountain chesnut oak, rock oak.
              acuminata — narrow leaf chesnut oak.
              pumila—Chinquapin oak.
              tomentosa—Illinois oak.
DIVISION 3.
Foliis—integris.
Species 6. Quercus virens.—Live oak of Carolina.
SECTION II.
Quercus, foliis adultæ plantæ setaceo-mucronatis; fructu subsessili; fructificatione bienni.
DIVISION 1.
Foliis integris.
Species 7. Q. Phellos—var. *sylvatica*, willow oak.
              maritima, sea willow oak.
              pumila, dwarf willow oak.
Species 8. Q. Cinerea—upland willow oak,
.. 9. Q. Imbricaria—shingle willow oak.
10. Q. Laurifolia—swamp willow oak.
              obtusiloba.
DIVISION 2.
Foliis—breviter lobatis.
Species 11. Q. Aquatica—water oak.
.. 12. Q. Nigra—black oak.
.. 13. Q. Tinctoria—var. *angulosa*, great black oak, Champlain black oak.
              sinuosa—quercitron oak.
Species 14. Q. Triloba—downy black oak.

DIVISION 3.
Foliis profunde multifidis.
Species 15. Q. Banisteri—running downy-oak.
.. 16. Q. Falcata—downy red-oak.
.. 17. Q. Catesbœi—sandy red-oak.
.. 18. Q. Coccinea—scarlet-oak.
.. 19. Q. Palustris—swamp red-oak.
.. 20. Q. Rubra—red-oak.
"We have been the more particular to exhibit this systematic arrangement of the oaks, because we believe it will be welcome to our readers, and enable them better to understand this difficult genus of plants."—*Med. Repos.* A.]

QUESNAY, Francis, was born near Paris in 1694. Though of humble parentage, and almost without education, he displayed an extraordinary zeal for knowledge, and after studying medicine in the French metropolis, he settled at Mantes. Having ably controverted the doctrines of Silva respecting blood-letting, he was appointed secretary to the Academy of Surgery; but the duties of this office having impaired his health, he graduated in physic, and was made consulting physician to the king. He was subsequently honoured with letters of nobility, and other marks of royal favour; and became a member of several learned societies. He died in 1774. He left several works, which display much research and observation, but with too great partiality to hypothesis. Besides the essays in favour of bleeding in many diseases, his preface to the Memoirs of the Academy of Surgery, gained him considerable applause: as likewise his Researches into the Progress of Surgery in France, though the accuracy of some of his statements was controverted.

Quick-grass. See *Triticum repens.*
Quick-lime. See *Lime.*
QUICKSILVER. See *Mercury.*
Quid pro quo. These words are applied the same as *succedaneum*, when one thing is made use of to supply the defect of another.
QUIESCENT. *Quiescens.* At rest.
Quiescent affinity. See *Affinity quiescent.*
Quina quina. The Peruvian bark.
QUINCE See *Pyrus cydonia.*
Quince, Bengal. See *Erateva marmelos.*
QUINCY. See *Cynanche.*
QUINIA. See *Cinchonina.*
QUININA. See *Cinchonina.*
Quininæ sulphas. Sulphate of quinine. Sulphate of cinchonia. A saline combination of sulphuric acid, with the active principle of cinchona bark. See *Cinchonina.*
Quinine, sulphate of. See *Quininæ sulphas.*
QUINQUEFO'LIUM. (From *quinque*, five, and *folium*, a leaf: so called because it has five leaves on each foot-stalk.) *Pentaphyllum.* Cinquefoil, or fi leaved grass. See *Potentilla reptans.*
Quinquina. See *Cinchona.*
QUOTIDIAN. See *Febris intermittens.*

R

R. or ℞. This letter is placed at the beginning of a prescription, as a contraction of *recipe*, take: thus, ℞ *Magnes,* ʒj. signifies, Take a drachm of magnesia. "In ancient times, such was the supposed importance," says Dr. Paris, in his most excellent work on pharmacology, "of planatory influence, that it was usual to prefix a symbol of the planet under whose reign the ingredients were to be collected; and it is not perhaps generally known, that the character which we at this day place at the head of our prescriptions, and which is understood and is supposed to mean *recipe*, is a relict of the astrological symbol of Jupiter, as may be seen in many of the older works on pharmacy."

RABBIT. A well known animal of the hare kind: the *Lepus cuniculus* of Linnæus, the flesh of which is tender, and easy of digestion.

RA'BIES. (From *rabio*, to be mad.) Madness. Generally applied to that disease of a dog, under which the saliva has the property of producing hydrophobia in man. See *Hydrophobia.*

Rabies canina. See *Hydrophobia.*

RACE'MUS. (*Racemus, i. m.*; from *ramus*.) A raceme or cluster. A species of inflorescence, consisting of a cluster of flowers, rather distant from each other, each on its own proper stalk, the tops of the lower ones not coming near to the tops of the upper ones, as in a corymb, and all connected by one common stalk; as a bunch of currants. It is therefore a kind of pedunculated spike.

From the *division* of the common stalk, it is denominated,
1. *Simple*, not having any branches; as in Ribes rubra, and Acer pseudo-platanus.
2. *Compound*, being branched; as in Vitis vinifera.
3. *Conjugate*, two clusters going from the end of the common peduncle.

4. *Aggregate*, several being gathered together; as in Actæa racemosa.

5. *Unilateral*, the proper stalks of the flowers proceeding from one side only of the common stalk; as in Pyrola secunda.

6. *Second*, the proper stalks of the flowers come from every part of the common stalk, yet they all look to one side only; as in Andromeda racemosa, Teucrium scorodonia, &c.

From the *direction* of the racemus,

7. *Erectus;* as in Chenopodium album, Ribes alpinum, and Astragalus austriacus.

8. *Pendulus;* as in Cytisus laburnum.

9. *Laxus,* easily bent; as in Celosia trigynia, and Solanum carolinense.

10. *Strictus,* bent with difficulty; as in Ononis cernua.

From its *vesture,*

11. *Nudus;* as in Vaccinium legustrinum.

12. *Pilosus;* as in Ribes nigrum.

13. *Foliatus;* as in Chenopodium ambrosioides.

14. *Bracteatus;* as in Andromeda racemosa.

RACHIA'LGIA. (From ραχις, the spine, and αλγος, pain.) A pain in the spine. It was formerly applied to several species of colic which induced pain in the back.

RACHIS. See *Rhachis.*

RACHI'TIS. (*Rachitis, idis.* f.; from ραχις, the spine of the back: so called because it was supposed to originate in a fault of the spinal marrow.) *Cyrtonosus.* The English disease. The rickets. A genus of disease in the Class *Cachexiæ,* and Order *Intumescentiæ,* of Cullen; known by a large head, prominent forehead, protruded sternum, flattened ribs, big belly, and emaciated limbs, with great debility. It is usually confined in its attack between the two periods of nine months and two years of age, seldom appearing sooner than the former, or showing itself for the first time, after the latter period. The muscles become flaccid, the head enlarges, the carotids are distended, the limbs waste away, and their epiphyses increase in bulk. The bones and spine of the back are variously distorted; disinclination to muscular exertion follows; the abdomen swells and grows hard; the stools are frequent and loose; a slow fever succeeds, with cough and difficulty of respiration; atrophy is confirmed, and death ensues. Frequently it happens that nature restores the general health, and leaves the limbs distorted.

After death, the liver and the spleen have been found enlarged and scirrhous; the mesenteric glands indurated, and the lungs either charged with vomicæ, or adhering to the pleura; the bones soft, the brain flaccid, or oppressed with lymph, and the distended bowels loaded most frequently with slime, sometimes with worms.

It is remarkable, that in the kindred disease, which Hoffman and Sauvages call the atrophy of infants, we have many of the same symptoms and the same appearances nearly after death. They who perish by this disease, says Hoffman, have the mesenteric glands enlarged and scirrhous; the liver and spleen obstructed, and increased in size; the intestines are much inflated, and are loaded with black and fœtid matters, and the muscles, more especially of the abdomen, waste away.

In the treatment of rickets, besides altering any improprieties in the regimen, which may have co-operated in producing it, those means should be employed, by which the system may be invigorated. Tonic medicines are therefore proper, particularly chalybeates, which are easily given to children; and the cold-bath may be essentially beneficial. The child should be regularly well exercised, kept clean and dry, and a pure air selected; the food nutritious and easy of digestion. When the appetite is much impaired, an occasional gentle emetic may do good; more frequently tonic aperients, as rhubarb, will be required to regulate the bowels; or sometimes a dose of calomel in gross habits. Of late, certain compounds of lime have been strongly recommended, particularly the phosphate, which is the earthy basis of the bones; though it does not appear likely to enter the system, unless rendered soluble by an excess of acid. Others have conceived the disease to arise from an excess of acid, and therefore recommended alkalies; which may certainly be useful in correcting the morbid prevalence of acid in the primæ viæ so frequent in children. When the bones are

inclined to bend, care must be taken not to throw the weight of the body too much upon them.

RACKA'SIRA BALSAMUM. See *Balsamum rackasira.*

RACO'SIS. (From ρακος, a rag.) A ragged excoriation of the relaxed scrotum.

RADCLIFFE, JOHN, was born at Wakefield, Yorkshire, in 1650. He went to Oxford at the age of 15; and having determined upon the medical profession, he passed rapidly through the preliminary studies, though with very little profoundness of research; and having taken the degree of bachelor of medicine in 1675, he immediately began to practise there. He professed to pay very little regard to the rules generally followed, which naturally drew upon him the enmity of the old practitioners; yet his vivacity and talents procured him a great number of patients, even of the highest rank. In 1684, he removed to London, having taken his doctor's degree two years before, and his success was unusually rapid; in the second year he was appointed physician to the princess Anne of Denmark; and after the Revolution, he was consulted by king William. By his rough independence of spirit and freedom of language, however, he ultimately lost all favour at court; though he is said to have been still privately consulted in cases of emergency. In 1703, he had an attack of pleurisy, which had nearly proved fatal from his own imprudence. He continued, after his recovery, in very extensive practice, notwithstanding the caprice which he continually displayed: but his declining to attend queen Anne in her last illness, though it does not appear that he was sent for officially, excited the popular resentment strongly against him; and his apprehensions of the consequences are supposed to have accelerated his own death, which happened about three months after, in 1714. He was buried in St. Mary's church at Oxford. He founded a noble library and infirmary at that university; and also endowed two travelling medical fellowships, with an annual income of 300*l.* attached to each. It does not appear that he ever attempted to write; and, indeed, he is believed to have been very little conversant with books; yet the universal reputation which he acquired and maintained, notwithstanding his capricious conduct, seem to sanction the testimony of Dr. Mead, that "he was deservedly at the head of his profession, on account of his great medical penetration and experience."

RADIAL. (*Radialis;* from *radius,* the name of a bone.) Belonging to the radius.

RADIAL ARTERY. *Arteria radialis.* A branch of the humeral artery that runs down the side of the radius.

RADIALIS EXTERNUS BREVIOR. See *Extensor carpi radialis brevior.*

RADIALIS EXTERNUS LONGIOR. See *Extensor carpi radialis longior.*

RADIALIS EXTERNUS PRIMUS. See *Extensor carpi radialis longior.*

RADIALIS INTERNUS. See *Flexor carpi radialis.*

RADIALIS SECUNDUS. See *Extensor carpi radialis brevior.*

RADICAL. In chemistry, this term is applied to that which is considered as constituting the distinguishing part of an acid, by its union with the acidifying principle or oxygen, which is common to all acids. Thus sulphur is the radical of the sulphuric and sulphurous acids. It is sometimes called the base of the acid; but base is a term of more extensive application.

Radical vinegar. See *Acetum.*

RADICALIS. Radical: applied to leaves. *Folia radicalia* are such as spring from the root, like those of the cowslip.

RADICANS. A botanical term, applied to a stem which clings to any other body for support, by means of fibres which do not imbibe nourishment; as the ivy Hedera helix.

RADI'CULA. (Diminutive of *radix,* a root.) 1. A radicle, rootlet, or little root. It probably means the fibres which come from the main root, and which are the most essential to the life of the plant, they only imbibing the nourishment.

2. Applied to the origin of vessels and nerves.

3. The common radish is sometimes so called See *Raphanus sativus.*

RADISH. See *Cochlearia* and *Raphanus.*

Radish, garden. See *Raphanus sativus*

Radish, horse. See *Cochlearia armoracia.*

RA'DIUS. .. A bone of the forearm, which has gotten its name from its supposed resemblance to the spoke of a wheel, or to a weaver's beam; and sometimes, from its supporting the hand, it has been called *manubrium manus.* Like the ulna, it is of a triangular figure, but it differs from that bone, in growing larger as it descends, so that its smaller part answers to the larger part of the ulna, and *vice versâ.* Of its two extremities, the uppermost and smallest is formed into a small rounded head, furnished with cartilage, and hollowed at its summit, for an articulation with the little head at the side of the pulley of the os humeri. The round border of this head, next the ulna, is formed for an articulation with the 'ess sigmoid cavity of that bone. This little head of the radius is supported by a neck, at the bottom of which, laterally, is a con siderable tuberosity, into the posterior half of which is inserted the posterior tendon of the biceps, while the interior half is covered with cartilage, and surrounded with a capsular ligament, so as to allow this tendon to slide upon it as upon a pulley. Immediately below this tuberosity, the body of the bone may be said to begin. We find it slightly curved throughout its whole length, by which means a greater space is formed for the lodgment of muscles, and it is enabled to cross the ulna without compressing them. Of the three surfaces to be distinguished on the body of the bone, the external and internal ones are the broadest and flattest. The anterior surface is narrower and more convex. Of its angles, the external and internal ones are rounded; but the posterior angle, which is turned towards the ulna, is formed into a sharp spine, which serves for the attachment of the interosseous ligament, of which mention is made in the description of the ulna. This strong ligament, which is a little interrupted above and below, serves not only to connect the bones of the forearm to each other, but likewise to afford a greater surface for the lodgment of muscles. On the forepart of the bone, and at about one-third of its length from its upper end, we observe a channel for vessels, slanting obliquely upwards. Towards its lower extremity, the radius becomes broader, of an irregular shape, and somewhat flattened, affording three surfaces, of which the posterior one is the smallest; the second, which is a continuation of the internal surface of the body of the bone, is broader and flatter than the first; and the third, which is the broadest of the three, answers to the anterior and external surface of the body of the bone. On this last, we observe several sinuosities, covered with a thin layer of cartilage, upon which slide the tendons of several muscles of the wrist and fingers. The lowest part of the bone is formed into an oblong articulating cavity, divided into two by a slight transverse rising. This cavity is formed for an articulation with the bones of the wrist. Towards the anterior and convex surface of the bone, this cavity is defended by a remarkable eminence, called the *styloid* process of the radius, which is covered with a cartilage that is extended to the lower extremity of the ulna; a ligament is likewise stretched from it to the wrist. Besides this large cavity, the radius has another much smaller one, opposite its styloid process, which is lined with cartilage, and receives the rounded surface of the ulna. The articulation of the radius with the less sigmoid cavity of the ulna, is strengthened by a circular ligament which is attached to the two extremities of that cavity, and from thence surrounds the head of the radius. This ligament is narrowest, but thickest at its middle part. But, besides this ligament, which connects the two bones of the forearm with each other, the ligaments which secure the articulation of the radius with the os humeri, are common both to it and to the ulna, and therefore cannot. well be understood till both these bones are described. These ligaments are a capsular and two lateral ligaments. The capsular ligament is attached to the anterior and posterior surface of the lower extremity of the os humeri, to the upper edges and sides of the cavities, we remarked, at the bottom of the pulley and little head, and likewise to some part of the condyles: from thence it is spread over the ulna, to the edges of the greater sigmoid cavity, so as to include in it the end of the olecranon and of the coronoid process; and it is likewise fixed round the neck of the radius, so as to include the head of that bone within it. The

lateral ligaments may be distinguished into external and internal, or, according to Winslow, into *brachio-radialis* and *brachio-cubitalis.* They both descend laterally from the lowest part of each condyle of the os humeri, and, from their fibres spreading wide as they descend, have been compared to a goose's foot. The internal ligament or brachio-cubitalis, which is the longest and thickest of the two, is attached to the coronoid process of the ulna. The external ligament, or brachio-radialis, terminates in the circular ligament of the radius. Both these ligaments adhere firmly to the capsular ligament, and to the tendons of some of the adjacent muscles. In considering the articulation of the forearm with the os humeri, we find that when both the bones are moved together upon the os humeri, the motion of the ulna upon the pulley allows only of flexion and extension; whereas, when the palm of the hand is turned downwards or upwards, or, in other words, in pronation and supination, we see the radius moving upon its axis, and in these motions its head turns upon the little head of the os humeri at the side of the pulley, while its circular edge rolls in the less sigmoid cavity of the ulna. At the lower end of the forearm the edge of the ulna is received into a superficial cavity at the side of the radius. This articulation, which is surrounded by a loose capsular ligament, concurs with the articulation above, in enabling the radius to turn with great facility upon its axis; and it is chiefly with the assistance of this bone that we are enabled to turn the palm of the hand upwards or downwards, the ulna having but a very inconsiderable share in these motions.

2. The term radius, in botany, is applied to the marginal part of the corolla of compound flowers; thus, in the daisy, the marginal white flowrets form the rays or radius, and the yellow central ones the discus or disk. See *Discus.*

The radii of a peduncle of a compound umbel are the *common stalks* of the umbel, and *pedicelli* are the stalks of the flowrets.

RA'DIX. (*Radix, dicis.* f.) A root. I. In botany, that part of a plant which imbibes its nourishment, producing the herbaceous part and the fructification, and which consists of the *caudex,* or body, and *radicles.*—Linnæus.

That part of the plant by which it attaches itself to the soil in which it grows, or to the substance on which it feeds, and is the principal organ of nutrition. —Keith.

In all plants, the primary root is a simple elongation of that part which, during the germination of the seed, is first protruded, and is denominated the radicle; and as the plant continues to grow, the root gradually assumes a determinate form and structure, which differs materially in different plants, but always is found similar in all the individuals of the same species. From the figure, duration, direction, and insertion, roots are arranged into,

From their *figure,*

1. *Radix fusiformis,* spindle-shaped, of an oblong, tapering form, pointed at its extremity; as in *Daucus carota,* the carrot; *Beta vulgaris,* beet; *Pastinaca sativa,* parsnip, &c.

2. *Radix ramosa,* branched, which consists of a *caudex,* or main root, divided into lateral branches, which are again subdivided; so that it resembles in its divisions the stem and branches inverted. Most trees, shrubs, and many herbaceous plants, have this form of root.

3. *Radix fibrosa,* fibrous, consisting wholly of small radicles; as the *Hordeum vulgare,* common barley, and most grasses.

4. *Radix præmorsa,* abrupt or truncated, appearing as if bitten off close to the top; as in *Scabiosa succisa,* the devil's bite; *Plantago major,* larger plantain; *Hieracium præmorsum,* &c.

5. *Radix globosa,* globose, having the caudex round, or subrotund, sending off radicles in many places; as in *Cyclamen europeum,* sow-bread; *Brassica rapa,* turnip, &c.

6. *Radix tuberosa,* tuberose, furnished with farinaceous tubers; as in *Solanum tuberosum,* the potato: *Helianthus tuberosus,* Jerusalem artichoke, &c.

7. *Radix pendula,* pendulous, consisting of tubers connected to the plant by thin, or filiform portions; as in *Spiræa filipendula,* common dropwort; *Pæonia officinalis* pæony, &c.

8. *Radix granulata*, granulated, formed of many small globules; as in *Saxifraga granulata*, meadow saxifrage, &c.

9. *Radix articulata*, articulated, or jointed, apparently formed of distinct pieces united, as if one piece grew out of another, with radicles proceeding from each joint: as in *Oxalis acetocella*, woodsorrel; *Asarum canadense*, wild ginger, &c.

10. *Radix dentata*, toothed, which has a fleshy caudex, with teeth like prolongations; as in *Ophrys corallorhiza*.

11. *Radix squamosa*, scaly, covered with fleshy scales; as in *Lathræa squamaria*, toothwort, &c.

12. *Radix fascicularis*, bundled, or fasciculate: as in *Ophrys, nidus avis*, &c.

13. *Radix cava*, hollow; as in *Fumaria cava*. There are other distinctions of modern botanists derived from the form; as conical, subrotund, napiform, placentiform, filiform, capillary, tufted, funiliform, geniculate, contorted, moniliform, &c.

From the *direction*, roots are distinguished into,

14. *Radix perpendicularis*, perpendicular, which descends in a straight direction; as in *Daucus corota*, *Beta vulgaris, Scorzonera hispanica*, &c.

15. *Radix horizontalis*, horizontal, which is extended under the earth transversely; as in *Laserpitium pruthenium*, &c.

16. *Radix obliqua*, oblique, descending obliquely; as in *Iris germanica*, &c.

17. *Radix repens*, creeping, descending transversely, but here and there sending off new plants; as in *Sambucus ebulus; Glycyrrhiza glabra; Ranunculus repens*, &c.

The *duration* affords,

18. *Radix annua*, yearly, which perishes the same year with the plant; as *Draba verna*, and all annuals.

19. *Radix biennis*, biennial, which vegetates the first year, flowers the next, and then perishes; as the *Œnothera biennis, Beta vulgaris*, &c.

20. *Radix perennis*, perennial, which lives for many years; as trees and shrubs.

Roots are also distinguished from their *situation* into,

21. *Terrena*, earth-root, which grow only in the earth; as the roots of most plants.

22. *Aquatica*, water-root, which grow only in the water, and perish when out of it; as *Trapa natans*, *Nymphæa alba*.

23. *Parasitica*, parasitical, which inserts the root into another plant; as in *Epidendrum vanilla*, &c.

24. *Arrhiza*, which does not insert radicles, but coheres to other plants by an anastomosis of vessels; as in *Viscum album, Horanthus europæus*, &c.

II. In anatomy, the term radix is applied to some parts which are inserted into others, as the root of a plant is in the earth; as the fangs of the teeth, the origin of some of the nerves, &c.

RADIX BENGALE. See *Cassumuniar*.

RADIX BRASILIENSIS. See *Callicocca ipecacuanha*.

RADIX DULCIS. See *Glycyrrhiza*.

RADIX INDIANA. See *Callicocca ipecacuanha*.

RADIX ROSEA. See *Rhodiola*.

RADIX RUBRA. See *Rubia tinctorum*.

RADIX URSINA. See *Æthusa meum*.

RA'DULA. (From *rado*, to scrape off.) A wooden spatula, or scraper.

RAGWORT. See *Senecio Jacobæa*.

RAISIN. See *Vitis vinifera*.

RAMA'LIS VENA. (From *ramale*, a dead bough.) Applied to the vena portæ, from its numerous ramifications, which resemble a bough stripped of its leaves.

RAMAZZINI, BERNARDIN, was born at Carpi, in Italy, in 1633. He graduated at Parma at the age of 26, and, after studying some time longer at Rome, settled in the dutchy of Castro: but ill health obliged him speedily to return to his native place. His reputation increasing, he removed to Modena in 1671, where he met with considerable success; and, in 1682, he was appointed professor of the theory of medicine in the university recently established there, which office he filled for eighteen years with great credit. He was then invited to a similar appointment at Padua, and exerted himself with laudable ardour for three years; when he was attacked with a disease of the eyes, which ultimately deprived him of sight. In 1708, the senate of Venice appointed him President of the College of Physicians of that capital, and in the following year raised him to the first professorship of the practice of medicine. He continued to perform the duties of these offices with great diligence and reputation till his death, in 1714. He was a member of many of the academies of science, established in Germany, &c.; and left several works in the Latin language, remarkable for the elegance of their style, and other merits. The principal of these, and which will be ever held in estimation, is entitled "De Morbus Artificum Diatriba," giving an account of the diseases peculiar to different artists and manufacturers.

RAMENTUM. A species of pubescence of plants, consisting of hairs in form of flat, strap-like portions, resembling shavings, seen on the leaves of some of the genus Bigonia. See *Pilus*.

RAMEUS. Of or belonging to a bough or branch; applied to branch leaves, which are so distinguished, because they sometimes differ from those of the main stem; as is the case in *Melampyrum arvense*; and also to a leaf-stalk when it comes directly from the main branch; as in *Eugenia malaccensis*.

RA'MEX. (From *ramus*, a branch: from its protruding forwards, like a bud.) An obsolete term for a rupture.

RAMOSISSIMUS. Much branched. Applied to a stem which is repeatedly subdivided into a great many branches, without order; as those of the apple, pear, and gooseberry-tree.

RAMOSUS. Branched. Applied to the roots, and especially those of trees.

RAMUS. A branch, or primary division of a stem into lateral stems. In the language of botanists rami, or branches, are denominated,

1. *Oppositi*, when they go off, or pair opposite to each other, as they do in Mentha arvensis.

2. *Alterni*, one after another, alternately; as in Althæa officinalis.

3. *Verticillati*, when more than two go from the stem in a whirlwind manner; as in Pinus abies.

4. *Sparsi*, without any order.

5. *Erecti*, rising close to the stem; as in Populus di latata.

6. *Patentes*, descending from the stalk at an obtuse angle; as in Galium mollugo, and Cistus italicus.

7. *Patentissimi*, descending at a right angle; as in Ammania ramosior.

8. *Brachiati*, the opposite spreading branches crossing each other; as in Pisonia aculeata, and Panisteria brachiata.

9. *Deflexi*, arched, with the apex downwards; as in Pinus larix.

10. *Reflexi*, hanging perpendicularly from the trunk; as in the Salix babylonica.

11. *Retroflexi*, turned backwards; as in Solanum dulcamara.

12. *Fastigiati*, forming a kind of pyramid; as in Chrysanthemum corymbosum.

13. *Vergati*, twig-like, long and weak; as in Salix vimialis.

RA'NA. The name of a genus of animals. Class, *Amphibia;* Order, *Reptilia*. The frog.

RANA ESCULENTA. The French frog. The flesh of this species of frog, very common in France, is highly nutritious and easily digested.

RANCID. Oily substances are said to have become rancid, when, by keeping, they acquire a strong, offensive smell, and altered taste.

RANCIDITY. The change which oils undergo by exposure to air, which is probably an effect analogous to the oxidation of metals.

RANINE. (*Raninus*, from rana, a frog.) 1. Appertaining to a frog.

2. The name of an artery, called also *Arteria ranina*. Sublingual artery. The second branch of the external carotid.

RA'NULA. (From *rana*, a frog: so called from its resemblance to a frog, or because it makes the patient croak like a frog.) *Batrachos; Hypoglossus; Hypoglossum; Rana*. An inflammatory or indolent tumour, under the tongue. These tumours are of various sizes and degrees of consistence, seated on either side of the frænum. Children, as well as adults, are sometimes affected with tumours of this kind; in the former, they impede the action of sucking; in the latter of mastication, and even speech. The contents of them are various; in some, they resemble the saliva, in others, the glairy matter found in the cells of swelled joints. Sometimes it is said that a fatty matter has been found in them; but from the nature and structure of the parts, we are sure that this can seldom happen; and, in by far the greatest number of cases, we find that the contents resemble the saliva itself. This, indeed, might naturally be expected, for the cause of these tumours is universally to be looked for in an obstruction of the salivary ducts. Obstructions here may arise from a cold, inflammation, violent fits of the toothache, attended with swelling in the inside of the mouth; and, in not a few cases, we find the ducts obstructed by a stony matter, seemingly separated from the saliva, as the calculous matter is from the urine; but where inflammation has been the cause, we always find matter mixed with the other contents of the tumour. As these tumours are not usually attended with much pain, they are sometimes neglected; till they burst of themselves, which they commonly do when arrived at the bulk of a large nut. As they were produced originally from an obstruction in the salivary duct, and this obstruction cannot be removed by the bursting of the tumour, it thence happens that they eave an ulcer extremely difficult to heal, nay, which cannot be healed at all till the cause is removed.

RANUNCULOI'DES. (From *ranunculus*, and ειδος, resemblance: so named from its resemblance to the ranunculus.) The marsh marigold. See *Caltha palustris*.

RANU'NCULUS. (Diminutive of *rana*, a frog: because it is found in fenny places, where frogs abound.) The name of a genus of plants in the Linnæan system. Class, *Polyandria*; Order, *Polygynia*.

The great acrimony of most of the species of ranunculus is such, that, on being applied to the skin, they excite itching, redness, and inflammation, and even produce blisters, tumefaction, and ulceration of the part. On being chewed, they corrode the tongue; and, if taken into the stomach, bring on all the deleterious effects of an acrid poison. The corrosive acrimony which this family of plants possesses, was not unknown to the ancients, as appears from the writings of Dioscorides; but its nature and extent had never been investigated by experiments, before those instituted by C. Krapf, at Vienna, by which we learn that the most virulent of the Linnæan species are the bulbosus, sceleratus, acris, arvensis, thora, and illyricus.

The effects of these were tried, either upon himself or upon dogs, and show that the acrimony of the different species is often confined to certain parts of the plants, manifesting itself either in the roots, stalks, leaves, flowers, or buds; the expressed juice, extract, decoction, and infusion of the plants, were also subjected to experiments. In addition to these species mentioned by Krapf, we may also notice the R. Flammula, and especially the R. Alpestris, which, according to Haller, is the most acrid of this genus. Curtis observes, that even pulling up the ranunculus acris, the common meadow species, which possesses the active principle of this tribe, in a very considerable degree, throughout the whole herb, and carrying it to some little distance, excited a considerable inflammation in the palm of the hand in which it was held. It is necessary to remark, that the acrimonious quality of these plants is not of a fixed nature; for it may be completely dissipated by heat; and the plant, on being thoroughly dried, becomes perfectly bland. Krapf attempted to counteract this venomous acrimony of the ranunculus by means of various other vegetables, none of which was found to answer the purpose, though he thought that the juice of sorrel, and that of unripe currants, had some effect in this way; yet these were much less availing than water; while vinegar, honey, sugar, wine, spirit, mineral acids, oil of tartar, p. d. and other sapid substances, manifestly rendered the acrimony more corrosive. It may be also noticed, that the virulency of most of the plants of this genus depends much upon the situation in which they grow, and is greatly diminished in the cultivated plant.

RANUNCULUS ABORTIVUS. The systematic name of a species of ranunculus, which possesses acrid and vesicating properties.

RANUNCULUS ACRIS. The systematic name of the meadow crow-foot. *Ranunculus pratensis*. This, and some other species of ranunculus, have, for medical purposes, been chiefly employed externally as a vesicatory, and are said to have the advantage of a common blistering plaster, in producing a quicker effect, and never causing a strangury; but, on the other

hand, it has been observed, that the ranunculus is less certain in its operation, and that it sometimes occasions ulcers, which prove very troublesome and difficult to heal. Therefore their use seems to be applicable only to certain fixed pains, and such complaints as require a long-continued topical stimulus or discharge from the part, in the way of an issue, which, in various cases, has been found to be a powerful remedy.

RANUNCULUS ALBUS. The plant which bears this name in the pharmacopœias is the *Anemone nemorosa*, of Linnæus. See *Anemone nemorosa*.

RANUNCULUS BULBOSUS. Bulbous-rooted crow-foot. The roots and leaves of this plant, *Ranunculus—calycibus retroflexis, pedunculis sulcatis, caule erecto multifloro, foliis compositis*, of Linnæus, have no considerable smell, but a highly acrid and fiery taste. Taken internally, they appear to be deleterious, even when so far freed from the caustic matter by boiling in water, as to discover no ill quality to the palate. The effluvia, likewise, when freely inspired, are said to occasion headaches, anxieties, vomitings, &c. The leaves and roots, applied externally, inflame and ulcerate, or vesicate the parts, and are liable to affect also the adjacent parts to a considerable extent.

RANUNCULUS FICARIA. The systematic name of the pilewort. *Chelidonium minus; Scrophularia minor; Chelidonia rotundifolia minor · Cursuma hæmorrhoidalis herba; Ranunculus vernus*. Less celandine, and pilewort. The leaves and root of this plant, *Ranunculus—foliis cordatis angulatis petiolatis, caule unifloro*, of Linnæus, are used medicinally. The leaves are deemed anti-scorbutic, and the root reckoned a specific, if beat into cataplasms, and applied to the piles.

RANUNCULUS FLAMMULA. The systematic name of the smaller water crow-foot, or spearwort. *Surrecta alba*. The roots and leaves of this common plant, *Ranunculus—foliis ovatis-lanceolatis, petiolatis, caule declinato*, of Linnæus, taste very acrid and hot, and when taken in a small quantity, produce vomiting, spasms of the stomach, and delirium. Applied externally, they vesicate the skin. The best antidote, after clearing the stomach, is cold water acidulated with lemon-juice, and then mucilaginous drinks.

RANUNCULUS PALUSTRIS. Water crow-foot. See *Ranunculus sceleratus*.

RANUNCULUS PRATENSIS. Meadow crow-foot. See *Ranunculus acris*.

RANUNCULUS SCELERATUS. The systematic name of the marsh crow-foot. *Ranunculus palustris*. The leaves of this species of crow-foot are so extremely acrid, that the beggars in Switzerland are said, by rubbing their legs with them, to produce a very fœtid and acrimonious ulceration.

RA'PA. See *Brassica rapa*.

RAPE. See *Brassica rapa*.

RAPHA'NIA. (From *raphanus*, the radish, or charlock; because the disease is said to be produced by eating the seeds of a species of raphanus.) *Convulsio ab ustilagine; Convulsio raphania; Eclampsia typhodes; Convulsio soloniensis; Necrosis ustilaginea*. Cripple disease. A genus of disease in the class *Neuroses*, and order *Spasmi*, of Cullen; characterized by a spasmodic contraction of the joints, with convulsive motions, and a most violent pain returning at various periods. It begins with cold chills and lassitude, pain in the head, and anxiety about the præcordia. These symptoms are followed by spasmodic twitchings in the tendons of the fingers and of the feet, discernible to the eye, heat, fever, stupor, delirium, sense of suffocation, aphonia, and horrid convulsions of the limbs. After these, vomiting and diarrhœa come on, with a discharge of worms, if there are any. About the eleventh or the twentieth day, copious sweats succeed, or purple exanthema, or tabes, or rigidity of all the joints.

RAPHANISTRUM. The trivial name of a species of raphanus.

RA'PHANUS. (Ραφανος παρα το ραδιως φαινεσθαι: from its quick growth.) 1. A genus of plants in the Linnæan system. Class, *Tetradynamia*; Order, *Siliculosa*.

2. The radish. See *Raphanus sativus*.

RAPHANUS HORTENSIS. See *Raphanus sativus*.

RAPHANUS NIGER. See *Raphanus sativus*.

RAPHANUS RUSTICANUS. See *Cochlearia armoracia*

RAPHANUS SATIVUS. The systematic name of the

radish plant. *Raphanus hortensis ; Radicula ; Rapha-nus niger.* The radish. The several varieties of this plant, are said to be employed medicinally in the cure of calculous affections. The juice, made into a syrup, is given to relieve hoarseness. Mixed with honey or sugar, it is administered in pituitous asthma; and as antiscorbutics, their efficacy is generally acknowledged.

RAPHANUS SYLVESTRIS. See *Lepidium sativum.*

RA'PHE. (Ραφη, a suture.) A suture. Applied to parts which appear as if they were sewed together; as the *Raphe scroti, cerebri,* &c.

RAPHE CEREBRI. The longitudinal eminence of the corpus callosum of the brain is so called, because it appears somewhat like a suture.

RAPHE SCROTI. The rough eminence which divides the scrotum, as it were, in two. It proceeds from the root of the penis inferiorly towards the perinæum.

RAPI'STRUM. (From *rapa,* the turnip; because its leaves resemble those of turnip. Originally, the wild turnip: so called from its affinity to *Rapa,* the cultivated one.) 1. The name of a genus of plants. Class, *Tetradynamia ;* Order, *Siliculosa.*
2. The name of two species of *Crambe,* the *orientalis* and *hispanica.*

RA'PUM. (*Etymology* uncertain.)
1. The turnip. See *Brassica rapa.*
2. The *Campanula rapunculus.*

RAPUNCULUS. (Diminutive of *rapa,* the turnip.) The trivial name of a species of *Campanula.*

RAPUNCULUS CORNICULATUS. See *Phyteuma orbiculare.*

RAPUNCULUS VIRGINIANUS. The name given by Morrison to the blue cardinal flower. See *Lobelia.*

RA'PUS. See *Brassica rapa.*

RASH. See *Exanthema.*

RASPATO'RIUM. (From *rado,* to scrape.) A surgeon's rasp.

RASPBERRY. See *Rubus idæus.*

RASU'RA. (From *rado,* to scrape.)
1. A rasure or scratch.
2. The raspings or shavings of any substance.

RATIFIA. A liquor prepared by imparting to ardent spirits the flavour of various kinds of fruits.

RATTLESNAKE. See *Crotalus horridus*

Rattlesnake-root. See *Polygala senega.*

RAUCE'DO. (From *raucus,* hoarse.) *Raucitas.* Hoarseness. It is always symptomatic of some other disease.

Ray of a flower. See *Radius.*

REAGENT. Test. A substance used in chemistry to detect the presence of other bodies. In the application of tests there are two circumstances to be attended to, viz. to avoid deceitful appearances, and to have good tests.

The principal tests are the following :
1. *Litmus.* The purple of litmus is changed to red by every acid; so that this is the test generally made use of to detect excess of acid in any fluid. It may be used either by dipping into the water a paper stained with litmus, or by adding a drop of the tincture to the water to be examined, and comparing its hue with that of an equal quantity of the tincture in distilled water.

Litmus already reddened by an acid will have its purple restored by an alkali; and thus it may also be used as a test for alkalies, but it is much less active than other direct alkaline tests.

2. *Red cabbage* has been found by Watt to furnish as delicate a test for acids as Litmus, and to be still more sensible to alkalies. The natural colour of an infusion of this plant is blue, which is changed to red by acids, and to green by alkalies in very minute quantities.

3. *Brazil wood.* When chips of this wood are infused in warm water they yield a red liquor, which readily turns blue by alkalies, either caustic or carbonated. It is also rendered blue by the carbonated earths held in solution by carbonic acid, so that it is not an unequivocal test of alkalies till the earthy carbonates have been precipitated by boiling. Acids change to yellow the natural red of Brazil wood, and restore the red when changed by alkalies.

4. *Violets.* The delicate blue of the common scented violet is readily changed to green by alkalies, and this affords a delicate test for these substances. Syrup of violets is generally used as it is at hand, being used in

medicine. But a tincture of the flower will answer as well.

5. *Turmeric.* This is a very delicate test for alkalies, and on the whole, perhaps, is the best. The natural colour either in watery or spirituous infusion is yellow, which is changed to a brick or orange-red by alkalies, caustic or carbonated, but not by carbonated earths, on which account it is preferable to Brazil wood.

The pure earths, such as lime and barytes, produce the same change.

6. *Rhubarb.* Infusion or tincture of rhubarb undergoes a similar change with turmeric, and is equally delicate.

7. *Sulphuric acid.* A drop or two of concentrated sulphuric acid, added to water that contains carbonic acid, free or in combination, causes the latter to escape with a pretty brisk effervescence, whereby the presence of this gaseous acid may be detected.

8. *Nitric and oxymuriatic acid.* A peculiar use attends the employment of these acids in the sulphuretted waters, as the sulphuretted hydrogen is decomposed by them, its hydrogen absorbed, and the sulphur separated in its natural form.

9. *Oxalic acid and oxalate of ammonia.* These are the most delicate tests for lime and all soluble calcareous salts. Oxalate of lime, though nearly insoluble in water, dissolves in a moderate quantity in its own or any other acid, and hence in analysis oxalate of ammonia is often preferred, as no excess of this salt can redissolve the precipitated oxalate of lime. On the other hand, the ammonia should not exceed, otherwise it might give a false indication.

10. *Gallic acid and tincture of galls.* These are tests of iron. Where the iron is in very minute quantities, and the water somewhat acidulous, these tests do not always produce a precipitate, but only a slight reddening, but their action is much heightened by previously adding a few drops of any alkaline solution

11. *Prussiate of potassa or lime.* The presence of iron in water is equally well indicated by these prussiates, causing a blue precipitate: and if the prussiate of potassa is properly prepared, it will only be precipitated by a metallic salt, so that manganese and copper will also be detected, the former giving a white precipitate, the latter a red precipitate.

12. *Lime-water* is the common test for carbonic acid ; it decomposes all the magnesian salts, and likewise the aluminous salts ; it likewise produces a cloudiness with most of the sulphates, owing to the formation of selenite.

13. *Ammonia.* This alkali when perfectly caustic serves as a distinction between the salts of lime and those of magnesia, as it precipitates the earth from the latter salts, but not from the former. There are two sources of error to be obviated, one is that of carbonic acid being present in the water, the other is the presence of aluminous salts.

14. *Carbonated alkalies.* These are used to precipitate all the earths ; where carbonate of potassa is used, particular care should be taken of its purity, as it generally contains silex.

15. *Muriated alumine.* This test is proposed by Mr. Kirwan to detect carbonate of magnesia, which cannot, like carbonated lime, be separated by ebullition, but remains till the whole liquid is evaporated

16. *Barytic salts.* The nitrate, muriate, and acetate of barytes are all equally good tests of sulphuric acid in any combination.

17. *Salts of silver.* The salts of silver are the most delicate tests of muriatic acid, in any combination, producing the precipitated luna cornea. All the salts of silver likewise give a dark-brown precipitate with the sulphuretted waters, which is as delicate a test as any that we possess.

18. *Salts of lead.* The nitrate and acetate of lead are the salts of this metal employed as tests. They will indicate the sulphuric, muriatic, and boracic acids, and sulphuretted hydrogen or sulphuret of potassa.

19. *Soap.* A solution of soap in distilled water or in alkohol is curdled by water containing any earthy or metallic salt.

20. *Tartaric acid.* This acid is of use in distinguishing the salts of potassa (with which it forms a precipitate of cream of tartar), from those of soda, from which it does not precipitate. The potassa, however, must exist in some quantity to be detected by the test

21 *Nitro muriate of platinum.* This sort is still more discriminative between potassa and the other alkalies, than acid of tartar, and will produce a precipitate with a very weak solution of any salt with potassa.

22. *Alkohol.* This most useful reagent is applicable in a variety of ways in analysis. As it dissolves some substances found in fluids, and leaves others untouched, it is a means of separating them into two classes, which saves considerable trouble in the further investigation. Those salts which it does not dissolve, it precipitates from their watery solution, but more or less completely according to the salt contained, and the strength of the alkohol, and as a precipitant it also assists in many decompositions.

REA'LGAR. *Arlada; Arladar; Auripigmentum rubrum; Arsenicum rubrum factitium; Abessi.* A native ore of sulphuret of arsenic.

RECEIVER. A chemical vessel adapted to the neck or beak of a retort, alembic and other distillatory vessel, to receive and contain the product of distillation.

RECEPTA'CULUM. (From *recipio,* to receive.)
1. A name given by the older anatomists to a part of the thoracic duct. See *Receptaculum chyli.*
2. In botany, the common basis or point of connexion of the other parts of the fructification of plants; by some called the *Thalamus* and the *Placenta.*

It is distinguished by botanists into *proper* and *common;* one flower only belongs to the *former,* and it is formed mostly from the apex of the peduncle or scape; as in *Tulipa gesneriana,* and *Lilium candidum.* The *latter* has many flowers; as in Helianthus annuus.

The proper receptacle or apex of the peduncle swells in some flowers, and becomes the fruit: thus the *Fragaria vesca* is not a berry, but a *fleshy receptacle,* with its naked seeds nestling on its surface: so, in the *Hovenia dulcis,* the peduncles swell into a thick *fleshy receptacle* on which there are small capsules; and, in the *Anacardium occidentale,* the peduncle swells into a receptacle, on which the nut rests.

The varieties of the common receptacle are,
1. *Planum;* as in *Helianthus annuus.*
2. *Convexum;* as in *Leontodon taraxacum.*
3. *Conicum;* as in *Billis perennis.*
4. *Punctatum;* as in *Leontodon taraxacum.*
5. *Globosum;* as in *Cephalanthus.*
6. *Ovale;* as in *Dorstenia drakenia.*
7. *Ovatum;* as in *Omphalea.*
8. *Favosum,* cellular on the surface, honeycomb-like; as in *Onopordium.*
9. *Scrobiculatum,* having round and deep holes; as in *Helianthus annuus.*
10. *Subulatum;* as in *Scabiosa atropurpurea.*
11. *Quadrangulum;* as in *Dorstenia houstonii,* and *Contrayerva.*
12. *Turbinatum;* as in *Ficus carica.*
13. *Digitiforme;* as in *Arum maculatum,* and *Calla æthiopica.*
14. *Filiforme,* thread-like; as in the catkins and corylus.
15. *Occlusum.* The *Ficus carica* is a connivent fleshy receptacle enclosing the florets.
16. *Nudum,* without any vesture; as in *Lactuca,* and *Leontodon taraxacum.*
17. *Pilosum;* as in *Carthamus tinctorius.*
18. *Villosum;* as in *Artemisia absynthium.*
19. *Setosum;* as in *Echynops sphærocephalus,* and *Centaurea.*
20. *Paleaceum,* covered with chaffy scales; as in *Zeranthemum, Dipsacus,* &c.

On the receptacle and seed-down are founded the most solid generic characters of syngenesious plants, admirably illustrated by the inimitable Gærtner.

The term receptacle is sometimes extended by Linnæus to express the base of a flower, or even its internal part between the stamens and pistils, provided there be any thing remarkable in such parts, without reference to the foundation of the whole fructification. It also expresses the part to which the seeds are attached in a seed vessel, and the common stalk of a spike, or spikelet, in grasses.

RECEPTACULUM CHYLI. *Receptaculum pecqueti,* because Pécquet first attempted to demonstrate it; *Diversorium; Sacculus chyliferus.* The existence of such a receptacle in the human body is doubted. In brute animals the receptacle of the chyle is situated on the dorsal vertebræ where the lacteals all meet. See *Absorbents.*

Reciprocal affinity. See *Affinity, reciprocal.*

RECLINATUS. Reclining: applied to stems, leaves, &c. which are curved towards the ground; as the stem of the bramble, and leaves of the *Leonurus cardiaca.*

RECTIFICATION (*Rectificatio;* from *rectifico,* to make clear.) A second distillation, in which substances are purified by their more volatile parts being raised by heat carefully managed; thus, spirit of wine, æther, &c. are rectified by their separation from the less volatile and foreign matter which altered or debased their properties.

RE'CTOR SPIRITUS. The aromatic part of plants. See *Aroma.*

RE'CTUM. (*Rectum intestinum:* so named from an erroneous opinion that it was straight.) *Apeuthysmenos; Longanon; Longaon; Archos; Cyssaros.* The last portion of the large intestines terminating in the anus. See *Intestine.*

RE'CTUS. Straight. Several parts of the body, particularly muscles, are so called from their direction.

Parts of plants also have this term; as *Caulis rectus,* the straight stem of the garden-lily, *spinarecta,* &c.

RECTUS ABDOMINIS. *Pubio-sternal,* of Dumas. A long and straight muscle situated near its fellow, at the middle and forepart of the abdomen, parallel to the linea alba, and between the aponeuroses of the other abdominal muscles. It arises sometimes by a single broad tendon from the upper and inner part of the os pubis, but more commonly by two heads, one of which is fleshy, and originates from the upper edge of the pubis, and the other tendinous, from the inside of the symphysis pubis, behind the pyramidalis muscle. From these beginnings, the muscle runs upwards the whole length of the linea alba, and becoming broader and thinner as it ascends, is inserted by a thin aponeurosis into the edge of the cartilago ensiformis, and into the cartilages of the fifth, sixth, and seventh ribs. This aponeurosis is placed under the pectoral muscle, and sometimes adheres to the fourth rib. The fibres of this muscle are commonly divided by three tendinous intersections, which were first noticed by Berenger, or as he is commonly called, Carpi, an Italian anatomist, who flourished in the sixteenth century. One of these intersections is usually where the muscle runs over the cartilage of the seventh rib; another is at the umbilicus; and the third is between these two. Sometimes there is one, and even two, between the umbilicus and the pubes. When one or both of these occur, however, they seldom extend more than half way across the muscle. As these intersections seldom penetrate through the whole substance of the muscle, they are all of them most apparent on its anterior surface, where they firmly adhere to the sheath; the adhesions of the rectus to the posterior layer of the internal oblique, are only by means of cellular membrane, and of a few vessels which pass from one to another.

Albinus and some others have seen this muscle extending as far as the upper part of the sternum.

The use of the rectus is to compress the forepart of the abdomen, but more particularly the lower part; and according to the different positions of the body, it may likewise serve to bend the trunk forwards, or to raise the pelvis. Its situation between the two layers of the internal oblique, and its adhesions to this sheath, secure it in its place, and prevent it from rising into a prominent form when in action: and, lastly, its tendinous intersections enable it to contract at any of the intermediate spaces.

RECTUS ABDUCENS OCULI. See *Rectus externus oculi.*

RECTUS ADDUCENS OCULI. See *Rectus internus oculi.*

RECTUS ANTERIOR BREVIS. See *Rectus capitis internus minor.*

RECTUS ANTERIOR LONGUS. See *Rectus capitis internus major.*

RECTUS ATTOLLÉNS OCULI. See *Rectus superior oculi.*

RECTUS CAPITIS ANTICUS LONGUS. See *Rectus capitis internus major.*

RECTUS CAPITIS INTERNUS MAJOR. A muscle situated on the anterior part of the neck, close to the vertebræ. *Rectus internus major,* of Albinus, Douglas, and Cowper *Trachelobasilaire,* of Dumas. *Rectus*

235

anterior longus, of Winslow. It was known to most of the ancient anatomists, but was not distinguished by any particular name until Cowper gave it the present appellation, and which has been adopted by most writers except Winslow. It is a long muscle, thicker and broader above than below, where it is thin, and terminates in a point. It arises, by distinct and flat tendons, from the anterior points of the transverse processes of the five inferior vertebræ of the neck, and ascending obliquely upwards is inserted into the anterior part of the cuneiform process of the occipital bone. The use of this muscle is to bend the head forwards.

RECTUS CAPITIS INTERNUS MINOR. Cowper, who was the first accurate describer of this little muscle, gave it the name of *rectus internus minor,* which has been adopted by Douglas and Albinus. Winslow calls it *rectus anterior brevis,* and Dumas *petit-trachelo-basilaire.* It is in part covered by the rectus major. It arises fleshy from the upper and forepart of the body of the first vertebra of the neck, near the origin of its transverse process, and, ascending obliquely inwards, is inserted near the root of the condyloid process of the occipital bone, under the last described muscle. It assists in bending the head forwards.

RECTUS CAPITIS LATERALIS. *Rectus lateralis Fallopii,* of Douglas. *Transversalis anticus primus,* of Winslow. *Rectus lateralis,* of Cowper; and *Tracheli-altoido basilaire,* of Dumas. This muscle seems to have been first described by Fallopius. Winslow calls it *transversalis anticus primus.* It is somewhat larger than the rectus minor, but resembles it in shape, and is situated immediately behind the internal jugular vein; at its coming out of the cranium. It arises fleshy from the upper and forepart of the transverse process of the first vertebra of the neck, and, ascending a little obliquely upwards and outwards, is inserted into the occipital bone, opposite to the stylo-mastoid hole of the os temporis. This muscle serves to pull the head to one side.

RECTUS CAPITIS POSTICUS MAJOR. This muscle, which is the *rectus major* of Douglas and Winslow, the *rectus capitis posticus minor* of Albinus, and the *spine-axoido-occipital* of Dumas, is small, short, and flat, broader above than below, and is situated, not in a straight direction, as its name would insinuate, but obliquely, between the occiput and the second vertebra of the neck, immediately under the complexus. It arises, by a short, thick tendon, from the upper and posterior part of the spinous process of the second vertebra of the neck; it soon becomes broader, and, ascending obliquely outwards, is inserted, by a flat tendon, into the external lateral part of the lower semicircular ridge of the os occipitis. The use of this is to extend the head, and pull it backwards.

RECTUS CAPITIS POSTICUS MINOR. This is the *rectus minor* of Douglas and Winslow, and the *tuber-altoido-occipital* of Dumas. It is smaller than the last-described muscle, but resembles it in shape, and is placed close by its fellow, in the space between the recti majores. It arises, by a short, thick tendon, from the upper and lateral part of a little protuberance in the middle of the back part of the first vertebra of the neck, and, becoming broader and thinner as it ascends, is inserted, by a broad, flat tendon, into the occipital bone, immediately under the insertion of the last-described muscle. The use of it is to assist the rectus major in drawing the head backwards.

RECTUS CRURIS. See *Rectus femoris.*

RECTUS DEPRIMENS OCULI. See *Rectus inferior oculi.*

RECTUS EXTERNUS OCULI. The outer straight muscle of the eye. *Abductor oculi; Iracundus; Indignabundus.* It arises from the bony partition between the foramen opticum and lacerum, being the longest of the straight muscles of the eye, and is inserted into the sclerotic membrane, opposite to the outer canthus of the eye. Its use is to move the eye outwards.

RECTUS FEMORIS. A straight muscle of the thigh, situated immediately at the forepart. *Rectus cive Gracilis anterior,* of Winslow. *Rectus cruris,* of Albinus; and *Ilio-rotulien,* of Dumas. It arises from the os ilium by two tendons. The foremost and shortest of these springs from the outer surface of the inferior and anterior spinous process of the ilium; the posterior tendon, which is thicker and longer than the other, arises from the posterior and outer part of the edge of the cotyloid cavity, and from the adjacent capsular liga-

ment. These two tendons soon unite, and form an aponeurosis, which spreads over the anterior surface of the upper part of the muscle; and through its whole length we observe a middle tendon, towards which its fleshy fibres run on each side in an oblique direction, so that it may be styled a penniform muscle. It is inserted tendinous into the upper edge and anterior surface of the patella, and from thence sends off a thin aponeurosis, which adheres to the superior and lateral part of the tibia. Its use is to extend the leg.

RECTUS INFERIOR OCULI. The inferior of the straight muscles of the eye. *Depressor oculi; Deprimens; Humilis; Amatorius.* It arises within the socket from below the optic foramen, and passes forwards to be inserted into the sclerotic membrane of the bulb on the under part. It pulls the eye downwards.

RECTUS INTERNUS FEMORIS. See *Gracilis.*

RECTUS INTERNUS OCULI. The internal straight muscle of the eye. *Adducens oculi; Adductor oculi; Bibitorius.* It arises from the inferior part of the foramen opticum, between the obliquus superior, and the rectus inferior, being, from its situation, the shortest muscle of the eye, and is inserted into the sclerotic membrane opposite to the inner angle. Its use is to turn the eye towards the nose.

RECTUS LATERALIS FALLOPII. See *Rectus capitis lateralis.*

RECTUS MAJOR CAPITIS. See *Rectus capitis posticus major.*

RECTUS SUPERIOR OCULI. The uppermost straight muscle of the eye. *Attollens oculi. Levator oculi. Superbus.* It arises from the upper part of the foramen opticum of the sphenoid bone below the levator palpebræ superioris, and runs forward to be inserted into the superior and forepart of the sclerotic membrane by broad and thin tendon.

RECURRENT. (*Recurrens:* so named from direction.) Reflected.

RECURRENT NERVE. Two branches of the par vagum in the cavity of the thorax are so called. The right is given off near the subclavian artery, which surrounds, and is reflected upwards to the thyroid gland; the left a little lower, and reflected around the aorta to the œsophagus, as far as the larynx. They are both distributed to the muscles of the larynx and pharynx.

RECURVUS. Recurved; reflexed; turned backward: applied to the leaves of the *Erica retorta.*

Red saunders. See *Pterocarpus santalinus.*

REDDLE. A species of ochre or argillaceous earth, of a dark red colour, which has been used medicinally as a tonic and antacid.

REDUCTION. Revivification. This word, in its most extensive sense, is applicable to all operations by which any substance is restored to its natural state, or which is considered as such: but custom confines it to operations by which metals are restored to their metallic state, after they have been deprived of this, either by combustion, as the metallic oxides, or by the union of some heterogeneous matters which disguise them, as fulminating gold, luna cornea, cinnabar, and other compounds of the same kind. These reductions are also called revivifications.

REFLEXUS. Reflected; recurved; bent backward: applied to the leaves of plants, as the *Erica retorta,* and to the border of the flower-cup of the *Œnothera biennis,* and the petals of the *Pancratium zeylanicum.*

REFRIGERANT. (*Refrigerans;* from *refrigero,* to cool.) Medicines which allay the heat of the body or of the blood.

REFRIGERATO'RIUM. (From *refrigero,* to cool.) A vessel filled with water to condense vapours, or to make cool any substance which passes through it.

RE'GIMEN. (From *rego,* to govern.) A term employed in medicine to express the plan or regulation of the diet.

REGI'NA. A queen. A name given by way of excellence to some plants.

REGINA PRATI. See *Spiræa ulmaria.*

REGION. (*Regio, onis.* f. *à rego.*) A part of the body; generally applied to external parts, under which is some particular viscus, that the particular place may be known. Anatomists have divided the regions, or several parts of the body when entire, as follows:

Into *caput,* or head; *truncus,* or trunk; and *extremitates,* or extremities.

A. The head is divided into

1. *Facies*, the face.

2. *Pars capillata*, the scalp.

The regions of the scalp are,

a *Vertex* the top or crown of the head.

b. *Synciput*, the forepart of the scalp.

c. *Occiput*, the back part of the head.

d. *Partes laterales*, the sides.

The regions of the face are,

a. *Frons*, the forehead.

b. *Tempora*, the temples.

c. *Nasus*, the nose, on which are, the *radix*, or root; the *dorsum* or bridge; the *apex*, or tip; and the *alœ*, or sides.

d. *Oculus*, the eye.

e. *Os*, the mouth, the external parts of which are, *labia*, the lips; *anguli oris*, where the lips meet; *philtrum*, an oblong depression in the middle of the upper lip.

f. *Mentum*, the chin, the hair of which is called *barba*, whereas that of the upper lip is termed *mistax*.

g. *Buccæ*, the cheeks.

h. *Auris*, the ear, on which are the *auricula*, *helix*, *antihelix*, *tragus*, *antitragus*, *concha*, *scapha*, and *lobulus*.

B. The trunk is divided into the *collum*, or neck; the *thorax*, or chest; the *abdomen*, or belly.

1. *Collum*, the neck, which has,

a. *Pars antica*, in which is the *pomum adami*, or *arynx*.

b. *Pars postica*, in which is the *fossa*, and *nucha*, or nape of the neck.

2. *Thorax*, the chest, which is divided into,

a. The front, on which are *mammæ*, the breasts, and *scrobiculus cordis*, the pit of the stomach.

b. The back part, or *dorsum*.

c. The sides.

3. *Abdomen*, is divided into the forepart, which is strictly the abdomen, or belly; the hindpart, or *lumbi*, the loins; the lateral parts or sides.

On the abdomen, or forepart, are the following regions:—

The *Epigastric*, the sides of which are termed *hypochondria*.

The *Umbilical*, the sides of which are termed *epicolic* regions.

The *Hypogastric*, the sides of which are the *ilia*.

The *Pubes* is the region below the abdomen, covered with hair; in women, termed *mons veneris*: the sides are *inguina*, or groins.

Below the pubes are the parts of generation in men, the *scrotum* and *penis*; in women, the *labia pudendi*, and the *rima vulvæ*. The space between the genitals and *anus* is called *perinæum*, or fork.

C. The extremities are the *superior* and the *inferior*. The upper extremity has,

1. The shoulder or top, under which is the *axilla*, or arm-pit.

2. The *brachium*, or arm.

3. The *antibrachium*, or fore-arm, in which are the bend, or *flexura*, and elbow.

4. The *manus*, or hand, which has *vola*, the palm; and *dorsum*, the back; and is divided into the *carpus*, or wrist, the *metacarpus*, and fingers.

The lower extremity embraces,

1. The *femur*, or thigh, the upper and outer part of which is called *coxa*, or the *regio ischiadica*.

2. The *crus*, or leg, in which are the *genu*, or knee, *cavum popletis*, or ham, and the *sura*, or calf.

3. The *pes*, or foot, which is divided into the *tarsus*, *metatarsus*, and toes.

The upper part of the tarsus laterally has the *malleolus externus* and *internus*, or the inner and outer ankle.

RE′GIUS. (From *rex*, a king.) Royal: applied to a disease, and to a chemical preparation; to the former, the jaundice, because in it the colour of the skin is like gold; and to the latter, because it dissolves gold.

REGULAR. *Regularis*. A term applied to diseases, which observe their usual course, in opposition to irregular, in which the course of symptoms deviate from what is usual, as regular gout, regular small-pox, &c.

Regular gout. See *Arthritis*.

RE′GULUS. (Diminutive of *rex*, a king: so called because the alchemist expected to find gold, the king of metals, collected at the bottom of the crucible after fusion.) The name regulus was given by chemists to metallic matters when separated from other substances by fusion. This name was introduced by alchemists, who, expecting always to find gold in the metal collected at the bottom of their crucibles after fusion, called this metal, thus collected, regulus, as containing gold, the king of metals. It was afterward applied to the metal extracted from the ores of the semi-metals, which formerly bore the name that is now given to the semi-metals themselves. Thus we had regulus of antimony, regulus of arsenic, and regulus of cobalt.

Regulus of antimony. See *Antimony.*

Regulus of arsenic. See *Arsenic.*

REME′DIUM. (*A re*, and *medeor*, to cure.) A remedy, or that which is employed with a view to prevent, palliate, or remove a disease.

REMEDIUM DIVINUM. See *Imperatoria.*

REMEDY. See *Remedium.*

REMINISCENCE. See *Memory.*

REMITTENT. (*Remittens*; from *remitto*, to assuage or lessen.) Any disorder, the symptoms of which diminish very considerably, and return again, so as not to leave the person ever free.

Remittent fever. See *Febris intermittens.*

RE′MORA ARATRI. (From *remoror*, to hinder, and *aratrum*, a plough.) See *Ononis spinosa.*

Remote cause. See *Exciting cause.*

REN. (*Ren*, *nis*, m. *Ren*, απο τoυ ρειν; because through them the urine flows.) The kidney. See *Kidney.*

RENAL. (*Renalis*; from *ren*, the kidney.) Appertaining to the kidney.

Renal artery. See *Emulgent artery.*

RENAL GLAND. *Glandulæ renalis.* Renal capsule. Supra-renal gland. The supra-renal glands are two hollow bodies, like glands in fabric, and placed, one on each side, upon the kidney. They are covered by a double tunic, and their cavities are filled with a liquor of a brownish red colour. Their figure is triangular; and they are larger in the fœtus than the kidneys; but, in adults, they are less than the kidneys. The right is affixed to the liver, the left to the spleen and pancreas, and both to the diaphragm and kidneys. They have arteries, veins, lymphatics, and nerves; their arteries arise from the diaphragmatic, the aorta, and the renal arteries. The vein of the right supra-renal gland empties itself into the vena cava; that of the left into the renal vein; their lymphatic vessels go directly into the thoracic duct; they have nerves common alike to these glands and the kidneys. They have no excretory duct, and their use is at present unknown. It is supposed they answer one use in the fœtus, and another in the adult, but what these uses are is uncertain. Boerhaave supposed their use to consist in their furnishing lymph to dilute the blood returned, after the secretion of the urine, in the renal vein; but this is very improbable, since the vein of the right supra-renal gland goes to the vena cava, and the blood carried back by the renal vein wants no dilution. It has also been said, that these glands not only prepare lymph, by which the blood is fitted for the nutrition of the delicate fœtus; but that in adults they serve to restore to the blood of the vena cava the irritable parts which it loses by the secretion of bile and urine. Some, again, have considered them as diverticula in the fœtus, to divert the blood from the kidneys, and lessen the quantity of urine. The celebrated Morgagni believed their office to consist in conveying something to the thoracic duct. It is singular, that in children who are born without the cerebrum, these glands are extremely small, and sometimes wanting.

Renal vein. See *Emulgent vein.*

Renal vessels. See *Emulgent.*

RENIFORMIS. Kidney-shaped. 1. In anatomy, this term is applied to any deviations of parts assuming a kidney-like form.

2. In botany, leaves, seeds, &c. are so called from their shape; it is a short, broad, roundish leaf, the base of which is hollowed out, as that of the *Asarum europæum*, and *Sibthorpia europæa*, and the seeds of *Beta* and *Phaseolus*.

RENNET. Runnet. The gastric juice and contents of the stomach of calves. It is much employed in preparing cheese, and in pharmacy, for making whey. To about a pound of milk, in a silver or earthen basin, placed on hot ashes, add three or four grains of rennet, diluted with a little water; as it becomes cold, the milk curdles, and the whey, or serous part, separates itself from the caseous part. When these parts appear perfectly distinct, pour the whole upon a strainer, through which the whey will pass, while the curds remain behind. This whey is always rendered somewhat whitish, by a very small and much divided portion of the caseous part; but it may be separated in such a manner, that the whey will remain limpid and colourless, and this is what is called clarifying it. Put into a basin the white of an egg, a glass of the serum of milk, and a few grains of tartaric acid in powder; whip the mixture with an ozier twig, and, having added the remainder of the unclarified whey, place the mixture again over the fire until it begins to boil. The tartaric acid completes the coagulation of the white part of the milk which remains; the white of egg, as it becomes hot, coagulates and envelopes the caseous part. When the whey is clear, filter it through paper: what passes will be perfectly limpid, and have a greenish colour. This is clarified whey.

RE′NUENS. (From *renuo*, to nod the head back in sign of refusal: so called from its office of jerking back the head.) A muscle of the head.

REPANDUS. Repand; wavy: a leaf is so called which is bordered with many acute angles, and small segments of circles alternately; as that of the Menyanthes nymphæoides.

REPELLE′NT. (*Repellens ; from repello*, to drive back.) Applications are sometimes so named which make diseases recede, as it were, from the surface of the body.

REPENS. Creeping; often used in botany: *caulis repens*, one that creeps along the earth, as that of the Ranunculus repens. Applied to a root, it means running transversely, and here and there giving off new plants ; as that of the Glycyrrhiza glabra, and Sambucus ebulus.

REPULSION. All matter possesses a power which is in constant opposition to attraction. This agency, which is equally powerful and equally obvious, acts an important part in the phenomena of nature, and is called *the power of repulsion.*

That such a force exists, which opposes the approach of bodies towards each other, is evident from numberless facts.

Newton has shown, that when a convex lens is put upon a flat glass, it remains at a distance of the one-hundred-and-thirty-seventh part of an inch, and a very considerable pressure is required to diminish this distance; nor does any force which can be applied bring them into actual mathematical contact. A force may indeed be applied sufficient to break the glasses into pieces, but it may be demonstrated that it does not diminish their distance much beyond the one-thousandth part of an inch. There is, therefore, a repulsive force, which prevents the two glasses from touching each other.

Boscovich has shown, that when an ivory billiard-ball sets another in motion, by striking against it, an equal quantity of its own motion is lost, and the ball at rest begins to move while the other is still at a distance.

There exists, therefore, a repulsion between bodies; this repulsion takes place while they are yet at a distance from each other ; and it opposes their approach towards each other.

The cause or the nature of this force is equally inscrutable with that of attraction, but its existence is undoubted: it increases, as far as has been ascertained, inversely as the square of the distance, consequently at the point of contact it is infinite.

The following experiments will serve to prove the energy of repulsion more fully.

Experiment.—When a glass tube is immersed in water, the fluid is attracted by the glass, and drawn up into the tube; but, if we substitute mercury instead of water, we shall find a different effect. If a glass tube of any bore be immersed in this fluid, it does not rise, but the surface of the mercury is considerably below the level of that which surrounds it, when the diameter of the tube is very small.

In this case, therefore, a repulsion takes place between the glass and the mercury, which is even considerably greater than the attraction existing between the particles of the mercury; and hence the latter cannot rise in the tube, but is repelled, and becomes depressed.

239

Experiment.—When we present the north pole of a magnet A, to the same pole of another magnet B, suspended on a pivot, and at liberty to move, the magnet B will recede as the other approaches; and, by following it with A, at a proper distance, it may be made to turn round on its pivot with considerable velocity.

In this case, there is evidently some agency, which opposes the approach of the north poles of A and B, which acts as an antagonist, and causes the moveable magnet to retire before the other. There is, therefore, a *repulsion* between the two magnets, a repulsion which increases with the power of the magnets, which may be made so great, that all the force of a strong man is insufficient to make the two north poles touch each other. The same repulsion is equally obvious in electrical bodies, for instance:

Experiment.—If two small cork balls be suspended from a body, so as to touch one another, and if we charge the body in the usual manner with electricity, the two cork balls separate from each other, and stand at a distance proportional to the quantity of electricity with which the body is charged; the balls, of course, repel each other.

Experiment.—If we rub over the surface of a sheet of paper the fine dust of lycopodium, or puff-ball, and then let water fall on it in small quantities, the water will instantly be repelled, and form itself into distinct drops, which do not touch the lycopodium, but roll over it with uncommon rapidity. That the drops do not touch the lycopodium, but are actually kept at a distance above it, is obvious from the copious reflection of white light.

Experiment.—If the surface of water contained in a basin be covered over with lycopodium, a solid substance, deposited at the bottom of the fluid, may be taken out of it with the hand, without wetting it. In this case, the repulsion is so powerful as to defend the hand completely from the contact of the fluid.

RES. A thing.

RES NATURALES. The naturals. According to Boerhaave, these are life, the cause of life, and its effects These, he says, remain in some degree, however disordered a person may be.

RES NON-NATURALES. See *Non-naturals.*

RESE′DA. (From *resedo*, to appease: so called from its virtue of allaying inflammation.) The name of a genus of plants in the Linnæan system. Class, *Dodecandria; Order, Trigynia.*

2. The name, in some pharmacopœias, of the dyers' weed. See *Reseda luteola.*

RESEDA LUTEOLA. The systematic name of the dyers' weed. Dioscorides mentions it as useful in jaundice.

RESIN. *Resina.* The name *resin* is used to denote solid inflammable substances, of vegetable origin, soluble in alkohol, usually affording much soot by their combustion. They are likewise soluble in oils, but not at all in water; and are more or less acted upon by the alkalies.

All the resins appear to be nothing else but volatile oils rendered concrete by their combination with oxygen. The exposure of these to the open air, and the decomposition of acids applied to them, evidently prove this conclusion.

There are some among the known resins which are very pure, and perfectly soluble in alkohol, such as the balsam of Mecca and of Capivi, turpentines, tacamahaca, elemi : others are less pure, and contain a small portion of extract, which renders them not totally soluble in alkohol ; such are mastic, sandarach, guaiacum, labdanum, and dragon's blood.

The essential properties of resin are, being in the solid form, insoluble in water, perfectly soluble in alkohol, and in essential and expressed oils, and being incapable of being volatilized without decomposition.

Resins are obtained chiefly from the vegetable kingdom, either by spontaneous exudation, or from incisions made into vegetables affording juices which contain this principle. These juices contain a portion of essential oil, which, from exposure to the air, is either volatilized or converted into resinous matter, or sometimes the oil is abstracted by distillation. In some plants the resin is deposited, in a concrete state, in the interstices of the wood, or other parts of the plant.

Resins, when concrete, are brittle, and have generally a smooth and conchoidal fracture; their lustre is peculiar, they are more or less transparent and of a colour which is usually some shade of yellow, or brown; they are of a greater specific gravity than water; they are often odorous and sapid, easily fusible, and, on cooling, become solid.

Resin, black. See *Resina nigra.*
Resin, elastic. See *Caoutchouc.*
Resin-tree, elastic. See *Caoutchouc.*
Resin, white. See *Resina alba.*
Resin, yellow. See *Resina flava.*

RESI'NA. (From ρεω, to flow: because it flows spontaneously from the tree.) See *Resin.*

RESINA ALBA. The inspissated juice of the *Pinus sylvestris,* &c. is so called; and sometimes the residuum of the distillation of oil of turpentine. See *Resina flava.*

RESINA ELASTICA. See *Caoutchouc.*

RESINA FLAVA. *Resina alba.* Yellow resin, what remains in the still after distilling oil of turpentine, by adding water to the common turpentine. It is of very extensive use in surgery as an active detergent, and forms the base of the *unguentum resinæ flavæ.*

RESINA NIGRA. *Colophonia.* What remains in the retort after distilling the oil of turpentine from the common turpentine. This name is also given, in the London Pharmacopœia, to pitch.

RESINA NOVI BELGII. See *Botany-bay.*

RESOLUTION. (*Resolutio;* from *resolvo,* to loosen.) A termination of inflammation in which the disease disappears without any abscess, mortification, &c. being occasioned.

The term is also applied to the dispersion of swellings, indurations, &c.

RESOLVENT. (*Resolvens;* from *resolvo,* to loosen.) This term is applied by surgeons to such substances as discuss inflammatory and other tumours.

RESPIRATION. (*Respiratio;* from *respiro,* to take breath.) To comprehend the important function of breathing or respiration, it is not only necessary to have a knowledge of the structure of the thoracic viscera, the form of the parietes, of the chest, and to comprehend the mechanism by which the air enters and passes out of it, but also to be well acquainted with the chemical and physical properties of the air, and the circulation of the blood.

The lungs are two spongy and vascular organs of a considerable size, situated in the lateral parts of the chest. Their parenchyma is divided and subdivided into lobes and lobules, the forms and dimensions of which it is difficult to determine.

We learn, by the careful examination of a pulmonary lobule, that it is formed of a spongy tissue, the *areolæ* of which are so small that a strong lens is necessary to observe them distinctly; these *areolæ* all communicate with each other, and they are surrounded by a thin layer of cellular tissue which separates them from the adjoining lobules.

Into each lobule enters one of the divisions of the bronchia, and one of the pulmonary artery; this last is distributed in the body of the lobule in a manner that is not well known; it seems to be transformed into numerous radicles of the pulmonary veins. Dr. Magendie believes that these numerous small vessels, by which the artery terminates and the pulmonary veins begin, by crossing and joining in different manners, form the *areolæ* of the tissue of the lobules. The small bronchial division that ends in the lobule, does not enter into the interior of it, but breaks off as soon as it has arrived at the parenchyma.

This last circumstance appears remarkable: because, since the bronchia do not penetrate into the spongy tissue of the lungs, it is not probable that the surface of the cells with which the air is in contact is covered by the mucous membrane. The most minute anatomy cannot prove its existence in this place.

A part of the nerve of the eighth pair, and some filaments of the sympathetic, are expended on the lungs, but it is not known how they are distributed; the surface of the organ is covered by the pleura, a serous membrane, similar to the *peritonæum* in its structure and functions.

Round the *bronchia,* and near the place where they enter into the tissue of the lungs, a certain number of lymphatic glands exist, the colour of which is almost black, and to which the small number of lymphatic vessels which spring from the surface and from the interior of the pulmonary tissue are directed.

With regard to the lungs, we receive from the art of delicate injections some information that we ought not to neglect.

If we inject mercury, or even coloured water, into the pulmonary artery, the injected matter passes immediately into the pulmonary veins, but at the same time a part enters the *bronchia,* and goes out by the *trachea.* If the matter be injected into a pulmonary vein, it passes partly into the artery and partly into the bronchia. Lastly, if it be introduced into the trachea, it very soon penetrates into the artery, into the pulmonary veins, and even into the *bronchial* artery and vein.

The lungs fill up a great part of the cavity of the chest, and enlarge and contract with it; and as they communicate with the external air by the trachea and the larynx, every time that the chest enlarges it is distended by the air, which is again expelled when the chest resumes its former dimensions. We must then necessarily stop to examine this cavity.

The breast, or the thorax, is of the form of a *cone,* the summit of which is above, and the base below.

The apparent form and dimensions of the breast are determined by the length, disposition, and motions of the ribs upon the vertebra.

The chest is capable of being dilated vertically, transversely, forward and backward, that is, in the direction of its principal diameters.

The principal, and almost the only, agent of the vertical dilatation, is the diaphragm, which, in contracting, tends to lose its vaulted form, and to become a plane; a motion which cannot take place without the pectoral motion of the thorax increasing, and the abdominal portion diminishing.

The sides of this muscle, which are fleshy, and correspond with the lungs, descend farther than the centre, which, being aponeurotic, can make no effort by itself, and which is, besides, retained by its union with the *sternum* and the *pericardium.*

In most cases this lowering of the diaphragm is sufficient for the dilatation of the breast; but it often happens that the sternum and the ribs, in changing the position between them and the vertebral column, produce a sensible augmentation in the pectoral cavity.

In the general elevation of the thorax, its form necessarily changes, as well as the relations of the bones of which it is composed: the cartilages of the ribs seem particularly intended to assist these changes; as soon as they are ossified, and consequently lose their elasticity, the breast becomes immoveable.

While the sternum is carried upwards, its inferior extremity is directed a little forward: it thus undergoes a slight swinging motion; the ribs become less oblique upon the vertebral column; they remove a little from each other, and their inferior edge is directed outward by a small tension of the cartilage. All these phenomena are not very apparent except in the superior ribs.

A general enlargement of the thorax takes place by its elevation, as well from front to back, as transversely, and upwards.

This enlargement is called *inspiration.* It presents three degrees: 1st, ordinary *inspiration,* which takes place by the depression of the diaphragm, and an almost insensible elevation of the thorax; 2dly, the *great* inspiration, in which there is an evident elevation of the thorax, and, at the same time, a depression of the diaphragm; 3dly, *forced* inspiration, in which the dimensions of the thorax are augmented in every direction, as far as the physical disposition of this cavity will permit.

Expiration succeeds to the dilatation of the thorax; that is, the return of the thorax to its ordinary position and dimensions.

The mechanism of this motion is the reverse of what we have just described. It is produced by the elasticity of the cartilages, and by the ligaments of the ribs, which have a tendency to resume their former shape, by the relaxation of the muscles that had raised the thorax, and by the contraction of a great number of muscles, so disposed that they lower and contract the chest.

The contraction of the thorax, or expiration, presents also three degrees: 1st, *ordinary expiration;* 2d, *great expiration;* 3d, *forced expiration.*

In ordinary expiration, the relaxation of the diaphragm, pressed upwards by the abdominal viscera, which are themselves urged by the anterior muscles of this cavity, produces the diminution of the vertical diameter; vehement expiration is produced by the relaxation of the inspiring muscles, and a slight contraction of those of expiration, which permits the ribs to assume their ordinary relations with the vertebral column. But the contraction of the chest may go still farther. If the abdominal and other expiratory muscles contract forcibly, a greater depression of the diaphragm takes place, the ribs descend lower, the base of the *conoid* shrinks, and there is, consequently, a greater diminution of the capacity of the thorax. This is called forced expiration.

We shall now consider the air as an elastic fluid, which possesses the property of exerting pressure upon the bodies it surrounds, and upon the sides of the vessels that contain it. This property supposes, in the particles of air, a continual tendency to repulse each other.

Another property of the air is *compressibility;* that is, its volume changes with the pressure which it supports.

The air expands by heat like all other bodies; its volume augments 1-480, by an increase of one degree of Fahrenheit's thermometer.

The air has weight: this is ascertained by weighing a vessel full of air, and then weighing the same vessel after the air has been taken out by the air-pump.

The air is more or less charged with humidity.

Air, notwithstanding its thinness and transparency, refracts, intercepts, and reflects the light.

The air is composed of two gases that are very different in their properties.

1st, Oxygen: this gas is a little heavier than air, in the proportion of 11 to 10, and it combines with all the simple bodies; it is an element of water, of vegetable and animal matters, and of almost all known bodies; it is essential for combustion and respiration. 2dly, Azote: this gas is a little lighter than air; it is an element of ammonia and of animal substances; it extinguishes bodies in combustion.

It has been thus found that 100 parts in weight of air contain 21 parts of oxygen and 79 of azote. These proportions are the same in every place and at all heights, and have not sensibly changed for these fifteen years, since they were positively established by chemistry.

Besides oxygen and azote, the air contains a variable quantity of the vapour of water, as we have already observed, and a *small quantity* of carbonic acid, the proportion of which has not yet been positively fixed.

The air is decomposed by almost all combustible bodies, at a temperature which is peculiar to each. In this decomposition they combine with the oxygen, and set the azote at liberty.

Of inspiration and expiration.—If we call to mind the disposition of the pulmonary lobules, the extensibility of their tissue, their communication with the external air by means of the bronchia, of the trachea, and of the larynx, we will easily conceive that every time the breast dilates, the air immediately enters the pulmonary tissue, in a quantity proportionate to the degree of dilatation. When the breast contracts, a part of the air that it contains is expelled, and passes out by the glottis.

In order to arrive at the glottis in inspiration, or to go outwards in expiration, the air sometimes traverses the nasal canal and sometimes the mouth: the position of the velum of the palate, in these two cases, deserves to be described. When the air traverses the nasal canals and the pharynx to enter or to pass out of the larynx, the velum of the palate is vertical, and placed with its anterior surface against the posterior part of the base of the tongue, so that the mouth has no communication with the larynx. When the air traverses the mouth in inspiration or expiration, the velum of the palate is horizontal, its posterior edge is embraced by the concave surface of the pharynx, and all communication is cut off between the inferior parts of the pharynx and the superior part of this canal, as well as with the nasal canals. Thence the necessity of making the sick breathe by the mouth, if it is necessary to examine the tonsils or the pharynx.

These two ways for the air to arrive at the glottis were necessary, for they assist each other: thus when the mouth is full of food, the respiration takes place by the nose; it takes place by the mouth when the nasal canals are obstructed by mucus, by a slight swelling of the membrane, or any other cause. The

glottis opens in the instant of inspiration, and, on the contrary, it shuts in the expiration.

It appears that in a given time the number of inspirations made by one person are very different from those of another. Haller thinks there are twenty in the space of a minute. A man upon whom Menzies made experiments respired only fourteen times in a minute. Sir H. Davy informs us that he respires in the same period twenty-six or twenty-seven times, Dr. Thomson says that he respires generally nineteen times; and Dr. Magendie only respires fifteen times. Taking twenty times in a minute for the mean, this will give 28,800 inspirations in twenty-four hours. But this number probably varies according to many circumstances, such as the state of sleep, motion, distention of the stomach by food, the capacity of the chest, moral affections, &c. What quantity of air enters the chest at each inspiration? What quantity goes out at each expiration? How much generally remains?

According to Menzies, the mean quantity of air that enters the lungs at each inspiration, is 40 cubic inches. Goodwin thinks that the quantity remaining after a complete expiration is 109 cubic inches; Menzies affirms that this quantity is greater, and that it amounts to 179 cubic inches.

According to Davy, after a forced expiration, his lungs contained 41 cubic inches.

After a natural expiration 118
After a natural inspiration 135
After a forced inspiration............... 254
By a forced expiration, after a forced inspiration, there passed out of the lungs 190
After a natural inspiration............... 78.5
After a natural expiration .... 67.5 c. i.

Dr. Thomson thinks that we should not be far from the truth in supposing that the ordinary quantity of air contained in the lungs is 280, and that there enter or go out at each inspiration, or expiration, 40 inches Thus, supposing 20 inspirations in a minute, the quantity of air that would enter and pass out in this time would be 800 inches; which makes 48,000 in the hour, and in 24 hours 1,152,000 cubic inches. A great number of experiments have been made by chemists to determine if the volume of air diminishes while it remains in the lungs. In considering the latest experiments, it appears, that in most cases there is no diminution; that is, a volume of expired air is exactly the same as one of inspired air. When this diminution takes place it appears to be only accidental.

By successively traversing the mouth or the nasal cavities, the pharynx, the larynx, the trachia, and the bronchia, the inspired air becomes of a similar temperature with the body. It most generally becomes heated, and consequently rarified, so that the same quantity in weight of air occupies a much greater space in the lungs than it occupied before it entered them. Besides this change of volume, the inspired air is charged with the vapour that it carries away from the mucous membranes of the air-passages, and in this state always, hot and humid, it arrives in the pulmonary lobules; also this portion of air of which we treat mixes with that which the lungs contained before.

But expiration soon succeeds to inspiration: an interval, only of a few seconds, passes in general between them; the air contained by the lungs, pressed by the powers of expiration, escapes by the expiratory canal in a contrary direction to that of the inspired air.

We must here remark that the portion of air expired is not exactly that which was inspired immediately before, but a portion of the mass which the lungs contained after inspiration; and if the volume of air that the lungs usually contain is compared with that which is inspired and expired at each motion of respiration, we will be inclined to believe that inspiration and expiration are intended to renew in part the considerable mass of air contained by the lungs.

This renewal will be so much more considerable as the quantity of air expired is greater, and as the following inspiration is more complete.

Physical and chemical changes that the air undergoes in the lungs.—The air, in its passage from the lungs has a temperature nearly the same as that of the body; there escapes with it from the breast a great quantity of vapour called *pulmonary transpiration;* besides, its chemical composition is different from that of the inspired air. The proportion of azote is much the same, but that of oxygen and carbonic acid is quite different.

In place of 0.21 of oxygen, and a trace of carbonic acid, which the atmospheric air presents, the expired air gives 0.18 or 0.19 of oxygen, and 0.3 to 0.4 of carbonic acid: generally, the quantity of carbonic acid exactly represents the quantity of oxygen which has disappeared; nevertheless, the last experiments of Gay Lussac and Davy give a small excess of acid; that is, there is a little more acid formed than the oxygen absorbed.

In order to determine the quantity of oxygen consumed by an adult in 24 hours, we have only to know the quantity of air respired in this time. According to Lavoisier, and Sir H. Davy, 32 cubic inches are consumed in a minute, which gives for 24 hours 46,037 cubic inches.

It is not difficult to appreciate the quantity of carbonic acid that passes out of the lungs in the same time, since it nearly represents the volume of oxygen that disappears. Thomson values it at 40,000 cubic inches, though he says it is probably a little less: now this quantity of carbonic acid represents nearly 12 ounces avoirdupois of carbon.

Some chemists say that a small quantity of azote disappears during respiration; others think, on the contrary, that its quantity is sensibly augmented; but there is nothing positive in this respect.

We are informed of the degree of alteration that the air undergoes in our lungs by a feeling which inclines us to renew it: though this is scarcely sensible in ordinary respiration, because we always continue it, it nevertheless becomes very painful if we do not satisfy it quickly; carried to this degree, it is accompanied with anxiety and fear, an instinctive warning of the importance of respiration.

While the air contained in the lungs is thus modified in its physical and chemical properties, the venous blood traverses the ramifications of the pulmonary artery, of which the tissue of the lobules of the lungs is partly formed: it passes into the radicles of the pulmonary veins, and very soon into these veins themselves; but in passing from the one to the other, it changes its nature from venous to arterial blood.

Rest-harrow. See *Ononis spinosa.*

RE'STA BOVIS. The plant named in English restharrow: so called because it hinders the plough; and hence *resta bovis.* See *Ononis spinosa.*

RESUPINATUS. *Resupinato.* Reversed: applied to leaves, &c. when the upper surface is turned downwards; as in the leaf of the *Pharus latifolius.*

RESUSCITATION. (*Resuscitatio; from resuscito,* to rouse and awake.) Revivification. The restoring of persons, apparently dead, to life. Under this head, strictly speaking, is considered the restoring of those who faint, or have breathed noxious air; yet it is chiefly confined to the restoring of those who are apparently dead from being immersed in a fluid, or by hanging. Dr. Curry has written a very valuable treatise on this subject; from which the following account is taken.

"From considering," he observes, "that a drowned person is surrounded by water instead of air, and that in this situation he makes strong and repeated efforts to breathe, we should expect that the water would enter and completely fill the lungs. This opinion, indeed, was once very general, and it still continues to prevail among the common people. Experience, however, has shown, that unless the body lies so long in the water as to have its living principle entirely destroyed, the quantity of fluid present in the lungs is inconsiderable; and it would seem that some of this is the natural moisture of the part accumulated; for, upon drowning kittens, puppies, &c. in ink, or other coloured liquors, and afterward examining the lungs, it is found that very little of the coloured liquor has gained admittance to them. To explain the reason why the lungs of drowned animals are so free from water, it is necessary to observe, that the muscles which form the opening into the wind-pipe are exquisitely sensible, and contract violently upon the least irritation, as we frequently experience when any part of the food or drink happens to touch that part. In the efforts made by a drowning person, or animal, to draw in air, the water rushes into the mouth and throat, and is applied to these parts, which immediately contract in such a manner as to shut up the passage into the lungs. This con-

tracted state continues as long as the muscles retain the principle of life, upon which the power of muscular contraction depends; when that is gone, they become relaxed, and the water enters the wind-pipe, and com pletely fills it. On dissecting the body of a recently drowned animal, no particular fulness of the vessels within the skull, nor any disease of the brain or its membranes, are visible. The lungs are also sound, and the branches of the wind-pipe generally contain more or less of a frothy matter, consisting chiefly of air, mixed with a small quantity of colourless fluid. The *right* cavity of the heart, and the trunks of the large internal veins which open into it, and also the trunk and larger branches of the artery which carries the blood from this cavity through the lungs, are all distended with dark-coloured blood, approaching almost to blackness. The *left* cavity of the heart, on the contrary, is nearly, or entirely empty, as are likewise the large veins of the lungs which supply it with blood, and the trunk and principal branches of the great artery which conveys the blood from hence to the various parts of the body. The external blood-vessels are empty; and the fleshy parts are as pale as if the animal had been bled to death. When a body has lain in the water for some time, other appearances will also be observable; such as, the skin livid, the eyes bloodshot, and the countenance bloated and swoln; but these appearances, though certainly unfavourable, do not absolutely prove that life is irrecoverably gone. It is now known, that in the case of drowning, no injury is done to any of the parts essential to life; but that the *right* cavity of the heart, together with the veins and arteries leading to and from that cavity, are turgid with blood, while every other part is almost drained of this fluid. The practice of holding up the bodies of drowned persons by the heels, or rolling them over a cask, is unnecessary; the lungs not being filled with any thing that can be evacuated in this way. Therefore such a practice is highly dangerous, as the violence attending it may readily burst some of those vessels which are already overcharged with blood, and thus convert what was only suspended animation, into absolute and permanent death. The operation of inflating the lungs is a perfectly safe, and much more effectual method of removing any frothy matter they may contain; and while it promotes the passage of the blood through them, also renders it capable of stimulating the *left* cavity of the heart, and exciting it to contrac tion. As soon as the body is taken out of the water, it should be stripped of any clothes it may have on, and be immediately well dried. It should then be wrapped in dry, warm blankets, or in the spare clothes taken from some of the by-standers, and be removed as quickly as possible to the nearest house that can be got convenient for the purpose. The fittest will be one that has a tolerably large apartment, in which a fire is ready or can be made. The body may be carried in men's arms, or laid upon a door; or, in case the house be at a distance from the place, if a cart can be procured, let the body be placed in it, on one side, upon some straw, with the head and upper part somewhat raised; and in this position a brisk motion will do no harm Whatever be the mode of conveyance adopt ed, particular care should be taken that the head be neither suffered to hang backwards, nor to bend down with the chin upon the breast. When arrived at the house, lay the body on a matrass, or a double blanket, spread upon a low table, or upon a door supported by stools; the head and chest being elevated by pillows. As the air of a room is very soon rendered impure by a number of people breathing in it, for this reason, as well as to avoid the confusion and embarrassment attending a crowd, no more persons should be admitted into the apartment where the body is placed, than are necessary to assist immediately in the recovery: in general *six* will be found sufficient for this purpose, and these should be the most active and intelligent of the by-standers. It will be found most convenient to divide the assistants into two sets; one set being employed in restoring the heat of the body, while the other institutes an artificial breathing in the best manner they are able. Every skilful person should be provided with a flexible tube made of elastic gum, half a yard in length, to introduce into the wind-pipe, and also with a similar tube to which a syringe can be affixed, to be put into the œsophagus. Should there not be at hand, air should be thrown into the lungs in the best manner that can be suggested at the time. Should it still be found that the air does not pass readily into the lungs, immediate recourse must be had to another and more effectual method for obtaining that object. As this method, however, requires address, and also some knowledge of the parts about the throat, we would recommend that when there is not a medical gentleman present, the mode already described, be tried repeatedly before this be attempted. As a quantity of frothy matter occupying the branches of the wind-pipe, and preventing the entrance of the air into the lungs, is generally the circumstance which renders this mode of inflation necessary, the mouth should be opened from time to time to remove this matter as it is discharged. While one set of the assistants are engaged in performing artificial respiration, the other should be employed in communicating heat to the body. The warm bath has been usually recommended for this purpose; but wrapping the body in blankets, or woollen cloths, strongly wrung out of warm water, and renewing them as they grow cold, besides being a speedier and more practicable method of imparting heat, has this great advantage, that it admits of the operation of inflating the lungs being carried on without interruption. Until a sufficient quantity of warm water can be got ready, other methods of restoring warmth may be employed; such as the application of dry warm blankets round the body and limbs; bags of warm grains or sand, bladders or bottles of hot water, or hot bricks applied to the hands, feet, and under the arm-pits, the bottles and bricks being covered with flannel: or the body may be placed before the fire, or in the sunshine, if strong at the time, and be gently rubbed by the assistants with their warm hands, or with cloths heated at the fire by a warming-pan. The restoration of heat should always be gradual, and the warmth applied ought never to be greater than can be comfortably borne by the assistants. If the weather happen to be cold, and especially if the body has been exposed to it for some time, heat should be applied in a very low degree at first: and if the weather be under the freezing point, and the body, when stripped, feel cold and nearly in the same condition with one that is frozen, it will be necessary at first to rub it well with snow, or wash it with cold water; the sudden application of heat in such cases having been found very pernicious. In a short time, however, warmth must be gradually applied. To assist in rousing the activity of the vital principle, it has been customary to apply various stimulating matters to different parts of the body. But as some of these applications are in themselves hurtful, and the others serviceable only according to the time and manner of their employment, it will be proper to consider them particularly. The application of all such matters in cases of apparent death, is founded upon the supposition that the skin still retains sensibility enough to be affected by them. It is well known, however, that even during life, the skin loses sensibility in proportion as it is deprived of heat, and does not recover it again until the natural degree of warmth be restored. Previous to the restoration of heat, therefore, to a drowned body, all stimulating applications are useless, and so far as they interfere with the other measures, are also prejudicial. The practice of rubbing the body with salt or spirits is now justly condemned. The salt quickly frets the skin, and has, in some cases, produced sores, which were very painful and difficult to heal after recovery. Spirits of all kinds evaporate fast, and thereby, instead of creating warmth, as they are expected to do, carry off a great deal of heat from the body. Spirit of hartshorn, or of sal volatile, are liable to the same objection as brandy or other distilled spirits, and are besides very distressing to the eyes of the assistants. When there is reason to think the skin has in any degree recovered its sensibility, let an assistant moisten his hand with spirit of hartshorn, or eau de luce, and hold it closely applied to one part: in this way evaporation is prevented, and the full stimulant effect of the application obtained. A liniment composed of equal parts of spirit of hartshorn and sallad oil, well shaken together, would appear to be sufficiently stimulating for the purpose, and as it evaporates very slowly, will admit of being rubbed on without producing cold. The places to which such remedies are usually applied, are, the wrists, ankles, temples, and the parts opposite the stomach and heart. The intestines, from their internal situation and peculiar constitution,

retain their irritability longer than the other parts of the body, and, accordingly, various means have been proposed for increasing the action of their fibres in order to restore the activity of the whole system Tobacco-smoke, injected by way of clyster, is what has been generally employed with this view, and the fumigator, or instrument for administering it, makes a part of the apparatus which is at present distributed by the different societies established for the recovery of drowned persons. Of late, however, the use of tobacco-smoke has been objected to, and upon very strong grounds; for when we consider that the same remedy is successfully employed with the very opposite intention, namely, that of lessening the power of contraction in the muscles, and occasioning the greatest relaxation consistent with life, it must be acknowledged to be a very doubtful, if not dangerous remedy, where the powers of life are already nearly exhausted. Instead of tobacco-smoke, then, we would recommend a clyster, consisting of a pint or more of water, moderately warmed, with the addition of one or two table-spoonfuls of spirit of hartshorn, a heaped tea-spoonful of strong mustard, or a table-spoonful of essence of peppermint; in defect of one or other of these, half a gill or more of rum, brandy, or gin may be added, or the warm water given alone. This step, however, need not be taken, until artificial respiration has been begun; for it will answer but little purpose to stimulate the heart through the medium of the intestines, unless we at the same time supply the left cavity with blood fitted to act upon it; which we cannot do without first removing the collapsed state of the lungs, and promoting the passage of the blood through them by a regular inflation. As the stomach is a highly sensible part, and intimately connected with the heart and brain, the introduction of some moderately warm and stimulating liquor into it, seems well calculated to rouse the dormant powers of life. This is very conveniently done by means of the syringe and flexible tube. The quantity of fluid thrown in ought not to exceed half a pint, and may be either warm negus, or water with the addition of one or other of the stimulating matters recommended above, using, however, only half the quantities mentioned there. As soon as the pulse or beating of the heart can be felt, the inside of the nostrils may be occasionally touched with a feather dipped in spirit of hartshorn, or sharp mustard; it being found by experience, that any irritation given to the nose, has considerable influence in exciting the action of the muscles concerned in respiration. When the natural breathing commences, the flexible tube and canula should be withdrawn, and any farther inflation that may be necessary, performed by blowing into the nostril. Letting blood has been generally thought requisite in every case of suspended animation. The practice, however, does not appear to have been founded upon any rational principle at first, and it has been continued from the force of custom, rather than from any experience of its good effects. In the case of drowned persons there is not, as in those who suffer from hanging or apoplexy, any unusual fulness of the vessels of the brain; and the quantity of blood that can be drawn from the external veins, will not sensibly diminish the accumulation of it in those near the heart. Besides, blood-letting, which always tends to *lessen* the action of the heart and arteries in the living body, cannot be supposed to have a directly opposite effect in cases of apparent death; on the contrary, if employed here, it will hazard the entire destruction of those feeble powers which yet remain, and to increase and support which all our endeavours should be directed. When the several measures recommended above have been steadily pursued for an hour or more, without any appearance of returning life, electricity should be tried; experience having shown it to be one of the most powerful stimuli yet known, and capable of exciting contraction in the heart and other muscles of the body, after every other stimulus had ceased to produce the least effect. Moderate shocks are found to answer best, and these should, at intervals, be passed through the chest in different directions, in order, if possible, to rouse the heart to act. Shocks may likewise be sent through the limbs, and along the spine; but we are doubtful how far it is safe or useful to pass them through the brain, as some have recommended. The body may be conveniently insulated, by placing it on a door, supported by a number of quart-bottles, whose sides are previously wiped with a towel, to remove any moisture they may have contracted. By experiments made on different animals, it is found that the blood passes through the lungs most readily when they are fully distended with air; consequently, that if the lungs of a drowned person are inflated, and kept in the expanded state while the electric shock is passed through the chest, the blood accumulated in the *right* cavity of the heart and its vessels will move forward without any resistance, should the heart be brought to contract upon it. As soon as the shock is given, let the lungs be emptied of the air they contain, and filled again with fresh air; then pass another shock, and repeat this until the heart is brought into action, or until it appear that all farther attempts are useless. In order more certainly to pass the shock through the heart, place the knob of one discharging rod above the collar-bone of the right side, and the knob of the other above the short ribs of the left: the position of the discharging rods, however, may be changed occasionally, so as to vary the direction of the shock. Two thick brass wires, each about eighteen inches long, passed through two glass tubes, or wooden cases, well varnished, and having at one end a knob, and at the other a ring to fasten the brass chain to, form very convenient discharging rods; and by means of them, the shock may be administered without the risk of its being communicated to the assistants, or carried off by the skin being wet. When the patient is so far recovered as to be able to swallow, he should be put into a warm bed, with his head and shoulders somewhat raised by means of pillows. Plenty of warm wine-whey, ale-posset, and other light and moderately nourishing drink, should now be given, and gentle sweating promoted, by wrapping the feet and legs in flannels well wrung out of hot water. If the stomach and bowels feel distended and uneasy, a clyster, consisting of a pint of warm water, with a table-spoonful of common salt, or an ounce or more of Glauber's or Epsom salt, dissolved in it, may be administered. The general practice in this case, is to give an emetic; but considering that the powers of the machine are still very weak, the agitation of vomiting is certainly hazardous. The patient should on no account be left alone, until the senses are perfectly restored, and he be able to assist himself; several persons having relapsed and been lost from want of proper attention to them, after the vital functions were, to all appearance, completely established. Either from the distention which the arteries of the lungs have suffered, or from the sudden change from great coldness to considerable warmth, it now and then happens, that the patient is attacked soon after recovery, with inflammation of some of the parts within the chest. This occurrence is pointed out by pain in the breast or side, increased on inspiration, and accompanied with frequent, and full or hard pulse, and sometimes with cough. Here the taking away some blood from the arm, or the application of cupping-glasses, leeches, or a blister, over the seat of the pain, will be very proper; but the necessity for these measures, as well as the times for putting them in practice, should be left to the judgment and discretion of a medical person. Dull pain in the head, lasting sometimes for two or three days, is by no means an unfrequent complaint in those who are recovered from this and from the other states of suspended animation; and here also a moderate bleeding from the neck, either with the lancet or with cupping-glasses may prove serviceable.

In hanging, the external veins of the neck are compressed by the cord, and the return of the blood from the head thereby impeded, from the moment that suspension takes place; but as the heart continues to act for a few seconds after the wind-pipe is closed, the blood which is sent to the head during this interval, is necessarily accumulated there. Hence it is, that in hanged persons the face is greatly swoln, and of a dark red or purple colour: the eyes are commonly suffused with blood, enlarged, and prominent. On dissection, the blood-vessels of the brain are found considerably distended, but, in general, no further marks of disease appear within the skull. The lungs are found generally quite collapsed, and free from frothy matter. The heart, and the large blood-vessels adjoining to it exhibit the same appearances as in the bodies of drowned persons. From the great accumulation of blood in the vessels of the head, many have been of opinion, that hanging kills chiefly by inducing apo-

plexy; but the following experiment made at Edinburgh several years ago, by an eminent medical professor there, clearly proves that in hanging as well as in drowning, the exclusion of air from the lungs is the immediate cause of death. A dog was suspended by the neck with a cord, an opening having been previously made in the wind pipe, below the place where the cord was applied so as to admit air into the lungs. In this state he was allowed to hang for three-quarters of an hour, during which time the circulation and breathing went on. He was then cut down without appearing to have suffered much from the experiment. The cord was now shifted below the opening into the wind-pipe, so as to prevent the ingress of air to the lungs; and the animal being again suspended, he was completely dead in a few minutes. Upon the whole, then, it appears, that the same measures recommended for drowned persons, are also necessary here; with this addition, that opening the jugular veins, or applying cupping-glasses to the neck, will tend considerably to facilitate the restoration of life, by lessening the quantity of blood contained in the vessels of the head, and thereby taking off the pressure from the brain. Except in persons who are very full of blood, the quantity taken away need seldom exceed an ordinary tea-cupful, which will in general be sufficient to unload the vessels of the head without weakening the powers of life."

RE'TE. A net. Applied to cellular membranes, vessels, nerves, parts of plants, &c. which are formed of meshes, like a net.

RETE MALPIGHII. The fine net-work of the extremities of the pulmonary arteries.

RETE MIRABILE. A network of blood-vessels in the basis of the brain of quadrupeds.

RETE MUCOSUM. *Corpus reticulare; Corpus mucosum; Mucus malpigii.* A mucous substance, deposited in a net-like form, between the epidermis and cutis, which covers the sensible cutaneous papillæ, connects the epidermis with the cutis, and gives the colour to the body: in Europeans it is of a white colour, in Ethiopians black. See *Skin.*

RETICULAR. (*Reticularis; from rete,* a net.) Interwoven like a net.

RETIFORM. (*Retiformis; from rete,* a net, and *forma,* resemblance.) Net-like.

RE'TINA. (From *rete,* a net.) *Amphiblestroides.* The third, or innermost membrane of the eye, ex panded round the choroid coat, to the ciliary ligament. It is the true organ of vision, and is formed by an expansion of the pulp of the optic nerve. See *Vision.*

RETINA'CULUM. (From *retineo,* to prop or restrain.) An instrument for keeping the bowels in their place.

RETIN-ASPHALTUM. See *Retinite.*

RETINITE. Retin-asphalt of Hatchet. A yellowish and reddish-brown coloured mineral, composed of resin, asphalt, and earth; found at Bovey Tracy, in Devonshire, adhering to coal.

RETORT. (*Retorta; from retorqueo,* to bend back again: probably so called, because its neck was curved and bent back, again.) A chemical vessel employed for many distillations, and most frequently for those which require a degree of heat superior to that of boiling water. They differ in form and materials: when pierced with a little hole in their roof, they are called tubulated retorts. They are made of common glass, stone-ware, and iron.

RETRA'CTOR. A muscle, the office of which is to retract the part into which it is inserted.

RETRACTOR ANGULI ORIS. See *Buccinator.*

RETRAHENS. Drawing back.

RETRAHENS AURIS. *Posterior auris,* of Winslow. *Retrahens auriculæ,* of Albinus. *Deprimens auricula,* of Douglas. *Retrahens auriculam,* of Cowper; and *Mastoido-conchinien,* of Dumas. Two small bundles of muscular fibres which arise from the external and posterior part of the mastoid process of the temporal bone immediately above the insertion of the sterno-cleido-mastoideus muscle. They are inserted into that part of the back of the ear which is opposite to the septum which divides the concha and scapha. Their use is to draw the ear backwards, and stretch the concha.

RETROCEDENT. *Retrocedens. Retrogradus* When a disease that moves about from one part to another, and is sometimes fixed, has been some time in its more common situation, and retires from it, it is said to be retrocedent.

RETROGRADE. See *Retrocedent*.

Retrocedent gout. See *Arthritis*.

RETROVERSION. *Retroversio.* See *Uterus, retroversion of.*

RETUSUS. Retuse. Applied to a leaf, which ends in a broad shallow notch, as in the *Rumex digynus.*

REUSSITE. A vegetable compound saline, found as an efflorescence on the surface, in the country round Seidlitz and Seidschutz.

REVERBERATORY. See *Furnace.*

REVOLUTUS. Revolute, rolled back. Applied to a leaf, the margin of which is turned or rolled backwards, as in *Andromeda polifolia.*

REVULSION. (*Revulsio ;* from *revello*, to draw away.) An old term used by the humoral pathologists, signifying the drawing of humours a contrary way.

RHABA'RBARUM. (From *Rha*, and *barbarus*, wild : so called because it was brought from the banks of the Rha, now called the Wolga, in Russia.) See *Rheum.*

RHABARBARUM ALBUM. See *Convolvulus mechoacanna.*

RHABARBARUM ANTIQUORUM. See *Rheum rhaponticum.*

RHABARBARUM DIOSCORIDIS. See *Rheum rhaponticum.*

RHABARBARUM MONACHORUM. See *Rumex patientia.*

RHABARBARUM RHAPONTICUM. See *Rheum rhaponticum.*

RHABARBARUM SIBERICUM. See *Rheum undulatum.*

RHABARBARUM TARTARICUM. See *Rheum.*

RHABARBARUM VERUM. See *Rheum.*

RHACHIA'LGIA. (From ραχις, the spine of the back, and αλγος, pain.) A pain in the spine of the back.

RHA'CHIS. (Ραχις, the spine of the back.) 1. In anatomy, the spine.

2. In botany, the common stalk or receptacle of the florets in the spikelets of grasses, or of the spikelets themselves ; as in *Lolium, Triticum, Hordeum,* &c. It also means the rib or leaf-stalk of ferns, which is often winged or bordered.

RHACHISA'GRA. (From ραχις, the spine of the back, and αγρα, a prey.) A sudden pain in the spine, applied to gout fixed in the spine of the back.

RHACHITA. (From ραχις, the spine of the back.) A muscle belonging to the spine of the back.

RHACHITIS. See *Rachitis.*

RHACO'SIS. (From ρακος, a rag.) A ragged excoriation.

RHA'GAS. (*Rhagas, adis.* f.; from ρηγνυμι, to break or bruise.) *Fissura.* A chap or cleft. A malignant, dry, and deep cutaneous fissure.

RHAGOIDES. (From ραξ, a grape-stone, and ειδος, a likeness : so called from its likeness in colour to a grape-seed.) Applied to the retiform tunic of the eye.

RHA'MNUS. (From ραιω, to destroy ; because of its many thorns.) 1. The name of a genus of plants in the Linnæan system. Class, *Pentandria ;* Order, *Monogynia.* Buckthorn.

2. The pharmacopœial name of the purging buckthorn. See *Rhamnus catharticus.*

RHAMNUS CATHARTICUS. The systematic name of the buckthorn. *Spina cervina ; Rhamnus solutivus ; Spina infectoria; Cervispina.* Purging buckthorn. The fruit or berries of this shrub, *Rhamnus—spinis terminalibus floribus quadrifidis dioicis, foliis ovatis, caule erecto,* of Linnæus, have been long received into the materia medica : they contain a pulpy, deep green juice, of a faint unpleasant smell, a bitterish, acrid, nauseous taste, which operates briskly by stool, producing thirst, dryness of the mouth and fauces, and severe gripings, unless some diluting liquor be drank plentifully after it : at present it is rarely prescribed except as a drastic purge. The dose is said to be about twenty of the fresh berries in substance ; twice or thrice that number in decoction ; a drachm or a drachm and a half of the dried berries ; an ounce of the expressed juice, or half an ounce of the rob or extract, obtained by inspissating the juice.

RHAMNUS FRANGULA. The systematic name of the black alder. *Frangula alnus ; Alnus nigra ; Rhamnus—inermis floribus monogynis hermaphroditis, foliis integerrimis,* of Linnæus.

244

All the parts of this tree, as well as of the common alder, are astringent and bitter. The bark is most astringent ; a decoction of it has cured agues, and is often used to repel inflammatory tumours of the throat, by way of gargle. The inner yellow bark of the trunk, or root, given to 3 ij, vomits, purges, and gripes ; but joined with aromatics, it operates more agreeably. An infusion, or decoction in water, inspissated to an extract, acts yet more mildly than these. It is mostly employed by the common people in dropsy and other disorders. The berries of alder are purgative. They are not in use under their own name, but are often substituted for buckthorn berries ; to discover which, it should be observed, that the berries of the black alder have a black skin, a blue juice, and two seeds in each of them ; whereas the buckthorn berries have a green juice, and commonly four seeds. The substitution of one for the other is not of material consequence, as the plants belong to the same genus, and the berries do not differ greatly.

Dr. Murray, of Gottingen, recommends, from his own experience, the leaves of alder chopped in small pieces, and heated over the fire, as the best remedy with which he is acquainted for dispersing milk in the breasts.

RHAMNUS ZIZYPHUS. The systematic name of the tree which affords the jujubes. A half-dried fruit of the plum kind, about the size and shape of an olive. Jujubes, when in perfection, have an agreeable, sweet taste, and in the southern parts of Europe, where they are common, they make an article of food in their recent state, and of medicine when half dried.

RHA'PHANUS. See *Raphanus.*

RHAPO'NTICUM. (The Rha of Pontus, *i. e.* the Rha, in Russia, a river on the banks of which it grew.) See *Rheum rhaponticum.*

Rhapontic rhubarb. See *Rheum rhaponticum.*

RHAPONTICUM VULGARE OFFICINARUM. See *Cen taurea.*

RHATA'NIA. See *Krameria.*

RHAZES, was born at Rhei, in the province of Khorasan, about the year 852. He is said not to have commenced the study of medicine till more than thirty years old, having previously removed to Bagdad : but by indefatigable application he obtained the highest reputation ; and was selected to superintend the celebrated hospital of that city. He has been considered as the Galen of the Arabians ; and from his assiduous attention during the rest of a long life, to the varieties of disease, he obtained the appellation of *the experienced.* He travelled much in pursuit of knowledge, particularly into his native country ; and was much consulted by Almanzor, the chief of that province, to whom several of his writings are dedicated, as well as by other princes. Abi Osbaia enumerated 226 treatises composed by Rhazes, but only a few of these are preserved through the medium of Latin translations. The ten books dedicated to Almanzor, were designed by him as a complete body of physic, and indeed may be regarded as the great magazine of all the Arabian medicine ; the ninth book in particular, treating of the cure of diseases, was in such general estimation for several centuries, as to be used as a text-book by professors. However, they contain little more than the substance of the writings of the Greek physicians ; though certainly the small-pox, and a few other diseases, are first distinctly described by Rhazes. He was author also of the first treatise on the diseases of children. The use of chemical preparations in medicine appears likewise to have originated with him, or at least with some of the Arabians. He died in the year 932. Besides the ten books above mentioned, and the tract on small-pox, there are extant by him a sort of commonplace book, entitled "Continens ;" and six books of Aphorisms, under the title of "De Secretis,"

RHE'UM. (From *Rha*, a river in Russia, now called the Wolga, from the banks of which it was first brought.) 1. The name of a genus of plants in the Linnæan system. Class, *Enneandria ;* Order, *Trigynia.* Rhubarb.

2. The pharmacopœial name of the official rhubarb. See *Rheum palmatum.*

RHEUM PALMATUM. The systematic name of the official rhubarb. *Rhabarbarum ; Rheon ; Rhæum ; Barbaria ; Lapathum orientale ; Lapathum chinense; Rhabarbarum verum ; Rhabarbarum tartaricum.* Rhubarb. It was not until the year 1732 that naturalits became acquainted with any plant which seemed to afford the rhabarbarum officinale; when some plants received from Russia by Jussieu at Paris, and Rhaud at Chelsea, were said to supply this important desideratum, and as such were adopted by Linnæus, in his first edition of the Species Plantarum, under the name of *Rheum rhabarbarum*. This, however, was not generally received as the genuine rhubarb plant; and with a view to ascertain this matter more completely Kaw Boerhaave procured from a Tartarian rhubarb merchant the seeds of those plants whose roots he annually sold, and which were admitted at Petersburgh to be the true rhubarb. These seeds were soon propagated, and were discovered by De Gorter to produce two distinct species, viz. the *Rheum rhabarbarum* of Linnæus, or as it has since been called, the *Rheum undulatum*, and another species, a specimen of which was presented to Linnæus, who declared it to be a new one; and it was first mentioned in the second edition of the Species Plantarum, in 1762, by the name of *Rheum palmatum*. Previous to this time, De Gorter had repeatedly sent its seeds to Linnæus, but the young plants which they produced constantly perished; at length he obtained the fresh root, which succeeded very well at Upsal, and afterward enabled the younger Linnæus to describe this plant, ann. 1767. But two years antecedent to this, Dr. Hope's account of the *Rheum palmatum*, as it grew in the Botanic Garden near Edinburgh, had been read before the Royal Society at London; and of the great estimation in which this plant was held by him, we have the following proof:—"From the perfect similarity of this root with the best foreign rhubarb, in taste, smell, colour, and purgative qualities, we cannot doubt of our being at last possessed of the plant which produces the true rhubarb, and may reasonably entertain the agreeable expectation of its proving a very important acquisition to Britain."

But from the relation we have given, it appears that both the seeds of the R. palmatum, and the R. undulatum, were transmitted to Petersburgh, as those of the true rhubarb; we are therefore to conclude, that the former species has an equal claim to this importance with the latter; and from further inquiries made in Russia, there is the best authority for believing that the R. compactum also affords this very useful drug. The seeds of the R. palmatum were first introduced into Britain in 1762, by Dr. Hounsy (who sent them from Russia), and were supposed to be a part of that already mentioned; and since their prosperous cultivation by the late professor of botany at Edinburgh, the propagation of this plant has been gradually extended to most of our English gardens, and with a degree of success which promises, in time, to supersede the importation of the foreign root. Two sorts of rhubarb roots are usually imported into this country for medical use; viz. the Chinese and the Tartary rhubarb.; the first is in oblong pieces, flattish on one side, and convex on the other; compact, hard, heavy, internally of a dull-red colour, variegated with yellow and white, and when recently powdered, appears yellow, but on being kept becomes gradually redder. The second is the most valuable, and is brought to us in roundish pieces, with a large hole through the middle of each; it is more soft and friable than the former sort, and exhibits, when broken, many streaks of a bright red colour. "The marks of the goodness of rhubarb are, the liveliness of its colour when cut; its being firm and solid, but not flinty or hard; its being easily pulverable, and appearing when powdered of a fine bright yellow colour; its imparting to the spittle when chewed a deep saffron tinge, and not proving slimy or mucilaginous in the mouth; its taste is subacrid, bitterish, and somewhat styptic; the smell lightly aromatic."

The purgative qualities of rhubarb are extracted more perfectly by water than by rectified spirit: the part remaining after the action of water is almost, if not wholly, inactive; whereas after repeated digestion in spirit, it proves still very considerably purgative. The virtue of a watery infusion, on being inspissated by a gentle heat, is so much diminished, that a drachm of the extract is said to have scarcely any greater effect than a scruple of the root in substance. The spirituous tincture loses less; half a drachm of this extract proving moderately purgative. The qualities of this root, says Dr. Cullen, are that of a gentle purgative, and so gentle that it is often inconvenient on. account of the bulk of the dose required, which in adults, must be from 3 ss.

to 3 j. When given in a large dose it will occasion some griping, as other purgatives do; but it is hardly ever heating to the system, or shows the other effects of the more drastic purgatives. The purgative quality is accompanied with a bitterness, which is often useful in restoring the tone of the stomach when it has been lost; and, for the most part, its bitterness makes it sit better on the stomach than many other purgatives do. Its operation joins well with neutral laxatives; and both together operate in a less dose than either of them would singly. Some degree of stypticity is always evident in this medicine; and as this quality acts when that of the purgative has ceased, so in cases of diarrhœa, when any evacuation is proper, rhubarb has been considered as the most proper remedy to be employed. It must, however, be remarked here, that, in many cases of diarrhœa, no further evacuation than what is occasioned by the disease, is necessary or proper. The use of rhubarb, in substance, for keeping the belly regular, for which it is frequently employed, is by no means proper, as the astringent quality is ready to undo what the purgative has done; but it is found that the purpose mentioned may be obtained by it, if the rhubarb is chewed in the mouth, and no more is swallowed than what the saliva has dissolved. And it must be remarked, that in this way employed it is very useful to dyspeptic persons. Analogous to this, is the use of rhubarb in solution, in which it appears to me, that the astringent quality is not so largely extracted as to operate so powerfully as when the rhubarb was employed in substance.

The officinal preparations of this drug are, a watery and a vinous infusion, a simple and a compound tincture. It is also an ingredient in different compositions.

RHEUM RHAPONTICUM. The systematic name of the rhapontic rhubarb. *Rhaponticum ; Rhabarbarum dioscoridis ; Rhabarbarum antiquorum.* The root of this species appears to have been the true rhubarb of the ancients. By some it is confounded with the modern rhubarb, though considerably different from that root in appearance, as well as in quality. The rhapontic is of a dusky colour on its surface, and a loose spongy texture ; is more astringent than rhubarb, and less purgative; in this last intention, two or three drachms are required for a dose.

RHEUM UNDULATUM. The systematic name of the Siberian rhubarb. The *Rheum—foliis subvillosis undulatis petiolis æqualibus*, of Linnæus. It possesses similar virtues to those of the palmate species, and is in common use in Russia.

RHE'UMA. (From ρεω, to flow.) The discharge from the nostrils or lungs arising from cold ; hence the following lines of the school of Salernum :

Si fluit ad pectus, dicatur rheuma catarrhus,
Ad fauces branchus, ad nares esto coryza!

RHEUMATI'SMUS. (From ρευματιζω, to be afflicted with defluxions.) *Dolores rheumatici et arthritici*, of Hoffman. *Myositis*, of Sagar. This is a genus of disease in the Class *Pyrexiæ*, and Order *Phlegmasiæ*, of Cullen; characterized by pyrexia, pains in the joints, increased by the action of the muscles belonging to the joint, and heat of the part. The blood, after venesection, exhibits an inflammatory crust. Rheumatism is distinguished into *acute* and *chronic*. The acute is preceded by shivering, heat, thirst, and frequent pulse; after which the pain commences, and soon fixes on the joints. The chronic rheumatism is distinguished by pain in the joints, without pyrexia, and is divided into three species; *lumbago*, affecting the loins; *sciatica*, affecting the hip; and *arthrodynia*, or pains in the joints. The acute rheumatism mostly terminates in one of these species.

Rheumatism may arise at all times of the year, when there are frequent vicissitudes of the weather, from heat to cold, but the spring and autumn are the seasons in which it is most prevalent; and it attacks persons of all ages ; but very young people are less subject to it than adults.

Obstructed perspiration, occasioned either by wearing wet clothes, lying in damp linen, or damp rooms, or by being exposed to cool air when the body has been much heated by exercise, is the cause which usually produces rheumatism. Those who are much afflicted with this complaint, are very apt to be sensible of the approach of wet weather, by finding wandering pains about them at that period.

Acute rheumatism usually comes on with lassitude

and rigours, succeeded by heat, thirst, anxiety, restlessness, and a hard pulse; soon after which, excruciating pains are felt in different parts of the body, but more particularly in the joints of the shoulder, wrist, knees, and ankles, or perhaps in the hip; and these keep shifting from one joint to another, leaving a redness and swelling in every part they have occupied, as likewise a great tenderness to the touch. Towards evening there is usually an exacerbation, or increase of fever; and during the night, the pains become more severe, and shift from one joint to another.

Early in the course of the disease, some degree of sweat ng usually occurs; but it is seldom so copious as either to remove the pains or to prove critical. In the beginning, the urine is without sediment; but as the disease advances in its progress, and the fever admits of considerable remissions, a lateritious sediment is deposited; but this by no means proves critical.

Chronic rheumatism is attended with pains in the head, shoulders, knees, and other large joints, which, at times, are confined to one particular part, and at others shift from one joint to another, without occasioning any fever; and in this manner the complaint continues often for a considerable time, and at length goes off.

No danger is attendant on chronic rheumatism; but a person having been once attacked with it, is ever afterward more or less liable to returns of it; and an incurable anchylosis is sometimes formed, in consequence of very frequent relapses. Neither is the acute rheumatism frequently accompanied with much danger; but, in a few instances, the patient has been destroyed by general inflammation, and now and then by a metastasis to some vital part, such as the head and lungs. Acute rheumatism, although accompanied with a considerable degree of inflammation in particular parts, has seldom been known to terminate in suppuration; but a serous or gelatinous effusion takes place.

Rheumatism seldom proving fatal, very few opportunities have offered for dissections of the disease. In the few which have occurred, the same appearances have been observed as in inflammatory fever, effusion within the cranium, and now and then affections of some of the viscera.

In the acute rheumatism the general antiphlogistic plan of treatment is to be pursued, so long as the febrile and inflammatory symptoms are severe. It may be sometimes proper to begin by a moderate abstraction of blood, where the patient is young and plethoric; and if the disease attacks any important part, this measure must be more actively pursued; but in general it does not appear necessary. Even the l ocal abstraction of blood is hardly advisable, unless the affection be very much fixed to one part, and the symptoms urgent: and it may be said, that most local applications are rather likely to drive the disease from one part to another, than to afford permanent relief. After freely opening the bowels, the chief object is to endeavour to procure a general and mild diaphoresis by antimonial and mercurial preparations, assisted by opium, or other narcotic, which may also alleviate the pain, and occasionally by the warm bath, where the skin is particularly harsh and dry. Digitalis, by moderating the circulation, will sometimes be usefully conjoined with these medicines. As the fever abates, and the strength appears impaired, tonics should be given to promote the convalescence of the patient, and obviate a relapse: and where the inflammation remains fixed in a particular joint, after the pyrexia has ceased, fomentations and other local measures, according to the state of the part, may be employed for its removal. In the *arthrodynia*, or chronic rheumatism, as it is commonly called, the remedies of chief efficacy are stimulant diaphoretics in moderate doses regularly persevered in, assisted by various local means of promoting the circulation through the affected part. Anodynes may be also used with advantage both internally and locally: and attention should be paid to support the strength, and correct any observable deficiency in the several functions.

RHE'UME. (From ρεω, to flow.) A defluxion, a common cold or catarrh.

RHEUMIC ACID. An acid said to be peculiar to rhubarb, but not yet sufficiently examined.

RHIBE'SIA. (From *ribes*, a currant.) See *Ribes*.

RHINÆ'US. (*Rhinæus*, sc. *musculus*: from ριν the nose.) See *Compressor n*^{aris}.

RHINENCHY'TES. (From ριν, the nose, and εγχυω, to pour in.) A syringe for the nose.

RHINOPHO'NIA. (From ριν, the nose, and φωνη, the voice.) A nasal voice.

RHIZA'GRA. (From ριζα, the root, and αγρευω, to seize.) An instrument for taking out the roots or stumps of teeth.

RHODIA. See *Rhodiola*.

RHODIOLA. (A diminutive of *Rhodia;* from οσδον, a rose; so called because its root smells like the damask rose.) The name of a genus of plants. Class, *Diœcia;* Order, *Octandria*.

RHODIOLA ROSEA. The radix rhodiæ of some pharmacopœias is the produce of the *Rhodiola rosea*, of Linnæus, called rosewort. When dry, it has a very pleasant smell, resembling that of the damask rose. In this odorous matter the medical virtue of the root resides. Poultices in which this root enters as a chief ingredient are said to allay violent pains of the head.

RHO'DIUM. (From ροδον, a rose; a wood which smells like roses.) 1. Rhodium, or rosewood.

2. A new metal discovered among the grains of crude platina, by Dr. Wollaston. The mode of obtaining it in the state of a triple salt combined with muriatic acid and soda, has been given under the article *Palladium*. This may be dissolved in water, and the metal precipitated from it in a black powder by zinc.

This powder, exposed to heat, continues black; but with borax it acquires a white metallic lustre, though it remains infusible. Sulphur, or arsenic, however, renders it fusible, and may afterward be expelled by continuing the heat. The button, however, is not malleable. Its specific gravity appears not to exceed 11.

Rhodium unites easily with every metal that has been tried except mercury. With gold or silver it forms a very malleable alloy, not oxidated by a high degree of heat, but becoming incrusted with a black oxide when slowly cooled. One-sixth of it does not perceptibly alter the colour of gold, but renders it much less fusible. Neither nitric nor nitro-muriatic acid acts on it in either of these alloys; but if it be fused with three parts of bismuth, lead, or copper, the alloy is entirely soluble in a mixture of nitric acid with two parts of muriatic.

The oxide was soluble in every acid Dr. Wollaston tried. The solution in muriatic acid did not crystallize by evaporation. Its residuum formed a rose-coloured solution with alkohol. Muriate of ammonia and of soda, and nitrate of potassa, occasioned no precipitate in the muriatic solution, but formed with the oxide triple salts, which were insoluble in alkohol. Its solution in nitric acid likewise did not crystallize, but silver, copper, and other metals precipitated it.

The solution of the triple salt with muriate of soda was not precipitated by nuriate, carbonate, or hydrosulphuret of ammonia, by carbonate or ferroprussiate of potassa, or by carbonate of soda. The caustic alkalies however throw down a yellow oxide, soluble in excess of alkali; and a solution of platina occasions in it a yellow precipitate.

The title of this product to be considered as a distinct metal was at first questioned; but the experiments of Dr. Wollaston have since been confirmed by Descotils.

RHODIUM LIGNUM. See *Aspulathus canariensis*.

RHODODE'NDRON. (From ροδον, a rose, and δενδρον, a tree: so called because its flowers resemble the rose.) 1. The name of a genus of plants in the Linnæan system. Class, *Decandria;* Order, *Mono gynia*.

2. The pharmacopœial name of the oleander. See *Rhododendron chrysanthemum*.

RHODODENDRON CHRYSANTHEMUM. The systematic name of the oleander, rosebay, or yellow rhododendron. This species of rhododendron, *foliis oblon gis impunctis supra scabris venosissimis, corolla rotata irregulari gemma florifera ferrugineo-tomentosa* has not yet been introduced in Britain; it is a native of Siberia, affecting mountainous situations, and flowering in June and July.

This plant and its medical virtues were first described in 1747, by Gmelin and Haller. Little attention, however, was paid to it, till the year 1779, when it was strongly recommended by Koelpin as an efficacious medicine, not only in rheumatism and gout, but even in venereal cases; and it is now very generally employed in chronic rheumatisms, in various parts of Europe. The leaves, which are the part directed for medicina. use, have a bitterish subadstringent taste. Taken in a large dose, they prove a narcotic poison; and, in moderate doses they are said to occasion heat, thirst, a degree of delirium, and a peculiar sensation of the parts affected.

As a powerful and active medicine, this shrub, says Dr. Woodville, may probably be found an addition to the materia medica. Dr. Home, who tried it unsuccessfully in some cases of acute rheumatism, says, "It appears to be one of the most powerful sedatives which we have, as, in most of the case, it made the pulse remarkably slow, and in one patient reduced it to thirty-eight beats. And in other cases, in which the rhododendron has been used at Edinburgh, it has been productive of good effects, and accordingly it is now introduced into the Edinburgh Pharmacopœia. The manner of using this plant by the Siberians, was by putting two drachms of the dried leaves in an earthen pot, with about ten ounces of boiling water, keeping it near a boiling heat for a night; and this they took in the morning, and by repeating it three or four times, generally effected a cure.

RHODO'MELI. (From ροδον, the rose, and μελι, honey.) Honey of roses.

RHŒADEÆ. (From rhœas, the red poppy.) The name of an order in Linnæus's Fragments of a Natural Method, consisting of poppy and similar plants, the calyx of which is caducous, and the fruit a capsule or selyna.

RHŒ'AS. (Rhœas, ados. m.; from ρεω, to flow.) The wild poppy is sometimes so called. See Papaver rhœas.

RHŒTIZITE. A glistening and pearly white mineral, which is found in primitive rocks, with quartz Psitzsci, in the Tyrol.

RHOMBOIDE'US. (From ρομβος, a geometrical figure, whose sides are equal but not right-angled, and ειδος, resemblance.) Rhomboideus major and minor. Rhomboides, of Douglas, Winslow, and Cowper; and Cervici dorso scapulaire, of Dumas. This muscle, which is so named from its shape, is situated immediately under the trapezius. We find it usually, though not always, divided into two portions, which Albinus describes as two distinct muscles. The uppermost of these, or rhomboideus minor, arises tendinous from the spinous processes of the three inferior vertebræ of the neck, and from the ligamentum colli; the lowermost, or rhomboideus major, arises tendinous from the spinous processes of the back: the former is inserted into the basis of the scapula, opposite to its spine; the latter into all the basis of the scapula, below its spine. Its use is to draw the scapula obliquely upwards, and directly backwards.

RHOMBSPAR. See Bitterspar.

RHOMBUS. Diamond-shaped, approaching to a square: applied to leaves, &c.; as those of the Chenopodium olidum, and to the pod of Cicer arientinum.

RHONCHUS. (Ρογχος, rhonchus, stertor.) Snoring.

RHOPALO'SIS. (From ροπαλον, a club.) A disorder in which the hair cleaves together; and hangs down in clusters resembling clubs. The plaited hair. See Plica.

RHUBARB. See Rheum.

Rhubarb, monk's. See Rumex patientia.

Rhubarb, rhapontic. See Rheum rhaponticum.

RHUS. (From ρεω, to flow: so called because it stops fluxes.) The name of a genus of plants in the Linnæan system. Class, Pentandria; Order, Trigynia. The sumach-tree.

RHUS BELGICA. The Dutch myrtle is sometimes so termed. See Myrica gale.

RHUS CORIARIA. Sumach. Elm-leaved sumach. This plant, Rhus—foliis pinnatis obtusiuscule serratus ovalibus subtus villosis, of Linnæus, is a small tree, a native of the south of Europe. It is singular that this is the only species of the genus rhus which is perfectly innocent; the others being active poisons. Both the leaves and berries of this plant are used medicinally, as astringents and tonics; the former are the most powerful, and have been long in common use, where they may be easily obtained in various complaints indicating this class of remedies. The berries, which are red, and of a roundish compressed figure, contain a pulpy matter, in which is lodged a brown, hard, oval seed, manifesting a considerable degree of

adstringency. The pulp, even when dry, is grateful, and has been discovered to contain an essential salt, similar to that of wood-sorrel. An infusion of the dried fruit is not rendered black by a solution of iron; hence it appears to be destitute of adstringency. But its acidity is extremely grateful; therefore, like many other fruits, these berries may be advantageously taken to allay febrile heat, and to correct bilious putrescency.

[RHUS GLABRUM. The berries of this, and several other American species of sumach, have a strong, acid taste, and at times exhibit crystallized or saline particles on their surface. Dr Harsefield supposes the acid they contain to be tartaric; but it is, not improbably, an acid sui generis. The acidulous infusion of these berries is used as a refrigerant in fevers, and a gargle in sore throats. The bark and leaves of the shrub are highly astringent, and are used in tanning leather. Big. Mat. Med. A.]

RHUS RADICANS. See Rhus vernix.

RHUS TIPHINUM. The systematic name of the Virginian sumach, the seeds of which are said to be useful in stopping hæmorrhages.

RHUS TOXICODENDRON. Poison oak, or sumach. This plant is a native of North America. The stems, if cut, exude a milky juice, which inflames the skin. The leaves, now inserted in the pharmacopœia, are inodorous, and have a mawkish, subacrid taste. Their virtues are extracted more perfectly by water than by alkohol. They prove stimulant and narcotic, when taken internally. Dr. Alderson, of Hull, found them successful in several cases of paralysis. They excite a sense of heat and pricking, and irregular twitches in the affected limbs. They have been sometimes useful, also, in herpetic eruptions. The dose may be from half a grain, gradually increased, to four grains, two or three times a-day.

RHUS VERNIX. Rhus radicans. The systematic name of a poisonous plant, the efficacy of which Dr. Fresnoi has endeavoured to prove, in the disease called paralysis, and herpetic affections. He, in order that others should not suffer by his experiments, began by taking an infusion of one of the three foliola of which each leaf of this plant consists; and, as this dose produced no sensible effect, he increased the number to twelve. His urine and perspiration were increased in quantity, and he had some pains in his belly. He relates seven cases, in which he thinks he can remove all doubt of the efficacy of this infusion, in herpetic affections. From these, the following are selected:

"A countrywoman," says Dr. Fresnoi, "came to me in the month of July, 1780, to consult me about the herpes farinosa, with which her face had been covered for more than a year. She was ordered to take an infusion of this plant; and, in six weeks, was entirely free from the disease."

He likewise relates five cases of paralysis, which were cured by the use of this plant.

The leaves of this plant are to be cut when in the greatest vigour, about the month of June. "Those who cut this plant," says Dr. F., "wear leathern gloves, on account of its poisonous qualities." The same gentleman observes, he saw one case in which inflammation of the eyelids was produced by the vapour from the plant. Four pounds of the leaves, being distilled with thirty-two pounds of water, give it a slight odour, although the plant is entirely free from it. Its taste is pungent, and inflames the mouth. The decoction which remains in the still is brown, and is generally covered with a light brown pellicle. When strained and evaporated, it gives a shining black extract. The leaves inflame and swell the hands and arms of those who take them out of the still, and bring on an itching, which remains for several days. Forty-two pounds of the leaves afford twenty ounces of extract, of a proper consistence for pills.

"A girl, in Flanders," says Dr. Fresnoi, "already subject to fits, laid down some flowers in her bedroom. Next day she told me that she had undergone a great change: that she had had no fits, and slept much better. It occurred to me," says Dr. F. "that the flowers occasioned this change. Next day, the flowers being removed, and the window opened, the convulsions reappeared; on their being again introduced, the fits disappeared; which proved plainly it was the effect of the flowers. The success of the extract, in tussis convulsiva, exceeded my hopes; forty-two children being cured of this disorder in Valenciennes, during the end of the year 1786. Four grains of extract are to be dissolved in four ounces of syrup, of which one table-spoonful, given to the child every third hour, generally abates the cough, and mostly leaves them."

RHY'AS. ('Ρυας, a disease of the eye.) A decrease or defect of the lachrymal caruncle. The proximate cause is a native defect; or it may originate from excision, erosion, or acrimony. This disorder is commonly incurable, and it induces an incurable *epiphora*, or a continual weeping.

RHYPIA. (From 'Ρυπος, *sordes*.) Foul, sordid, ill-conditioned.

RHYTIDO'SIS. See *Rutidosis*.

RIB. *Costa*. The ribs are the long curved bones which are placed in an oblique direction at the sides of the chest. Their number is generally twelve on each side; but, in some subjects, it has been found to be thirteen, and in others, though more rarely, only eleven. They are distinguished into true and false ribs. The seven upper ribs, which are articulated to the sternum, are called *true* ribs; and the five lower ones, which are not immediately attached to that bone, are called *false* ribs. At the posterior extremity of each rib, we observe a small head, divided by a middle ridge into two articulating surfaces, covered with cartilage, which are received into two cavities, contiguous to each other, and formed in the upper and lower part of each dorsal vertebra, as we have observed in our description of the spine. This articulation, which is secured by a capsular ligament, is a species of ginglymus, and allows only of motion upwards and downwards. The head of each rib is supported by a short neck, and immediately beyond this we find a flattened tubercle, affording an oblong and slightly convex surface, which is articulated with the transverse process of the lowest of the two dorsal vertebræ, with which its head is articulated. At some little distance from this tuberosity, the rib makes a considerable curve, which is usually called its angle. From the tubercle to the angle, the ribs are of considerable thickness, and approaching to a cylindrical shape; but, from the angle to their anterior extremity, they become thinner and flatter. To this anterior extremity is fixed a long, broad, and strong cartilage, which, in each of the true ribs, reaches to the sternum, where its articulation is secured by a capsular ligament, and by other ligamentous fibres. The cartilages of the sixth and seventh ribs being longer than the rest, are extended upwards, in order to reach the sternum, the inferior portion of which is about on a level with the fifth rib. The cartilages of these two ribs are usually united into one, so as to leave no space between them. The false ribs are supported in a different manner; their cartilages terminate in an acute point before they reach the sternum, the eighth rib being attached by its cartilage to the lower edge of the cartilage of the seventh, or last of the true ribs; the ninth in the same manner to the eighth; and the tenth to the ninth; the cartilages of each rib being shorter than that of the rib above it. The eleventh and twelfth, which are the two lowermost ribs, are not fixed at their anterior extremities like the other ribs, but hang loose, and are supported only by their ligamentous fibres, and by muscles and other soft parts.

The external surface of each rib is somewhat convex, and its internal surface slightly concave. On the inferior and interior surface of these bones we observe a long fossa, for the lodgment of the intercostal vessels and nerves. This channel, however, does not extend through the whole length of the rib, being observable neither at the posterior extremity, where the vessels have not yet reached the bone, nor at the fore-end, where they are distributed to the parts between the ribs. We seldom see any marks of it in the short ribs, as in the first, second, eleventh, and twelfth.

Thus far we have given a description which is applicable to the ribs in general; but, as we find them differing from each other in shape, length, situation, and other respects, it will be right to speak of each rib in particular.

The *first* rib, which is the shortest of any, is likewise the most curved. It is broader than the other ribs, and, instead of being placed, as they are, obliquely, and with its edges upwards and downwards, it is situated nearly in a transverse direction, one of its edges being placed inwards, or nearly so. Of these edges, the inner one is sharp, and the outer one

somewhat rounded. Its inner surface is smooth, and its superior surface is sometimes slightly depressed anteriorly by the clavicle. The head of this rib, instead of being angular, is flattened, and slightly convex, being received into a cavity, which is formed wholly in the first vertebra, and not by two vertebræ, as in the case with the other ribs.

The *second* rib is longer than the first, but shorter than the ribs below it. Its angle is placed at a small distance from its tuberosity, and its head is articulated with two vertebræ, like the other ribs. The other ten ribs, the last two only excepted, differ from the general description we have given, chiefly in the difference of their length, which goes on gradually increasing, from the first or uppermost, to the seventh or last of the true ribs, and as gradually diminishing from that to the twelfth. Their obliquity, in respect to the spine, likewise increases as they descend, as does the distance between the head and angle of each rib, from the first rib to the ninth. The two lowest ribs differ from all the rest in the following particulars:—Their heads, like that of the first rib, are rounded, and received into a cavity formed entirely in the body of one vertebra; they have no tubercle for their articulation with the transverse processes, to which they are only loosely fixed by ligaments, and, in this respect, the tenth rib is sometimes found to agree with them: they are much shorter than the rest of the false ribs, and the twelfth is still shorter than the eleventh. The length of the latter, however, is different in different subjects, and is not always found to be the same on both sides. Anteriorly, as we have already observed, their cartilages are short and loose, not being attached to the cartilages of the other ribs; and this seems to be, because the most considerable motions of the trunk are not performed on the lumbar vertebræ alone, but likewise on the lower vertebræ of the back; so that if these two ribs had been confined anteriorly, like the rest, and likewise united to the bodies of two vertebræ, and to the transverse process, this disposition would have impeded the motion of the two last vertebræ of the back, and consequently would have affected the motion of the trunk in general.

The use of the ribs is to give form to the thorax, and to cover and defend the lungs; also to assist in breathing; for they are joined to the vertebræ by regular hinges, which allow of short motions, and to the sternum by cartilages, which yield to the motion of the ribs, and return again when the muscles cease to act.

Ribbed-leaf. See *Nervosus*.

RI'BES. The name of a genus of plants in the Linnæan system. Class, *Pentandria;* Order, *Monogynia.* The currant-tree.

RIBES NIGRUM. Black currant. This indigenous plant, *Ribes—racemis pilosis, floribus oblongis,* of Linnæus, affords larger berries than those of the red, which are said to be peculiarly useful in sore throats, and to possess a diuretic power in a very considerable degree. The leaves of the black currant are extremely fragrant, and have been likewise recommended for their medicinal virtue, which Bergius states to be mundificans, pellens, diuretica. The officinal preparations of the berries are the *syrupus ribis nigri,* and the *succus ribis nigri inspissatus.*

RIBES RUBRUM. *Grossularia non spinosa.* The red currant. *Ribes—inerme; racemis glabris pendulis, floribus planiusculis,* of Linnæus. The white currant-tree is merely a variety of the red, the fruit of both is perfectly analogous; therefore, what is said of the one applies to the other. The red currant is abundantly cultivated in gardens, and, from its grateful acidity, is universally acceptable, either as nature presents it, or variously prepared by art, with the addition of sugar. Considered medicinally, it is esteemed to be moderately refrigerant, antiseptic, attenuant, and aperient. It may be used with considerable advantage to allay thirst, in most febrile complaints, to lessen an increased secretion of bile, and to correct a putrid and scorbutic state of the fluids, especially in sanguine temperaments; but, in constitutions of a contrary kind, it is apt to occasion flatulency and indigestion

RIBWORT. See *Plantago lanceolata*.

RICE. See *Oryza*.

RI'CINUS. (*Quasi,* ριν κυνος, a dog's nose: because they stick to the noses of dogs.) 1. The name of a genus of plants in the Linnæan system. Class, *Monœcia;* Order, *Monadelphia*.

2. The pharmacopœial name of the plant that affords the seed from which the castor-oil is prepared.

RICINUS COMMUNIS. The systematic name of the castor-oil plant. *Cataputia major; Kerva; Ricinus vulgaris; Palma christi Ricinus—foliis peltatis subpalmatis serratis*, of Linnæus. This plant appears to be the Κικι, or Κροτων, of Dioscorides, who observes, that the seeds are powerfully cathartic; it is also mentioned by Aëtius, Paulus Ægineta, and Pliny. The ricinus was first cultivated in England, in the time of Turner, and is now annually reared in many gardens in the neighbourhood of London; and in that of Dr. Saunders, at Highbury, the plant grew to a state of great perfection. An oil extracted from the seeds of this plant, and known by the name of oleum ricini, palma christi, or castor-oil, is the drug to which the pharmacopœias refer, and which has lately come into frequent use, as a quick but gentle purgative. The London College directs this oil to be expressed from the seeds in the same way as that of the oil of almonds, and without the assistance of heat, by which the oil would seem to be obtained in the purest state. However, we have some reason to believe that this method is seldom practised, and that the oil usually employed here is imported from the West Indies, where it is commonly prepared in the following manner :—"The seeds being freed from the husks, or pods, which are gathered upon their turning brown, and when beginning to burst open, are first bruised in a mortar, afterward tied up in a linen bag, and then thrown into a large pot, with a sufficient quantity of water (about eight gallons, to one gallon of the seeds), and boiled till the oil is risen to the surface, when it is carefully skimmed off, strained, and kept for use. Thus prepared, the oil is entirely free from acrimony, and will stay upon the stomach when it rejects all other medicines." Mr. Long remarks, that the oil intended for medicinal use, is more frequently cold drawn, or extracted from the bruised seeds by means of a handpress. But this is thought more acrimonious than that prepared by coction. Dr. Brown is also of this opinion, and prefers the oil prepared by coction to that by expression; he attributes its greater mildness to the action of the fire, observing that the expressed oil, as well as the mixed juices of the seeds, are far more active and violent in their operation.

Dr. Cullen observes, that "this oil, when the stomach can be reconciled to it, is one of the most agreeable purgatives we can employ. It has this particular advantage, that it operates sooner after its exhibition than any other purgative I know of, as it commonly operates in two or three hours. It seldom gives any griping, and its operation is generally moderate, producing one, two, or three stools only. It is particularly suited to cures of costiveness, and even to cases of spasmodic colic.

In the West Indies, it is found to be one of the most certain remedies in the dry belly-ache, or colica pictonum. It is seldom found heating or irritating to the rectum; and, therefore, is sufficiently well suited to hæmorrhoidal persons.

The only inconvenience attending the use of this medicine is, that as an oil it is nauseous to some persons; and that, when the dose is large, it occasions sickness at the stomach for some time after it is taken. To obviate these inconveniences, several means have been tried; and it is found that the most effectual means is the addition of a little ardent spirit. In the West Indies, they employ rum; but that I might not withdraw any part of the purgative, I employed the *Tinc. sennæ comp.* This, added in the proportion of one to three parts of the oil, and very intimately mixed, by being shaken together in a phial, both makes the oil less nauseous to the taste, and makes it sit more easy on the stomach. The common dose of this oil is a table spoonful, or half an ounce; but many persons require a double quantity."

RICINUS MAJOR. See *Jatropha curcas*.

RICINUS VULGARIS. See *Ricinus*.

RICKETS. See *Rachitis*.

RICTUS. This term is applied by botanists to the grinning mouth or opening between the two lips of a ringent or personate flower.

RI'GOR. A sudden coldness, attended by a shivering, more or less perfect.

RI'MA. A fissure, or opening; as the *rima laryngis, rima vulvæ*.

RIMA GLOTTIDIS. The opening of the larynx, through which the air passes in and out of the lungs.

RI'MULA. (Diminutive of *rima*, a fissure.) A small fissure.

RINÆ'US. (From ριν, the nose.) See *Compressor naris*.

RING-WORM. A species of herpes. See *Herpes*.

RINGENS. Ringent: a term applied to flowers or their corolla, which are irregular and gaping, like the mouth of an animal; as those of the nettle, &c. A ringent flower is also called a lipped or labiate by some botanists.

RI'SAGON. See *Cassumuniar*.

RISIGALLUM. The auripigmentum was so called. See *Arsenious acid*.

RI'SUS. Laughter; laughing.

RISUS CANINUS. A kind of laughter in which the lips are contracted, so as to show all the teeth.

RISUS SARDONICUS. See *Sardonic laugh*.

RIVERIUS, LAZARUS, was born at Montpelier, in 1589. Being naturally slow in his attainments, he failed in his first examinations for a degree; but this only stimulated him to redoubled exertions, so that in the following spring he accomplished his object at the age of 22. His attachment to study became then very great, and eleven years after that period he was appointed to the professorship of medicine in the university; which office he filled with great honour till his death in 1655. Riverius published some valuable works, especially one, entitled "Praxis Medica;" which appeared at first in a concise form, as a sort of text-book; but finding it very favourably received by the public, he enlarged and improved it considerably: and it added greatly to his reputation, having passed through numerous editions, as well in the original, as translated into French and English.

RIVINUS, AUGUSTUS QUIRINUS, was son of a learned physician and critic, Andrew Bachmann, whose name was Latinized into Rivinus, and born at Leipsic, in 1652. He graduated at the age of 24, and fifteen years after obtained the professorships of physiology and botany in his native university; he was also associated with many learned bodies; and he filled these appointments with honour to himself till his death, in 1723. Rivinus distinguished himself chiefly as a systematic botanist; but his arrangement was very defective, being founded on the number of the petals, and their being regular, or irregular. Though by no means eminent as a practical anatomist, he is said to have discovered a new salivary duct. As a medical writer, he has the merit of faithful observation and description in his treatise "De Peste Lipsiensi," published in 1680. He wrote also on dyspepsia, on intermittents, and various other subjects. His "Censura Medicamentorum officinalium," ranks very high, on account of the freedom with which he attacked opinions, however generally received, which he believed erroneous; and to the prevalence of this spirit we owe the great simplification, and other improvements, which the Materia Medica exhibits at present.

ROASTING. A chemical process, generally performed in crucibles, by which mineral substances are divided, some of their principles being volatilized, and others changed, so as to prepare them for other operations.

ROB. (*Rob*, dense, Arabian.) An old term for an inspissated juice.

ROBORANT. (*Roborans;* from *roboro*, to strengthen.) That which is strengthening. See *Tonic*.

ROCCE'LLA. See *Lichen roccella*.

Rochelle-salt. See *Soda tartarisata*.

ROCKAMBOLE. The *Allium scorodoprasum*, of Linnæus. The root is used for pickles and high-seasoned dishes.

ROCK-BUTTER. A greasy mineral which oozes out of rocks that contain alum, at the Hurlet alumwork, near Paisley.

Rock cork. See *Asbestos*.

ROCK-CRYSTAL. A white and brown-coloured crystallized silicious mineral, found of great size and beauty in some parts of Scotland, and Dauphiny affords most magnificent groupes.

Rock-oil. See *Petroleum*.

ROCK-SALT. Of this there are two kinds, the *foliated* and the *fibrous*. The principal deposite of this salt in Great Britain is in Cheshire. In 1000 parts are contained, according to Henry, 983 of muriate of soda,

64 sulphate of lime, a little muriate of lime and muriate of magnesia, and 10 parts insoluble matter.

Rock-samphire. See *Crithmum maritimum.*

Rock, wood. The ligniform abestos.

ROCKET. See *Brassica eruca.*

Rocket, Roman. See *Brassica eruca.*

Rocket, wild. See *Brassica erucastrum.*

[ROMAYNE, NICHOLAS, M. D. was born in the city of New-York in September, 1756, and obtained his elementary education at Hackensack in New-Jersey, under the instruction of Dr. Peter Wilson, the late professor of languages in Columbia College. About the commencement of the revolutionary war he went abroad, and completed his medical studies at Edinburgh. He also visited the continent, and spent two years in Paris. Upon his return to New-York he commenced his professional career. He was advantageously known as an able private lecturer on many branches of medical science, and it is with pleasure I bear witness to his efficient instrumentality, in the foundation of the College of Physicians and Surgeons. He was its first president, and gave instructions in that institution on Anatomy and the Institutes of Medicine. His address as president, delivered at the first opening of the college in November, 1807, is an honourable specimen of his diversified attainments and talent. He died in New-York in 1817.

"Dr. Romayne," says Dr. M'Leod, "was a man of strong mind, well cultivated and much improved by reading, by the society of learned men, and by travelling. I knew him in health and in the midst of disease; in affluence and in adversity. He had much self-command, though naturally of powerful passions, and very tender sensibilities. Bereaved of all his children in their infancy, he could not endure the recollection of their endearment. On the last evening of his life he gave testimony to a dear friend, of his respect for the Scriptures. He departed too suddenly for me to see him on his death bed."—*Thach. Med. Biog.* A.]

RORE'LLA. See *Drosera rotundifolia.*

ROS. Dew.

ROS CALABRINUS. The official manna is sometimes so termed.

ROS SOLIS. See *Drosera rotundifolia.*

RO'SA. 1. The name of a genus of plants in the Linnæan system. Class, *Icosandria;* Order, *Polygynia.* The rose.

2. A name sometimes given to the erysipelas, because it begins with a redness like that of a rose.

ROSA ALBA. The white rose. The flowers of this species possess similar but inferior virtues to those of the damask.

ROSA CANINA. *Rosa sylvestris; Cynorrhodon; Cynosbatos.* The dog rose, or wild-brier, or hip-tree. *Rosa—germinibus ovatis pedunculisque glabris, caule petiolisque aculeatis,* of Linnæus. The fruit of this tree, called heps, or hips, has a sourish taste, and obtains a place in the London pharmacopœia, in the form of conserve. It is seldom employed but to give form to more active remedies, in pills, boluses, linctuses, &c.

ROSA CENTIFOLIA. The pharmacopœial and systematic name of the damask rose. *Rosa damasceda; Rosa pallida.* The damask rose. The pharmacopœias direct a syrup to be prepared from the petals of this rose, *Rosa—germinibus ovatis pedunculisque hispidis, caule hispido aculeato petiolis inermibus,* of Linnæus; which is found to be a pleasant and useful laxative for children, or to obviate costiveness in adults. Most of the roses, though much cultivated in our gardens, are far from being distinctly characterized. Those denominated varieties are extremely numerous, and often permanently uniform; and the specific differences, as hitherto pointed out, are in many respects so inadequate to the purpose of satisfactory discrimination, that it becomes a difficult matter to distinguish which are species and which are varieties only. The damask rose seems to be another species widely different from the centifolia, as appears from the description given of it by Du Roi and Miller.

The petals are directed for medical use; they are of a pale red colour, and of a very fragrant odour, which, to most people, is extremely agreeable; and therefore this and most of the other roses are much used as nosegays. We may remark, however, that in some instances, they have, under certain circumstances, produced alarming symptoms. The petals "impart

250

their odorous matter to watery liquors, both by infusion and distillation. Six pounds of fresh roses impregnate, by distillation, a gallon, or more, of water, strongly with their fine flavour. On distilling large quantities, there separates from the watery fluid a small portion of a fragrant butyraceous oil, which liquefies by heat, and appears yellow, but concretes in the cold into a white mass. A hundred pounds of the flowers, according to the experiments of Tachenius and Hoffman, afforded scarcely half an ounce of oil." The smell of the oil exactly resembles that of roses, and is therefore much used as a perfume. It possesses very little pungency, and has been highly recommended for its cordial and analeptic qualities. These flowers also contain a bitterish substance, which is extracted by water along with the odorous principle, and remains entire in the decoction after the latter has been separated by distillation, or evaporation.

This fixed sapid matter of the petals manifests a purgative quality; and it is on this account that the flowers are received in the Materia Medica.

ROSA DAMASCENA. See *Rosa centifolia.*

ROSA GALLICA. The pharmacopœial and systematic name of the red rose. *Rosa rubra.* The flowers of this species, *Rosa—germinibus ovatis pedunculisque hispidis, caule petiolisque hispido aculeatis,* of Linnæus, are valued for their adstringent qualities, which are most considerable before the petals expand; and therefore in this state they are chosen for medicinal use, and ordered by the pharmacopœias in different preparations, as those of a conserve, or confection, a honey, an infusion, and a syrup. The infusion of roses is a grateful cooling subadstringent, and useful in hæmoptysis, and other hæmorrhagic complaints: its efficacy, however, depends chiefly on the sulphuric acid added.

ROSA PALLIDA. See *Rosa centifolia.*

ROSA RUBRA. See *Rosa gallica.*

ROSA SYLVESTRIS. See *Rosa canina.*

ROSA'CEUS. Rose-like. 1. Applied to corolla which spread like a rose, as those of the *Dryas.*

2. The term *gutta rosacea* is applied to little rosy-coloured spots upon the face and nose.

ROSACIC ACID. There is deposited from the urine of persons, labouring under gout and inflammatory fevers, a sediment of a rose colour, occasionally in reddish crystals. This was first discovered to be a peculiar acid by M. Proust, and afterward examined by M. Vauquelin. This acid is solid, of a lively cinnabar hue, without smell, with a faint taste, but reddening litmus very sensibly. On burning coal it is decomposed into a pungent vapour, which has not the odour of burning animal matter. It is very soluble in water, and it even softens in the air. It is soluble in alkohol It forms soluble salts with potassa, soda, ammonia, barytes, strontites, and lime. It gives a slight rose-coloured precipitate with acetate of lead. It also combines with lithic acid, forming so intimate a union, that the lithic acid in precipitating from urine, carries the other, though a deliquescent substance, down along with it. It is obtained pure by acting on the sediment of urine with alkohol.

ROSALIA. A name in some authors for the measles, or a disease very like the measles.

ROSE. See *Rosa.*

Rose, damask. See *Rosa centifolia.*

Rose, dog. See *Rosa canina.*

ROSEA RADIX. See *Rhodiola.*

Rose, red. See *Rosa gallica.*

ROSE ROOT. See *Rhodiola.*

Rose, white. See *Rosa alba.*

Rosebay willow herb. See *Epilobium angustifolium.*

ROSEMARY. See *Rosmarinus.*

ROSEOLA. (From *rosa,* a rose: so called from the colour of the rash.) A rose-coloured efflorescence, variously figured, without wheals, or papulæ, and not contagious. It is mostly symptomatic, occurring in connexion with different febrile complaints, and requiring no deviation from the treatment respectively adapted to them.

Its principal varieties are comprised under the seven following heads:

1. The *Roseola æstiva* appears first on the face and neck, and in the course of a day or two is distributed over the whole body, producing a considerable degree of itching and tingling. It is distributed into separate small patches, of various figure, but larger and more irregular forms than in the measles. It is at first red,

but soon assumes its deep roseate hue. The fauces are tinged with the same colour, and a slight roughness of the tonsils is felt in swallowing.

The rash continues vivid through the second day; after which it declines in brightness, slight specks only remaining of a dark hue, on the fourth day; which, with the constitutional affection, wholly disappear on the fifth.

The efflorescence sometimes is partial, extending only over portions of the face, neck, and upper part of the breast and shoulders, in patches, slightly-elevated, and itching considerably, but in this form the disease continues a week or longer, the rash appearing and disappearing several times; sometimes from taking warm liquors, and sometimes without any apparent cause. The retrocession is usually accompanied with disorder of the stomach, headache, and faintness; which are immediately relieved on its appearance. It commonly occurs in females of irritable constitution in summer. Light diets and acidulated drinks, with occasional laxatives, palliate the symptoms.

2. The *Roseola autumnalis* occurs in children, in the autumn, in distinct circular or oval patches, which gradually increase to the size of a shilling, and are of a dark damask rose hue. It appears chiefly on the arms, sometimes desquamating, and its decline seems to be expedited by the internal use of sulphuric acid.

3. The *Roseola annulata* occurs on almost every part of the body, in rose-coloured rings, with central areas of the usual colour of the skin. When accompanied with fever its duration is short: at other times, without any constitutional disorder, it continues for a considerable and uncertain period. The rings are, at first, from a line to two lines in diameter, but gradually dilating leave a larger central space, sometimes of the diameter of half an inch. The efflorescence is less vivid (and in the chronic form usually fades) in the morning, but increases in the evening or night, and produces a heat and itching in the skin. When it becomes very faint in colour for several days, the stomach is disordered, and languor, giddiness, and pains of the limbs ensue, which are relieved by the use of the warm bath.

Sea-bathing and the mineral acids afford much relief in the chronic forms of this rash.

4. *Roseola infantilis* is a closer rash occurring in infants during the irritation of dentition, of disordered bowels, and in fevers. It is very irregular in its appearances, sometimes continuing only for a night, sometimes appearing and disappearing for several successive days with violent disorder, and sometimes arising in single patches in different parts of the body successively. It is alleviated by the remedies adapted to relieve bowel complaints, painful dentition and other febrile affections with which it is connected.

5. *Roseola variolosa* occurs previously to the eruption both of the natural and inoculated small-pox, but seldom before the former. It appears in the inoculated disease, on the second day of the eruptive fever, which is generally the ninth or tenth after inoculation. It is first seen on the arms, breast, and face; and on the following day it extends over the trunk, and extremities. Sometimes it is distributed in oblong irregular patches, sometimes diffused with numerous interstices, and sometimes it forms an almost continuous redness over the whole body, being in some parts slightly elevated. It continues about three days, on the second or last of which, the variolous pustules may be distinguished, in the general redness, by their rounded elevation, hardness, and whiteness of their tops.

6. *Roseola vaccina* appears generally in a congeries of dots and small patches, but sometimes diffuse like the former; takes place on the ninth or tenth day after vaccination, at the place of inoculation, and at the same time with the areola that is formed round the vesicle, from whence it spreads irregularly over the whole surface of the body.

It is usually attended with a very quick pulse, white tongue, and great restlessness.

7. *Roseola miliaris* often accompanies an eruption of miliary vesicles after fever. It is sometimes connected with attacks of the gout and of the febrile rheumatism, accompanied with considerable fever, extreme languor and depression of spirits, total loss of appetite, and torpid bowels, and terminates on the seventh day by desquamation.

ROSEWOOD. See *Rhodium lignum.*

ROSEWORT. See *Rhodiola*

ROSIN. See *Resina.*

ROSMARI'NUS. (*Quasi rosá, ϱμυρνα,* because it smells like myrrh.) 1. The name of a genus of plants in the Linnæan system. Class, *Diandria;* Order, *Monogynia.*

2. The pharmacopæial name of the common rosemary.

ROSMARINUS HORTENSIS. See *Rosmarinus officinalis.*

ROSMARINUS OFFICINALIS. The systematic name of the common rosemary. *Rosmarinus hortensis; Libanotis coronaria; Dendrolibanus; Rosmarinus,* of Linnæus. The leaves and tops of this plant have a fragrant aromatic smell, and a bitterish pungent taste. Rosemary is reckoned one of the most powerful of those plants which stimulate and corroborate the nervous system; it has therefore been recommended in various affections supposed to proceed from debility, or defective excitement of the brain and nerves, as in certain headaches, deafness, giddiness, and in some hysterical and dyspeptic symptoms. The officinal preparations of rosemary are, an essential oil from their leaves, or from the herb in flower, a conserve of the flowers, and a spirit formerly called Hungary water, from the flowery tops. The tops are also used in the compound spirit of Lavender, and soap liniment.

ROSMARINUS SYLVESTRIS. See *Ledum palustre.*

ROSTELLUM. A little beak. Applied to that part of the seed which is pointed, penetrates the earth, and becomes the root. See *Corculum.*

ROSTRATUS. Rostrate. Applied to the pod of the *Sinapis alba.*

ROSTRUM. (From *rodo,* to gnaw; because birds use it to tear their food with.) 1. A beak.

2. The piece of flesh which hangs between the division of the hare-lip is called rostrum leporinum.

3. Applied in botany to some elongation of a seed-vessel, originating from the permanent style; as in *Geranium:* though it is also used for naked seeds; as *Scandix.*

ROTACEÆ. (From *rota,* a wheel.) The name of an order of plants in Linnæus's Fragments of a Natural Method, consisting of those which have one flat wheel-shaped petal.

ROTACISMUS. The harsh or asperated vibration of the letter *r* or *ρο,* which is very common in the northern parts of England.

ROTANG. See *Calamus rotang.*

ROTA'TOR. (From *róto,* to turn.) A muscle the office of which is to wheel about the thigh.

ROTATUS. Rotate, or wheel-like; salver-shaped Applied to the corolla, nectary, &c.; as the nectary of the *Cyssampelos,* the corolla of the *Borago officinalis.*

RO'TULA. (Diminutive of *rota,* a wheel: so called from its shape.) See *Patella.*

ROTUNDUS. See *Round.*

ROUGE. See *Carthamus tinctorius.*

ROUND. *Rotundus.* Many parts of animals and vegetables receive this trivial name from their shape; as round ligaments, round foramen, &c.; and leaves, stems, seeds, &c. as the *seed* of the *Pisum Brassica,* &c.

Round-leaved sorrel. See *Rumex scutatus.*

ROUND LIGAMENTS. *Ligamenta rotunda.* A bundle of vessels and fibres contained in a duplicature of the peritonæum, that proceed from the sides of the uterus, through the abdominal rings, and disappear in the pudenda.

RUBE'DO. (From *ruber,* red.) A diffused, but not spotted, redness in any part of the skin; such as that which arises from blushing.

RUBEFACIENT. (*Rubefaciens;* from *rubefacio,* to make red.) That substance which, when applied a certain time to the skin, induces a redness without blistering.

RUBELITE. Red tourmalin.

RUBE'OLA. (From *ruber,* red; or from *rubeo,* to become red.) *Morbili.* The measles. A genus of disease in the Class *Pyrexiæ,* and Order *Exanthemata,* of Cullen; known by synocha, hoarseness, dry cough, sneezing, drowsiness; about the fourth day, eruption or small red points, discernible by the touch, which, after three days, ends in mealy desquamation. The blood, after venæsection, exhibits an inflammatory crust. In addition to the symptoms already related, it is remarkable, that the eyes and eyelids always show the presence of this disease, being somewhat inflamed and suffused with tears. The synocha continues during the whole progress of the disease. In systems of nosology, several varieties of measles are mentioned, but they may be all comprehended under two heads; the one attended with more or less of the symptoms of general inflammation; the other accompanied by a putrid diathesis.

The measles may prevail at all seasons of the year as an epidemic, but the middle of winter is the time they are usually most prevalent; and they attack persons of all ages, but children are most liable to them. They prove most unfavourable to such as are of a plethoric or scrofulous habit. Like the small-pox, they never affect persons but once in their life; their contagion appears to be of a specific nature. The eruption is usually preceded by a general uneasiness, chilliness, and shivering, pain in the head, in grown persons; but in children a heaviness and soreness in the throat; sickness and vomiting, with other affections, such as happen in most fevers; but the chief characteristic symptoms are, a heaviness about the eyes, with swelling, inflammation, and a defluxion of sharp tears, and great acuteness of sensation, so that they cannot bear the light without pain, together with a discharge of such serous humour from the nostrils, which produce sneezing. The heat and other febrile symptoms, increase very rapidly; to which succeeds a frequent and dry cough, a stuffing, great oppression, and oftentimes retching to vomit, with violent pains in the loins, and sometimes a looseness; at other times there is great sweating, the tongue foul and white, the thirst very great, and, in general, the fever runs much higher than in the milder sort of the regular small-pox. The eruptions appear about the fourth or fifth day, and sometimes about the end of the third. On the third or fourth day from their first appearance, the redness diminishes, the spots, or very small papulæ, dry up, the cuticle peels off, and is replaced by a new one. The symptoms do not go off on the eruption, as in the small-pox, except the vomiting; the cough and headache continue, with the weakness and defluxion on the eyes, and a considerable degree of fever. On the ninth or eleventh day, no trace of redness is to be found, but the skin assumes its wonted appearance; yet, without there have been some considerable evacuations either by the skin, or by vomiting, the patient will hardly recover strength, but the cough will continue, the fever return with new violence, and bring on great distress and danger.

In the more alarming cases, spasms of the limbs, subsultus, tendinum, delirium, or what more frequently happens, coma, supervene. This last symptom so frequently attends the eruptive fever of measles, that by some practitioners it is regarded as one of its diagnostics.

In measles, as in other febrile diseases, the symptoms generally suffer some remission towards the morning, returning however towards the evening with increased severity.

The measles, even when violent, are not usually attended with a putrid tendency; but it sometimes happens, that such a disposition prevails both in the course of the disease and at its termination. In such cases, petechiæ are to be observed interspersed among the eruptions, and these last become livid, or assume almost a black colour. Hæmorrhages break out from different parts of the body, the pulse becomes frequent, feeble, and perhaps irregular, universal debility ensues, and the patient is destroyed.

In those cases where there is much fever, with great difficulty of breathing, and other symptoms of pneumonic inflammation, or where there is great debility, with a tendency to putrescency, there will always be considerable danger; but the consequences attendant on the measles are in general more to be dreaded than the immediate disease; for although a person may get through it, and appear for a time to be recovered, still hectic symptoms and pulmonary consumption shall afterward arise, and destroy him, or an ophthalmia shall ensue.

Measles, as well as small-pox, not unfrequently call into action a disposition to scrofula, where such happens to exist in the habit. Another bad consequence of the measles is, that the bowels are often left by them in a very weak state; a chronic diarrhœa remaining, which has sometimes proved fatal. Dropsy has also been known as a consequence of measles.

252

The morbid appearances to be observed on dissections of those who die of measles are pretty much confined to the lungs and intestines: the former of which always show strong marks of inflammation, and sometimes a tendency to sphacelus. Where the patient dies under the eruption, the trachea and larger branches of the bronchia, as in the small-pox, are often covered with it, which may account for the increase of the cough after the appearance of the eruption.

In the treatment of this disorder, as it usually appears, the object is to moderate the accompanying synocha fever, and attend to the state of certain organs, particularly the lungs and the bowels. When there are no urgent local symptoms, it will be commonly sufficient to pursue the general antiphlogistic plan, (avoiding, however, too free or sudden exposure to cold,) keeping the bowels open, and encouraging diaphoresis by mild antimonials, &c. Sometimes, however, in plethoric habits, especially where the lungs are weak, it will be proper to begin by a moderate abstraction of blood. Where the eruption has been imprudently checked, much distress usually follows, and it will be advisable to endeavour to bring it out again by the warm bath, with other means of increasing the action of the cutaneous vessels. Should an inflammatory determination of the lungs occur, more active evacuations must be practised, as explained under the head of *Pneumonia.* The cough may be palliated by opium, joined with expectorants, demulcents, &c.: and an occasional emetic will be proper, when there is much wheezing. Where diarrhœa takes place, it is better not to attempt to suppress it at once; but if troublesome, moderate it by small doses of opium, assisted perhaps by astringents. At the decline of the disorder, much attention is often required to prevent phthisis pulmonalis supervening. Should the disorder ever put on a putrid character, the general plan pointed out under *Typhus* must be pursued.

RU'BIA. (From *ruber,* red: so called from its red roots.) 1. The name of a genus of plants in the Linnæan system. Class, *Tetrandria;* Order, *Monogynia.*

2. The pharmacopœial name of the madder plant, *Rubia tinctorum.*

RUBIA TINCTORUM. The systematic name of the madder plant. *Erythrodanum; Rubia major; Radix rubra.* Dyers' madder. *Rubia—foliis annuis, caule aculeato,* of Linnæus. The roots of this plant have a bitterish, somewhat austere taste, and a slight smell, not of the agreeable kind. It was formerly considered as a deobstruent, detergent, and diuretic, but it is now very seldom used.

RUBI'GO. (*Rubigo, inis.* f.; *à colore rubro,* from its red colour.) Rust.

RUBIGO CUPRI. See *Verdigris.*

RUBIGO FERRI. See *Ferri subcarbonas.*

RUBI'NUS. (From *ruber,* red: so named from its colour.) A carbuncle. See *Anthrax.*

RUBINUS VERUS. See *Anthrax.*

RUBULI. (From *rubus,* a blackberry or raspberry.) The specific name in Good's Nosology of the yaws.

RU'BUS. (From *ruber,* red: so called from its red fruit.) The name of a genus of plants in the Linnæan system. Class, *Icosandria;* Order, *Polygynia.*

RUBUS ARCTICUS. The systematic name of the shrubby strawberry. *Rubus—foliis alternatis, caule inermi uniflora.* The berries, *Baccæ norlandicæ,* are recommended by Linnæus as possessing antiseptic, refrigerant, and antiscorbutic qualities.

RUBUS CÆSIUS. The systematic name of the dewberry plant, the fruit of which resembles the blackberry in appearance and qualities.

RUBUS CHAMÆMORUS. The systematic name of the cloudberry-tree. *Chamæmorus; Chamærubus foliis ribis Anglicæ; Rubus palustris humilis; Vaccinium Lancastrense; Rubus alpinus humilis Anglicus.* Cloudberries and knotberries. The ripe fruit of this plant, *Rubus —foliis simplicibus lobatis, caule interno unifloro,* of Linnæus, is prepared into a jam; and is recommended to allay thirst, &c. in fevers, phthisical diseases, hæmoptysis, &c. As an antiscorbutic, it is said to excel the scurvy-grass and other vegetables of that tribe in common use.

RUBUS FRUTICOSUS. The systematic name of the common bramble, which affords blackberries. The berries are eaten in abundance by children, and are wholesome and gently aperient. Too large quantities, however, when the stomach is weak, produce vomit ing and great distention of the belly, from flatus. See *Fruits, summer.*

RUBUS IDÆUS. The systematic name of the raspberry. *Batinon; Moron. Rubus—foliis quinato-pinnatis ternatisque, caule aculeato, petiolis canaliculatis,* of Linnæus. The fruit of this plant has a pleasant sweet taste, accompanied with a peculiar grateful flavour, on account of which it is chiefly valued. Its virtues consist in allaying heat and thirst, and promoting the natural excretions. A grateful syrup prepared from the juice is directed for officinal use.

[RUBUS TRIVIALIS. See *Blackberry.* A.]
[RUBUS VILLOSUS. See *Blackberry.* A.]

RUBY. See *Sapphire.*

RU'CTUS. An eructation.

RUE. See *Ruta graveolens.*

Rue, goats. See *Galega.*

RUFI PILULÆ. Rufus's pills. A compound very similar to the aloëtic pills with myrrh. See *Pilula aloes cum myrrha.*

RUFUS, the Ephesian a physician and anatomist of considerable eminence in the reign of Trajan, esteemed by Galen one of the most able of his predecessors. He traced the origin of the nerves in the brain by dissecting brutes, and considered some of them as contributing to motion, others to sensation. He even observed the capsule of the crystalline lens in the eye. He considered the heart as the seat of life, and of the animal heat, and as the origin of the pulse, which he ascribed to the *spirit* of its left ventricle and of the arteries. There is a very respectable treatise by him on the Diseases of the Urinary Organs, and the Method of curing them. He also wrote a good work on Purgative Medicines; and a little treatise on the Names given by the Greeks to the different Parts of the Body. Galen affirms also, that Rufus was the author of an Essay on the Materia Medica, in verse; and Suidas mentions others on the *Atra bilis,* &c., but these are all lost.

R U G O S U S. Rugged. A term applied to a leaf, when the veins are tighter than the surface between them, causing the latter to swell into little inequalities, as the various species of sage. The seeds of the Lithospermum arvense are rugose.

RUM. A spirituous liquor, well known, the produce of the sugar-cane.

RU'MEX. (*Rumex, icis.* m.; a sort of pike, spear, or halberd, which the shape of the leaves in various species much resembles.) The name of a genus of plants in the Linnæan system. Class, *Hexandria;* Order, *Trigynia.* The dock.

RUMEX ACETOSA. The systematic name of the common sorrel. *Acetosa; Acetosa vulgaris; Acetosa pratensis; Acetosa arvensis.* Sorrel; sour-dock. *Rumex—foliis oblongis sagittatis, floribus diæciis,* of Linnæus. The leaves of this plant are sour, but not the root, which is bitter. It grows in the meadows and common fields.

RUMEX ACUTUS. The systematic name of the sharppointed wild-dock. *Oxylapathum; Lapathum. Rumex—floribus hermaphroditis; valvulis dentatis graniferis, foliis cordato oblongis acuminatis,* of Linnæus. The decoction of the root of this plant is used in Germany to cure the itch; and it appears to have been used in the time of Dioscorides, in the cure of leprous and impetiginous affections, both alone and boiled with vinegar.

RUMEX ALPINUS. The systematic name of the plant which affords the monk's rhubarb. See *Rumex patientia.*

RUMEX AQUATICUS. See *Rumex hydrolapathum.*

["RUMEX BRITANNICA. The common American water-dock, which grows in wet, boggy soils, and upon the margin of ditches, is a moderately stimulating and astringent plant. It is esteemed by many country practitioners as a local application to indolent and ill-conditioned ulcers. A strong decoction of the root is usually employed as a wash in these cases. Sometimes an ointment, formed by simmering the root in hog's lard, is beneficially applied in herpes. The use of this plant, according to Colden, was learned from the Indians."—*Big. Mat. Med.* A.]

RUMEX CRISPUS. The systematic name of the crispleaved dock.

RUMEX HYDROLAPATHUM. The systematic name of the water-dock. *Hydrolapathum; Rumex aquaticus; Herba Britannica; Lapathum aquaticum.* The wa-

ter-dock. *Rumex—floribus hermaphroditis, valvulis integris graniferis, foliis lanceolatis,* of Linnæus. The leaves of this plant manifest considerable acidity, and are said to possess a laxative quality. The root is strongly astringent, and has been much employed, both externally and internally, for the cure of some diseases of the skin, as scurvy, lepra, lichen, &c. The root powdered is said to be an excellent dentifrice.

["RUMEX OBTUSIFOLIUS. This species of dock is a foreign plant, naturalized as a weed in the cultivated grounds in this country. The root is bitterish and astringent. A decoction, taken internally, is laxative Externally it is applied for the cure of ulcers and cutaneous diseases, and sometimes with very good effect. The *Rumex crispus,* or *curled dock,* another important weed, resembles this in its qualities, and, in the form of ointment or decoction, is found to cure mild cases of psora and other eruptions."—*Big. Mat. Med.* A.]

RUMEX PATIENTIA. The systematic name of the garden patience. *Rhabarbarum monachorum; Hip polapathum; Patientia.* Monk's rhubarb. The root of this plant, and that of the *Rumex alpinus,* according to Professor Murray, is supposed to possess the virtues of rhubarb, but in an inferior degree. It is obviously more astringent than rhubarb, but comes very far short of its purgative virtue.

RUMEX SANGUINEUS. The systematic name of the bloody dock, the root of which has an austere and astringent taste, and is sometimes given by the vulgar in the cure of dysentery.

RUMEX SCUTATUS. The systematic name of the French sorrel, sometimes called *acetosa rotundifolia,* in the shops. *Acetosa romana; Acetosa rotundifolia hortensis.* Roman, or garden sorrel. *Rumex—foliis cordato-hastatis, ramis divergentibus, floribus hermaphroditis,* of Linnæus. It is common in our gardens, and in many places is known by the culinary name of Green-sauce. Its virtues are similar to those of common sorrel. See *Rumex acetosa.*

RUNCINA'TUS. Runcinate: applied to leaves which are shaped like the tooth of a lion: that is, cut into several transverse, acute segments, pointing backwards; as in *Leontodon taraxacum,* called from the shape of its leaf, dens de lion, and hence Dandelion.

RUPELLENSIS SAL. (From *Rupella, Rochella,* where it was first made.) Rochelle salt. See *Soda tartarizata.*

RUPTU'RA. See *Hernia.*

RUPTURE. See *Hernia.*

RUPTURE-WORT. See *Herniaria.*

RU'SCUS. (*A russo colore,* from the carnation colour of its berries.) 1. The name of a genus of plants in the Linnæan system. Class, *Diœcia;* Order, *Syngenesia.*

2. The pharmacopœial name of the butcher's broom. *Ruscus aculeatus.*

RUSCUS ACULEATUS. The systematic name of butcher's broom, or knee holly. *Bruscus; Oxymyrrhine; Oxymyrsine; Myrtacantha; Myacantha; Scopa regia.* Wild myrtle. A small evergreen shrub, the *Rucus foliis supra floriferis nudis* of Linnæus. It grows in woods and thickets in this country. The root, which is somewhat thick, knotty, and furnished with long fibres, externally brown, internally white, and of a bitterish taste, has been recommended as an aperient and diuretic in dropsies, urinary obstructions, and nephritic cases. It is seldom used in this country. See *Ruscus.*

RUSCUS HYPOGLOSSUM. The systematic name of he uvularia. This plant was formerly used against relaxation of the uvula, but is now laid aside for more adstringent remedies.

RUSH. See *Arundo.*

["RUSH, BENJAMIN, M. D., was born in December, 1745, near the city of Philadelphia, in Pennsylvania, and he died in that city in April, 1813, aged 68 years. Dr. Rush was a man of small stature, but of a strong and vigorous mind. During the eventful period of his life, he occupied the distinguished consideration of his countrymen, as one of the patriots of the American Revolution, as an able physician, as a professor in the medical school of Philadelphia, as a philanthropist, and as an exemplary Christian. His writings, on subjects connected with his professional pursuits, are numerous, and worthy the attention of members of the profession. Such as were printed during his life-time, treat on the following subjects, viz.:—"An Inquiry into the Natural History of Medicine among the Indians of North America, and a comparative View of their Diseases and Remedies, with those of civilized Nations."—" An Account of the Climate of Pennsylvania, and its Influence upon the Human Body."—" An Account of the Bilious Remitting Fever, as it appeared in Philadelphia in the Summer and Autumn of 1780."—" An Account of the Scarlatina Anginosa, as it appeared in Philadelphia in 1783 and 1784."—" An Inquiry into the Cause and Cure of the Cholera Infantum."—" Obsert vations on the Cynanche Trachealis."—" An Account of the Efficacy of Blisters and Bleeding in the Cure of obstinate Intermitting Fevers."—" An Account of the Disease occasioned by drinking Cold Water in Warm Weather, and the Method of curing it."—" An Account of the Efficacy of common Salt in the cure of Hæmoptysis."—" Thoughts on the Cause and Cure of Pulmonary Consumption."—"Observations upon Worms in the alimentary Canal, and upon anthelmintic Medicines."—" An Account of the external use of Arsenic in the cure of Cancers."—"Observations on the Tetanus."—" The Result of Observations made upon the Diseases which occurred in the Military Hospitals of the United States, during the Revolutionary War."—" An Account of the Influence of military and political Events of the American Revolution upon the Human Body."—" An Inquiry into the Relations of Tastes and Aliments on each other, and upon the Influence of this Relation upon Health and Pleasure."—"The new Method of inoculating for the Small-pox."—" An Inquiry into the Effects of ardent Spirits upon the Human Mind and Body, with an Account of the Means of preventing, and the Remedies for curing them."—"Observations on the Duties of Physicians, and the Methods of improving Medicines; accommodated to the present State of Society and Manners in the United States."—" An Inquiry into the Causes and Cure of sore Legs."—" An Account of the State of the Body and Mind in Old Age, with Observations on its Diseases and their Remedies."—" An Inquiry into the Influence of Physical Causes upon the Moral Faculty."—"Observations upon the Cause and Cure of Pulmonary Consumption."—"Observations upon the Symptoms and Cure of Dropsies."—" Inquiry into the Cause and Cure of Gout."—"Observations on the Nature and Cure of Hydrophobia."—" An Account of the Measles as they appeared in Philadelphia in the Spring of 1789."—" An Account of the Influenza, as it appeared in Philadelphia in the years 1790 and 1791."—"An Inquiry into the Cause of Animal Life."—"Outlines of a Theory of Fever."—" An Account of the Bilious Yellow Fever, as it appeared in Philadelphia in 1793, and of each successive year till 1805."—" An Inquiry into the various Sources of the usual Forms of the Summer and Autumnal Diseases in the United States, and the Means of preventing them."—" Facts intended to prove the Yellow Fever not contagious."—" Defence of Bloodletting, as a Remedy in certain Diseases.—" An Inquiry into the comparative States of Medicine in Philadelphia, between the years 1760 and 1766 and 1805."—" A Volume of Essays: Literary, Moral, and Philosophical, in which the following Subjects are discussed:—A Plan for establishing Public Schools in Philadelphia, and for conducting Education agreeably to a Republican Form of Government. Addressed to the Legislature and Citizens of Pennsylvania, in the year 1786.—Of the Mode of Education proper in a Republic.—Observations upon the Study of the Latin and Greek Languages, as a Branch of liberal Education; with Hints of a Plan of liberal Instruction without them, accommodated to the present State of Society, Manners, and Government, in the United States.—Thoughts upon the Amusements and Punishments which are proper for Schools.—Thoughts upon Female Education, accommodated to the present State of Society, Manners, and Government, in the United States of America.—A Defence of the Bible as a School-book.—An Address to the Ministers of the Gospel of every denomination in the United States, upon Subjects interesting to Morals.—An Inquiry into the Consistency of the Punishment of Murder by Death, with Reason and Revelation.—A Plan of a Peace Office for the United States.—Information to Europeans who are disposed to emigrate to the United States of America.—An Account of the Progress of Population, Agriculture, Manners, and Government, in Pennsylvania.—An Account of the Manners of the German Inhabitants of Pennsyl-

vania.—Thoughts on Common Sense.—An Account of the Vices peculiar to the Indians of North America.—Observations upon the Influence of the Habitual Use of Tobacco, upon Health, Morals, and Property.—An Account of the Sugar Maple-tree of the United States.—An Account of the Life and Death of Edward Drinker, who died on the 17th of November, 1782, in the one hundred and third year of his age.—Remarkable Circumstances in the Constitution and Life of Ann Woods, an old Woman of ninety-six years of age.—Biographical Anecdotes of Benjamin Lay.—Biographical Anecdotes of Anthony Benezet.—Paradise of Negro Slaves, a Dream.—Eulogium upon Dr. William Cullen.—Eulogium upon David Rittenhouse."—" A Volume of Lectures," most of which were introductory to his annual Course of Lectures on the Institutes and Practice of Medicine.—" Medical Inquiries and Observations on the Diseases of the Mind."—*Thach. Med. Biog. A.]*

Rush-nut. See *Cyperus esculentus.*

Rush, sweet. See *Andropogon schœnanthus,* and *Acorus calamy.*

RUSSELL, ALEXANDER, was a native of Edinburgh, where he received his medical education, and after ward became physician to the English factory at Aleppo, where he resided several years. He soon obtained a proud pre-eminence above all the practitioners there, and was consulted by persons of every description. The pacha particularly distinguished him by his friendship, and sought his advice on every act of importance. In 1755, he published his " Natural History of Aleppo," a valuable and interesting work, containing especially some important observations relative to the Plague. On his return to England four years after, he settled in London, and was elected physician to St. Thomas's hospital, which office he retained till his death in 1770. He presented several valuable communications to the Royal Society, as also to the Medical Society.

RUSSELL, PATRICK, was brother of the preceding, and his successor as physician to the English factory at Aleppo. He published a copious treatise on the Plague, having had ample opportunities of treating that disease during 1760, and the two following years. In this work he has fully discussed the important subject of Quarantine, Lazarettoes, and the Police to be adopted in times of Pestilence. He likewise gave to the public a new edition of his brother's work on a very enlarged scale.

Russia ashes. The impure potassa, as imported from *Russia.*

Rust. A carbonate of iron.

RUTA. (From ρυω, to preserve, because it preserves health.) 1. The name of a genus of plants in the Linnæan system. Class, *Decandria;* Order, *Monogynia.*

2. The pharmacopœial name of the common rue. See *Ruta graveolens.*

RUTA GRAVEOLENS. The systematic name of the common rue. *Ruta—foliis decompositis, floribus lateralibus quadrifidis,* of Linnæus. Rue has a strong ungrateful smell, and a bitter, hot, penetrating taste, the leaves are so acrid, that by much handling they have been known to irritate and inflame the skin; and the plant, in its natural or uncultivated state, is said to possess these sensible qualities still more powerfully. The imaginary quality of the rue, in resisting and expelling contagion, is now disregarded. It is doubtless a powerful stimulant, and is considered, like other medicines of the fœtid kind, as possessing attenuating, deobstruent, and antispasmodic powers. In the former London Pharmacopœia it was directed in the form of an extract; and was also an ingredient in the *pulvis e myrrha comp.,* but these are now omitted. The dose of the leaves is from fifteen grains to two scruples.

RUTA MURARIA. See *Asplenium ruta muraria.*

RUTIDO′SIS. A corrugation and subsiding of the cornea of the eye. The species are,

1. *Rutidosis,* from a wound or puncture penetrating the cornea.

2. *Rutidosis,* from a fistula penetrating the cornea.

3. *Rutidosis,* from a deficiency of the aqueous humour, which happens from old age, fevers, great and continued evacuations, and in extreme dryness of the air.

4. *Rutidosis,* of dead persons, when the aqueous humour exhales through the cornea, and no fresh hu-

mour is secreted ; so that the cornea becomes obscure and collapsed : this is a most certain sign of death.

RUTILE. An ore of titanium.

RUTULA. (From *ruta*, rue.) A small species of rue

RUYSCH, FREDERICK, was born at the Hague, in 1638. After going through the preliminary studies with great zeal, he graduated at Leyden in 1664, and then settled in his native city. In the following year he published his treatise on the lacteal and lymphatic vessels ; in consequence of which he was invited to the chair of anatomy at Amsterdam. From that period his attention was chiefly devoted to anatomical researches, both human and comparative ; and he contributed materially to the improvement of the art of injecting, for the purpose of demonstrating minute structure, and preserving the natural appearance of parts. His museum became ultimately the most magnificent that any private individual had ever accumulated ; and being at length purchased by the czar Peter for thirty thousand florins, he immediately set about a new collection. He appears not to have paid sufficient attention to inform himself of the writings of others, whence he sometimes arrogated to himself what was really before known, which led him into several controversies ; but his indefatigable researches in anatomy were certainly rewarded with many discoveries. In 1685, he was appointed professor of physic, and received subsequently several marks of distinction, as well in his own as from foreign countries. In 1728, he had the misfortune to break his thigh by a fall in his chamber, and the remainder of his life, for about three years, was chiefly occupied in proceeding with his new museum, in which his youngest daughter assisted him. Besides his controversial tracts, he published several other works, chiefly anatomical ; " Observationum Anat. Chirurg. Centuria ;" twelve essays under the title of " Thesaurus Anatomicus," at different periods, the last containing Remarks on the Anatomy of Vegetables ; a " Thesaurus Animalium," with plates ; three decades of " Adversaria Anat. Chirurg. Medica," &c.

RUYSCHIANA TUNICA. The internal surface of the choroid membrane of the human eye, which this celebrated anatomist imagined was a distinct lamina from the external surface.

RYAS. See *Rhœas*.

RYE. See *Secale cereale*.

S

S. A. The contraction of *secundum artem*.

S, or *ss*. Immediately following any quantity, imports *semis*, or half.

SABADILLA. See *Cevadilla*.

SABI'NA. Named from the Sabines, whose priests used it in their religious ceremonies. See *Juniperus sabina*.

SABULOUS. (*Sabulosis ;* from *sabulum,* fine gravel.) Gritty, sandy. Applied to the calcareous matter in urine.

SABU'RRA. Dirt, sordes, filth. Foulness of the stomach, of which authors mention several kinds, as the acid, the bitter, the empyreumatic, the insipid, the putrid.

SACCATED. (*Saccatus,* encysted.) Encysted or contained in a bay-like membrane, applied to tumours, &c. See *Ascites saccatus*.

SACCHARI ACIDUM. See *Mucic acid*.

SA'CCHARUM. (Σακχαρον, from *sachar,* Arabian.) 1. The name of a genus of plants in the Linnæan system. Class, *Triandria ;* Order, *Digynia.* The sugar-cane.

2. The sweet substance called sugar. See *Saccharum officinale*.

SACCHARUM ACERNUM. See *Acer saccharinum*.

SACCHARUM ALBUM. Refined sugar.

SACCHARUM ALUMINIS. Alum mixed with dragon's blood and dried.

SACCHARUM CANADENSE. See *Acer pseudo platanus*.

SACCHARUM CANDIDUM. Sugar-candy.

SACCHARUM NON PURIFICATUM. Brown sugar.

SACCHARUM OFFICINALE. (*Arundo saccharifera* of Sloane. The systematic name of the cane from which sugar is obtained. *Suchar ; Succhar ; Sutter ; Zuchar ; Zucaro ; Zozar* of the Arabians. Σακχαρ η σακχαρον, of the Greeks.) Sugar is prepared in the West and East Indies from the expressed juice of this plant boiled with the addition of quick-lime or common vegetable alkali. It may be extracted also from a number of plants, as the maple, birch, wheat, corn, beet-root, skirret, parsnips, and dried grapes, &c. by digesting in alcohol. The alcohol dissolves the sugar, and leaves the extractive matter untouched, which falls to the bottom. It may be taken into the stomach in very large quantities, without producing any bad consequences, although proofs are not wanting of its mischievous effects, by relaxing the stomach, and thus inducing disease. It is much used in pharmacy, as it forms the basis of syrups, lozenges, and other preparations. It is very useful as a medicine, although it cannot be considered to possess much power, to favour the solution or suspension of resins, oils, &c. in water, and is given as a purgative for infants. Dr. Cullen classes it with the attenuantia, and Bergius states it to be saponacea, edulcorans, relaxans, pectoralis, vulneraria, antiseptica, nutriens. In catarrhal affections, both sugar and honey are frequently employed : it has also been advantageously used in calculous complaints ; and from its known power in preserving animal and vegetable substances from putrefaction, it has been given with a view to its antiseptic effects. Sugar candy, by dissolving slowly in the mouth, is well suited to relieve tickling coughs and hoarseness. Sugar is every where the basis of that which is called sweetness. Its presence is previously necessary in order to the taking place of vinous fermentation. Its extraction from plants, which afford it in the greatest abundance, and its refinement for the common uses of life, in a pure state, are among the most important of the chemical manufactures.

The following is the mode of its manufacture in the West Indies : The plants are cultivated in rows, on fields enriched by such manures as can most easily be procured, and tilled with the plough. They are annually cut. The cuttings are carried to the mill. They are cut into short pieces, and arranged in small bundles. The mill is wrought by water, wind, or cattle. The parts which act on the canes are inserted, compressed till all their juice is obtained from them, and themselves, sometimes, even reduced to powder. One of these mills, of the best construction, bruises canes to such a quantity as to afford, in one day, 10,000 gallons of juice, when wrought with only ten mules. The expressed juice is received into a leaden bed. It is thence conveyed into a vessel called the receiver. The juice is found to consist of eight parts of pure water, one part of sugar, one part of oil and gummy mucilage. From the greener parts of the canes there is apt to be at times derived an acid juice, which tends to bring the whole unseasonably into a state of acid fermentation. Fragments of the ligneous part of the cane, some portions of mud or dirt which unavoidably remain on the canes, and a blackish substance called the crust, which coated the canes at the joints, are also apt to enter into contaminating mixture with the juice. From the receiver the juice is conducted along a wooden gutter lined with lead, to the boiling-house. In the boiling-house it is received into copper pans or caldrons, which have the name of clarifiers. Of these clarifiers the number and the capacity must be in proportion to the quantity of canes, and the extent of the sugar plantation on which the work is carried on. Each clarifier has a syphon or cock, by which the liquor is to be drawn off. Each hangs over a separate fire ; and this fire must be so confined, that by the drawing of an iron slider fitted to the chimney, the fire may be at any time put out. In the progress of the operations the stream of juice from

255

the receiver fills the clarifiers with fresh liquor. Lime in powder is added in order to take up the oxalic acid, and the carbonaceous matters which are mingled with the juice. The lime also in the new salts, into the composition of which it now enters, adds itself to the sugar, as a part of that which is to be obtained from the process. The lime is to be put in the proportion of somewhat less than a pint of lime to every hundred gallons of liquor. When it is in too great quantities, however, it is apt to destroy a part of the pure saccharine matter. Some persons employ alkaline ashes, as preferable to lime, for the purpose of extracting the extraneous matter; but it is highly probable that lime, judiciously used, might answer better than any other substance whatsoever. The liquor is now to be heated almost to ebullition. The heat dissolves the mechanical union, and thus favours the chemical changes in its different parts. When the proper heat appears from a rising scum on the surface of the liquor to have been produced, the fire is then extinguished by the application of the damper. In this state of the liquor, the greater part of the impurities, being different in specific gravity from the pure saccharine solution, and being also of such a nature as to yield more readily to the chemical action of heat, are brought up to the surface in a scum. After this scum has been sufficiently formed on the cooling liquor, this liquor is carefully drawn off, either by a syphon, which raises a pure stream through the scum, or by a cock drawing the liquor at the bottom from under the scum. The scum, in either case, sinks down unbroken, as the liquor flows; and is now, by cooling, of such tenacity, as not to tend to any intermixture with the liquor. The liquor drawn, after this purification from the boiler, is received into a gutter or channel, by which it is conveyed to the grand copper, or evaporating boiler. If made from good canes, and properly clarified, it will now appear almost transparent. In this copper the liquor is heated to actual ebullition. The scum raised to the surface by the boiling is skimmed off as it rises. The ebullition is continued till there be a considerable diminution in the quantity of the liquor. The liquor now appears nearly of the colour of Madeira wine. It is at last transferred into a second and smaller copper. An addition of lime-water is here made, both to dilute the thickening liquor, to detach the super-abundant acid, and to favour the formation of the sugar. If the liquor be now in its proper state, the scum rises in large bubbles, with very little discoloration. The skimming and the evaporation together produce a considerable diminution in the quantity of the liquor. It is then transferred into another smaller boiler. In this last boiler, the evaporation is renewed, and continued till the liquor is brought to that degree of thickness at which it appears fit to be finally cooled. In the cooler, (a shallow wooden vessel of considerable length and wideness, commonly of such a size as to contain a hogshead of sugar,) the sugar, as it cools, granulates, or runs into an imperfect crystallization, by which it is separated from the molasses, a mixed saccharine matter too impure to be capable even of this imperfect crystallization. To determine whether the liquor be fit to be taken from the last boiler to be finally cooled, it is necessary to take out a portion from the boiler, and try separately, whether it does not separate into granulated sugar and melasses. From the cooler, the sugar is removed to the curing-house. This is a spacious, airy building. It is provided with a capacious cistern for the reception of melasses, and over the cistern is erected a frame of strong joist-work, unfilled and uncovered. Empty hogsheads open at the head, bored at the bottom with a few holes, and having a stalk of plantain leaf thrust through each of the holes, while it rises at the same time through the inside of the hogshead, are disposed upon the frames. The mass of the saccharine matter from the coolers is put into these hogsheads. The melasses drip into the cistern through the spongy plantain stalks in the holes. Within the space of three weeks the melasses are sufficiently drained off, and the sugar remains dry. By this process it is at last brought into the state of what is called muscovado or raw sugar. This is the general process in the British West Indies. In this state our West India sugar is imported into Britain. The formation of loaves of white sugar is a subsequent process. In the French West India isles it has long been customary to perform the last part of this train of processes in a manner somewhat different,

and which affords the sugar in a state of greater purity This preparation, taking the sugar from the coole then puts it, not into hogsheads with holes in the bot tom as above, but into conical pots, each of which has at its bottom a hole half an inch in diameter, that is, in the commencement of the process, stopped with a plug After remaining sometime in the pot, the sugar becomes perfectly cool and fixed. The plug is then re moved out of the hole; the pot is placed over a large jar, and the melasses are suffered to drip away from it. After as much of the melasses as will easily run off has been thus drained away, the surface of the sugar in the jar is covered with a stratum of fine clay, and water is poured upon the clay. The water, oozing gently through the pores of the clay, pervades the whole mass of sugar redissolves the melasses, still remaining in it, with some parts of the sugar itself, and carrying these off by the holes in the bottom of the pot, renders that which resists the solution much purer than the muscovado sugar made in the English way. The sugar prepared in this manner is called clayed sugar. It is sold for a higher price in the European market than the muscovado sugar; but there is a loss of sugar in the process by claying, which deters the British planters from adopting this practice so generally as do the French.

The raw sugars are still contaminated and debased by a mixture of acid, carbonaceous matter, oil, and colouring resin. To free them from these is the business of the European sugar-bakers. A new solution; clarification with alkaline substances fitted to attract away the oil, acid, and other contaminating matters; slow evaporation; and a final cooling in suitable moulds, are the processes which at last produce loaves of white sugar.

The melasses being nothing else but a very impure refuse of the sugar from which they drip, are susceptible of being employed in a new ebullition, by which a second quantity of sugar may be obtained from them The remainder of the melasses is employed to yield rum by distillation. In rum, alkohol is mixed with oil, water, oxalic acid, and a mixture of empyreumatic matter. The French prepare, from the mixture of melasses with water, a species of wine of good quality. In its preparation, the solution is brought into fermentation; then passed through strainers to purify it, then put in casks; after clearing itself in these, transferred into others, in which it is to be preserved for use. The ratio of these processes is extremely beautiful; they are all directed to purify the sugar from contaminating mixtures, and to reduce it into that state of dryness or crystallization, in which it is susceptible of being the most conveniently preserved for agreeable use. The heat in general acts both mechanically to effect a sufficient dissolution of the aggregation of the parts of the cane juice, and chemically to produce in it new combinations into which caloric must enter as an ingredient. The first gentle heat is intended chiefly to operate with the mechanical influence, raising to the surface impurities, which are more easily removed by skimming, than by any other means; a gentle, not a violent heat, is in this instance employed, because a violent heat would produce empyreumatic salts, the production of which is to be carefully avoided. A boiling heat is, in the continuation of the processes, made use of, because, after the first impurities have been skimmed off, contaminating empyreumatic salts are less readily formed, because a boiling heat is necessary to effect the complete developement of the saccharine matter, and because the gradual concentration of the sugar is, by such a heat, to be best accomplished. Lime is employed, because it has a stronger affinity than sugar with all the contaminating matters, and particularly because it attracts into a neutral combination that excess of oxalic acids which is apt to exist in the saccharine solution. Skimming removes the new salts, which the most easily assume a solid form. The drippings carries away a mixture of water, oil, earth, and sugar, from the crystallized sugar: for, in all our crystallizations, we can never perform the process in the great way, with such nicety as to preserve it free from an inequality of proportions that must necessarily occasion a residue. Repeated solution, clarification, evaporation, are requisite to produce pure white sugar from the brown and raw sugars; because the complete purification of this matter from acid and colouring matter, is an operation of great difficulty, and not to be finally completed without processes which are longer than can be conveniently performed, at the first, upon the sugar plantation. From vegetables of European growth, sugar is not to be easily obtained, unless the process of germination be first produced in them ; or unless they have been penetrated by intense frost. Germination, or thorough freezing, developes sugar into all vegetables in which its principles of hydrogen and carbon, with a small proportion of oxygen, exist in any considerable plenty. It is not improbable, but that if penetration by a freezing cold could be commanded at pleasure with sufficient cheapness, it would enable us to obtain saccharine matter in a large proportion, from a variety of substances, from which even generation does not yield a sufficient quantity. In the beet, and some other European vegetables, sugar is naturally formed by the functions of vegetation to perfect combination. From these the sugar is obtained by rasping down the vegetable, extracting by water its saccharine juice, evaporating the water charged with the juice to the consistency of syrup, clarifying, purifying, and crystallizing it, just in the same manner as sugar from the sugar-cane. It is afforded by the maple, the birch, wheat, and Turkey corn. Margraaf obtained it from the roots of beet, red beet, skirrit, parsnips, and dried grapes.

In Canada, the inhabitants extract sugar from the maple. At the commencement of spring, they heap snow in the evening at the foot of the tree, in which they previously make apertures for the passage of the returning sap. Two hundred pounds of this juice afford, by evaporation, fifteen of a brownish sugar. The quantity prepared annually amounts to fifteen thousand weight.

The Indians likewise extract sugar from the pith of the bamboo.

The beet has lately been much cultivated in Germany, for the purpose of extracting sugar from its root. For this the roots are taken up in autumn, washed clean, wiped, sliced lengthwise, strung on threads, and hung up to dry. From these the sugar is extracted by maceration in a small quantity of water ; drawing off this upon fresh roots, and adding fresh water to the fresh roots, which is again to be employed the same way, so as to get out all their sugar, and saturate the water as much as possible with it. This water is to be strained and boiled down for the sugar.

Some merely express the juice from the fresh roots, and boil this down ; others boil the roots ; but the sugar extracted in either of these ways is not equal in quality to the first.

Professor Lampadius obtained from 110 lbs. of the roots, 4 lbs. of well-grained white powder sugar ; and the residuums afforded 7 pints of a spirit resembling rum. Achard says, that about a ton of roots produced him 100 lbs. of raw sugar, which gave 55 lbs. of refined sugar, and 25 lbs. of treacle.

Sugar is very soluble in water, and is a good medium for uniting that fluid with oily matters. It is much used for domestic purposes, and appears on the whole to be a valuable and wholesome article of food, the uses of which are most probably restricted by its high price.

It appears that sugar has the property of rendering some of the earths soluble in water.

The union of sugar with the alkalies has been long known ; but this is rendered more strikingly evident, by carbonated potassa or soda, for instance, decomposing the solutions of lime and strontia in sugar, by double affinity.

In making solutions of unrefined sugar for culinary purposes, a gray-coloured substance is found frequently precipitated. It is probable that this proceeds from a superabundance of lime which has been used in clarifying the juice of the sugar-cane at the plantations abroad. Sugar with this imperfection is known among the refiners of this article by the name of *weak*. And it is justly termed so, the precipitated matter being nothing but lime which has attracted carbonic acid from the sugar (of which there is a great probability), or from the air of the atmosphere. A bottle, in which Dr. Ure kept a solution of lime in sugar for at least four years, closely corked, was entirely incrusted with a yellowish-coloured matter, which on examination was found to be entirely carbonate of lime.

Kirchoff, an ingenious Russian chemist, accidentally discovered, that starch is convertible into sugar, by being boiled for some time with a very dilute sulphuric

acid. Saussure showed, that 100 parts of starch yield 110 of sugar.

Braconnot has recently extended our views concerning the artificial production of sugar and gum. Sulphuric acid (sp. gr. 1.827) mixed with well-dried elm dust, became very hot, and on being diluted with water, and neutralized with chalk, afforded a liquor which became gummy on evaporation. Shreds of linen, triturated in a glass mortar, with sulphuric acid, yield a similar gum. Nitric acid has a similar power. If the gummy matter from linen be boiled for some time with dilute sulphuric acid, we obtain a crystallizable sugar, and an acid, which Braconnot calls the vegeto-sulphuric acid. The conversion of wood also into sugar, will no doubt appear remarkable ; and when persons not familiarized with chemical speculations are told, that a pound weight of rags can be converted into more than a pound weight of sugar, they may regard the statement as a piece of pleasantry, though nothing, says Braconnot, can be more real.

Silk is also convertible into gum by sulphuric acid Twelve grammes of glue, reduced to powder, were digested with a double weight of concentrated sulphuric acid without artificial heat. In twenty hours the liquid was not more coloured than if mere water had been employed. A decilitre of water was then added, and the whole was boiled for five hours, with renewal of the water, from time to time, as it wasted. It was next diluted, saturated with chalk, filtered, and evaporated to a syrupy consistence, and left in repose for a month. In this period a number of granular crystals had separated, which adhered pretty strongly to the bottom of the vessel, and had a very decided saccharine taste. This sugar crystallizes much more easily than cane sugar. The crystals are gritty under the teeth, like sugarcandy ; and in the form of flattened prisms or tabular groupes. Its taste is nearly as saccharine as grape sugar ; its solubility in water scarcely exceeds that of sugar of milk. Boiling alkohol, even when diluted, has no action on this sugar By distillation it yields ammonia, indicating the presence of azote. This sugar combines intimately with nitric acid, without sensibly decomposing it, even with the assistance of heat, and there results a peculiar crystallized acid, to which the name nitro-saccharine has been given. *Annales de Chimie,* xii., or *Tillock's Magazine,* vols. lv. and lvi.

The varieties of sugar are ; cane sugar, maple sugar, liquid sugar of fruits, sugar of figs, sugar of grapes, starch sugar, the mushroom sugar of Braconnot, manna, sugar of gelatin, sugar of honey, and sugar of diabetes.

Sugar of grapes does not affect a peculiar form. It is deposited, from its alkoholic solution, in small grains, which have little consistence, are grouped together, and which constitute tubercles, similar to those of cauliflowers. When put in the mouth, it produces at first a sensation of coolness, to which succeeds a saccharine taste, not very strong. Hence to sweeten to an equal degree the same quantity of water, we must employ two and a half times as much sugar of grapes as of that of the cane. In other respects, it possesses all the properties of cane sugar. Its extraction is very easy. The expressed juice of the grapes is composed of water, sugar, mucilage, bitartrate of potassa, tartrate of lime, and a small quantity of other saline matters. We pour into it an excess of chalk in powder, or rather of pounded marble. There results, especially on agitation, an effervescence, due to the unsaturated tartaric acid. The liquor is then clarified with whites of eggs or blood. It is next evaporated in copper pans, till it marks a density of 1.32 at the boiling temperature. It is now allowed to cool. At the end of some days, it concretes into a crystalline mass, which, when drained, washed with a little cold water, and strongly compressed, constitutes sugar.

In the south of France, where this operation was some years back carried on on the great scale, to prevent fermentation of the *must*, there was added to this a little sulphate of lime, or it was placed in tuns in which sulphur matches had been previously made to burn. The oxygen of the small quantity of air left in the tuns being thus abstracted by the sulphurous acid, fermentation did not take place. By this means the *must* can be preserved a considerable time ; whereas, in the ordinary way, it would lose its saccharine taste at the end of a few days and become vinous

Must thus treated, is said to be *muted.* The syrup was evaporated to the density of only 1.285.—*Proust. Ann. de Chimie,* lvii. 131.; and the *Collection of Memoirs published by Parmentier in* 1813.

It is this species of sugar which is obtained from starch and woody fibre by the action of dilute sulphuric acid.

Sugar of diabetes has sometimes the sweetening force of sugar of grapes; occasionally much less.

Braconnot's mushroom sugar is much less sweet than that of the cane. It crystallizes with remarkable facility, forming long quadrilateral prisms with square bases. It yields alkohol by fermentation.

All honeys contain two species of sugar; one similar to sugar of the grape, another like the uncrystallizable sugar of the cane (melasses). These combined and mingled in different proportions with an odorant matter, constitute the honeys of good quality. Those

of inferior quality contain, besides, a certain quantity of wax and acid : the honeys of Britanny contain even an animal secretion (*esuvain*) to which they owe their putrescent quality. A slight washing with a little alkohol separates the uncrystallizable sugar, and leaves the other, which may be purified by washing with a very little more alkohol.

"The relation" says Dr. Prout, "which exists between urea and sugar, seems to explain in a satisfactory manner the phenomena of diabetes, which may be considered as a depraved secretion of sugar. The weight of the atom of sugar, is just half that of the weight of the atom of urea ; the absolute quantity of hydrogen in a given weight of both is equal; while the absolute quantities of carbon and oxygen in a given weight of sugar, are precisely twice those of urea."

The constituents of these two bodies and lithic acid, are thus expressed by that ingenious philosopher —

Elements	Urea.			Sugar.			Lithic Acid.		
	No.	Per. Atom.	Per Cent.	No.	Per Atom.	Per Cent.	No.	Per Atom.	Per Cent.
Hydrogen .	2	2.5	6.66	1	1.25	6.66	1	1.25	2.85
Carbon . .	1	7.5	19.99	1	7.50	39.99	2	15.00	34.28
Oxygen . .	1	10.0	26.66	1	10.00	53.33	1	10.00	22.85
Azote . .	1	17.5	46.66				1	17.50	40.00
	5	37.5	100.10	3	18.75	100.10	5	43.75	100.10

The above compounds appear to be formed by the union of more simple compounds ; as sugar, of carbon and water ; urea, of carburetted hydrogen and nitrous oxide ; lithic acid, of cyanogen and water, &c. ; whence it is inferred, that their artificial formation falls within the limits of chemical operations.

SACCHARUM OFFICINARUM. The systematic name in some pharmacopœias of the sugar-cane. See *Saccharum.*

SACCHARUM PURIFICATUM. Double refined, or loaf-sugar. See *Saccharum.*

SACCHARUM SATURNI. See *Plumbi acetas.*

SACCHO-LACTIC. So called, because it is sugar prepared from milk.

Saccho-lactic acid. Acidum saccholacticum. See *Mucic acid.*

SACCHOLATE. *Saccholas.* A salt formed by the combination of the saccholactic acid with salifiable bases, as saccholate of iron, saccholate of ammonia, &c. &c.

SACCULUS. (Dim. of *saccus,* a bag.) A little bag.

SACCULUS ADIPOSUS. The bursæ mucosæ of the joints.

SACCULUS CHYLIFERUS. See *Receptaculum chyli.*

SACCULUS CORDIS. The pericardium.

SACCULUS LACHRYMALIS. See *Saccus lachrymalis.*

SA'CCUS. A bag.

SACCUS LACHRYMALIS. The lachrymal sac is situated in the internal canthus of the eye, behind the lachrymal caruncle, in a cavity formed by the os unguis. It receives the tears from the puncta lachrymalia, and conveys them into the ductus lachrymalis.

SA'CER. (From *sagur,* secret, Heb.) Sacred. Applied to some diseases which were supposed to be immediately inflicted from heaven ; as *sacer morbus,* the epilepsy, *sacer ignis, erysipelas,* &c. A bone is called the *os sacrum,* because it was once offered in sacrifices. Sacer also means belonging to the os sacrum.

SACK. A wine used by our ancestors, which some have taken to be Rhenish, and others Canary wine. Probably it was what is called dry mountain, or some Spanish wine of that sort. Howel, in his French and English Dictionary, 1650, translates sack by the words *vin d'Espagne.* Vin. sec.

SACLA'CTATE. A combination of saccholactic acid with a salifiable basis.

SACLACTIC ACID. See *Mucic acid.*

SACRA HERBA. Common vervain.

SACRA TINCTURA. Made of aloes canella, alba, and mountain wine

SACRAL. Of or belonging to the sacrum; as sacra arteries, veins, nerves, &c.

SA'CRO. Words compounded of this belong to the sacrum.

SACRO-COCCYGÆUS. A muscle arising from the sacrum, and inserted into the os coccygis.

SACRO-LUMBALIS. *Sacro-lumbaris,* of authors. *Lumbo-costo trachelien* of Dumas. A long muscle, thicker and broader below than above, and extending from the os sacrum to the lower part of the neck, under the serrati postici rhomboideus, trapezius, and latissimus dorsi. It arises in common with the longissimus dorsi, tendinous without, and fleshy within, from the posterior part of the os sacrum; from the posterior edge of the spine of the ilium; from all the spinous process; and from near the roots of the transverse processes of the lumbar vertebræ. At the bottom of the back it separates from the longissimus dorsi, with which it had before formed, as it were, only one muscle, and ascending obliquely outwards, gradually diminishes in thickness, and terminates above in a very narrow point. From the place where it quits the longissimus dorsi, to that of its termination, we find it fleshy at its posterior, and tendinous at its anterior edge. This tendinous side sends off as many long and thin tendons as there are ribs. The lowermost of these tendons are broader, thicker, and shorter than those above ; they are inserted into the inferior edge of each rib, where it begins to be curved forwards towards the sternum, excepting only the uppermost and last tendon, which ends in the posterior and inferior part of the transverse process of the last vertebra of the neck. From the upper part of the five, six, seven, eight, nine, ten, or eleven lower ribs, (for the number, though most commonly seven or eight, varies in different subjects,) arise as many thin bundles of fleshy fibres, which, after a very short progress, terminate in the inner side of this muscle, and have been named by Steno, *musculi ad sacro lumbalem accessorii.* Besides these we find the muscle sending off a fleshy slip from its upper part, which is inserted into the posterior and inferior part of the transverse processes of the five inferior vertebræ of the neck, by as many distinct tendons. This is generally described as a distinct muscle. Diemerbroeck, and Douglas, and Albinus after him, call it *cervicalis descendens.* Winslow names it *transversalis collateralis colli* Morgagni considers it as an appendage to the sacro lumbalis. The uses of this muscle are to assist in erecting the trunk of the body, in turning it upon its axis or to one side, and in drawing the ribs downwards. By means of its upper slip, it serves to turn the neck obliquely backwards or to one

SACRO-SCIATIC LIGAMENTS. The ligaments which connect the ossa innominata with the os sacrum.

SA'CRUM. (So called from *sacer*, sacred; because it was formerly offered in sacrifices.) *Os sacrum ; Os basilare.* The os sacrum derives its name from its being offered in sacrifice by the ancients, or perhaps from its supporting the organs of generation, which they considered as sacred. In young subjects it is composed of five or six pieces, united by cartilage; but in more advanced age it becomes one bone, in which, however, we may still easily distinguish the marks of the former separation. Its shape has been sometimes compared to an irregular triangle ; and sometimes, and perhaps more properly, to a pyramid, flattened before and behind, with its basis placed towards the lumbar vertebræ, and its point terminating in the coccyx. We find it convex behind, and slightly concave before, with its inferior portion bent a little forwards. Its anterior surface is smooth, and affords four, and sometimes five transverse lines, of a colour different from the rest of the bone. These are the remains of the intermediate cartilages by which its several pieces were united in infancy. Its posterior convex surface has several prominences, the most remarkable of which are its spinous processes; these are usually three in number, and gradually become shorter, so that the third is not so long as the second, nor the second as the first. This arrangement enables us to sit with ease. Its transverse processes are formed into one oblong process, which becomes gradually smaller as it descends. At the superior part of the bone we observe two oblique processes, of a cylindrical shape, and somewhat concave, which are articulated with the last of the lumbar vertebræ. At the base of each of these oblique processes is a notch, which, with such another in the vertebra above it, forms a passage for the twenty-fourth spinal nerve. In viewing this bone, either before or behind, we observe four, and sometimes five holes on each side, situate at each extremity, of the transverse lines which mark the divisions of the bone. Of these holes, the anterior ones, and of these again the uppermost, are the largest, and afford a passage to the nerves. The posterior holes are smaller, covered with membranes, and destined for the same purpose as the former. Sometimes at the bottom of the bone there is only a notch, and sometimes there is a hole common to it and the os coccygis. The cavity between the body of this bone and its processes, for the lodgment of the spinal marrow, is triangular, and becomes smaller as it descends, till at length it terminates obliquely on each side at the lower part of the bone. Below the third division of the bone, however, the cavity is no longer completely bony, as in the rest of the spine, but is defended posteriorly only by a very strong membrane; hence a wound in this part may be attended with the most dangerous consequences. This bone is articulated above, with the last lumbar vertebra : laterally it is firmly united, by a broad irregular surface, to the ossa innominata, or hipbones : and below it is joined to the os coccygis. In women the os sacrum is usually shorter, broader and more curved than in men, by which means the cavity of the pelvis is more enlarged.

SAFFLOWER. See *Carthamus.*

SAFFRON. See *Crocus.*

Saffron, bastard. See *Carthamus.*

Saffron, meadow. See *Colchicum.*

Saffron of steel. A red oxide of iron.

SAGAPE'NUM. (The name is derived from some eastern dialect.) *Serapinum.* It is conjectured that this concrete gummi-resinous juice is the production of an oriental umbelliferous plant. Sagapenum is brought from Persia and Alexandria in large masses, externally yellowish, internally paler, and of a horny clearness. Its taste is hot and biting, its smell of the alliaceous and fœtid kind, and its virtues are similar to those which have been ascribed to asafœtida, but weaker, and consequently it is less powerful in its effects.

SAGE. See *Salvia.*

Sage of Bethlehem. See *Pulmonaria.*

Sage of Jerusalem. See *Pulmonaria officinalis.*

Sage of virtue. See *Salvia hortensis minor.*

SAGENITE. Acicular rutile.

SAGITTAL. (*Sagittalis ;* from *sagitta*, an arrow.) Shaped like an arrow.

SAGITTAL SUTURE. *Satura sagittalis, virgata, obelæa, rhabdoides.* The suture which unites the two

parietal bones. It has been named *sagittal*, from its lying between the coronal and lambdoidal sutures, as an arrow between the string and the bow.

SAGITTA'RIA. (So called from *sagitta*, an arrow, in allusion to the shape of the leaves in the original species and some others.) The name of a genus of plants in the Linnæan system. Class, *Monœcia ·* Order, *Polyandria.*

SAGITTARIA ALEXIPHARMICA. *Malacca ; Canna indica ; Arundo indica.* The systematic name of the plant cultivated with great care in the West Indies, for its root, which is supposed to be a remedy for the wounds of poisonous arrows. The root of this species, called *radix malacca*, is sometimes used medicinally.

SAGITTARIA SAGITTIFOLIA. The systematic name of the common arrow-head, the roots of which are esculent, but not very nutritious.

SAGITTATUS. (From *sagittas*, an arrow.) Arrow-shaped : applied to leaves, &c. which are triangular and hollowed out very much at the base ; as the leaves of the Sagittaria sagittifolia.

SAGO. See *Cycas circinalis.*

SAGU. See *Cycas circinalis.*

SAHLITE. Malacholite. A sub-species of oblique-edged augite, of a greenish colour, and found in Unst in Shetland, in Tiree, and Glentilt.

Saint Anthony's fire. See *Erysipelas.*

Saint Ignatius's bean. See *Ignatia amara.*

Saint James's wort. See *Senecio jacobæa.*

Saint John's wort. See *Hypericum.*

Saint Vitus's dance. See *Chorea sancti viti.*

SAL. (*Sal, salis.* m. and, rarely, neut. from the Greek, ἅλς, salt.) Salt. See *Saline.*

SAL ABSINTHII. See *Potassæ subcarbonas.*

SAL ACETOSELLÆ. See *Oxalis acetocella.*

Sal alembroth. A compound muriate of mercury and ammonia.

SAL ALKALINUS FIXUS. See *Alkali fixum.*

SAL ALKALINUS VOLATILIS. See *Ammonia.*

SAL AMMONIAC. (So called because it was found in Egypt, near the temple of Jupiter Ammon.) *Murias ammoniæ.* A saline concrete formed by the combination of the muriatic acid with ammonia. This salt is obtained from several sources.

1. It is found in places adjacent to volcanoes. It appears in the form of an efflorescence, or groupes of needles, separate or compacted together, generally of a yellow or red colour, and mixed with arsenic and orpiment ; but no use is made of that which is procured in this way. This native sal ammoniac is distinguished by mineralogists, into, 1. *Volcanic*, which occurs in efflorescences, imitative shapes, and crystallized in the vicinity of burning beds of coal, both in Scotland and England, at Solfaterra, Vesuvius, Ætna, &c. 2. *Conchoidal*, which occurs in angular pieces, it is said, along with sulphur, in beds of indurated clay, or clay-slate, in the country of Bucharia.

2. In Egypt it is made in great quantities from the soot of camel's dung, which is burned at Cairo instead of wood. This soot is put into large round bottles, a foot and a half in diameter, and terminating in a neck two inches long. The bottles are filled up with this matter to within four inches of the neck. Each bottle holds about forty pounds of soot, and affords nearly six pounds of salt. The vessels are put into a furnace in the form of an oven, so that only the necks appear above. A fire of camel's dung is kindled beneath it, and continued for three days and three nights. On the second and the third days the salt is sublimated. The bottles are then broken, and the salt is taken out in cakes. These cakes, which are sent just as they have been taken out of the bottles in Egypt, are convex, and unequal on the one side ; on the middle of this side they exhibit each a turbercle corresponding to the neck of the bottle in which it was prepared. The lower side is concave, and both are sooty.

3. In this country, sal ammoniac is likewise prepared in great quantities. The volatile alkali is obtained from soot, bones, and other substances known to contain it. To this the sulphuric acid is added, and the sulphate of ammonia so formed, is decomposed by muriate of soda, or common salt, through a double affinity. The liquor obtained in consequence of this decomposition contains sulphate of soda and muriate of ammonia. The first is crystallized, and the second sublimated so as to form cakes, which are then exposed to sale.

Ammoniacal muriate has a poignant, acid, and urinous taste. Its crystals are in the form of long hexahedral pyramids; a number of them are sometimes united together in an acute angular direction, so as to exhibit the form of feathers. Rome de Lille thinks the crystals of ammoniacal muriate to be octahedrons bundled together. This salt is sometimes, but not frequently, found in cubic crystals in the middle of the concave hollow part of the sublimated cakes. It possesses one singular physical property, a kind of ductility or elasticity, which causes it to yield under the hammer, or even the fingers, and makes it difficult to reduce to a powder. Muriate of ammonia is totally volatile, but a very strong fire is requisite to sublime it. It is liable to no alteration from air; it may be kept for a long time without suffering any change; it dissolves very readily in water. Six parts of cold water are sufficient to dissolve one of the salt. A considerable cold is produced as the solution takes place, and this cold is still keener when the salt is mixed with ice. This artificial cold is happily applied to produce several phenomena, such as the congelation of water on certain occasions, the crystallization of certain salts, the fixation and preservation of certain liquids, naturally very subject to evaporation; &c.

SAL AMMONIACUM ACETOSUM. See *Ammonia acetatis liquor.*

SAL AMMONIACUM LIQUIDUM. See *Ammoniæ acetatis liquor.*

SAL AMMONIACUM MARTIALE. See *Ferrum ammoniatum.*

SAL AMMONIACUM SECRETUM GLAUBERI. See *Sulphas ammoniæ.*

SAL AMMONIACUM VEGETABILE. See *Ammoniæ acetatis liquor.*

SAL AMMONIACUS FIXUS. The muriate of lime was formerly so termed.

SAL AMMONIACUS NITROSUS. See *Nitras ammoniæ.*

SAL ANTIMONII. Tartar emetic.

SAL ARGENTI. See *Argenti nitras.*

SAL CATHARTICUS AMARUS. See *Magnesiæ sulphas.*

SAL CATHARTICUS ANGLICANUS. See *Magnesiæ sulphas.*

SAL CATHARTICUS GLAUBERI. See *Sodæ sulphas.*

SAL COMMUNIS. See *Sodæ murias.*

SAL CORNU CERVI VOLATILE. See *Ammonia subcarbonas.*

SAL CULINARIS. See *Sodæ murias.*

SAL DE DUOBUS. See *Potassæ sulphas*

SAL DIURETICUS. See *Potassæ acetas.*

SAL DIGESTIVUS SYLVII. See *Murias potassæ.*

SAL EPSOMENSIS. See *Magnesiæ sulphas.*

SAL FEBRIFUGUS SYLVII. See *Murias potassæ.*

SAL FONTIUM. See *Sodæ murias.*

SAL FOSSILIS. See *Sodæ murias.*

SAL GEMMÆ. See *Sodæ murias.*

SAL GLAUBERI. See *Sodæ sulphas.*

SAL HERBARUM. See *Potassæ subcarbonas.*

SAL MARINUS. See *Sodæ murias.*

SAL MARTIS. See *Ferri sulphas.*

SAL MARTIS MURIATICUM SUBLIMATUM. See *Ferrum ammoniatum.*

SAL MICROCOSMICUS. The compound saline matter obtained by inspissating human urine.

SAL MIRABILIS GLAUBERI. See *Sodæ sulphas.*

SAL MURIATICUS. See *Sodæ murias.*

SAL PLANTARUM. See *Potassæ subcarbonas.*

SAL POLYCHRESTUS. See *Potassæ sulphas.*

SAL POLYCHRESTUS GLASERI. See *Potassæ sulphas.*

SAL POLYCHRESTUS SEIGNETTI. See *Soda tartarizata.*

SAL PRUNELLÆ. Nitrate of potassa cast into flat cakes or round balls.

SAL RUPELLENSIS. See *Soda tartarizata.*

SAL SATURNI. See *Plumbi acetas.*

SAL SEDATIVUS. See *Boracic acid.*

SAL SEIDLICENSIS. See *Magnesiæ sulphas.*

SAL SEIGNETTI. See *Soda tartarizata.*

SAL SUCCINI. See *Succinic acid.*

SAL TARTARI. See *Tartaric acid.*

SAL THERMARUM CAROLINARUM. See *Magnesiæ sulphas.*

SAL VEGETABILIS. See *Potassæ tartras.*

SAL VOLATILE. See *Spiritus ammoniæ aromaticus,* and *Ammoniæ subcarbonas.*

260

SAL VOLATILIS SALIS AMMONIACI. See *Ammoniæ subcarbonas.*

SALEP. *Salap.* See *Orchis morio.*

SALICARIA. (From *salix,* a willow; from the resemblance of its leaves to those of the willow.) See *Lythrum salicaria.*

SALICO'RNIA. The name of a genus of plants in the Linnæan system. Class, *Monandria;* Order, *Monogynia.*

SALICORNIA EUROPÆA. The systematic name of the jointed glass-wort, which is gathered by the country people and sold for samphire. It forms a good pickle with vinegar, and is little inferior to the samphire.

SALIFIABLE. Having the property of forming a salt. The alkalies, and those earths, and metallic oxides, which have the power of neutralizing acidity, entirely or in part, and producing salts, are called salifiable bases.

SALINE. (*Salinus;* from *sal,* salt.) Of a salt nature. The number of saline substances is very considerable; and they possess peculiar characters by which they are distinguished from other substances. These characters are founded on certain properties, which, it must be confessed, are not accurately distinctive of their true nature. All such substances, however, as possess several of the four following properties, are considered as saline: 1. A strong tendency to combination, or a very strong affinity of composition; 2. A greater or less degree of sapidity; 3. A greater or less degree of solubility in water; 4. Perfect incombustibility.

SALINUS. See *Saline.*

SALINUCA. See *Valeriana celtica.*

SALI'VA. (So called, *a salino sapore,* from its salt taste, or from σιαλος, spittle.) The fluid which is secreted by the salivary glands into the cavity of the mouth. The *secretory organ* is composed of three pair of salivary glands. 1. The *parotid glands,* which evacuate their saliva by means of the *Stenonian duct,* behind the middle dens molaris of the upper jaw. 2. The *submaxillary glands,* which pour out their saliva through the *Warthonian ducts* on each side of the frenulum of the tongue by a narrow osculum. 3. The *sublingual glands,* situated between the internal surface of the maxilla and the tongue, which pour out their saliva through numerous *Rivinian ducts* at the apex of the tongue.

The saliva in the cavity of the mouth has mixed with it, 1. The *mucus of the mouth,* which exhales from the labial and genal glands. 2. The *roscid vapour,* from the whole surface of the cavity of the mouth. The saliva is continually swallowed with or without masticated food, and some is also spit out. It has no *colour* nor *smell;* it is *tasteless,* although it contains a little salt, to which the nerves of the tongue are accustomed. Its *specific gravity* is somewhat greater than water. Its *consistence* is rather plastic and spumous, from the entangled atmospheric air. The *quantity* of twelve pounds is supposed to be secreted in twelve hours. During mastication and speaking, the secretion is augmented, from the mechanical pressure of the muscles upon the salivary glands. Those who are hungry secrete a great quantity, from the sight of agreeable food. It is imperfectly dissolved by water, somewhat coagulated by alcohol; and congealed with more difficulty than water. It is inspissated by a small dose, and dissolved in a large dose, of mineral acids. It is also soluble in carbonated alkali. Caustic alkali and quick-lime extract volatile alkali from saliva. It corrodes copper and iron; and precipitates silver and lead from containing muriatic acid. It assists the spirituous fermentation of farinaceous substances; hence, barbar ousnations prepare an inebriating drink from the chewed roots of the *Jatropha manihot* and *Piper methisticum* It possesses an antiseptic virtue, according to the experiments of the celebrated Pringle. It easily becomes putrid in warm air, and gives off volatile alkali.

Constituent Principles. Saliva appears to consist, in a healthy state of the body, of water, which constitutes at least four-fifths of its bulk, mucilage, albumen, muriate of soda, phosphate of lime, and phosphate of ammonia.

The use of the saliva is, 1. It augments the taste of the food, by evolution of sapid matter. 2. During mastication it fixes with, dissolves, and resolves into its principles, the food; and changes it into a pultaceous mass, fit to be swallowed: hence it commences chymification. 3. It moderates thirst, by moistening the cavity of the mouth and fauces.

SALIVAL. (*Salivalis*; from *saliva*, the spittle.) Of or belonging to the saliva.

SALIVAL DUCTS. The excretory ducts of the salival glands. That of the parotid gland is called the *Stenonian* duct; those of the submaxillary glands, the *Warthonian* ducts; and those of the sublingual, the *Rivinian* ducts.

SALIVAL GLANDS. Those glands which secrete the saliva are so termed. See *Saliva*.

SALIVA'NS. (From *saliva*, spittle.) That which excites salivation.

SALIVA'RIA. (From *saliva*, the spittle ; so called because it excites a discharge of saliva.) See *Anthemis pyrethrum*.

SALIVARIS HERBA. See *Anthemis pyrethrum.*

SALIVA'TIO. An increased secretion of saliva. See *Ptyalismus.*

SA'LIX. (From *sala*, Heb.) 1. The name of a genus of plants in the Linnæan system. Class, *Diœcia ;* Order, *Diandria.* The willow.

2. The pharmacopœial name of *Salix.* See *Salix fragilis.*

SALIX ALBA. See *Salix fragilis.*

SALIX CAPREA. The systematic name of a species of willow, the bark of the branches of which possess the same virtues with that of the fragilis. See *Salix fragilis.*

SALIX FRAGILIS. The systematic name of the common crack willow. *Salix.* The bark of the branches of this species manifests a considerable degree of bitterness to the taste, and is very adstringent. It is recommended as a good substitute for Peruvian bark, and is said to cure intermittents and other diseases requiring tonic and adstringent remedies. Not only the bark of this species of salix, but those also of several others, possess similar qualities, particularly of the *Salix alba* and *Salix pentandria*, both of which are recommended in the foreign pharmacopœias. But Dr. Woodville is of opinion that the bark of the Salix triandria is more effectual than that of any other of this genus; at least its sensible qualities give it a decided preference. The trials Dr. Cullen made were with the bark of the Salix pentandria, taken from its branches, the third of an inch diameter, and of four or five years' growth. Nevertheless, he adds, in intermittent fevers, Bergius always failed with this bark.

SALIX PENTANDRIA. The bark of the branches of this species of willow possesses the same virtues as that of the fragilis. See *Salix fragilis.*

SALIX VITULINA. The bark of the branches of this species of willow may be substituted for the fragilis. See *Salix fragilis*

SALMO. The name of a genus of fishes of the order *Abdominales.* The salmon.

SALMO ALPINUS. The red charr. This beautiful and delicate little fish, and the *Palmo carpio*, or gilt charr, are found in our lakes of Westmoreland, in Wales, and Scotland. They are very rich, and hard of digestion.

SALMO EPERLANUS. The smelt. A beautiful little fish, found in great abundance in the Thames and river Dee, and in the European seas, between November and February.

SALMO FARIO. The common fresh-water trout, the flesh of which is very delicate and rich.

SALMO LACUSTRIS. The lake-trout.

SALMO SALAR. The systematic name of the common salmon. This fish is considered as one of the greatest delicacies. It is rich, and of difficult digestion to weak stomachs, and with some, whose stomachs are not particularly feeble, it uniformly disagrees. The pickled, salted, and smoked, though much eaten, are only fitted for the very strong and active.

SALMO SALMULUS. The samlet: the least of the British species of the salmo-genus. It is found in the river Wye, and up the Severn.

SALMO THYMALLUS. The graling salmon, which is somewhat like our trout. It inhabits the rivers of Derbyshire, and some of the north, and near Christchurch in Hampshire. It is much esteemed for the delicacy of its flesh, which is white, firm, and of a fine flavour; and is considered as in the highest season in the depth of winter.

SALMO TRUTTA. The systematic name of the salmon trout, or bull trout.

SALMON. See *Salmo.*

SALPINGO. (From Σαλπιγξ *buccina*, a trumpet.)

Names compounded of this word belong to the palate, and are connected with the Eustachian tube.

SALPINGO-PHARYNGEUS. This muscle is composed of a few fibres of the palatopharyngeus, which it assists in dilating the mouth of the Eustachian tube.

SALPINGO-STAPHILINUS. See *Levator palati.*

SALPINGO-STAPHILINUS INTERNUS. See *Levator palati.*

SALSAFY. See *Tragopogon pratense.*

SALSO'LA. (So called from its saline properties; hence the English word saltwort, most of the species affording the fossile alkali.) The name of a genus of plants in the Linnæan system Class, *Pentandria ;* Order, *Digynia.*

SALSOLA KALI. *Kali spinosum cochleatum ; Tragus, sive Tragum Matthioli.* Snail-seeded glasswort or salt-wort. The systematic name of a plant which affords the mineral alkali. See *Soda.*

SALSOLA SATIVA. The systematic name of a plant, which affords the mineral alkali. See *Soda.*

SALSOLA SODA. The systematic name of a plant which affords mineral alkali. See *Soda.*

SALT. This term has been usually employed to denote a compound, in definite proportions, of acid matter, with an alkali, earth, or metallic oxide. When the proportions of the constituents are so adjusted, that the resulting substance does not affect the colour of infusion of litmus, or red cabbage, it is then called a neutral salt. When the predominance of acid is evinced by the reddening of these infusions, the salt is said to be acidulous, and the prefix, *super*, or *bi*, is used to indicate this excess of acid. If, on the contrary, the acid matter appears to be in defect, or short of the quantity necessary for neutralizing the alkalinity of the base, the salt is then said to be with excess of base, and the prefix *sub* is attached to its name. The discoveries of Sir H. Davy have, however, taught chemists to modify their opinions concerning saline constitution. Many bodies, such as culinary salt, and muriate of lime, to which the appellation of *salt* cannot be refused, have not been proved to contain either acid or alkaline matter; but must, according to the strict logic of chemistry, be regarded as compounds of chlorine with metals.

Salt, acid This is distinguished by its sour taste when diluted with water. See *Acid.*

Salt, alkaline. Possesses a urinous, burning, and caustic taste, turns the syrup of violets to a green, has a strong affinity for acids, dissolves animal substances, unites readily with water, combines with oils and fat, and renders them miscible with water, dissolves sulphur, and is crystallizable. See *Alkali.*

Salt, ammoniacal, fixed. Muriate of lime.

Salt, bitter purging. Sulphate of magnesia.

Salt, cathartic. See *Magnesia sulphas*, and *Sodæ sulphas.*

Salt, common. See *Sodæ murias.*

Salt, digestive. Acetate of potassa.

Salt, diuretic. Acetate of potassa.

Salt, Epsom. See *Magnesiæ sulphas*

Salt, febrifuge, of Sylvius. Muriate of potassa.

Salt, fossil. A salt found in the earth.

Salt, fusible. Phosphate of ammonia.

Salt, fusible, of urine. Triple phosphate of soda and ammonia.

Salt, microcosmic. Triple phosphate of soda and ammonia.

Salt, nitrous ammoniacal. Nitrate of ammonia.

Salt, neutral. Secondary salt. Under the name of neutral or secondary salts are comprehended such matters as are composed of two primitive saline substances combined together in a certain proportion. These salts are called neutral, because they do not possess the characters of primitive salts; that is to say, they are neither acid nor alkaline: such as Epsom salts, nitre, &c. But in many secondary salts the qualities of one ingredient predominate; as tartar, or supertartrate of potassa, has an excess of acid; borax, or subborate of soda, an excess of base. The former are termed acidulous, the latter sub-alkaline salts.

SALT-PETRE. See *Nitre.*

Salt of amber. Succinic acid.

Salt of benzoin. Benzoic acid.

Salt of colcothar. Sulphate of iron.

Salt of lemons. Superoxylate of potassa

Salt of Saturn. Acetate of lead.

Salt of Seidlitz. Sulphate of magnesia

Salt of sorrel. Superoxylate of potassa.

Salt, Rochelle. See *Soda tartarizata.*

Salt, sea. See *Sodæ murias.*

Salt of steel. See *Ferri sulphas.*

Salt, polychrest. Sulphate of potassa.

Salt, secondary. See *Neutral salt.*

Salt, sedative. Boracic acid.

Salt, spirit of. Muriatic acid.

Salt of vitriol. Purified sulphate of zinc.

Salt of wisdom. Sal alembroth.

Salt, primitive. Simple salt. Under this order is comprehended those salts which were formerly thought to be simple or primitive, and which are occasionally called simple salts. The accurate experiments of the moderns have proved that these are for the most part compounded; but the term is retained with greater propriety when it is observed, that these salts composed, when united, salts which are termed secondary. These salts are never met with perfectly pure in nature, but require artificial processes to render them so. This order is divided into three genera, comprehending saline terrestrial substances, alkalies, and acids.

SALTWORT. See *Salsola kali.*

SALVATE'LLA. (From *salus*, health, because the opening of this vein was formerly thought to be of singular use in melancholy.) This vein runs along the little finger, unites upon the back of the hand with the cephalic of the thumb, and empties its blood into the internal and external cubical veins.

SA'LVIA. (*A sálvendo.*) 1. The name of a genus of plants in the Linnæan system. Class, *Diandria;* Order, *Monogynia.* Sage.

2. The pharmacopœial name of the common sage. See *Salvia officinalis.*

SALVIA HORTENSIS MINOR The small sage, or sage of virtue. A variety of the officinal sage, possessing similar virtues.

SALVIA OFFICINALIS. The systematic name of the garden sage. *Elelisphacos.* *Salvia—foliis lanceolato ovatis integris crenulatis, floribus spicatis, calycibus acutis,* of Linnæus. In ancient times sage was celebrated as a remedy of great efficacy, as would appear from the following lines of the school of Salernum:

' *Cur moriatur homo, cui salvia crescit in horto?*
Contra vim mortis, non est medicamen in hortis?
Salvia salvatrix, naturæ conciliatrix.
Salvia cum ruta faciunt tibi pocula tuta."

But at present it is not considered as an article of much importance. It has a fragrant, strong smell; and a warm, bitterish, aromatic taste, like other plants containing an essential oil. It has a remarkable property in resisting the putrefaction of animal substances, and is in frequent use among the Chinese as a tonic, in the form of tea, in debility of the stomach and nervous system.

SALVIA SCLAREA. The systematic name of the garden clary, called *horminum* in the pharmacopœias. *Sclarea hispanica.* The leaves and seeds are recommended as corroborants and antispasmodics, particularly in leucorrhœas and hysterical weaknesses. They have a bitterish, warm taste, and a strong smell of the aromatic kind. The seeds are infused in white wine, and imitate muscadel.

SAMARA. (The name, according to Pliny, of the fruit of the elm.) 1. The name of a genus of plants in the Linnæan system. Class, *Tetrandria;* Order, *Monogynia.*

2. A species of capsule of a compressed form, and dry coriaceous texture, with one or two cells, never bursting, but falling off entire, and dilated into a kind of wing at the summit or sides. In *Fraxinus*, it goes from the summit of the seed: in *Acer* and *Batula*, from the side: in *Ulmus campestris*, it goes all round.

SAMBU'CUS. (From *sabucca*, Heb. a musical instrument formerly made of this tree.) Elder.

1. The name of a genus of plants in the Linnæan system. Class, *Pentandria;* Order, *Trigynia.*

2. The pharmacopœial name of the elder-tree. See *Sambucus nigra.*

SAMBUCUS EBULUS. The systematic name of the dwarf-elder. *Ebulus; Chamæacte; Sambucus humilis; Sambucus herbacea.* Dwarf elder, or dane-wort. The root, interior bark, leaves, flowers, berries, and seeds of this herbaceous plant, *Sambucus—cymis trifidis, stipulis foliaceis, caule herbaceo*, of Linnæus, have all been administered medicinally, in moderate

doses, as resolvents and deobstruents, and, in larger doses, as hydragogues. The plant is chiefly employed by the poor of this country, among whom it is in common use as a purgative, but Dr. Cullen speaks of it as a violent remedy.

SAMBUCUS NIGRA. The systematic name of the elder-tree. *Sambucus vulgaris; Sambucus arborea, Acte; Infelix lignum. Sambucus—cymis quinquepartitis, foliis pinnatis, caule arboreo,* of Linnæus. This indigenous plant has an unpleasant narcotic smell, and some authors have reported its exhalations to be so noxious, as to render it unsafe to sleep under its shade. The parts of this tree that are proposed for medicinal use in the pharmacopœias are the inner bark, the flowers, and the berries. The first has scarcely any smell, and very little taste; on first chewing, it impresses a degree of sweetness, which is followed by a very slight but durable acrimony, in which its powers seem to reside. From its cathartic property it is recommended as an effectual hydragogue by Sydenham and Boerhaave: the former directs three handfuls of it to be boiled in a quart of milk and water, till only a pint remains, of which one half is to be taken night and morning, and repeated for several days; it usually operates both upwards and downwards, and upon the evacuation it produces, its utility depends. Boerhaave gave its expressed juice in doses from a drachm to half an ounce. In smaller doses it is said to be a useful aperient and deobstruent in various chronic disorders. The flowers have an agreeable flavour; and infusions of them, when fresh, are gently laxative and aperient. When dry, they are said to promote chiefly the cuticu lar excretion, and to be particularly serviceable in erysipelatous and eruptive disorders. Externally they are used in fomentations, &c. and in the London pharmacopœia are directed in the form of an ointment. The berries in taste are somewhat sweetish, and not unpleasant; on expression they yield a fine purple juice, which proves a useful aperient and resolvent in sundry chronic diseases, gently loosening the belly, and promoting the urine and perspiration.

Samphire. See *Crithmum maritimum.*

SAMPSUCHUS. See *Thymus mastichina.*

SAMPSYCHUM. (From σαω, to preserve, and ψυχη the mind; because of its cordial qualities.) Marjoram.

SANATI'VE. (From *sano*, to cure.) That which heals diseases.

SANCTI ANTONII IGNIS. See *Erysipelas.*

SANCTORIUS, SANCTORIUS, was born in 1561, at Capo d'Istria. He studied medicine at Padua, where he took his degree, and then settled at Venice, and practised with considerable success. At the age of fifty, however, he was appointed professor of the theory of medicine at Padua; in which office he distinguished himself for thirteen years. He was then allowed to retire on his salary, finding his health impaired by the fatigue of the visits, which he was frequently obliged to make in his professional capacity, to Venice, where he passed the remainder of his life in great reputation. On his death, in 1636, a statue of marble was raised to his memory; and an annual oration was instituted by the College of Physicians, to whom he had bequeathed an annuity, in commemoration of his benevolence. Sanctorius first called the attention of physicians to the cutaneous and pulmonary transpiration, which he proved to exceed the other excretions considerably in weight; and he maintained that this function must have a material influence on the system, and was deserving of great consideration in the treatment of diseases. There is, no doubt, much truth, in this general observation; but in its application to practice, he appears to have gone to an extravagant length, and to have contributed much to prolong the reputation of the humoral pathology. His treatise, entitled "Ars de Statica Medicina," was first published in 1614, and passed through more than twenty editions, including translations, with various commentaries: it is written in an elegant and per spicuous Latin style. He was also author of a Method of avoiding Errors in Medicine, to which was after ward added an essay "De Inventione Remediorum;" and of Commentaries on some of the ancient physicians. Besides the statical chair, by which he con trived to determine the weight of the Ingesta and Egesta, he invented an instrument for measuring the force of the pulse, and several others for surgical use;

and he was the first who attempted to determine the temperature of the body by a thermometer, of which, indeed, he is considered as the inventor.

SANCTUM SEMEN. The worm-seed, or santonicum.

SA'NCTUS. Holy. A term formerly applied to diseases, herbs, &c. See *Chorea, Carduus benedictus,* &c.

SANDALIFORMIS. Sandal or slipper-like, Applied to the nectary of the *Cypripedium calceolus.*

SANDARA'CHA. (From *saghad narak,* Arabian.) 1. A gummy resin.

2. A sort of arsenic.

SANDARACHA ARABUM. Arabian sandarach. This rosinous juice appears to have been the produce of a large species of juniper-tree.

Sandbath. See *Bath.*

SANDERS. See *Pterocarpus santalinus.*

SANDRACK. (An Arabian word.) See *Juniperus communis.*

SANDYX. (From *sani duk,* red, Arabian.) Cerusse burnt till it becomes red.

SANGUIFICATION. (*Sanguificatio;* from *sanguis,* blood, and *faceo,* to make.) A natural function of the body, by which the chyle is changed into blood. The uses of sanguification are the generation of blood, which serves to fill the blood-vessels, to irritate and stimulate the heart and arteries, to generate or cause heat, to secrete the humours, and to excite the vital actions.

SANGUINALIS. (From *sanguis,* blood: so named from its use in stopping bleedings.) The *Polygonum aviculare,* or knot-grass, is sometimes so called.

SANGUINARIA. (From *sanguis,* blood: so named from its use in stopping bleedings.) See *Polygonum aviculare.*

[SANGUINARIA CANADENSIS. See *Blood-root.* A.]

SANGUINEOUS. Bloody. Appertaining to the blood. Applied to certain conditions of the body and diseases, and appearances of solids and fluids; as sanguineous temperament, sanguineous apoplexy.

Sanguineous apoplexy. See *Apoplexy.*

SANGUIPURGIUM. (From *sanguis,* blood, and *purgo,* to purge.) A gentle fever, or such a one as by its discharges is supposed to purify the blood.

SA'NGUIS. (*Sanguis, guinis.* m.) See *Blood.*

SANGUIS DRACONIS. See *Calamus rotang.*

SANGUIS HERCULIS. A name for the crocus.

SANGUISO'RBA. (Probably so named originally from the blood-red colour of its flowers, although the juices of this plant, being astringent, the medicinal properties it possesses of stopping hæmorrhages may be a better warrant for its name.) The name of a genus of plants in the Linnæan system. Class, *Triandria;* Order, *Monogynia.*

SANGUISORBA OFFICINALIS. The systematic name of the Italian pimpinel, which was formerly much esteemed as an astringent, but is not now in use.

SANGUISU'GA. (From *sanguis,* blood, and *sugo,* to suck.) The leech or blood-sucker. See *Leech.*

SANICLE. See *Sanicula.*

Sanicle, Yorkshire. See *Pinguicula.*

SANI'CULA. (From *sano,* to heal: so called from its virtues in healing.)

1. The name of a genus of plants in the Linnæan system. Class, *Pentandria;* Order, *Digynia.*

2. The pharmacopœial name of sanicle.

SANICULA EBORACENSIS. See *Pinguicula vulgaris.*

SANICULA EUROPEA. The systematic name of the sanicle. *Cucullata; Dodecatheon; Symphytum petræum; Sanicula mas; Diapensia cortusa.* This herb was formerly recommended as a mild adstringent, and is supposed to have received its name from its sanative power. Its sensible qualities are a bitterish and somewhat austere taste, followed by an acrimony which chiefly affects the throat. It is only in use in the present day among the country people.

SANICULA MAS. See *Sanicula europea.*

SA'NIES. *Ichor.* This term is sometimes applied to a thin, limpid, and greenish discharge; and at other times to a thick and bloody kind of pus.

SA'NTALUM. (From *zandal,* Arabian.) The name of a genus of plants in the Linnæan system. Class, *Tetrandria;* Order, *Monogynia.* Saunders.

SANTALUM ALBUM. The systematic name of the yellow saunders. *Santalum citrinum; Santalum pallidum.* Yellow saunders. White saunders wood is of a pale white colour, often with a yellowish tinge, and, being destitute of taste or odour, it is superseded by the santalum citrinum, which is of a brownish yellow colour, of a bitterish aromatic taste, and of a pleasant smell, approaching to that of the rose. Both kinds are brought from the East Indies in billets, consisting of large thick pieces, which, according to Rumphius, are sometimes taken from the same, and sometimes from different trees. For though the white and yellow saunders are the wood of the same species of tree, yet the latter, which forms the central part of the tree, is not always to be found in sufficient quantity to repay the trouble and expense of procuring it, especially, unless the trees be old; while the white, which is the exterior part of the wood, is always more abundant, and is consequently much cheaper.

Yellow saunders, distilled with water, yields a fragrant essential oil, which thickens in the cold into the consistence of a balsam, approaching in smell to ambergris, or a mixture of ambergris and roses; the remaining decoction, inspissated to the consistence of an extract, is bitterish, and slightly pungent. Rectified spirit extracts, by digestion, considerably more than water; the colour of the tincture is a rich yellow. The distilled spirit is slightly impregnated with the flavour of the wood; the remaining brownish extract has a weak smell, and a moderate balsamic pungency. The wood is valued highly on account of its fragrance; hence the Chinese are said to fumigate their clothes with it, and to burn it in their temples in honour of their gods. Though still retained in the Materia Medica, it cannot be thought to possess any considerable share of medicinal power. Hoffman considers its virtues as similar to those of ambergris; and some others have esteemed it in the character of a corroborant and restorative.

["The sandal-wood, which is found on some of the islands of the South Sea, has been a great article of commerce for the Chinese market. The following extract of a letter from Coles Fanning & Co. to Dr. Mitchill gives an account of the trade and employment of this wood as a perfume.

"In the month of August, 1806, we despatched the ship Hope, Capt. Brumley, from New-York, on a voyage to the Fejee islands, to procure a cargo of Sandal-wood, for the Canton market. The Hope having succeeded at the island of *Toconroba,* in procuring a full cargo for herself, and in part freighting an English brig that she met with at said island, arrived in November 1807, at Canton, where both cargoes were sold at about 25 cents per pound. While at the Fejee islands the Captain of the Hope contracted and paid in part to the chief of the island for about 270 tons more of sandal-wood, (this being about the whole quantity of good wood remaining on the islands) to be taken away in a certain time. In order therefore to seize so profitable a speculation while there were so few to participate in it, we built and sent the ship Tonquin, commanded by E. Fanning, in May, 1807, to meet the Hope at Canton; but the Hope not having arrived in time for Capt. Fanning to fulfil our original intentions, the season was so far wasted as to compel him to load the Tonquin for New-York, and he met the Hope in the mouth of the Tigris or (Canton river). Both vessels will, therefore, return to the United States under no expectations that the trespasses of European nations would compel our government to inhibit their departure again on said voyage. Being thus situated we have taken the liberty to address you for your advice, whether, under the embargo law, or the supplements, the Executive will not have sufficient authority to permit us to proceed immediately with a ship sufficient to bring the above quantity of wood, and by that means save to ourselves and our country at least $130,000, which will probably, if such permission is refused, fall into English hands; for you will please to observe, that there was in the first place but a small patch of the wood on one of the islands, that the Hope left four English vessels there, selecting from the refuse a little of very inferior quality, and in expectation too that some accident would prevent our ship from returning within the limited time, which would release the chief from his engagement, and leave him at liberty to sell the good wood purchased by Capt. Brumley to them. From the knowledge Capt. Brumley has of the chief's conduct, we rely as confidently on his keeping his engagement for the time limited as we would on the chief of the most civilized nation. You will no doubt recollect that the Chinese have long considered sandal-wood as possessing religious properties; they are accustomed to burn it on their altars as incense; their god Josh is supposed always out of humour, unless his nose is regaled with its delightful effluvia. We have enclosed a small piece of the wood, that you may have an opportunity of judging how far a Pagan god's taste may be deemed exquisite. The Hope is the first vessel, to the best of our knowledge, that ever proceeded from the United States on this voyage, and on her return, we presume she will pay about $40,000 into the Treasury for duties from the proceeds of the wood, which originally cost only about nine hundred dollars.'—*Med. Repos.* A.]

SANTALUM CITRINUM. See *Santalum album.*

SANTALUM PALLIDUM. See *Santalum album.*

SANTALUM RUBRUM. Red saunders. See *Pterocarpus santalinus.*

SANTOLI'NA. (From *santalum*, saunders; because it smells like the saunders-wood.) See *Artemisia santonica.*

SANTOLINA CHAMÆ-CYPARISSUS. The systematic name of the lavender cotton.

SANTONICUM. (From *Santonio*, its native place.) See *Artemisia santonica.*

SAPHE'NA. (From σαφης, visible.) *Vena saphena.* The large vein of the leg, which ascends along the little toe over the external ankle, and evacuates part of the blood from the foot into the popliteal veins.

SAPIENTIÆ DENTES. (*Sapientia*, wisdom, discretion: so called because they appear when the person is supposed to be at years of discretion.) See *Teeth.*

SAPI'NDUS. (That is, *Sapo Indus*, Indian soap: the rind of the fruit serving instead of soap to cleanse linen, but not without hazard of injury to the texture of the cloth.) The name of a genus of plants. Class, *Octandria*; Order, *Digynia*. The soap-tree.

SAPINDUS SAPONARIA. The systematic name of the plant which affords soap-nuts. *Saponariæ nuculæ; Baccæ bermudensis.* Soap-berries. A spherical fruit, about the size of a cherry, the cortical part of which is yellow, glossy, and so transparent as to show the spherical black nut which rattles within, and which includes a white kernel. The tree grows in Jamaica. It is said that the cortical part of this fruit has a bitter taste, and no smell; that it raises a soapy froth with water, and has similar effects with soap in washing; that it is a medicine of singular and specific virtue in chlorosis. They are not known in the shops of this country.

SA'PO. (*Sapo, nis.* m.) Soap. A compound, in definite proportions, of certain principles in oils, fats, or resin, with a salifiable base. When this base is potassa or soda, the compound is used as a detergent in washing clothes. When an alkaline earth, or oxide of a common metal, as litharge, is the salifiable base, the compound is insoluble in water. The first of these combinations is scarcely applied to any use, if we except that of linseed oil with lime-water, sometimes prescribed as a liniment against burns; and the last is known only in surgery as the basis of certain plasters. Concerning the chemical constitution of soaps and saponification, no exact ideas were entertained prior to Chevreuil's researches.

Fats are compounds of a solid and a liquid substance; the former called *stearine*, the latter resembling vegetable oil, and therefore called *elaïne.* When fat is treated with a hot ley of potassa or soda, the constituents react on one another, so as to generate the solid pearly matter *margaric acid*, and the fluid matter *oleic acid*, both of which enter into a species of saline combination with the alkali; while the third matter that is produced, the *sweet principle*, remains free. We must therefore regard our common soap as a mixture of an alkaline margarate and oleate, in proportions determined by the relative proportions of the two acids producible from the peculiar species of fat. It is probable, on the other hand, that the soap formed from vegetable oil is chiefly an *oleate*. No chemical researches have hitherto been made known, on the compounds of resin with alkalies, though these constitute the brown soaps so extensively manufactured in this country. All oils or fats do not possess in an equal degree the property of saponification. Those which saponify best, are,

1. Oil of olives, and of sweet almonds.

2. Animal oils; as hog's-lard, tallow, butter, and horse-oil.

3. Oil of colza, or rape-seed oil.

4. Oil of beech-mast and poppy-seed, when mixed with olive-oil or tallow.

5. The several fish-oils, mingled like the preceding.

6. Hempseed-oil.

7. Nut-oil and linseed-oil.

8. Palm oil.

9. Rosin.

In general, the only soaps employed in commerce, are those of olive-oil, tallow, lard, palm-oil, and rosin. A species of soap can also be formed by the union of beeswax with alkali; but this has no detergent application, being used only for painting in *encausto*.

The specific gravity of soap is in general greater than that of water. Its taste is faintly alkaline. When subjected to heat it speedily fuses, swells up, and is then decomposed. Exposed to the air in thin slices, it soon becomes dry; but the whole combined water does not leave it, even by careful desiccation on a sand-bath.

Soap is much more soluble in hot than in cold water. This solution is instantly disturbed by the greater number of acids, which seizing the alkali, either separate the fatty principles, or unite with them into an acido-soapy emulsion. The solution is likewise decomposed by almost all the earthy and metallic salts, which give birth to insoluble compounds of the oleic and margaric acids, with the salifiable bases.

Soap is soluble in alkohol, and in large quantity by the aid of heat. When boiling alkohol is saturated with soap, the liquid, on cooling, forms a consistent transparent mass of a yellow colour. When this mass is dried, it still retains its transparency, provided the soap be a compound of tallow and soda; and in this state it is sold by the perfumers in this country.

Good soap possesses the property of removing from linen and cloth the greater part of fatty substances which may have been applied to them.

The medicinal soap, *sapo amygdolinus*, is made with oil of sweet almonds, and half its weight of caustic alkali. Common or soft soap, *sapo mollis*, is made of potassa and oil, or tallow. Spanish, or Castile soap, *sapo durus*, of oil of olives and soda, or barilla. Black soap is a composition of train oil and an alkali; and green soap of hemp, linseed, or rape oil, with an alkali. The white Spanish soap, being made of the finer kinds of olive oil, is the best, and therefore, preferred for internal use. Soap was imperfectly known to the ancients. It is mentioned by Pliny as made of fat and ashes, and as an invention of the Gauls. Aretæus and others inform us, that the Greeks obtained their knowledge of its medical use from the Romans. Its virtues, according to Berglus, are detergent, resolvent, and aperient, and its use recommended in jaundice, gout, calculous complaints, and obstruction of the viscera. The efficacy of soap, in the first of these diseases, was experienced by Sylvius, and since recommended very generally by various authors who have written on this complaint; and it has also been thought of use in supplying the place of bile in the primæ viæ. The utility of this medicine in icterical cases was inferred chiefly from its supposed power of dissolving biliary concretions; but this medicine has lost much of its reputation in jaundice, since it is now known, that gall-stones have been found in many after death who had been daily taking soap for several months, and even years. Of its good effects in urinary calculous affections, we have the testimonies of several, especially when dissolved in lime-water, by which its efficacy is considerably increased; for it thus becomes a powerful solvent of mucus, which an ingenious modern author supposes to be the chief agent in the formation of calculi; it is, however, only in the incipient state of the disease that these remedies promise effectual benefit, though they generally abate the more violent symptoms where they cannot remove the cause. With Boerhaave, soap was a general medicine; for as he attributed most complaints to viscidity of the fluids, he, and most of the Boerhaavian school, prescribed it, in conjunction with different resinous and other substances, in gout, rheumatism, and various visceral complaints. Soap is also externally employed as a resolvent, and gives name to several officinal preparations.

[" The history of personal cleanliness is very important, and has been lamentably neglected. Pliny, in his Natural History, treating of strumous swellings, makes mention of Soap: *Prodet est sapo. Galliarum hoc inventum rutilandis capillis. Fit ex sebo et cinere.*

Optimus ex fagino et caprino : duobis modis, spissus ac liquidus : uterque apud Germanus majore in usu viris quam fœminis. " *Soap is good for them.* This was invented in Gaul, and used for reddening the hair. It is made of fat and ashes. The best is prepared from the ashes of the beach-tree and the suet of the goat. There are two sorts, the thick and the liquid. Among the Germans, both kinds are more used by the men than by the women." Priscian writes of "Sapo Gallicus," or *Gaulish soap ;* and Martial of "Spuma Batava," or *Dutch lather,* and " Spuma Caustica," or *Caustic foam.* The German soap was reckoned the best and cleanest. The *Gaulish* was next in quality and value.

It is clear, and President *Goguet* is of the same opinion, (in his history of the origin of laws, &c.) that the ancient Hebrews, Greeks, and Romans knew nothing of soap. These nations used to supply the want of it by various other means. From the barbarous people of the north, the knowledge and employment of soap passed to the Romans; and from the Romans was made known to the Greeks. A very remarkable fact!

When the Romans first became acquainted with soap, they called it " Unguentum Cineris," or *Ointment of ashes.* So prevalent was the idea of its origin, that several writers have treated of it under the denomination of " Cinis," or ASHES, itself. And those who consumed soap were in those days called " Cinerarii," or *Ashes users.*

After a while, however, this detergent ointment was distinguished among the Romans by the word " Sapo." This term probably is of Gothic or Barbarian origin. Some of the Parthian and other nations bordering on the frontier provinces of the Roman Empire, distinguished their rulers or chiefs by the name "Sapor" or " Sapores." The good they derived from the *Unguentum Cineris* was so great and excellent, and it was so powerful in overcoming bodily inconveniences, and so conducive to personal comfort, that they called this preserver of private health, by a name corresponding to, and derived from the sovereigns who presided over their public safety. From Sapor, thus was derived Sapo; two terms significant of the powers which protected the political and the individual bodies of the people. The Romans adopted Sapo, and naturalized it to their language. From them the Greeks borrowed their σαπων. The French have derived their " savon" from the same source, and so have the English their " soap."

But if soap was so late an invention, and learned from the rougher nations of the north of Europe at so advanced a period of the history of their southern neighbours, how comes it to pass the Hebrews were acquainted with it, as we read in the English version of the Bible, translated under the auspices of king James? The term "soap" does indeed occur there in *Jeremiah,* chap. ii. v. 22, and in *Malachi,* chap. iii. v. 2. Yet there can scarcely be entertained a doubt, that the translators were mistaken. This opinion of their having misinterpreted the text is supported by the Latin vulgate version, which expresses the former of these passages by the words, " herbam borith," and the latter by " herba fullonum." What, now, is the *plant Borith,* and what is the *Fuller's herb ? Calmet,* in his Dictionary of the Bible, states, that it is the kali or saline vegetable, of whose ashes "ley and soap are made." *Goguet* thinks it was salt-wort, a plant very common in Syria, Judea, Egypt, and Arabia; which, if burned to ashes, and the ashes mingled with water, formed a strong ley fit for cleansing and whitening cloths, and doubtless they were right.

Notwithstanding all this authority, *Beza* evidently issed the true meaning of the original, which he expresses in both the before-mentioned texts, by the substantive " smegma." But *John Jacob Schmidt,* in his *Biblischer Medicus,* mentions this cleansing article by the Hebrew name of "Bor." This substantive being derived from the root " ur" *fire,* plainly indicates that the purifying material in question was obtained *by* or *through fire. Borith* would thus seem to be the plant which, by the *action of the fire,* yielded *Bor,* that is, the detergent article of the washers and fullers. Or the two words might be used indifferently to signify the plant both before and after incineration. Hence, it may be inferred, the plant was a species of *Salsola* or *Glass-wort,* and that the saline residuum, after burn-

ing, was *kelp* or *barilla ;* a material possessing qualities similar to the oriental natron or mineral alkali. The same thing has been latterly called *Soda,* whence comes *La Soude* of the French, and the *Suds* or Alkaline lixivium of the English.—*New-York Med. Repos.* A.]

SAPO TEREBINTHINÆ. Starkey's soap.

℞. kali preparati calidi, ℥j. Olei terebinth, ℥ iij. The hot kali preparatum is to have the oil of turpentine gradually blended with it, in a heated mortar. Indolent swellings were formerly rubbed with this application, and perhaps some chronic affections of the joints might still be benefited by it.

SAPONA'RIA. (From *sapo,* soap: so called because its juice, like soap, cleans cloths.) 1. The name of a genus of plants in the Linnæan system. Class, *Decandria ;* Order, *Digynia.*

2. The pharmacopœial name of the soap-wort. See *Saponaria officinalis.*

SAPONARIA NUCULA. See *Sapindus saponaria.*

SAPONARIA OFFICINALIS. The systematic name of the soap-wort, called also bruise-wort. *Struthium ; Lanaria ; Lychnis sylvestris ; Ibixuma.* The root of this plant, *Saponaria—calycibus cylindricis, foliis ovato-lanceolatis,* of Linnæus, is employed medicinally ; it has no peculiar smell; its taste is sweetish, glutinous, and somewhat bitter. On being chewed for some time, it is said to discover a degree of acrimony, which continues to affect the mouth for a considerable time. According to Neuman, two ounces of the root yielded eleven drachms of watery extract; but Cartheuser, from a like quantity, only obtained six drachms, and twenty-four grains. This extract manifested a sweetish taste, followed by an acrid quality. The spirituous extract is less in quality, but of a more penetrating acrid taste. Decoctions of the root, on being sufficiently agitated, produces a saponaceous froth ; a similar soapy quality is observable also in the extract, and still more manifestly in the leaves, insomuch that they have been used by the mendicant monks as a substitute for soap in washing of their clothes; and Bergius, who made several experiments with the saponaria, declares that it had all the effects of soap itself.

From these peculiar qualities of the saponaria, there can be little doubt of its possessing a considerable share of medical efficacy, which Dr. Woodville says he could wish to find faithfully ascertained.

The diseases for which the saponaria is recommended, as syphilis, gout, rheumatism, and jaundice, are not, perhaps, the complaints in which its use is most availing; for a fancied resemblance of the roots of saponaria with those of sarsaparilla, seems to have led physicians to think them similar in their effects; and hence they have both been administered with the same intentions, particularly in fixed pains, and venereal affections. Bergius says, "in arthritide, cura mercuriale, &c. nullum aptiorem potum novi." However, according to several writers, the most inveterate cases of syphilis were cured by a decoction of this plant, without the use of mercury.

Haller informs us that Boerhaave entertained a high opinion of its efficacy in jaundice and other visceral obstructions.

SAPONULE. *Saponulus.* A combination of a volatile or essential oil with different bases; as *saponule of ammonia,* &c.

SAPOTA. (The West Indian name of several sorts of fruits of the plum kind.) See *Acras sapota.*

SAPPAN LIGNUM. See *Hæmatoxylon campechianum*

SAPPHIRE. *Telesie* of Haüy. *Perfect corundum* of Bournon. The oriental ruby and topaz are sapphires. Sapphire is a subspecies of rhomboidal corundum. It is one of the esteemed precious stones, a sapphire of ten carats' weight being worth fifty guineas. Its colours are blue, red, and also gray, white, green, and yellow. It is found in blunt-edged pieces, in roundish pebbles, and crystallized after the diamond. It is the hardest substance in nature.

SAPPHIRINA AQUA. (So called from its sapphire or blue colour.) *Aqua cupri ammoniati.* Made by a solution of sal ammoniac in lime-water, standing in a copper vessel.

Saracens consound. See *Solidago virga aurea.*

SARATOGA. The name of a county in the State of New-York, in America, celebrated for its springs of mineral water, which are numerous throughout a circuit of several miles near the centre of that county The ground throughout this circuit is, generally speaking, flat, and in two or three places is covered with extensive sheets of limpid water, which are fed by streams that take their origin in the neighbouring mountains of granite and gneiss. The soil in which the springs rise is sandy, and rests upon a bed of compact limestone, or argillaceous slate, or gray wacke; and they are apparently more numerous where these specimens of the transition and secondary formation are ascertained to meet. There is more variety in the degree of mineral impregnation at two points, about seven miles distant from each other, where accommodation has been more liberally provided for visiters, and which have taken the names of Saratoga and Ballston Spa. The former of these seems to have been known to the Indians before the formation of European settlements, and was pointed out by them to Sir William Johnson, in 1767. It was called in their language the *Spring of Life*, and is in temperature about 50° of Fahrenheit. Most of the American chemists have made the analysis of the Saratoga water an object of inquiry and publication, and though one or two of them differ as to the existence of some of the more trifling impregnations, they agree generally that it contains carbonic acid gas, muriate of soda, carbonate of soda, carbonate of lime, carbonate of iron, and carbonate of magnesia.

In two or three of the springs, there is, besides, sulphuretted hydrogen gas, and in one at least traces of silica and alumina. These incidental varieties give rise to slight differences in the medicinal effects of the springs; but, as a general rule for guiding strangers in their selection, it may be stated, that the more abundant the muriate of soda, and carbonates of soda, lime, and magnesia, the more aperient and diuretic will be the water; while the greater the quantity of carbonic acid and of iron, in proportion to the former ingredients, the more powerful will be its tonic effects.

The great superiority of these American mineral waters over every thing of the kind to be found in Europe, consists,

1st, In their containing a greater quantity of carbonic acid, or fixed air, by which they are capable of retaining in solution a much larger proportion of useful saline matter, of a particular character, than any European mineral water.

2dly, In their possessing more efficient purgative properties than any of the springs of Europe, with the exception of Harrowgate, and perhaps Cheltenham, which are both not only destitute of the refreshing taste given by the carbonic acid, but contain (Harrowgate in particular) matters which render them to the palate in some degree offensive.

3dly, In containing such a combination of materials, in the most eligible form, as fit them to become at once a most refreshing beverage to all, and to those suffering from the diseases about to be mentioned in particular, a more perfect union of what is agreeable with that which is necessary and useful in the way of medicine, than any that has hitherto been provided, either by nature or art.

The diseases in which the Saratoga waters have been found to be productive of the best effects, are, dyspepsia, cutaneous diseases, scrofulous affections, dropsy, chlorosis, and other affections peculiar to the female sex, nephritic affections and gravel.

SARCI'TES. (From σαρξ, flesh.) See *Anasarca.*

SA'RCIUM. (Diminutive of σαρξ, flesh.) A caruncle, or small fleshy excrescence.

SARCOCE'LE. (From σαρξ, flesh, and κηλη, a tumour.) *Hernia carnosa.* This is a disease of the body of the testicle, and as the term implies, consists, in general, in such an alteration made in the structure of it, as produces a resemblance to a hard fleshy substance, instead of that fine, soft, vascular texture, of which it is, in a natural and healthy state, composed.

The ancient writers have made a great number of distinctions of the different kinds of this disease, according to its different appearances, and according to the mildness, or malignity of the symptoms with which it may chance to be attended. Thus, the *sarcocele*, the *hydro-sarcocele*, the *scirrhus*, the *cancer*, the *caro adnata ad testem*, and the *caro adnata ad vasa*, which are really little more than descriptions of different states and circumstances of the same disease, are reckoned as so many different complaints, requiring a variety of treatment, and deriving their origin from a variety of different humours

Every species of sarcocele consists primarily in an enlargement, induration, and obstruction of the vas cular part of the testicle; but this alteration is, in different people, attended with such a variety of circumstances, as to produce several different appearances, and to occasion the many distinctions which have been made.

If the body of the testicle, though enlarged, and indurated to some degree, be perfectly equal in its surface, void of pain, has no appearance of fluid in its tunica vaginalis, and produces very little uneasiness, except what is occasioned by its mere weight, it is usually called a simple sarcocele, or an indolent scirrhus; if, at the same time that the testis is enlarged and hardened, there be a palpable accumulation of fluid in the vaginal coat, the disease has by many been named a *hydro-sarcocele;* if the lower part of the spermatic vessels, and the epididymus were enlarged, hard, and knotty, they supposed it to be a fungous, or morbid accretion, and called it the *caro adnata ad vasa;* if the testicle itself was unequal in its surface, but at the same time not painful, they distinguish it by the title of *caro adnata ad testem;* if it was tolerably equal, not very painful, nor frequently so, but at the same time hard and large, they gave it the appellation of an occult or benign cancer; if it was ulcerated, subject to frequent acute pain, to hæmorrhage, &c. it was known by that of a malignant or confirmed cancer. These different appearances, though distinguished by different titles, are really no more than so many stages (as it were) of the same kind of disease, and depend a great deal on several accidental circumstances, such as age, habit, manner of living, &c. It is true, that many people pass several years with this disease, under its most favourable appearances, and without encountering any of its worst; but, on the other hand, there are many who, in a very short space of time, run through all its stages. They who are most conversant with it, know how very convertible its mildest symptoms are into its most dreadful ones, and how very short a space of time often intervenes between the one and the other.

There is hardly any disease affecting the human body, which is subject to more variety than this is, both with regard to its first manner of appearance, and the changes which it may undergo.

Sometimes the first appearance is a mere simple enlargement and induration of the body of the testicle; void of pain, without inequality of surface, and producing no uneasiness, or inconvenience, except what is occasioned by its mere weight. And some people are so fortunate to have it remain in this state for a very considerable length of time without visible or material alteration. On the other hand, it sometimes happens that very soon after its appearance in this mild manner, it suddenly becomes unequal and knotty, and is attended with very acute pains darting up to the loins and back, but still remaining entire, that is, not bursting through the integuments. Sometimes the fury of the disease brooks no restraint, but making its way through all the membranes which envelope the testicle it either produces a large, foul, stinking, phagedenic ulcer, with hard edges, or it thrusts forth a painful gleeting fungus, subject to frequent hæmorrhage.

Sometimes an accumulation of water is made in the tunica vaginalis, producing that mixed appearance, called the *hydro-sarcocele.*

Sometimes there is no fluid at all in the cavity of the tunica vaginalis: but the body of the testicle itself is formed into cells, containing either a turbid kind of water, a bloody sanies, or a purulent fœtid matter. Sometimes the disorder seems to be merely local, that is, confined to the testicle, not proceeding from a tainted habit, nor accompanied with diseased viscera, the patient having all the general appearances and circumstances of health, and deriving his local mischief from an external injury. At other times, a pallid, leaden countenance, indigestion, frequent nausea, colicky pains, sudden purgings, &c. sufficiently indicate a vitiated habit, and diseased viscera, which diseased viscera may also sometimes be discovered and felt.

The progress also which it makes from the testis upward, toward the process, is very uncertain; the disease occupying the testicle only, without affecting the spermatic process, in some subjects, for a great length of time; while, in others, it totally spoils the testicle very soon, and almost as soon seizes on the spermatic chord.

SARCOCOLLA. (From σαρξ, flesh, and κολλα, glue; because of its supposed power of gluing together wounds.) A spontaneous exudation from a tree of the fur kind, which grows in Persia, supposed to be similar to olibanum or frankincense.

SARCOEPIPLOCE'LE. Enlarged testicle, with rupture, containing omentum.

SARCOLITE. A variety of analcime.

SARCO'LOGY. (*Sarcologia;* from σαρξ, flesh, and λογος, a discourse.) The doctrine of the muscles and soft parts.

SARCO MA. (*Sarcoma, atis.* n.; from σαρξ, flesh.) *Sarcosis; Porrus; Sarcophyia Nævus.* A fleshy excrescence. A genus of disease in the Class *Locales,* and Order *Tumores,* of Cullen.

SARCO'MPHALUS. (From σαρξ, flesh, and ομφαλος, the navel.) A fleshy excrescence about the navel.

SARCOPHYIA. (From σαρξ, flesh, and φυω, to grow.) A fleshy excrescence.

SARCOPYODES. (From σαρξ, flesh, and πυον, pus.) Applied to the purulent, fleshy discharge, which is thrown up in some stages of consumption.

SARCO'SIS. (From σαρξ, flesh.) 1. A fleshy tumour.

2. The generation of flesh.

SARCOTICA. (From σαρξ, flesh.) Medicines which promote the generation of flesh in wounds.

SARDE.. Sardoin. A variety of cornelian of a deep blood-red colour.

SARDIASIS. (From σαρδωνιη, the sardonia, or herb, which, being eaten, causes convulsive laughter.) See *Sardonic laugh.*

SARDONIA. (From *Sardonia,* its native soil.) A kind of smallage.

SARDONIC LAUGH. (*Risus sardonicus:* so called from the herb *sardonia,* which being eaten is said to cause a deadly convulsive laughter.) A kind of convulsive laugh, or spasmodic grin. See *Spasmus cynicus.*

SARDONICUS RISUS. See *Sardonic laugh.*

SARDONYX. A variety of cornelian composed of layers of white and red.

SARMENTACEÆ. The name of a natural order of Linnæus's *Fragmenta:* embracing the plants with twining or trailing stems.

SARMENTOSUS. (From *sarmentum,* a twig, or trailing stalk.) Trailing. Applied to a creeping stem, barren of flowers, thrown out from the root for the purpose of increase.

SARMENTUM. (*Sarmen;* from *sarpio,* to prune, lop, or cut off.) A twig, a runner.

SARSAPARI'LLA. (This word is of Spanish origin, signifying a red tree.) See *Smilax sarsaparilla.*

SARSAPARILLA GERMANICA. See *Carex arenaria.*

SAR'TORIUS. (From *sartor,* a tailor; because tailors cross their legs with it.) *Sartorius seu longissimus femoris,* of Cowper; *Ilio cresti tibial* of Dumas. This flat and slender muscle, which is the longest of the human body, and from an inch and a half to two inches in breadth, is situated immediately under the integuments, and extends obliquely from the upper and anterior part of the thigh, to the upper, anterior, and inner part of the tibia, being enclosed by a thin membranous sheath, which is derived from the adjacent *fascia lata.* It arises, by a tendon of about half an inch in breadth, from the outer surface and inferior edge of the anterior superior spinous process of the ilium, but soon becomes fleshy, and runs down a little way obliquely inwards, and then for some space upon the rectus, nearly in a straight direction, after which it passes obliquely over the vastus internus, and the lower part of the adductor longus, and then running down between the tendons of the adductor magnus, and the gracilis, is inserted, by a thin tendon, into the inner part of the tibia, near the inferior part of its tuberosity, and for the space of an inch or two below it. This tendon sends off a thin aponeurosis, which is spread over the upper and posterior part of the leg. This muscle serves to bend the leg obliquely inwards, or to roll the thigh outwards, and at the same time to bring one leg across the other, on which account Spigelius first gave it the name of *sartorius,* or the tailor's muscle.

SA'SSAFRAS. (*Quasi saxifraga;* from *saxum,* a stone, and *frango,* to break; so called because a decoction of its wood was supposed good for the stone; or, which is most probable, from the river Sassafras, in America, on the banks of which it grows in abundance.) See *Laurus sassafras.*

SASSOLINE. Native boracic acid, found on the edges of hot springs near Sasso in Florence. It consists of boracic acid 86, ferruginous sulphate of manganese 11, and sulphate of lime 3.

SATELLITE. The veins which accompany the brachial artery as far as the bend of the cubit, are so called.

SATIN SPAR. A species of fibrous limestone.

SATURANTIA. Medicines which neutralize the acid in the stomach.

SATURATION. *Saturatio.* A term employed in pharmacy and chemistry to express the state of a body which has a power of dissolving another, to a certain extent only, in which it has effected that degree of solution. Some substances unite in all proportions. Such, for example, are acids in general, and some other salts with water; and many of the metals with each other. But there are likewise many substances which cannot be dissolved in a fluid, at a certain temperature, in any quantity beyond a certain proportion. Thus water will dissolve only about one-third of its weight of common salt, and, if more be added, it will remain solid. A fluid, which holds in solution as much of any substance as it can dissolve, is said to be saturated with it. But saturation with one substance does not deprive the fluid of its power of acting on and dissolving some other bodies, and in many cases it increases this power. For example, water saturated with salt will dissolve sugar; and water saturated with carbonic acid will dissolve iron, though without this addition its action on this metal is scarcely perceptible.

The word saturation is likewise used in another sense by chemists: The union of two principles produces a body, the properties of which differ from those of its component parts, but resemble those of the predominating principle. When the principles are in such proportion that neither predominates, they are said to be saturated with each other; but if otherwise, the most predominant principle is said to be subsaturated or undersaturated, and the other supersaturated or over saturated.

SATUREI'A. (From *satyri,* the lustful satyrs; because it makes those who eat it lascivious. Blanch.) 1. The name of a genus of plants in the Linnæan system. Class, *Didynamia;* Order, *Gymnospermia.*

2. The pharmacopœial name of the summer savory.

SATUREIA CAPITATA. The systematic name of the ciliated savory. *Thymus creticus.* It possesses similar virtues to our thyme, but in a stronger degree.

SATUREIA HORTENSIS. The systematic name of the summer savory. *Satureia sativa; Culina sativa Plinii; Thymbra.* This low shrub is cultivated in our gardens for culinary purposes. It has a warm, aromatic, penetrating taste, and smells like thyme, but milder. It is an ingredient in most of the warm stews and made dishes.

SATUREIA SATIVA. See *Satureia hortensis.*

SATU'RNUS. (From the planet or heathen god, of that name.) The chemical name of lead.

SATYRI'ASIS. (From σατυρος, a satyr; because they are said to be greatly addicted to venery.) *Satyriasmus; Priapismus; Salacitas; Brachuna; Aras con.* Excessive and violent desire for coition in men. A genus of disease in the Class *Locales,* and Order *Dysorexiæ,* of Cullen.

SATY'RION. (From σατυρος, an animal given to venery : so called because it was supposed to excite venery if only held in the hand.) See *Orchis mascula*

SATYRIUM. See *Orchis mascula.*

Sauce alone. See *Erysimum alliaria.*

SAUNDERS. See *Santalum album.*

Saunders, red. See *Pterocarpus.*

SAUR KRAUT. Cabbage preserved in brine. An article of food common in Germany, like our pickled cabbage.

SAUSSURITE. A hard mineral, placed by Jameson near Andalusite, of white and gray or green colour, found at the foot of Mount Rosa.

SAUVAGES, FRANCIS BOISSIER DE, was born at Alais, in Lower Languedoc, in 1706. He graduated at Montpelier when only 20, but still continued his studies, and four years after went for farther improvement to Paris. On his return to Montpelier he obtained a professorship in 1734; but his reputation for ingenuity of speculation is said to have obstructed his success in practice. In 1752 he was made professor of botany, having for twelve years before officiated as demonstrator of the plants in the botanic garden. His death occurred in 1767. He was a member of several of the learned societies of Europe, and obtained the prizes given by many public bodies for the best essays on given subjects. Among his earlier publications was one, entitled "Nouvelles Classes des Maladies," the outline of the system of Nosology, which has rendered his name illustrious, but which did not appear in its complete form, till after an additional labour of thirty years had been bestowed upon it. This work, consisting of five octavo volumes, contains an immense body of information, indeed, almost every thing then known concerning the species of disease; but the whole is very loosely arranged. He had collected many new observations and descriptions, with a view to incorporate them in a second edition; which, however, he did not live to accomplish. These materials were used by Dr. Cramer after his death. Besides this valuable work, Sauvages was author of numerous others on different subjects relating to medicine.

SAVIN. See *Juniperus sabina.*

Savin ointment. See *Ceratum sabinæ.*

SAVINA. See *Juniperus sabina.*

SAVOURY. See *Satureia.*

SAXI'FRAGA. (From *saxum,* a stone, and *frango,* to break: so called because it was supposed to be good against the stone in the bladder.) The name of a genus of plants in the Linnæan system. Class, *Decandria;* Order, *Digynia.*

SAXIFRAGA ALBA. See *Saxifraga granulata.*

SAXIFRAGA ANGLICA. See *Peucedanum.*

SAXIFRAGA CRASSIFOLIA. The root of this species of saxifrage is extolled by professor Pallas as an antiseptic.

SAXIFRAGA GRANULATA. The systematic name of the white saxifrage. *Saxifraga alba.* Called by Oribasius *Besto. Sanicula sedum.* Linnæus describes the taste of this plant to be acrid and pungent, which we have not been able to discover; neither the tubercles of the root nor the leaves manifest to the organs of taste any quality likely to be of medicinal use, and therefore, though this species of saxifrage has been long employed as a popular remedy in nephritic and gravelly disorders, yet we do not find either from its sensible qualities, or from any published instances of its efficacy, that it deserves a place in the Materia Medica. The superstitious doctrine of signatures suggested the use of the root, which is a good example of what Linnæus has termed radix granulata. The bulbs or tubercles of such roots answer an important purpose in vegetation, by supplying the plants with nourishment and moisture, and thereby enabling them to resist the effects of that drought to which the dry soils they inhabit peculiarly expose them.

SAXIFRAGA RUBRA. See *Spiræa filipendula.*

SAXIFRAGA VULGARIS. Seu *Peucedanum silaus.*

SAXIFRAGE. See *Saxifraga.*

Saxifrage, burnet. See *Pimpinella saxifraga.*

Saxifrage, English. See *Peucedanum silaus.*

Saxifrage, meadow. See *Peucedanum silaus.*

Saxifrage, white. See *Saxifraga granulata.*

Saxon blue. See *Blue, saxon.*

SCAB. A hard substance covering superficial ulcerations, and formed by a concretion of the fluid discharged from them.

SCABER. Rough to the touch from any little rigid inequalities: applied to several parts of plants.

SCA'BIES. (*Scabies, ei.* f.; from *scabo,* to scratch.) See *Psora.*

SCABIO'SA. (From *scaber,* rough: so called from its rough hairy surface.) 1. The name of a genus of plants in the Linnæan system. Class, *Tetrandria;* Order, *Monogynia.*

2. The pharmacopœial name of the common scabious. See *Scabiosa arvensis.*

SCABIOSA ARVENSIS. The systematic name of the common field scabious. This herb, *Scabiosa—corollis quadrifidis radiantibus; foliis pinnatifidis, incisis; caule hispido,* of Linnæus, and its flowers are sometimes used medicinally. The whole plant possesses a bitter and subadstringent taste, and was formerly much employed in the cure of some leprous affections and diseases of the lungs.

SCABIOSA SUCCISA. The systematic name of the devil's bit scabious.

SCABRIDE'Æ. (From *scaber,* rough.) The name of an order of plants in Linnæus's Fragments of a Natural Method, consisting of plants with rough leaves, incomplete and inelegant flowers.

SCA'LA. A ladder or staircase.

SCALA TYMPANI. The superior spiral cavity of the cochlea.

SCALA VESTIBULI. The inferior spiral cavity of the cochlea.

SCALD. See *Ambustio.*

Scald head. See *Tinea capitis.*

SCALE. *Squama.* A lamina of morbid cuticle, hard, thickened, whitish, and opake, of a very small size, and irregular, often increasing into layers, denominated crusts. Both scales and crusts repeatedly fall off, and are reproduced in a short time.

SCALE'NUS. (*Scalenus,* sc. *Musculus;* from σκαληνος, irregular or unequal.) A muscle about which anatomical writers have differed greatly in their descriptions. It is situated at the side of the neck, between the transverse processes of the cervical vertebræ and the upper part of the thorax. The ancients who gave it its name from its resemblance to an irregular triangle, considered it as one muscle. Vesalius and Winslow divide it into two, Fallopius and Cowper into three, Douglas into four, and Albinus into five portions, which they describe as distinct muscles. Without deviating in the least from anatomical accuracy, it may be considered as one muscle divided into three portions. The anterior portion arises commonly from the transverse processes of the six inferior vetebræ of the neck, by as many short tendons, and descending obliquely outward, is inserted tendinous and fleshy, into the upper side of the first rib, near its cartilage. The axillary artery passes through this portion, and sometimes divides it into two slips, about an inch and a half above its insertion. The middle portion arises by distinct tendons, from the transverse processes of the four last vertebræ of the neck, and descending obliquely outwards and a little backwards, is inserted tendinous into the outer and upper part of the first rib, from its root to within the distance of an inch from its cartilage. The space between this and the anterior portion, affords a passage to the nerves going to the upper extremities. It is in part covered by the third or posterior portion, which is the thinnest and longest of the three. This arises from the transverse processes of the second, third, fourth, and fifth vertebræ of the neck, by distinct tendons, and is inserted into the upper edge of the second rib, at the distance of about an inch and a half from its articulation, by a broad flat tendon. The use of the scalénus is to move the neck to one side, when it acts singly, or to bend it forwards, when both muscles act; and when the neck is fixed, it serves to elevate the ribs, and dilate the chest.

SCALENUS PRIMUS. See *Scalenus.*

SCALENUS SECUNDUS. See *Scalenus.*

SCALENUS TERTIUS. See *Scalenus.*

SCALPE'LLUM. A scalpel or common dissecting knife.

SCALPRUM. A denticular raspetory, used in trepanning.

Scaly. See *Squamosus.*

SCAMMO'NIUM. (A corruption of the Arabian word *chamozah.*) See *Convolvulus scammonia.*

SCAMMONY. See *Convolvulus scammonia.*

SCANDENS. Climbing, either with spiral tendrils for its support, or by adhesive fibres. Applied to stems, &c. as that of the *Vitis vinifera,* and *Bryonia dioica.*

SCA'NDIX. The name of a genus of plants in the Linnæan system. Class *Pentandria;* Order, *Digynia.*

SCANDIX CEREFOLIUM. The systematic name of the officinal chervil. *Cerefolium; Chærophyllum; Chærefolium.* Chervil. This plant, *Scandix—semi nibus nitidis, ovato-subulatis; umbellis sessilibus lateralibus,* of Linnæus, is a salubrious culinary herb sufficiently grateful both to the palate and stomach, slightly aromatic, gently aperient, and diuretic.

SCANDIX ODORATA. The systematic name of the sweet cicely, *myrrhis,* which possesses virtues similar to the common chervil. See *Scandix cerefolium.*

SCA'PHA. (A skiff, or cock-boat; from σκαπτω, to make hollow: because formerly it was made by excavating a large tree.) 1. The excavation or cavity of the auricula, or external ear, between the helix and antihelix.

2. The name of a double-headed roller.

SCAPHOID. See *Scaphoides*.

SCAPHOI'DES: (From σκαφη, a little vessel, or boat, and ειδος, resemblance.) Boat-like. See *Naviculare os*.

SCAPOLITE. Pyramidal felspar. Professor Jameson divides this into four subspecies:

1 *Radiated*, of a gray colour, resinous, and pearly in distinct concretions, and crystallized, found in the neighbourhood of Arendal, in Norway, associated with magnetic ironstone, and felspar.

2. *Foliated scapolite*, crystallized and of a gray, green, and black colour, found in granular granite, or whitestone, in the Saxon Erzegebirge.

3. *Compact scapolite*, of a red colour, found with the former species.

4. *Elæolite*.

SCA'PULA. (From the Hebrew *schipha*.) *Omoplata; Os homoplatæ; Scoptula; Epinotion.* The shoulder-blade. This bone, which approaches nearly to a triangular figure, is fixed, not unlike a buckler, to the upper, posterior, and lateral part of the thorax, extending from the first to about the seventh rib. The anterior and internal surface is irregularly concave, from the impression, not of the ribs, as the generality of anatomists have supposed, but of the subscapularis muscle. Its posterior and external surface is convex and divided into two unequal fossæ by a considerable spine, which, rising small from the posterior edge of the scapula, becomes gradually higher and broader, as it approaches the anterior and superior angle of the bone, till at length it terminates in a broad and flat process, at the top of the shoulder, called the *processus acromion*. On the anterior edge of this processus acromion, we observe an oblong, concave, articulating surface covered with cartilage, for the articulation of the scapula with the clavicle. At its lower part, the acromion is hollowed, to allow a passage to the supra and infra spinati muscles. The ridge of the spine affords two rough, flat surfaces, for the insertion of the trapezius and deltoid muscles. Of the two fossæ into which the external surface of the bone is divided by the spine, the superior one, which is the smallest, serves to lodge the supra spinatus muscle; and the inferior fossa, which is much larger than the other, gives origin to the infra spinatus. The triangular shape of the scapula leads us to consider its angles and its sides. The upper posterior angle is neither so thick, nor has so rough a surface, as the inferior one; but the most remarkable of the three angles of this bone is the anterior one, which is of great thickness, and formed into a glenoid cavity of an oval shape, the greatest diameter of which is from below upwards. This cavity, in the recent subject, is furnished with cartilage, and receives the head of the os humeri. The cartilaginous crust, which surrounds its brims, makes it appear deeper in the fresh subject than in the skeleton. A little beyond this glenoid cavity, the bone becomes narrower, so as to give the appearance of a neck: and above this rises a considerable process, which, from being thick at its origin, becomes thinner, and, in some degree, flattened at its extremity. This process projects considerably, and is curved downwards. From its supposed resemblance to a beak of a bird, it is called the *coracoid* process. From the whole external side of this process, a strong and broad ligament is stretched to the processus acromion, becoming narrower as it approaches the latter process, so as to be of a somewhat triangular shape. This ligament, and the two processes with which it is connected, are evidently intended for the protection of the joint, and to prevent a luxation of the os humeri upwards. Of the three sides of the scapula, the posterior one, which is the longest, is called the *basis*. This side is turned towards the vertebræ. Its other two sides are called *costæ*. The superior costa, which is the upper and shortest side, is likewise thinner than the other two, having a sharp edge. It is nearly horizontal, and parallel with the second rib; and is interrupted near the basis of the coracoid process, by a semicircular niche, which is closed by a ligament that extends from one end of it to the other, and affords a passage to vessels and nerves. Besides this passage, there are other niches in the scapula for the transmission of vessels; viz. one between the coracoid process and the head of the bone, and another between its neck and the processus acromion. The third side of the scapula, or the inferior costa, as it is called, is of considerable thickness, and

extends obliquely from the neck of the bone to its inferior angle, reaching from about the third to the eighth rib. The scapula has but very little cellular substance, and is of unequal thickness, being very thin at its middle part, where it is covered by a great number of muscles, and having its neck, the acromion, and coracoid process, of considerable strength. In the fœtus, the basis and the neck of the scapula, together with its glenoid cavity, acromion, coracoid process, and the ridge of the spine, are so many epiphyses with respect to the rest of the bone, to which they are not completely united till a considerable time after birth. The scapula is articulated to the clavicle and os humeri, to which last it serves as a fulcrum; and, by altering its position, it affords a greater scope to the bones of the arm in their different motions. It likewise affords attachment to a great number of muscles, and posteriorly serves as a defence to the thorax.

SCAPULAR. (*Scapularis;* from *scapula*, the shoulder bone.) Belonging to the scapula; as the scapulary arteries and veins, which are branches of the subclavian and axillary.

SCAPULA'RIA. (From *scapula*, the shoulder-bone.) A scapulary. A bandage for the shoulder-blade.

SCAPUS. (*Scapus, i. m.*; from σκαπτω, to lean or rest upon: because it rests as it were on the root or base.) A stalk which springs from the root, and bears the flowers and fruit, but not the leaves. The primrose and cowslip are good examples of it.

The following are the principal varieties:

1. *Teres;* as in Plantago major.
2. *Angulosus;* as in Plantago lanceolata.
3. *Ventricosus*, hollow at the bottom; as in Allium cepa.
4. *Flexuosus;* as in Orchis flexuosa.
5. *Anceps;* as Alium angulosum.
6. *Filiformis;* as Bellis bellidoides.
7. *Triquetrus;* as Allium triquetrum.
8. *Spiralis;* as Anthericum spirale, and that wonderful plant, Vallsneria spiralis.
9. *Pentagonus;* as Ophris paludosa.
10. *Articulatus;* as Statice echioides.
11. *Erectus;* in Tulipa gesneriana.
12. *Ascendens;* in Silymbrium vimineum.
13. *Declinatus;* as Astragalus incanus.
14. *Decumbens;* as Potentilla sabacaulis.
15. *Dichotomus;* as Statice tartarica.
16. *Nudus;* as Convallaria majalis.
17. *Foliosus;* as Ophris insectifera.
18. *Bracteatus*, and most of the Orchides.
19. *Imbricatus;* as Tussilago farfara.
20. *Setaceus;* as Schænus bulbosus.
21. *Vaginatus;* as Arethusa bulbosa.

When several species of the same plant have a scapus, and it is wanting in one of the same species, it is termed *exscapus;* as in Astragalus exscapus.

SCARBOROUGH. 1. The name of a town in Yorkshire, noted for its ferruginous spring. There are two species of chalybeate water found in this spot, and they differ considerably in their composition, though they rise nearly contiguous to each other. The one is a simple carbonated chalybeate, similar to the Tunbridge water; the other, which is better known and more frequented, and more particularly distinguished as Scarborough water, has, in conjunction with the iron, a considerable admixture of a purging salt, which adds much to its value. The diseases in which it is ordered are similar to those in which Cheltenham water is prescribed, only it is necessary to increase the purgative effect of this water by adding similar salts It is, therefore, chiefly as an alterative that this water can be employed in its natural state.

Scarborough has an advantage belonging to its situation which Cheltenham does not possess, that of affording an opportunity for sea-bathing, the use of which will, in many cases, much assist in the plan of cure for many of the disorders for which the mineral water is resorted to.

2. The name of a physician. Sir CHARLES, born about the year 1616. Intending to follow the medical profession, he went to study at Cambridge, and applied himself particularly to the mathematics, in which he made great proficiency. During the civil wars he was obliged to remove to Oxford, where he entered under the celebrated Harvey, then warden of Merton College, who, being employed in writing his treatise " De

Generatione Animalium," gladly accepted the assistance of Mr. Scarborough. Upon taking the degree of doctor of medicine, he settled in the metropolis, where he practised with great reputation. He became a fellow of the college of physicians, in which he was much respected for his talents; and being appointed to introduce the Marquis of Dorchester, who was admitted into that body in 1658, he made an elegant Latin speech on that occasion. In the mean time he began to deliver anatomical lectures at Surgeons' Hall, which were highly approved, and continued for sixteen or seventeen years. In 1669 the order of knighthood was conferred upon him by Charles II., who also appointed him his chief physician; and he enjoyed the same office under the two succeeding monarchs. He was likewise made physician to the Tower of London, which appointment he retained till his death about the year 1702. The works left by him were chiefly mathematical.

SCARF-SKIN. See *Cuticle* and *Skin*.

SCARIFICATION. (*Scarificatio;* from *scarifico*, to scarify.) A superficial incision made with a lancet, or a chirurgical instrument called a scarificator, for the purpose of taking away blood, or letting out fluids, &c.

SCARIFICATOR. An instrument used by surgeons and cuppers to evacuate blood. It is made in form of a box, in which are fitted, ten, twelve, or more lancets, all perfectly in the same plane; which being, as it were, cocked, by means of a spring are all discharged at the same time, by pulling a kind of trigger, and driven equally within the skin.

SCARI'OLA. See *Lactuca scariola*.

SCARIOLA GALLORUM. See *Lactuca scariola*.

SCARLATI'NA. (From *scarlatto*, the Italian for a deep red.) The scarlet fever. A genus of disease in the Class *Pyrexiæ*, and Order *Exanthemata*, of Cullen; characterized by contagious synocha; the fourth day the face swells; a scarlet eruption appears on the skin in patches; which, after three or four days, ends in the desquamation of the cuticle, and is often succeeded by anasarca. It has two species:

1. *Scarlatina simplex*, the mild.
2. *Scarlatina cynanchica*, or *anginosa*, with ulcerated sore throat.

Dr. Willan has added to these a third, called *maligna*, agreeing with the cynanche maligna, of Cullen.

Some have asserted that scarlatina never attacks the same person a second time; more extensive observation has confuted this opinion. It seizes persons of all ages, but children and young persons are most subject to it, and it appears at all seasons of the year; but it is more frequently met with towards the end of autumn, or beginning of winter, than at any other periods, at which time it very often becomes a prevalent epidemic. It is, beyond all doubt, a very contagious disease.

The one to which it bears the greatest resemblance is the measles; but from this it is readily to be distinguished by the absence of the cough, watery eye, running at the nose and sneezing, which are the predominant symptoms in the early stage of the measles, but which do not usually attend on the scarlatina, or at least in any high degree.

It begins, like other fevers, with languor, lassitude, confusion of ideas, chills, and shiverings, alternated by fits of heat. The thirst is considerable, the skin dry, and the patient is often incommoded with anxiety, nausea, and vomiting. About the third day, the scarlet efflorescence appears on the skin, which seldom produces, however, any remission of the fever. On the departure of the efflorescence, which usually continues out only for three or four days, a gentle sweat comes on, the fever subsides, the cuticle or scarf-skin then falls off in small scales, and the patient gradually regains his former strength and health.

On the disappearance of the efflorescence in scarlatina, it is, however, no uncommon occurrence for an anasarcous swelling to affect the whole body, but this is usually of a very short continuance.

Scarlatina anginosa, in several instances, approaches very near to the malignant form. The patient is seized not only with a coldness and shivering, but likewise with great languor, debility, and sickness, succeeded by heat, nausea, vomiting of bilious matter, soreness of the throat, inflammation, and ulceration in the tonsils, &c., a frequent and laborious breathing, and a quick and small depressed pulse. When the efflorescence appears, which is usually on the third day, it

brings no relief; on the contrary, the symptoms are much aggravated, and fresh ones arise.

In the progress of the disease, one universal redness unattended, however, by any pustular eruption, pervades the face, body, and limbs, which parts appear somewhat swollen. The eyes and nostrils partake likewise more or less of the redness, and, in proportion as the former have an inflamed appearance, so does the tendency to delirium prevail.

On the first attack, the fauces are often much inflamed; but this is usually soon succeeded by grayish sloughs, which give the parts a speckled appearance, and render the breath more or less fœtid. The patient is often cut off in a few days: and even if he recovers, it will be by slow degrees; dropsical swellings, or tumours of the parotid, and other glands, slowly suppurating, being very apt to follow. In the malignant form of the disease the symptoms at first are pretty much the same; but some of the following peculiarities are afterward observable. The pulse is small, indistinct, and irregular; the tongue, teeth, and lips, covered with a brown or black incrustation; a dull redness of the eyes, with a dark-red flushing of the cheeks, deafness, delirium, or coma; the breath is extremely fœtid; the respiration rattling and laborious, partly from viscid phlegm clogging the fauces; the deglutition is constricted and painful; and there is a fulness and livid colour of the neck, with retraction of the head. Ulcerations are observed on the tonsils and adjoining parts, covered with dark sloughs, and surrounded by a livid base; and the tongue is often so tender as to be excoriated by the slightest touch. An acrid discharge flows from the nostrils, causing soreness, or chaps, nay, even blisters, about the nose and lips; the fluid discharged being at first thin, but afterward thick and yellowish. The rash is usually faint, except in a few irregular patches; and it presently changes to a dark, or livid red colour: it appears late, is very uncertain in its duration, and often intermixed with petechiæ; it sometimes disappears again a few hours after it is formed, and comes out again at the expiration of two or three days. In an advanced stage of the disease, where petechiæ, and other symptoms characteristic of putrescency, are present, hæmorrhages frequently break forth from the nose, mouth, and other parts.

When scarlatina is to terminate in health, the fiery redness abates gradually, and is succeeded by a brown colour, the skin becomes rough, and peels off in small scales, the tumefaction subsides, and health is gradually restored. On the contrary, when it is to terminate fatally, the febrile symptoms run very high from the first of its attack, the skin is intensely hot and dry, the pulse is very frequent but small, great thirst prevails, the breath is very fœtid, the efflorescence makes its appearance on the second day, or sooner, and about the third or fourth is probably interspersed with large livid spots; and a high degree of delirium ensuing, or hæmorrhages breaking out, the patient is cut off about the sixth or eighth day. In some cases a severe purging arises, which never fails to prove fatal. Some, again, where the symptoms do not run so high, instead of recovering, as is usual, about the time the skin begins to regain its natural colour, become dropsical, fall into a kind of lingering way, and are carried off in the course of a few weeks.

Scarlatina, in its inflammatory form, is not usually attended with danger, although a considerable degree of delirium sometimes prevails for a day or two; but when it partakes much of the malignant character, or degenerates into typhus putrida, which it is apt to do, it often proves fatal. On dissection of those who die of this disease, the fauces are inflamed, suppurated, and gangrenous; and the trachea and larynx are likewise in a state of inflammation, and lined with a viscid fœtid matter. In many instances the inflammatory affection extends to the lungs themselves. Large swellings of the lymphatic glands about the neck, occasioned by an absorption of the acrid matter poured out in the fauces, are now and then to be found. The same morbid appearances which are to be met with in putrid fever, present themselves in other parts of the body.

The plan to be pursued will differ according to the form of the disease. In the scarlatina simplex little is required, except clearing the bowels, and observing the antiphlogistic regimen. But where the throat is affected, and the fever runs higher, more active means become necessary, varying according to the type of this, whether synochal, or typhoid. In general, we may begin by exhibiting a nauseating emetic, which, besides its effect on the fever, may be useful in checking inflammation in the throat ; and occasionally the repetition, of such a remedy after a time, may answer a good purpose: but commonly it will be better to follow up the first by some cathartic remedy of sufficient activity. Then, so long as the strength will allow, we may endeavour to moderate the fever by mercurial and antimonial preparations, or other medicines promoting the several secretions, by steadily pursuing the antiphlogistic regimen, and occasionally applying cold water to the skin, when this is very hot and dry. Sometimes severe inflammation in the throat at an early period may render it advisable to apply a few eeches externally, or blisters behind the ears; and gargles of nitrate of potassa, the mineral acids, &c. should be used from time to time. But where the disorder exhibits the typhoid character, with ulcers in the throat, tending perhaps to gangrene, it is necessary to support the system by a nutritious diet, with a moderate quantity of wine, and tonic or stimulant medicines, as the cinchona, calumba, ammonia, capsicum, &c.; the acids will also be very proper from their antiseptic, as well as tonic power; and stimulant antiseptic gargles should be frequently employed, as the mineral acids sufficiently diluted, with the addition of tincture of myrrh, or these mixed with the decoction of bark, &c. Besides the general measures, thus varied according to the character of the disease, particular alarming symptoms may require to be palliated ; as vomiting by the effervescing draught, and occasionally a blister to the stomach, if there be tenderness on pressure; diarrhœa by small doses of opium, &c. The management of these, however, as well as of the dropsical swellings, and other sequels of the disease, will be understood from what is said under those heads respectively.

SCARLATINA ANGINOSA. See *Scarlatina.*
SCARLATINA CYNANCHICA. See *Scarlatina.*
SCARLATINA SIMPLEX. See *Scarlatina.*
Scarlet fever. See *Scarlatina.*
SCELOTYRBE. (From σκελος, the leg, and τυρβη, riot, intemperance.) A debility of the legs from scurvy, or an intemperate way of life.
Schaalstein. See *Tabular spar.*
Schaum earth. See *Aphrite.*
SCHERO′MA. A dryness of the eye from the want of the lachrymal fluid. The effects of this lachrymal fluid being deficient are, the eyes become dry, and in their motions produce a sensation as though sand, or some gritty substances, were between the eye and the eyelid ; the vision is obscured, the globe of the eye appears foulish and dull, which is a bad omen in acute diseases. The species are,
1. *Scheroma febrile,* or a dryness of the eyes, which is observed in fevers complicated with a phlogistic density of the humours.
2. *Scheroma exhaustorum,* which happens after great evacuations, and in persons dying.
3. *Scheroma inflammatorum,* which is a symptom of the ophthalmia sicca.
4. *Scheroma itinerantium,* or the dryness of the eyes, which happens in sandy places, to travellers, as in hot Syria, or from dry winds, which dry up the humidity necessary for the motion of the eyes.
SCHIDACE′DON. (From σχιδαξ, a splinter.) A longitudinal fracture of the bone.
SCHILLER SPAR. This mineral contains two subspecies :
1. See *Bronzite.*
2. The *common Schiller spar,* which is of an olive green colour, and occurs imbedded in serpentine in Shetland, Cornwall, &c.
SCHINELÆUM. (From σχινος, mastich, and ελαιον, oil.) Oil of mastich.
SCHNEIDER, CONRAD VICTOR, was born at Bitterfeld, in Misnia. He filled the offices of professor of anatomy, botany, and medicine, at Wittemberg, with great reputation : and was father of the faculty when he died in 1680. He wrote many treatises ; those on anatomical subjects relating chiefly to the bones of the cranium, and to the pituitary membrane of the nostrils, to which his name is still attached. He refuted an ancient error, that the mucus in catarrh distilled through the cribriform bone from the brain, showing that it was

secreted by the pituitary membrane. In other respects, his writings, except in anatomy, are diffuse and obscure, and full of ancient hypothetical doctrines.
SCHNEIDER′S MEMBRANE. So called from its discoverer. See *Membrana Schneideriana.*
SCHŒNA′NTHUS. (From σχοινος, a rush, and ανθος, a flower.) See *Andropogon schænanthus.*
SCHŒNOLÀGURUS. (From σχοινος, a rush, λαγως, a hare, and ουρα, a tail: so called from its resemblance to a hare's-tail.) Hare's-tail. The *Trifolium arvense.*
SCHORL. A sub-species of rhomboidal tourmaline, of a velvet black colour, found imbedded in granite, gneiss, &c. in Scotland and Cornwall.
Schorl, blue. A variety of Haüyne.
Schorl, red and titanic. Rutile.
SCHORLITE. Schorlous topaz. Pycnite of Werner. This mineral is of a straw-yellow colour, and becomes electric by heating. It is found at Altenberg in Saxony, in a rock of quartz and mica in porphyry.
SCIATIC. (*Sciaticus;* from *ischiaticus.*) Belonging to the ischium.
SCIATIC ARTERY. *Arteria sciatica.* Ischiatic retery. A branch of the internal iliac.
SCIATIC NERVE. *Nervus sciaticus.* Ischiatic nerve. A branch of a nerve of the lower extremity, formed by the union of the lumbar and sacral nerves. It is divided near the popliteal cavity into the tibial and peroneal, which are distributed to the leg and foot.
SCIATIC NOTCH. Ischiatic notch. See *Innominatum os.*
SCIATIC VEIN. *Vena sciatica.* The vein which accompanies the sciatic artery in the thigh.
SCIATICA. A rheumatic affection of the hip-joint.
Sciatica cresses. See *Lepidium iberis.*
SCI′LLA. (From σκιλλω, to dry : so called from its property of drying up humours.) 1. The name of a genus of plants in the Linnæan system. Class, *Hexandria;* Order *Monogynia.*
2. The pharmacopœial name of the medicinal squill. See *Scilla maritima.*
SCILLA HISPANICA. The Spanish squill.
SCILLA MARITICA. The systematic name of the officinal squill. *Ornithogalum maritimum; Squilla Scilla—nudiflora, bracteis refractis,* of Linnæus. A native of Spain, Sicily, and Syria, growing on the sea coast. The red-rooted variety has been supposed to be more efficacious than the white, and is, therefore, still preferred for medicinal use. The root of the squill, which appears to have been known as a medicine in the early ages of Greece, and has so well maintained its character ever since, as to be deservedly in great estimation, and of very frequent use at this time, seems to manifest a poisonous quality to several animals. In proof of this, we have the testimonies of Hillefield, Bergius, Vogel, and others. Its acrimony is so great, that even if much handled, it exulcerates the skin, and if given in large doses, and frequently repeated, it not only excites nausea, torminæ, and violent vomiting, but it has been known to produce strangury, bloody urine, hypercatharsis, cardialgia, hæmorrhoids, convulsions, with fatal inflammation, and gangrene of the stomach and bowels. But as many of the active articles of the Materia Medica, by injudicious administration, become equally deleterious, these effects of the scilla do not derogate from its medicinal virtues; on the contrary, we feel ourselves fully warranted, says Dr. Woodville, in representing this drug, under proper management, and in certain cases and constitutions, to be a medicine of great practical utility and real importance in the cure of many obstinate diseases. Its effects, as stated by Bergius, are incidens, diuretica, emetica, subpurgans, hydragoga, expectorans, emmenagoga. In dropsical cases it has long been esteemed the most certain and effectual diuretic with which we are acquainted ; and in asthmatic affections, or dyspnœa, occasioned by the lodgement of tenacious phlegm, it has been the expectorant usually employed. The squill, especially in large doses, is apt to stimulate the stomach, and to prove emetic ; and it sometimes acts on the intestines, and becomes purgative ; but when these operations take place, the medicine is prevented from reaching the blood vessels and kidneys, and the patient is deprived of its diuretic effects, which are to be obtained by giving the squill in smaller doses, repeated at more distant intervals, or by the joining of an

opiate to this medicine, which was found by Dr. Cullen to answer the same purpose. The Doctor further observes, that from a continued repetition of the squill, the dose may be gradually increased, and the interval of its exhibitions shortened; and when in this way the dose becomes to be tolerably large, the opiate may be most conveniently employed to direct the operation of the squill more certainly in the kidneys. "In cases of dropsy, that is, when there is an effusion of water into the cavities, and therefore less water goes to the kidneys, we are of opinion that neutral salt, accompanying the squill, may be of use in determining this fluid more certainly to the kidneys; and whenever it can be perceived that it takes this course, we are persuaded that it will be always useful, and generally safe, during the exhibition of the squills, to increase the usual quantity of diuretic."

The diuretic effects of squills have been supposed to be promoted by the addition of some mercurial; and the less purgative preparations of mercury, in the opinion of Dr. Cullen, are best adapted to this purpose; he therefore recommends a solution of corrosive sublimate, as being more proper than any other, because most diuretic. Where the primæ viæ abound with mucous matter, and the lungs are oppressed with viscid phlegm, this medicine is likewise in general estimation.

As an expectorant, the squill may be supposed not only to attenuate the mucus in the follicles, but also to excite a more copious secretion of it from the lungs, and thereby lessen the congestion, upon which the difficulty of respiration very generally depends. Therefore in all pulmonic affections, excepting only those of actual or violent inflammation, ulcer, and spasm, the squill has been experienced to be a useful medicine. The officinal preparations of squills are, a conserve, dried squills, a syrup, and vinegar, an oxymel, and pills. Practitioners have not, however, confined themselves to these. When this root was intended as a diuretic, it has most commonly been used in powder, as being, in this state, less disposed to nauseate the stomach; and to the powder it has been the practice to add neutral salts, as nitre, or crystals of tartar, especially if the patient complained of much thirst; others recommend calomel; and with a view to render the squills less offensive to the stomach, it has been usual to conjoin an aromatic. The dose of dried squills is from one to four or six grains once a day, or half this quantity twice a day; afterward to be regulated according to its effects. The dose of the other preparations of this drug, when fresh, should be five times this weight; for this root loses in the process of drying four-fifths of its original weight, and this loss is merely a watery exhalation.

SCILLITES. (From σκιλλα, the squill.) A wine impregnated with squills.

SCILLITIN. A white transparent, acrid substance, extracted by Vosel from squills.

SCI'NCUS. (From sheque, Hebrew.) The skink. This amphibious animal is of the lizard kind, and caught about the Nile, and thence brought dried into this country, remarkably smooth and glossy, as if varnished. The flesh of the animal, particularly of the belly, has been said to be diuretic, alexipharmic, aphrodisiac, and useful in leprous disorders.

SCIRRHO'MA. (From σκιρροω, to harden.) See Scirrhus.

SCI'RRHUS. (From σκιρροω, to harden.) Scirrhoma; Scirrhosis. A genus of disease in the Class Locales, and Order Tumores, of Cullen; known by a hard tumour of a glandular part, indolent, and not readily suppurating. The following observations of Pearson are deserving of attention. A scirrhus, he says, is usually defined to be a hard, and almost insensible tumour, commonly situated in a glandular part, and accompanied with little or no discoloration of the surface of the skin. This description agrees with the true or exquisite scirrhus: but when it has proceeded from the indolent to the malignant state, the tumour is then unequal in its figure, it becomes painful, the skin acquires a purple or livid hue, and the cutaneous veins are often varicose. Let us now examine whether this enumeration of symptoms be sufficiently accurate for practical purposes.

It is probable, that any gland in the living body may be the seat of a cancerous disease, but it appears more frequently as an idiopathic affection in those glands
272

that form the several secretions than in the absorbent glands; and of the secreting organs, those which separate fluids that are to be employed in the animal economy, suffer much oftener than the glands which secrete the excrementitious parts of the blood. Indeed, it may be doubted whether an absorbent gland be ever the primary seat of a true scirrhus. Daily experience evinces, that these glands may suffer contamination from their connexion with a cancerous part; but under such circumstances, this morbid alteration being the effect of a disease in that neighbouring part, it ought to be regarded as a secondary or consequent affection. I never yet met with an unequivocal proof of a primary scirrhus in an absorbent gland; and if a larger experience shall confirm this observation, and establish it as a general rule, it will afford material assistance in forming the diagnosis of this disease. The general term scirrhus hath been applied, with too little discrimination, to indurated tumours of lymphatic glands. When these appendages of the absorbent system enlarge in the early part of life, the disease is commonly treated as strumous; but as a similar alteration of these parts may, and often does, occur at a more advanced period, there ought to be some very good reasons for ascribing malignity to one rather than the other. In old people the tumour is indeed often larger more indurated, and less tractable than in children, but when the alteration originated in the lymphatic glands, it will very rarely be found to possess any thing cancerous in its nature.

If every other morbid alteration in a part were attended with pain and softness, then induration and defective sensibility might point out the presence of a scirrhus. But this is so far from being the case, that even encysted tumours, at their commencement, frequently excite the sensation of impenetrable hardness.

All glands are contained in capsulæ, not very elastic, so that almost every species of chronic enlargement of these bodies must be hard; hence this induration is rather owing to the structure of the part, than to the peculiar nature of the disease; and as glands in their healthy state are endowed with much sensibility, every disease that gradually produces induration, will rather diminish than increase their perceptive powers. Induration and insensibility may, therefore, prove that the affected part does not labour under an acute disease; but these symptoms alone can yield no certain information concerning the true nature of the morbid alteration. Those indolent affections of the glands that so frequently appear after the meridian of life, commonly manifest a hardness and want of sensation, not inferior to that which accompanies a true scirrhus; and yet these tumours will often admit of a cure by the same mode of treatment which we find to be successful in scrofula; and when they prove unconquerable by the powers of medicine, we generally see them continue stationary and innocent to the latest period of life. Writers have indeed said much about certain tumours changing their nature, and assuming a new character; but I strongly suspect that the doctrine of the mutation of diseases into each other, stands upon a very uncertain foundation. Improper treatment may, without doubt, exasperate diseases, and render a complaint, which appeared to be mild and tractable, dangerous, or destructive; but to aggravate the symptoms, and to change the form of the disease, are things that ought not to be confounded. I do not affirm, that a breast which has been the seat of a mammary abscess, or a gland that has been affected with scrofula, may not become cancerous: for they might have suffered from this disease had no previous complaint existed; but these morbid alterations generate no greater tendency to cancer than if the parts had always retained their natural condition. There is no necessary connexion between the cancer and any other disease, nor has it been proved that one is convertible into the other.

Chirurgical writers have generally enumerated tumour as an essential symptom of the scirrhus; and it is very true, that this disease is often accompanied with an increase of bulk in the part affected. From long and careful observation, I am however induced to think, that an addition to the quantity of matter is rather an accidental than a necessary consequence of the presence of this affection.

When the breast is the seat of a scirrhus, the altered part is hard, perhaps unequal in its figure, and definite;

but these symptoms are not always connected with an actual increase in the dimensions of the breast. On the contrary, the true scirrhus is frequently accompanied with a contraction and diminution of bulk, a retraction of the nipple, and a puckered state of the skin.

The irritation produced by an indurated substance lying in the breast, will very often cause a determination of blood to that organ, and a consequent enlargement of it; but I consider this as an inflammatory state of the surrounding parts, excited by the scirrhus, acting as a remote cause, and by no means essential to the original complaint. From the evident utility of topical blood-letting under these circumstances, a notion has prevailed that the scirrhus is an inflammatory disease; but the strongly-marked dissimilarity of a phlegmon and an exquisite scirrhus, in their appearances, progress, and mode of termination, obliges me to dissent from that opinion. That one portion of the breast may be in a scirrhous state, while the other parts are in a state of inflammation, is agreeable to reason and experience; but that an inflammation, which is an acute disease, and a scirrhus, whose essential characters are almost directly the reverse of inflammation, shall be coexistent in the same part, is not a very intelligible proposition. Tumour and inflammation are commonly met with on a variety of other occasions, and in this particular instance they may be the effects of the disease, but are not essentially connected with its presence.

An incipient scirrhus is seldom accompanied with a discoloration of the skin; and a dusky redness, purple, or even livid appearance of the surface, is commonly seen when there is a malignant scirrhus. The presence or absence of colour can, however, at the best, afford us but a very precarious criterion of the true nature of the complaint. When the disease is clearly known, an altered state of the skin may assist us in judging of the progress it has made; but as the skin may suffer similar variations in a number of very dissimilar diseases, it would be improper to found an opinion upon so delusive a phenomenon.

SCITAMINEÆ. (From scitamentum, a dainty.) The name of an order of plants in Linnæus's Fragments of a Natural Method, consisting of those which have an herbaceous stalk, broad leaves, and the germen obtusely angled under an irregular corolla; as amomum, canna, musa, &c.

SCLA′REA. (From σκληρος, hard; because its stalks are hard and dry, Blanch.) See Salvia sclarea.

SCLAREA HISPANICA. See Salvia sclarea.

SCLERI′ASIS. (From σκληροω, to harden.) Scleroma; Sclerosis. A hard tumour or induration; a scirrhus.

SCLEROPHTHA′LMIA. (From σκληρος, hard, and οφθαλμος, the eye.) A protrusion of the eyeball. An inflammation of the eye, attended with hardness of the parts.

SCLEROSARCOMA. (From σκληρος, and σαρκωμα, a fleshy tumour.) A hard fleshy excrescence on the gums.

SCLEROSIS. See Scleriasis.

SCLERO′TIC. (Scleroticus; from σκληροω, to harden.) The name of one of the coats of the eye. See Sclerotic acid.

SCLEROTIC COAT. Tunica sclerotica; Membrana sclerotica; Sclerotis. The outermost coat of the eye, of a white colour, dense, and tenacious. Its anterior part, which is transparent, is termed the cornea transparens. It is into this coat of the eye that the muscles of the bulb are inserted.

SCLERO′TIS. See Sclerotic coat.

SCLOPETARIA AQUA. (From sclopetum, a gum: so called from its supposed virtues in healing gun-shot wounds.) Arquebusade. It is made of sage, mugwort, and mint, distilled in wine.

SCLOPETOPLA′GA. (From sclopetum, a gun, and plaga, a wound.) A gun-shot wound.

SCOLI′ASIS. (From σκολιοω, to twist.) A distortion of the spine.

SCOLOPE′NDRIA. See Asplenium ceterach.

SCOLOPE′NDRIUM. (From σκολοπενδρα, the earwig: so called because its leaves resemble the earwig.) See Asplenium ceterach.

SCOLOPOMACHÆRIUM. (From σκολωπαξ, the woodcock, and μαχαιρα, a knife: so called because it is bent a little at the end like a woodcock's bill.) An incisionknife.

SCO′LYMUS. (From σκολος, a thorn: so named from its prickly leaves.) See Cinara scolymus.

SCOMBER. The name of a genus of fishes of the order Thoracici.

SCOMBER SCOMBER. The systematic name of the common mackarel, a beautiful fish, of easy digestion, which frequents our shore in vast shoals, between the months of April and July.

SCOMBER THYNNUS. The systematic name of the tunny-fish, which frequents the shore of the Mediterranean, and, though a coarse fish, was much esteemed by the Greeks and Romans, and is still considered a delicacy by some.

SCOPA REGIA. See Ruscus aculeatus.

SCORBU′TIA. (From scorbutus, the scurvy.) Medicine for the scurvy.

SCORBU′TUS. (From schorboet, Germ.) Gingibrachium, when the gums and arms, and gingipedium, when the gums and legs, are affected by it. The scurvy. A genus of disease in the Class Cachexia, and Order Impetigines, of Cullen; characterized by extreme debility; complexion pale and bloated; spongy gums; livid spots on the skin; breath offensive; œdematous swellings in the legs; hæmorrhages; foul ulcers; fœtid urine; and extremely offensive stools. The scurvy is a disease of a putrid nature, much more prevalent in cold climates than in warm ones, and which chiefly affects sailors, and such as are shut up in besieged places, owing, as is supposed, to their being deprived of fresh provisions, and a due quantity of acescent food, assisted by the prevalence of cold and moisture, and by such other causes as depress the nervous energy, as indolence, confinement, want of exercise, neglect of cleanliness, much labour and fatigue, sadness, despondency, &c. These several debilitating causes, with the concurrence of a diet consisting principally of salted or putrescent food, will be sure to produce this disease. It seems, however, to depend more on a defect of nourishment, than on a vitiated state; and the reason that salted provisions are so productive of the scurvy, is, most probably, because they are drained of their nutritious juices, which are extracted and run off in brine. As the disease is apt to become pretty general among the crew of a ship when it has once made its appearance, it has been supposed by many to be of a contagious nature; but the conjecture seems by no means well founded.

A preternatural saline state of the blood has been assigned as its proximate cause. It has been contended, by some physicians, that the primary morbid affection in this disease is a debilitated state of the solids, arising principally from the want of aliment. The scurvy comes on gradually, with heaviness, weariness, and unwillingness to move about, together with dejection of spirits, considerable loss of strength, and debility. As it advances in its progress, the countenance becomes sallow and bloated, respiration is hurried on the least motion, the teeth become loose, the gums are spongy, the breath is very offensive, livid spots appear on different parts of the body, old wounds which have been long healed up break out afresh, severe wandering pains are felt, particularly by night, the skin is dry, the urine small in quantity, turning blue vegetable infusions of a green colour; and the pulse is small, frequent, and, towards the last, intermitting; but the intellects are, for the most part, clear, and distinct. By an aggravation of the symptoms, the disease, in its last stage, exhibits a most wretched appearance. The joints become swelled and stiff, the tendons of the legs are rigid and contracted, general emaciation ensues, hæmorrhages break forth from different parts, fœtid evacuations are discharged by stool, and a diarrhœa or dysentery arises, which soon terminates the tragic scene.

Scurvy, as usually met with on shore, or where the person has not been exposed to the influence of the remote causes before enumerated, is unattended by any violent symptoms, as slight blotches, with scaly eruptions on different parts of the body, and a sponginess of the gums, are the chief ones to be observed.

In forming our judgment as to the event of the disease, we are to be directed by the violence of the symptoms, by the situation of the patient with respect to a vegetable diet, or other proper substitutes, by his former state of health and by his constitution, not having been impaired by previous diseases.

Dissections of scurvy have always discovered the

blood to be in a very dissolved state, The thorax usually contains more or less of a watery fluid, which, in many cases, possesses so high a degree of acrimony, as to excoriate the hands by coming in contact with it; the cavity of the abdomen contains the same kind of fluid; the lungs are black and putrid; and the heart itself has been found in a similar state, with its cavity filled with a corrupted fluid. In many instances, the epiphyses have been found divided from the bones, the cartilages separated from the ribs, and several of the bones themselves dissolved by caries. The brain seldom shows any disease.

In the cure, as well as the prevention of scurvy, much more is to be done by regimen, than by medicines, obviating as far as possible the several remote causes of the disease, but particularly providing the patient with a more wholesome diet, and a large proportion of fresh vegetables; and it has been found that those articles are especially useful, which contain a native acid, as oranges, lemons, &c. Where these cannot be procured, various substitutes have been proposed, of which the best appear to be the inspissated juices of the same fruits, or the crystallized citric acid. Vinegar, sour crout, and farinaceous substances made to undergo the acetous fermentation, have likewise been used with much advantage: also brisk fermenting liquors, as spruce beer, cider, and the like Formerly many plants of the Class *Tetradynamia*, as mustard, horse-raddish, &c. likewise garlic, and others of a stimulant quality, promoting the secretions, were much relied upon, and, no doubt, proved useful to a certain extent. The spongy state of the gums may be remedied by washing the mouth with some of the mineral acids sufficiently diluted, or perhaps mixed with decoction of cinchona. The stiffness of the limbs by fomentations, cataplasms, and friction; and sometimes in hot climates, the earth-bath has afforded speedy relief to this symptom.

SCO'RDIUM. (From σκοροδον, garlic: so called because it smells like garlic.) See *Teucrium scordium.*

SCO'RIÆ. (*Scoria*; from σκω, excrement.) Dross. The refuse or useless parts of any substance.

SCORODOPRASUM. (From σκοροδον, garlic, and πρασον, the leek.) The wild garlic, or leek shalot.

SCO'RODUM. (Απο του σκωρ οξειν, from its filthy smell.) Garlic.

SCORPIACA. (From σκορπιος, a scorpion.) Medicines against the bite of serpents.

SCORPIOI'DES. (From σκορπιος, a scorpion, and ειδος, a likeness: so called because its leaves resemble the tail of a scorpion.) *Scorpiurus.* The *Myosurus scorpioides.*

SCORPIU'RUS. See *Scorpioides.*

SCORZA. A variety of epidote.

SCORZONE'RA. (From *escorza*, a serpent, Spanish: so called because it is said to be effectual against the bite of all venomous animals.) 1. The name of a genus of plants in the Linnæan system. Class, *Syngenesia*; Order, *Polygamia æqualis.*

2. The pharmacopœial name of the viper grass. See *Scorzonera humilis.*

SCORZONERA HISPANICA. The systematic name of the esculent vipers' grass. *Serpentaria hispanica.* The root of this plant is mostly sold for that of the *humilis.*

SCORZONERA HUMILIS. The systematic name of the officinal vipers' grass. *Escorzonera; Viperaria; Serpentaria hispanica.* Goats' grass; Vipers' grass. The roots of this plant, *Scorzonera—caule subnudo, unifloro; foliis lato-lanceolatis, nervosis, planis,* of Linnæus, have been sometimes employed medicinally as alexipharmics, and in hypochondriacal disorders and obstructions of the viscera. The *Scorzonera hispanica* mostly supplies the shops, whose root is esculent, oleraceous, and against diseases inefficacious.

SCOTODINE. See *Scotodinus.*

SCOTODI'NUS. (From σκοτος, darkness, and δινος, a giddiness.) *Scotodinia; Scotodinos; Scotoma; Scotodine; Scotomia.* Giddiness, with impaired sight.

SCOTOMA. (From σκοτος, darkness.) Blindness. See *Scotodinus.*

SCRIBONIUS, LARGUS, a Roman physician in the reign of Claudius, who wrote a treatise, "De Compositione Medicamentorum." Many of these formulæ are perfectly trifling and superstitious; and the whole work displays a great attachment to empiricism. The style is also very deficient in elegance for the time in

which he lived, whence he appears to have been a person of inferior education.

SCROBICULATUS. (*Scrobiculus*, a ditch, or furrow.) Hollowed; having a deep, round foramina: applied to the receptacle of the *Helianthus annuus.*

SCROBI'CULUS CO'RDIS. (Diminutive of *scrobs*, a ditch.) The pit of the stomach.

SCRO'FULA. (From *scrofa*, a swine; because this animal is said to be much subject to a similar disorder.) *Scrophula; Struma; Coiras; Chræas; Ecruelles;* Fr. Scrofula. The king's evil. A genus of disease in the Class *Cachexiæ*, and Order *Impetigines*, of Cullen. He distinguishes four species. 1. Scrofula vulgaris, when it is without other disorders external and permanent. 2. Scrofula mesenterica, when internal, with loss of appetite, pale countenance, swelling of the belly, and an unusual fœtor of the excrements. 3. Scrofula fugax. This is of the most simple kind; it is seated only about the neck, and for the most part is caused by absorption from sores on the head. 4. Scrofula americana, when it is joined with the yaws. Scrofula consists in hard indolent tumours of the conglobate glands in various parts of the body; but particularly in the neck; behind the ears, and under the chin, which, after a time, suppurate and degenerate into ulcers, from which, instead of pus, a white curdled matter, somewhat resembling the coagulum of milk is discharged.

The first appearance of the disease is most usually between the third and seventh year of the child's age; but it may arise at any period between this and the age of puberty; after which it seldom makes its first attack. It most commonly affects children of a lax habit, with smooth, fine skins, fair hair, and rosy cheeks. It likewise is apt to attack such children as show a disposition to rachitis, marked by a protuberant forehead, enlarged joints, and a tumid abdomen. Like this disease, it seems to be peculiar to cold and variable climates, being rarely met with in warm ones. Scrofula is by no means a contagious disease, but, beyond all doubt, is of an hereditary nature, and is often entailed by parents on their children. There are, indeed, some practitioners who wholly deny that this, or any other disease, can be acquired by an hereditary right; but that a peculiar temperament of body, or predisposition in the constitution of some diseases, may extend from both father and mother to their offspring, is observed by Dr. Thomas, very clearly proved. For example, we very frequently meet with gout in young persons of both sexes, who could never have brought it on by intemperance, sensuality, or improper diet, but must have acquired the predisposition to it in this way.

Where there is any predisposition in the constitution to scrofula, and the person happens to contract a venereal taint, this frequently excites into action the causes of the former; as a venereal bubo not unfrequently becomes scrofulous, as soon as the virus is destroyed by mercury. The late Dr. Cullen supposed scrofula to depend upon a peculiar constitution of the lymphatic system. The attacks of the disease seem much affected or influenced by the periods of the seasons. They begin usually some time in the winter and spring, and often disappear, or are greatly amended in summer and autumn. The first appearance of the disorder is commonly in that of small oval, or spherical tumours under the skin, unattended by any pain or discoloration. These appear, in general, upon the sides of the neck, below the ear, or under the chin; but, in some cases, the joints of the elbows or ankles, or those of the fingers and toes, are the parts first affected. In these instances, we do not, however, find small moveable swellings; but, on the contrary, a tumour almost uniformly surrounding the joint, and interrupting its motion.

After some length of time the tumours become larger and more fixed, the skin which covers them acquires a purple or livid colour, and, being much inflamed, they at last suppurate, and break into little holes, from which, at first, a matter somewhat puriform oozes out; but this changes by degrees into a kind of viscid serous discharge, much intermixed with small pieces of a white substance, resembling the curd of milk.

The tumours subside gradually, while the ulcers at the same time open more, and spread unequally in various directions. After a time some of the ulcers heal; but other tumours quickly form in different parts of the body, and proceed on, in the same slow manner as the former ones, to suppuration. In this manner the disease goes on for some years, and appearing at last to have exhausted itself, all the ulcers heal up, without being succeeded by any fresh swellings; but leaving behind them an ugly puckering of the skin, and a scar of considerable extent. This is the most mild form under which scrofula ever appears. In more virulent cases, the eyes are particularly the seat of the disease, and are affected with ophthalmia, giving rise to ulcerations in the tarsi, and inflammation of the tunica adnata, terminating not unfrequently in an opacity of the transparent cornea.

In similar cases, the joints become affected, they swell and are incommoded by excruciating deep-seated pain, which is much increased upon the slightest motion. The swelling and pain continue to increase, the muscles of the limb become at length much wasted. Matter is soon afterward formed, and this is discharged at small openings made by the bursting of the skin. Being, however, of a peculiar acrimonious nature, it erodes the ligaments and cartilages, and produces a caries of the neighbouring bones. By an absorption of the matter into the system, hectic fever at last arises, and, in the end, often proves fatal.

When scrofula is confined to the external surface, it is by no means attended with danger, although on leaving one part, it is apt to be renewed in others; but when the ulcers are imbued with a sharp acrimony, spread, erode, and become deep, without showing any disposition to heal; when deep-seated collections of matter form among the small bones of the hands and feet, or in the joints, or tubercles in the lungs, with hectic fever, arise, the consequences will be fatal.

On opening the bodies of persons who have died of this disease, many of the viscera are usually found in a diseased state, but more particularly the glands of the mesentery, which are not only much tumified, but often ulcerated. The lungs are frequently discovered beset with a number of tubercles or cysts, which contain matter of various kinds. Scrofulous glands, on being examined by dissection, feel somewhat softer to the touch than in their natural state, and when laid open, they are usually found to contain a soft curdy matter, mixed with pus. The treatment consists chiefly in the use of those means, which are calculated to improve the general health; a nutritious diet, easy of digestion, a pure dry air, gentle exercise, friction, cold bathing, especially in the sea, and strengthening medicines, as the preparations of iron, myrrh, &c.; but, particularly the Peruvian bark, with soda. Various mineral waters, and other remedies which moderately promote the secretions, appear also to have been often useful. In irritable states of the system, hemlock has been employed with much advantage. Mercury is generally injurious to scrofulous persons, when carried so far as to affect the mouth; yet they have sometimes improved under the use of the milder preparations of that metal, determined principally towards the skin. Moderate antimonials also, decoctions of sarsaparilla, mezereon, guaiacum, &c., burnt sponge, muriate of lime, and other such remedies, have been serviceable in many cases, perhaps chiefly in the same way. The application to scrofulous tumours and ulcers must vary according to the state of the parts, whether indolent or irritable: where the tumours show no disposition to enlarge, or become inflamed, it is, perhaps, best to interfere little with them; but their inflammation must be checked by leeches, &c., and when ulcers exist, stimulant lotions or dressings must be used to give them a disposition to heal; but if they are in an irritable state, a cataplasm, made, perhaps, with hemlock, or other narcotic.

SCROPHULA. See *Scrofula.*

SCROPHULA'RIA. (From *scrofula*, the king's evil: so called from the unequal tubercles upon its roots, like scrofulous tumours.) The name of a genus of plants in the Linnæan system. Class, *Didynamia ;* Order, *Angiospermia.* The fig-wort.

SCROPHULARIA AQUATICA. *Betonica aquatica.* Greater water fig-wort. Water-betony. The leaves of this plant, *Scrophularia—foliis cordatis obtusis, petiolatis, decurrentibus; caule membranis angulato; racemis terminalibus*, of Linnæus, are celebrated as correctors of the ill-flavour of senna. They were, also, formerly in high estimation against piles, tumours of a scrofulous nature, inflammations, &c.

SCROPHULARIA MINOR. The pile-wort is sometimes so called. See *Ranunculus ficaria.*

SCROPHULA'RIA NODOSA. The systematic name of the fig-wort. *Scrophularia vulgaris ; Millemorbia ; Scrophularia.* Common fig-wort or kernel-wort. The root and leaves of this plant, *Scrophularia—foliis cordatis, trinervatis; caule obtusangulo*, of Linnæus, have been celebrated both as an internal and external remedy against inflammations, the piles, scrofulous tumours and old ulcers; but they are now only used in this country by the country people.

SCROPHULARIA VULGARIS. See *Scrophularia nodosa.*

SCROTAL. Belonging to the scrotum.

SCROTAL HERNIA.' *Scrotocele.* A protrusion of any part of an abdominal viscus or viscera into the scrotum. See *Hernia.*

SCROTIFORMIS. Bag-like: applied to the nectary of the genus *Satyrium.*

SCROTOCE'LE. (From *scrotum*, and κηλη, a tumour.) A rupture or hernia in the scrotum.

SCRO'TUM. (*Quasi scrotum*, a skin or hide.) *Bursa testium; Oscheus ; Oscheon; Orchea*, of Galen The common integuments which cover the testicles.

SCRU'PULUS. (Dim. of *scrupus*, a small stone.) A scruple or weight of 20 grains.

SCULTETUS, JOHN, was born at Ulm, in 1595, and, after the requisite studies, graduated at Padua. He then practised with considerable reputation in his native city, as well in surgery as in physic, and he appears to have been very bold in his operations. He was carried off by an apoplectic stroke, in 1645. His principal work is entitled, "Armamentarium Chirurgicum," with plates of the instruments; which was published after his death, and has passed through many editions, and been translated into most European languages.

SCURF. *Furfura.* Small exfoliations of the cuticle, which take place after some eruptions on the skin, a new cuticle being formed underneath during the exfoliation.

SCURVY. See *Scorbutus.*

Scurvy-grass. See *Cochlearia officinalis.*

Scurvy-grass, lemon. See *Cochlearia officinalis.*

Scurvy-grass, Scotch. See *Convolvulus soldanella.*

SCUTIFORM. (*Scutiformis;* from σκυτος, a shield, and ειδος, resemblance.) Shield-like. See *Thyroid cartilage.*

SCUTIFORM CARTILAGE. See *Thyroid cartilage.*

SCUTELLA. A little dish or cup. Applied to the round, flat, or shallow fruit, of the calyculate algæ, seen in *Lichen stellaris.*

SCUTELLA'RIA. (From *scutella*, a small dish or saucer, apparently in allusion to the little concave appendage which crowns the calyx. Some have thought it to be more directly derived from *scutellum*, a little shield, to which they have compared the shield.) The name of a genus of plants in the Linnæan system Class, *Didynamia ;* Order, *Gymnospermia.*

SCUTELLARIA GALERICULATA. The systematic name of the skull-cap. *Tertianaria.* The *Scutellaria, foliis cordato lanceolatis, crenatis ; floribus axillaribus*, of Linnæus, which is common in the hedges and ditches of this country. It has a bitter taste and a garlic smell, and is said to be serviceable against that species of ague which attacks the patient every other day.

SCY'BALUM. Σκυβαλα. Dry hard excrement, rounded like nuts or marbles.

SCYTHICUS. (From *Scythia*, its native soil.) An epithet of the liquorice root, or any thing brought from Scythia.

SEA. *Mare.* The air of the sea, the motion of the vessels, the exhalation from the tar as well as the water of the ocean, and its contents all come under the attention of the physician.

1. *Sea-air* is prescribed in a variety of complaints, being considered as more medicinal and salubrious than that on land, though not known to possess in its composition a greater quantity of oxygen. This is a most powerful and valuable remedy. It is resorted to with the happiest success against most cases of debility, and particularly against scrofulous diseases affecting the external parts of the body. See *Bath, cold.*

2. *Sea-sickness.* A nausea or tendency to vomit which varies, in respect of duration, in different persons upon their first going to sea. With some it continues only for a day or two; while with others it remains throughout the voyage. The diseases in which sea-sickness is principally recommended are asthma and consumption.

3. *Sea-water.* This is arranged among the simple saline waters. Its chemical analysis gives a proportion of one of saline contents to about twenty-three and one-fourth of water; but on our shores it is not greater than one of salt to about thirty of water. Sea-water on the British coast may therefore be calculated to contain in the wine pint of muriated soda 186.5 grains, of muriated magnesia fifty-one, of selenite six grains; total 243 one-half grains; or half an ounce and three and one-half grains of saline contents. The disorders for which the internal use of sea-water has been and may be resorted to, are in general the same for which all the simple saline waters may be used. The peculiar power of sea-water and sea-salt as a discutient, employed either internally or externally in scrofulous habits, is well known, and is attended with considerable advantage when judiciously applied.

Sea-holly. See *Eryngium.*
Sea-moss. See *Fucus helminthocorton.*
Sea-oak. See *Fucus vesiculosus.*
Sea-onion. See *Scilla.*
SEA-SALT. Muriate of Soda. See *Sodæ murias.*
SEA-WAX. Maltha. A white, solid, tallowy-looking fusible substance, soluble in alkohol, found on the Baikal lake, in Siberia.

Sea-wrack. See *Fucus vesiculosus.*
Sealed earths. See *Sigillata terra.*
SEARCHING. The operation of introducing a metallic instrument through the urethra into the bladder for the purpose of ascertaining whether the patient has the stone or not.

SEBACEOUS. (*Sebaceus;* from *sebum,* suet.) A term applied to glands, which secrete a suetty humour.

SEBACIC ACID. Subject to a considerable heat, 7 or 8 pounds of hog's lard, in a stoneware retort capable of holding double the quantity, and connect its oeak by an adopter with a cooled receiver. The condensible products are chiefly fat, altered by the fire, mixed with a little acetic and sebacic acids. Treat this product with boiling water several times, agitating the liquor, allowing it to cool, and decanting each time. Pour at last into the watery liquid, solution of acetate of lead in excess. A white flocculent precipitate of sebate of lead will instantly fall, which must be collected on a filter, washed, and dried. Put the sebate of lead into a phial, and pour upon it its own weight of sulphuric acid, diluted with five or six times its weight of water. Expose this phial to a heat of about 212°. The sulphuric acid combines with the oxide of lead, and sets the sebacic acid at liberty. Filter the whole white hot. As the liquid cools, the sebacic acid crystallizes, which must be washed to free it completely from the adhering sulphuric acid. Let it be then dried at a gentle heat.

The sebacic acid is inodorous; its taste is slight, but it perceptibly reddens litmus paper; its specific gravity is above that of water, and its crystals are small white needles of little coherence. Exposed to heat, it melts like fat, is decomposed, and partially evaporated. The air has no effect upon it. It is much more soluble in hot than in cold water; hence boiling water saturated with it, assumes a nearly solid consistence on cooling. Alkohol dissolves it abundantly at the ordinary temperature.

With the alkalies it forms soluble neutral salts; but if we pour into their concentrated solutions, sulphuric, nitric, or muriatic acids, the sebacic is immediately deposited in large quantity. It affords precipitates with the acetates and nitrates of lead, mercury, and silver.

Such is the account given by Thenard of this acid, in the third volume of his Traité de Chimie, published in 1815. Berzelius, in 1806, published an elaborate dissertation, to prove that Thenard's new sebacic acid was only the benzoic contaminated by the fat, from which however it may be freed, and brought to the state of common benzoic acid. Thenard takes no notice of Berzelius whatever, but concludes his account by stating that it has been known only for twelve or thirteen years, and that it must not be confounded with the acid formerly called sebacic, which possesses a strong disgusting odour, and was merely acetic or muriatic acid; or fat which had been changed in some way or other according to the process used in the preparation.

SEBADILLA. See *Cevadilla.*
SEBATE. (*Sebas;* from *sebum,* suet.) The name

in the neutral compound of the acid of fat, with a saltifiable base.

SEBESTEN. (An Egyptian word.) See *Cordia myxa.*
SECA'LE. (*Secale,* i. neut. A name in Pliny which some etymologists, among whom is De Theis, de rive from the Celtic *segal.* This, says he, comes from *sega,* a sickle in the same language, and thence *seges,* the Latin appellation of all grain that is cut with a similar instrument. Those who have looked no farther for an etymology than the Latin *seco,* to cut or mow, have come to the same conclusion.) 1. The name of a genus of plants in the Linnæan system. Class, *Triandria;* Order, *Digynia.* Rye.
2. The common name of the seed of the *Secale cereale,* of Linnæus.

SECALE CEREALE. The systematic name of the rye-plant. Rye-corn is principally used as an article of diet, and in the northern countries of Europe is employed for affording an ardent spirit. Rye-bread is common among the northern parts of Europe; it is less nourishing than wheat, but a sufficiently nutritive and wholesome grain. It is more than any other grain strongly disposed to acescency; hence it is liable to ferment in the stomach, and to produce purging, which people on the first using it commonly experience.

SECALE CORNUTUM. *Secale corniculatum; Clavius secalinus. Mutterkom kornzapfeu,* of the Germans. *Ergot; Seigle ergote* of the French. A black, curved, morbid excrescence, like the spur of a fowl, which is found in the spike of the *Secale cereale* of Linnæus, especially in hot climates, when a great heat suddenly succeeds to much moisture. The seed, which has this diseased growth, gives off, when powdered, an odour which excites sneezing, and titilates the nose, like tobacco. It has a mealy, and then a rancid, nauseous, and biting taste, which remains a long time, and causes the mouth and fauces to become dry; which sensation is not removed by watery fluids, but is soon relieved by milk. The cause of this excrescential disease in rye appears to be an insect which penetrates the grain, feeds on its amylaceous part, and leaves its poison in the parenchyma; hence it is full of small foramina or perforations made by the insect.

The secale cornutum has a singular effect on the animal economy. The meal or flour sprinkled on a wound coagulates the blood, excites a heat and then a numbness in the part, and soon after in the extremities. Bread which contains some of it, does not ferment well, nor bake well, and is glutinous and nauseous. The bread when eaten produces intoxication, lassitude, a sense of something creeping on the skin, weakness of the joints, with convulsive movements occurring periodically. This state is what is called *raphanio,* and *convulsiones cerealiæ.* Of those so affected, some can only breathe in an upright posture, some become maniacal, others epileptic, or tabid, and some have a thirst not to be quenched; and livid eruptions and cutaneous ulcers are not uncommon. The disease continues from ten days to two or three months and longer. Those who have formication, pain, and numbness of the extremities in the commencement, generally lose the feeling in these parts, and the skin, from the fingers to the fore-arm, or from the toes to the middle of the tibia, becomes dry, hard, and black, as if covered with soot. This species of mortification is called *Necrosis cerealis.*

As a medicine, the secale cornutum is given internally to excite the action of the uterus in an atonic state of that organ, producing amenorrhœa, &c. and during parturition. Given in the dose of ten grains, it soon produces a desire to make water, and the labour pains quickly follow; but it is a dangerous medicine, the effect not being controllable.

The antidote to the ill effects produced in the mouth and fauces by eating bread which has this poison, is milk. Against the convulsions, vomits, saline purgatives, clysters, submuriate of mercury as a purgative, are first to be given, and after the primæ viæ have been duly cleaned, stimulants of camphire, ammonia, and æther with opium. To the necrosis, rectified oil of turpentine is very beneficial in stopping its progress, and then warm stimulating fomentations and poultices. [See *pulvis parturiens.* A.]

SECONDARY. This term denotes something that acts as second or in subordination to another. Thus, in diseases, we have *secondary symptoms.* See *Primary.*

Secondary fever. That febrile affection which arises after a crisis, or the discharge of some morbid matter, as after the declension of the small-pox or the measles.

SECRETION. *Secretio.* "The generic name of *secretion* is given to a function, by which a part of the blood escapes from the organs of circulation, and diffuses itself without or within; either preserving its chemical properties, or dispersing after its elements have undergone another order of combinations.

The secretions are generally divided into three sorts; the *exhalations*, the *follicular secretions*, and the *glandular secretions.*

Exhalations.—The exhalations take place as well within the body as at the skin, or in the mucous membranes; thence their divisions into *external* and *internal.*

Internal exhalations.—Wherever large or small surfaces are in contact, an exhalation takes place; wherever fluids are accumulated in a cavity without any apparent opening, they are deposited there by exhalations: the phenomenon of exhalation is also manifested in almost every part of the animal economy. It exists in the serous, the synovial, the mucous membranes; in the cellular tissue, the interior of vessels, the adipose cells, the interior of the eye, of the ear, the parenchyma of many of the organs, such as the thymus, thyroid glands, the *capsulæ suprarenales*, &c. &c. It is by exhalation that the watery humour, the vitreous numour, the liquid of the labyrinth, are formed and renewed. The fluids exhaled in these different parts have not all been analyzed; among those that have been, several approach more or less to the elements of the blood, and particularly to the serum; such are the fluids of the serous membranes of the cellular tissue, of the chambers of the eye; others differ more from it, as the synovia, the fat, &c.

Serous exhalation.—All the viscera of the head, of the chest, and the abdomen, are covered with a serous membrane, which also lines the sides of these cavities, so that the viscera are not in contact with the sides, or with the adjoining viscera, except by the intermediation of the same membrane; and as its surface is very smooth, the viscera can easily change their relation with each other, and with the sides. The principal circumstance which keeps up the polish of their surface is the exhalation of which they are the seat; a very thin fluid constantly passes out of every point of the membrane, and mixing with that of the adjoining parts, forms with it a humid layer that favours the frictions of the organs.

It appears that this facility of sliding upon each other is very favourable to the action of the organs, for as soon as they are deprived of it by any malady of the serous membrane, their functions are disordered, and they sometimes cease entirely.

In the state of health, the fluid secreted by the serous membranes appears to be the serum of the blood, a certain quantity of albumen excepted.

Serous exhalation of the cellular tissue.—This tissue, which is called *cellular*, is generally distributed through animal bodies; it is useful at once to separate and unite the different organs, and the parts of the organs. The tissue is every where formed of a great number of small thin plates, which, crossing in a thousand different ways, form a sort of felt. The size and arrangement of the plates vary according to the different parts of the body. In one place they are larger, thicker, and constitute large cells; in another, they are very narrow and thin, and form extremely small cells; in some points the tissue is capable of extension; in others, it is little susceptible of it, and presents a considerable resistance. But whatever is the disposition of the cellular tissue, its plates, by their two surfaces, exhale a fluid which has the greatest analogy with that of the serous membranes, and which appears to have the same uses; these are to render the frictions of the plates easy upon each other, and therefore to favour the reciprocal motions of the organs, and even the relative changes of the different parts of which they are composed.

Fatty exhalation.—Independently of the serosity, a fluid is found in many parts of the cellular tissue of a very different nature, which is the fat.

Under the relation of the presence of the fat, the cellular tissue may be divided into three sorts; that which contains it always, that which contains it some-times, and that which never contains it. The orbit, the sole of the foot, the pulp of the fingers, that of the toes, always present fat; the subcutaneous cellular tissue, and that which covers the heart, veins, &c. present it often; lastly, that of the scrotum, of the eyelids, of the interior of the skull, never contain it.

The fat is contained in distinct cells that never communicate with the adjoining ones. It has been supposed, from this circumstance, that the tissue that contains, and that forms the fat, was not the same as that by which the serosity is formed; but as these fatty cells have never been shown, except when full of fat, this anatomical distinction seems doubtful. The size, the form, the disposition of these cells, are not less variable than the quantity of fat which they contain. In some individuals scarcely a few ounces exist, while in others there are several hundred pounds.

According to the last researches, the human fat is composed of two parts, the one fluid, the other concrete, which are themselves compounded, but in different proportions, of two new proximate principles.

Synovial exhalations.—Round the moveable articulations a thin membrane is found, which has much analogy with the serous membranes; but which, however, differs from them by having small reddish prolongations that contain numerous blood-vessels. These are called *synovial fringes*; they are very visible in the great articulations of the limbs.

Internal exhalation of the eye.—The different humours of the eye are also formed by exhalation; they are each of them separately enveloped in a membrane that appears intended for exhalation and absorption.

The humours of the eye are, the aqueous humour, the formation of which is at present attributed to the ciliary processes; the vitreous humour, secreted by the hyaloid; the crystalline, the black matter of the choroid; and that of the posterior surface of the iris.

Bloody exhalations.—In all the exhalations of which we have spoken, it is only a part of the principle of the blood that passes out of the vessels; the blood itself appears to spread in several of the organs, and fill in them the sort of cellular tissue which forms their parenchyma; such are the cavernous bodies of the penis and of the clitoris, the urethra and the glans, the spleen, the mamilla, &c. The anatomical examination of these different issues seems to show that they are habitually filled with venous blood, the quantity of which is variable according to different circumstances, particularly according to the state of action or inaction of the organs.

Many other interior exhalations exist also, among those of the cavities of the internal ear, of the parenchyma, of the thymus, of the thyroid gland; that of the cavity of the *capsulæ suprarenales*, &c.: but the fluids formed in these different parts are scarcely understood; they have never been analyzed, and their uses are unknown.

External exhalations.—These are composed entirely of the exhalations of the *mucous membranes*, and of that of the skin, or *cutaneous transpiration.*

Exhalation of the mucous membranes.—There are two mucous membranes; the one covers the surface of the eye, the lachrymal ducts, the nasal cavities, the sinuses, the middle ear, the mouth, all the intestinal canal, the excretory canals which terminate in it, lastly, the larynx, the trachea, and the bronchia.

The other mucous membrane covers the organs of generation and of the urinary apparatus.

Cutaneous transpiration.—A transparent liquid, of an odour more or less strong, salt, acid, usually passes through the innumerable openings of the epidermis See *Perspiration.* This liquid is generally evaporated as soon as it is in contact with the air, and at other times it flows upon the surface of the skin. In the first case it is imperceptible, and bears the name of *insensible transpiration;* in the second it is called *sweat.*

Follicular secretions.—The follicles are small hollow organs lodged in the skin or mucous membranes, and which on that account are divided into *mucous* and *cutaneous.*

The follicles are, besides, divided into simple and compound. The simple mucous follicles are seen upon nearly the whole extent of the mucous membranes, where they are more or less abundant; however, there are points of considerable extent of these membranes where they are not seen.

The bodies that bear the name of *fungous papillæ* of the tongue the amygdalæ, the glands of the cardia, the prostate, &c. are considered by anatomists as collections of simple follicles. Perhaps this opinion is not sufficiently supported.

The fluid that they secrete is little known ; it appears analogous to the mucous, and to have the same uses. In almost all the points of the skin, little openings exist, which are the orifices of small hollow organs, with membranous sides, generally filled with an albuminous and fatty matter, the consistence, the colour, the odour, and even the savour of which are variable, according to the different parts of the body, and which is continually spread upon the surface of the skin.

These small organs are called the follicles of the skin ; one of them at least exists at the base of each hair, and generally the hairs traverse the cavity of a follicle in their direction outwards.

The follicles form that mucous and fatty matter which is seen upon the skin of the cranium, and on that of the pavillion of the ear ; the follicles also secrete the *cerumen* in the auditory canal ; that whitish matter, of considerable consistence, that is pressed out of the skin of the face, in the form of small worms, is also contained in follicles ; it is the same matter which, by its surface being in contact with the air, becomes black, and produces the numerous spots that are seen upon some persons' faces, particularly on the sides of the nose and cheeks.

The follicles also appear to secrete that odorous, whitish matter, which is always renewed at the external surface of the genital parts.

By spreading on the surface of the epidermis, of the hair of the head, of the skin, &c., the matter of the follicles supports the suppleness and elasticity of those parts, renders their surface smooth and polished, favours their frictions upon one another. On account of its unctuous nature, it renders them less penetrable by humidity, &c.

Glandular Secretions.—The name of gland is given to a secreting organ which sheds the fluid that it forms upon the surface of a mucous membrane, or of the skin, by one or more excretory glands.

The number of glands is considerable , the action of each bears the name of glandular secretion. There are six secretions of this sort, that of the tears, of the saliva, of the bile, of the pancreatic fluid, of the urine, of the semen, and lastly, that of the milk. We may add the action of the mucous glands, and of the glands of Cowper.

Secretion of Tears.—The gland that forms the tears is very small ; it is situated in the orbit of the eye, above and a little outward ; it is composed of small grains, united by cellular tissues ; its excretory canals, small and numerous, open behind the external angle of the upper eyelid : it receives a small artery, a branch of the ophthalmic, and a nerve, a division of the fifth pair.

In a state of health, the tears are in small quantity ; the liquid that forms them is limpid, without odour, of a salt savour. Fourcroy and Vauquelin, who analyzed it, found it composed of much water, of some centesimals of mucus, muriate and phosphate of soda, and a little pure soda and lime. What are called *tears*, are not, however, the fluid secreted entirely by the lachrymal gland ; it is a mixture of this fluid with the matter secreted by the conjunctiva, and probably with that of the glands of Meibomius.

The tears form a layer before the conjunctiva of the eye, and defend it from the contact of air ; they facilitate the frictions of the eyelids upon the eye, favour the expulsion of foreign bodies, and prevent the action of irritating bodies upon the conjunctiva ; in this case the quantity rapidly augments. They are also a means of expressing the passions : the tears flow from vexation, pain, joy, and pleasure. The nervous system has therefore a particular influence upon their secretion. This influence probably takes place by means of the nerve that the fifth pair of cerebral nerves sends to the lachrymal gland.

Secretion of the Saliva.—The salivary glands are, 1st, the two parotids, situated before the ear and behind the neck, and the branch of the jaw ; 2d, the submaxillaries, situated below and on the front of the body of this bone ; 3d, lastly, the sublinguals, placed immediately below the tongue. The parotids and the submaillxaries have only one excretory canal : the sublin-

guals have several. All these glands are formed by the union of the granulations of different forms and dimensions ; they receive a considerable quantity of arteries relatively to their mass. Several nerves are distributed to them, which proceed from the brain or the spinal marrow.

The saliva which these glands secrete flows constantly into the mouth, and occupies the lower part of it ; it is at first placed between the anterior and lateral part of the tongue and the jaw ; and when the space is filled, it passes into the space between the lower lip, the cheek, and the external side of the jaw. Being thus deposited in the mouth, it mixes with the fluids secreted by the membranes and the mucous follicles.

Secretion of the Pancreatic Juice.—The pancreas is situated transversely in the abdomen, behind the stomach. It has an excretory canal, which opens into the duodenum, beside that of the liver. The granulous structure of this gland has made it be considered a salivary gland ; but it is different from them by the smallness of the arteries that it receives, and by not appearing to receive any cerebral nerve.

It is impossible to explain the use of the pancreatic juice.

Secretion of the Bile.—The liver is the largest of all the glands ; it is also distinguished by the singular circumstance among the secretory organs, that it is constantly traversed by a great quantity of venous blood, besides the arterial blood, which it receives as well as every other part. Its parenchyma does not resemble, in any respect, that of the other glands, and the fluid formed by it is not less different from that of the other glandular fluids.

The excretory canal of the liver goes to the duodenum ; before entering it, it communicates with a small membranous bag, called *vesicula fellis*, and on this account, that it is almost always filled with bile.

Few fluids are so compound, and so different from the blood, as the bile. Its colour is greenish, its taste very bitter ; it is viscous, thready, sometimes limpid, and sometimes muddy. It contains water, albumen, a matter called resinous by some chemists, a yellow colouring principle, soda, and some salts, viz. muriate, phosphate, and sulphate of soda, phosphate of lime and oxide of iron. These properties belong to the bile contained in the gall bladder. That which goes out directly from the liver, called *hepatic bile*, has never been analyzed ; it appears to be of a less deep colour, less viscous, and less bitter than the *cystic bile*. The formation of the bile appears constant.

The liver receiving venous blood at the same time by the vena porta, and arterial blood by the hepatic artery physiologists have been very eager to know which of the two it is that forms the bile. Several have said that the blood of the vena porta, having more carbon and hydrogen than that of the hepatic artery, is more proper for furnishing the elements of the bile. Bichat has successfully contested this opinion ; he has shown, that the quantity of arterial blood which arrives at the liver is more in relation with the quantity of bile formed than that of the venous blood ; that the volume of the hepatic canal is not in proportion with the vena porta ; that the fat, a fluid much hydrogenated, is secreted by the arterial blood, &c. He might have added, that there is nothing to prove that the blood of the vena porta has more analogy with the bile than the arterial blood. We shall take no part in this discussion ; both opinions are equally destitute of proof. Besides, nothing repels the idea, that both sorts of blood serve in the secretion. This seems even to be indicated by anatomy ; for injections show that all the vessels of the liver, arterial, venous, lymphatic, and excretory, communicate with each other.

The bile contributes very usefully in digestion, but the manner is unknown. In our present ignorance relative to the causes of diseases, we attribute noxious properties to the bile, which it is probably far from possessing.

Secretion of the Urine.—This secretion is different in several respects from the preceding. The liquid which results from it is much more abundant than that of any other gland ; in place of serving in any internal uses, it is expelled ; its retention would be attended by the most dangerous consequences. We are advertised of the necessity of its expulsion by a particular feeling, which, like the instinctive phenomena of this sort beco - very painful if not quickly attended to.

In explaining the glandular secretions, physiologists have given full scope to their imagination. The glands have been successively considered as sieves, filters, as a focus of fermentation. Bordeu, and, more recently, Bichat, have attributed a peculiar motion and sensibility to their particles, by which they choose, in the blood which traverses them, the particles that are fit to enter into the fluids that they secrete. Atmospheres and compartments have been allotted to them; they have been supposed susceptible of erection, of sleep, &c. Notwithstanding the efforts of many learned men, the truth is, that what passes in a gland when it acts, is entirely unknown. Chemical phenomena necessarily take place.

Several secreted fluids are acid, while the blood is alkaline. The most of them contain proximate principles which do not exist in the blood, and which are formed in the glands, but the particular mode of these combinations is unknown.

We must not, however, confound among these suppositions upon the action of the glands, an ingenious conjecture of Dr. Wollaston. This learned man supposes that very weak electricity may have a marked influence upon the secretions. He rests his opinion upon a curious experiment, of which we will here give an account.

Dr. Wollaston took a glass tube, two inches long, and three quarters of an inch diameter: he closed one of its extremities with a bit of bladder. He poured a little water into the tube, with 1-240 parts of its weight of muriate of soda. He wet the bladder on the outside, and placed it on a piece of silver. He then bent a zinc wire, so that one of its ends touched the silver, and the other entered the tube the length of an inch. In the same instant the external face of the bladder gave indications of the presence of pure soda; so that, under the influence of this very weak electricity, there was a decomposition of muriate of soda, and a passage of the soda, separated from the acid, through the bladder. Dr. Wollaston thinks it is not impossible that something analogous may happen in the secretions; but, before admitting this idea, many other proofs are necessary.

Several organs, such as the thyroid and thymus bodies, the spleen, the supra-renal capsules, have been called glands by many anatomists. Professor Chaussier has substituted for this denomination that of the *glandiform ganglions*. The use of these parts is entirely unknown. As they are generally more numerous in the fœtus, they are supposed to have important functions, but there exists no proof of it. Works of physiology contain a great many hypotheses intended to explain their functions."—*Magendie's Physiology*.

SECTIO CÆSAREA. See *Cæsarian operation*.

SECTIO FRANCONIA. See *Lithotomy*.

SECUNDINES. The after-birth, and membranes which are expanded from its edge, and which form a complete involucrum of the fœtus and its waters, go under the term of secundines. See *Placenta*.

SECUNDUM ARTEM. According to art. A term frequently used in prescription, and denoted by the letters S. A., which are usually affixed, when the making up of the recipe in perfection requires some uncommon care and dexterity.

SECUNDUS. Applied by botanists to leaves and parts of the fructification which are unilateral, all leaning towards one side; as the leaves and flowers of the *Convallaria majalis*.

SECURIDACA. (From *securis*, an axe: so called because its leaves resemble a small axe.) See *Hyoscyamus niger*.

SEDATIVE. (*Sedativus*; from *sedo*, to ease or assuage.) *Sedantia*. Medicines which have the power of diminishing the animal energy, without destroying life. They are divided into *sedativa soporifica*, as opium, poppies, hyoscyamus; and *sedativa refrigerantia*, as neutral salts, acids, &c.

Sedative salt. See *Boracic acid*.

SEDENTARIA OSSA. The bones on which we sit. The os coccygis and ischia.

SEDGE. See *Iris pseudacorus*.

SEDIMENT. The heavy parts of liquids which fall to the bottom.

Sediment, lateritious. See *Lateritious sediment*.

SEDLITZ. *Seydschutz*. The name of a village of Bohemia, in the circle of Saartz, where Hoffman discovered a simple mineral water, *Aqua Sedlitziana*.

From chemical analysis it appears, that it is strongly impregnated with sulphate of magnesia or Epsom salt, and it is to this, along with, probably, the small quantity of muriate of magnesia, that it owes its bitter and saline taste, and its purgative properties. The diseases in which this water is recommended are, crudities of the stomach, hypochondriasis, amenorrhœa, and the anomalous complaints succeeding the cessation of the catamenia, œdematous tumours of the legs in literary men, hæmorrhoidal affections, and scorbutic eruptions.

SE'DUM. (From *sedo*, to assuage: so called because it allays inflammation.) The name of a genus of plants in the Linnæan system. Class, *Decandria*; Order, *Pentagynia*.

SEDUM ACRE. *Illecebra*; *Vermicularis*; *Piper murale*; *Sedum minus*. Wall-pepper; Stone-crop. The plant thus called is, in its recent state, extremely acrid, like the hydropiper; hence, if taken in large doses, it acts powerfully on the primæ viæ, proving both emetic and cathartic; applied to the skin as a cataplasm, it frequently produces vesications and erosions. Boerhaave therefore imagines, that its internal employment must be unsafe; but experience has discovered, that a decoction of this plant is not only safe, but of great efficacy in scorbutic complaints. For which purpose, a handful of the herb is directed, by Below, to be boiled in eight pints of beer, till they are reduced to four, of which three or four ounces are to be taken every, or every other morning. Milk has been found to answer this purpose better than beer. Not only ulcers simply scorbutic, but those of a scrofulous or even cancerous tendency, have been cured by the use of this plant; of which Marquet relates several instances. He likewise found it useful as an external application in destroying fungous flesh, and in promoting a discharge in gangrenes and carbuncles. Another effect for which this plant is esteemed, is that of stopping intermittent fevers.

SEDUM LUTEUM MURALE. Navel-wort.

SEDUM MAJUS. See *Sempervivum tectorum*.

SEDUM MINUS. See *Sedum acre*.

SEDUM TELEPHIUM. The systematic name of the orpine. *Faba crassa*; *Telephium*; *Fabaria crassula*; *Anacampseros*. The plant which bears these names in various pharmacopœias, is the *Sedum—foliis planiusculis serratis, corymbo folioso, caule erecto*, of Linnæus. It was formerly ranked as an antiphlogistic, but now forgotten.

SEED. See *Semen*.

Seed vessel. See *Pericarpium*.

SEEING. See *Vision*.

SEIGNETTE'S SALT. A neutral salt: first prepared and made known by Peter Seignette, who lived at Rochelle, in France, towards the end of the seventeenth century. See *Soda tartarizata*.

SELENITES. (From σεληνη, the moon.) 1. Sparry gypsum, a sulphate of lime.

2. A white stone having a figure on it resembling a moon.

SELENIUM. (From σεληνη, the moon. so called from its usefulness in lunacy.) 1. A kind of peony.

2. A new elementary body extracted by Berzelius from the pyrites of Fahlun, which, from its chemical properties, he places between sulphur and tellurium, though it has more properties in common with the former, than with the latter substance.

SELF-HEAL. See *Prunella*.

SELINE. (From σεληνη, the moon; because they are opake, and look like little moons.) A disease of the nails, in which white spots are occasionally seen in their substance.

SELINIC ACID. *Acidum selinicum*. If selinium be heated to dryness it forms with nitric acid, a volatile and crystallizable compound, called selinic acid, which unites to some of the metallic oxides producing salts, called *seleniates*.

SELI'NUM. (The ancient generic name of Theophrastus and Dioscorides, whose Σελιον is said to be derived from παρα το εν ελει φυεσθαι, on account of its growing in mud; whence Homer's ελεοθρεπ]ον σελινον. De Theis says, that *selinum* is derived from σεληνη the moon, because of the shape of its growing seeds; and that it is the foundation of many other compound names of umbelliferous plants among the Greeks, as ορεοσελινον, πετροσελινον, &c.) The name of a genus of plants. Class, *Pentandria*; Order, *Digynia*.

SELLA. (*Sella, quasi sedda ; from sedeo, to sit.*) A saddle.

SE′LLA TURCICA. (So called from its supposed resemblance to a Turkish saddle.) *Ephippium.* A cavity in the sphenoid bone, containing the pituitary gland, surrounded by the four clinoid processes.

SELTZER. The name of a place in Germany, Neider Seltzer, about ten miles from Frankfort on the Mayne, where a saline mineral water rises, which is slightly alkaline, highly acidulated with carbonic acid, containing more of this volatile principle than is sufficient to saturate the alkali, and the earths which it holds in solution. It is particularly serviceable in relieving some of the symptoms that indicate a morbid affection of the lungs ; in slow hectic fever, exanthematous eruptions of the skin, foulness of the stomach, bilious vomiting, acidity, and heartburn, spasmodic pains in any part of the alimentary canal, and bloody or highly offensive stools. On account of its property in relieving spasmodic pains, and from its rapid determination to the kidneys, and perhaps its alkaline contents, it has been sometimes employed with great advantage in diseases of the urinary organs, especially those that are attended with the formation of calculus. A large proportion of the Seltzer water, either genuine or artificial, that is consumed in this country, is for the relief of these disorders. Even in gonorrhœa, either simple or venereal, Hoffmann asserts, that advantage is to be derived from this medicine. The usual dose is from half a pint to a pint.

SEMECA′RPUS. (From σημειω, to mark, and καρπος, a fruit: a name evidently derived from the use that is made of its nut in the East Indies to mark table linen and articles of apparel.) The name of a genus of plants, Class *Pentandria ;* Order, *Trigynia.*

SEMECARPUS ANACARDIUM. The marking nut-tree. The systematic name, according to some, of the tree which is supposed to afford the Malacca bean. See *Avicenna tomentosa.*

SEMEIO′SIS. (From σημειοω, to notify.) See *Semiotice.*

SE′MEN. (*Semen, inis.* n. ; *sero,* to sow.) A. The seed or prolific liquor of animals secreted in the testicles, and carried through the epididymis and vas deferens into the vesiculæ seminales, to be emitted *sub coitu* into the female vagina, and there, by its aura, to penetrate and impregnate the ovulum in the ovarium.

In castrated animals, and in eunuchs, the vesiculæ seminales are small, and contracted ; and a little lymphatic liquor, but no semen, is found in them. The semen is detained for some time in the vesiculæ seminales, and rendered thicker from the continual absorption of its very thin part, by the oscula of the lymphatic vessels. In lascivious men, the semen is sometimes, though rarely, propelled by nocturnal pollution from the vesiculæ seminales, through the ejaculatory ducts (which arise from the vesiculæ seminales, perforate the urethra transversely, and open themselves by narrow and very nervous mouths at the sides of the caput gallinaginis), into the urethra, and from it to some distance. But in chaste men, the greatest part is again gradually absorbed from the vesiculæ seminales through the lymphatic vessels, and conciliates strength to the body. The smell of semen is specific, heavy, affecting the nostrils, yet not disagreeable. The same odour is observed in the roots of the orchis, the iuli of chesnuts, and the antheræ of many plants. The smell of the semen of quadrupeds, when at heat, is so penetrating, as to render their flesh fœtid and useless, unless castrated. Thus the flesh of the stag, *tempore coitus,* is unfit to eat. The taste of semen is fatuous, and somewhat acrid. In the testes, its consistence is thin and diluted ; but in the vesiculæ seminales, viscid, dense, and rather pellucid ; and by venery and debility it is rendered thinner.

Specific gravity. The greatest part of the semen sinks to the bottom in water, yet some part swims on its surface, which it covers like very fine threads mutually connected together in the form of a cobweb.

Colour. In the testicles it is somewhat yellow, and in the vesiculæ seminales it acquires a deeper hue. That emitted by pollution or coition, becomes white from its mixture with the whitish liquor of the prostate gland during its passage through the urethra. In those people who labour under jaundice, and from the abuse of saffron, the semen has been seen yellow, and, in an atrabilary young man black.

Quality. Semen, exposed to the atmospheric air, loses its pellucidity, and becomes thick, but after a few hours it is again rendered more fluid and pellucid than it was immediately after its emission. This phenomenon cannot arise from water or oxygen attracted from the air. At length it deposites phosphate of lime, and forms a corneous crust.

Experiments with semen prove, that it turns the syrup of violets green, and dissolves earthy, neutral, and metallic salts. Fresh semen is insoluble in water, until it has undergone the above changes in atmospheric air. It is dissolved by alkaline salts. By æthereal oil it is dried into a pellucid pellicle, like the cortex of the brain.

It is dissolved by all acids, except the oxymuriatic, by which it is coagulated in the form of white flakes. It is also acted upon by alkohol of wine.

Vauquelin, who analyzed it, found it composed of

1. Water.....................	900
2. Animal mucilage............	60
3. Soda......	10
4. Phosphate of lime...........	30

5. Examined by the microscope, a multitude of animalcula are observed in it, which appear to have a round head and a long tail ; these animalcula move with considerable rapidity ; they seem to fly the light, and to seek the shade. 6. *The odorous principle,* which flies off immediately from fresh semen. It appears to consist of a peculiar vital principle, and by the ancients was called *aura seminis.*

Use. 1. Emitted into the female vagina, *sub coitu,* it possesses the wonderful and stupendous power of impregnating the ovulum in the female ovarium. The odorous principle, or aura spermatica only, appears to penetrate through the cavity of the uterus and Fallopian tubes to the female ovarium, and there to impregnate the albuminous latex of the mature ovulum by its vital power. The other principles of the semen appear to be only a vehicle of the seminal aura. 2. In chaste men, the semen returning through the lymphatic vessels into the mass of the blood, gives strength to the body and mind ; hence the bull is so fierce and brave, the castrated ox so gentle and weak ; hence every animal languishes *post coitum ;* and hence tabes dorsalis from onanism. 3. It is by the stimulus of the semen absorbed, at the age of puberty, into the mass of the humours, that the beard and hair of the pubes, but in animals, the horns, are produced ; and the weeping voice of the boy changed into that of a man.

B. The seed of plants or nucleus formed in the germen of a plant, for the purpose of propagating its species, the sole "end and aim" of all the organs of fructification. Every other part is in some manner subservient to the forming, perfecting, or dispersing of these.

A seed consists of several parts, some of which are more essential than others, viz.

1. The *hilum,* or scar.
2. The *funiculus umbilicalis,* or filament, by which the immature seed is connected to the receptacle.
3. The *testa,* or *tunica seminis.*
4. The seed lobes, or *cotyledons.* These parts are beautifully seen by macerating the seeds of a kidney or other bean, or gourd, in water.

The less essential parts are,
1. The *arillus.*   4. The *capsula.*
2. The *pappus.*   5. The *ala.*
3. The *cauda.*

From the difference in the form, surface, situation, and number, rise the following distinctions of seeds.
1. *Semina arillata ;* as in *Jasminum.*
2. *Paposa ;* as in *Leontodon taraxacum.*
3. *Caudata ;* as in *Clematis vitalba.*
4. *Calyculata,* covered with a bony calyx ; as in *Coix lachryma.*
5. *Alata ;* as in *Bignonia.*
6. *Hamosa,* furnished with one or three hooks ; as in *Daucus muricatus.*
7. *Lanata,* covered with wool ; as in *Bombax Gossipium,* and *Anemone hortensis.*
8. *Rotuda ;* as in *Pisum,* and *Brassica*
9. *Rotunda-compressa ;* as *Ervum lens.*
10. *Oblonga ;* as in *Boerhavia diffusa.*
11. *Conica ;* as in *Bellium.*
12. *Ovata ;* as in *Quercus robur.*
13. *Triquetra ;* as in *Rheum,* and *Rumex.*
14. *Lanceolata ;* as in *Fraxinus.*
15. *Acuminata ;* as *Cucumis sativus.*
16. *Reniformia ;* as in *Phaseolus.*

17. *Aculeata;* as *Ranunculus arvensis.*
18. *Cochleata;* as in *Salsola.*
19. *Cymbiformia;* as in *Calendula officinalis.*
20. *Linearia;* as in *Crucianella.*
21. *Aristata;* as in *Holcus saccharatus.*
22. *Echinata;* as in *Verbena lapulacea.*
23. *Hispida;* as *Daucus carota.*
24. *Hirsuta;* as in *Scandix trichosperma.*
25. *Muricata;* as *Ranunculus parviflorus.*
26. *Glabra;* as in *Galium montanum.*
27. *Rugosa;* as in *Lithospermum arvense.*
28. *Callosa;* as in *Citrus medica.*
29. *Lapidea;* as in *Lithospermum.*
30. *Colorata;* as in *Chærophyllum aureum.*
31. *Striata;* as in *Conium maculatum.*
32. *Sulcata;* as in *Scandix odorata.*
33. *Transversim sulcatu;* as *Picris.*
34. *Nuda;* as in the Gymnospermial plants.
35. *Tecta;* as in Angiospermial plants.
36. *Nidulantia,* adhering to the external surface; as in *Fragaria vesca.*
37. *Pendula,* suspended by a filament external to the seed vessel; as in *Magnolia grandiflora.*
38. *Pauca,* when few in number.
39. *Plurima,* many; as in *Papaver.*

The parts of a seed when germinating are,
1. Cotyledones.
2. Corculum.

The variety of forms of seeds are not without their uses, and the various modes by which seeds are dispersed, cannot fail to strike an observing mind with admiration. "Who has not listened," says Sir James Smith, "in a calm and sunny day, to the crackling of furze bushes, caused by the explosion of their little elastic pods; nor watched the down of innumerable seeds floating on the summer breeze, till they are overtaken by a shower, which, moistening their wings, stops their further flight, and at the same time accomplishes its final purpose, by immediately promoting the germination of each seed in the moist earth? How little are children aware, as they blow away the seeds of dandelion, or stick burs, in sport, on each other's clothes, that they are fulfilling one of the greatest ends of nature. Sometimes the calyx, beset with hooks, forms the bur; sometimes hooks encompass the fruit itself. Pulpy fruits serve quadrupeds and birds as food, while their seeds, often small, hard, and indigestible, pass uninjured by them through the intestines, and are deposited far from their original place of growth, in a condition peculiarly fit for vegetation. Even such seeds as are themselves eaten, like the various sorts of nuts, are hoarded up in the cracked ground, and occasionally forgotten, or the earth swells and encloses them. The ocean itself serves to waft the larger kinds of seeds from their native soil to far distant shores."

SEMEN ADJOWAEN. A seed imported from the East, of a pleasant smell, a grateful aromatic taste, somewhat like savory. It possesses exciting, stimulating, and carminative virtues, and is given in the East in nervous weakness, dyspepsia, flatulency, and heartburn.

SEMEN AGAVE. An East Indian seed, exhibited there in atonic gout.

SEMEN CONTRA. See *Artemisia santonica.*

SEMEN SANCTUM. See *Artemisia santonica.*

SEMI. (From *ημισυ,* half.) *Semi,* in composition, universally signifies half; as *semicupium,* a half-bath, or bath up to the navel; *semilunaris,* in the shape of a half-moon.

SEMICIRCULAR. *Semicircularis.* Of the shape of half a circle.

SEMICIRCULAR CANALS. These canals are three in number, and take their name from their figure. They belong to the organ of hearing, and are situated in the petrous portion of the temporal bone, and open into the vestibulum.

SEMICU'PIUM. A half-bath, or such as receives only the hips, or extremities.

SEMICYLINDRACEUS. Semicylindrical; flat on one side, round on the other, as the leaves of the *Conchium gibbosum.*

SEMI INTEROSSEUS INDICIS. See *Abductor indicis manus.*

SEMILUNAR. *Semilunaris.* Half-moon shaped.

SEMILUNAR VALVES. The three valves at the beginning of the pulmonary artery and aorta are so termed, from their half-moon shape.

SEMI-MEMBRANO'SUS. *Ischio-popliti-femoral,* of Dumas. This muscle arises from the outer surface of the tuberosity of the ischium, by a broad flat tendon which is three inches in length. From this tendon it has gotten the name of semi-membranosus. It then begins to grow fleshy, and runs at first under the long head of the biceps, and afterward between that muscle and the semi-tendinosus. At the lower part of the thigh it becomes narrower again, and terminates in a short tendon, which is inserted chiefly into the upper and back part of the head of the tibia, but some of its fibres are spread over the posterior surface of the capsular ligament of the knee. Between this cupsular ligament and the tendon of the muscle, we find a small bursa mucosa. The tendons of this and the last-described muscle form the inner ham-string. This muscle bends the leg, and seems likewise to prevent the capsular ligament from being pinched.

SEMI-NERVOSUS. See *Semitendinosus.*

SEMINIS CAUDA. See *Cauda seminis.*

SEMINIS EJACULATOR. See *Accelerator urinæ.*

Semiopal. See *Opal.*

SEMI-ORBICULARIS ORIS. See *Orbicularis oris.*

SEMIO'TICE. (From *σημειον,* a sign.) *Cemeiosis.* That part of pathology which treats on the signs of diseases.

SEMI-SPINALIS COLDI. *Semi-spinalis sive transverso-spinalis colli,* of Winslow; *Spinalis transverso-spinalis colli,* of Albinus; *Spinalis colli,* of Douglas; *Transversalis colli,* of Cowper; and *Transverso-spinal,* of Dumas. A muscle situated on the posterior part of the neck, which turns the neck obliquely backwards, and a little to one side. It arises from the transverse processes of the uppermost six vertebræ of the back by as many distinct tendons, ascending obliquely under the complexus, and is inserted into the spinous processes of all the vertebræ of the neck, except the first and last.

SEMI-SPINALIS DORSI. *Semi-spinalis externus seu transverso-spinalis dorsi,* of Winslow. *Semi-spinatus,* of Cowper; and *Transverso-spinal,* of Dumas. A muscle situated on the back, which extends the spine obliquely backwards. It arises from the transverse processes of the seventh, eighth, ninth, and tenth vertebræ of the back, by as many distinct tendons, which soon grow fleshy, and then become tendinous again, and are inserted into the spinous processes of all the vertebræ of the back above the eighth, and into the lowermost of the neck, by as many tendons.

SEMI-SPINALIS EXTERNUS. See *Semi-spinalis dorsi.*

SEMI-SPINATUS. See *Semi-spinalis dorsi.*

SEMI-TENDINOSUS. This muscle, which is the *semi-nervosus,* of Douglas and Winslow; and *Ischio-creti-tibial,* of Dumas, is situated obliquely along the back part of the thigh. It arises tendinous and fleshy from the inferior, posterior, and outer part of the tuberosity of the ischium, in common with the long head of the biceps cruris, to the posterior edge of which it continues to adhere, by a great number of oblique fibres, for the space of two or three inches. Towards the lower part of the os femoris, it terminates in a round tendon, which passes behind the inner condyle of the thigh bone, and, becoming flat, is inserted into the upper and inner part of the ridge of the tibia, a little below its tuberosity. This tendon sends off an aponeurosis, which helps to form the tendinous fascia that covers the muscles of the leg. This muscle assists in bending the leg, and at the same time draws it a little inwards.

SEMPERVIRENS. Evergreen. Applied to leaves which are permanent through one, two, or more winters, so that the branches are never stripped; as the ivy, fir, laurel, bay, &c.

SEMPERVI'VUM. (From *semper,* always, and *vivo,* to live: so called because it is always green.)
1. The name of a genus of plants in the Linnæan system. Class, *Dodecandria;* Order, *Polygynia.*
2. The pharmacopœial name of some plants.

SEMPERVIVUM ACRE. The stone-crop is occasionally so termed. See *Cedum acre.*

SEMPERVIVUM TECTORUM. The systematic name of the houseleek. *Cedum majus; Æonion; Aizoum; Aizoon; Barba jovis.* Houseleek, or sengreen. The leaves of this plant have no remarkable smell, but discover to the taste a mild subacid austerity; they are frequently applied by the vulgar to bruises and old ulcers.

SENAC, John, was born in Gascony, about the close of the seventeenth century. He is stated to have received the degree of doctor at Rheims, and that of bachelor of physic at Paris. He was a man of profound erudition, united with great modesty; and by his industry acquired much experience. His merits procured him the favour of Louis XV. who appointed him his consulting, and afterward his chief physician, which office he retained till his death in 1770. He was also a member of the Royal Academy of Sciences at Paris, and of the Royal Society of Nancy. He left some works, which will probably maintain a lasting reputation, particularly his treatise on the Structure, Function, and Diseases of the Heart. An edition of Heister's Anatomy, with some interesting Observations, was published by him when young. A paper on Drowning, in the Memoirs of the Academy of Sciences, refuting certain erroneous opinions respecting the Cause of Death, and the Treatmen founded upon them, is also due to him; as well as some other minor publications.

SENE'CIO. (*Senecio;* from *senesco,* to grow old: so called because it has a grayish down upon it, like the beard of old men.)

1. The name of a genus of plants in the Linnæan system. Class, *Syngenesia;* Order, *Polygamia superflua.*

2. The pharmacopœial name also of the groundsel. See *Senecio vulgaris.*

SENECIO JACOBÆA. The systematic name of the *Jacobæa,* of old writers. St. James's wort. Ragwort. The leaves of this common plant have a roughish, bitter, sub-acrid taste, extremely nauseous. A decoction is said to have been of infinite service in the cure of epidemic camp dysentery. A poultice made of the fresh leaves is said to have a surprising effect in removing pains of the joints, and to remove the sciatica, or hip gout, in two or three applications when ever so violent. The root is of an adstringent nature. A decoction of it was formerly good for wounds and bruises.

SENECIO MADRASPATANUS. See *Senecio pseudochina.*

SENECIO PSEUDO-CHINA. *China supposita; Senecio madraspatanus.* Bastard China. It grows in Malabar. The root greatly resembles the China root in appearance and qualities.

SENECIO VULGARIS. *Erigerum; Senecio; Erigeron.* Groundsel. This very common plant is frequently applied bruised to inflammations and ulcers, as a refrigerant and antiscorbutic.

SENECTA ANGUIUM. The cast skin of a serpent; its decoction is said to cure deafness.

SENECTUS. See *Age.*

[SENECA OIL. See *Genessee oil.*]

SE'NEGA. (So called because the Seneca or Senegaw Indians use it against the bite of the rattlesnake.) See *Polygala senega.*

Senegal gum. See *Mimosa senegal.*

Senegaw milkwort. See *Polygala senega.*

SE'NEKA. See *Senega.*

SENGREEN. See *Sempervivum tectorum.*

SE'NNA. (From *senna,* an Arabian word, signifying acute: so called from its sharp-pointed leaves.) See *Cassia senna.*

SENNA ALEXANDRINA. See *Cassia senna.*

SENNA ITALICA. Pee *Cassia senna*

SENNA PAUPERUM. Bastard senna, or milk-vetch.

SENNA SCORPIUM. The scorpion senna.

SENNÆ EXTRACTUM. Extract of senna.

SENNERTUS, Daniel, was born at Breslaw in 1572. He was sent to Wittemberg at the age of twenty-one, and exhibited such marks of talent, that every opportunity was afforded him of visiting the other celebrated universities of Germany. On his return in 1601, he received the degree of doctor, and the next year was appointed to a professorship of medicine. He distinguished himself greatly by his eloquence and sound knowledge, and his publications concurred in raising his fame, insomuch that he was consulted by patients from all parts of the world; towards whom he evinced great disinterestedness. The plague prevailed seven times at Wittemberg, while he was professor there, yet he never quitted his post, nor declined his services, even to the poorest sick: however, he was at last a victim to that disease in 1637. Sennertus was a voluminous writer, and has been represented by

some as a mere compiler; but his works are valuable, as containing a full and clear epitome of ancient learning; and besides, display much judgment, and freedom, in criticising their doctrines, which indeed involved him in many controversies. He first introduced the study of chemistry at Wittemberg; and in his writings he maintained the propriety of admitting chemical as well as Galenical theories and remedies into medicine.

SENSATION. *Sensatio.* Sensation, or feeling, is the consciousness of a change taking place in any part, from the contact of a foreign body with the extremities of our nerves. The seat of sensation is in the pulp of the nerves.

The impression produced on any organ by the action of an external body constitutes sensation. This sensation, transmitted by nerves to the brain, is perceived, that is, felt by the organ; the sensation then becomes *perception;* and this first modification implies, as must be evident, the existence of a central organ, to which impressions produced on the senses are conveyed. The cerebral fibres are acted on with greater or less force by the sensations propagated by all the senses influenced at the same time; and we could only acquire confused notions of all bodies that produce them, if one particular and stronger perception did not obliterate the others, and fix our attention. In this collective state of the mind on the same subject, the brain is weakly affected, by several sensations which leave no trace behind. It is on this principle that, having read a book with great attention, we forget the different sensations produced by the paper and character.

When a sensation is of short duration, the knowledge we have of it is so weak, that soon afterward there does not remain any knowledge of having experienced it. In proportion as a sensation, or an idea, which is only a sensation transformed or perceived by the cerebral organ, has produced in the fibres of this organ a stronger or weaker impression, the remembrance of it becomes more or less lively and permanent. Thus we have a *reminiscence* of it, that is, call to mind that we have already been affected in the same manner; a *memory,* or the act of recalling the object of the sensation with some of its attributes, as colour, volume, &c.

When the brain is easily excitable, and, at the same time, accurately preserves impressions received, it possesses the power of representing to itself ideas with all their connexions, and all the accessory circumstances by which they are accompanied, of reproducing them in a certain degree, and of recalling an entire object, while the memory only gives us an idea of its qualities. This creative faculty is called *imagination.* When two ideas are brought together, compared, and their analogy considered, we are said to form a *judgment;* several judgments connected together constitute reasoning. Besides the sensations that are carried from the organs of sense to the brain, there are others, internal, that seem to be transmitted to it by a kind of sympathetic reaction. It is well known what uneasiness the affection of certain organs conveys to the mind, how much an habitual obstruction of the liver is connected with a certain order of ideas; these internal sensations are the origin of our moral faculties, in the same manner as impressions that are conveyed by the organs of sense are the source of intellectual faculties. We are not on that account to place the seat of the passions of the mind in the viscera; it is only necessary to remember that the appetites, whence arise the passions, reside in their respective organs, and are a phenomenon purely physical, while passion consists, at the same time, in the intellectual exertion. Thus an accumulation of semen in the cavities that are employed as a reservoir for it, excites the appetite for venery, very distinct from the passion of love, although it may be frequently the determinate cause of it.

The senses may be enumerated under the following heads, viz. the sense of vision, hearing, smelling, tasting, touching.

SENSIBILITY. *Sensibilitas.* That action of the brain by which we receive impressions, either from within, or from without.

"What is said of sensation generally, is applicable to sensibility; for this reason, we only mention here that this faculty exerts itself in two ways very different. In the first, the phenomena happens, unknown to us; in the second, we are aware of it, we perceive the sensation. It is not enough that a body may act upon one of our senses, that a nerve transmits to the brain the impression which is produced—it is not enough that this organ receive the impression: in order that there may be really a sensation, the brain must perceive the impression received. An impression thus perceived is called, in *Ideology*, a Perception, or an Idea.

These two modes of sensibility may be easily verified upon ourselves. For example, it is easy to see that a number of bodies have a continual action upon our senses without our being aware of it: this depends in a great measure upon habit.

Sensibility is infinitely variable: in certain persons it is very obtuse; in others it is very elevated: generally a good organization keeps between the extremes.

Sensibility is vivid in infancy and youth; it continues in a degree something less marked until past the age of manhood; in old age it suffers an evident diminution; and very old persons appear quite insensible to all the ordinary causes of sensations."

All parts possessed of a power of producing a change, so as to excite a sensation, are called *sensible;* those which are not possessed of this property, *insensible.* To the insensible parts by nature belong all our fluids, the blood, bile, saliva, &c. and many of the solids, the hair, epidermis, nails, &c.; but the sensible parts are the skin, eyes, tongue, ear, nose, muscles, stomach, intestines, &c.

SENSO'RIUM. The organ of any of the senses. See *Cerebrum.*

SENSORIUM COMMUNE. See *Cerebrum.*

SENSUS. (*Sensus, ûs.* m.; *à sentiendo.*) The senses are distinguished into external and internal. The external senses are seeing, hearing, tasting, smelling, and feeling. The internal, imagination, memory, judgment, attention, and the passions.

SENTICOSÆ. (From *sentis,* a brier.) The name of an order of plants in Linnæus's Fragments of a Natural Method, consisting of such as resemble the bramble, rose, &c.

SENTIENT. This term is applied to those parts which are more susceptible of feeling than others, as the sentient extremities of the nerves, &c.

SENTIS CANINUS. (*Sentis,* a thorn; from its being prickly like a thorn.) See *Rosa canina.*

SEPARA'TORIUM. (From *separo,* to separate.) An instrument for separating the pericranium from the skull, and a chemical vessel for separating essential parts of liquids.

SE'PIA. The name of a genus of fish, of the Class, *Vernes;* Order, *Molusca.* The cuttle-fish.

SEPIA OFFICINALIS. *Sepium; Præcipitans magnum.* The cuttle-fish. The systematic name of the fish, the shell of which is a phosphate of lime, and is often mixed into tooth-powders.

SEPIÆ os. See *Sepia officinalis.*

SEPIARIÆ. (From *sepes,* a hedge.) The name of an order of plants in Linnæus's Fragments of a Natural Method, consisting of woody plants, which form a hedge-like appearance; the flowers are mostly a thymus or panicle.

SE'PIUM. See *Sepia officinalis.*

SEPTARIA. *Ludi helmontii.* Spheroidal concretions that vary from a few inches to a foot in diameter. When broken in a longitudinal direction, the interior of the mass is observed intersected by a number of fissures, sometimes empty, sometimes filled with calcareous spar. The body of the concretion is ferruginous marle. From these septaria is manufactured that excellent material for building under water, called Parke's cement, or Roman cement.

Septenary years. Climacteric years. A period, or succession of years in human life, at which, important constitutional changes are supposed to take place; and the end of this period is therefore judged critical. This period is fixed at every seventh year. The grand climacteric is fixed at 63, and, passing that time, age, it is considered, may be protracted to 90. So general is this belief, that the passing of 60 generally gives much anxiety to most people.

SEPTFOIL. See *Tormentilla.*

SEPTIC. (*Septicus;* from σηπω, to putrefy.) Relating to putrefaction.

SEPTIFO'LIA. (From *septem,* seven, and *folium,* a leaf: so named from the number of its leaves.) Coralwort, or septfoil toothwort.

SEPTINE'RVIA. (From *septem,* seven, and *nervus,*

a string: so called from the seven strings upon its leaf. A species of plantain.

SE'PTUM. A partition.

SEPTUM CEREBELLI. A process of the dura mater, dividing the cerebellum perpendicularly into two principal parts.

SEPTUM CEREBRI. The falciform process of the dura mater is sometimes so called. See *Falciform process.*

SEPTUM CORDIS. (*Septum;* from *sepio,* to separate.) The partition between the two ventricles of the heart.

SEPTUM LUCIDUM. *Septum pellucidum.* The thin and tender portion of the brain, dividing the lateral ventricles from each other.

SEPTUM NARIUM. *Interseptum.* The partition between the nostrils.

SEPTUM PALATI. The partition of the palate.

SEPTUM PELLUCIDUM. See *Septum lucidum.*

SEPTUM THORACIS. See *Mediastinum.*

SEPTUM TRANSVERSUM. See *Diaphragm.*

SERA'PIAS. (From *Serapis,* a lascivious idol: so called because it was thought to promote venery; or from the testiculated shape of its roots.) The name of a genus of plants in the Linnæan system. Class, *Gynandria;* Order, *Diandria.*

SERAPI'NUM. The gum-resin sagapenum is sometimes so called. See *Sagapenum.*

SERAPION, of Alexandria, lived about 280 years before Christ, and is affirmed by Celsus to have been the founder of the empiric sect of physicians; though others have attributed the origin of this sect to Philinus.

SERAPION, JOHN, an Arabian physician who lived between the time of Mesue and Rhazes, towards the middle of the ninth century, and is supposed to have been the first writer on physic in the Arabic language. Haly Abbas describes his writings as containing only the cure of diseases, without any precepts concerning the preservation of health, or relating to surgery: and they are frequently quoted by Rhazes. He often transcribes the remarks of Alexander Trallian, with whom the other Arabians appear to be little acquainted. Some confusion appears to exist respecting another Serapion, who is supposed to have lived 180 years later, and to have been the author of a work on the Materia Medica, entitled "De Medicamentistam simplicibus, quam compositis;" in which authors are quoted, much posterior to Rhazes, Avenzoar for instance, so that it must have been written towards the latter part of the eleventh century.

SERICUM. Silk. A species of hairy pubescence of plants, which consists of a white shining silkiness: hence the leaves of the Potentilla anserina, Alchemilla alpina, &c. are called *Folia sericea.*

SERI'PHIUM. (Seems to have been applied to this genus on account of the analogy in its habit and foliage with the *Artemisia pontica* of Pliny, called by the Greeks Σερεφιον. The origin of this name may be traced to *Seriphion,* or, as it is now called, *Serpho,* an island in the Ægean sea, the soil of which is of so dry and sterile a nature, as only to abound in plants of this rough kind.) The name of a genus of plants. Class *Syngenesia;* Order, *Polygamia segregata.*) Flix-weed.

SE'RIS. Σερις. Endive.

SERMOUNTAIN. See *Laserpitium siler.*

SEROUS. (*Serosus;* from *serum.*) Relating to serum.

Serous apoplexy. See *Apoplexia.*

SERPENTA'RIA. (*Serpentaria, e. f.:* so called from the resemblance of the roots of the plant which first bore this name to the tail of the rattle-snake.) See *Aristolochia serpentaria.*

SERPENTARIA GALLORUM. See *Arum dracunculus.*

SERPENTARIA HISPANICA. The viper's grass. See *Scorzonera hispanica.*

SERPENTARIA VIRGINIANA. See *Aristolochia serpentaria.*

SERPENTINE. A hard mineral, of which there are two kinds, the common and precious. The common is of a green colour, and is found in various mountains in Scotland and England. Of the precious, there are two species; the splintery, found in Corsica, and is cut into snuff boxes; and the conchoidal, which is of a leek green colour.

SERPENTUM LIGNUM. See *Ophioxylum serpentinum.*

SERPENTUM RADIX. See *Ophiorrhiza mungos.*

SERPI'GO. (From *serpo,* to creep; because it

creeps on the surface of the skin by degrees.) A ringworm, or tetter. See *Herpes.*

SERPY'LLUM. (From ερπω, to creep, or à *serpendo,* by reason of its creeping nature.) See *Thymus serpyllum.*

SERPYLLUM CITRATUM. See *Thymus serpyllum.*

SERPYLLUM VULGARE MINUS. See *Thymus serpyllum.*

SERRATA. (From *serra,* a saw: so called from its serrated leaves.) See *Serratula.*

SERRA'TULA. (From *serra,* a saw: so called from its serrated leaves.) The name of a genus of plants in the Linnæan system. Class, *Syngenesia;* Order, *Polygamia æqualis.*

SERRATULA AMARA. The systematic name of a species of saw-wort, which is said to cure agues.

SERRATULA ARVENSIS. The common creeping waythistle. *Carduus arvensis; Carduus hæmorrhoidalis; Circium arvense.* This plant was formerly used in an application to resolve scirrhous tumours, and is now considered useful against piles.

SERRA'TUS. (From *serra,* a saw.) Serrated; a botanical term applied to leaves when the teeth are sharp, and resemble those of a saw, pointing towards the extremity of the leaf, as in Urtica; and the *petals* of the Dianthus arboreus, and Cystus polyfolius.

Some leaves are called *duplicato-serrate;* these are doubly serrate, having a series of smaller serratures intermixed with the larger; as in Campanula trachelium.

SERRATUS ANTICUS. See *Pectoralis minor.*

SERRATUS MAGNUS. (So called from its saw-like appearance.) *Serratus major anticus,* of Douglas and Cowper. *Serratus major,* of Winslow; and *Costo basi-scapulaire,* of Dumas. This muscle is so named by Albinus. Douglas calls it *Serratus major anticus,* but improperly, as it is seated at the side, and not at the anterior part of the thorax. It is a broad fleshy muscle, of a very irregular shape, and is in part covered by the subscapularis, pectoralis, and latissimus dorsi. It arises, by fleshy digitations, from the eight superior ribs, and is inserted fleshy into the whole basis of the scapula internally, between the insertion of the rhomboides, and the origin of the sub-scapularis, being folded, as it were, about the two angles of the scapula. This muscle may easily be divided into two and even three portions. The latter division has been adopted by Winslow. The first of these portions is the thick and short part of the muscle that arises from the first and second ribs, and is inserted into the upper angle of the scapula, its fibres ascending obliquely backwards. The second portion arises from the second rib, behind the origin of the first portion, and likewise from the third and fourth ribs; this portion is thin and short, and its fibres run nearly in a horizontal direction, to be inserted into the basis of the scapula. The third, and most considerable portion, is that which arises from the fifth, sixth, seventh, and eighth ribs, and is inserted into the lower angle of the scapula. The serratus magnus serves to move the scapula forwards, and it is chiefly by the contraction of this muscle that the shoulder is supported, when loaded with any heavy weight. The ancients, and even many of the moderns, particularly Douglas and Cowper, supposed its chief use to be to dilate the thorax, by elevating the ribs; but it can only do this when the scapula is forcibly raised.

SERRATUS MAJOR ANTICUS. See *Serratus magnus.*

SERRATUS MINOR ANTICUS. See *Pectoralis minor.*

SERRATUS POSTICUS INFERIOR. *Dorso-lumbo-costal,* of Dumas. This is a thin muscle of considerable breadth, situated at the bottom of the back, under the middle part of the latissimus dorsi. It arises by a broad thin tendon, in common with that of the last-mentioned muscle from the spinous processes of the two, and sometimes of the three inferior dorsal vertebræ, and from three, and sometimes four of those of the lumbar vertebræ. It then becomes fleshy, and, ascending a little obliquely outwards and forwards, divides into three, and sometimes four fleshy slips, which are inserted into the lower edges of the three or four inferior ribs, at a little distance from their cartilages. Its use seems to be to pull the ribs downwards, backwards, and outwards.

SERRATUS SUPERIOR POSTICUS. *Cervici-dorso-costal,* of Dumas. This is a small, flat, and thin muscle, situated at the upper part of the back, immediately under the rhomboideus. It arises, by a broad thin tendon, from the lower part of the ligamentum colli,

from the spinous process of the last vertebræ of the neck, and the two or three uppermost of the back, and is inserted into the second, third, fourth, and sometimes fifth ribs, by as many distinct slips. Its use is to expand the thorax, by pulling the ribs upwards and outwards.

SERRULATUS. Minutely serrate: applied to such saw-like edged leaves which have their teeth very fine; as in Polygonum amphibium.

SERTULA CAMPANA. See *Trifolium melilotus.*

SE'RUM. (From *serus,* late; because it is the remainder of the milk, after its better parts have been taken from it.)

1. Whey.

2. The yellow and somewhat greenish fluid, which separates from the blood when cold and at rest. See *Blood.*

SERUM ALUMINOSUM. Alum whey.

SERUM LACTIS. Whey.

SERVETUS, MICHAEL, was born at Villanueva, in Arragon, in 1509. He first studied the law at Toulouse; but his attention was drawn to theology by the discussions of the reformers; and as he was disposed to carry his dissent from the church of Rome even to a greater length, he judged it prudent to retire into Switzerland, where he published his opinions concerning the Trinity. He afterward went to study physic at Paris, where he took his degree, and then gave mathematical lectures, while he followed the profession of a physician: but having quarrelled with the faculty, and his "Apology" being suppressed by the parliament, he removed to Charlieu, and soon after to Vienna, at the invitation of the archbishop. Here he published a more full account of his religious opinions under a feigned name; but Calvin, the reformer, in whom he had confided, betrayed him to the magistrates, so that he was thrown into prison, from which, however, he escaped. But as he was passing through Geneva, Calvin, whose treachery he did not suspect, procured his arrest, and a charge of blasphemy and heresy to be brought against him; of which, being found guilty, he was cruelly burnt alive in 1553. Servetus is numbered among those anatomists who made the nearest approach to the doctrine of the circulation of the blood: in the work already mentioned, which led to his death, the passage of the blood through the lungs is clearly stated. He was a man of great learning and unfeigned piety, and generally admired for his worth and talents, and the discoveries which he made in medicine, as well as other branches of knowledge.

Service-tree. See *Sorbus aucuparia.*

SESAMOID. (*Os sesamoideum;* from σησαμη, an Indian grain, and ειδος, likeness.) This term is applied to the little bones, which, from their supposed general resemblance to the seeds of the sesamum, are called *Ossa sesamoidea.* They are found at the articulation of the great toes, and sometimes at the joints of the thumbs; now and then we meet with them upon the condyles of the os femoris, at the lower extremity of the fibula, under the os cuboides of the tarsus, &c They do not exist in the fœtus; but as we advance in life, begin first to appear in a cartilaginous state, and, at length, in adult subjects, are completely ossified. Age and hard labour seem to add to the number and size of these bones, and being most commonly found wherever the tendons and ligaments are most exposed to pressure from the action of the muscles, they are now generally considered by anatomists as the ossified parts of tendons and ligaments. These bones are usually smooth and flat on the side of the bone on which they are placed: their upper surface is convex, and, in general, adheres to the tendon that covers it, and of which it may, in some measure, be considered as a part. Although their formation seems to be owing to accidental circumstances; yet, as the two at the first joint of the great toe are much larger than the rest, and are seldom wanting in an adult, it would seem as if these bones were of some utility; perhaps by removing the ten dons farther from the centre of motion, and thus increasing the power of the muscles. The ossa sesamoidea of the great toe and thumb seem likewise to be of use, by forming a groove for lodging the flexor tendons secure from compression.

Sesamoidal bones. See *Sesamoid.*

SE'SAMUM. (An Egyptian word.)

1. The name of a genus of plants in the Linnæan system.

2. The pharmacopœial name of the oriental sesamum. See *Sesamum orientale.*

Sesamum orientale. *Sesamum.* The seeds of this plant are in much esteem in South Carolina, where they are called *oily grain;* they are made into soups and puddings, after the manner of rice. Toasted over the fire, they are mixed with other ingredients, and stewed into a delicious food. The fresh seed affords a considerable quantity of a warm pungent oil, otherwise not unpalatable. In a year or two the pungency leaves it when the oil is used for salad, &c. The seeds of the *Sesamum indicum* are used in the same manner. The leaves are also used medicinally in some countries, being of a mucilaginous quality. [See *Benne seed* and *Benne oil.* A.]

SE'SELI. (Παρα τα σαωσαι ελλον; because it is salutary for young fawns.)

1. The name of a genus of plants. Class, *Pentandria;* Order, *Digynia.*

2. An old name of the hart-wort. See *Laserpitium siler.*

Seseli creticum. There is great confusion among the species of the seseli. The plant which bears this epithet in the pharmacopœias is the *Tordylium officinale,* of Linnæus. The seeds are said to be diuretic.

Seseli massiliense. See *Seseli tortuosum.*

Seseli tortuosum. The systematic name of the hart-wort of Marseilles. *Seseli masiliense.* The seeds of this plant are directed for medicinal use, and have a warm biting taste, and a greater degree of pungency than those of the *Laserpitium.*

SESQUI. This word, joined with any number, weight, measure, &c. signifies one integer and a half; as *sesqui granum,* a grain and a half.

SESSILIS. (*Sessilis,* that sitteth, as it were.) Sessile. This term is applied to many parts of plants, as flowers, leaves, and parts of the fructification, and implies that they are without footstalk, flowerstalk, or what often supports them: hence, *flores sessilis,* as in Centaurea calciptrapa; *folia sessilia,* as in Pinguicula vulgaris; stigma sessile, Tulipa gesneriana, &c.

SETA. (*Seta, œ.* f.; from χαιτα, a bristle.) A. The fruitstalk of mosses, which is either solitary, aggregate, terminal, axillary, or lateral.

B. A bristle, as applied in botanical language to a hollow, rigid, sharp-pointed pubescence, which either wounds the finger when it is pressed upon it, or gives a very harsh scabrous, or prickly character to the surface of the stem, or of the leaves when the finger is rubbed over them.

Bristles are often arranged into *aculei* in elementary works, but they have more affinity to hairs. They are simple and compound.

1. *Setæ simplices* are of two kinds, awl-shaped and spindle-shaped.

a. The *subulate* is the most common of the simple bristles; it is slightly curved, and gradually tapering from the base to the apex, which is rigid and very sharp. These bristles, when they all incline in the same direction, produce the scabrous character of some leaves, as in symphitum orientale. A variety of the awl-shaped bristle, found on the stem and branches of the sensitive plant, is barbed on its sides; and another variety, as exemplified on the leaves of the *Borago officinalis,* is seated on a vesicular tubercle containing a fluid, which is ejected through the bristle when it is compressed, so as to wound the finger, and which being left in the wound excites inflammation in the part. But the sting of the nettle is the best example of this form of bristle.

b. The *fusiform* is, as its name implies, thickest in the centre, and accumulated at each end. It lies parallel to the surface of the leaf, to which it is affixed by a very small footstalk, is hollow, and contains a coloured liquid, which apparently enters it through the footstalk. This form of bristle is peculiar to the genus *Malphigia.*

2. *Setæ compositæ.* These are almost always solid. The term comprehends two species of bristles, *furcatæ* and *fasciculatæ.*

a. The forked are, in some instances, merely rigid hair-like bodies terminating in two or three diverging points, as in *Thrincia hispida:* but in other instances, as the stems and leaves of the hop plant, the stalk of the bristle, which is supported on a firm cellular tubercle, is very short, and its forking extremities resemble two flattish, awl-shaped bristles, pointing in opposite directions.

b. The *fasciculated* consist of a number of simple, straight bristles, diverging from a papillary knob; as in *Cactus flagilliformis.*

There is still another species of pubescence which cannot properly be arranged with the pilus or seta: it is found on a species of house-leek, extending like a very fine thread, stretching from the tip of one leaf to that of another, and resembling so exactly a spider's web, that the plant has been named *Arachnoideum.—Thompson.*

Bristles are also distinguished into *erect,* as in Leontodon hirtum; *hamose,* as in the pericarp of the Arcti cum lappa; *stellate* and *plumose.* The bristles of plants have received other denominations.

1. *Striga,* that variety of the subulate which is seen in Borago officinalis.

2. *Hamus,* that which is hooked at its extremity; as in Galium aperine, Caucalis daucoides, &c.

3. *Glochis* when several sharp tooth-like processes are turned back from the apex of the bristle.

5. *Arista,* a long bristle proceeding from the husk of grasses; as in Hordeum vulgare.

SETACEUM. (From *seta,* a bristle; because horse-hairs were first used to keep open the wound.) A se ton. See *Seton.*

SETACEUS. Bristly. Applied to the petals of Trapæolum majus.

SETIFORMIS. Setiform: bristly. Applied to the nectary, as that of the *Periploea græca.*

SETON. *Setaceum.* An artificial ulcer made under the skin by means of an instrument called the seton needle, which carries with it a portion of thread or silk, that is moved backwards or forwards, and thus keeps up a constant irritation.

SETOSUS. Setose: bristly; applied to the receptacle of the Echynops sphærocephalus, and of Centaurea.

SETTERWORT. See *Helleborous fœtidus.*

SEVERINUS, Marcus Aurelius, was born in Calabria, in 1580. He graduated at Naples, where he became one of the most celebrated professors in anatomy and surgery. He was, however, somewhat harsh in his practice; and in his work, "De Efficaci Medicina," condemned his contemporaries for neglecting the use of the cautery, and of the knife, as practised by the ancients. He died in 1656. Many publications were written by him, evincing much boldness and originality of thought, but too great attachment to paradox. His treatise on abscesses, in eight books, passed through many editions. He paid considerable attention to comparative anatomy, on which subject some of his works are composed.

SE'VUM. Suet. See *Fat.*

Sevum ceti. See *Physeter macrocephalus.*

Sevum ovile. *Sevum ovillum.* Mutton suet.

SEXUAL. Appertaining to the sexes.

Sexual actions. Sexual functions. Those functions proper to each sex, by which the species is propagated, as the excretion of semen in men; menstruation, conception, the evolution of the fœtus, parturition, &c. in women.

Sexual organs. See *Generation, organs of, Sta men,* and *Pistillum.*

Sexual system. See *Plants.*

SEYDSCHUTZ. See *Sedlitz.*

[**SHAD.** See *Clupea alosa.* A.]

SHADDOCK. A variety of orange.

SHALLOT. A species of allium.

SHARP. 1. See *Acutus.*

2. **Samuel,** an able and distinguished surgeon in the middle of the last century, was a pupil of Cheselden, and afterward studied with great zeal at Paris. He is said to have commenced his profession rather late in life; nevertheless, after settling in London, and becoming surgeon to Guy's hospital, his genius and assiduity soon procured him great celebrity and extensive practice. He was elected a Fellow of the Royal Society and a Member of the Academy of Surgery at Paris He contributed to the improvement of his art by two valuable publications, which passed through many editions, and were translated into several foreign languages. The first of these was a "Treatise on the Operations of Surgery," with an Introduction on the Nature and Treatment of Wounds, &c. The other work was entitled "A Critical Inquiry into the present State of Surgery," first printed in 1750.

Sharp-pointed dock. See *Rumex acutus.*

SHAW, PETER, a physician of considerable reputation in the early part of the last century. His first publication was entitled "New Practice of Physic," in two volumes, 1726, containing a brief Description of Diseases, and their Treatment. He then published an "Inquiry into the Virtues of the Scarborough Spa Waters;" and about the same time his "Chemical Lectures," which was deemed a scientific work, and translated into French. He also edited the Edinburgh Dispensatory; and gave to the world some other minor publications.

SHEATH. See *Vagina*; and *Spatha.*

Sheathing leaves. See *Vaginans*

Shedding-teeth. The primary or milk-teeth. See *Teeth.*

SHELL. See *Testæ preparatæ.*

SHERBET. A compound liquor prepared for punch before the spirit is added.

SHINGLES. See *Erysipelas.*

Shistus, argillaceous. Clay-slate.

SHRUB. 1. A low bushy tree.

2. A spirituous liquor composed of the juice of oranges, mixed with brandy and rum.

SI'AGON. Σιαγων. The jaw.

SIAGONA'GRA. (From σιαγων, the jaw, and αγρα, a seizure.) The gout in the jaw.

SIALAGOGUE. (*Sialagogus*; from σιαλον, saliva, and αγω, to expel.) Those medicines are so called, which excite an uncommon flow of saliva: such are mercurial preparations, pyrethrum, &c. They are divided into *sialagoga topica*, as scilla, nicotiana, piper, &c.; and *sialagoga interna*, as the various preparations of mercury.

SIBBENS. A disease resembling syphilis.

SIBERITE. Red tourmaline.

SICCA'NTIA. (From *sicco*, to dry.) Drying medicines.

SICCHA'SIA. (From σικχος, weak, weary.) An unpleasant lassitude and debility peculiar to women with child.

SI'CULA. (Dim. of *sica*, a short sword: so called from its dagger-like root.) The beet.

SICYE'DON. (From σικυος, a cucumber.) A transverse fracture like a cucumber broken in two parts.

SICYO'NE. (From σικυος, a cucumber or gourd: so named from its resemblance to a gourd.) A cucurbit.

SIDERA'TIO. (From *sidus*, a planet; because it was thought to be produced by the influence of the planets.) An apoplexy; a blast; a slight erysipelas.

SIDE'RIUM. (From σιδηρος, iron.) An herb so called from its supposed virtues in healing wounds made by iron instruments.

SIDERUM. Phosphuret of iron.

SIENITE. Syenite. A compound granular aggregated rock, composed of felspar and hornblende, and sometimes quartz and black mica. The hornblende is the characteristic ingredient, and distinguishes it perfectly from granite, with which it is often confounded; but the felspar, which is almost always red, and seldom inclines to green, forms the most abundant and essential ingredient of the rock. Some varieties contain a very considerable portion of quartz and mica, but little hornblende. This is particularly the case with the Egyptian varieties, and hence these are often confounded with real granite.

SIGESBE'CKIA. (So named by Linnæus himself, in memory of his antagonist, Dr. J. G. Siegesbeck, Superintendent of the Physic Garden at Petersburgh, who raised various objections against the sexes of plants.) The name of a genus of plants, Class, *Syngenesia*; Order, *Polygamia superflua.*

SIGESBECKIA ORIENTALIS. The systematic name of a plant which is said to be useful in removing strangury, and in calculous diseases, gout, and fluor albus.

SIGHT. See *Vision.*

SIGILLA'TA TERRA. Sealed earth; a species of bolar earth made into cakes.

SIGI'LLUM. (Diminutive of *signum*, a sign.)

SIGILLUM BEATÆ MARIÆ. Black briony, or *Tamus communis.*

SIGILLUM HERMETICUM. An hermetic seal, made by closing the end of a glass tube by melting it.

SIGILLUM SOLOMONIS. (Called Solomon's seal, because it has upon its root the resemblance of an impression made by a seal.) See *Convallaria polygonatum.*

SIGMOID. (*Sigmoides*; from the Greek letter σιγμα, anciently written C, and ειδος, a likeness.) Resembling the Greek letter sigma. Applied to several parts, as the valves of the heart, the cartilages of the trachea, the semilunar apophysis of the bones, and the flexure or turn of the colon.

SIGMOIDE'A FLEXURA. The sigmoid flexure, or turn of the colon.

SIGMOI'DES PROCESSUS. Valves of the heart.

SIGNA CRITICA. Signs of the crisis of disease.

SIGNA DIAGNOSTICA. Diagnostic or distinguishing signs.

SI'GNUM. A sign: applied to symptoms. See *Semiotice.*

SI'LER MONTANUM. Common hartwort. See *Laserpitium siler.*

[SILEX, RESINITE. See *Halb-opal.* A.]

SI'LICA. (*Selag*, Hebrew.) *Silex.* One of the primitive earths is the principal constituent part of a very great number of the compound earths and stones forming the immense mass of the solid nucleus of the globe. It is the basis of almost all the scintillating stones, such as *flint, rock crystal, quartz, agate, calcedony, jasper*, &c. The sand of rivers, and of the seashore, chiefly consist of it. It is deposited in vegetable substances forming petrified wood, &c. It is likewise precipitated from certain springs in a stalactical form. It has been discovered in several waters in a state of solution, and is found in many plants, particularly grasses and equisetums. Professor Davy has proved that it forms a part of the epidermis of these vegetables. It is never met with absolutely pure in nature.

Properties.—Silica, when perfectly pure, exists in the form of a white powder. It is insipid and inodorous. It is rough to the touch, cuts glass, and scratches or wears away metals. Its specific gravity is about 2.66. It is unalterable by the simple combustible bodies. When mixed with water it does not form a cohesive mass. Its moleculæ, when diffused in water, are precipitated with the utmost facility. It is not acted on by any acid, except the fluoric. When in a state of extreme division it is soluble in alkalies; fused with them it forms glass. It melts with the phosphoric and boracic acids. It is unchangeable in the air, and unalterable by oxygen and the rest of the gaseous fluids. It has been considered as insoluble in water, but it appears when in a state of extreme division to be soluble in a minute quantity.

Method of obtaining Silex.—Silex may be obtained, tolerably pure, from flints, by the following process: Procure some common gun-flints; expose them in a crucible to a red heat, and then plunge them into cold water; by this treatment they will become brittle, and easily reducible to powder. Mix them, when pulverized, with three or four times their weight of carbonate of potassa, and let the mixture be fused, in a dull red heat, in a silver crucible. We shall thus obtain a compound of alkali and silex, called silicious potassa. Dissolve this compound in water, filter the solution, and add to it dilute sulphuric or muriatic acid. An immediate precipitation now ensues, and as long as this continues, add fresh portions of acid. Let the precipitate subside; pour off the fluid that floats above it; and wash the precipitate with hot water till it comes off tasteless. This powder when dry is silica.

In this process the acid added to the solution of flint unites to the potassa, and forms sulphate or nitriate of potassa; the silicious earth is therefore precipitated.

It is necessary to add an excess of acid, in order that all the foreign earths which are present may be separated.

If the solution of flints be diluted with a great quantity of water, as for instance, in the proportion of 24 parts to one, and in this state an acid be poured upon it, no perceptible precipitation will ensue; the silex continues suspended in the fluid, and is invisible on account of its transparency; but it may be made to appear by evaporating part of the water.

The solution of flint, on account of its affinity with the carbonic acid, is also in course of time decomposed by mere contact with air.

Another method of obtaining silica exceedingly pure is to separate it from fluoric acid. In consequence of Sir H. Davy's researches on the metallic bases of the alkalies and earths, this earth has been recently regarded as a compound of a peculiar combustible principle with oxygen. If we ignite powdered quartz with three parts of pure potassa in a silver crucible, dissolve the fused compound in water, add to the solution a quantity of acid, equivalent to saturate the alkali, and evaporate to dryness, we shall obtain a fine gritty powder, which being well washed with hot water, and ignited, will leave pure silica. By passing the vapour of potassium over silica in an ignited tube, Sir H. Davy obtained a dark-coloured powder, which apparently contained silicon, or silicium, the basis of the earth. Like boron and carbon, it is capable of sustaining a high temperature without suffering any change.

SILICON. The base of silica.

SILICULA. A pouch, or pod, that is scarcely longer than it is broad. It is,

1. *Orbiculate*, in *Thlaspi arvense.*
2. *Cordate*, in *Isatis armena.*
3. *Obcordate*, in *Thlaspi bursæ partoris, alpestre,* and *Myagrum perfoliatum.*
4. *Lanceolate*, in *Lepedium alpinum,* and *Isatis tinctoria.*
5. *Angulate*, in *Myagrum ægyptiacum.*
6. *Emarginate*, in *Alyssum,* and *Cochlearia.*
7. *Drupaceous*, if the membrane is double, soft externally, and hard within; as in *Erucago* and *Bunias.*

SILIGO. Σιλιγνις. Fine wheat or rye.

SI'LIQUA. (From *silo*, a nose turned up, a hooked nose.) A long, dry, membranaceous pericarpium, or seed-vessel, of two valves, separated by a linear receptacle, along the edges of each of which, the seeds are arranged alternately. The dissepiment is a partition dividing a siliqua and silicula into two loculaments, or cells. Botanists distinguish,

1. The *round* pod in *Fumaria lutea,* and *Cheiranthus tricus pidatus.*
2 The *compressed*, with level valves, in *Cheiranthus annuus.*
3. The *four-edged*, in *Erysimum; Cheiranthus erysimoides,* and *Brassica orientalis.*
4. *Articulate*, in *Raphanus raphanistrum.*
5. The *tortulose*, which has elevated nodes here and there, in *Raphanus sativus.*
6. *Rostra te*, having the partition very prominent at the apex; as in *Sinapis alba.*

SILIQUA DULCIS. See *Ceratonia siliqua.*

SILIQUA HIRSUTA. See *Dolichos pruriens.*

SILIQUA'STRUM. (From *siliqua*, a pod: named from its pods.) Judas-tree The Capsicum, or Guinea-pepper, was so termed by Pliny. See *Capsicum.*

SILIQUO'SÆ. (From *siliqua*, a pod.) *Cruciformis.* The name of an order of plants in Linnæus's Fragments of a Natural Method, consisting of such as have a siliqua or silicula, the flower tetradynamous and cruciate.

SOLIQUOSA INDICA. An American plant; its juice is alexipharmic.

SILK-WORM. See *Bombyx.*

Silk-worm, acid of. See *Bombic acid.*

SI'LPHIUM. (*Zalaph*, Arabian.) Asafœtida, or the plant which affords it.

SILVER. *Argentum.* This metal is found both native and mineralized, and combined with lead, copper, mercury, cobalt, sulphur, arsenic, &c. The principal ores of this metal are the following: *Native silver; antimoniated silver; sulphuret of silver; sulphuretted oxide of silver* and *antimony; muriate of silver; native oxide of silver,* &c. It is found in different parts of the earth. The mines of the Erzgebürge or the metalliferous rocks of Mexico and Potosi, Bohemia, Norway, Transylvania, &c. are the richest.

Native silver possesses all the properties of this metal, and it appears in series of octahedra inserted in one another; in small capillary flexible threads intwined together; in plates; or in masses. The colour of native silver is white, often tarnished. Silver alloyed with gold forms the *auriferous native silver ore.* The colour of this ore is a yellowish white. It has much metallic lustre. The *antimoniated silver ore* belongs to this class. Silver, combined with antimony, forms the *sulphuretted oxide of silver,* or *vitreous silver ore.* This ore occurs in masses, sometimes in threads, and sometimes crystallized in cubes or regular octahedra. Its colour is dark bluish gray, inclined to black. Its fracture is uneven, and its lustre metallic. It is soft enough to be cut with a knife. It is sometimes found alloyed with antimony (gray silver ore). Silver united with muriatic acid forms the *corneous silver ore*

(*muriate of silver*), which appears under different colours and shapes. Silver united to oxygen constitutes the *caliform silver ore,* of which there are several varieties. The colour of these ores is a lead gray, or grayish black. They occur massive, disseminated, and crystallized.

Germany, and other countries of Europe, but more especially Peru and Mexico in South America, contain the principal silver mines. There are, however, silver mines in Ireland, Norway, France, and many other parts in the world.

Method of obtaining silver.—Different methods are employed in different countries to extract silver from its ores. In Mexico, Peru, &c. the mineral is pounded, roasted, washed, and then triturated with mercury in vessels filled with water. A mill is employed to keep the whole in agitation. The silver combines by that means with the mercury. The alloy thus obtained is afterward washed, to separate any foreign matters from it, and then strained and pressed through leather This being done, heat is applied to drive off the mercury from the silver, which is then melted and cast into bars or ingots.

In order to extract silver from sulphuretted or vitreous silver ore, the mineral is roasted, and then melted with lead and borax, or some other flux to assist the fusion. By the first operation the sulphur is volatilized, and by the second the silver is obtained, though for the most part alloyed with other metals, from which it is separated by cupellation, or fusion with lead or bismuth.

"Silver is the whitest of all metals, considerably harder than gold, very ductile and malleable, but less malleable than gold; for the continuity of its parts begins to break when it is hammered out into leaves of about the hundred and sixty thousandth of an inch thick, which is more than one-third thicker than gold leaf; in this state it does not transmit the light. Its specific gravity is from 10.4 to 10.5. It ignites before melting, and requires a strong heat to fuse it. The heat of common furnaces is insufficient to oxidize it: but the heat of the most powerful burning lenses vitrifies a portion of it, and causes it to emit fumes, which when received on a plate of gold, are found to be silver in the metallic state. It has likewise been partly oxidized by twenty successive exposures to the heat of the porcelain furnace at Sevres. By passing a strong electric shock through a silver wire, it may be converted into a black oxide; and by a powerful galvanic battery, silver leaf may be made to burn with a beautiful green light. Lavoisier oxidized it by the blow-pipe and oxygen gas; and a fine silver wire burns in the kindled united stream of oxygen and hydrogen gases. The air alters it very little, though it is disposed to obtain a thin purple or black coating from the sulphureous vapours which are emitted from animal substances, drains, or putrifying matters. This coating, after a long series of years, has been observed to scale off from images of silver exposed in churches; and was found, on examination, to consist of silver united with sulphur.

There seems to be only one oxide of silver, which is formed either by intense ignition in an open vessel, when an olive-coloured glass is obtained; or by adding a solution of caustic barytes to one of the nitrate of silver, and heating the precipitate to dull redness. Sir H. Davy found that 100 of silver combined with 7.3 of oxygen in the above oxide; and if we suppose it to consist of a prime equivalent of each constituent, we shall have 13.7 for the prime of silver. Silver leaf burned with a voltaic battery, affords the same olive-coloured oxide.

Silver combines with chlorine, when the metal is heated in contact with the gas. This chloride is, however, usually prepared by adding muriatic acid or a muriate, to nitrate of silver. It has been long known by the name of *luna-cornea,* or *horn silver,* because though a white powder, as it falls down from the nitrate solution, it fuses at a moderate heat, and forms a horny-looking substance when it cools. It consists of 13.875 silver + 4.5 chlorine.

The sulphuret of silver is a brittle substance, of a black colour and metallic lustre. It is formed by heating to redness thin plates of silver stratified with sulphur. It consists of 13.875 silver + 2 sulphur.

Silver is soluble in the sulphuric acid when concentrated and boiling, and the metal in a state of division,

The muriatic acid does not act upon it, but the nitric acid, if somewhat diluted, dissolves it with great rapidity, and with a plentiful disengagement of nitrous gas ; which, during its extrication, gives a blue or green colour to the acid, and entirely disappears if the silver made use of be pure; if it contain copper, the solution remains greenish ; and if the acid contain either sulphuric or muriatic acid, these combine with a portion of the silver, and form scarcely soluble compounds, which fall to the bottom. If the silver contain gold, this metal separates in blackish-coloured flocks.

The nitric acid dissolves more than half its weight of silver; and the solution is very caustic, that is to say, it destroys and corrodes animal substances very powerfully.

The solution of silver, when fully saturated, deposites thin crystals as it cools, and also by evaporation. These are called *lunar nitre*, or *nitrate of silver*. A gentle heat is sufficient to fuse them, and drive off their water of crystallization. In this situation the nitrate, or rather subnitrate, for the heat drives off part of the acid, is of a black colour, may be cast into small sticks in a mould, and then forms the lapis infernalis, or lunar caustic used in surgery. A stronger heat decomposes nitrate of silver, the acid flying off, and the silver remaining pure. It is obvious that, for the purpose of forming the lunar caustic, it is not necessary to suffer the salt to crystallize, but that it may be made by evaporating the solution of silver at once to dryness; and as soon as the salt is fused, and ceases to boil, it may be poured out. The nitric acid driven off from nitrate of silver is decomposed, the products being oxygen and nitrogen.

The *sulphate of silver*, which is formed by pouring sulphuric acid into the nitric solution of silver, is sparingly soluble in water : and on this account forms crystals, which are so small, that they compose a white powder. The muriatic acid precipitates from nitric acid the saline compound called *luna-cornea*, or hornsilver ; which has been so distinguished, because, when melted and cooled, it forms a semitransparent and partly flexible mass, resembling horn. It is supposed that a preparation of this kind has given rise to the accounts of malleable glass. This effect takes place with aqua regia, which acts strongly on silver, but precipitates it in the form of muriate, as fast as it is dissolved.

If any salt with base of alkali, containing the muriatic acid, be added to the nitric solution of silver, the same effect takes place by double affinity; the alkaline base uniting with the nitric acid, and the silver falling down in combination with the muriatic acid.

Sulphur combines very easily with silver, if thin plates imbedded in it, be exposed to a heat sufficient to melt the sulphur. The sulphuret is of a deep violet colour, approaching to black, with a degree of metallic lustre, opake, brittle, and soft. It is more fusible than silver, and this in proportion to the quantity of sulphur combined with it. A strong heat expels part of the sulphur.

Sulphuretted hydrogen soon tarnishes the surface of polished silver, and forms on it a thin layer of sulphuret.

The alkaline sulphurets combine with it by heat, and form a compound, soluble in water. Acids precipitate sulphuret of silver from this solution.

Phosphorus left in a nitric solution of silver, becomes covered with the metal in a dendritic form. By boiling this becomes first white, then a light black mass, and is ultimately converted into a light brown phosphuret. The best method of forming a phosphuret of silver is Pelletier's, which consists in mixing phosphoric acid and charcoal with the metal, and exposing the mixture to heat.

Most metallic substances precipitate silver in the metallic state from its solution.

Silver unites with gold by fusion, and forms a pale alloy, as has been already mentioned in treating of that metal. With platina it forms a hard mixture, rather yellower than silver itself, and of difficult fusion.

Silver very readily combines with mercury. A very sensible degree of heat is produced, when silver leaf and mercury are kneaded together in the palm of the hand. With lead it forms a soft mass, less sonorous than pure silver. With copper it becomes harder and more sonorous, at the same time that it remains sufficiently ductile: this mixture is used in the British

288

coinage. 12½ parts of silver, alloyed with one of copper, form the compound called standard silver. The mixture of silver and iron has been little examined. With tin it forms a compound, which, like that of gold with the same metal, has been said to be brittle, however small the proportion ; though there is probably as little foundation for the assertion in the one case as in the other. With bismuth, arsenic, zinc, and antimony, it forms brittle compounds. It does not unite with nickel. The compound of silver and tungsten, in the proportion of two of the former to one of the latter, was extended under the hammer during a few strokes ; but afterward split in pieces.

The uses of silver are well known : it is chiefly applied to the forming of various utensils for domestic use, and as the medium of exchange in money. Its disposition to assume a black colour by tarnishing, and its softness, appear to be the chief objection to its use in the construction of graduated instruments for astronomical and other purposes, in which a good white metal would be a desirable acquisition. The nitrate of silver, besides its great use as a caustic, has been employed as a medicine."

SILVER-WEED. See *Potentilla anserina.*

SIMAROU'BA. (A patronymic name of America.) See *Quassia simarouba.*

SI'MIÆ LAPIS. See *Bezoar simiæ.*

Simple affinity. See *Affinity simple.*

Simple attraction. See *Affinity simple.*

Simple leaf. See *Leaf.*

Simple substance. See *Element.*

S'IMPLEX. Simple: applied very generally in every department of nature to designate that which is not compound.

SIMPLEX OCULUS. A bandage for the eye.

SINAPE. See *Sinapis.*

SINAPELÆ'UM. (From σιναπι, mustard, and ελαιον, oil.) Oil of mustard.

SINA'PI. See *Sinapis.*

SINA'PIS. (Οτι σινει τους ωπας, because it hurts the eyes.) 1. The name of a genus of plants in the Linnæan system. Class, *Tetradynamia ;* Order, *Siliquosa.* Mustard.

2. The pharmacopœial name of the black mustard See *Sinapis nigra.*

SINAPIS ALBA. The systematic name of the white mustard plant, which is directed for medicinal use in the Edinburgh pharmacopœia. It is somewhat less pungent than the black species. See *Sinapis nigra.*

SINAPIS NIGRA. The systematic name of the common black mustard. *Napus ; Eruca ; Sinape ; Sinapi.* Common black mustard. *Sinapis—siliquis glabris racemo appressis,* of Linnæus. The seeds of this species of mustard, which are directed by the London College, and those of the *Sinapis alba,* which are preferred by that of Edinburgh, manifest no remarkable difference to the taste, nor in their effects, and therefore, answer equally well for medicinal and culinary purposes. They have an acrid pungent taste and, when bruised, this pungency shows its volatility by powerfully affecting the organs of smell. Mustard is considered as capable of promoting appetite, assisting digestion, attenuating viscid juices, and, by stimulating the fibres, it proves a general remedy in paralytic affections. Joined to its stimulant qualities, it frequently, if taken in considerable quantity, opens the body, and increases the urinary discharge, and hence it has been found useful in dropsical complaints. Externally, flower of mustard is frequently used mixed with vinegar, as a stimulant or sinapism.

SINAPI'SMUS. *Sinapismum ; Cataplasma sinapios.* A sinapism or mustard poultice. A term given to a mixture of mustard and vinegar in form of poultice, generally applied to the calves of the legs, or soles of the feet, as a stimulant, and employed in low states of fevers and other diseases, and intended to supercede the use of a blister. See *Cataplasma sinapis.*

SINA'PIUM. (From σιναπι, mustard.) An infusion or decoction of mustard-seed.

SI'NCIPUT. The forepart of the head. See *Caput.*

SI'NE PARI. Several muscles, veins, arteries, &c. are so called which are without a fellow. See *Azygos.*

Single elective attraction. See *Affinity simple.*

SINGU'LTUS. *Lygmos.* The hiccough. A convulsive motion of the diaphragm and parts adjacent.

SINUATUS. Sinuated : applied to leaves which

are cut into rounded or wide openings; as in *Statice sinuata.*

SI'NUS. 1. A cavity or depression.

2. In surgery it means a long, narrow, hollow track, leading from some abscess, diseased bone, &c.

3. The veins of the dura mater are termed sinuses. They are several in number, the principal of which are, 1. The *longitudinal sinus*, which rises anteriorly from the crista galli, ascends and passes between the two laminæ of the falciform process to where this process ends. It then opens into, 2. *Two lateral sinuses*, distinguished into right and left, which lie in the crucial spine of the os occipitis: 3. The *inferior longitudinal*, which is a small sinus situated at the acute inferior margin of the falx.

Sinus coxæ. The acetabulum.

Sinus genæ pituitarius. See *Antrum of Highmore.*

Sinus lateral. See *Lateral sinuses.*

Sinus longitudinalis. See *Longitudinal sinus.*

Sinus maxillaris. See *Antrum of Highmore.*

Sinus muliebris. The vagina.

Sinus venæ portarum. The entrance into the liver.

SI'PHILIS. See *Syphilis.*

SIPHO'NIA. (From σιφων, a pipe; alluding to the uses made of the exudation of the tree, called Indian rubber.) The name of a genus of plants in the Linnæan system. Class, *Monœcia;* Order, *Monadelphia.*

Siphonia elastica. The systematic name of the elastic resin-tree. See *Caoutchouc.*

SIRI'ASIS. (From σιρος, a cavity.) An inflammation of the brain peculiar to children, and attended with a hollowness of the eyes and depression of the fontanella.

Si'rium myrtifolium. The systematic name of the tree which is supposed by some to afford the yellow saunders. See *Santalum album.*

SI'SARUM. (*Sisa*, Hebrew.) Siser or skirret. See *Sium sisarum.*

SI'SER. See *Sium sisarum.*

SI'SON. (Σισων. A name adopted by Dioscorides.) The name of a genus of plants. Class, *Pentandria,* Order, *Monogynia.*

Sison ammi. The systematic name of the plant which affords the ammi verum of the shops. The seeds of this plant, *Sison—foliis tripinnatis, radicalibus linearibus, caulinis setaceis stipularibus longioribus,* of Linnæus, have a grateful smell, somewhat like that of origanum, and were formerly administered as a carminative.

SISY'MBRIUM. (From σισυβος, *fringe:* so named from its fringed roots.) The name of a genus of plants in the Linnæan system. Class, *Tetradynamia;* Order, *Siliquosa.*

Sisymbrium nasturtium. The systematic name of the water-cress. *Nasturtium aquaticum; Laver odoratum; Cratevæ sium; Cressi; Cardumines.* Watercress. This indigenous plant, *Sisymbrium—siliquis declinatis, foliis pinnatis, foliolis subcordatis,* of Linnæus, grows plentifully in brooks and stagnant waters. The leaves have a moderately pungent taste, emit a quick penetrating smell, like that of mustardseed, but much weaker. Water-cresses obtain a place in the Materia Medica, for their antiscorbutic qualities, which have been long very generally acknowledged by physicians. The most pleasant way of administering them is in form of a salad.

Sisymbrium sophia. The systematic name of the herb sophia. *Sophia chirurgorum.* This plant is now almost banished from practice. It was formerly in high estimation in the cure of wounds. It has been given internally in hysterical affections and uterine hæmorrhages, and the seeds are said to be efficacious in destroying intestinal worms.

SITIOLOGY. (*Sitiologia:* from σιγος, aliment, and λογος, a discourse or treatise.) A doctrine or treatise on aliment.

SI'UM. (From σειω, to move; from its agitation in water. 1. The name of a genus of plants in the Linnæan system. Class, *Pentandria;* Order, *Digynia.*

2. The pharmacopœial name of the creeping waterparsnip.

Sium aromaticum. The amomum is sometimes so called.

Sium ninsi. The systematic name of the plant, the root of which is called *radix ninsi; Ninzin: Nindsin.*

This root was long supposed to be the same as ginseng. It now appears, however, to be the produce of this plant. It possesses similar, though weaker properties, than ginseng.

Sium nodiflorum. The systematic name of the creeping water-parsnip. This plant was admitted into the London pharmacopœia in the character of an antiscorbutic. It is not nauseous, and children take it readily if mixed with milk.

Sium sisarum. The siser or skirret. The root of this plant is eatable, but now out of use, though cultivated in the days of Gerarde and Parkinson. Its flavour is said to be aromatic, with a sweetness not acceptable to every palate, and of a flatulent and indigestible quality.

SKELETON. (*Sceletus*, from σκελλω, to dry.) Sceleton. When the bones of the body are preserved in their natural situation, and deprived of the flesh, the assemblage is called a skeleton. See *Bone.*

Skeleton, artificial. The assemblage of all the bones of the animal, when hung in their respective situations by means of wire. See *Bone.*

Skeleton, natural. A skeleton is so termed in opposition to an artificial one, when the bones are retained in their proper places by means of their natural ligaments.

SKIN. Δερμις. *Pellis; Cutis.* The skin, though apparently a simple membrane, is in reality laminated, consisting of several subdivisions; the outermost lamina is termed with us scarf skin, or cuticle; the second has no English name, is known only to anatomists, and is called *rete mucosum.* After these two are removed, we come to, as is commonly thought, the surface of the skin itself.

When a blister has been applied to the skin of a negro, if it has not been very stimulating, in twelve hours after a thin transparent grayish membrane is raised, under which we find a fluid. This membrane is the cuticle or scarf skin. When this, with the fluid, is removed, the surface under them appears black; but if the blister had been very stimulating, another membrane, in which this black colour resides, would also have been raised with the cuticle. This is the rete mucosum, which is itself double, consisting of another gray transparent membrane, and of a black web, very much resembling the *nigrum pigmentum* of the eye. When this membrane is removed, the surface of the true skin (as has hitherto been believed) comes in view, and is white, like that of a European. The *rete mucosum* gives the colour to the skin; is black in the Negro; white, brown, or yellowish, in the European. The reason why this membrane is black in the Negro, is, perhaps, that his body may be better able to defend itself against the sun's rays, and that the heat may be prevented from penetrating. The intention of a similar membrane behind the retina in the eye, appears to be not only that of absorbing the superfluous rays of light, but, like the *amalgam* behind the looking-glass, it may enable the retina to reflect the rays, in order to perfect vision. It is not very improbable that some such purpose, as enabling the cuticle to reflect the sun's rays in those warm climates, where the inhabitants originally go naked, may be the intention of nature, in giving them the black membrane. Perhaps, too, the circumstance of the countenance becoming brown, when exposed to the sun's rays in summer, in our own climate, may be a process of nature to defend herself against the access of external heat into the body.

Both cuticle and *rete mucosum* send innumerable processes into the pores of the true skin. The process of the *rete mucosum* is always within that of the cuticle, and in contact with the sides of the pore, as formed by the true skin. These processes are remarkable in the cuticle and *rete mucosum* of the elephant, some of them are almost an inch long; the cuticle, or *rete mucosum* or a membrane very similar, having the same properties with these, appears to be also continued into the inside of the mouth, over the tongue, internal surface of the lungs, œsophagus, stomach, and intestinal tube. In most of the last-named parts, the cuticle, however, forms sheaths for *villi,* and not processes which line pores. On viewing the surface of the skin, even with the naked eye, we find it porous; more so in some places than in others; and the pores are also larger in some parts than others. Some of these pores are ducts of sebaceous glands, and others serve not only to transmit hairs, but, it is supposed, the greatest part of the per

spirable matter itself. Absorption on the skin also, in all probability, begins on the sides of these pores. They are particularly remarkable about the mouth, nose, palms of the hands, soles of the feet, external ear, scalp, *mons veneris*, and around the nipple in women.

The skin itself was given to man not only for feeling in a general sense, but for perspiration, absorption, and particularly for *touch*, in which he excels all other animals, and which resides principally in the *tips of the fingers*. He was intended for examining, reasoning, forming a judgment, and acting accordingly; he was fitted by this sense to examine accurately the properties of surrounding bodies, not capable of being examined by his other senses. This, among other reasons, was one why he was made erect, that the point of his fingers should not be made callous, or less sensible, *by walking on them*.

When carefully dissected off and separated from all adventitious matter in a middle-sized man, the skin weighs about four pounds and a half.

The skin of human bodies is always of a white colour, in the dead body, let the colour of the *rete mucosum* be what it may; it is extremely full of pores, and extremely vascular; a child in full vigour comes into the world from this circumstance, *scarlet*; it is endowed with intense sensibility. Almost all the pain, in the different operations of surgery, is past when we have divided the skin. Some parts of the skin have more feeling than others; the lips, for example, as Haller says, "*ad basia destinata*." The *glans clitoridis*, and the *glans penis*, with a similar intention; there, though the nerves are not so large as in some other parts, they are longer, more numerous, and endowed with more exquisite feeling; but where the common offices of life merely are intended, the marks of superior feeling or touch, in the skin, are the projections, above the common surface, of those packets of arteries, veins, and absorbents, called *villi*. The nerves are there not only also longer, but larger, as in the points of the fingers and toes.

We are not certain that the skin is muscular, but it has properties very like those of muscle; it contracts, relaxes, and even vibrates in some places, on certain occasions. It is extremely distensible; the skin of the *perinæum* has stretched in labour from a quarter of an inch to six inches. It is also extremely elastic, and instantly after labour has returned again to the original quarter of an inch; it is thickest on those parts intended by nature to bear weight or pressure; of course it is thickest on the back, on the soles of the feet, and palms of the hands. It is thinner on the forepart of the body, on the insides of the arms and legs, and where its surfaces touch opposite surfaces. It is extremely thin on the lips, and allows the colour of the blood to shine through it. It is also extremely thin on the *glans penis* in men, *glans clitoridis* in women, and on the inside of the *labia pudendi*. Skin dried and dressed is extremely strong and durable, and therefore employed in making harness for horses, clothing for men, and a variety of other purposes.

Skin, scarf. See *Cuticle*, and *Skin.*

SKINK. See *Scincus.*

SKORODITE. An arsenate of iron, without copper, of a green colour, found in quartz and hornstone in primitive rocks in Saxony.

SKULL. *Cranium.* The skull, or that bony box which contains the brain. It forms the forehead, and every part of the head, except the face. It consists of eight bones, namely, one os frontis, one os occipitis, one os sphenoides, one os ethmoideum, two ossa temporalia, and two ossa parietalia.

[SKUNK CABBAGE. See *Dracontium.* A.]

Slaters. See *Oniscus asellus.*

SLEEP. *Somnus.* That state of the body in which the internal and external senses and voluntary motions are not exercised. The end and design of sleep is both to renew, during the silence and darkness of the night, the vital energy which has been exhausted through the day, and to assist nutrition.

"When the time of being awake has continued for sixteen or eighteen hours, we have a general feeling of fatigue and weakness; our motions become more difficult, our senses lose their activity, the mind becomes confused, receives sensations indistinctly, and governs muscular contraction with difficulty. We recognise, by these signs, the necessity of *sleep*; we choose such a position as can be preserved with little effort; we

seek obscurity and silence, and sink into the arms of oblivion. The man who slumbers loses successively the use of his senses. The sight first ceases to act by the closing of the eyelids, the smell becomes dormant only after the taste, the hearing after the smell, and the touch after the hearing: the muscles of the limbs, being relaxed, cease to act before those that support the head, and these before those of the spine. In proportion as these phenomena proceed, the respiration becomes slower and more deep; the circulation diminishes; the blood proceeds in greater quantity to the head; animal heat sinks; the different secretions become less abundant. Man, although plunged in this sopor, has not, however, lost the feeling of his existence; he is conscious of most of the changes that happen in him, and which are not without their charms; ideas, more or less incoherent, succeed each other in his mind; he ceases, finally, to be sensible of existence: he is *asleep.*

During sleep, the circulation and respiration are retarded, as well as the different secretions, and, in consequence, digestion becomes less rapid.

I know not on what foundation the most part of authors say that absorption alone acquires more energy. Since the nutritive functions continue in sleep, it is evident that the brain has ceased to act, only with regard to muscular contraction, and as an organ of intelligence; and that it continues to influence the muscles of respiration, the heart, the arteries, the secretions, and nutrition.

Sleep is *profound* when strong excitants are necessary to arrest it; it is *light* when it ceases easily.

Sleep, such as it has been described, is perfect, that is, it results from the suspension of the action of the relative organs of life, and from the diminution of the action of the nutritive functions; but it is not extraordinary for some of the relative organs of life to preserve their activity during sleep, as it happens when one sleeps standing; it is also frequent for one or more of the senses to remain awake, and transmit the impressions which it perceives to the brain; it is still more common for the brain to take cognizance of different internal sensations that are developed during sleep, as wants, desires, pain, &c. The understanding itself may be in exercise in man during sleep, either in an irregular and incoherent manner, as in most dreams, or in a consequent and regular manner, as it happens in some persons happily organized.

The turn which the ideas assume during sleep, or the nature of dreams, depends much on the state of the organs. If the stomach is overcharged with indigested food, the respiration difficult on account of position, or other causes, dreams are painful, fatiguing; if hunger is felt, the person dreams of eating agreeable food; if it is the venereal appetite, the dreams are erotic, &c. The character of dreams is no less influenced by habitual occupations of the mind; the ambitious dream of success or disappointment, the poet makes verses, the lover sees his mistress, &c. It is because the judgment is sometimes correctly exercised in dreams, with regard to future events, that in times of ignorance the gift of divination was attributed to them.

Nothing is more curious in the study of sleep than the history of *sleep-walkers.*

Those individuals being first profoundly asleep, rise all at once, dress themselves, see, hear, speak, employ their hands with ease, perform certain exercises, write, compose, then go to bed, and preserve, when they awake, no recollection of what happened to them. What difference is there, then, between a sleep-walker of this kind, and a man awake? A very evident difference,—the one is conscious of his existence, and the other is not.

Many hypotheses have been offered on the proximate cause of sleep, as the depression of the laminæ of the cerebrum, the afflux of blood to the brain, &c. Sleep, which is the immediate effect of the laws of organization, cannot depend on any physical cause of this kind. Its regular return is one of the circumstances that contributes the most to the preservation of health; its suppression, even for a short time, is often attended with serious inconvenience; and in no case can it be carried beyond certain limits.

The ordinary duration of sleep is variable; generally, it is from six to eight hours. Fatigue of the muscular system, strong exertions of the mind, lively and mulnplied sensations, prolong it, as well as habits of idleness, the immoderate use of wine, and of too strong aliments. Infancy and youth, whose life of relation is very active, have need of longer repose. Riper age, more frugal of time, and tortured with cares, devotes to it but a small portion. Very old people present two opposite modifications; either they are almost always slumbering, or their sleep is very light; but the reason of this latter is not to be found in the foresight they have of their approaching end.

By uninterrupted peaceable sleep, restrained within proper limits, the powers are restored, and the organs recover the facility of action; but if sleep is troubled by disagreeable dreams, and painful impressions, or even prolonged beyond measure, very far from repairing, it exhausts the strength, fatigues the organs, and sometimes becomes the occasion of serious diseases, as idiotism and madness."

SLICKENSIDES. The specular variety of galena is so called in Derbyshire.

SLOE. See *Prunus sylvestris*.

SMALLAGE. See *Apium graveolens*.

SMALL-POX. See *Variola*.

SMALT. See *Zaffre*.

SMARAGDITE. See *Diallage*.

SMARAGDUS. See *Emerald*.

SMELLIE, WILLIAM, was born in Scotland, where he practised midwifery for nineteen years, and then settled in London. He attained considerable reputation as a lecturer, which he appears to have merited by his assiduity and talents. He introduced many improvements in the instruments employed in that branch of the profession, and established some useful rules for their application. He was the first writer who, by accurately determining the shape and size of the pelvis, and of the head of the foetus, and considering its true position in utero, clearly pointed out the whole progress of parturition: and his opinions were subsequently confirmed, especially by his pupil, the celebrated Dr. W. Hunter. He abolished many superstitious notions, and erroneous customs, that prevailed in the management of parturient women, and of the children; and had the satisfaction of seeing most of these improvements adopted, as well in this as in other countries of Europe. In 1752, he published the substance of his lectures in an octavo volume; to which he added, two years after, a second volume of cases; and a third appeared about five years after his death, in 1768. In 1754, he also published a set of anatomical plates, of a large folio size, to elucidate his doctrines farther.

SMELL. "There escapes from almost every body in nature certain particles of an extreme tenuity, which are carried by the air often to a great distance. These particles constitute odours. There is one sense destined to perceive and appreciate them. Thus an important relation between animals and bodies is established.

All bodies of which the atoms are fixed are called inodorous.

The difference of bodies is very great relative to the manner in which odours are developed. Some permit them to escape only when they are heated; others only when rubbed. Some again produce very weak odours, while others produce only those which are highly powerful. Such is the extreme tenuity of odoriferous particles, that a body may produce them for a very long time without losing weight in any sensible degree.

Every odoriferous body has an odour peculiar to itself.

As these bodies are very numerous, there have been attempts made to class them, which have nevertheless all failed.

Odours can be distinguished only into weak and strong, agreeable and disagreeable. We can recognise odours which are musky, aromatic, foetid, rancid, spermatic, pungent, muriatic, &c. Some are fugitive, others tenacious. In most cases an odour cannot be distinguished but by comparing it with some known body. There have been attributed to odours properties which are nourishing, medical, and even venomous; but in the cases which have given rise to these opinions, might not the influence of odours have been confounded with the effects of absorption? A man who pounds jalap for some time will be purged in the same manner as if he had actually swallowed part of it. This ought not to be attributed to the effects of odours, but rather to

the particles which, being spread around, float in the air, and are introduced either with the saliva or with the breath. We ought to attribute to the same cause the drunkenness of persons who are exposed for some time to the vapours of spirituous liquors. The air is the only vehicle of odours; it transports them to a distance; they are also produced, however, *in vacuo*, and there are bodies which project odoriferous particles with a certain force. This matter has not yet been carefully studied; it is not known if, in the propagation of odours, there be any thing analogous to the divergence, the convergence, to the reflection, or the refraction of the rays of light. Odours mix or combine with many liquids, as well as solids. This is the means employed to fix or preserve them. Liquids, gases, vapours, as well as many solid bodies reduced to powder, possess the property of acting on the organs of smell.

Apparatus for smelling.—The olfactory apparatus ought to be represented as a sort of sieve, placed in the passage of the air, as it is introduced into the chest, and intended to stop every foreign body that may be mixed with the air, particularly the odours.

This apparatus is extremely simple; it differs essentially from that of the sight and the hearing; since it presents no part anterior to the nerve, destined for the physical modification of the external impulse, the nerve is to a certain degree exposed. The apparatus is composed of the pituitary membrane, which covers the nasal cavities, of the membrane which covers the *sinuses*, and of the olfactory nerve.

The pituitary membrane covers the whole extent of the nostrils, increases the thickness of the spongy bones very much, is continued beyond their edges and their extremities, so that the air cannot traverse the nostrils but in a long narrow direction. This membrane is thick, and adheres strongly to the bones and cartilages that it covers. Its surface presents an infinity of small projections, which have been considered by some as nervous *papillæ*, by others as mucous follicles, but which, according to all appearance, are vascular.

These small projections give to the membrane an appearance of velvet. The pituitary is agreeable and soft to the touch, and it receives a great number of vessels and nerves. The passages through which the air proceeds to arrive at the *fauces* deserve attention.

These are three in number. They are distinguished in anatomy by the names of Inferior, middle, and superior *meatus*. The inferior is the broadest and the longest, the least oblique and least crooked; the middle one is the narrowest, almost as long, but of greater extent from top to bottom. The superior is much shorter, more oblique, and narrower. It is necessary to add to these the interval, which is very narrow, and which separates the partition of the external side of the nostrils in its whole extent. These canals are so narrow, that the least swelling of the pituitary renders the passage of the air in the nostrils difficult, and sometimes impossible.

The two superior *meatus* communicate with certain cavities, of dimensions more or less considerable, which are hollowed out of the bones of the head, and are called *sinuses*. These *sinuses* are the *maxillary*, the *palatine*, the *sphenoidal*, the *frontal*; and those which are hollowed out of the *ethmoid bone*, better known by the name of ethmoidal cells.

The *sinuses* communicate only with the two superior *meatus*.

The *frontal*, the *maxillary sinus*, the anterior cells of the *ethmoid bone*, open into the middle *meatus*; the *sphenoidal*, the *palatine sinus*, the posterior cells of the *ethmoid*, open into the superior *meatus*. The *sinuses* are covered by other soft membranes, very little adherent to the sides, and which appear to be of the mucous kind. It secretes more or less abundantly a matter called *nasal mucus*, which is continually spread over the pituitary, and seems very useful in smelling. A more considerable extent of the *sinus* appears to coincide with a greater perfection of the smell. This is at least one of the most positive results of comparative physiology.

The olfactory nerve springs, by three distinct roots, from the posterior, inferior, and internal parts of the anterior lobe of the brain. Prismatic at first, it proceeds towards the perforated plate of the *ethmoid bone*. It swells all at once, and then divides itself into a great number of small threads, which spread themselves upon the *pituitary* membrane, principally on the superior part of it.

It is important to remark, that the filaments of the olfactory nerves have never been traced upon the inferior *spongy bones*, upon the internal surface of the middle *meatus*, nor in any of the *sinuses*. The *pituitary* membrane receives not only the nerves of the first pair, but also a great number of threads, which spring from the internal aspect of the *spheno-palatine ganglion*. These threads are distributed in the *meatus*, and in the inferior part of the membrane. It covers also, for a considerable length, the ethmoidal thread of the nasal nerve, and receives from it a considerable number of filaments. The membrane which covers the sinus receives also a number of nervous ramifications.

The *nasal fossæ* communicate outwardly by means of the nostrils, the form and size of which are very variable. The nostrils are covered with hair on the inside, and are capable of being increased in size by muscular action. The nasal fossæ open into the *pharynx* by the posterior nostrils.

Mechanism of Smelling.—Smell is exerted essentially at the moment when the air traverses the nasal fossæ in proceeding towards the lungs. We very rarely perceive any odour when the air proceeds from the lungs; it happens sometimes, however, particularly in organic diseases of the lungs.

The mechanism of smell is extremely simple. It is only necessary that the odoriferous particles should be stopped upon the pituitary membrane, particularly in the places where it receives the threads of the olfactory nerves.

As it is exactly in the superior part of the nasal fossæ, where the extremes are so narrow, that they are covered with mucus, it is also natural that the particles should stop there.

We may conceive the utility of mucus. Its physical properties are such that it appears to have a much greater affinity with the odoriferous particles than with air; it is also extremely important to the olfactory sense, that the *nasal mucus* should always preserve the same physical properties. Whenever they are changed, as it is observed in different degrees of *coryza*, the smell is either not exerted at all, or in a very imperfect manner.

After what has been said of the distribution of the olfactory nerves, it is evident that the odours that reach the upper part of the nasal cavities will be perceived with greater facility and acuteness: for this reason, when we wish to feel more acutely, and with greater exactness, the odour of any body, we modify the air in such a manner that it may be directed towards this point. For the same reason, those who take snuff endeavour also to make it reach the upper part of the nasal fossæ. The internal face of the *ossa spongiosa* appears well disposed to stop the odours at the instant the air passes. And, as there is an extreme sensibility in this point, we are inclined to believe that here the smell is exerted, though the filaments of the first pair have not been traced so far.

Physiologists have not yet determined the use of the external nose in smelling; it appears intended to direct the air charged with odours towards the superior part of the *nasal cavities*.

Those persons who have their noses deformed, particularly if broken; those who have small nostrils, directed forward, have in general almost no smell. The loss of the nose, either by sickness or accident, causes almost entirely the loss of smell. Such people recover the benefit of this sense by the use of an artificial nose.

The only use of the sinuses which is generally admitted, is that of furnishing the greater part of the nasal mucus. The other uses which are attributed to them are, to serve as a depôt to the air charged with odoriferous particles, to augment the extent of the surface which is sensible to odours, and to receive a portion of the air that we inspire for the purpose of putting the power of smell in action, &c. These are far from being certain.

Vapours and gases appear to act in the same manner upon the pituitary membrane as odours. The mechanism of it ought, however, to be a little different. Bodies reduced to a coarse powder have a very strong action on this membrane; even their first contact is painful; but habit changes the pain into pleasure, as is

seen in the case of taking snuff. In medicine, this property of the pituitary membrane is employed for the purpose of exciting a sharp instantaneous pain.

In the history of smell, the use of those hairs with which the nostrils and the nasal fossæ are provided, must not be forgotten. Perhaps they are intended to prevent the entrance of foreign bodies along with the air into the nasal fossæ. In this case, they would bear a strong analogy to the eyelashes, and the hairs with which the ear is provided.

It is generally agreed that the olfactory nerve is especially employed in transmitting to the brain the impressions produced by odoriferous bodies; but there is nothing to prove that the other nerves, which are placed upon the *pituitary*, as well as those near it, may not concur in the same function."—*Magendie's Physiology.*

SMELT. See *Salmo eperlanus.*

SMI'LAX. (From σμιλευω, to cut: so called from the roughness of its leaves and stalk.) The name of a genus of plants in the Linnæan system. Class, *Diœcia;* Order, *Octandria.* Rough bind-weed.

SMILAX CHINA. The systematic name of the China root tree. *China; China orientalis; Sankira; Guaquara; Smilax aspera Chinensis.* China root. It was formerly in esteem, as sarsaparilla now is, in the cure of the venereal disease, and cutaneous disorders.

Smilax, Chinese. See *Smilax china.*

SMILAX SARSAPARILLA. The systematic name of the plant which affords the sarsaparilla. *Sarsaparilla; Smilax aspera Peruviana; Sarsa; Carivillandi; Iva pecanga; Macapatli; Zarza; Zarzaparilla; Salsaparilla; Zarcaparilla.* The root of this plant, *Smilax—caule aculeato angulato, foliis inermibus ovatis re tuso mucronatis trinerviis,* of Linnæus, has a farina ceous, somewhat bitter taste, and no smell. About two centuries ago it was introduced into Spain, as an undoubted specific in syphilitic disorders; but owing to difference of climate, or other causes, it has not answered the character which it had acquired in the Spanish West Indies. It is now considered as capable of improving the general habit of body, after it has been reduced by the continued use of mercury.

To refute the opinion that sarsaparilla possesses antisyphilitic virtues, Mr. Pearson, of the Lock Hospital, divides the subject into two distinct questions. 1. Is the sarsaparilla root, when given alone, to be safely relied on in the treatment of lues venerea? The late Mr. Bloomfield, his predecessor, and during some years his colleague at the Lock Hospital, has given a very decided answer to this question: "I solemnly declare," says he, "I never saw a single instance in my life where it cured that disorder without the assistance of mercury, either at the same time with it, or when it had been previously taken before the decoction was directed." Pearson's experience, during many years, coincides entirely with the observations of Bloomfield. He has employed the sarsaparilla, in powder and in decoctions, in an almost infinite variety of cases, and feels himself fully authorized to assert, that this plant has not the power of curing any one form of the lues venerea. The sarsaparilla, indeed, like the guaiacum, is capable of alleviating symptoms derived from the venereal virus; and it sometimes manifests the power of suspending, for a time, the destructive ravages of that contagion; but where the poison has not been previously subdued by mercury, the symptoms will quickly return; and, in addition to them, we often see the most indubitable proofs that the disease is making an actual progress, during the regular administration of the vegetable remedy.

2. When the sarsaparilla root is given in conjunction with mercury, does it render the mercurial course more certain and efficacious? In replying to this query, it is necessary to observe that the phrase, "to increase the efficacy of mercury," may imply, that a smaller quantity of this mineral antidote will confer security on an infected person, when sarsaparilla is added to it; or it may mean, that mercury would be sometimes unequal to the cure, without the aid of sarsaparilla. If a decoction of this root did indeed possess so admirable a quality, that the quantity of mercury, necessary to effect a cure, might be safely reduced, whenever it was given during a mercurial course, it would form a most valuable addition to our Materia Medica. This opinion has been, however, unfortunately falsified by the most ample experience, and whoever shall be so un

wary as to act upon such a presumption, will be sure to find his own and his patient's expectations egregiously disappointed.

If the sarsaparilla root be a genuine antidote against the syphilitic virus, it ought to cure the disease administered alone; but, if no direct proof can be adduced of its being equal to this, any arguments founded on histories where mercury has been previously given, or where both the medicines were administered at the same time, must be ambiguous and undecisive.

It appears probable, that Sir William Fordyce, and some other persons, entertained a notion, that there were certain venereal symptoms which commonly resisted the potency of mercury, and that the sarsaparilla was an appropriate remedy in these cases. This opinion, it is presumed, is not correct, for it militates against all Mr. P. has ever observed of the progress and treatment of lues venerea. Indeed, those patients who have lately used a full course of mercury, often complain of nocturnal pains in their limbs; they are sometimes afflicted with painful enlargements of the elbow and knee-joints; or they have membranous nodes, cutaneous exulcerations, and certain other symptoms, resembling those which are the offspring of the venereal virus.

It may and does often happen, that appearances like these are mistaken for a true venereal affection, and, in consequence of this error, mercury is administered, which never fails to exasperate the disease. Now, if a strong decoction of sarsaparilla root be given to persons under these circumstances, it will seldom fail of producing the most beneficial effects; hence it has been contended, that symptoms derived from the contagion of lues venerea, which could not be cured by mercury, have finally yielded to this vegetable remedy. It must be acknowledged, that representations of this kind have a specious and imposing air; nevertheless, Mr. Pearson endeavours to prove, that they are neither exact nor conclusive. If any of the above-named symptoms should appear near the conclusion of a course of mercury, when that medicine was operating powerfully on the whole system, it would be a strange and inexplicable thing if they could possibly be derived immediately from the uncontrolled agency of the venereal virus.

This would imply something like a palpable contradiction that the antidote should be operating with sufficient efficacy to cure the venereal symptoms, for which it was directed, while, at the same time the venereal virus was proceeding to contaminate new parts, and to excite a new order of appearances.

One source, and a very common one, to which some of the mistakes committed upon this subject may be traced, is a persuasion that every morbid alteration which arises in an infected person is actually tainted with the venereal virus, and ought to be ascribed to it as its true cause.

Every experienced surgeon must, however, be aware, that very little of truth and reality exists in a representation of this kind. The contagious matter, and the mineral specific may jointly produce, in certain habits of body, a new series of symptoms, which, strictly speaking, are not venereal, which cannot be cured by mercury, and which are sometimes more to be dreaded than the simple and natural effects of the venereal virus.

Some of the most formidable of these appearances may be sometimes removed by sarsaparilla, the venereal virus still remaining in the system; and, when the force of that poison has been completely subdued by mercury, the same vegetable is also capable of freeing the patient from what may be called the sequelæ of a mercurial course.

The root of the sarsaparilla is sometimes employed in rheumatic affections, scrofula, and cutaneous complaints, where an acrimony of the fluids prevails.

["SMITH, ELIHU H., M. D. Dr. Smith was one of the first projectors of the New-York Medical Repository, uniting with Drs. Mitchill and Miller in establishing one of the first Medical and Scientific Journals in this country. He, however, survived but a short time after its commencing, having died of the Yellow-Fever in New-York, in 1798. Dr. E. H. Smith was born in Litchfield, in Connecticut, in 1771, and died in the 27th year of his age.

'In announcing the death of Dr. Smith, the surviving editors of the Medical Repository thus speak: As a Physician his loss is irreparable. He had explored

at his early age an extent of Medical learning, for which the longest lives are seldom found sufficient. The love of science, and the impulse of philanthropy, directed his whole professional career, and left little room for the calculations of emolument. He had formed vast designs of medical improvement, which embraced the whole family of mankind; was animated by the soul of benevolence, and aspired after every object of a liberal and a dignified ambition. He was ripe for the highest honours of his profession; his merits were every day becoming more conspicuous, and nothing but his premature fate deprived him of that extraordinary degree of public confidence which awaited a longer continuance of his life."—N. Y. Med. Repos. A.]

SMYRNION HORTENSE. See Imperatoria ostruthium.

SMY'RNIUM. (So called from σμυρνα, myrrh, the smell of the seed resembling that of myrrh very much.) The name of a genus of plants. Class, Pentandria; Order, Digynia.

SMYRNIUM OLUSATRUM. The systematic name of the plant called Alexanders. Hipposelinum; Smyrnium; Macerona; Macedonisium; Herba alexandrina; Grielum; Agrioselinum. Common Alexanders. This plant was formerly cultivated in our gardens, for culinary use, but is now superseded by scelery. The seeds are bitter and aromatic, and the roots are more powerfully bitter. They stand recommended as resolvents, diuretics, and emmenagogues, though seldom used in medical prescriptions.

SMYRNIUM ROTUNDIFOLIUM. The blanched leaves of this species are said to be more agreeable than those of the olusatrum.

SNAIL. See Limax.

Snail-seeded glasswort. See Salsola kali.

SNAKE. Anguis. The flesh was formerly made into broth as a restorative.

Snake, common. The Coluber natrix, of Linnæus.

Snake, rattle. See Coluber.

SNAKEROOT. See Aristolochia serpentaria, and Polygala senega.

[Snake-root, black. See Cimicifuga. A.

SNAKEWEED. See Polygonum bistorta.

SNAKEWOOD. See Colubrinum lignum.

Snake-killing birthwort. See Aristolochia anguicida.

SNAP-DRAGON. See Antirrhinum.

SNEEZEWORT. (So called, because the dried flowers and roots, when powdered, cause sneezing when applied to the nose.) See Achillea ptarmica.

SNEEZING. Snernutatio. A convulsive action of the muscles of the chest from irritation of the nostrils.

SNUFF. See Nicotiana.

SOAP. See Sapo.

SOAP-BERRY. See Saponaria officinalis.

SOAP, MOUNTAIN. A pale brownish black mineral, which has a greasy feel; writes, but does not soil: and occurs in trap rocks in the Isle of Skye. It is used in crayon painting.

SOAP-STONE. See Steatite.

SOAP-TREE. See Saponaria.

SOAP-WORT. See Saponaria.

Socotorine aloës. Aloës brought from Socotora See Aloë.

SO'DA. (An Arabian word.) The name now universally given by chemists and physicians to the mineral alkali.

It is obtained from several sources, but principally from plants growing on the sea coast. It occurs in the mineral kingdom, united with sulphuric, muriatic, and boracic acids; it is also found in large quantities in Egypt, combined with carbonic acid. It appears to be deposited in large impure masses, under the surface of the earth, in various countries, from which it is extracted by running waters. Thus it is found, after the spontaneous evaporation of the water, mixed with sand in the bottom of lakes in Hungary; in the neighbourhood of Bilin in Bohemia; and in Switzerland. It occurs also in China, and near Tripoli; in Syria, Egypt, Persia, and India. It frequently oozes out of walls and crystallizes on their surface. Like potassa, it is procured by lixiviation from the ashes of burnt plants, but only from those which grow upon the sea-shores. The variety of plants employed for this purpose is very considerable. In Spain, soda is procured from different species of the Salsola and Salicornia, and the Batis maritima. The Zostera maritima is burnt in some places on the borders of the Baltic. In this country we burn the various species of *fuci;* and in France they burn the *Chenopodium maritimum.* See *Soda impura.*

The alkali thus procured is more or less pure, according to the nature of the particular plant from which it is obtained. The greatest part, however, is a sub-carbonate of soda.

" To procure pure soda, we must boil a solution of the pure carbonate with half its weight of quicklime, and after subsidence decant the clear ley, and evaporate in a clean iron or silver vessel, till the liquid flows quietly like oil. It must then be poured out on a polished iron plate. It concretes into a hard white cake, which is to be immediately broken in pieces, and put up, while still hot, in a phial, which must be well corked. If the carbonate of soda be somewhat impure, then, after the action of lime, and subsequent concentration of the ley, alkohol must be digested on it, which will dissolve only the caustic pure soda, and leave the heterogeneous salts. By distilling of the alkohol in a silver alembic, the alkali may then be obtained pure.

This white solid substance is, however, not absolute soda, but a hydrate, consisting of about 100 soda + 28 water; or of nearly 77 + 23, in 100. If a piece of this soda be exposed to the air, it softens and becomes pasty; but it never deliquesces into an oily looking liquid, as potassa does. The soda in fact soon becomes drier, because by absorption of carbonic acid from the air it passes into an efflorescent carbonate. Soda is distinguishable from potassa by sulphuric acid, which forms a very soluble salt with the former, and a sparingly soluble one with the latter; by muriate of platina and tartaric acid, which occasions precipitates with potassa salts, but not with those of soda.

The basis of soda is a peculiar metal, called *sodium,* discovered by Sir H. Davy in 1807, a few days after he discovered potassium. It may be procured in exactly the same manner as potassium, by electrical or chemical decomposition of the pure hydrate. A rather higher degree of heat, and greater voltaic power, are required to decompose soda than potassa. Sodium resembles potassium in many of its characters. It is as white as silver, possesses great lustre, and is a good conductor of electricity. It enters into fusion at about 280° Fahr., and rises in vapour at a strong red heat. Its sp. gr. is, according to Gay Lussac and Thenard, 0.972, at the temperature of 59° Fahr. In the cold, it exercises scarcely any action on dry air, or oxygen. But when heated strongly in oxygen or chlorine, it burns with great brilliancy. When thrown upon water, it effervesces violently, but does not inflame, swims on the surface, gradually diminishes with great agitation, and renders the water a solution of soda. It acts upon most substances in a manner similar to potassium, but with less energy. It tarnishes in the air, but more slowly; and, like potassium, it is best preserved under naphtha.

Sodium forms two distinct combinations with oxygen; one is pure soda, whose hydrate is above described; the other is the orange oxide of sodium, observed, like the preceding oxide, first by Sir H. Davy in 1807, but of which the true nature was pointed out, in 1810, by Gay Lussac and Thenard.

Pure soda may be formed by burning sodium in a quantity of air, containing no more oxygen than is sufficient for its conversion into this alkali; *i. e.* the metal must be in excess: a strong degree of heat must be employed.

Pure soda is of a gray colour, it is a non-conductor of electricity, of a vitreous fracture, and requires a strong red heat for its fusion. When a little water is added to it, there is a violent action between the two bodies; the soda becomes white, crystalline in its appearance, and much more fusible and volatile. It is then the substance commonly called *pure* or *caustic soda;* but properly styled the *hydrate.*

The other oxide or peroxide of sodium may be formed by burning sodium in oxygen, in excess. It is of a deep orange colour, very fusible, and a non-conductor of electricity. When acted on by water, it gives off oxygen, and the water becomes a solution of soda. It deflagrates when strongly heated with combustible bodies

The proportions of oxygen in soda, and in the orange peroxide of sodium, are easily learned by the action of sodium on water and on oxygen. If a given weight of

sodium, in a little glass tube, be thrown by means of the finger under a graduated inverted jar filled with water, the quantity of hydrogen evolved will indicate the quantity of oxygen combined with the metal to form soda; and when sodium is slowly burned in a ray of platina (lined with dry common salt), in oxygen in great excess, from the quantity of oxygen absorbed the composition of the peroxide may be learned. From Sir H. Davy's experiments, compared with those of Gay Lussac and Thenard, it appears that the prime equivalent of sodium is 3.0, and that of dry soda, or protoxide of sodium, 4.0; while the orange oxide or deutoxide is 5.0. The numbers given by Thenard are, for the first, 100 metal + 33.995 oxygen; and for the second, 100 metal + 67.990 oxygen.

Another oxide is described containing less oxygen than soda; it is therefore a sub-oxide. When sodium is kept for some time in a small quantity of moist air, or when sodium in excess is heated with hydrate of soda, a dark grayish substance is formed, more inflammable than sodium, and which affords hydrogen by its action upon water.

Only one combination of sodium and chlorine is known. This is the important substance, *common salt.* It may be formed directly by combustion, or by decomposing any compound of chlorine by sodium. Sodium has a much stronger attraction for chlorine than for oxygen: and soda, or its hydrate, is decomposed by chlorine, oxygen being expelled from the first, and oxygen and water from the second.

Potassium has a stronger attraction for chlorine than sodium has; and one mode of procuring sodium easily, is by heating together to redness common salt and potassium. The chloride of sodium, improperly called the muriate, consists of 4.5 chlorine + 3.0 sodium. There is no known action between sodium and hydrogen or azote.

Sodium combines readily with sulphur and with phosphorus, presenting similar phenomena to those presented by potassium. The sulphurets and phosphurets of sodium agree in their general properties with those of potassium, except that they are rather less inflammable. They form, by burning, acidulous compounds of sulphuric and phosphoric acid and soda.

Potassium and sodium combine with great facility, and form peculiar compounds, which differ in their properties, according to the proportions of the constituents. By a small quantity of sodium, potassium is rendered fluid at common temperatures, and its sp. gr. is considerably diminished. Eight parts of potassium, and one of sodium, form a compound that swims in naphtha, and that is fluid at the common temperature of the air. Three parts of sodium, and one of potassium, make a compound fluid at common temperatures. A little potassium destroys the ductility of sodium, and renders it very brittle and soft. Since the prime of potassium is to that of sodium as 5 to 3, it will require the former quantity of potassium to eliminate the latter quantity of sodium from the chloride. The attractions of potassium, for all substances that have been examined, are stronger than those of sodium.

Soda is the basis of common salt, of plate and crown-glass, and of all hard soaps."

The compounds of soda used in medicine are the following:

1. Sodæ acetas.		6. Sodæ murias.	
2. —— boras.		7. —— phosphas	
3. —— carbonas.		8. —— sulphas.	
4. —— subcarbonas.		9. —— tartras.	
5. ——————ex-		10. Soda tartarizata.	
siccata.		11. Sapo durus.	

SODA ACETATA. A neutral salt formed of a combination of acetic acid with the mineral alkali. Its virtues are similar to those of the acetate of potassa.

SODA BORAXATA. See *Borax.*

Soda, carbonate of. See *Sodæ carbonas.*

SODA HISPANICA. See *Soda impura.*

SODA HISPANICA PURIFICATA. See *Sodæ subcarbonas.*

SODA IMPURA. Impure soda. *Soda; Barilla; Bariglia; Barillor; Anatron; Natron; Anaton; Nitrum antiquorum; Aphronitrum; Barrach; Sal alkalinus fixus fossilus; Carbonas sodæ impurus; Subcarbonas sodæ impura.* Soda. Barilla is the term given, in commerce, to the impure mineral alkali, or imperfect carbonate of soda, imported from Spain and the Levant It is made by burning to ashes different plants that grow on the sea-shore, chiefly of the genus *Salsola*. Many have referred it to the *Salsola kali*, of Linnæus; but various other plants, on being burned, are found to afford this alkali, and some in a greater proportion than this: these are,

1. The *Salsola sativa*, of Linnæus. *Salsola sonda*, of Losting. *Kali hispanicum supinum annuum sedifoliis brevibus. Kali d'alicante.* This grows abundantly on that part of the Spanish coast which is washed by the Mediterranean sea. This plant is deservedly first enumerated by Professor Murray, as it supplies all the best soda consumed in Europe, which by us is called Spanish or Alicant soda, and by the Spanish merchants Barilla de Alicante.

2. *Salsola soda*, of Linnæus. *Kali majus cochleato semine; Le Salicor.* This species, which grows on the French Mediterranean coast, is much used in Languedoc for the preparation of this salt, which is usually exported to Sicily and Italy.

3. *Salsola tragus*, of Linnæus, affords an ordinary kind of soda, with which the French frequently mix that made in Languedoc. This adulteration is also practised by the Sicilians, who distinguish the plant by the term salvaggia.

4. *Salicornia herbacea*, of Linnæus, is common in salt marshes, and on the sea-shore all over Europe. Linnæus prefers the soda obtained from this plant to that of all the others; but though the quantity of alkali which it yields is very considerable, it is mixed with much common salt.

5. *Salicornia arabica*, of Linnæus, and also the *Mesembryanthemum nodiflorum*, and *Plantago squarrosa*. All these, according to Alpinus, afford this alkali. It nas also been procured from several of the fuci, especially *F. vesicolosus*, and distinguished here by the name kelp. Various other marine plants might also be noticed as yielding an impure soda by combustion; but the principal are confined to the genus salsola, and that of salicornia. The salsola kali, on the authority of Rawolf, is the species from which the salt is usually obtained in eastern countries; which is brought to us in hard porous masses, of a speckled brown colour. Kelp, a still more impure alkali, made in this country by burning various sea-weeds, is sometimes called British barilla. The marine plants, collected for the purpose of procuring barilla in this country, are the *Salsola kali, Salicornia europæ, Zostera maritima, Triglochen maritimum, Chenopodium maritimum, Atriplex portulacoides et littoralis, Plantago maritima; Tamarix gallica, Eryngium maritimum, Sedum telephium, Dipsacus fullonum*, &c. &c.

It is to be regretted, that the different kinds of soda which are brought to European markets have not been sufficiently analyzed to enable us to ascertain with tolerable certainty the respective value of each; and, in deed, while the practice of adulterating this salt continues, any attempts of this kind are likely to prove fruitless. The best information on this subject is to be had from Jessica, Mascorelle, Cadet, Bolare, and Sestini. In those places where the preparation of soda forms a considerable branch of commerce, as on the coast of the Mediterranean, seeds of the salsola are regularly sown in a proper situation near the sea, which usually shoot above ground in the course of a fortnight. About the time the seeds become ripe, the plants are pulled up by the roots, and exposed in a suitable place to dry, where their seeds are collected; this being done, the plants are tied up in bundles, and burned in an oven constructed for the purpose, where the ashes are then, while hot, continually stirred with long poles. The saline matter, on becoming cold, forms a hard solid mass, which is broken in pieces of a convenient size for exportation.

According to chemical analysis, the impure sodas of commerce generally contain a portion of vegetable alkali, and neutral salts, as muriate of soda and sulphate of potassa, and not unfrequently some portion of iron is contained in the mass; they are, therefore, to be considered as more or less a compound, and their goodness to be estimated accordingly. The Spanish soda, of the best sort, is in dark-coloured masses, of a bluish tinge, very ponderous, sonorous, dry to the touch, and externally abounding with small cavities, without any offensive smell, and very salt to the taste; if long exposed to the air, it undergoes a degree of spontaneous calcination. The best French soda is also dry, sono-

rous, brittle, and of a deep blue colour, approaching to black. The soda which is mixed with small stones, which gives out a fœtid smell on solution, and is white soft, and deliquescent, is of the worst kind.

SODA MURIATA. See *Sodæ murias*.

SODA MURIATICA. See *Sodæ murias*.

SODA PHOSPHORATA. Phosphorated soda. *Alkali minerale phosphoratum*, of Bergman. This preparation is a compound of phosphoric acid and soda. It is cathartic in the dose of half an ounce to an ounce; dissolved in gruel it is not unpleasant, and it is said to be useful in scrofula, bronchocele, rachitis, and gout, in small doses.

Soda, subcarbonate of. See *Sodæ subcarbonas*.

Soda, subcarbonate of, dried. See *Sodæ subcarbonas exsiccata*.

Soda, sulphate of. See *Sodæ sulphas*.

SODA TARTARIZATA. Tartarized soda, formerly known by the names of *sal rupellensis, sal polychrestum Seignetti*, and lately by that of *natron tartarizatum*. Take of subcarbonate of soda twenty ounces; supertartrate of potassa, powdered, two pounds; boiling water ten pints. Dissolve the subcarbonate of soda in the water, and add gradually the supertartrate of potassa; filter the solution through paper, and evaporate it until a pellicle forms upon the surface; then set it by that crystals may form. Having poured away the water, dry these crystals upon bibulous paper. This salt consists of tartaric acid, soda, and potassa, the soda only combining with the superabundant acid of the super salt; it is therefore a triple salt, and it has been judged by the London College more convenient to express this difference by the adjective *tartarizata*, than to introduce the three words necessary to its description. It possesses mildly cathartic, diuretic, and deobstruent virtues, and is administered in doses from one drachm to an ounce, as a cathartic, and in the dose of twenty to thirty grains in abdominal physconia, and torpidity of the kidneys.

Soda tartarized. See *Soda tartarizata*.

SODÆ BORAS. See *Borax*.

SODÆ CARBONAS. Carbonate of soda. Take of subcarbonate of soda, a pound; subcarbonate of ammonia, three ounces; distilled water, a pint. Having previously dissolved the soda in water, add the ammonia, then by means of a sand bath apply a heat of 180° for three hours, or until the ammonia be driven off. Lastly, set the solution by to crystallize. The remaining solution may be evaporated and set by in the same manner, that crystals may again form. This salt, which is called also *aërated soda*, and *natron*, bears to the subcarbonate of soda the same relation that the carbonate of potassa does to its subcarbonate. It is prepared in the same way, possesses the same comparative advantages, and contains, in like manner, double the quantity of carbonic acid.

SODÆ MURIAS. Muriate of soda. *Alkali minerale salinum; Sal communis; Sal culinaris; Sal fontium; Sal gemmæ; Sal marinus; Natron muriatum; Soda muriata.* Common culinary salt. This salt is more abundant in nature than any other. It is found in prodigious masses in the internal part of the earth, in Calabria, in Hungary, in Muscovy, and more especially in Weilicska, in Poland, near Mount Capax, where the mines are very large, and afford immense quantities of salt. It is also obtained by several artificial means from sea-water. It possesses antiseptic, diuretic, and resolvent qualities, and is frequently employed in form of clyster, fomentation, lotion, pediluvium, and bath, in obstipation, against worms, gangrene, scrofulous tumours, herpetic eruptions, arthritis, &c.

SODÆ SUBBORAS. See *Borax*.

SODÆ SUBCARBONAS. Subcarbonate of soda, formerly called *natron præparatum* and *sal sodæ*. Take of impure soda, powdered, a pound; boiling distilled water, half a gallon. Boil the soda in the water for half an hour, and strain the solution; let the solution evaporate to two pints, and be set by, that crystals may form. Throw away the remaining solution. The pure crystals, thus formed of Alicant barilla, are colourless, transparent, lamellated, of a rhomboidal figure; and one hundred parts are found to contain twenty of alkali, sixteen of aërial acid, and sixty-four of water; but upon keeping the crystals for a length of time, if the air be not excluded, the water evaporates, and they assume the form of a white powder. According to Islin, one ounce of water, at the temperature 62° of Fahr. dissolves five drachms and fifteen grains of the crystals. This salt consists of soda imperfectly saturated with carbonic acid, and is therefore called *soda subcarbonas*. It is given in doses of from ten grains to half a drachm as an attenuant and antacid; and joined with bark and aromatics, it is highly praised by some in the cure of scrofula. It is likewise a powerful solvent of mucus, a deobstruent and diuretic; and has been thought an antidote against oxide of arsenic and corrosive sublimate. The other diseases in which it is administered are those arising from an abundance of mucus in the primæ viæ, calculous complaints, gout, some affections of the skin, rickets, tinea capitis, crusta lactea, and worms. Externally it is recommended by some in the form of lotion, to be applied to scrofulous ulcers.

SODÆ SUBCARBONAS EXSICCATA. Dried subcarbonate of soda. Take of subcarbonate of soda, a pound. Apply a boiling heat to the soda in a clean iron vessel, until it becomes perfectly dry, and constantly stir it with an iron rod. Lastly, reduce it into powder. Its virtues are similar to those of the subcarbonate.

SODÆ SULPHAS. Sulphate of soda, commonly known by the name of *natron vitriolatum*, and formerly *sal catharticus glauberi*. Take of the salt which remains after the distillation of muriatic acid, two pounds. Boiling water, two pints and a half. Dissolve the salt in the water, then add gradually as much subcarbonate of soda as may be required to saturate the acid; boil the solution away until a pellicle forms upon the surface, and, after having strained it, set it by, that crystals may form. Having poured away the water, dry these crystals upon bibulous paper. It possesses cathartic and diuretic qualities, and is in high esteem as a mild cathartic. It is found in the mineral kingdom formed by nature, but that which is used medicinally is prepared by art. The dose is from one drachm to one ounce.

SODALITE. A green-coloured mineral discovered in a bed of mica slate in West Greenland.

SODIUM. See *Soda.*

SOL. The sun. Gold was so called by the older chemists.

SOLA'MEN. (From *solor*, to comfort.) Aniseed is named solamen intestinorum, from the comfort it affords in disorders of the intestines.

SOLANO'IDES. (From *solanum*, night-shade, and ειδος, likeness.) Bastard night-shade.

SOLA'NUM. (From *solor*, to comfort, because it gives ease by its stupifying qualities.) 1. The name of a genus of plants in the Linnæan system. Class, *Pentandria*: Order, *Monogynia.*

2. The pharmacopœial name of the *solanum nigrum.*

SOLANUM DULCAMARA. The systematic name of the bitter-sweet. *Dulcamara; Solanum scandens; Glycypicros, sive amaradulcis; Solanum lignosum. Στρυχνος* of Theophrastus. Woody night-shade. *Solanum—caule inermi frutescente flexuosa; foliis superioribus hastatis; racemis cymosis,* of Linnæus. The roots and stalks of this night-shade, upon being chewed, first cause a sensation of bitterness, which is soon followed by a considerable degree of sweetness; and hence the plant obtained the name of bitter-sweet. The berries have not yet been applied to medical use; they seem to act powerfully upon the primæ viæ, exciting violent vomiting and purging. Thirty of them were given to a dog, which soon became mad, and died in the space of three hours; and, upon opening his stomach, the berries were discovered to have undergone no change by the powers of digestion; there can, therefore, be little doubt of the deleterious effects of these berries; and, as they are very common in the hedges, and may be easily mistaken, by children, for red currants, which they somewhat resemble, this circumstance is the more worthy of notice. The stipites, or younger branches, are directed for use in the Pharm., and they may be employed either fresh or dried, making a proportionate allowance in the dose of the latter for some diminution of its powers by drying. In autumn, when the leaves are fallen, the sensible qualities of the plant are said to be the strongest; and, on this account, it should be gathered in autumn rather than spring. Dulcamara does not manifest those strong narcotic qualities which are common to many of the night-shades; it is, however, very generally admitted to be a medicine of considerable efficacy. Murray says it promotes all the secretions; Haller observes, that it partakes of the milder powers of the night-shade joined to a resolvent

and saponaceous quality; and the opinion of Bergius seems to coincide with that of Murray :—" Virtus : pellens urinam, sudorum, menses, lochia, sputa ; mundificans." The diseases in which we find it recommended by different authors, are extremely various ; but Bergius confines its use to rheumatisms, retentio mensium, et lochiorum. Dulcamara appears, also, by the experiments of Razoux and others, to have been used with advantage in some obstinate cutaneous affections. Dr. Cullen says, " We have employed only the stipites, or slender twigs of this shrub; but, as we have collected them, they come out very unequal, some parcels of them being very mild and inert, and others of them considerably acrid. In the latter state, we have employed a decoction of them in the cure of rheumatism, sometimes with advantage, but at other times without any effect. Though the dulcamara is here inserted in the catalogue of diuretics, it has never appeared to us as powerful in this way ; for, in all the trials made here, it has hardly ever been observed to be in any measure diuretic." This plant is generally given in decoction, or infusion, and, to prevent its exciting nausea, it is ordered to be diluted with milk, and to begin with small doses, as large doses have been found to produce very dangerous symptoms. Razoux directs the following : ℞. Stipitum dulcam. rec. drac. ss in aquæ font. unc. 16 coquater ad unc. 8. This was taken in the dose of three or four drachms, diluted with an equal quantity of milk, every four hours. Linnæus directs two drachms, or half an ounce of the dried stipites, to be infused half an hour in boiling water, and then to be boiled ten minutes ; and of this decoction he gives two teacups full morning and evening. For the formula of a decoction of this plant, according to the London Pharm. See *Decoctum dulcamaræ.*

SOLANUM FŒTIDUM. The thorn-apple plant. See *Datura stramonium.*

SOLANUM LETHALE. See *Atropa belladonna.*

SOLANUM LIGNOSUM. See *Solanum dulcamara.*

SOLANUM LYCOPERSICUM. The love-apple plant. The fruit of this, called *Tomata* and *love-apple*, is so much esteemed by the Portuguese and the Spaniards, that it is an ingredient in almost all their soups and sauces, and is by them considered as cooling and nutritive.

SOLANUM MELONGENA. The systematic name of the mad-apple plant. Its oblong egg-shaped fruit is often boiled in their native places, in soups and sauces, the same as the love-apple; is accounted very nutritive, and is much sought after by the votaries of Venus.

SOLANUM NIGRUM. The systematic name of the garden night-shade, which is highly deleterious.

SOLANUM SANCTUM. The systematic name of the Palestine night-shade. The fruit of which is globular, and in Egypt much eaten by the inhabitants.

SOLANUM TUBEROSUM. *Batatas; Solanum esculentum; Kippa; Kelengu; Papas Americanus; Papus Americanus; Convolvulus Indicus.* The potato plant, a native of Peru, first brought into Europe by Sir Francis Drake, 1486, and planted in London. See *Potato.*

SOLANUM VESICARIUM. The winter-cherry plant is so called by Caspar Bauhin. See *Physalis alkekengi.*

SOLDANELLA. (*A solidando;* from its uses in healing fresh wounds.) The sea convolvulus. See *Convolvulus soldanella.*

SO'LEN. Σωλην. A tube or channel. A cradle for a broken limb.

SOLENA'RIUM. (Diminutive of σωλην, a tube.) A catheter.

SO'LEUS. (From *solea,* a sole: from its shape being like the sole-fish.) See *Gastrocnemius internus.*

SOLIDA'GO. (From *solido,* to make firm: so called from its uses in consolidating wounds.) The name of a genus of plants in the Linnæan system. Class, *Syngenesia;* Order, *Polygamia superflua.* The herb comfrey.

SOLIDAGO VIRGAUREA. The systematic name of the golden rod. *Virga aurea; Herba dorea; Conyza coma aurea; Symphytum; Petræum; Elichrysum; Consolida saracenica* and *aurea.* Golden rod. The leaves and flowers of this plant are recommended as aperients and corroborants in urinary obstructions, ulcerations of the kidneys and bladder, and it is said by some to be particularly useful in stopping internal hæmorrhages.

SOLIDS. In anatomy, are the bones, ligaments, membranes, muscles, nerves, and vessels.

SOLITARIUS. Solitary. Applied to worms in the body, and to leaves, stems, footstalk, &c. when either single on a plant, or only one in the same place.

SO'LIUM. (From *solus*, alone: so called because it infests the body singly.) The tape-worm. See *Tænia*.

Solomon's seal. See *Convallaria polygonatum.*

SOLSE'QUIUM. (From *sol*, the sun, and *sequor*, to follow: so called because it turns its flowers toward the sun.) Marigold or turnsole. See *Heliotropium*.

SOLVENT. See *Menstruum.*

SOLUTION. *Solutio.* An intimate commixture of solid bodies with fluids, into one seemingly homogeneous liquor. The dissolving fluid is called a menstruum or solvent.

SOLUTIVA. (From *solvo*, to loosen.) Laxative medicines, gentle purgatives.

SOMMITE. See *Nepheline.*

SOMNAMBULISM. See *Oneirodynia.*

SOMNI'FEROUS. (*Somniferus;* from *somnus*, sleep, and *fero*, to bring.) Having the power of inducing sleep.

[SOMNIUM. This is a term introduced by Dr. Mitchill, to designate the state between sleeping and waking, in which persons perform acts of which they are unconscious. It includes all those states of the system in which persons walk, talk, sing, dream, &c. during which they are neither perfectly asleep nor awake. This state of *Somnium* may be divided into Symptomatic, and Idiopathic,

I. Symptomatic Somnium.

1. Somnium, from indigestion (a dyspepsia), when from too much food, or too feeble a condition of the stomach, there is a fermentation with acidity, eructations, and pain or uneasiness, followed by troublesome dreams.

2. Somnium from the nightmare (ab incubo), supposed to arise from some impediment to the free circulation of the blood through the heart and lungs; always unpleasant and sometimes frightful. The memory here is active, but the will is suspended, and the efforts to exert it fails. Persons are supposed to have died in fits of incubus.

3. Somnium from effusions of water in the chest (ab hydrothorace), believed to proceed from anxiety about the vital parts, caused by lymph in the pericardium or thorax. Terrifying dreams rousing the patient suddenly are the common consequences of this disorder. This and the preceding are the Oneirodynia of Nosologists.

4. Somnium from a feverish state of the body (a febre), caused by an undue and irregular excitement of the brain. This is known by the name of high delirium, or sometimes furor.

5. Somnium from debility (cum debilitate), where there is not excitement enough to embody ideas in steady trains. Memory and imagination act in a confused and irregular manner. Low delirium.

6. Somnium from fainting (cum asphyxia), where, though there is an exhaustion of vital power, and the individual appears to be dead, there is life enough in the body to prevent putrefaction. The animal functions do not seem to be so much depressed as the vital ; for, on recovery, the individual relates what he witnessed during the *trance* in which he lay, while in the very lowest ebb of life.

7. Somnium from fresh and vivid occurrences (a recentibus), as when dreams can be traced to some conversation or occurrence of the day, or to some actual condition of the body. Common dreaming.

8. Somnium from old and forgotten occurrences (ab obsoletis), when long-lost images are renewed to the memory, and dead friends are brought before us.

9. Somnium from an overloaded brain (a plethora), with symptoms bordering on epilepsy, apoplexy, and catalepsy. Sometimes called typhomania.

10. Somnium of a prospective character (a prophetia), when the dreamer is engaged in seeing funeral processions, and foretelling events by a sort of *second sight*, as it is called. This disease is symptomatic of a peculiar state of body, running in families like gout, consumption and insanity.

11. Somnium, from vivid impressions on the internal organ of sight (a visione), where visual images are so strong, that the dreamers are called *Seers*, because they see so much, and their sights are termed *Visions*, inasmuch as the eyes are so peculiarly concerned.

12. Somnium from the conditions of other corporeal organs (a sexu velpruritu), causing dreams.

13. Somnium (a respiratione) from inhaling nitrous oxide gas, depriving the person of consciousness and will, and inspiring delightful sensations.

14. Somnium (a toxico) from doses of opium, hyoscyamus datura, and other narcotic plants, taken into the stomach, disturbing the will and exciting strange fancies.

15. Somnium from drunkenness (ab ebrietate), caused by drinking spirituous liquors, overcoming consciousness and spontaneity.

II. Idiophathic Somnium.

1. Somnium, from abstraction, where the internal senses are so engaged that there is no knowledge, or an imperfect one, of the passing events, constituting what is termed *Reverie ;* where fanciful trains of the thought are indulged at considerable length.

2. Somnium, with partial or universal lunacy (cum insanitate), vitiating the mind with some fundamental error on a particular subject, or disturbing and confounding all the operations of the animal mind. This characterizes some forms of *madness* and melancholy.

3. Somnium, with talking (cum sermone), where the ideas of the mind are uttered in audible words, as in a wakeful state : called frequently, Somniloquism, or sleep talking on ordinary subjects.

4. Somnium, with walking (cum ambulatione), where the person rises from bed, walks about, frequently goes abroad, without the smallest recollection that any volition had been exerted on the occasion : the whole affair is forgotten, and not a trace left in the memory : this is called somnambulism.

5. Somnium, with invention (cum inventione), as when unbidden ideas rise in the mind in a methodical series, and form a poetical sonnet, different from any thing known before, and unattainable by the waking powers. These are sometimes reduced to writing at the time and found afterward, though the act of committing them to paper is generally forgotten. On other occasions the memory preserves the particulars of such dreams.

6. Somnium, (cum hallucinatione) with mistaken impressions of sight, and sometimes of hearing, so strong as to enforce a conviction of their reality. Many visions, conversations, and mistaken representations gain currency in this way. The patients being unwittingly deceived themselves, propagate with an honest zeal their delusions, and labour to gain the assent of their friends and acquaintances.

7. Somnium, with singing (cum musica), wherein the person, though unable to raise a note when awake, becomes capable in the somnial condition of uttering sounds in most melodious accents.

8. Somnium, with ability to pray and preach (cum religione), or to address the Supreme Being and human auditors in an instructive and eloquent manner, without any recollection of having been so employed, and with utter incompetency to perform such exercises of devotion and instruction when awake.

See these states of Somnium, illustrated by cases, published in New-York, in 1815, under the title of "DEVOTIONAL SOMNIUM," &c. containing the account of RACHEL BAKER, &c. Notes from Dr. M.'s lectures on *Mat. Med.* A.]

SONCHI'TES. (From *σογχος*, the sow-thistle: so named from its resemblance to the sonchus.) The herb hawkweed.

SO'NCHUS. (Παρα το σωον, χεειν ; from its wholesome juice.) The name of a genus of plants in the Linnæan system. Class, *Syngenesia;* Order, *Polygamia æqualis.* The sow-thistle.

SONCHUS OLERACEUS. The systematic name of the sow-thistle. Most of the species of sonchus abound with a milky juice, which is very bitter, and said to possess diuretic virtues. This is sometimes employed with that intention. Boiled it may be eaten as a sub stitute for cabbage.

SOOT. See *Fuligo.*

SO'PHIA. (From *σοφος*, wise: so named from its great virtues in stopping fluxes.) Flix-weed or flux-weed. See *Sisymbrium.*

SOPHIA CHIRURGORUM. See *Sisymbrium sophia.*

SOPHISTICATION. A term employed in pharmacy, to signify the counterfeiting or adulterating any medicine. This practice unhappily obtains with most dealers in drugs, &c. ; and the cheat is carried on so artificially by many as to prevent a discovery even by persons of the most discerning faculties.

SOPHO'RA. (A name of most whimsical origin. *Sophera* is, according to Prosper Alpinus, the Egyptian denomination of a species of cassia, the *Cassia sophera* of Linnæus, nearly related to this genus. Linnæus, spelling it *sophora*, calls it a *genus sophorum*, or of wise men ; as teaching that separate stamens, in the papilionaceous family, if ever the limits of that family can be determined, afford so decisive a mark of discrimination, as almost to exclude the plants furnished with such, from the same natural class, or order, with those the filaments of which are combined.) The name of a genus of plants. Class, *Decandria ;* Order, *Monogynia.*

SOPHORA HEPTAPHYLLA. The systematic name of the shrub, the root and seeds of which are sometimes called *anticholerica ;* they are both intensely bitter, and said to be useful in cholera, colic, and dysury.

SOPHRONISTE'RES. (From σωφρονιζω, to become wise: so called because they do not appear till after puberty.) The last of the grinding-teeth.

SOPIE'NTIA. (From *sopio*, to make sleep.) Medicines which procure sleep.

SO'POR. Profound sleep.

SOPORIFEROUS. (*Soporiferus ;* from *sopor*, sleep, and *fero*, to bear.) A term given to whatever induces sleep. See *Anodyne.*

So'RA. (Arabian.) The nettle-rash.

SORBASTRE'LLA. (From *sorbeo*, to suck up; because it stops hæmorrhages.) The herb burnet. See *Pimpinella saxifraga.*

SORBATE. A compound of sorbic or malic acid, with the salifiable basis.

SORBIC ACID. (*Acidum sorbicum ;* from *sorbus*, the mountain ash, from the berries of which it is obtained.) "The acid of apples called malic, may be obtained most conveniently and in greatest purity from the berries of the mountain ash, called *sorbus*, or *pyrus aucuparia*, and hence the present name, sorbic acid. This was supposed to be a new and peculiar acid by Donovan and Vauquelin, who wrote good dissertations upon it. But it now appears that the sorbic and pure malic acids are identical.

Bruise the ripe berries in a mortar, and then squeeze them in a linen bag. They yield nearly half their weight of juice, of the specific gravity of 1.077. This viscid juice, by remaining for about a fortnight in a warm temperature, experiences the vinous fermentation, and would yield a portion of alkohol. By this change, it has become bright, clear, and passes easily through the filter, while the sorbic aci ı itself is not altered. Mix the clear juice with filtered solution of acetate of lead. Separate the precipitate on a filter, and wash it with cold water. A large quantity of boiling water is then to be poured upon the filter, and allowed to drain into glass jars. At the end of some hours, the solution deposites crystals of great lustre and beauty. Wash these with cold water, dissolve them in boiling water, filter, and crystallize. Collect the new crystals, and boil them for half an hour in 2.3 times their weight of sulphuric acid, specific gravity 1.090, supplying water as fast as it evaporates, and stirring the mixture diligently with a glass rod. The clear liquor is to be decanted into a tall narrow glass jar, and while still hot, a stream of sulphuretted hydrogen is to be passed through it. When the lead has been all thrown down in a sulphuret, the liquor is to be filtered, and then boiled in an open vessel to dissipate the adhering sulphuretted hydrogen. It is now a solution of sorbic acid.

When it is evaporated to the consistence of a syrup, it forms manimelated masses of a crystalline structure. It still contains a considerable quantity of water, and deliquesces when exposed to the air. Its solution is transparent, colourless, void of smell, but powerfully acid to the taste. Lime and barytes waters are not precipitated by solution of the sorbic acid, although the sorbate of lime is nearly insoluble. One of the most characteristic properties of this acid, is the precipitate which it gives with the acetate of lead, which is at first white and flocculent, but afterward assumes a brilliant crystalline appearance. With potassa, soda, and ammonia, it forms crystallizable salts containing an excess of acid."

SO'RBUS. (From *sorbeo*, to suck up; because its fruit stops fluxes.) The name of a genus of plants in the Linnæan system. Class, *Icosandria ;* Order, *Trigynia.* The service-tree.

SORBUS AUCUPARIA. The wild service-tree. The

berries of this plant are adstringent, and, it is said, have been found serviceable in allaying the pain of calculous affections in the kidneys.

SO'RDES. When the matter discharged from ulcers is rather viscid, glutinous, of a brownish-red colour, somewhat resembling the grounds of coffee, or grumous blood mixed with water, it is thus named. *Sordes, Saines*, and *Ichor*, are all of them much more fœtid than purulent matter, and none of them are altogether free from acrimony; but that which is generally termed *Ichor*, is by much the most acrid of them, being frequently so sharp and corrosive as to destroy large quantities of the neighbouring parts.

Sore, bay. A disease which Dr. Mosely considers as a true cancer, commencing with an ulcer. It is endemic at the Bay of Honduras.

SORE-THROAT. See *Cynanche.*

SORREL. See *Rumex acetosa.*

Sorrel, French. See *Rumex scutatus.*

Sorrel, round-leaved. See *Rumex scutatus.*

Sorrel, wood. See *Oxalis acetosella.*

SOUND. 1. An instrument which surgeons introduce through the urethra into the bladder, to discover whether there is a stone in this viscus or not.

2. See *Hearing.*

SOUR DOCK. See *Rumex acetosa.*

SOUTHERNWOOD. See *Artemisia abrotanum.*

SOW-BREAD. See *Cyclamen.*

SPA. A town in France, in the department of the Ourte, famous for its mineral water, which appears to be a very strongly acidulous chalybeate, containing more iron and carbonic acid than any other mineral spring. What applies to the use of chalybeates will apply to this water.

SPADIX. An elongated receptacle or flower-bearing column, which emerges, mostly, from a spathe or sheath, as it does in *Arum maculatum, Calla æthiopica*, and *palustris ;* but the *Acorus calamus* has a spadix without any sheath.

The inflorescence of palms, and some other plants, is a *branched spadix ;* as the *Chamærops humilis, Musa*, &c.

Spain, pellitory of. See *Anthemis pyrethrum.*

Spanish fly. See *Cantharis.*

Spanish liquorice. See *Glycyrrhiza.*

Spar, fluor. See *Fluor.*

Spar, ponderous. See *Heavy-spar*, and *Barytes.*

Spar, tabular. See *Tabular spar.*

SPARGANO'SIS. (From σπαργαω, to swell.) A milk abscess.

Sparry anhydrite. A sulphate of lime. See *Anhydrite.*

SPARRY IRON. A carbonate of iron, of a pale yellowish gray colour, found in limestone in England, Scotland, and Ireland, and in large quantities in Hessia.

SPARSUS. Dispersed, irregularly scattered. Frequently used in medicine, anatomy, and botany, to eruptions, glands, leaves, flower-stalks.

SPA'RTIUM. (Σπαρδιον of Dioscorides : so called from σπαρ]η, a rope; because of the use of the long, slender, tough branches, or bark, in making cordage.) The name of a genus of plants in the Linnæan system. Class, *Diadelphia ;* Order, *Decandria.*

SPARTIUM SCOPARIUM. The systematic name of the common broom. *Genista.* The tops and leaves of this indigenous plant, *Spartium—foliis ternatis solitariisque, ramis inermibus angulatis*, of Linnæus, are the parts that are employed medicinally ; they have a bitter taste, and are recommended for their purgative and diuretic qualities, in hydropic cases.

SPASMI Spasmodic diseases. The third order of the Class *Neuroses*, of Cullen; characterized by a morbid contraction or motion of muscular fibres.

SPASMODIC. *Spasmodicus.* Belonging to a spasm, or convulsion.

Spasmodic colic. See *Colica.*

SPASMOLOGY. (*Spasmologia ;* from σπασμος, a spasm, and λογος, a discourse.) A treatise on convulsions.

SPASMUS. (*Spasmus ;* from σπαω, to draw.) A cramp, spasm, or convulsion. An involuntary contraction of the muscular fibres, or that state of the contraction of muscles which is not spontaneously disposed to alternate with relaxation, is properly termed spasm. When the contractions alternate with relaxation, and are frequently and preternaturally repeated, they are called convulsions. Spasms are distinguished by authors into clonic and tonic spasms. In *clonic* spasms, which are the true convulsions, the contractions and relaxations are alternate, as in epilepsy ; but in *tonic* spasms the member remains rigid, as in locked jaw. See *Convulsion, Tonic, spasm*, and *Tetanus*.

SPASMUS CYNICUS. Sardonic laugh. A convulsive affection of the muscles of the face and lips on both sides, which involuntarily forces the muscles of those parts into a species of grinning distortion. If one side only be affected, the disorder is nominated tortura oris. When the masseter, buccinator, temporal, nasal, and labial muscles, are involuntarily excited to action, or contorted by contraction or relaxation, they form a species of malignant sneer. It sometimes arises from eating hemlock, or other acrid poisons, or succeeds to an apoplectic stroke.

SPATHA. (From σπαθη, a slice, or ladle.) A botanical term. A sheath, or covering of an immature flower which bursts longitudinally, and is more or less remote from the flower. From the number of membranes, which are called valves, and of the flowers, and their duration, it is named,

1. *Spatha univalvis*, having only one membranous leaf; as in *Arum maculatum*, and *Crocus sativus*.

2. *Bivalvis*, in *Stratiates alioides*.

3. *Dimidiata*, or *lacera*, there being only one valve, and that covering the flower only partially ; as in *Ixia uniflora*, and *africana*.

4. *Vaga*, the common sheath enclosing several partial ones ; as in *Iris germanica*, and *helonica*.

5. *Uniflora*, containing only one flower; as the *Narcissus poeticus, Pseudo-narcissus*, and *Amaryllis formosissima*.

6. *Biflora*, with two; as in *Alpina racemosa*, and *Moraea vegeta*.

7. *Multiflora* ; as in *Allium, Narcissus jonquilla*, and *Pancreatium carabeum*.

8. *Spatha persistens*, remaining with the fruit; as in *Heliconia bihai*.

9. *Marcescens*, withering before or soon after the flowering ; as in *Allia* and *Leucojum vernum*.

SPATHOME'LE. (From σπαθη, a sword, and μηλη, a probe.) An edged probe.

SPA'TULA. (Diminutive of *spatha*, a broad instrument.) An instrument for spreading salve. Also a name of the herb spurgewort, from its broad leaves.

SPATULATUS. Spatulate: applied to leaves, &c. of a roundish figure, tapering into an oblong base; as in *Silene otites*.

SPEARMINT. See *Mentha viridis*.

Spearwort, water. See *Ranunculus flammula*.

SPECIFIC. *Specificus*. A remedy that has an infallible efficacy in the cure of disorders. The existence of such remedies is doubted.

Specific gravity. See *Gravity, specific*.

SPECI'LLUM. (From *specio*, to examine.) A probe.

SPE'CULUM. (From *specio*, to view.) An instrument for opening or obtaining a view of parts within each other ; as *Speculum oculi, Speculum oris, Speculum ani*, &c.

SPECULUM ANI. An instrument for distending the anus, while an operation is performed upon the parts within.

SPECULUM MATRICIS. An instrument to assist in any manual operation belonging to the womb.

SPECULUM OCULI. An instrument used by oculists to keep the eyelids open and the eye fixed.

SPECULUM ORIS. An instrument to force open the mouth.

SPECULUM VENERIS. See *Achillea millefolium*.

SPEECH. See *Voice*.

SPEEDWELL. See *Veronica*.

Speedwell, female. See *Antirrhinum elatine*.

Speedwell, mountain. See *Veronica*.

SPERMA-CETI. (From σπερμα, seed, and *cete*, or *cetus*, the whale.) See *Physeter macrocephalus*.

SPERMA'TIC. (*Spermaticus*; from σπερμα, seed.) Belonging to the testicle and ovary ; as the spermatic artery, chord, and veins.

SPERMATOCE'LE. (From σπερμα, seed, and κηλη, a tumour.) *Epididymis distensa*. A swelling of the testicle or epididymis from an accumulation of semen. It is known by a swelling of those organs, pain extending to the loins without inflammation.

SPERMATOPOE'TICA. (From σπερμα, and ποιεω, to make.) Medicines which increase the generation of seed.

SPERMORRHŒ'A. (From σπερμα, *semen*, and ρεω, *fluo*.) The name of a genus of diseases in Good's Nosology. Class, *Genetica* ; Order, *Cenotica*. Semi nal flux. It has two species, viz. *Spermorrhœa ento nica*, and *atonica*.

SPHACELI'SMUS. (From σφακελιζω, to gangrene.) 1. A gangrene:

2. A phrenitis.

SPHA'CELUS. (From σφακω, to destroy.) A mortification of any part. See *Gangrene*.

SPHÆ'NOIDES. See *Sphenoides*.

SPHÆRI'TIS. (From σφαιρα, a globe: so called from its round head.) *Sphærocephalia elatior. Sphærocephalus*. The globe-thistle.

SPHÆROCE'PHALUS. See *Sphæritis*.

SPHÆRO'MA. (From σφαιρα, a globe.) A fleshy, globular protuberance.

SPHÆRULITE. A brown and gray-coloured mineral, found in imbedded roundish balls and grains, in pearlstone and pitchstone porphyries, near Schemnitz.

SPHE'NO. Names compounded of this word belong to the sphenoid bone.

SPHENO-MAXILLARIS. An artery, and a fissure of the orbit of the eye, is so called.

SPHENO-SALPINGO-STAPHYLINUS. See *Circumflexus*.

SPHENO-STAPHYLINUS. See *Levator palati*.

SPHENOIDALIS. *Sphenoidalis*. Belonging to the sphenoid bone.

SPHENOIDAL SUTURE. *Sutura sphenoidalis*. The sphenoidal and ethmoidal sutures are those which surround the many irregular processes of these two bones, and join them to each other and to the rest.

SPHENOI'DES OS. (From σφην, a wedge, and ειδος, a likeness ; because it is fixed in the cranium like a wedge.) *Os cuneiforme ; Os multiforme ; Os azygos ; Papillare os ; Basilare os ; Os polymorphos*. Pterygoid bone. The os sphenoides, or cuneiforme, as it is called from its wedge-like situation amidst the other bones of the head, is of a more irregular figure than any other bone. It has been compared to a bat with its wings extended. This resemblance is but faint, but it would be difficult perhaps to find any thing it resembles more.

We distinguish, in this bone, its body or middle part, and its wings or sides, which are much more extensive than its body.

Each of its wings or lateral processes is divided into two parts. Of these, the uppermost and most consi derable portion, helping to form the deepest part of the temporal fossa on each side, is called the *temporal process*. The other portion makes a part of the orbit, and is therefore named the *orbitar process*. The back part of each wing, from its running out sharp to meet the os petrosum, has been called the *spinous process* ; and the two processes, which stand out almost perpendicular to the basis of the skull, have been named *pterygoid* or *aliform* processes, though they may be said rather to resemble the legs than the wings of the bat. Each of these processes has two plates and a middle fossa facing backwards ; of these plates, the external one is the broadest, and the internal one the longest. The lower end of the internal plate forms a kind of hook, over which passes the round tendon of the *musculus circumflexus palati*. Besides these, we observe a sharp middle ridge, which stands out from the middle of the bone. The forepart of it, where it joins the nasal lamella of the ethmoidal bone, is thin and straight ; the lower part of it is thicker, and is re ceived into the vomer.

The cavities, observable on the external surface of the bone, are where it helps to form the temporal, nasal, and orbitar fossæ.

It has likewise two fossæ in its pterygoid processes. Behind the edge, which separates these two fossæ, we observe a small groove, made by a branch of the superior maxillary nerve, in its passage to the temporal muscle. Besides these, it has other depressions, which serve chiefly for the origin of the muscles.

Its foramina are four on each side. The three first serve for the passage of the optic, superior maxillary, and inferior maxillary nerves ; the fourth transmits the largest artery of the dura mater. On each side we observe a considerable fissure, which, from its situa tion, may be called the superior orbitar fissure. Through it pass the third and fourth pair of nerves, a branch of the fifth, and likewise the sixth pair. Lastly, at the basis of each pterygoid process, we observe a foramen which is named *pterygoidean*, and sometimes *Vidian*, from Vidius, who first described it. Through it passes a branch of the external carotid, to be distributed to the nose.

The os sphenoides, on its internal surface, affords three fossæ. Two of these are considerable ones; they are formed by the lateral processes, and make part of the lesser fossæ of the basis of the skull. The third, which is smaller, is on the top of the body of the bone, and is called *sella turcica*, from its resemblance to a Turkish saddle. In this the pituitary gland is placed. At each of its four angles is a process. They are called the *clinoid* processes, and are distinguished by their situation into anterior and posterior processes. The two latter are frequently united into one.

Within the substance of the os sphenoides, immediately under the sella turcica, we find two cavities, separated by a thin bony lamella. These are the sphenoidal sinuses. They are lined with the pituitary membrane, and, like the frontal sinuses, separate a mucus which passes into the nostrils. In some subjects, there is only one cavity; in others, though more rarely, we find three.

In infants, the os sphenoides is composed of three pieces, one of which forms the body of the bone and its pterygoid processes, and the other two its lateral processes. The clinoid processes may even then be perceived in a cartilaginous state, though some writers have asserted the contrary; but we observe no appearance of any sinus.

This bone is connected with all the bones of the cranium, and likewise with the ossa maxillaria, ossa malarum, ossa palati, and vomer. Its uses may be collected from the description we have given of it.

SPHI'NCTER. (From σφιγγω, to shut up.) The name of several muscles, the office of which is to shut or close the aperture around which they are placed.

SPHINCTER ANI. *Sphincter externus*, of Albinus and Douglas. *Sphincter cutaneus*, of Winslow; and *coccigio-cutané-sphincter*, of Dumas. A single muscle of the anus, which shuts the passage through the anus into the rectum, and pulls down the bulb of the urethra, by which it assists in ejecting the urine and semen. It arises from the skin and fat that surrounds the verge of the anus on both sides, nearly as far as the tuberosity of the ischium; the fibres are gradually collected into an oval form, and surround the extremity of the rectum. It is inserted by a narrow point into the perineum, acceleratores urinæ, and transversi perinei; and behind into the extremity of the os coccygis, by an acute termination.

SPHINCTER ANI CUTANEUS. See *Sphincter ani*.
SPHINCTER ANI EXTERNUS. See *Sphincter ani*.
SPHINCTER ANI INTERNUS. Albinus and Douglas call the circular fibres of the muscular coat of the rectum, which surround its extremity, by this name.
SPHINCTER CUTANEUS. See *Sphincter ani*.
SPHINCTER EXTERNUS. See *Sphincter ani*.
SPHINCTER GULÆ. The muscle which contracts the top of the throat.
SPHINCTER LABIORUM. See *Orbicularis oris*.
SPHINCTER ORIS. See *Orbicularis oris*.
SPHINCTER VAGINÆ. *Constrictor cunni*, of Albinus. *Second muscle of the clitoris*, of Douglas; and *anulo-syndesmo-clitoridien*, of Dumas. This muscle arises from the sphincter ani and from the posterior side of the vagina, near the perineum; from thence it runs up the side of the vagina near its external orifice, opposite to the nymphæ, covers the corpus cavernosum, and is inserted into the crus and body, or union of the crura clitoridis. Its use is to contract the mouth of the vagina.

SPHINGO'NTA. (From σφιγγω, to bind.) Astringent medicines.

SPHONDY'LIUM. (From σπονδυλος, vertebra; named from the shape of its root, or probably because it was used against the bite of a serpent, called σπονδυλις.) This is supposed to be the branckursine. See *Acanthus mollis*.

SPHRAGIDE. A species of Lemnian earth.
SPHRONGIDIUM. See *Columnula*.
SPICA. A spike. I. A species of inflorescence, consisting of one common stalk bearing numerous flowers, all ranged along it without any, or having very
300

small partial stalks, as the flower-stalk of the greater plantain. From its figure, the situation of the flowers, and its vesture, it is called,

1. *Cylindrica*; as in *Plantago media*, and *albicans*.
2. *Ovata*, in *Sanguisorba officinalis*.
3. *Articulata*, with joints; as in *Salicornea herbacea*, and *Polygonum articulatum*.
4. *Conjugata*, two spikes going from the summit of the peduncle; as in *Heliotropium europæum* and *parviflorum*.
5. *Ramosa*, divided into branches; as in *Chenopodium bonus henricus*, and *Osmunda*.
6. *Imbricata*; as in *Salvia hispanica*.
7. *Secunda*, the flowers leaning all to one side; as in *Anchusa officinalis*.
8. *Interrupta*, in separate groupes; as in *Betonica officinalis*, and *Gomphrena interrupta*.
9. *Disticha*, two series of spikes; as in *Gladiolus alopecuroides*.
10. *Terminalis*; as in *Lavendula*.
11. *Axillares*; as in *Justitia spinosa*.
12. *Foliosa*, leaflets between the flowers; as in *Agrimonia eupatoria*.
13. *Comosa*, having a leafy bundle at the apex; as in *Lavendula stæchas*, and *Bromelia ananas*.
14. *Ciliata*, hairs between the flowers; as in *Nardus ciliaris*.

II. An ear of corn.

III. A bandage resembling an ear of corn.
SPICA BREVIS. The *Alopecuris pratensis*
SPICA CELTICA. See *Valeriana celtica*.
SPICA FÆMINA. Common lavender.
SPICA INDICA. See *Nardus indica*.
SPICA INGUINALIS. A bandage for ruptures in the groin.
SPICA INGUINALIS DUPLEX. Double bandage for ruptures.
SPICA MAS. Broad-leaved 'avender.
SPICA NARDI. See *Nardus indica*.
SPICA SIMPLEX. A common roller or bandage.
SPICULA. A spikelet. A term applied exclusively to grasses that have many florets on one calyx, such florets ranged on a little stalk, constituting the spikelet, which is therefore a part of the flower itself, and not of the efflorescence; as in *Briza minor*, and *Poa aquatica*. *Locusta* means the same as *spicula*.

SPIGE'LIA. (So called by Linnæus in commemoration of an old botanist, Adrian Spigelius, who wrote *Isagoge in rem herbariam*, in 1606.) 1. The name of a genus of plants in the Linnæan system. Class, *Pentandria*; Order, *Monogynia*.

2. The name in some pharmacopœias for the *Spigelia marilandica*.

SPIGELIA ANTHELMIA. The systematic name of the spigelia of some pharmacopœias. It is directed as an anthelmintic; its virtues are very similar to those of the Indian pink. See *Spige liamarilandica*.

SPIGELIA LONICERA. See *Spigelia marilandica*.
SPIGELIA MARILANDICA. *Spigelia lonicera*. Perennial worm-grass, or Indian pink. *Spigelia—caule tetragono, foliis omnibus, oppositis*, of Linnæus. The whole of this plant, but most commonly the root, is employed as an anthelmintic by the Indians, and inhabitants of America. Dr. Hope has written in favour of this plant, in continued and remitting low worm fevers. Besides its property of destroying the worms in the primæ viæ, it acts as a purgative.

Spigelion lobe. See *Liver*.

SPIGELIUS, ADRIAN, was born at Brussels, in 1578. He studied at Louvain, and afterward at Padua, where he took his degree. He became thoroughly skilled in every branch of his profession, particularly in anatomy and surgery; and after travelling some time to the different schools in Germany, he settled in Moravia, where he was soon appointed physician to the States of the Province. In 1616 he was invited to occupy the principal professorship in anatomy and surgery at Padua, where he acquitted himself with so much success, that he was created a knight of St. Mark, and presented with a collar of gold. He died in 1625. His writings evince him to have possessed very extensive medical knowledge. The first, which he published, contains some interesting information concerning the virtues of plants, respecting which he appears to have learned much from the Italian peasantry. He wrote also concerning some diseases and other matters. But the most valuable of his works are those composed on anatomical subjects, published after his death, by his son-in-law, Crema.

SPIGNEL. See *Æthusa meum.*

SPIKELET. See *Spicula.*

SPIKENARD. See *Nardus indica.*

SPILA'NTHUS. (From σπιλος, a spot, and ανθος, a flower; because of its dotted or speckled flowers.) The name of a genus of plants. Class, *Syngenesia;* Order, *Polygamia æqualis.*

SPILANTHUS ACMELLA. *Achmella. Achamella.* The systematic name of the balm-leaved spilanthus, which possesses a glutinous bitter taste, and a fragrant smell. The herb and seed are said to be diuretic and emmenagogue, and useful in dropsies, jaundice, fluor albus, and calculous complaints, given in infusion.

SPI'NA. (*Quasi spiculina*, diminutive of *spica.*) A thorn.

A. The back-bone: so called from the thorn-like processes of the vertebræ. See *Vertebræ*, and *Spine.*

B. The shin-bone.

C. A thorn of a plant. A prickly armature of plants, not easily removed by the finger, and proceeding from the woody part of the plant. It is either,

1. *Culine;* as in Prunus spinosa.

2. *Terminal*, at the end of a branch: as in Rhamnus catharticus.

3. *Foliar*, on the surface of the leaf; as in Carduus marianus.

4. *Marginal*, on the margin of the leaf; as in Ilex aquifolium.

5. *Axillary*, going from the axilla of the leaf; as in Gleditschia triacanthos.

6. *Calycine*, on the calyx; as in Carduus marianus.

7. *Pericarpial*, on the pod; as in Datura stramonium.

8. *Stipular*, on the stipule; as in Mimosa nilotica, and horrida.

9. *Straight;* as in Mimosa nigra.

10. *Recurve;* as in Costus nobilis.

11. *Decussate;* as in Genista lucitanica.

12. *Setaceous;* as in Cactus opuntia.

13. *Subulate;* as in Cactus tuna.

14. *Inerm*, covered with soft and not prickly spines, also called *muricate;* as in Convolvulus muricatus, and Mimosa muricata.

15. *Simple*, when not divided; as Genista anglica.

16. *Germinal;* as in Limonia trifoliata.

17. *Ternate;* as in Zanthium spinosum.

18. *Ramose;* as in Gleditschia horrida.

SPINA ACIDA. See *Berberis.*

SPINA ACUTA. The hawthorn.

SPINA ÆGYPTIACA. The Egyptian thorn or sloe-tree. See *Acacia vera.*

SPINA ALBA. The white-thorn tree.

SPINA ARABICA. The chardon, or Arabian thistle.

SPINA BIFIDA. *Hydrops medullæ spinalis; Hydrocele spinalis; Hydrorachytis spinosa.* A tumour upon the spine of new-born children, immediately about the lower vertebræ of the loins, and upper parts of the sacrum; at first, it is of a dark blue colour; but in proportion as it increases in size, approaches nearer and nearer to the colour of the skin, becoming perfectly diaphanous.

From the surface of this tumour a pellucid watery fluid sometimes exudes, and this circumstance has been noticed by different authors. It is always attended with a weakness, or more properly speaking, a paralysis of the lower extremities. The opening of it rashly has proved quickly fatal to the child. Tulpius, therefore, strongly dissuades us from attempting this operation. Acrel mentions a case where a nurse rashly opened a tumour, which, as he described it, was a blood bag on the back of the child at the time of its birth, in bigness equal to a hen's egg, in two hours after which, the child died. From the dissection it appeared, that the bladder lay in the middle of the os sacrum, and consisted of a coat, and some strong membrane, which proceeded from a long fissure of the bones. The extremity of the spinal marrow lay bare, and the spinal duct, in the os sacrum, was uncommonly wide, and distended by the pressure of the waters. Upon tracing it to the head, the brain was found nearly in its natural state, but the ventricles contained so much water, that the infundibulum was quite distended with it, and the passage between the third and fourth ventricle was greatly enlarged.

He likewise takes notice of another case, where a child lived about eight years labouring under this complaint, during which time it seemed to enjoy tolerable health, though pale. Nothing seemed amiss in him, but such a degree of debility as rendered him incapable to stand on his legs.

The tumour, as in the former case, was in the middle of the os sacrum, of the bigness of a man's fist, with little discolouring; and upon pressing it became less. When opened it was found full of water, and the coats were the same as in the former, but the separation of the bones was very considerable. The spinal marrow, under the tumour, was as small as a packthread, and rigid; but there were no morbid appearances in the brain.

SPINA BURGHI MONSPELIENSIS. Evergreen privet.

SPINA CERVINA. (So called from its thorns resembling those of the stag.) See *Rhamnus catharticus.*

SPINA HIRCI. The goat's-thorn of France, yielding gum-tragacanth.

SPINA INFECTORIA. See *Rhamnus catharticus.*

SPINA PURGATRIX. The purging thorn.

SPINA SOLSTITIALIS. The *calcitrapa officinalis* Barnaby's thistle.

SPINA VENTOSA. (The term of spina seems to have been applied by the Arabians to this disorder, because it occasions a prickling in the flesh like the puncture of thorns; and the epithet ventosa is added, because, upon touching the tumour, it seems to be filled with wind, though this is not the cause of the distention.) *Spinæ ventositas; Teredo; Fungus articuli; Arthrocace: sideratio ossis; Cancer ossis; Gangræna ossis*, and some French authors term it *exostosis.* When children are the subjects of this disease, Severinus calls it *Pædarthrocace.* A tumour arising from an internal caries of a bone. It most frequently occurs in the carpus and tarsus, and is known by a continual pain in the bone, and a red swelling of the skin, which has a spongy feel.

SPINA'CHIA. See *Spinacia.*

SPINA'CIA. (From Ισπανια, Spain, whence it originally came; or from its spinous seed.) The name of a genus of plants. Class, *Diæcia;* Order, *Pentandria.* Spinage

SPINACIA OLERACEA. The systematic name of the *Spinachia.* Spinach. Spinage. This plant is sometimes directed for medicinal purposes in the cure of phthisical complaints; made into a poultice, by boiling the leaves and adding some oil, it forms an excellent emollient. As an article of food it may be considered as similar to cabbage and other oleraceous plants. See *Brassica capitata.*

SPINÆ CRATES. The spine of the back.

SPINÆ VENTOSITAS. A caries, or decay of a bone. See *Spina ventosa.*

SPINAL. *Spinalis.* Belonging to the spine of the back.

Spinal-marrow. See *Medulla spinalis.*

SPINA'LIS. See *Spinal.*

SPINALIS CERVICIS. This muscle, which is situated close to the vertebræ at the posterior part of the neck and upper part of the back, arises, by distinct tendons, from the transverse processes of the five or six uppermost vertebræ of the back, and ascending obliquely under the complexus, is inserted, by small tendons, into the spinous processes of the sixth, fifth, fourth, third, and second vertebræ of the neck. Its use is to extend the neck obliquely backwards.

SPINALIS COLLI. See *Semi-spinalis colli.*

SPINALIS DORSI. *Transversalis dorsi*, of Winslow; and *inter-épineux*, of Dumas. This is the name given by Albinus to a tendinous and fleshy mass, which is situated along the spinous processes of the back and the inner side of the longissimus dorsi.

It arises tendinous and fleshy from the spinous processes of the uppermost vertebræ of the loins, and the lowermost ones of the back, and is inserted into the spinous processes of the nine uppermost vertebræ of the back.

Its use is to extend the vertebræ, and to assist in raising the spine.

SPINALES LUMBORUM. Muscles of the oins.

SPINE. (*Spina;* from *spina, thorn:* so called from the spine-like processes of the vertebræ.) 1. *Spina dorsi; Columna spinæ; Columna vertebralis.* A bony column or pillar extending in the posterior part of the trunk from the great occipital foramen to the sacrum. It is composed of twenty-four bones called vertebræ. See *Vertebræ.*

2. An armature of plants. See *Spina.*

SPINEL. A sub-species of octohedral corundum, of a red colour, and equal value with a diamond. It comes from Pegu and Ceylon.

SPINELLANE. A plumb, blue-coloured crystallized mineral, found on the shores of the lake of Laach.

SPINESCENS. Spinescent. Becoming thorny, applied to the leaf-stalk, when it hardens into a thorn, and the leaf falls, as is the case in Rhamnus catharticus, and Robinia spinosa, and to the stipulæ of the Robinia pseudacacia, which also become thorns.

Spi'nosa. See *Spina bifidi.*

Spino'sum syriacum. The Syrian broom.

SPINTHERE. A greenish gray-coloured mineral, believed to be a variety of prismatic titanium ore.

SPIRÆ'A. (From *Spira,* a pillar: so named from its spiral stalk.) Meadow-sweet. The name of a genus of plants in the Linnæan system. Class, *Icosandria;* Order, *Pentagynia.*

Spiræa africana. African meadow-sweet.

Spiræa filipendula. The systematic name of the officinal dropwort. *Filipendula; Saxifraga rubra.* Dropwort. The root of this plant, *Spiræa—foliis pennatis, foliolis uniformibus serratis ; caule herbaceo ; floribus corymbosis,* of Linnæus, possesses adstringent, and, it is said, lithontriptic virtues. It is seldom used in the practice of the present day.

Spiræa ulmaria. The systematic name of the meadow-sweet. *Ulmaria; Regina prati; Barba capræ.* Meadow-sweet. Queen of the meadows. This is a beautiful and fragrant plant. The leaves are recommended as mild adstringents. The flowers have a strong smell, resembling that of May; they are supposed to possess antispasmodic and diaphoretic virtues, and as they are very rarely used in medicine, Linnæus suspects that the neglect of them has arisen from the plant being supposed to be possessed of some noxious qualities, which it seemed to betray by its being left untouched by cattle. It may be observed, however, that the cattle also refuse the Angelica and other herbs, whose innocence is apparent from daily experience.

[Spiræa trifoliata. See *Gillenia.* A.]

SPI'RITUS. (*Spiritus, us.* m. ; spirit.) This name was formerly given to all volatile substances collected by distillation. Three principal kinds were distinguished: inflammable or ardent spirits, acid spirits, and alkaline spirits. The word spirit is now almost exclusively confined to alkohol.

Spiritus ætheris nitrici. *Spiritus ætheris nitrosi : Spiritus nitri dulcis.* Take of rectified spirits, two pints; nitric acid, by weight, three ounces; add the acid gradually to the spirit, and mix them, taking care that the heat do not exceed 120°; then with a gentle heat distil twenty-four fluid ounces. A febrifuge, diaphoretic, and diuretic compound mostly administered in asthenia, nervous affections, dysuria, and calculous complaints.

Spiritus ætheris aromaticus. Take of cinnamon-bark, bruised, three drachms; cardamom seeds powdered, a drachm and a half; long pepper powdered, ginger-root sliced, each a drachm; spirit of sulphuric æther, a pint; macerate for fourteen days, in a closed glass vessel, and strain. An excellent stimulating and stomachic compound, which is administered in debility of the stomach and nervous affections.

Spiritus ætheris sulphurici. *Spiritus vitrioli dulcis ; Spiritus ætheris vitriolici.* Take of sulphuric æther, half a pint; rectified spirit, a pint: mix them. A diaphoretic, antispasmodic, and tonic preparation, mostly exhibited in nervous debility and weakness of the primæ viæ.

Spiritus ætheris sulphurici compositus. Take of spirit of sulphuric æther a pint; ætherial oil, two fluid drachms; mix them. A stimulating anodyne, supposed to be similar to the celebrated *liquor mineralis anodynus,* of Hoffman. It is exhibited in fevers, nervous affections, hysteria, &c.; and in most cases of fever where medicines are rejected by the stomach, this is of infinite service.

Spiritus ammoniæ. Spirit of ammonia. Formerly called *Spiritus salis ammoniaci dulcis ; Spiritus salis ammoniaci.* Take of proof spirit, three pints ; muriate of ammonia, four ounces; subcarbonate of potassa, six ounces; mix them, and, with a gentle fire, let a pint and a half be distilled into a cooled receiver. A stimulating antispasmodic, occasionally exhibited in cases of asphyxia, asthenia, and in nervous diseases, but mostly

302

used as an external stimulant against rheumatism, sprains, and bruises.

Spiritus ammoniæ aromaticus. Aromatic spirit of ammonia. Formerly known by the name of *Spiritus ammoniæ compositus : Spiritus volatilis aromaticus : Spiritus salis volatilis oleosus.* Take of cinnamon-bark bruised, cloves bruised, each two drachms; lemon-peel, four ounces; subcarbonate of potassa, half a pound; muriate of ammonia, five ounces; rectified spirit, four pints; water, a gallon; mix and distil six pints. A stimulating antispasmodic and sudorific in very general use, to smell at in faintings and lowness of spirits. It is exhibited internally in nervous affections, hysteria, and weakness of the stomach. The dose is from half a drachm to a drachm.

Spiritus ammoniæ fœtidus. Fœtid spirit of ammonia. Formerly called *spiritus volatilis fœtidus.* Take of spirit of ammonia, two pints; asafœtida, two ounces. Macerate for twelve hours, then by a gentle fire distil a pint and a half into a cooled receiver. A stimulating antispasmodic, often exhibited to children against convulsions, and to gouty and asthmatic persons. The dose is from half to a whole fluid drachm.

Spiritus ammoniæ succinatus. Succinated spirit of ammonia. Formerly known by the names of *Eau de luce ; Spiritus salis ammoniaci succinatus ; Liquor cornu cervi succinatus.* Take of mastich, three drachms; rectified spirit, nine fluid drachms; oil of lavender, fourteen minims; oil of amber, four minims, solution of ammonia, ten fluid ounces. Macerate the mastich in the spirit that it may dissolve, and pour oil the clear tincture; to this add the remaining articles, and shake them together. This preparation is much esteemed as a stimulant and nervine medicine, and is employed internally and externally against spasms, hysteria, syncope, vertigo, and the stings of insects. The dose is from ten minims to half a fluid drachm.

Spiritus anisi. Spirit of aniseed. Formerly called *Spiritus anisi compositus ; Aqua seminum anisi composita.* Take of aniseed, bruised, half a pound ; proof spirit, a gallon ; water sufficient to prevent empyreuma. Macerate for twenty-four hours, and distil a gallon by a gentle fire. A stimulating carminative and stomachic calculated to relieve flatulency, borborygmus, colic, and spasmodic affections of the bowels. The dose is from half to a whole fluid drachm.

Spiritus armoraciæ compositus. Compound spirit of horse-radish, formerly called *Spiritus raphani compositus ; Aqua raphani composita.* Take of horse-radish root, fresh and sliced, dried orange-peel, of each a pound ; nutmegs, bruised, half an ounce; proof spirit, a gallon ; water sufficient to prevent empyreuma. Macerate for twenty-four hours, and distil a gallon by a gentle fire. A very warm stimulating compound, given in gouty, rheumatic, and spasmodic affections of the stomach, and in scorbutic disorders. The dose is from half a fluid drachm to half a fluid ounce.

Spiritus camphoræ. Spirit of camphor. Formerly known by the names of *Spiritus camphoratus ; Spiritus vinosus camphoratus ; Spiritus vini camphoratus.* Take of camphor, four ounces ; rectified spirit, two pints. Mix, that the camphor may be dissolved. A stimulating medicine, used as an external application against chilblains, rheumatism, palsy, numbness, and gangrene.

Spiritus carui. Spirit of caraway. Formerly called *Aqua seminum carui.* Take of caraway seed, bruised, a pound and a half; proof spirit a gallon ; water sufficient to prevent empyreuma. Macerate for 24 hours, and distil a gallon by a gentle fire. The dose is from a fluid drachm to half a fluid ounce.

Spiritus cinnamomi. Spirit of cinnamon. For merly called *Aqua cinnamomi spirituosa; Aqua cinnamomi fortis.* Take of cinnamon-bark, bruised, a pound ; proof spirit a gallon ; water sufficient to prevent empyreuma. Macerate for 24 hours, and distil a gallon by a gentle fire. Spirit of cinnamon is mostly used in conjunction with other carminatives to give a pleasant flavour; it may be exhibited alone as a car minative and stimulant. The dose is from a fluid drachm to half a fluid ounce.

Spiritus cornu cervi. See *Ammoniæ subcarbonas.*

Spiritus juniperi compositus. Compound spirit of juniper. Formerly called *Aqua juniperi composita.* Take of juniper-berries, bruised, a pound ; caraway-seeds, bruised, fennel-seeds, bruised, of each an ounce and a half; proof spirits, a gallon; water sufficient to prevent empyreuma. Macerate for 24 hours, and distil a gallon by a gentle fire.

SPIRITUS LAVENDULÆ. Spirit of lavender. Formerly called *Spiritus lavendulæ simplex.* Take of fresh lavender flowers, two pounds; rectified spirit, a gallon; water sufficient to prevent empyreuma. Macerate for 24 hours, and distil a gallon by a gentle fire. Though mostly used as a perfume, this spirit may be given internally as a stimulating nervine and antispasmodic. The dose is from a fluid drachm to half a fluid ounce.

SPIRITUS LAVENDULÆ COMPOSITUS. Compound spirit of lavender. Formerly called *Spiritus lavendulæ compositus matthiæ.* Take of spirit of lavender, three pints; spirit of rosemary, a pint; cinnamon-bark, bruised, nutmegs, bruised, of each half an ounce; red saunders wood, sliced, an ounce. Macerate for fourteen days, and strain. An elegant and useful antispasmodic and stimulant in very general use against nervous diseases, lowness of spirits, and weakness of the stomach, taken on a lump of sugar.

SPIRITUS LUMBRICORUM. The spirit obtained by the distillation of the earth-worm is similar to hartshorn.

SPIRITUS MENTHÆ PIPERITÆ. Spirit of peppermint. Formerly called *Spiritus menthæ piperitidis; Aqua menthæ piperitidis spirituosa.* Take of peppermint, dried, a pound and a half; proof spirit, a gallon; water sufficient to prevent empyreuma. Macerate for 24 hours, and distil a gallon by a gentle fire. This possesses all the properties of the peppermint, with the stimulating virtues of the spirit. The dose from one fluid drachm to a fluid ounce.

SPIRITUS MENTHÆ VIRIDIS. Spirit of spearmint. Formerly called *Spiritus menthæ sativæ; Aqua menthæ vulgaris spirituosa.* Take of spearmint, dried, a pound and a half; proof spirit, a gallon; water sufficient to prevent empyreuma. Macerate for 24 hours, and distil a gallon. This is most commonly added to carminative or antispasmodic draughts, and seldom exhibited alone. The dose from one fluid drachm to a fluid ounce.

SPIRITUS MILLEPEDARUM. A volatile alkali, the virtues of which are similar to hartshorn.

SPIRITUS MINDERERI. See *Ammonia acetatis liquor.*

SPIRITUS MYRISTICÆ. Spirit of nutmeg. Formerly called *Aqua nucis moschatæ.* Take of nutmegs, bruised, two ounces; proof spirit, a gallon; water sufficient to prevent empyreuma. Macerate for twenty-four hours, and distil a gallon by a gentle fire. A stimulating and agreeable spirit possessing the virtues of the nutmeg. The dose from one fluid drachm to a fluid ounce.

SPIRITUS NITRI DULCIS. See *Spiritus ætheris nitrici.*

SPIRITUS NITRI DUPLEX. The nitrous acid. See *Acidum nitrosum,* and *Nitric acid.*

SPIRITUS NITRI FUMANS. See *Acidum nitrosum,* and *Nitric acid.*

SPIRITUS NITRI GLAUBERI. See *Acidum nitrosum,* and *Nitric acid.*

SPIRITUS NITRI SIMPLEX. The dilute nitrous acid. See *Acidum nitricum dilutum.*

SPIRITUS NITRI VULGARIS. This is now called acidum nitricum dilutum.

SPIRITUS PIMENTÆ. Spirit of pimento. Formerly called *Spiritus pimento.* Take allspice, bruised, two ounces; proof spirit, a gallon; water sufficient to prevent empyreuma. Macerate for 24 hours, and distil a gallon by a gentle fire. A stimulating aromatic tincture mostly employed with astringent and carminative medicines. The dose is from half a fluid drachm to half a fluid ounce.

SPIRITUS PULEGII. Spirit of pennyroyal. Formerly called *Aqua pulegii spirituosa.* Take of pennyroyal, dried, a pound and a half; proof spirit, a gallon; water, sufficient to prevent empyreuma. Macerate for 24 hours, and distil a gallon by a gentle fire. This is in very general use as an emmenagogue among the lower orders. It possesses nervine and carminative virtues. The dose is from half a fluid drachm to half a fluid ounce.

SPIRITUS RECTOR. Boerhaave and other chemists give this name to a very attenuated principle, in which the smell of odorant bodies peculiarly reside. It is now called *aroma.*

SPIRITUS ROSMARINI. Spirit of rosemary. Take of rosemary tops, fresh, two pounds; proof spirit, a gallon; water sufficient to prevent empyreuma. Macerate for 24 hours, and distil a gallon by a gentle fire. A very fragrant spirit, mostly employed for external purposes in conjunction with other resolvents.

SPIRITUS SALIS AMMONIACI AQUOSUS. See *Ammoniæ subcarbonas.*

SPIRITUS SALIS AMMONIACI DULCIS. See *Spiritus ammoniæ.*

SPIRITUS SALIS AMMONIACI SIMPLEX. See *Ammoniæ subcarbonas.*

SPIRITUS SALIS GLAUBERI. See *Muriatic acid.*

SPIRITUS SALIS MARINI. See *Muriatic acid.*

SPIRITUS VINI RECTIFICATUS. See *Alkohol.* Rectified spirit of wine is in general use to dissolve resinous and other medicines. It is seldom exhibited internally, though it exists in the diluted state in all vinous and spirituous liquors.

SPIRITUS VINI TENUIOR. Proof spirit, which is about half the strength of rectified, is much employed for preparing tinctures of resinous juices, barks, roots, &c.

SPIRITUS VITRIOLI. See *Sulphuric acid.*

SPIRITUS VITRIOLI DULCIS. See *Spiritus ætheris sulphurici.*

SPIRITUS VOLATILIS FŒTIDUS. See *Spiritus ammoniæ fœtidus.*

SPISSAME'NTUM. (From *spisso,* to thicken.) A substance put into oils and ointments to make them thick.

Spitting of blood. See *Hæmatemesis* and *Hæmoptysis.*

SPLANCHNIC. (*Splanchnicus;* from σπλαγχνον, an entrail.) Belonging to the viscera.

SPLANCHNIC NERVE. The great intercostal nerve. See *Intercostal nerve.*

SPLA'NCHNICA. (From σπλαγχνον, an intestine.) Remedies for diseased bowels.

SPLANCHNOLOGY. (*Splanchnologia;* from σπλαγχνον, an entrail, and λογος, a discourse.) The doctrine of the viscera.

SPLEEN. Σπλην. *Lien.* The spleen or milt is a spongy viscus of a livid colour, and so variable in form, situation, and magnitude, that it is hard to determine either. Nevertheless, in a healthy man it is always placed on the left side, in the left hypochondrium, between the eleventh and twelfth false ribs. Its circumference is oblong and round, resembling an oval figure. It is larger, to speak generally, when the stomach is empty, and smaller when it is compressed, or evacuated by a full stomach.

It should particularly be remembered of this viscus, that it is convex towards the ribs, and concave internally: also, that it has an excavation, into which vessels are inserted.

It is connected with the following parts: 1. With the stomach by a ligament and short vessels. 2. With the omentum, and the left kidney. 3. With the diaphragm, by a portion of the peritonæum. 4. With the beginning of the pancreas, by vessels. 5. With a colon, by a ligament.

In man the spleen is covered with one simple, firm membrane, arising from the peritonæum, which adheres to the spleen, very firmly, by the intervention of cellular structure.

The vessels of the spleen are, the splenic artery coming from the cœliac artery, which, considering the size of the spleen, is much larger than is requisite for the mere nutrition of it. This goes by serpentine movements, out of its course, over the pancreas, and behind the stomach, and after having given off branches to the adjacent parts, it is inserted into the concave surface of the spleen. It is afterward divided into smaller branches, which are again divided into other yet smaller, delivering their blood immediately to the veins, but emitting it nowhere else. The veins, at length, come together into one, called the splenic vein, and having received the larger coronary vein of the stomach, besides others, it constitutes the left principal branch of the vena portæ.

The nerves of the spleen are small; they surround the arteries with their branches; they come from a particular plexus, which is formed of the posterior branches of the eighth pair, and the great intercostal nerve.

Lymphatic vessels are almost only seen creeping along the surface of the human spleen.

303

The use of the spleen has not hitherto been determined; yet if the situation and fabric be regarded, one would imagine its use to consist chiefly in affording some assistance to the stomach during the progress of digestion.

SPLEEN-WORT. See *Asplenium ceterach*, and *Asplenium trichomanes.*

SPLENA'LGIA. (From σπλην, the spleen, and αλγος, pain.) A pain in the spleen or its region.

SPLENETIC. (*Spleneticus*; from σπλην, the spleen.) Belonging to the spleen.

SPLENI'TIS. (From σπλην, the spleen.) Inflammation of the spleen. A genus of disease in the Class *Pyrexiæ*, and Order *Phlegmasiæ*, of Cullen; characterized by pyrexia, tension, heat, tumour, and pain in the left hypochondrium, increased by pressure. This disease, according to Juncker, comes on with a remarkable shivering, succeeded by a most intense heat, and very great thirst; a pain and tumour are perceived in the left hypochondrium, and the paroxysms for the most part assume a quartan form; when the patients expose themselves for a little to the free air, their extremities immediately grow very cold. If a hæmorrhagy happen, the blood flows out of the left nostril. The other symptoms are the same with those of the hepatitis. Like the liver, the spleen is also subject to a chronic inflammation, which often happens after agues, and is called the ague cake, though that name is also frequently given to a scirrhous tumour of the liver succeeding intermittents. The causes of this disease are in general the same with those of other inflammatory disorders; but those which determine the inflammation to that particular part more than another, are very much unknown. It attacks persons of a very plethoric and sanguine habit of body rather than others.

During the acute stage of splenitis, we must follow the antiphlogistic plan, by general and topical bleedings, by purging frequently, and by the application of blisters near the part affected. If it should terminate in suppuration, we must endeavour to discharge the pus externally, by fomentations or poultices. When the organ is in an enlarged scirrhous state, mercury may be successful in preventing its farther progress, or even producing a diminution of the part: but proper caution is required in the use of it, lest the remedy do more harm than the disease.

SPLE'NIUM. (From σπλην, the spleen: so called from its efficacy in disorders of the spleen.) 1. Spleenwort.

2. A compressed shape like the spleen.

SPLE'NIUS. (From σπλην, the spleen: so named from its resemblance in shape to the spleen, or, according to some, it derives its name from *splenium*, a *ferula*, or splint, which surgeons apply to the sides of a fractured bone.) *Splenius capitus*, and *splenius colli*, of Albinus; and *cervico-dorsi-mastoidien et dorso-trachelien*, of Dumas. The splenius is a flat, broad, and oblong muscle, in part covered by the upper part of the trapezius, and obliquely situated between the back of the ear, and the lower and posterior part of the neck.

It arises tendinous from the four or five superior spinous processes of the dorsal vertebræ; tendinous and fleshy from the last of the neck, and tendinous from the ligamentum colli, or rather the tendons of the two splenii unite here inseparably; but about the second or third vertebræ of the neck they recede from each other, so that part of the complexus may be seen.

It is inserted, by two distinct tendons, into the transverse processes of the two first vertebræ of the neck, sending off some few fibres to the complexus and levator scapulæ; tendinous and fleshy into the upper and posterior part of the mastoid process, and into a ridge on the occipital bone, where it joins with the root of that process.

This muscle may easily be separated into two parts. Eustachius and Fallopius were aware of this; Winslow has distinguished them into the *superior* and *inferior* portions; and Albinus has described them as two distinct muscles, calling that part which is inserted into the mastoid process and os occipitis, *splenius capitis*, and that which is inserted into the vertebræ of the neck, *splenius colli*. We have here followed Douglas, and the generality of writers, in describing these two portions as one muscle, especially as they are intimately united near their origin.

When this muscle acts singly, it draws the head and upper vertebræ of the neck obliquely backwards when both act, they pull the head directly backwards.

SPLENIUS CAPITIS. See *Splenius.*

SPLENIUS COLLI. See *Splenius.*

SPLENOCE'LE. (From σπλην, the spleen, and κηλη, a tumour.) A hernia of the spleen.

SPLINT. A long piece of wood, tin, or strong pasteboard employed for preventing the ends of broken bones from moving, so as to interrupt the process by which fractures unite.

SPO'DIUM. Σποδιον. The *spodium* of Dioscorides and of Galen are now not known in the shops. It is said to have been produced by burning cadmia alone in the furnace; for having thrown it in small pieces into the fire, near the nozzle of the bellows, they blow the most fine and subtle parts against the roof of the furnace: and what was reflected from thence was called *spodium*. It differed from the pompholyx in not being so pure, and in being more heavy. Pliny distinguishes several kinds of it, as that of copper, silver, gold, and lead.

SPODIUM ARABUM. Burnt ivory, or ivory black. See *Abaisir.*

SPODIUM GRÆCORUM. The white dung of dogs.

SPODUMENE. Prismatic triphane spar of Mohs. A mineral of a greenish white colour, first found in the island of Uton, in Sudermannland, and lately in the vicinity of Dublin. It contains the new alkali called *lethia.*

SPOLIA'RIUM. A private room at the baths.

SPONDY'LIUM. (From σπονδυλος, a vertebra: so named from the shape of its root, or probably because it was used against the bite of a serpent called σπονδυλις.) See *Heracleum spondylium.*

SPO'NDYLUS. Σπονδυλος. Some have thought fit to call the spine or backbone thus, from the shape and fitness of the vertebræ, to move every way upon one another.

SPONGE. See *Spongia.*

SPONGE-TENT. See *Spongia præparata.*

SPO'NGIA. Σπογγος; Σπογγια. Sponge. See *Spongia officinalis.*

SPONGIA OFFICINALIS. The systematic name of the sponge. A sea-production; the habitations of insects. A soft, light, very porous and compressible substance, readily imbibing water, and distending thereby. It is found adhering to rocks, particularly in the Mediterranean sea, about the islands of the Archipelago. It was formerly supposed to be a vegetable production, but is now classed among the zoophytes; and analyzed, it yields the same principles with animal substances in general. Burnt sponge is said to cure effectually the bronchocele, and to be of infinite utility in scrofulous complaints. Sponge tents are employed by surgeons to dilate fistulous ulcers, &c.

SPONGIA PRÆPARATA. Prepared sponge. Sponge tent. This is formed by dipping pieces of sponge in hot melted emplastrum ceræ compositum, and pressing them between two iron plates. As soon as cold, the substance thus formed may be cut into pieces of any shape. It was formerly used for dilating small openings, for which it was well adapted, as when the wax melted, the elasticity of the sponge made it expand and distend the opening, in which it had been put. Sir Ashley Cooper informs us that the best modern surgeons seldom employ it.

SPONGIA USTA. Burnt sponge. Cut the sponge into pieces, and beat it, that any extraneous matters may be separated; then burn it in a close iron vessel until it becomes black and friable; lastly, rub it to a very fine powder. This preparation is exhibited with bark in the cure of scrofulous complaints, and forms the basis of a lozenge, which has been known to cure the bronchocele in many instances. The dose is from a scruple to a drachm.

SPONGIOSA OSSA. *Ossa turbinata inferiora; Ossa convoluta.* These bones are situated in the under part of the side of the nose; they are of a triangular form and spongy appearance, resembling the os spongiosum superius; externally they are convex; internally they are concave; the convexity is placed towards the septum nasi, and the concavity outwards. The under edge of each bone is placed horizontally near the outer part of the nose, and ending in a sharp point behind. At the upper part of the bone are two processes, the anterior of which ascends and forms part of the lachry mal groove, and the posterior descends and forms a hook to make part of the maxillary sinus.

The connexion of this bone is to the os maxillare, os palati, and os unguis, by a distinct suture in the young subject; but in the adult, by a concretion of substance.

The ossa spongiosa afford a large surface for extending the organ of smell by allowing the membrane of the nose to be expanded, on which the olfactory nerves are dispersed.

In the fœtus, these bones are almost complete.

SPONGIO'SUM OS. 1. The ethmoid bone.

2. See *Spongiosa ossa.*

SPONGIO'SUS. Spongy.

SPONGOI'DES. (Σωογγοειδης; from σωογγος, a sponge, and ειδος, *forma,* shape: so called because it is hollow and porous, like a sponge or sieve.) See *Ethmoid bone.*

SPORA'DIC. (*Sporadicus;* from σπειρω, to sow.) An epithet for such infectious and other diseases as seize a few persons at any time or season.

Spotted lung-wort. See *Pulmonaria.*

SPRAIN. See *Subluxatio.*

SPRAT. The *Clupea sprattus,* of Linnæus. A small herring-like fish which comes to us between November and March, and are eaten fried and pickled. They are strong and hard of digestion.

SPRONGIDIUM. See *Columnula.*

SPRUCE. 1. A particular species of fir. See *Pinus abies.*

2. A fermented liquor called spruce beer prepared from the spruce fir. From the quantity of carbonic acid it contains, it is found a useful antiscorbutic.

Spurge flax. See *Daphne gnidium.*

Spurge laurel. See *Daphne laureola.*

Spurge olive. See *Daphne mezereum.*

[*Spurge, large flowering.* See *Euphorbia corollata.*

Spurred rye. See *Pulvis parturiens.* A.]

SPUTA'MEN. See *Sputum.*

SPU'TUM. (From *spuo,* to spit.) *Sputamen.* Saliva. Any kind of expectoration.

SQUAMA'RIA. (From *squama,* a scale: so called from its scaly roots.) The great tooth-wort, or *Plumbago europea.*

SQUAMATUS. Scaly: applied to the nectary of the *Ranunculus* genus, &c. See *Nectarium.*

SQUAMOSE. (*Squamosus;* from *squama,* a scale, because the bones lie over each other like scales.) Scaly.

SQUAMOSE SUTURE. The suture which unites the squamose portion of the temporal bone with the parietal.

SQUAMOSUS. Squamose. Scaled: applied to roots which are covered with fleshy scales; as in *Lathræa squamaria.*

SQUARROSUS. (From *squarra;* rough.) Squarrose. Rough, scabby, scaly. Applied to plants, &c.; as *Juncus squarrosus.*

SQUILL. See *Scilla.*

SQUI'LLA. See *Scilla.*

Squills, vinegar of. See *Acetum scillæ.*

SQUINA'NTHUS. (From *squinanthia,* the quinsy: so named from its uses in the quinsy.) See *Andropogon schœnanthus.*

STA'CHYS. (Σταχυς, a spike: so named from its spicated stalk and seed.) 1. The name of a genus of plants in the Linnæan system. Class, *Didynamia; Order, Gymnospermia.*

2. Some species of wild sage, and hoarhound, nettle, &c. were formerly so called.

STACHYS FŒTIDA. Yellow archangel. Hedge-nettle, or *Ballote nigra.*

STACHYS PALUSTRIS. Clown's woundwort or allheal.

STA'CTE. (Στακτη from ςαζω, to distil.) This term signifies that kind of myrrh which distils or falls in drops from the trees. It is also used by some writers for a more liquid kind of amber than what is commonly met with in the shops; whence in Scribonius Largus, Paulus Ægineta, and some others, we meet with a collyrium, and several other forms, wherein this was the the chief ingredient, distinguished by the name of *Stactica.*

STA'CTICON. Instillation: also an eye-water.

STA'GMA. (From ςαζω, to distil.) 1. Any distilled liquor.

2. The vitriolic acid.

STAHL, GEORGE ERNEST, was born at Anspach,

in 1660. He graduated at Jena, at the age of twenty four, and immediately commenced a course of private lectures there; and about three years after, he was made physician to the duke of Saxe-Weimar. On the establishment of the university of Halle, in 1694, he was appointed to a medical professorship, at the solicitation of Hoffman: and he became the leader of a sect of physicians, in opposition to the mechanical theorists, in which he was followed by many eminent persons as well in Germany as in other countries, notwithstanding the very fanciful nature of the hypothesis, on which his system was founded. It had been always observed, that there is a certain power in the animal body of resisting injuries, and correcting some of its disorders; and Van Helmont had ascribed some degree of intelligence to this power: but it was reserved for Stahl to refer it entirely to the rational soul, which, he affirmed, not only originally formed the body, but is the sole cause of all its motions, in the constant ex citement of which life consists. Whence diseases were generally regarded as salutary efforts of the presiding soul, to avert the destruction of the body. This hypothesis, besides its visionary character, was justly deprecated, as leading to an inert practice, and the neglect of the collateral branches of medical science, even of anatomical researches, which Stahl maintained, had little or no reference to the art of healing. And in fact both he and his followers, trusting principally to the operations of nature, zealously opposed the use of some of the most efficacious remedies, as opium, cinchona, and mercury; and were extremely reserved in the employment of bleeding, vomiting, &c., although their system led them to refer most diseases to plethora This hypothesis was maintained by Stahl with much ingenuity in several publications, particularly in his "Theoria Medica vera," printed in 1708. The merits of Stahl, as a chemical philosopher, are of a much higher character; and the school, which he founded in this science, has only been superseded of late by farther discoveries. He was the inventor of the celebrated theory of phlogiston, which appeared to account for the phenomenon of combustion, and was received every where with high applause. His chief chemical work was entitled "Fundamenta Chemiæ dogmaticæ et Experimentalis," first printed in 1729 : but this had been preceded more than thirty years, by others, in which his doctrine was fully displayed. Stahl was elected a member of the Academy Naturæ Curiosorum: and he was called, in 1716, to visit the king of Prussia at Berlin, whither he went also on several subsequent occasions, and on one of these he was attacked with a disease, which proved fatal, in the 74th year of his age.

STALACTITES. The calcareous substances found suspended from vaults, being formed by the oozing of water charged with calcareous particles gradually evaporating, and leaving these particles behind.

STALAGMI'TIS. (From ςαλαγμος, a dropping or distillation, because the gum which it yields escapes in that manner.) The name of a genus of plants. Class, *Polygamia; Order, Monœcia.*

STALAGMITIS CAMBOGIOIDES. This is now ascertained to be the tree which affords gamboge. This drug, from its supposed virtues, is also called *gummi ad podagram; gummi gutta;* and, by corruption, *gotta; gutta gamba; gamon; germandra; catagemu; gam boidea,* &c.; and, from its gold colour, *chrysopus;* and, from its purgative quality, *succus laxativus; succus Indicus purgans;* and *scammonium orientale.* Gamboge is a concrete vegetable juice, which was supposed to be the produce of two trees, both called by the Indians, *Caracapulli,* and by Linnæus, *Gambogia gutta;* but Kœnig ascertained its true source. It is partly of a gummy, and partly of a resinous nature. It is brought to us chiefly from Gambaja, in the East Indies, either in form of orbicular masses, or of cylindrical rolls of various sizes; and is of a dense, compact, and firm texture and of a beautiful yellow colour. In medi cine it is chiefly used as a drastic purge; it operates powerfully both upwards and downwards. Some condemn it as acting with too great violence, while others are of a contrary opinion. The dose is from two to four grains, as a cathartic; from four to eight grains it proves emetic and purgative. The roughness of its operation is said to be diminished, by giving it in a liquid form sufficiently diluted. Rubbed with almonds from its want of taste, it is a good laxative for children

It has been given in dropsy, with cream of tartar, to correct its operation. It has also been recommended by some, to the extent of fifteen grains, joined with an equal quantity of vegetable alkali, to destroy the tapeworm. This dose is ordered in the morning, and if the worm is not expelled in two or three hours, it is repeated even to the third time, with safety and efficacy. It is asserted, that it has been given to this extent even in delicate habits. This is said to be the remedy alluded to by Dr. Van Swieten, which was employed by Dr. Herenchwand, and with him proved so successful in the removal of the tænia lata. It is an ingredient, and probably the active one, in most of the nostrums for expelling tæniæ.

Dr. Cullen says, that, on account of the quick passage of gamboge through the intestines, he was induced to give it in small, and frequently repeated doses, as three or four grains, rubbed with a little sugar, every three hours; and thus found it operate without griping or sickness; and, in three or four exhibitions, evacuate a great quantity of water, both by stool and urine.

STALA′GMUS. (From ςαλαζω, to distil.) Distillation.

STA′LTICA. (From ςελλω, to contract.) Healing applications.

STAMEN. The male genital organ of plants, found generally within the corolla, near the pistil. Stamens were formerly called *chives.* They are various in number in different flowers, from one to some hundreds. This organ is essential to a plant, no one having yet been discovered, after the most careful research, that is destitute of it, either in the same flower with the pistils, or a separate one of the same species.

A stamen consists of three parts.

1. The *filamentum*, or *filament,* the part which supports the anther.

2. The *anthera,* placed on the filament, and the most essential part of all.

3. The *pollen,* or powder adhering to the anther.

STANNI PULVIS. Tin finely divided is exhibited internally as a vermifuge. It acts mechanically, and the fine filings are more effectual than the powder.

STANNIC ACID. A name which has been given to the peroxide of tin, because it is soluble in alkalies.

STA′NNUM. See *Tin.*

STAPE′DIS MUSCULUS. See *Stapedius.*

STAPE′DIUS. (*Stapedius,* sc. *musculus;* from *stapes,* one of the bones of the ear.) *Musculus stapes,* of Cowper; and *pyramidal-stapedien,* of Dumas. A muscle of the internal ear, which draws the stapes obliquely upwards towards the cavern, by which the posterior part of its base is moved inwards, and the anterior part outwards.

STA′PES. (*In quo pes stat,* a stirrup.) A bone of the internal ear, so called from its resemblance to a stirrup.

STAPHILI′NUS. See *Azygos uvulæ.*

STAPHILINUS EXTERNUS. See *Circumflexus.*

STA′PHIS. Σταφις, is strictly a grape, or a bunch of grapes; whence, from their likeness thereunto, it is applied to many other things, especially the glands of the body, whether natural or diseased.

STAPHISA′GRIA, Σταφις αγρια, wild vine; from the resemblance of its leaves to those of the vine.) See *Delphinium.*

STAPHYLE. (Σταφυλη. A grape or raisin: so called from its resemblance.) The uvula.

STAPHYLI′NUS. (*Staphylinus;* from ςαφυλη, the uvula.) See *Azygos uvulæ.*

STAPHYLINUS EXTERNUS. See *Circumflexus.*

STAPHYLINUS GRÆCORUM. *Staphylinus sylvestris.* The wild carrot.

STAPHYLO′MA. (From ςαφυλη, a grape: so named from its being thought to resemble a grape.) *Staphylosis.* A disease of the eyeball in which the cornea loses its natural transparency, rises above the level of the eye, and successively even projects beyond the eyelids, in the form of an elongated, whitish, or pearl-coloured tumour, which is sometimes smooth, sometimes uneven, and is attended with a total loss of sight. The proximate cause is an effusion of thick humour between the lamellæ of the cornea, so that the internal and external superfices of the cornea, very much protuberate. The remote causes are, an habitual ophthalmia, great contusion, and frequently a deposition of the variolous humour in the small-pox. The species are:

1st. *Staphyloma totale,* which occupies the whole transparent cornea; this is the most frequent species. The symptoms are, the opaque cornea protuberates, and if in the form of a cone, increasing in magnitude it pushes out and inverts the lower eyelid; and sometimes the morbid cornea is so elongated, as to lie on the cheek, causing friction and excoriation. The bulb of the eye being exposed to the air, sordes generate, the inferior palpebra is irritated by the cilia, and very painful red and small papillæ are observable.

2d. *Staphyloma racemosum,* is a staphyloma formed by carnous tubercles, about the size of a small pin's head.

3d. *Staphyloma partiale,* which occupies some part of the cornea: it exhibits an opaque tumour prominent from the cornea, similar to a small bluish grape.

4th. *Staphyloma scleroticæ* is a bluish tumour attached to some part of the sclerotica, but arises from the tunica albuginea.

5th. *Staphyloma pellucidum,* in which the cornea is not thickened or incrassated, but very much extended and pellucid.

6th. *Staphyloma complicatum,* which is complicated with an ulcer, ectropium, caruncles, or any other disorder of the eye.

7th. *Staphyloma iridis.* For this species, see *Ptosis iridis.*

Star thistle. See *Carlina acaulis.*

STARCH. *Amylum.* A white, insipid, combustible substance, insoluble in cold water, but forming a jelly with boiling water. It exists chiefly in the white and brittle parts of vegetables, particularly in tuberose roots, and the seeds of the gramineous plants. It may be extracted by pounding these parts, and agitating them in cold water; when the parenchyma, or fibrous parts, will first subside; and these being removed, a fine, white powder, diffused through the water, will gradually subside, which is the starch. Or the pounded or grated substance, as the roots of arum, potatoes, acorns, or horse-chesnuts, for instance, may be put into a hair-sieve, and the starch washed through with cold water, leaving the grosser matters behind. Farinaceous seeds may be ground and treated in a similar manner. Oily seeds require to have the oil expressed from them before the farina is extracted.

Starch is one of the constituent parts in all mealy farinaceous seeds, fruits, roots, and other parts of plants. Our common starch is made from wheat. It is not necessary that the grain be first bruised in mills. The entire corn, well cleansed, is soaked in cold water until the husks separate; and the grains, having become quite soft, give out, by pressure, a milky fluid. The grains are then taken out of the water by means of a sieve, put into a coarse linen sack, and transferred into the treading-tub; where they are trodden, after cold water has been poured upon them.

By this operation the starchy part is washed out, and, mingling with the water, makes it milky. The water is now drawn off, running through a sieve into the settling-tub. Fresh water is again effused upon the grains, and the same operation is continued till the water in the treading-tub is no longer rendered milky. The starch here precipitates by repose from the water that held it suspended; during which, especially in a warm season, the mucilaginous saccharine matter of the flour, that was dissolved by the water, goes into the acetous fermentation. From this cause the starch grows still purer and whiter. The water is next let off from the starch, which is several times more washed with clear fresh water; the remaining part of which is suffered to drip through linen cloths, supported by hurdles, upon which the wet starch is placed. When the starch has fully subsided, it is wrapped in, wrung between these cloths, or pressed, to extort still more of the remaining liquid.

It is afterward cut into pieces, which are laid in airy places, on slightly burnt bricks, to be completely dried, partly by the free currency of air, and partly by the bricks imbibing their moisture. Lastly, the outer crust is scraped off, and they are broken into smaller pieces.

If starch be subjected to distillation, it gives out water impregnated with empyreumatic acetous acid, a little red or brown oil, a great deal of carbonic acid, and carburetted hydrogen gas. Its coal is bulky, easily burned, and leaves a very small quantity of potassa and phosphate of lime If when diffused in water it

be exposed to a heat of 60° F., or upward, it will ferment, and turn sour; but much more so if it be not
freed from the gluten, extract, and colouring matter.
Thus, in starch-making, the farina ferments and becomes sour, but the starch that does not undergo fermentation is rendered the more pure by this process.
Some water, already soured, is mixed with the flour
and water, which regulates the fermentation, and prevents the mixture from becoming putrid; and in this
state it is left about ten days in summer, and fifteen in
winter, before the scum is removed, and the water
poured off. The starch is then washed out from the
bran, and dried, first in the open air, and finally in an
oven.

With boiling water, starch forms a nearly transparent mucilage, emitting a peculiar smell, neither disagreeable nor very powerful. This mucilage may be
dried, and will then be semitransparent, and much
resembling gum, all the products of which it affords.
When dissolved, it is much more easily digested and
nutritious than before it has undergone this operation.

Both acids and alkalies, combined with water, dissolve it. It separates the oxides of several metals from
their solutions, and takes oxygen from many of them.
It is found naturally combined with all the immediate
principles of vegetables, and may easily be united with
most of them by art.

When starch is triturated with iodine, it forms combinations of various colours. When the proportion of
iodine is small, these compounds are violet; when
somewhat greater, blue; and, when still greater, black.

We can always obtain the finest blue colour, by
treating starch with an excess of iodine, dissolving the
compound in liquid potassa, and precipitating by a
vegetable acid. The colour is manifested even at the
instant of pouring water of iodine into a liquid which
contains starch diffused through it. Hence iodine becomes an excellent test for detecting starch; and starch
for detecting iodine. Besides these combinations, it
appears that there is another of a white colour, in
which the iodine exists in very small quantity. All of
them possess peculiar properties.

Starch is not affected in the cold, by water, alkohol,
or ether. But it dissolves readily, when triturated
with potassa water.

Starch is convertible into sugar by dilute sulphuric
acid. To produce this change we must take 2000 parts
of starch, diffuse them in 8000 parts of water, containing 40 parts of strong oil of vitriol; and boil the
mixture for 36 hours in a basin of silver or lead, taking
care to stir the materials with a wooden rod, during
the first hour of ebullition. At the end of this time,
the mass having become liquid, does not require to be
stirred, except at intervals. In proportion as the
water evaporates, it ought to be replaced. When the
liquid has been sufficiently boiled, we must add to it
chalk and animal charcoal, then clarify with white of
egg, filter the mixture through a flock of wool, and
then concentrate the liquid till it has acquired a syrupy
consistence. After this, the basin must be removed
from the fire, in order that, by cooling, the greater part
of the sulphate of lime may fall down. The pure
syrup is now to be decanted off, and evaporated to the
proper dryness. The greater the quantity of acid employed, the less ebullition is required to convert the
starch into the saccharine matter.

The discovery of the preceding process is due to
Kirchhoff, of St. Petersburgh.

The presence of sulphuric acid is not indispensable
for obtaining sugar from starch. It may also be obtained by leaving the starch to itself, either with or
without contact of air, or by mixing it with dried
gluten. At the same time, indeed, several other products are formed. M. Theod. de Saussure's interesting observations on this subject are published in the
Annales de Chemie et de Physique, xi. 379. The starch,
brought to the state of a pulpy mass, must be left to
spontaneous decomposition. The products are, 1st, a
sugar, like the sugar of grapes; 2d, Gum, like that
from roasted starch; 3d, Amidine, a body whose properties are intermediate between those of starch and
gum: and 4th, an insoluble substance, like ligneous
matter. In these experiments, the mass on which he
operated was made by pouring 12 parts of boiling
water on 1 of starch. When it was fermented by
dried gluten, he obtained—

	Without contact of air.	With contact of air.
Sugar	47.4	49.7
Gum	23.0	9.7
Amadine	8.9	5.2
Amalaceous lignin	10.3	9.2
Lignin with charcoal	A trace	0.3
Undecomposed starch	4.0	3.8

Potato starch differs perceptibly from that of wheat;
it is more friable; is composed of ovoïd grains, about
twice the size of the other.

As starch forms the greatest part of flour, it cannot
be doubted but that it is the principal alimentary substance contained in our bread. In a medical point of
view, it is to be considered as a demulcent; and, accordingly, it forms the principal ingredient of an offi
cinal lozenge in catarrhs, and a mucilage prepared
from it often produces excellent effects, both taken by
the mouth and in the form of clyster, in dysenteries
and diarrhœa, from irritation of the intestines. Milk
and starch, with the addition of suet finely shred, and
incorporated by boiling, was the soup employed by Sir
John Pringle, in dysenteries, where the mucous membrane of the intestines had been abraded. Externally,
surgeons apply it as an absorbent in erysipelas.

STA'TICE. (From ςατιζω, to stop: so named from
its supposed property of restraining hæmorrhages.)
The name of a genus of plants in the Linnæan system. Class, *Pentandria;* Order, *Pentagynia.* The
herb sea-thrift.

STATICE LIMONIUM. The systematic name of the
sea-thrift. Sea-lavender, or red behen. *Behen rubrum; Limonium: Limonium majus; Behen.* The
roots possess astringent and strengthening qualities,
but not in a very remarkable degree.

STATIONA'RIA FEBRIS. A stationary fever. So
Sydenham called those fevers which happen when
there are certain general constitutions of the years,
which owe their origin neither to heat, cold, dryness,
nor moisture; but rather depend on a certain secret
and inexplicable alteration in the bowels of the earth,
whence the air becomes impregnated with such kinds
of effluvia as subject the body to particular distempers,
so long as that kind of constitution prevails, which,
after a certain course of years, declines and gives way
to another.

STAUROLITE. Grenatite, or prismatic garnet.

STAUROTIDE. Grenatite. Prismatic garnet. A
crystallized, dark, reddish-brown garnet, found in Scotland, and Ireland.

STA'VESACRE. See *Delphinium staphisagria.*

STEARINE. See *Fat.*

STEATITE. Soapstone. A subspecies of rhomboidal mica.

STEATOCE'LE. (From ςεαρ, suet, and κηλη, a
tumour.) A collection of a suety substance in the
scrotum.

STEATOMA. (From ςεαρ, suet.) An encysted
tumour, the contents of which are of a suety consistence.

STEEL. *Chalybs.* The best, hardest, finest, and
closest grained iron, combined with carbon by a particular process.

STEINHEILITE. The blue quartz of Finland.

STELOCHI'TES. See *Osteocolla.*

STE'LLA. (From ςελλω, to arise.) A star. A
bandage with many crossings, like a star.

STELLA'RIA. (From *stella,* a star: so named
from the star-like appearance of its flowers.) The
name of a genus of plants. Class, *Decandria;* Order, *Trigynia.* Stitchwort.

STELLATUS. (From *stella,* a star.) Stellate.
Starlike. Applied to the nectary of the *Stapelia,* &c.

STELLATÆ. The name of an order of plants in
Linnæus's Fragments of a Natural Method, consisting
of such as have stellate leaves, and quadrified corolla
mostly tetrandrous; as Galium, Asperula, Rubea tinc
torum, &c

STE'MA. (From ςημι, to stand.) The penis.
Stemless milkvetch. See *Astragalus excapus.*

STENO, NICHOLAS, was born at Copenhagen, in
1638. Having studied with great diligence, under the
celebrated Bartholin, he passed several years in visiting
the best schools in different parts of Europe. His reputation was then increased, so that about the age of
29 he was appointed Physician to Ferdinand II. Grand
Duke of Tuscany, with a liberal salary. He was

afterward honoured with the esteem of Cosmo III. who selected him as preceptor to his son. He had been led, by the eloquence of Bossuet, to change from the Protestant to the Roman Catholic persuasion; which proved an obstacle to his accepting the invitation of Frederick III. to return to Copenhagen; but the succeeding King of Denmark, not imposing any religious restraint, he was induced about the year 1672 to go to his native city, where he was appointed professor of anatomy. But finding his situation less agreeable than he had expected, he resumed the education of the young prince at Florence. Some time after this he embraced the ecclesiastical profession, was speedily appointed a bishop, and then vicar apostolical to all the states of the north, in which capacity he became a zealous preacher in various parts of Germany, and died in the course of his labours in 1686. The works extant by him relate principally to medical subjects. He was a diligent cultivator of anatomy, and made some discoveries relative to the minute structure of the eye, and other parts; which are detailed in papers communicated to the academy of Copenhagen, and in some small works published by himself.

STENOTHORA'CES. (From ςενος, narrow, and θωραξ, the chest.) Those who have narrow chests are so called.

STERILITY. *Sterilitas.* Barrenness. In women this sometimes happens from a miscarriage, or violent labour, injuring some of the genital parts; but one of the most frequent causes is the suppression of the menstrual flux. There are other causes, however, arising from various diseases incident to those parts; by which the uterus may be unfit to receive or retain the male seed;—from the tubæ Fallopianæ being too short, or having lost their erective power; in either of which cases no conception can take place;—from universal debility and relaxation; or a local debility of the genital system; by which means the parts having lost their tone, or contractile power, the semen is thrown off immediately *post coitum;*—from imperforation of the vagina, of the uterus, or tubæ, or from diseased ova, &c.

STERNO. Names compounded of this word belong to muscles which are attached to the sternum; as, STERNO-CLEIDO-HYOIDEUS. See *Sterno-hyoideus.*

STERNO-CLEIDO MASTOIDEUS. *Sterno-mastoideus,* and *cleido-mastoideus,* of Albinus. *Mastoideus,* of Douglas and Cowper; and *sterno-clavio-mastoidicn,* of Dumas. A muscle, on the anterior and lateral part of the neck, which turns the head to one side, and bends it forward. It arises by two distinct origins; the anterior tendinous and fleshy, from the top of the sternum near its junction with the clavicle; the posterior fleshy, from the upper and anterior part of the clavicle. Both unite a little above the anterior articulation of the clavicle, to form one muscle, which runs obliquely upwards and outwards to be inserted, by a thick strong tendon, into the mastoid process of the temporal bone, which it surrounds; and gradually becoming thinner, is inserted as far back as the lambdoidal suture.

STERNO-COSTALES. Vesalius considered these as forming a single muscle on each side of a triangular shape; hence we find the name of *triangularis* adopted by Douglas and Albinus; but Verheyen, who first taught that they ought to be described as four or five distinct muscles, gave them the name of *sterno costales ;* and in this he is very properly followed by Winslow, Haller, and Lieutaud.

These muscles are situated at each side of the under surface of the sternum, upon the cartilages of the third, fourth, fifth, and sixth ribs. Their number varies in different subjects; very often there are only three, sometimes five, and even six, but most usually we find only four.

The lowermost of the sterno-costales, or what would be called the inferior portion of the triangularis, arises tendinous and fleshy from the edge and inner surface of the lower part of the cartilago ensiformis, where its fibres intermix with those of the diaphragm and transversalis abdominis. Its fibres run nearly in a transverse direction, and are inserted, by a broad thin tendon, into the inner surface of the cartilage of the sixth rib, and lower edge of that of the fifth.

The second and largest of the sterno-costales, arises tendinous from the cartilago ensiformis and lower part of the sternum, laterally, and, running a little obliquely outwards, is inserted into the lower edge of the cartilage of the fifth, and sometimes of the fourth rib.

The third arises tendinous from the sides of the middle part of the sternum, near the cartilages of the fourth and fifth ribs, and ascending obliquely outwards, is inserted into the cartilage of the third rib.

The fourth and uppermost, which is the most frequently wanting, arises tendinous from the beginning of the cartilage of the third rib and the adjacent part of the sternum, and running almost perpendicularly upwards, is inserted by a thin tendon (which covers a part of the second internal intercostal,) into the cartilage and beginning of the bony part of the second rib.

All these muscles are more or less intermixed with one another at their origin, and this probably occasioned them to be considered as one muscle. Fallopius informs us, that the plate Vesalius has given of them was taken from a dog, in which animal they are much larger than in man. Douglas has endeavoured to account for this difference, but his explanation is far from being satisfactory.

STERNO-HYOIDEUS. As this muscle arises from the clavicle, as well as from the sternum, Winslow calls it *sterno-cleido-hyoideus.* It is a long, flat, and thin muscle, situated obliquely between the sternum and os hyoides, behind the lower part of the mastoideus, and covering the *sterno-thyroideus* and the *hyo-thyroideus.* It arises, by very short tendinous fibres, from the cartilaginous part of the first rib, from the upper and inner part of the sternum, from the capsular ligament that connects that bone with the clavicle, and commonly from a small part of the clavicle itself; from thence, ascending along the anterior and lateral part of the neck, we see it united to its fellow, opposite to the inferior part of the larynx, by means of a thin membrane, which forms a kind of *linea alba.* After this the two muscles separate again, and each passing over the side of the thyroid cartilage, is inserted into the basis of the os hyoides, immediately behind the insertion of the last described muscle.

Its use is to draw the os hyoides downwards.

STERNO-MASTOIDEUS. See *Sterno-cleido-mastoideus.*

STERNO-THYROIDEUS. *Sterno-thyroidien,* of Dumas. This is flat and thin, like the sterno-hyoideus but longer and broader. It is situated at the forepart of the neck, between the sternum and thyroid cartilage, and behind the sterno-hyoideus. It arises broad and fleshy from the upper and inner part of the sternum, between the cartilages of the first and second ribs, from each of which it receives some few fibres, as well as from the clavicle, where it joins with the sternum. From thence, growing somewhat narrower, it ascends, and, passing over the thyroid gland and the cricoid cartilage, is inserted tendinous into the lower and posterior edge of the rough line of the thyroid cartilage, immediately under the insertion of the sterno-hyoideus. Now and then a few of its fibres pass on to the os hyoides. Its use is to draw the thyroid cartilage, and consequently the larynx, downwards.

STE'RNUM. *Pectoris os.* The breast-bone. The sternum, os pectoris, or breast-bone, is the oblong, flat bone, placed at the forepart of the thorax. The ossification of this bone in the fœtus begins from many different points at the same time, we find it, in young subjects, composed of several bones united by cartilages; but as we advance in life, most of these cartilages ossify, and the sternum, in the adult state, is found to consist of three, and sometimes only of two pieces, the two lower portions being united into one; and very often, in old subjects, the whole is formed into one bone. But, even in the latter case, we may still observe the marks of its former divisions; so that, in describing the bone, we may very properly divide it into its upper, middle, and inferior portions.

The upper portion forms an irregular square, which, without much reason, has, by many writers, been compared to the figure of a heart as it is painted on cards. It is of considerable thickness, especially at its upper part. Its anterior surface is irregular, and slightly convex; posteriorly, it is somewhat concave. Its upper middle part is hollowed, to make way for the trachea. On each side, superiorly, we observe an oblong articulating surface, covered with cartilage in the recent subject, for receiving the ends of the clavicles. Immediately below this, on each side, the bone becomes thinner, and we observe a rough surface for receiving the cartilage of the first rib, and, almost close to the inferior edge of this, we find the half of such another surface, which, combined with a similar surface in the middle portion of the sternum, serves for the articulation of the cartilage of the second rib.

The middle portion is much longer, narrower, and thinner than the former; but is somewhat broader and thinner below than above, where it is connected with the upper portion. The whole of its anterior surface is slightly convex, and within it is slightly concave. Its edge, on each side, affords four articulating surfaces, for the third, fourth, fifth, and sixth ribs; and parts of articulating surfaces at its upper and lower parts, for the second and seventh ribs. About the middle of this portion of the sternum we sometimes find a considerable hole, large enough in some subjects to admit the end of the little finger. Sylvius seems to have been the first who described it. Riolanus and some others after him have, without reason, supposed it to be more frequent in women than in men. In the recent subject it is closed by a cartilaginous substance; and, as it does not seem destined for the transmission of vessels, as some writers have asserted, we may, perhaps very properly, with Hunauld, consider it as an accidental circumstance, occasioned by an interruption of the ossification, before the whole of this part of the bone is completely ossified.

The third and inferior portion of the sternum is separated from the former by a line, which is seldom altogether obliterated, even in the oldest subjects. It is smaller than the other parts of the bone, and descends between the ribs, so as to have been considered as an appendix to the rest of the sternum. From its shape, and its being constantly in a state of cartilage in young subjects, it has been commonly named *cartilago xiphoides, ensiformis*, or sword-like cartilage; though many of the ancients gave the name of xiphoides to the whole sternum; comparing the first two bones to the handle, and this appendix to the blade of the sword. The shape of this appendix varies in different subjects; in some it is longer and more pointed, in others shorter and more obtuse. Veslingius has seen it reaching as low as the navel, and incommoding the motion of the trunk forwards. In general it terminates obtusely, or in a single point; sometimes, however, it is bifurcated, and Eustachius and Haller have seen it trifid. Very often we find it perforated, for the transmission of branches of the mammary artery. In the adult it is usually ossified and tipped with cartilage, but it very often continues cartilaginous through life, and Haller once found it in this state in a woman who died in her hundredth year.

The substance of the sternum, internally, is of a light, spongy texture, covered externally with a thin bony plate; hence it happens that this bone is easily fractured. From the description we have given of it, its uses may be easily understood. We have seen it serving for the articulation of seven true ribs on each side, and hence we shall find it of considerable use in respiration. We likewise observed, that it is articulated with each of the clavicles. It serves for the origin and insertion of several muscles; it supports the mediastinum; and lastly, defends the heart and lungs; and it is observable, that we find a similar bone in almost all animals that have lungs, and even in such as have no ribs, of which latter we have an instance in the frog.

STERNUTAMENTO RIA. So called because the powdered flowers and roots have the property of exciting sneezing. See *Achillea ptarmica.*

STE'RTOR. A noisy kind of respiration, as is observed in apoplexy. A snoring or snorting.

STHE'NIA. A term employed by the followers of Dr. Brown, to denote that state of the body which disposes to inflammatory diseases, in opposition to those of debility, which arise from asthenia.

STIBIA'LIS. (From *stibium*, antimony.) An antimonial or medicine, the chief ingredient of which is antimony.

STIBIC ACID. Berzelius's name of the yellow oxide of antimony.

STIBII ESSENTIA. Antimonial wine.

STIBIOUS ACID. So Berzelius calls the white oxide of antimony.

STI'BIUM. (Στιβιον : from ςιλβω, to shine.) An ancient name of antimony. See *Antimony.*

STI'GMA. (Στιγμα : from ςιζω, to inflict blows.) I. A small red speck in the skin, occasioning no elevation of the cuticle. Stigmata are generally distinct, or

apart from each other. They sometimes assume a livid colour, and are then termed *petechiæ.*

II. A natural mark or spot on the skin. See *Nævus maternus.*

III. That part of the female organ of a plant which is placed at the summit of the style. It is an indispensable part of the fructification, and consists of a vast number of absorbing papillæ, rarely observable by the naked eye, but best seen in the *Mirabilis jalapa.* Botanists distinguish the following differences in the form of stigmas:

1. *Globose;* as in *Trachelium.*
2. *Capitate,* round, but flat below; as in *Sorbus* and *Vinca.*
3. *Acute,* ending in a point; as in *Piscidia.*
4. *Obtuse;* as in *Nigrina.*
5. *Clubbed;* as in *Genipi.*
6. *Emarginate,* cut; as in *Dentaria.*
7. *Peltate;* as in *Garcinia.*
8. *Uncinate,* acute and reflected; as in *Lantana.*
9. *Triangular;* as in *Lilium candidum.*
10. *Trilobed;* as in *Tulipa gesneriana.*
11. *Petaliform;* as in *Iris germanica.*
12. *Convolute;* as in *Crocus.*
13. *Revolute;* as in *Leontodon.*
14. *Pennicilliform,* resembling a pencil-brush; as in *Milium paspalium.*
15. *Perforatum;* as in *Sloanea*
16. *Concave;* as in *Viola.*
17. *Bifid;* as in *Menyanthes.*
18. *Trifid;* as in *Amaryllis.*
19. *Multifid;* as in *Castus.*
20. *Striate;* as in *Papaver.*
21. *Plumose,* on each side, like a hairy pen; as in grasses.
22. *Four-sided;* as in *Amyris.*
23. *Pubescent,* covered with hair; as in *Vicia.*
24. *Simple,* not differing from the stile at its summit; as in *Galanthus* and *Hippuris.*
25. *Sessile,* on the germen; there being no stile.

The stigma is always more or less moist with a peculiar viscid fluid, which in some plants is so conspicuous as to form a large drop, though never big enough to fall to the ground. This moisture is designed for the reception of the pollen, which explodes on meeting with it; and hence the seeds are rendered capable of. ripening, which, though in many plants fully formed, they would not otherwise be.

STILBITE. See *Zeolite.*

STI'LBO'MA. (From ςιλβω, to polish.) A cosmetic

STILLICI'DIUM. (From *stilla,* to drop, and *cado,* to fall.) A strangury, or discharge of the urine drop by drop. Also the pumping upon a part.

STILPNOSIDERITE. A brownish black-coloured mineral, said to contain phosphoric acid. It occurs along with brown iron in Saxony and Bavaria.

STI'MMI. Στιμμι. Antimony.

STIMULANT. (*Stimulans;* from *stimulo,* to stir up.) That which possesses a power of exciting the animal energy. Stimulants are divided into,

1. *Stimulantia tonica;* as *sinapi,* cantharides, *hydrargyri præparationes.*
2. *Stimulantia diffusibilia;* as alkali *volatile,* electricity, heat, &c.
3. *Stimulantia cardiaca;* as cinnamomum, nux moschata, wine, &c.

STI'MULUS. (*Stimulus, i.* m.; from ςτιγμος, *stigmulus,* per sync. *stimulus,* a sting or spur.) That which rouses the action or energy of a part.

Stinking lettuce. See *Lactuca virosa.*

STINKSTONE. Swinestone. A variety of compact luculite, a subspecies of limestone.

STIPES. (*Stipes, itis.* m.; from the Greek, ςυπος.) A stipe, or stem of a fungus, fern, or palm.

STIPULA. A leafy appendage to the proper leaves, or to their footstalks. In some instances they are so like unto leaves, that they are believed to be so, and can only be distinguished from leaves by their situation on the footstalk. Stipulæ are,

1. *Solitary;* as in *Astragalus onobrychis.*
2. *In pairs;* as in *Lathyrus annuus.*
3. *Lateral,* on the side of the footstalk; as in *Lotus tetraphyllus.*
4. *Oppositifoliar,* in the side of the opposite leaves; as in *Trifolium pratense.*
5. *Extrafoliaceous,* external with respect to the leaf or footstalk; as in *Astragalus onobrichis.*

6. *Intrafoliaceous*, internal; as in *Morus nigra* and *alba*.

7. *Caducous*, falling off before the leaves are expanded; as in *Prunus avium*.

8. *Persistent*, remaining after the fall of the leaf; as in *Trifolium pratense*.

9. *Deciduous*, falling with the leaves; as in many stipulated plants.

10. *Spinescent*, becomes thorns; as in *Robinia pseudacacia*.

11. *Sessile;* as in *Pisum sativum*.

12. *Adnate;* as in *Rosa canina*.

13. *Decurrent;* as in *Crotullaria sagittalis*.

14. *Sheathed;* as in *Hedysum vaginale*.

15. *Lanceolate;* as in *Cistus helianthemum*.

16. *Subulate;* as in *Cassia glandulosa*.

17. *Sagittate;* as in *Pisum maritimum*.

18. *Lunate;* as in *Lathyrus tingitanus*.

19. *Ovate;* in *Ononis repens*.

20. *Cordate;* in *Ocymum sanctum*.

21. *Filiform;* in *Ononis mauritanica*.

22. *Foliaceous;* in *Sambucus ebulus*.

23. *Entire;* in *Vicia cracca*.

24. *Serrate;* in *Pisum sativum*.

25. *Ciliate;* in *Passiflora fœtida*.

26. *Toothed;* in *Orobus lathyroides*.

27. *Pinnatifid;* in *Viola tricolor*.

STIPULARIS. Stipular: belonging to the stipula of plants; as the *spina stipularis* of the Mimosa nilotica and horrida.

STIZOLO'BIUM. The cowage. See *Dolichos*.

STOE'CHAS. (From ςοιχαδες, the islands on which it grew.) See *Lavendula stœchas*.

STOECHAS ARABICA. See *Lavendula stœchas*.

STOECHAS CITRINA. See *Gnaphalium stœchas*.

STOLO. (*Stolo, onis.* m.; a shoot, branch, or twig.) A sucker or scyon. A runner which proceeds from the roots of some plants, and takes root in the earth. It is distinguished into a *supraterraneous*, which runs on the surface above ground; as in *Fagaria vesca*, and *Potentilla reptans*; and *subterraneous*, which runs under the surface, as in *Triticum repens*, the stolos of which are erroneously taken for the roots.

STOMACA'CE. (*Stomacace, es.* f.; from ςομα, the mouth, and κακος, evil.) Canker. A fetor in the mouth, with a bloody discharge from the gums. It is generally a symptom of the scurvy. It is also a name for the scurvy.

STOMACH. (*Stomachus, chi.* m.; from ςομα, the mouth, and χεω, to pour.) *Ventriculus;* called also *Anocœlia; Gaster; Nedys*. A membraneous receptacle, situated in the epigastric region, which receives the food from the œsophagus; its figure is somewhat oblong and round: it is largest on the left side, and gradually diminishes towards its lower orifice, where it is the least. Its superior orifice, where the œsophagus terminates, is called the *cardia:* the inferior orifice, where the intestine begins, the *pylorus*. The anterior surface is turned towards the abdominal muscles, and the posterior opposite the lumbar vertebræ. It has two curvatures: the first is called the great curvature of the stomach, and extends downwards from one orifice to the other, having the omentum adhering to it; the second is the small curvature, which is also between both orifices, but superiorly and posteriorly. The stomach, like the intestinal canal, is composed of three coats, or membranes: 1. The *outermost*, which is very firm, and from the peritonæum. 2. The *muscular*, which is very thick, and composed of various muscular fibres; and, 3. The *innermost*, or *villous coat*, which is covered with exhaling and inhaling vessels, and mucus. These coats are connected together by cellular membrane. The glands of the stomach which separate the mucus are situated between the villous and muscular coat, in the cellular structure. The arteries of the stomach come chiefly from the cœliac artery, and are distinguished into the coronary, gastro-epiploic, and short arteries; they are accompanied by veins which have similar names, and which terminate in the vena portæ. The nerves of the stomach are very numerous, and come from the eighth pair and intercostal nerves. The lymphatic vessels are distributed throughout the whole substance, and proceed immediately to the thoracic duct. The use of the stomach is to excite hunger and partly thirst, to receive the food from the œsophagus, and to retain it, till, by the motion of the stomach, the admixture of various fluids and many

310

other changes, it is rendered fit to pass the right orifice of the stomach, and afford chyle to the intestines

Stomach, inflammation of. See *Gastritis*.

[STOMACH PUMP. This is an instrument introduced of late for the purpose of emptying the stomach of its contents, when poison has been swallowed. It is a long catheter made of gum elastic, which being introduced into the mouth, is passed into the œsophagus and pressed forwards, until the point reaches the stomach A syringe adapted to the upper end is then applied, and the stomach is emptied of its fluid contents. If poison be swallowed in a liquid state, it may thus be most effectually removed, and rendered harmless. A.]

STOMACHIC. (*Stomachicus;* from ςομαχος, the stomach.) That which excites and strengthens the action of the stomach.

STOMA'CHICA· PASSIO. A disorder in which there is an aversion to food; even the thought of it begets a nausea, anxiety, cardialgia, and effusion of saliva, and often a vomiting. Fasting is more tolerable than eating; if obliged to eat, a pain follows that is worse than hunger itself.

STO'MACHUS. See *Stomach*.

STONE. See *Calculus*.

STONE-CROP. See *Sedum acre*.

STO'RAX. Στοραξ. See *Styrax*.

Storax, liquid. See *Liquidambra*.

STORAX LIQUIDA. See *Liquidambra*.

STORAX RUBRA OFFICINALIS. Cascarilla bark was so called.

Storax, white. See *Myroxylon peruiferum*.

STORCK, ANTHONY, a medical professor of considerable note at Vienna, who succeeded the celebrated Van Swieten as president and director of the faculty of medicine in that university, and was also honoured with the appointment of principal consulting physician to the Empress Maria Theresa. He distinguished himself chiefly by a long and assiduous course of experiments, with various narcotic vegetables, as hemlock, henbane, stramonium, aconite, colchicum, &c.; of which, though he appears to have overrated the efficacy, yet certainly he had the merit of calling the attention of practitioners to a class of active remedies, which may often be highly useful under prudent management. His various tracts on these subjects were printed between 1760 and 1771, and they have since passed through several editions and translations. He was also author of a collection of cases, which occurred under his observation in the hospital at Vienna; and this work was afterward continued by his successor, Dr. Collin.

STRABI'SMUS. See *Strabismus*.

STRABI'SMUS. (From ςραβιζω, to squint.) *Stra balismus : Strabositas*. Squinting. An affection of the eye by which a person sees objects in an oblique manner, from the axis of vision being distorted. Cullen arranges this disease in the Class *Locales*, and Order *Dyscinesiæ*. He distinguishes three species:—

1. *Strabismus habitualis*, when from a custom of using only one eye.

2. *Strabismus commodis*, when one eye in comparison with the other, from greater weakness, or mobility, cannot accommodate itself to the other.

3. *Strabismus necessarius*, when some change takes place in the situation or figure of the eye, or a part of it.

STRABO'SITAS. See *Strabismus*.

STRAHLSTEIN. See *Actinolite*.

STRA'MEN CAMELORUM. Camel's hay. See *Andropogon schœnanthus*.

STRAMMO'NIUM. See *Stramonium*.

STRAMO'NIUM. (From *stramen*, straw: so called from its fibrous roots.) See *Datura stramonium*.

STRAMONIUM OFFICINALE. See *Datura stramonium*.

STRAMONIUM SPINOSUM. See *Datura stramonium*.

STRA'NGALIS. (From ςραγγευω, to torment.) A hard, painful tumour in the breast, from milk.

STRANGURIA. See *Strangury*.

STRA'NGURY. (*Stranguria, æ.* f.; from ςραγξ, a drop, and ουρον, urine.) A difficulty in making water, attended with pain and dripping. See *Ischuria*.

STRATIO'TES. (From ςρα]ος, an army: so named from its virtues in healing fresh wounds, and its usefulness to soldiers.) See *Achillea millefolium*.

STRATIO'TICUM. See *Achillea millefolium*.

STRAWBERRY. See *Fragaria*.

STREATHAM. A village in Surrey, where is a

weak purging water, drunk to the amount of one, two, or more pints in a morning.

STRE'MMA. (Στρεμμα; from ςρεφω, to turn.) A strain or sprain of the parts about a joint.

STRIA'TUS. Striate. Applied to stems, seeds, &c.; as the stem of the Œnanthe fistula, and seeds of the Conium maculatum.

STRICTURE. *Strictura.* A diminution, or contracted state of some tube, or duct, of the body, as the œsophagus, intestines, urethra, vagina, &c. They are either organic or spasmodic.

STRICTUS. In botanical language it means straight, as *Caulis strictus.*

STRI'DOR. A noise of crashing.

STRIDOR DENTIUM. Grinding of the teeth.

STRIGA. A species of pubescence of plants, white, bristle-like, with broad bases mostly decumbent; as in *Borago officinalis.*

STRI'GIL. *Strigilis.* An instrument to scrape off the sweat during the gymnastic exercises of the ancients, and in their baths: *strigils* were made of metal, horn, or ivory, and were curved. Some were made of linen.

STRIGME'NTUM. The strigment, filth, or sordes, scraped from the skin, in baths and places of exercises.

STROBILUS. A cone. A species of pericarpium, or seed-vessel. A catkin hardened and enlarged into a seed-vessel; an example of which is in the *pinus,* or fir. It is either *conic, cylindric, ovate, globose, squamose,* or *spurious,* consisting of membraneous and not woody scales; as in *Origanum marjorana.*

STRONTIA. (So called because it was first found in a lead mine at Strontian, in Scotland.) A grayish white-coloured earth, found in combination with carbonic acid in the mineral called Strontianite.

Pure strontia is of a grayish-white colour; a pungent, acrid taste; and when powdered in a mortar, the dust that rises irritates the lungs and nostrils. Its specific gravity approaches that of barytes. It requires rather more than 160 parts of water at 60° to dissolve it; but of boiling water much less. On cooling, it crystallizes in thin, transparent, quadrangular plates, generally parallelograms, seldom exceeding a quarter of an inch in length, and frequently adhering together. The edges are most frequently bevelled from each side. Sometimes they assume a cubic form. These crystals contain about .68 of water; are soluble in 51.4 times their weight of water at 60°, and in little more than twice their weight of boiling water. They give a blood-red colour to the flame of burning alkohol. The solution of strontia changes vegetable blues to a green. Strontia combines with sulphur either in the wet or dry way, and its sulphuret is soluble in water.

In its properties, strontia has a considerable affinity to barytes. It differs from it chiefly in being infusible, much less soluble, of a different form, weaker in its affinities, and not poisonous. Its saline compounds afford differences more marked.

The basis of strontia is *strontium,* a metal first procured by Sir H. Davy, in 1808, precisely in the same manner as barium, to which it is very analogous, but has less lustre. It appeared fixed, difficultly fusible, and not volatile. It became converted into strontia by exposure to air, and when thrown into water, decomposed it with great violence, producing hydrogen gas, and making the water a solution of strontia. By igniting the mineral strontianite intensely with charcoal powder, strontia is cheaply procured.

Strontianite. See *Heavy spar.*

STRONTIUM. The metallic base of strontia. See *Strontia.*

STROPHIOLUM. A little curved gland-like part near the scar or base of some seeds; as that of *Asarum,* but especially in several papilionaceous genera, as *Ulex, Spartium,* &c.

STRO'PHOS. (From ςρεφω, to turn.) A twisting of the intestines.

STRO'PHULUS. A papulous eruption peculiar to infants, and exhibiting a variety of forms, which are described by Dr. Willan, under the titles of *intertinctus, albidus, confertus, volaticus,* and *candidus.*

1. *Strophulus inte-tinctus,* usually called the *red gum,* and, by the French, *Effloresce-ce benigne.* The papulæ characterizing this affection, rise sensibly above the level of the cuticle, are of a vivid red colour, and commonly distinct from each other. Their number and extent vary much in different cases. They ap-pear most constantly on the cheeks, forearm, and back of the hand, but are sometimes diffused over the whole body. The papulæ are, in many places, intermixed with stigmata, and often with red patches of a larger size, which do not, however, occasion any elevation of the cuticle. A child's skin thus variegated, somewhat resembles a piece of red printed linen; and hence this eruption was formerly called the *red gown,* a term which is still retained in several counties of England, and may be found in old dictionaries. Medical writers have changed the original word for one of a similar sound, but not more significant. The *strophulus intertinctus* has not, in general, any tendency to become pustular; a few small pustules, containing a straw-coloured watery fluid, occasionally appear on the back of the hand, but scarcely merit attention, as the fluid is always reabsorbed in a short time, without breaking the cuticle. The eruption usually terminates in scurf, or exfoliation of the cuticle; its duration, however, is very uncertain; the papulæ and spots sometimes remain for a length of time without an obvious alteration; sometimes disappear and come out again daily; but, for the most part, one eruption of them succeeds another, at longer intervals, and with more regularity. This complaint occurs chiefly within the first two months of lactation. It is not always accompanied with, or preceded by any disorders of the constitution, but appears occasionally in the strongest and most healthy children. Some authors connect it with aphthous ulcerations common in children, supposing the latter to be a part of the same disease diffused along the internal surfaces of the mouth and intestines. The fact, however, seems to be, that the two affections alternate with each other: for those infants who have the papulous eruption on the skin are less liable to aphthæ; and when the aphthæ take place to a considerable degree, the skin is generally pale and free from eruption. The *strophulus intertinctus* is, by most writers, said to originate from an acidity, or acrimonious quality of the milk taken into a child's stomach, communicated afterward to the blood, and stimulating the cutaneous excretories. This opinion might, without difficulty, be proved to have little foundation. The predisposition to the complaint may be deduced from the delicate and tender state of the skin, and from the strong determination of blood to the surface, which evidently takes place in infants. The papulous eruption is, in many cases, connected with a weak, irritable state of the alimentary canal, and consequent indigestion. For if it be by any means suddenly repelled from the surface, diarrhœa, vomiting, spasmodic affections of the bowels, and often general disturbance of the constitution succeed; but as soon as it reappears, those internal complaints are wholly suspended. Dr. Armstrong and others have particularly noted this reciprocation, which makes the red gum, at times, a disease of some importance, though in its usual form it is not thought to be in any respect dangerous. On their remarks a necessary caution is founded, not to expose infants to a stream of very cold air, nor to plunge them unseasonably in a cold bath. The most violent, and even fatal symptoms, have often been the consequence of such imprudent conduct.

2. The *Strophulus albidus,* by some termed the *white gum,* is merely a variety of strophulus intertinctus, but deserves some notice on account of the different appearance of its papulæ. In place of those described as characterizing the red gum, there is a number of minute whitish specks, a little elevated, and sometimes, though not constantly, surrounded by a slight redness. These papulæ, when their tops are removed, do not discharge any fluid; it is, however, probable, that they are originally formed by the deposition of a fluid, which afterward concretes under the cuticle. They appear chiefly on the face, neck, and breast, and are more permanent than the papulæ of the red gum. In other respects, they have the same nature and tendency, and require a similar plan of treatment. Although a distinctive name has been applied to this eruption, when occurring alone, yet it is proper to observe, that, in a great number of cases, there are red papulæ and spots intermixed with it, which prove its connexion with the strophulus intertinctus.

3. The *Strophulus confertus.* An eruption of numerous papulæ, varying in their size, appears on different parts of the body in infants, during dentition, and has thence been denominated the *tooth-rash.* It

is sometimes also termed the *rank red gum*. About the fourth or fifth month after birth, an eruption of this kind usually takes place on the cheeks and sides of the nose, extending sometimes to the forehead and arms, but rarely to the trunk or body. The papulæ on the face are smaller, and set more closely together than in the red gum; their colour is not so vivid, but they are generally more permanent. They terminate at length with slight exfoliations of the cuticle, and often appear again in the same places, a short time afterward. The papulæ which, in this complaint, occasionally appear on the back or loins, are much larger, and somewhat more distant from each other, than those on the face. They are often surrounded by an extensive circle of inflammation, and a few of them contain a semi-pellucid watery fluid, which is reabsorbed when the inflammation subsides. In the seventh or eighth month, the strophulus confertus assumes a somewhat different form; one or two large irregular patches appear on the arms, shoulder, or neck; in which the papulæ are hard, of a considerable size, and set so close together, that the whole surface is of a high red colour. Most commonly the forearm is the seat of this eruption, the papulæ rising first on the back of the hand, and gradually extending upwards along the arm. Sometimes, however, the eruption commences at the elbow, and proceeds a little upwards and downwards on the outside of the arm. It arrives at its height in about a fortnight; the papulæ then begin to fade, and become flat at the top; afterward the cuticle exfoliates from the part affected, which remains discoloured, rough, and irregular, for a week or two longer.

An obstinate and very painful modification of this disease takes place, though not often, on the lower extremities. The papulæ spread from the calves of the legs to the thighs, nates, loins, and round the body, as high as the navel: being very numerous and close together, they produce a continuous redness over all these parts.

The cuticle, presently, however, shrivelled, cracks in various places, and finally separates from the skin in large pieces. During this process a new cuticle is formed, notwithstanding which the complaint recurs in a short time, and goes through the same course as before. In this manner successive eruptions take place, during the course of three or four months, and perhaps do not cease till the child is one year old, or somewhat more. Children necessarily suffer great uneasiness from the heat and irritation occasioned by so extensive an eruption, yet while they are affected with it, they often remain free from any internal or febrile complaint. This appearance should be distinguished from the intertrigo of infants, which exhibits a uniform, red, smooth, shining surface, without papulæ; and which affects only the lower part of the nates and inside of the thighs, being produced by the stimulus of the urine, &c. with which the child's clothes are almost constantly wetted. The strophulus confertus, where the child is otherwise healthy, is generally ascribed to a state of indigestion, or some feverish complaint of the mother or nurse. Dr. Willan, however, asserts, that he has more frequently seen the eruption when no such cause was evident. It may, with more probability, be considered as one of the numerous symptoms of irritation, arising from the inflamed and painful state of the gums in dentition; since it always occurs during that process, and disappears soon after the first teeth have cut the gums.

4. The *Strophulus volaticus* is characterized by an appearance of small circular patches, or clusters of papulæ, arising successively on different parts of the body. The number of papulæ in each cluster is from six to twelve. Both the papulæ and their interstices are of a high red colour. These patches continue red, with a little heat, or itching, for about four days, when they turn brown, and begin to exfoliate. As one patch declines, another appears at a small distance from it; and in this manner the complaint often spreads gradually over the face, body, and limbs, not terminating in less than three or four weeks. During that time the child has sometimes a quick pulse, a white tongue, and seems uneasy and fretful. In many cases, however, the eruption takes place without any symptoms of internal disorder. The above complaint has been by some writers denominated *ignis volaticus infantum*; under this title Astruc and Lowry have described one of the forms of crusta lactea, in which a successive

eruption of pustules takes place on the same spot generally about the mouth or eyes, in children of different ages, and sometimes in adults. The *maculæ volaticæ infantum* mentioned by Wittichius, Sennertus, and Scbizeus, agree in some respects with the strophulus volaticus; but they are described by other German authors as a species of erysipelas, or as irregular efflorescences affecting the genitals of infants, and often proving fatal. The strophulus volaticus is a complaint by no means frequent. In most cases which have come under Dr. Willan's observation, it appeared between the third and sixth month; in one instance, however, it occurred about ten days after birth, and continued three weeks, being gradually diffused from the cheeks and forehead to the scalp, afterward to the trunk of the body and to the extremities; when the patches exfoliated, a red surface was left, with a slight border of detached cuticle.

5. *Strophulus candidus.* In this form of strophulus, the papulæ are larger than in any of the foregoing species. They have no inflammation round their base; their surface is very smooth and shining, whence they appear to be of a lighter colour than the adjoining cuticle. They are diffused, at a considerable distance from each other, over the loins, shoulders, and upper part of the arms; in any other situation they are seldom found.

This eruption affects infants about a year old, and most commonly succeeds some of the acute diseases to which they are liable. Dr. Willan has observed it on their recovery from a catarrhal fever, and after inflammation of the bowels, or lungs. The papulæ continue hard and elevated for about a week, then gradually subside and disappear.

STRU′MA. (*Struma, æ. f.*; from *struo*, to heap up, or *à struendo*, because they grow insensibly.) This term is generally applied to scrofula, and by some to bronchocele, or an induration of the thyroid gland.

STRU′MEN. (From *struma*, a scrofulous tumour.) An herb so called from its uses in healing strumous tumours.

STRUMOUS. (*Strumosus*; from *struma*, a wen or scrofula.) Of the nature of scrofula.

STRUMUS. An obsolete name of the berry bearing chickweed, which was supposed to be efficacious in the cure of scrofula. See *Cucubalas bacciferus.*

STRU′THIUM. (From ϛρυθος, a sparrow: so named from the resemblance of its flowers to an unfledged sparrow.) The master-wort. See *Imperatoria ostruthium.*

STRYCHNIA. *Strychnine.* An alkaline substance obtained from the bean of the strychnos ignatia by the following process: The bean was rasped down as small as possible. It was then exposed to the action of nitric æther in a Fapin's digester. The residue, thus deprived of a quantity of fatty matter, was digested in alkohol as long as that reagent was capable of dissolving any thing. The alkoholic solutions were evaporated to dryness, and the residue redissolved in water. Caustic potassa being dropped into the solution, a white crystalline precipitate fell, which was strychnia. It was purified by washing it in cold water, dissolving it in alkohol, and crystallizing it. Strychnia was obtained likewise from the bean of the strychnos ignatia, by boiling the infusion of the bean with magnesia, in the same manner as Robiquet had obtained morphia from the infusion of opium.

The properties of strychnia, when in a state of purity, are as follows:

It is crystallized in very small four-sided prisms, terminated by four-sided low pyramids. It has a white colour; its taste is intolerably bitter, leaving a metallic impression in the mouth. It is destitute of smell. It is not altered by exposure to the air. It is neither fusible nor volatile, except at temperatures at which it undergoes decomposition. It is charred at the temperature at which oil enters into ebullition (about 580°). When strongly heated, it swells up, blackens, gives out empyreumatic oil, a little water, and acetic acid; carbonic acid and carburetted hydrogen gases are disengaged, and a bulky charcoal remains behind. When heated with peroxide of copper, it gives out only carbonic acid gas and water. It is very little soluble in cold water, 100,000 parts of that liquor dissolving only 15 parts of strychnia; but it dissolves in 2,500 times its weight of boiling water. A cold solution of strychnia in water may be diluted with 100 times its volume of that liquid, without losing its bitter taste.

When strychnia is introduced into the stomach, it acts with prodigious energy. A locked jaw is induced in a very short time, and the animal is speedily destroyed. Half a grain of strychnia blown into the throat of a rabbit proved fatal in five minutes, and brought on locked jaw in two minutes.

Sulphate of strychnia is a salt which crystallizes in transparent cubes, soluble in less than ten times its weight of cold water. Its taste is intensely bitter, and the strychnia is precipitated from it by all the soluble salifiable bases. It is not altered by exposure to the air.

Muriate of strychnia crystallizes in very small needles, which are grouped together, and before the microscope exhibit the form of quadrangular prisms. When exposed to the air it becomes opaque. It is more soluble in water than the sulphate, has a similar taste, and acts with the same violence upon the animal economy as all the other salts of strychnia.

Phosphate of strychnia crystallizes in four-sided prisms. It can only be obtained neutral by double decomposition.

Nitrate of strychnia can be obtained only by dissolving strychnia in nitric acid, diluted with a great deal of water. The saturated solution, when cautiously evaporated, yields crystals of neutral nitrate in pearly needles. This salt is much more soluble in hot than in cold water. Its taste is exceedingly bitter, and it acts with more violence upon the animal economy than pure strychnia. It seems capable of uniting with an excess of acid. When heated, it becomes yellow, and undergoes decomposition. It is slightly soluble in alkohol, but is insoluble in æther.

When concentrated nitric acid is poured upon strychnia, it immediately strikes an amaranthine colour, followed by a shade similar to that of blood. To this colour succeeds a tint of yellow, which passes afterward into green. By this action the strychnia seems to be altered in its properties, and to be converted into a substance still capable of uniting with acids.

Carbonate of strychnia is obtained in the form of white flocks, little soluble in water, but soluble in carbonic acid.

Acetic, oxalic, and tartaric acids form with strychnia neutral salts, which are very soluble in water, and more or less capable of crystallizing. They crystallize best when they contain an excess of acid. The neutral acetate is very soluble, and crystallizes with difficulty.

Hydrocyanic acid dissolves strychnia, and forms with it a crystallizable salt.

Strychnia combines neither with sulphur nor carbon. When boiled with iodine, a solution takes place, and iodate and hydriodate of strychnia are formed. Chlorine acts upon it precisely in the same way.

Strychnia, when dissolved in alkohol, has the property of precipitating the greater number of metallic oxides from their acid solutions. It is precipitated by the alkalies and alkaline earths; but the effect of the earths proper has not been tried.

STRYCHNINE. See *Strychnia*.

STRYCHNOMANIA. (From ϛρυχνος, nightshade, and μανια, madness.) So the ancients called the disorder produced by eating the deadly nightshade.

STRY'CHNOS. (*Strychnos, i.* m.; an ancient name which occurs in Pliny and Dioscorides derived from ϛρωννυμι, to overthrow, and applied most probably from the overpowering narcotic quality of the plant to which it was assigned, ϛρυχνος of the Greeks being a kind of nightshade. Linnæus adopted this name for the present genus, on account of the analogy of its narcotic properties with the plant of the ancients. Some derive it from ϛρυχω, to torment: from its properties of producing insanity.) The name of a genus of plants in the Linnæan system. Class, *Pentandria*; Order, *Monogynia*.

STRYCHNOS NUX VOMICA. The systematic name of the tree, the seed of which is called the poison-nut. *Nux vomica*; *Nux metella*. The nux vomica, lignum colubrinum, and faba sancti Ignatii, have been long known in the Materia Medica as narcotic poisons, brought from the East Indies, while the vegetables which produced them were unknown, or at least not botanically ascertained.

By the judicious discrimination of Linnæus, the nux vomica was found to be the fruit of the tree described and figured in the *Hortus malabaricus*, under the name

of *Caniram cucurbitifera malabarensis*, of Plukenet, now called *Strychnos nux vomica*.

To this genus also, but upon evidence less conclusive, he likewise justly referred the colubrinum. But the fabi sancti Ignatii he merely conjectured might belong to this family, as appears by the query, *An Strychni species?* which subsequent discoveries have enabled us to decide in the negative; for in the Supp. Plant. it constitutes the new genus *Ignatia*, which Loureiro has lately confirmed, changing the specific name *amara* to that of *philippinica*. The strychnos and ignatia are, however, nearly allied, and both rank under the Order *Solanaceæ*.

Dr. Woodville has inquired thus far into the botanical origin of these productions, from finding that, by medical writers, they are generally treated of under the same head, and in a very confused and indiscriminate manner. The seed of the fruit, or berry of this tree, *Strychnos nux vomica*, is the officinal nux vomica: it is flat, round, about an inch broad, and near a quarter of an inch thick, with a prominence in the middle on both sides, of a gray colour, covered with a woolly matter; and internally hard and tough like horn. To the taste it is extremely bitter, but has no remarkable smell. It consists chiefly of a gummy matter, which is moderately bitter; the resinous part is very inconsiderable in quantity, but intensely bitter; hence rectified spirit has been considered as its best menstruum.

Nux vomica is reckoned among the most powerful poisons of the narcotic kind, especially to brute animals; nor are instances wanting of its deleterious effects upon the human species. It proves fatal to dogs in a very short time, as appears by various authorities. Hillefield and others found that it also poisoned hares, foxes, wolves, cats, rabbits, and even some birds, as crows and ducks; and Loureiro relates, that a horse died in four hours after taking a drachm of the seed in a half-roasted state.

The effects of this baneful drug upon different animals, and even upon those of the same species, appear to be rather uncertain, and not always in proportion to the quantity of the poison given. With some animals it produces its effects almost instantaneously; with others, not till after several hours, when laborious respiration, followed by torpor, tremblings, coma, and convulsions, usually precede the fatal spasms, or tetanus, with which this drug commonly extinguishes life.

From four cases related of its mortal effects upon human subjects, we find the symptoms corresponded nearly with those which we have here mentioned of brutes; and these, as well as the dissections of dogs killed by this poison, not showing any injury done to the stomach or intestines, prove that the nux vomica acts immediately upon the nervous system, and destroys life by the virulence of its narcotic influence.

The quantity of the seed necessary to produce this effect upon a strong dog, as appears by experiments, need not to be more than a scruple; a rabbit was killed by five, and a cat by four, grains: and of the four persons to whom we have alluded, and who unfortunately perished by this deleterious drug, one was a girl ten years of age, to whom fifteen grains were exhibited at twice for the cure of an ague. Loss, however, tells us, that he took one or two grains of it in substance, without discovering any bad effect; and that a friend of his swallowed a whole seed without injury.

In Britain, where physicians seem to observe the rule *Saltem non nocere*, more strictly than in many other countries, the nux vomica has been rarely, if ever, employed as a medicine. On the Continent, however, and especially in Germany, they have certainly been guided more by the axiom, "What is incapable of doing much harm, is equally unable to do much good." The truth of this remark was very fully exemplified by the practice of Baron Störck, and is farther illustrated by the medicinal character given of nux vomica, which, from the time of Gesner till that of a modern date, has been recommended by a succession of authors as an antidote to the plague, as a febrifuge, as a vermifuge, and as a remedy in mania, hypochondriasis, hysteria, rheumatism, gout, and canine madness. In Sweden, it has of late years been successfully used in dysentery; but Berguis, who tried its effects in this disease, says, that it suppressed the flux for twelve hours, which afterward returned again. A woman who took a scruple of this drug night and morning, two successive days, is said to have been seized with convulsions and vertigo, notwithstanding which the dysenteric symptoms returned, and the disorder was cured by other medicines; but a pain in the stomach, the effect of the nux vomica, continued afterward for a long time.

Bergius, therefore, thinks it should only be administered in the character of a tonic and anodyne, in small doses (from five to ten grains), and not till after proper laxatives have been employed. Loureiro recommends it as a valuable internal medicine in fluor albus; for which purpose he roasts it till it becomes perfectly black and friable, which renders its medicinal use safe, without impairing its efficacy. It is said to have been used successfully in the cure of agues, and has also been reckoned a specific in pyrosis, or water-brash.

STRYCHNOS VOLUBILIS. The systematic name of the tree which was supposed to afford the Jesuit's bean. See *Ignatia amara.*

STUPEFACIENT. (*Stupefaciens*; from *stupefacio*, to stupify.) Of a stupifying quality.

STU'PHA. (From ςυφω, to bind.) *Stupa*; *Stuppa*. A stupe, or fomentation.

STU'POR. (From *Stupeo*, to be senseless.) Insensibility.

STU'PPA. See *Stupha.*

STYE. See *Hordeolum.*

STY'GIA. (From *Styx*, a name given by the poets to one of the rivers in hell.) A water made from sublimate, and directed in old dispensatories, was so called from a supposition of its poisonous qualities. A name of the *Aqua regia* also. from its corrosive qualities.

STYLIFORM. (*Styliformis*; from *stylus*, a bodkin, and *forma*, a likeness.) Shaped like a bodkin, or style.

STYLISCUS. (From ςυλος, a bodkin.) A tent made in the form of a bodkin.

STYLO. Names compounded of this word belong to muscles which are attached to the styloid process of the temporal bone; as,

STYLO-CERATO-HYOIDEUS. See *Stylo-hyoideus.*

STYLO-CHONDRO-HYOIDEUS. See *Stylo-hyoideus.*

STYLO-GLOSSUS. *Stylo-glosse*, of Dumas. A muscle situated between the lower jaw and os hyoides laterally, which draws the tongue aside and backwards. It arises tendinous and fleshy from the styloid process, and from the ligament which connects that process to the angle of the lower jaw, and is inserted into the root of the tongue, runs along its sides, and is insensibly lost near its tip.

STYLO-HYOIDEUS. *Stylo-hyoidien*, of Dumas. A muscle situated between the lower jaw, and os hyoides laterally, which pulls the os hyoides to one side and a little upwards. It is a small, thin, fleshy muscle, situated between the styloid process and os hyoides, under the posterior belly and middle tendon of the digastricus, near the upper edge of that muscle. It arises by a long thin tendon, from the basis and posterior edge of the styloid process, and, descending in an oblique direction, is inserted into the lateral and anterior part of the os hyoides, near its horn. The fleshy belly of this muscle is usually perforated on one or both sides, for the passage of the middle tendon of the digastricus. Sometimes, though not always, we find another smaller muscle placed before the stylo-hyoideus, which, from its having nearly the same origin and insertion, and the same use, is called *stylo-hyoideus-alter*. It seems to have been first known to Eustachius: so that Douglas was not aware of this circumstance when he placed it among the muscles discovered by himself. It arises from the apex of the styloid process, and sometimes by a broad and thin aponeurosis, from the inner and posterior part of the angle of the lower jaw, and is inserted into the appendix, or little horn, of the os hyoides. The use of these muscles is to pull the os hyoides to one side, and a little upwards.

STYLO-HYOIDEUS-ALTER. See *Stylo-hyoideus.*

STYLO-MASTOID FORAMEN. *Foramen stylo-mastoideum.* A hole between the styloid and mastoid process of the temporal bone, through which the portio dura of the auditory nerve passes to the temples.

STYLO-PHARYNGEUS. *Stylo-thyro-pharyngien*, of Dumas. A muscle situated between the lower jaw and os hyoides laterally, which dilates and raises the pharynx and thyroid cartilage upwards. It arises fleshy from the root of the styloid process, and is inserted into

the side of the pharynx and back part of the thyroid cartilage.

STYLUS. The style of a flower is the column which proceeds from the germen, and bears the stigma It is,

1. *Filiform*, in Jasminum, and Zea mays.
2. *Linear*, in Orobus.
3. *Subulate*, thicker below than towards apex; as in Geranium.
4. *Clavate*, thicker at its summit than towards its base; as in Leucojum vernum.
5. *Triangular*, in Pisum.
6. *Bifid*, in Polygonum persicaria.
7. *Trifid*, in Bryonia and Momordica.
8. *Dichotomous*, divided into two, which again bifurcate; as in Cordia.
9. *Long*, much more so than the stamina; as in Campanula and Dianthus.
10. *Persistent*, not going off after the fecundation of the germen; as Synapis.

STYMATO'SIS. (From ςυω, to have a priapism.) A violent erection of the penis, with a bloody discharge.

STYPTE'RIA. (From ςυφω, to bind: so called from its astringent properties.) Alum.

STYPTIC. (*Stypticus*; from ςυφω, to adstringe.) A term given to those substances which possess the power of stopping hæmorrhages such as turpentine, alum, &c.

STYRACI'FLUA. (From *styrax*, storax, and *fluo*, to flow.) See *Liquidambra.*

STY'RAX. (*Styrax*, *acis*. m. and f.; from ςυραξ, a reed in which it was used to be preserved.) 1. The name of a genus of plants in the Linnæan system. Class, *Decandria* ; Order, *Monogynia.*

2. The pharmacopœial name of the *Styrax calamita.*

STYRAX ALBA. See *Myroxylon peruiferum.*

STYRAX BENZOIN. The systematic name of the tree which affords the gum benzoin. *Benzoë* ; *Benjoinum* ; *Assa dulcis* ; *Assa odorata* ; *Liquor cyreniacus* ; *Balzoinum* ; *Benzoin* ; *Benjui* ; *Benjuin*. Gum-benja min. This substance is classed, by modern chemists, among the balsams. There are two kinds of benzoin; *benzoe amygdaloides*, which is formed of white tears. resembling almonds, united together by a brown matter; and *common benzoin*, which is brown and without tears. The tree which affords this balsam, formerly called *Laurus benzoin* ; *Benzoifera* ; *Arbor benici*, is the *Styrax—foliis oblongis acuminatis, subtus tomentosis, racemis compositis longitudine foliorum*, of Dryander, from which it is obtained by incisions. The benzoin of the shops is usually in very large brittle masses. When chewed it imparts very little taste, except that it impresses on the palate a slight sweetness; its smell, especially when rubbed or heated, is extremely fragrant and agreeable. Gum-benjamin was analyzed by Brande. The products obtained by distillation were, from 100 grains, benzoic acid, 9 grains; acidulated water, 5.5; butyraceous and empyreumatic oil, 60; brittle coal, 22; and a mixture of carburetted hydrogen and carbonic acid gas, computed at 3.5. On treating the empyreumatic oil with water, however, 5 grains more of acid were extracted, making 14 in the whole.

From 1500 grains of benzoin, Bucholz obtained 1250 of resin; 187 benzoic acid; 25 of a substance similar to balsam of Peru; 8 of an aromatic substance soluble in water and alkohol; and 30 of woody fibres and impurities.

Æther, sulphuric and acetic acids, dissolve benzoin; so do solutions of potassa and soda. Nitric acid acts violently on it, and a portion of artificial tannin is formed. Ammonia dissolves it sparingly. It hrs rarely been used medicinally in a simple state, but its preparations are much esteemed against inveterate coughs and phthisical complaints, unattended with much fever; it has also been used as a cosmetic, and in the way of fumigation, for the resolution of indolent tumours. The acid of benzoin is employed in the *tinctura camphoræ composita*, and a tincture is directed to be made of the balsam.

STYRAX CALAMITA. Storax in the cane, because it was formerly brought to us in reeds, or canes. See *Styrax officinalis.*

STYRAX COLATA. Strained storax.

STYRAX LIQUIDA. Liquid storax. See *Liquid ambra.*

STYRAX OFFICINALIS. The systematic name of the tree which affords the solid storax. Officinal storax. *Styrax—foliis ovatis, subtus villosis, racemis simplicibus folio brevioribus,* of Linnæus. There are two kinds of storax to be found in the shops; the one is usually in irregular compact masses, free from impurities, of a reddish-brown appearance, and interspersed with whitish tears, somewhat like gum ammoniac, or benzoin; it is extremely fragrant, and upon the application of heat readily melts. This has been called *storax in lump, red storax,* and, when in separate tears, *storax in tears.* The other kind, which is called the *common storax,* is in large masses, very light, and bears no external resemblance whatever to the former storax, as it seems almost wholly composed of dirty saw-dust, caked together by resinous matter. Storax was formerly used in catarrhal complaints, coughs, asthmas, obstructions, &c. In the present practice it is almost totally disregarded, notwithstanding it is an efficacious remedy in nervous diseases.

STYRAX RUBRA. Red storax, or storax in the tear.

SUB. 1. In anatomy, it is applied to parts which lie under the other word or name, which sub precedes; as *subscapularis,* under the scapula, &c.

2. In pathology, it is used to express an imperfect disease, or a feeble state of a disease; as subluxation, subacute, &c.

3. In botany, when shape, or any other character, cannot be precisely defined, *sub* is prefixed to the term used; as *subrotundus,* roundish; *subsessiles,* not quite destitute of a footstalk, &c.

4. In chemistry, this term is applied, when a salifiable base is predominant in a compound, there being a deficiency of the acid; as *subcarbonate of potassa, subcarbonate of soda.*

SUBACE'TAS CUPRI. See *Verdigris.*

SUBACETATE. *Subacetas.* An imperfect acetate.

Subacetate of copper. See *Verdigris.*

SUBALA'RIS VENA. The vein of the axilla or arm-pit.

SUBCARBO'NAS POTASSÆ. See *Potassæ subcarbonas.*

SUBCARBONAS FERRI. See *Ferri subcarbonas.*

SUBCARBONAS PLUMBI. See *Plumbi subcarbonas.*

SUBCARBONATE. *Subcarbonas.* An imperfect carbonate.

SUBCARTILAGI'NOUS. (*Subcartilaginosus;* from *sub,* under, and *cartilago,* a cartilage.) Of a structure approaching to that of cartilage.

SUBCLA'VIAN. (*Subclaviculus;* from *sub,* beneath, and *clavicula,* the clavicle.) That which is, or passes, under the clavicle.

SUBCLAVIAN ARTERY. The right subclavian arises from the arteria innominata, and proceeds under the clavicle to the axilla. The left subclavian arises from the arch of the aorta, and ascends under the left clavicle to the axilla. The subclavians in their course give off the internal mammary, the cervical, the vertebral, and the superior intercostal arteries.

SUBCLAVIAN VEIN. This receives the blood from the veins of the arm, and runs into the vena cava superior.

SUBCLA'VIUS. (From *sub,* under, and *clavicula,* the channel bone: as being situated under the clavicle, or channel bone.) *Subclavianus. Costo-claviculaire,* of Dumas. A muscle, situated on the anterior part of the thorax, which pulls the clavicle downwards and forwards. It arises tendinous from the cartilage that joins the first rib to the sternum, is inserted after becoming fleshy into the inferior part of the clavicle, which it occupies from within half an inch of the sternum as far outwards as to its connexion, by a ligament, with the coracoid process of the scapula.

SUBCRURÆ'US. A name of two little muscular slips sometimes found under the cruræus; they are inserted into the capsular ligament which they pull up.

SUBCUTANEOUS. (*Subcutaneus;* from *sub,* under, and *cutis,* the skin.) Under the skin; a name given to some nerves, vessels, glands, &c. which are very superficial.

SUBCUTANEOUS GLANDS. *Glandulæ subcutaneæ.* These are sebaceous glands lying under the skin, which they perforate by their excretory ducts.

SUBCUTA'NEUS. See *Platysma myoides.*

SUBER. Cork. See *Quercus suber.*

SUBERIC ACID. *Acidum subericum.* This acid was obtained by Brugnatelli from cork, and afterward more fully examined by Bouillon la Grange. To pro-

cure it, pour on cork, grated to powder, six times its weight of nitric acid, of the specific gravity of 1.26, in a tubulated retort, and distil the mixture with a gentle heat as long as any red fumes arise. As the distillation advances, a yellow matter, like wax, appears on the surface of the liquid in the retort. While its contents continue hot, pour them into a glass vessel, placed on a sand heat, and keep them continually stirring with a glass rod; by which means the liquid will gradually grow thicker. As soon as white penetrating vapours appear, let it be removed from the sand heat, and kept stirring till cold. Thus an orange-coloured mass will be obtained, of the consistence of honey, of a strong sharp smell while hot, and a peculiar aromatic smell when cold. On this, pour twice its weight of boiling water, apply heat till it liquefies, and filter. As the filtered liquor cools, it deposites a powdery sediment, and acquires a thin pellicle. Separate the sediment by filtration, and evaporate the fluid nearly to dryness. The mass thus obtained is the suberic acid, which may be purified by saturating with an alkali, and precipitating by an acid, or by boiling it with charcoal powder.

Chevreuil obtained the suberic acid by mere digestion of the nitric acid on the grated cork, without distillation, and purified it by washing with cold water. 12 parts of cork may be made to yield one of acid. When pure, it is white and pulverulent, having a feeble taste, and little action on litmus. It is soluble in 80 parts of water at 55½° F. and in 38 parts at 140°. It is much more soluble in alkohol, from which water throws down a portion of the suberic acid. It occasions a white precipitate when poured into acetate of lead, nitrates of lead, mercury, and silver, muriate of tin, and protosulphate of iron. It affords no precipitate with solutions of copper or zinc. The suberates of potassa, soda, and ammonia are very soluble. The two latter may be readily crystallized. Those of barytes, lime, magnesia, and alumina, are of sparing solubility.

SUBLIMAME'NTUM. (From *sublimo,* to lift up.) The pendulous substance which floats in the middle of the urine.

SUBLIMATE. See *Hydrargyri oxymurias.*

Sublimate, corrosive. See *Hydrargyri oxymurias.*

SUBLIMATION. (*Sublimatio;* from *sublimo,* to raise or sublime.) A process by which volatile substances are raised by heat, and again condensed in a solid form. This chemical process differs from evaporation only in being confined to solid substances. It is usually performed either for the purpose of purifying certain substances, and disengaging them from extraneous matters; or else to reduce into vapour, and combine, under that form, principles which would have united with greater difficulty if they had not been brought to that state of extreme division.

As all fluids are volatile by heat, and consequently capable of being separated, in most cases, from fixed matters, so various solid bodies are subjected to a similar treatment. Fluids are said to distil, and solids to sublime, though sometimes both are obtained in one and the same operation. If the subliming matter concretes into a solid, hard mass, it is commonly called a sublimate; if into a powdery form, flowers.

The principal subjects of this operation are, volatile alkaline salts; neutral salts, composed of volatile alkali and acids, as sal ammoniac; the salt of amber, and flowers of benzoin, mercurial preparations, and sulphur. Bodies of themselves not volatile are frequently made to sublime by the mixture of volatile ones; thus iron is carried over by sal ammoniac in the preparation of the flores martiales, or ferrum ammoniatum.

The fumes of solid bodies in close vessels rise but a little way, and adhere to that part of the vessel where they concrete.

SUBLI'MIS. See *Flexor brevis digitorum pedis,* and *Flexor sublimis perforatus.*

SUBLINGUAL. (*Sublingualis;* from *sub,* under, and *lingua,* the tongue.) A name given to parts immediately under the tongue.

SUBLINGUAL GLANDS. *Glandulæ sublinguales,* vel *Bartholinianæ,* vel *Rivinianæ.* The glands which are situated under the tongue, and secrete saliva. Their excretory ducts are called *Rivinian* from their discoverer.

SUBLUXA'TIO. A sprain.

SUBMERSION. (*Submersio;* from *sub,* under, and *mergo,* to sink.) Drowning. A variety of the apoplexia suffocata. Sauvages terms it asphyxia immersorum.

SUBMERSUS. Plunged under water: applied to leaves which are naturally under water, while others of the plants are above; as in Ranunculus aquatilis.

SUBMU′RIAS HYDRARGYRI. See *Hydrargyri submurias.*

SUBMURIATE. *Submurias.* An imperfect muriate.

SUBORBITA′RIUS. The suborbitary nerve; a branch of the fifth pair.

Subphosphuretted hydrogen. See *Phosphorus.*

SUBROTUNDUS. Roundish: applied to several parts of plants. The leaf of the Pyrola is subrotund.

SUBSALT. A salt having an excess of base beyond what is requisite for saturating the acid, as *supersalt* is one with an excess of the acid. The sulphate of potassa is the neutral compound of sulphuric acid and potassa; subsulphate of potassa, a compound of the same ingredients, in which there is an excess of base; supersulphate of potassa, a compound of the same acid and the same base, in which there is an excess of acid.

SUBSCAPULA′RIS. (From *sub*, under, and *scapula*, the shoulder-blade.) *Sous-scapulo-trochinien*, of Dumas. *Infra-scapularis.* The name of this muscle sufficiently indicates its situation. It is composed of many fasciculi of tendinous and fleshy fibres, the marks of which we see imprinted on the under surface of the scapula. These fasciculi, which arise from all the basins of that bone internally, and likewise from its superior, as well as from one-half of its inferior costa, unite to form a considerable flat tendon which adheres to the capsular ligament, and is inserted into the upper part of the less tuberosity at the head of the os humeri.

The principal use of this muscle is to roll the arm inwards. It likewise serves to bring it close to the ribs; and, from its adhesion to the capsular ligament, it prevents that membrane from being pinched.

SUBSU′LTUS. (From *subsulto*, to leap.) *Subsultus tendinum.* Weak convulsive motions or twitchings of the tendons, mostly of the hands, generally observed in the extreme stages of putrid fever.

SUBU′BERES. (From *sub*, under, and *ubera*, the breasts.) This term hath been used by some writers for those infants who yet suck, in distinction from those who are weaned, and then are called *exuberes.*

SUBULATUS. Subulate. Awl-shaped: applied in botany to leaves, receptacles, &c. which are tapering from a thick base to a point like an awl; as the leaf of the *Salsola kali*, and receptacle of the *Scabiosa atropurpurea.*

SUCCA′GO. The rob of any fruit.

SUCCEDA′NEUM. A medicine substituted for another.

SUCCENTURIA′TI MUSCULI. The pyramidal muscles of the belly.

SUCCENTURIATI RENES. Two glands lying above the kidneys.

SU′CCI SCORBUTICI. The juice of English scurvy-grass, &c.

SUCCINATE. *Succinas.* A salt formed by the combination of the acid of amber, or succinic acid, with a salifiable base, *succinate of potassa, succinate of copper,* &c.

SUCCI′NGENS MEMBRANA. The diaphragm.

SUCCINIC. (*Succinicus*; from *Succinum*, amber.) Of or belonging to amber.

SUCCINIC ACID. *Acidum succinicum. Sal succini.* It has long been known that amber, when exposed to distillation, affords a crystallized substance, which sublimes into the upper part of the vessel. Before its nature was understood it was called *salt of amber*; but it is now known to be a peculiar acid, as Boyle first discovered. The crystals are at first contaminated with a little oil, which gives them a brownish colour; but they may be purified by solution and crystallization, repeated as often as necessary, when they will become transparent and shining. Pott recommends to put on the filter, through which the solution is passed, a little cotton previously wetted with oil of amber. Their figure is that of a triangular prism. Their taste is acid, and they redden the blue colour of litmus, but not that of violets. They are soluble in less than two parts of boiling alkohol, in two parts of boiling water, and in twenty-five of cold water.

Planche, of Paris, observes, that a considerable quantity might be collected in making amber varnish, as it sublimes while the amber is melting for this purpose, and is wasted.

Several processes have been proposed for purifying this acid: that of Richter appears to be the best. The acid being dissolved in hot water, and filtered, is to be saturated with potassa or soda, and boiled with charcoal, which absorbs the oily matter. The solution being filtered, nitrate of lead is added; whence results an insoluble succinate of lead, from which, by digestion in the equivalent quantity of sulphuric acid, pure succinic acid is separated. Nitrate or muriate of barytes will show whether any sulphuric acid remains mixed with the succinic solution; and if so, it may be withdrawn by digesting the liquid with a little more succinate of lead. Pure succinic acid may be obtained by evaporation, in white transparent prismatic crystals. Their taste is somewhat sharp, and they redden powerfully tincture of turnsole. Heat melts, and partially decomposes succinic acid. Air has no effect upon it. It is soluble in both water and alkohol, and much more so when they are heated.

SU′CCINUM. (*Succinum, i. n.*; from *succus*, juice: because it was thought to exude from a tree.) See *Amber.*

SUCCINUM CINEREUM. Ambergris is so called by some authors. See *Ambergris.*

SUCCINUM GRISEUM. Ambergris is sometimes so called. See *Ambergris.*

SUCCINUM OLEUM. See *Oleum succini.*

SUCCINUM PREPARATUM. Prepared amber. See *Amber.*

SUCCI′SA. (From *succido*, to cut: so named from its being indented, and, as it were, cut in pieces.) Applied to a species of the genus *Scabiosa.*

SUCCORY. See *Cichorium.*

SU′CUBUS. See *Incubus.*

SUCCULENS. Succulent, juicy, rich. Applied to fruits, pods, soils, &c.

SUCCULENT′Æ. The name of an order of Linnæus's Fragments of a Natural Method, containing those which have fleshy and succulent leaves; a Csactus, Sedum, Sempervivum, &c.

SUCCULENTUS. Juicy: full of juice. Applied to pods, leaves, &c.

SU′CCUS. Juice.

SUCCUS COCHLEARIÆ COMPOSITUS. A warm aperient and diuretic, mostly exhibited in the cure of diseases of the skin, arising from scurvy.

SUCCUS CYRENIACUS. Juice of laserwort.

SUCCUS GASTRICUS. See *Gastric juice.*

SUCCUS HELIOTROPII. See *Croton tinctorium*

SUCCUS INDICUS PURGANS. Gamboge.

SUCCUS LIQUORITIÆ. See *Glycyrrhiza glabra.*

SUDA′MINA. (*Sudamen, inis.* n.; from *sudor* sweat.) *Hidroa. Boa.* Vesicles resembling milletseeds, in form and magnitude, which appear suddenly, without fever, especially in the summer-time, after much labour and sweating.

SUDA′TIO. (From *sudor*, sweat.) A sweating. See *Ephidrosis.*

SUDATO′RIUM. (From *sudo*, to sweat.) A stew or sweating-house.

SUDOR. Sweat or perspiration.

SUDOR ANGLICUS. *Hydronosus; Gargeatio.* The sweating sickness of England; and endemic fever. Dr. Cullen thinks it a species of typhus. This disorder is thus named from its first appearing in this island, and acquires the title of sudor, from the patient suddenly breaking out into a profuse sweat, which forms the great character of the disease.

SUDORI′FIC. (*Sudorificus*: from *sudor*, sweat, and *facio*, to make.) A synonyme of diaphoretic. See *Diaphoretics.*

SUFFIME′NTUM. (From *suffimen*, a perfume) A perfume.

SUFFI′TUS. A perfume.

SUFFOCA′TIO. Suffocation.

SUFFOCATIO STRIDULA. The croup.

SUFFRUTICES PLANTÆ. Under shrubby plants. Such ligneous or somewhat woody vegetables that are of a nature, in some degree, between that of the shrubby, and the herbaceous; as thyme, sage, hyssop, &c.

SUFFUMIGATION. (*Suffumigatio*; from *sub*, under, and *fumigo*, to smoke.) The burning odorous substances to remove an evil smell, or destroy miasma.

SUFFUSIO. (From *suffundo*, to pour down: so called because the ancients supposed the opacity proceeded from something running under the crystalline humour.)

1. A cataract.

2. An extravasation of some humour, as the blood: thus we say, a suffusion of blood in the eye, when it is what is vulgarly called bloodshot.

SUFFUSIO AURIGINOSA. A jaundice.

SUGAR. See *Saccharum.*

Sugar of lead. See *Plumbi acetas.*

Sugar of milk. A substance produced from whey, which, if not sour, contains a saline substance, to which this name has been given.

SUGILLATION. (*Sugillatio ;* from *sugillo,* to stain.) A bruise. A spot or mark made by a leech or cupping-glass.

SULCATUS. Furrowed: applied to stems, leaves, seeds, &c. of plants; as the seeds of the *Scandix odorata,* and *australis.*

SU'LCUS. A groove or furrow; generally applied to the bones.

SU'LPHAS. (*Sulphas, atis.* m.; from *sulphur,* brimstone.) A sulphate or salt formed by the union of the sulphuric acid with a salifiable base.

SULPHAS ALUMINOSUS. Alum. See *Alumen.*

SULPHAS AMMONIÆ. *Alkali volatile vitriolatum,* of Bergman. *Sal ammoniacum secretum,* of Glauber. *Vitriolum ammoniacale.* This salt has been found native in the neighbourhood of some volcanoes. It is esteemed diuretic and deobstruent, and exhibited in the same diseases as the muriate of ammonia.

SULPHAS CUPRI. See *Cupri sulphas.*

SULPHAS FERRI. See *Ferri sulphas.*

SULPHAS HYDRARGYRI. See *Hydrargyrus vitriolatus.*

SULPHAS MAGNESIÆ. See *Magnesiæ sulphas.*

SULPHAS POTASSÆ. See *Potassæ sulphas.*

SULPHAS QUININÆ. See *Cinchonina.*

SULPHAS SODÆ. See *Sodæ sulphas.*

SULPHAS ZINCI. See *Zinci sulphas.*

SULPHATE. See *Sulphas.*

SU'LPHITE. *Sulphis.* A salt formed by the combination of a definite quantity of the sulphurous acid with a salifiable base; as *sulphite of potassa, ammoniacal sulphite,* &c.

SULPHOVINIC ACID. Sulphovinous acid. The name given by Vogel to an acid, or a class of acids, which may be obtained by digesting alkohol and sulphuric acid together by heat. It seems probable that this acid is merely the hyposulphuric, combined with a peculiar oily matter.—*Ure's Chem. Dict.*

SU'LPHUR. (*Sulphur, uris.* n.; from *sal* or *sul,* and πυρ, fire: so named from its great combustibility.) *Abric; Alcubrith; Anpater; Appebrioc; Aquala; Aquila; Chibur; Chybur; Cibur.* Sulphur, which is also known by the name of brimstone, is the only simple combustible substance which nature offers pure and in abundance. It was the first known of all. It is found in the earth, and exists externally in depositions, in sublimed incrustations, and on the surface of certain waters, principally near burning volcanoes It is found combined with many metals. It exists in vegetable substances, and has lately been discovered in the albumen of eggs.

Sulphur, in the mineral kingdom, is either in a loose powder, or compact; and then either detached or in veins. It is found in the greatest plenty in the neighbourhood of volcanoes, or pseudo-volcanoes, whether modern or extinct, as at *Solfatara,* &c. and is deposited as a crust on stones contiguous to them, either crystallized or amorphous. It is frequently met with in mineral waters, and in caverns adjacent to volcanoes; sometimes also in coal-mines. It is found in combination with most of the metals. When united to iron, it forms the mineral called *martial pyrites,* or *iron pyrites.* All the ores known by the name of *pyrites,* of which there are a vast variety, are combinations of sulphur with different metals; and hence the names of copper, tin, arsenical, &c. pyrites. It exists likewise in combination with alumine and lime; it then constitutes different kinds of schistus, or alum ores.

Method of obtaining Sulphur.—A prodigious quantity of sulphur is obtained from Solfatara, in Italy.

This volcanic country every where exhibits marks of the agency of subterraneous fires; almost all the ground is bare and white; and is every where sensibly warmer than the atmosphere, in the greatest heat of summer; so that the feet of persons walking there are burnt through their shoes. It is impossible not to observe the sulphur, for a sulphurous vapour which rises through different apertures is every where perceptible, and gives reason to believe that there is a subterraneous fire underneath, from which that vapour proceeds.

From pyrites, sulphur is extracted in the large way by the following process:

Pyrites is broken into small pieces, and put into large earthen tubes, which are exposed to the heat of a furnace. A square vessel of cast iron, containing water, is connected as a receiver with the tube in the furnace. The action of the fire proceeds, and the sulphur, being thus melted, is gradually accumulated on the water in the receiver. It is then removed from this receiver, and melted in large iron ladies; in consequence of which, the earthy parts with which it was contaminated are made to subside to the bottom of the ladle, leaving the purified sulphur above. It is then again melted, and suffered to cool gradually, in order to free it from the rest of the impurities. It is then tolerably pure, and constitutes the sulphur we meet with, in large masses or lumps, in the market.

In order to form it into rolls, it is again melted, and poured into cylindrical wooden moulds; in these it takes the form in which we usually see it in commerce, as roll sulphur.

Flowers of sulphur, as they are called, are formed by subliming purified sulphur with a gentle heat, in close rooms, where the sublimed sulphur is collected, though the article met with in general, under that name, is nothing but sulphur finely powdered.

Method of purifying sulphur.—Take one part of flowers of sulphur, boil it in twenty parts of distilled water, in a glass vessel, for about a quarter of an hour; let the sulphur subside, decant the water, and then wash the sulphur repeatedly in distilled water. Having done this, pour over it three parts of pure nitro-muriatic acid, diluted with one part of distilled water, boil it again in a glass vessel for about a quarter of an hour, decant the acid, and wash the sulphur in distilled water till the fluid passes tasteless, or till it does not change the blue colour of tincture of cabbage or litmus. The sulphur, thus carefully treated, is *pure sulphur,* fit for philosophical experiments.

Physical properties.—"Sulphur is a combustible, dry, and exceedingly brittle body, of a pale lemon-yellow colour. Its specific gravity is 1.990. It is destitute of odour, except when rubbed or heated. It is of a peculiar faint taste. It frequently crystallizes in entire or truncated octahedra, or in needles. If a piece of sulphur, of a considerable size, be very gently heated, as, for example, by holding it in the hand and squeezing it firmly, it breaks to pieces with a crackling noise. It is a non-conductor of electricity, and hence it becomes electric by friction. When heated, it first softens before it melts, and its fusion commences at 218° Fahr.; it is capable of subliming at a lower temperature; and takes fire at 560°. In the beginning of fusion it is very fluid, but by continuing the heat it grows tough, and its colour changes to a reddish-brown. If, in this condition, it be poured into water, it remains as soft as wax, and yields to any impression. In time, however, it hardens again, and recovers its former consistence.

When a roll of sulphur is suddenly seized in a warm hand, it crackles, and sometimes falls in pieces. This is owing to the unequal action of heat on a body which conducts that power slowly, and which has little cohesion. If a mass of sulphur be melted in a crucible, and after the surface begins to concrete, if the liquid matter below be allowed to run out, fine acicular crystals of sulphur will be obtained.

Sulphur is insoluble in water; but in small quantity in alkohol and ether, and more largely in oil.

Sulphur combines with oxygen in four definite proportions, constituting an interesting series of acids. See *Sulphuric acid.*

Sulphur combines readily with chlorine. This compound was first made by Dr. Thomson, who passed chlorine gas through flowers of sulphur. It may be made more expeditiously by heating sulphur in a retort containing chlorine. The sulphur and chlorine unite, and form a fluid substance, which is volatile below 200° F.; and distils into the cold part of the retort. This substance, seen by reflected light, appears of a red colour, but is yellowish-green when seen by transmitted light. It smokes when exposed to air, and has an odour somewhat resembling that of seaweed, but much stronger; it affects the eyes like the smoke of peat. Its taste is acid, hot, and bitter. Its sp. gr is 1.7.

It does not redden perfectly dry paper tinged with litmus; when it is agitated in contact with water, the water becomes cloudy from the appearance of sulphur, and strongly acid, and it is found to contain oil of vitriol.

Iodide of sulphur is easily formed by mixing the two ingredients in a glass tube, and exposing them to such a heat as melts the sulphur. It is grayish-black, and has a radiated structure like that of sulphuret of antimony. When distilled with water, iodine is disengaged.

Sulphur and hydrogen combine. Their union may be effected, by causing sulphur to sublime in dry hydrogen in a retort. There is no change of volume; but only a part of the hydrogen can be united with the sulphur in this mode of operating.

The usual way of preparing *sulphuretted hydrogen* is to pour a dilute sulphuric or muriatic acid on the black sulphuret of iron or antimony in a retort. For accurate experiments it should be collected over mercury. It takes fire when a lighted taper is brought in contact with it, and burns with a pale blue flame, depositing sulphur. Its smell is extremely fœtid, resembling that of rotten eggs. Its taste is sour. It reddens vegetable blues. It is absorbable by water, which takes up more than an equal volume of the gas. Its sp. gr., according to Gay Lussac and Thenard, is to that of air as 1.1912 to 1.0.

Of all the gases, sulphuretted hydrogen is perhaps the most deleterious to animal life. A greenfinch, plunged into air, which contains only 1-1500th of its volume, perishes instantly. A dog of middle size is destroyed in air that contains 1-800th; and a horse would fall a victim to an atmosphere containing 1-250th.

Dr. Chaussier proves, that to kill an animal, it is sufficient to make the sulphuretted hydrogen gas act on the surface of its body, when it is absorbed by the inhalants. He took a bladder having a stop-cock at one end, and at the other an opening, into which he introduced the body of a rabbit, leaving its head outside, and securing the bladder air-tight round the neck by adhesive plaster. He then sucked the air out of the bladder, and replaced it by sulphuretted hydrogen gas. A young animal in these circumstances usually perishes in 15 or 20 minutes. Old rabbits resist the poison much longer.

When potassium or sodium is heated, merely to fusion, in contact with sulphuretted hydrogen, it becomes luminous, and burns with extrication of hydrogen, while a metallic sulphuret remains, combined with sulphuretted hydrogen, or a sulphuretted hydrosulphuret.

Sulphuretted hydrogen combines with an equal volume of ammonia; and unites to alkalies and oxides, so that it has all the characters of an acid. These compounds are called *hydrosulphurets.*

All the *hydrosulphurets*, soluble in water, have an acrid and bitter taste, and, when in the liquid state, the odour of rotten eggs. All those which are insoluble are, on the contrary, insipid, and without smell. There are only two coloured hydrosulphurets, that of iron, which is black, and of antimony, which is chestnut-brown.

All the hydrosulphurets are decomposed by the action of fire. That of magnesia is transformed into sulphuretted hydrogen and oxide of magnesium; those of potassa and soda, into sulphuretted hydrogen, hydrogen, and sulphuretted alkalies; those of manganese, zinc, iron, tin, and antimony, into water and metallic sulphurets.

When we put in contact with the air, at the ordinary temperature, an aqueous solution of a hydrosulphuret, there results, in the space of some days, 1st, water, and a sulphuretted hydrosulphuret, which is yellow and soluble; 2d, water, and a colourless hydrosulphite, which, if its base be potassa, soda, or ammonia, remains in solution in the water; but which falls down

in acicular crystals, if its base be barytes, strontia, or lime.

The acids in general combine with the base of the hydrosulphurets, and disengage sulphuretted hydrogen with a lively effervescence, without any deposition of sulphur, unless the acid be in excess, and be capable, like the nitric and nitrous acid, of yielding a portion of its oxygen to the hydrogen of the sulphuretted hydrogen.

The hydrosulphurets of potassa, soda, ammonia, lime, and magnesia, are prepared directly, by transmitting an excess of sulphuretted hydrogen gas through these bases, dissolved or diffused in water.

The composition of the hydrosulphurets is such, that the hydrogen of the sulphuretted hydrogen is to the oxygen of the oxide in the same ratio as in water. Hence, when we calcine the hydrosulphurets of iron, tin, &c. we convert them into water and sulphurets.

Hydrosulphuret of potassa crystallizes in four-sided prisms, terminated by four-sided pyramids. Its taste is acrid and bitter. Exposed to the air, it attracts humidity, absorbs oxygen, passes to the state of a sulphuretted hydrosulphuret, and finally to that of a hydrosulphite. It is extremely soluble in water. Its solution in this liquid occasions a perceptible refrigeration. Subjected to heat, it evolves much sulphuretted hydrogen, and the hydrosulphuret passes to the state of a sub-hydrosulphuret.

Hydrosulphuret of soda crystallizes with more difficulty than the preceding.

Hydrosulphuret of ammonia is obtained by the direct union of the two gaseous constituents in a glass balloon at a low temperature. As soon as the gases mingle, transparent white or yellowish crystals are formed. When a mere solution of this hydrosulphuret is wished for medicine or analysis, we pass a current of sulphuretted hydrogen through aqueous ammonia till saturation.

The pure hydrosulphuret is white, transparent, and crystallized in needles or fine plates. It is very volatile. Hence, at ordinary temperatures, it gradually sublimes into the upper part of the phials in which we preserve it. We may also by the same means separate it from the yellow sulphuretted hydrosulphuret, with which it is occasionally mixed. When exposed to the air, it absorbs oxygen, passes to the state of a sulphuretted hydrosulphuret, and becomes yellow. When it contains an excess of ammonia, it dissolves speedily in water, with the production of a very considerable cold.

Sub-hydrosulphuret of barytes is prepared by dissolving, in five or six parts of boiling water, the sulphuret of the earth obtained by igniting the sulphate with charcoal. The solution being filtered while hot, will deposite, on cooling, a multitude of crystals, which must be drained, and speedily dried by pressure between the folds of blotting-paper. It crystallizes in white scaly plates. It is much more soluble in hot than in cold water. Its solution is colourless, and capable of absorbing, at the ordinary temperature, a very large quantity of sulphuretted hydrogen.

Sub-hydrosulphuret of strontites crystallizes in the same manner as the preceding. The crystals obtained in the same way must be dissolved in water; and the solution being exposed to a stream of sulphuretted hydrogen, and then concentrated by evaporation in a retort, will afford, on cooling, crystals of pure sub-hydrosulphuret.

Hydrosulphurets of lime and magnesia have been obtained only in aqueous solutions. The metallic hydrosulphurets of any practical importance are treated of under their respective metals.

When we expose sulphur to the action of a solution of a hydrosulphuret, saturated with sulphuretted hydrogen, as much more sulphuretted hydrogen is evolved as the temperature is more elevated. But when the solution of hydrosulphuret, instead of being saturated, has a sufficient excess of alkali, it evolves no perceptible quantity of sulphuretted hydrogen, even at a boiling heat; although it dissolves as much sulphur as in its state of saturation. It hence follows, 1st, That sulphuretted hydrogen, sulphur, and the alkalies, have the property of forming very variable triple combinations; 2d, That all these combinations contain less sulphuretted hydrogen than the hydrosulphurets; and, 3d, That the quantity of sulphuretted hydrogen is inversely as the sulphur they contain, and reciprocally. These compounds have been called, in general, sulphuretted

hydrosulphurets; but the name of hydrogenated sulphurets is more particularly given to those combinations which are saturated with sulphur at a high temperature, because, by treating them with acids, we precipitate a peculiar compound of sulphur and hydrogen, of which we shall now treat.

This compound of hydrogen and sulphur, the proportions of the elements of which have not yet been accurately ascertained, is also called hydruret of sulphur. It is formed by putting flowers of sulphur in contact with nascent sulphuretted hydrogen. With this view, we take an aqueous solution of the hydrogenated sulphuret of potassa, and pour it gradually into liquid muriatic acid, which seizes the potassa, and forms a soluble salt, while the sulphur and sulphuretted hydrogen unite, fall down together, collecting by degrees at the bottom of the vessel, as a dense oil does in water. To preserve this hydruret of sulphur, we must fill with it a phial having a ground stopper, cork it, and keep it inverted in a cool place. We may consider this substance either as a combination of sulphur and hydrogen, or of sulphur and sulphuretted hydrogen; but its properties, and the mode of obtaining it, render the latter the more probable opinion. The proportion of the constituents is not known.

The most interesting of the hydrogenated sulphurets, is that of ammonia. It was discovered by the Hon. Robert Boyle, and called his fuming liquor. To prepare it, we take one part of muriate of ammonia and of pulverized quicklime, and half a part of flowers of sulphur. After mixing them intimately, we introduce the mixture into an earthen or glass retort, taking care that none of it remains in the neck. A dry cooled receiver is connected to the retort by means of a long adopter-tube. The heat must be urged slowly almost to redness. A yellowish liquor condenses in the receiver, which is to be put into a phial with its own weight of flowers of sulphur, and agitated with it seven or eight minutes. The greater part of the sulphur is dissolved, the colour of the mixture deepens remarkably, and becomes thick, constituting the hydrogenated sulphuret.

The distilled liquor diffuses, for a long time, dense vapour in a jar full of oxygen or common air, but scarcely any in azote or hydrogen; and the dryness or humidity of the gases makes no difference in the effects. It is probably owing to the oxygen converting the liquor into a hydrogenated sulphuret, or perhaps to the state of sulphite, that the vapours appear.

Hydrogenated sulphurets are frequently called hydroguretted sulphurets.

Sulphur combines with carbon, forming an interesting compound, to which the name of sulphuret of carbon is sometimes given.

Sulphur has been long an esteemed article of the Materia Medica; it stimulates the system, loosens the belly, and promotes the insensible perspiration. It pervades the whole habit, and manifestly transpires through the pores of the skin, as appears from the sulphurous smell of persons who have taken it, and from silver being stained in their pockets of a blackish colour. In the stomach it is probably combined with hydrogen. It is a celebrated remedy against cutaneous diseases, particularly psora, both given internally and applied externally. It has likewise been recommended in rheumatic pains, flying gout, rickets, atrophy, coughs, asthmas, and other disorders of the breast and lungs, and particularly catarrhs of the chronic kind, also in solica pictonum, worm cases, and to lessen salivation.

In hæmorrhoidal affections it is almost specific; but in most of these cases it is advantageously combined with some cooling purgative, especially supertartrate of potassa.

The preparations of sulphur directed to be used by the London and Edinburgh Colleges, are the Sulphur lotum, Sulphur præcipitatum, and Sulphur sublimatum.

SULPHUR ANTIMONII PRÆCIPITATUM. *Sulphur auratum antimonii.* This preparation of antimony appears to have rendered that called *kermes mineral* unnecessary. It is a yellow hydrosulphuret of antimony, and therefore called *hydro-sulphuretum stibii luteum.* As an alterative and sudorific it is in high estimation, and given in diseases of the skin and glands; and joined with calomel, it is one of the most powerful and penetrating alteratives we are in possession of.

SULPHUR AURATUM ANTIMONII. See *Sulphur antimonii præcipitatum.*

SULPHUR LOTUM. Washed sulphur; *Flores sulphuris loti.* Take of sublimed sulphur, a pound. Pour on boiling water so that the acid, if there be any may be entirely washed away; then dry it. The dose is from half a drachm to two drachms.

SULPHUR PRÆCIPITATUM. *Lac sulphuris.* Take of sublimed sulphur, a pound; fresh lime, two pounds; water, four gallons: boil the sulphur and lime together in the water, then strain the solution through paper, and drop in it as much muriatic acid as may be necessary to precipitate the sulphur; lastly, wash this by repeated effusions of water until it is tasteless. This preparation is mostly preferred to the flowers of sulphur, in consequence of its being freed from its impurities. The dose is from half a drachm to three drachms.

Sulphur, precipitated. See *Sulphur præcipitatum.*

SULPHUR SUBLIMATUM. Sublimed sulphur. See *Sulphur.*

SULPHUR VIVUM. Native sulphur.

Sulphur, washed. See *Sulphur lotum.*

SULPHURWORT. See *Peucedanum.*

Sulphurated hydrogen gas. See *Hydrogen gas, sulphuretted.*

SULPHURE. See *Sulphuret.*

Sulphureous acid. See *Sulphurous acid.*

Sulphuretted chyazic acid. See *Sulphuroprussic acid.*

SULPHURETTED HYDROGEN. See *Hydrogen, sulphuretted.*

SULPHURE'TUM. Sulphuret. Sulphure. A combination of sulphur with an alkali, earth, or metal.

SULPHURETUM AMMONIÆ. *Hepar sulphuris volatile.* Boyle's or Beguine's fuming spirit. Sulphuret of ammonia is obtained in the form of a yellow fuming liquor, by the ammonia and sulphur uniting while in a state of gas during distillation. It excites the action of the absorbent system, and diminishes arterial action, and is given internally in diseases arising from the use of mercury, phthisis, diseases of the skin, and phlegmasiæ: externally it is prescribed in the form of bath in paralysis, contractura, psora, and other cutaneous diseases.

SULPHURETUM ANTIMONII PRÆCIPITATUM. See *Antimonii sulphuretum præcipitatum.*

SULPHURETUM CALCIS. *Hepar calcis.* Sulphuret of lime. It is principally used as a bath in various diseases of the skin.

SULPHURETUM HYDRARGYRI NIGRUM. See *Hydrargyri sulphuretum nigrum.*

SULPHURETUM HYDRARGYRI RUBRUM. See *Hydrargyri sulphuretum rubrum.*

SULPHURETUM POTASSÆ. See *Potassæ sulphuretum.*

SULPHURETUM SODÆ. A combination of soda and sulphur.

SULPHURETUM STIBII NATIVUM. *Sulphuretum stibii nigrum; Antimonium crudum.* Native sulphuret of antimony. It is from this ore that all our preparations of antimony are made. See *Antimony.*

SULPHURIC. *Sulphuricus.* Belonging to sulphur.

SULPHURIC ACID. *Acidum sulphuricum.* Oil of vitriol. Vitriolic acid. "When sulphur is heated to 180° or 190° in an open vessel, it melts, and soon afterward emits a bluish flame, visible in the dark, but which, in open daylight, has the appearance of a white fume. This flame has a suffocating smell, and has so little heat that it will not set fire to flax, or even gunpowder, so that in this way the sulphur may be entirely consumed out of it. If the heat be still augmented the sulphur boils, and suddenly bursts into a much more luminous flame, and the same suffocating vapour still continuing to be emitted.

The suffocating vapour of sulphur is imbibed by water, with which it forms the fluid formerly called *volatile vitriolic,* now sulphurous acid. If this fluid be exposed for a time to the air, it loses the sulphurous smell it had at first, and the acid becomes more fixed. It is then the fluid which was formerly called the *spirit of vitriol.* Much of the water may be driven off by heat, and the dense acid which remains is the sulphuric acid commonly called *oil of vitriol;* a name which was probably given to it from the little noise it makes when poured out, and the unctuous feel it has when rubbed between the fingers, produced by its corroding

and destroying the skin, with which it forms a soapy compound.

The stone or mineral called martial pyrites, which consists for the most part of sulphur and iron, is found to be converted into the salt vulgarly called *green vitriol*, but more properly sulphate of iron, by exposure to air and moisture. In this natural process the pyrites breaks and falls in pieces; and if the change takes place rapidly, a considerable increase of temperature follows, which is sometimes sufficient to set the mass on fire. By conducting this operation in an accurate way, it is found that oxygen is absorbed. The sulphate is obtained by solution in water and subsequent evaporation; by which the crystals of the salt are separated from the earthy impurities, which were not suspended in the water.

The sulphuric acid was formerly obtained in this country by distillation from sulphate of iron, as it still is in many parts abroad: the common green vitriol is made use of for this purpose, as it is to be met with at a low price, and the acid is most easily to be extracted from it. With respect to the operation itself, the following particulars should be attended to: First, the vitriol must be calcined in an iron or earthen vessel, till it appears of a yellowish-red colour: by this operation it will lose half its weight. This is done in order to deprive it of the greater part of the water which it has attracted into its crystals during the crystallization, and which would otherwise, in the ensuing distillization, greatly weaken the acid. As soon as the calcination is finished, the vitriol is to be put immediately, while it is warm, into a coated earthen retort, which is to be filled two-thirds with it, so that the ingredients may have sufficient room upon being distended by the heat, and thus the bursting of the retort be prevented. It will be most advisable to have the retort immediately enclosed in brick-work in a reverberatory furnace, and to stop up the neck of it till the distillation begins, in order to prevent the materials *from* attracting fresh humidity from the air. At the beginning of the distillation the retort must be opened, and a moderate fire is to be applied to it, in order to expel from the vitriol all that part of the phlegm which does not taste strongly of the acid, and which may be received in an open vessel placed under the retort. But as soon as there appear any acid drops, a receiver is to be added, into which has been previously poured a quantity of the acidulous fluid which has come over, in the proportion of half a pound of it to twelve pounds of the calcined vitriol; when the receiver is to be secured with a proper luting. The fire is now to be raised by little and little to the most intense degree of heat, and the receiver carefully covered with wet cloths, and, in winter time, with snow or ice, as the acid rises in the form of a thick white vapour, which towards the end of the operation becomes hot, and heats the receiver to a great degree. The fire must be continued at this high pitch for several days, till no vapour issues from the retort, nor any drops are seen trickling down its sides. In the case of a great quantity of vitriol being distilled, Bernhardt has observed it to continue emitting vapours in this manner for the space of ten days. When the vessels are quite cold, the receiver must be opened carefully, so that none of the luting may fall into it; after which the fluid contained in it is to be poured in a bottle, and the air carefully excluded. The fluid that is thus obtained is the German sulphuric acid, of which Bernhardt got sixty-four pounds from six hundredweight of vitriol; and, on the other hand, when no water had been previously poured into the receiver, fifty-two pounds only of a dry concrete acid. This acid was formerly called *glacial oil of vitriol*, and its consistence is owing to a mixture of sulphurous acid, which occasions it to become solid at a moderate temperature.

It has been lately stated by Vogel, that when this fuming acid is put into a glass retort, and distilled by a moderate heat into a receiver cooled with ice, the fuming portion comes over first, and may be obtained in a solid state by stopping the distillation in time. This has been supposed to constitute absolute sulphuric acid, or acid entirely void of water. It is in silky filaments, tough, difficult to cut, and somewhat like asbestos. Exposed to the air, it fumes strongly, and gradually evaporates. It does not act on the skin so readily as concentrated oil of vitriol. Up to 66°, it continues solid, but at temperatures above this it becomes a

colourless vapour, which whitens on contact with air. Dropped into water in small quantities, it excites a hissing noise, as if it were red-hot iron; in larger quantities it produces a species of explosion. It is said to be convertible into ordinary sulphuric acid, by the addition of a fifth of water. It dissolves sulphur, and assumes a blue, green, or brown colour, according to the proportion of sulphur dissolved. The specific gravity of the black fuming sulphuric acid, prepared in large quantities from copperas, at Nordhausen, is 1.896. Its constitution is not well ascertained.

The sulphuric acid made in Great Britain is produced by the combustion of sulphur. There are three conditions requisite in this operation. Oxygen must be present to maintain the combustion; the vessel must be so close as to prevent the escape of the volatile matter which rises, and water must be present to imbibe it. For these purposes, a mixture of eight parts of sulphur with one of nitre is placed in a proper vessel enclosed within a chamber of considerable size, lined on all sides with lead, and covered at bottom with a shallow stratum of water. The mixture being set on fire, will burn for a considerable time by virtue of the supply of oxygen which nitre gives out when heated, and the water imbibing the sulphurous vapours, becomes gradually more and more acid after repeated combustions, and the acid is afterward concentrated by distillation.

Such was the account usually given of this operation, till Clement and Desormes showed, in a very interesting memoir, its total inadequacy to account for the result. 100 parts of nitre, judiciously managed, will produce, with the requisite quantity of sulphur, 2000 parts of concentrated sulphuric acid. Now these contain 1200 parts of oxygen, while the hundred parts of nitre contain only 39½ of oxygen; being not 1-30th part of what is afterward found in the resulting sulphuric acid. But after the combustion of the sulphur, the nitre is converted into sulphate and bisulphate of potassa, which mingled residuary salts contain nearly as much oxygen as the nitre originally did. Hence the origin of the 1200 parts of the oxygen in the sulphuric acid is still to be sought for. The following ingenious theory was first given by Clement and Desormes. The burning sulphur or sulphurous acid, taking from the nitre a portion of its oxygen, forms sulphuric acid, which unites with the potassa, and displaces a little nitrous and nitric acids in vapour. These vapours are decomposed by the sulphurous acid, into nitrous gas, or deutoxide of azote. This gas, naturally little denser than air, and now expanded by the heat, suddenly rises to the roof of the chamber: and might be expected to escape at the aperture there, which manufacturers were always obliged to leave open, otherwise they found the acidification would not proceed. But the instant that nitrous gas comes in contact with atmospherical oxygen, nitrous acid vapour is formed, which being a very heavy aëriform body, immediately precipitates on the sulphurous flame, and converts it into sulphuric acid; while itself resuming the state of nitrous gas, reascends for a new charge of oxygen, again to redescend, and transfer it to the flaming sulphur. Thus we see, that a small volume of nitrous vapour, by its alternate metamorphoses into the states of oxide and acid, and its consequent interchanges, may be capable of acidifying a great quantity of sulphur.

This beautiful theory received a modification from Sir H. Davy. He found that nitrous gas had no action on sulphurous gas, to convert it into sulphuric acid, unless water be present. With a *small* proportion of water, four volumes of sulphurous acid gas, and three of nitrous gas, are condensed into crystalline solid, which is instantly decomposed by *abundance* of water; oil of vitriol is formed, and nitrous gas given off; which with contact of air becomes nitrous acid gas, as above described. The process continues, according to the same principle of combination and decomposition, till the water at the bottom of the chamber is become strongly acid. It is first concentrated in large leaden pans, and afterward in glass retorts heated in a sandbath. Platinum alembics, placed within pots of cast-iron of a corresponding shape and capacity, have been lately substituted in many manufactories for glass, and have been found to save fuel, and quicken the process of concentration.

The proper mode of burning the sulphur with the nitre, so as to produce the greatest quantity of oil

of vitriol, is a problem, concerning which chemists hold a variety of opinions. Thenard describes the following as the best. Near one of the sides of the leaden chamber, about a foot above its bottom, an iron plate, furnished with an upright border, is p'aced horizontally over a furnace, whose chimney passes across, under the bottom of the chamber, without having any connexion with it. On this plate, which is enclosed in a little chamber, the mixture of sulphur and nitre is laid. The whole being shut up, and the bottom of the large chamber covered with water, a gentle fire is kindled in the furnace. The sulphur soon takes fire, and gives birth to the products described. When the combustion is finished, which is seen through a little pane adapted to the trap-door of the chamber, this is opened, the sulphate of potassa is withdrawn, and is replaced by a mixture of sulphur and nitre. The air in the great chamber is meanwhile renewed by opening its lateral door, and a valve in its opposite side. Then, after closing these openings, the furnace is lighted anew. Successive mixtures are thus burned till the acid acquires a specific gravity of about 1.390, taking care never to put at once on the plate more sulphur than the air of the chamber can acidify. The acid is then withdrawn by stop-cocks, and concentrated.

The following details are extracted from a paper on sulphuric acid, which Dr. Ure published in the fourth volume of the Journal of Science and the Arts.

"The best commercial sulphuric acid that I have been able to meet with," says he, "contains from one-half to three quarters of a part in the hundred, of solid saline matter, foreign to its nature. These fractional parts consist of sulphate of potassa and lead, in the proportion of four of the former to one of the latter. It is, I believe, difficult to manufacture it directly, by the usual methods, of a purer quality. The ordinary acid sold in the shops contains often three or four per cent. of saline matter. Even more is occasionally introduced, by the employment of nitre, to remove the brown colour given to the acid by carbonaceous matter. The amount of these adulterations, whether accidental or fraudulent, may be readily determined by evaporating, in a small capsule of porcelain, or rather platinum, a definite weight of the acid. The platinum cup placed on the red cinders of a common fire, will give an exact result in five minutes. If more than five grains of matter remain from five hundred of acid, we may pronounce it sophisticated.

Distillation is the mode by which pure oil of vitriol is obtained. This process is described in chemical treatises as both difficult and hazardous; but since adopting the following plan, I have found it perfectly safe and convenient. I take a plain glass retort, capable of holding from two to four quarts of water, and put into it about a pint-measure of the sulphuric acid, (and a few fragments of glass,) connecting the retort with a large globular receiver, by means of a glass tube four feet long, and from one to two inches in diameter. The tube fits very loosely at both ends. The retort is placed over a charcoal fire, and the flame is made to play gently on its bottom. When the acid begins to boil smartly, sudden explosions of dense vapour rush forth from time to time, which would infallibly break small vessels. Here, however, these expansions are safely permitted, by the large capacity of the retort and receiver, as well as by the easy communication with the air at both ends of the adopter tube. Should the retort, indeed, be exposed to a great intensity of flame, the vapour will no doubt be generated with incoercible rapidity, and break the apparatus. But this accident can proceed only from gross imprudence. It resembles in suddenness, the explosion of gunpowder, and illustrates admirably Dr. Black's observation, that, but for the great latent heat of steam, a mass of water, powerfully heated, would explode on reaching the boiling temperature. I have ascertained, that the specific caloric of the vapour of sulphuric acid is very small, and hence the danger to which rash operators may be exposed during its distillation. Hence, also, it is unnecessary to surround the receiver with cold water, as when alkohol and most other liquids are distilled. Indeed, the application of cold to the bottom of the receiver generally causes it, in the present operation, to crack. By the above method, I have made the concentrated oil of vitriol flow over in a continuous slender stream, without the globe becoming sensibly hot

I have frequently boiled the *distilled* acid till only one-half remain in the retort; yet at the temperature of 60° Fahrenheit, I have never found the specific gravity of acid so concentrated, to exceed 1.8455. It is, I believe, more exactly 1.8452. The number 1.850, which it has been the fashion to assign for the density of pure oil of vitriol, is undoubtedly very erroneous, and ought to be corrected. Genuine *commercial* acid should never surpass 1.8485; when it is denser we may infer sophistication, or negligence, in the manufacture."

The sulphuric acid strongly attracts water, which it takes from the atmosphere very rapidly, and in larger quantities, if suffered to remain in an open vessel, imbibing one-third of its weight in twenty-four hours, and more than six times its weight in a twelvemonth. If four parts by weight be mixed with one of water at 50°, they produce an instantaneous heat of 300° F.; and four parts raise one of ice to 212°: on the contrary, four parts of ice, mixed with one of acid, sink the thermometer to 4 below 0. When pure it is colourless, and emits no fumes. It requires a great degree of cold to freeze it; and if diluted with half a part or more of water, unless the dilution be carried very far, it becomes more and more difficult to congeal; yet at the specific gravity of 1.78, or a few hundredths above or below this, it may be frozen by surrounding it with melting snow. Its congelation forms regular prismatic crystals with six sides. Its boiling point, according to Bergman, is 540°; according to Dalton, 590°.

Pure sulphuric acid is without smell and colour, and of an oily consistence. Its action on litmus is so strong, that a single drop of acid will give to an immense quantity of water the power of reddening. It is a most violent caustic; and has sometimes been administered with the most criminal purposes. The person who unfortunately swallows it, speedily dies in dreadful agonies and convulsions. Chalk, or common carbonate of magnesia, is the best antidote for this, as well as for the strong nitric and muriatic acids

When transmitted through an ignited porcelain tube of one fifth of an inch diameter, it is resolved into two parts of sulphurous acid gas, and one of oxygen gas, with water. Voltaic electricity causes an evolution of sulphur at the negative pole; while a sulphate of the metallic wire is formed at the positive. Sulphuric acid has no action on oxygen gas or air. It merely abstracts their aqueous vapour.

If the oxygenized muriatic acid of Thenard be put in contact with the sulphate of silver, there is immediately formed insoluble chloride of silver, and oxygenized sulphuric acid. To obtain sulphuric acid in the highest degree of oxygenation, it is merely necessary to pour barytes water into the above oxygenized acid, so as to precipitate only a part of it, leaving the rest in union with the whole of the oxygen. Oxygenized sulphuric acid partially reduces the oxide of silver, occasioning a strong effervescence.

All the simple combustibles decompose sulphuric acid, with the assistance of heat. About 400° Fahr. sulphur converts sulphuric into sulphurous acid. Several metals at an elevated temperature decompose this acid, with evolutions of sulphuric acid gas, oxidizement of the metal, and combination of the oxide with the undecomposed portion of the acid.

The sulphuric acid is of very extensive use in the art of chemistry, as well as in metallurgy, bleaching, and some of the processes for dying; in medicine, it is given as a tonic and stimulant, and is sometimes used externally as a caustic.

The combinations of this acid with the various bases are called *sulphates*, and most of them have long been known by various names. With barytes it is found native and nearly pure in various forms, in coarse powder, rounded masses, stalactites, and regular crystallizations, which are in some lamellar, in others needly, in others prismatic or pyramidal.

This salt, if at all deleterious, is less so than the carbonate of barytes, and is more economical for preparing the muriate for medicinal purposes. It requires 43,000 parts of water to dissolve it at 60°.

Sulphate of strontian has a considerable resemblance to that of barytes in its properties. It is found native in considerable quantities at Aust Passage and other places in the neighbourhood of Bristol. It requires 3840 parts of boiling water to dissolve it.

Eee

Its composition is 5 acid + 6.5 base.

The *sulphate of potassa, vitriolated kali,* formerly *vitriolated tartar, sal de duobus,* and *arcanum duplicatum,* crystallizes in hexahedral prisms, terminated by hexagonal pyramids, but susceptible of variations. Its crystallization by quick cooling is confused. Its taste is bitter, acrid, and a little saline. It is soluble in 5 parts of boiling water, and 16 parts at 60°. In the fire it decrepitates, and is fusible by a strong heat. It is decomposable by charcoal at a high temperature. It may be prepared by direct mixture of its component parts; but the usual and cheapest mode is to neutralize the acidulous sulphate left after distilling nitric acid, the *sal enixen* of the old chemists, by the addition of carbonate of potassa. The *sal polychrest* of old dispensatories, made by deflagrating sulphur and nitre in a crucible, was a compound of the sulphate and sulphite of potassa. The acidulous sulphate is sometimes employed as a flux, and likewise in the manufacture of alum. In medicine, the neutral salt is sometimes used as a deobstruent, and in large doses as a mild cathartic; dissolved in a considerable portion of water, and taken daily in such quantity as to be gently aperient, it has been found serviceable in cutaneous affections, and is sold in London for this purpose as a nostrum; and certainly it deserves to be distinguished from the generality of quack medicines, very few indeed of which can be taken without imminent hazard.

It consists of 5 acid + 6 base; but there is a compound of the same constituents, in the proportion of 10 acid + 6 potassa, called the bisulphate.

The *sulphate of soda* is the *vitriolated natron* of the college, the well known *Glauber's salt,* or *sal mirabile.* It is commonly prepared from the residuum left after distilling muriatic acid, the superfluous acid of which may be saturated by the addition of soda, or precipitated by lime; and is likewise obtained in the manufacture of the muriate of ammonia. Scherer mentions another mode by Funcke, which is, making 8 parts of calcined sulphate of lime, 5 of clay, and 5 of common salt, into a paste with water; burning this in a kiln; and then powdering, lixiviating, and crystallizing. It exists in large quantities under the surface of the earth in some countries, as Persia, Bohemia, and Switzerland; is found mixed with other substances in mineral springs and sea-water; and sometimes effloresces on walls. Sulphate of soda is bitter and saline to the taste. It is soluble in 2.85 parts of cold water, and 0.8 at a boiling heat. It crystallizes in hexagonal prisms bevelled at the extremities, sometimes grooved longitudinally, and of very large size, when the quantity is great. These effloresce completely into a white powder if exposed to a dry air, or even if kept wrapped up in a paper in a dry place, yet they retain sufficient water of crystallization to undergo the aqueous fusion on exposure to heat, but by urging the fire, melt. Barytes and strontian take its acid from it entirely, and potassa partially; the nitric and muriatic acids, though they have a weaker affinity for its base, combine with a part of it when digested on it. Heated with charcoal, its acid is decomposed. As a purgative, its use is very general; and it has been employed to furnish soda. Pajot des Charmes has made some experiments on it in fabricating glass; with sand alone it would not succeed, but equal parts of carbonate of lime, sand, and dried sulphate of soda, produced a clear, solid, pale yellow glass.

It is composed of 5 acid + 4 base + 11.25 water in crystals; when dry, the former two primes are its constituents.

Sulphate of soda and sulphate of ammonia form together a *triple salt.*

Sulphate of lime, selenite, gypsum, plaster of Paris, or sometimes *alabaster,* forms extensive strata in various mountains. The *specular gypsum,* or *glacies Maria,* is a species of this salt, and affirmed by some French travellers to be employed in Russia, where it abounds, as a substitute for glass in windows. Its specific gravity is from 1.872 to 2.311. It requires 500 parts of cold water, and 450 of hot, to dissolve it. When calcined, it decrepitates, becomes very friable and white, and heats a little with water, with which it forms a solid mass. In this process it loses its water of crystallization. In this state it is found native in Tyrol, crystallized in rectangular parallelopipeds, or octahedral or hexahedral prisms, and is called *anhydrous sulphate of lime.* Both the natural and artificial anhydrous sulphate consists of 56.3 lime, and 43.6 acid, according to Chenevix. The calcined sulphate is much employed for making casts of anatomical or ornamental figures as one of the bases of stucco; as a fine cement for making close and strong joints between stone, and joining rims or tops of metal to glass; for making moulds for the Staffordshire potteries; for cornices, mouldings, and other ornaments in building. For these purposes, and for being wrought into columns, chimney-pieces, and various ornaments, about eight hundred tons are raised annually in Derbyshire, where it is called alabaster. In America, it is laid on grass land as a manure.

[*Sulphate of lime, gypsum,* or *plaster of Paris,* is extensively and beneficially employed in some parts of the United States as a manure. It is reduced to a fine powder, and applied by the spoonful to a hill of Indian corn (maize), or it is thinly scattered over grass land, and it has a most powerful and fertilizing effect. The gypsum of Nova Scotia afforded the principal supply for this and other purposes some time since, but the states of New-York and Pennsylvania now furnish large quantities, and of an excellent quality, from their own quarries. Gypsum, as a manure, will not answer on the sea-coast, or within the influence of a saline atmosphere. It begins to produce fertilizing effects about 40 or 50 miles from the sea-shore. A.]

Ordinary crystallized gypsum consists of 5 sulphuric acid + 3.5 lime + 2.25 water; the anhydrous variety wants of course the last ingredient.

Sulphate of magnesia, the *vitriolated magnesia* of the late, and *sal catharticus amarus* of former London Pharmacopœias, is commonly known by the name of *Epsom salt,* as it was furnished in considerable quantity by the mineral water at that place, mixed however with a considerable portion of sulphate of soda. It is afforded, however, in greater abundance and more pure from the bittern left after the extraction of salt from sea-water. It has likewise been found efflorescing on brick walls, both old and recently erected, and in small quantity in the ashes of coals. The capillary salt of Idria, found in silvery crystals mixed with the aluminous schist in the mines of that place, and hitherto considered as a feathery alum, has been ascertained by Klaproth to consist of sulphate of magnesia, mixed with a small portion of sulphate of iron. When pure, it crystallizes in small quadrangular prisms, terminated by quadrangular pyramids or dihedral summits. Its taste is cool and bitter. It is very soluble, requiring only an equal weight of cold water, and three-fourths its weight of hot. It effloresces in the air, though but slowly. If it attract moisture it contains muriate of magnesia, or of lime. Exposed to heat it dissolves in its own water of crystallization, and dries, but is not decomposed nor fused, but with extreme difficulty. It consists, according to Bergman, of 33 acid, 19 magnesia, 48 water. A very pure sulphate is said to be prepared in the neighbourhood of Genoa, by roasting a pyrites found there; exposing it to the air in a covered place for six months; watering it occasionally, and then lixiviating.

Sulphate of magnesia is one of our most valuable purgatives; for which purpose only it is used, and for furnishing the carbonate of magnesia.

It is composed of 5 acid + 2.5 magnesia + 7.875 water, in the state of crystals.

Sulphate of ammonia crystallizes in slender, flattened, hexahedral prisms, terminated by hexagonal pyramids; it attracts a little moisture from very damp air, particularly if the acid be in excess; it dissolves in two parts of cold and one of boiling water. It is not used, though Glauber, who called it his *secret ammoniacal salt,* vaunted its excellence in assaying.

It consists of 5 acid + 2.125 ammonia + 1.125 water in its most desiccated state; and in its crystalline state of 5 acid + 2.125 ammonia + 3.375 water.

If sulphate of ammonia and sulphate of magnesia be added together in solution, they combine into a *triple salt* of an octahedral figure, but varying much; less soluble than either of its component parts; unalterable in the air; undergoing on the fire the watery fusion; after which it is decomposed, part of the ammonia flying off, and the remainder subliming with an excess of acid. It contains, according to Fourcroy, 68 sulphate of magnesia, and 32 sulphate of ammonia.

Sulphate of glucina crystallizes with difficulty, its solution readily acquiring and containing a syrupy consistence; its taste is sweet, and slightly astringent; it is not alterable in the air; a strong heat expels its acid, and leaves the earth pure; heated with charcoal, it forms a sulphuret; infusion of galls forms a yellowish-white precipitate with its solution.

Yttria is readily dissolved by sulphuric acid; and as the solution goes on, the sulphate crystallizes in small brilliant grains, which have a sweetish taste, but less so than sulphate of glucina, and are of a light amethyst-red colour. They require 30 parts of cold water to dissolve them, and to give up their acid when exposed to a high temperature. They are decomposed by oxalic acid, prussiate of potassa, infusion of galls, and phosphate of soda.

Sulphate of alumina in its pure state is but recently known, and it was first attentively examined by Vauquelin. It may be made by dissolving pure alumina in pure sulphuric acid, heating them for some time, evaporating the solution to dryness, drying the residuum with a pretty strong heat, redissolving it, and crystallizing. Its crystals are soft, foliaceous, shining, and pearly; but these are not easily obtained without cautious evaporation and refrigeration. They have an astringent taste; are little alterable in the air; are pretty soluble, particularly in hot water; give out their acid on exposure to a high temperature: are decomposable by combustible substances, though not readily; and do not form a pyrophorus like alum.

If the evaporation and desiccation directed above be omitted, the alumina will remain supersaturated with acid, as may be known by its taste, and by its reddening vegetable blue. This is still more difficult to crystallize than the neutral salt, and frequently thickens into a gelatinous mass.

A compound of acidulous sulphate of alumina, with potassa or ammonia, has long been known by the name of alum.

Sulphate of zircon may be prepared by adding sulphuric acid to the earth recently precipitated, and not yet dry. It is sometimes in small needles, but commonly pulverulent; very friable; insipid; insoluble in water, unless it contain some acid; and easily decomposed by heat."—*Ure's Chem. Dict.*

Sulphuric acid is a powerful antiseptic and tonic: it is given, properly diluted, in the dose of from one to three drops with cinchona and other medicines in the cure of fevers and debilities, and it is often applied externally, when very much diluted, against psora and some chronic affections of the skin.

SULPHURIS FLORES. See *Sulphur sublimatum.*

SULPHUROPRUSSIC ACID. The sulphuretted chyazic acid of Porrett.

Dissolve in water one part of sulphuret of potassa, and boil it for a considerable time with three or four parts of powdered Prussian blue added at intervals. Sulphuret of iron is formed, and a colourless liquid containing the new acid combined with potassa, mixed with hyposulphate and sulphate of potassa. Render this liquid sensibly sour, by the addition of sulphuric acid. Continue the boiling for a little, and when it cools, add a little peroxide of manganese in fine powder, which will give the liquor a fine crimson colour. To the filtered liquid add a solution containing persulphate of copper, and protosulphate of iron, in the proportion of two of the former salt to three of the latter, until the crimson colour disappears. Sulphuroprussiate of copper falls. Boil this with a solution of potassa, which will separate the copper. Distil the liquid mixed with sulphuric acid in a glass retort, and the peculiar acid will come over. By saturation with carbonate of barytes, and then throwing down this by the equivalent quantity of sulphuric acid, the sulphuroprussic acid is obtained pure.

It is a transparent and colourless liquid, possessing a strong colour, somewhat resembling acetic acid. Its specific gravity is only 1.032. It dissolves a little sulphur at a boiling heat. It then blackens nitrate of silver; but the pure acid throws down the silver white. By repeated distillations sulphur is separated and the acid is decomposed.

SULPHUROUS ACID. "Sulphur burned at a low temperature absorbs less oxygen than it does when exposed to greater heat, and is consequently acidified in a slighter degree, so as to form sulphurous acid. This in the ordinary state of the atmosphere is a gas; but on reducing its temperature very low by artificial cold, and exposing it to strong compression, it becomes a liquid. To obtain it in the liquid state, however, for

practical purposes, it is received into water, by which it is absorbed.

As the acid obtained by burning sulphur in this way is commonly mixed with more or less sulphuric acid, when sulphurous acid is wanted it is commonly made by abstracting part of the oxygen from sulphuric acid by means of some combustible substance. Mercury or tin is usually preferred. For the purposes of manufactures, however, chopped straw or saw-dust may be employed. If one part of mercury and two of concentrated sulphuric acid be put into a glass retort with a long neck, and heat applied till an effervescence is produced, the sulphurous acid will arise in the form of gas, and may be collected over quicksilver, or received into water, which, at the temperature of 61°, will absorb thirty-three times its bulk, or nearly an eleventh of its weight.

Water thus saturated is, intensely acid to the taste, and has the smell of sulphur burning slowly. It destroys most vegetable colours, but the blues are reddened by it previous to their being discharged. A pleasing instance of its effect on colours may be exhibited by holding a red rose over the blue flame of a common match, by which the colour will be discharged wherever the sulphurous acid comes into contact with it, so as to render it beautifully variegated, or entirely white. If it be then dipped into water, the redness after a time will be restored.

Sulphurous acid is used in bleaching, particularly for silks. It likewise discharges vegetable stains, and iron-moulds from linen.

In combination with the salifiable bases, it forms sulphites which differ from the sulphates in their properties. The alkaline sulphites are more soluble than the sulphates, the earthy less. They are converted into sulphates by an addition of oxygen, which they acquire even by exposure to the air."

Sultan flower. The *Centaurea moschata*, of Linnæus.

SUMACH. (*Sumak;* from *samak,* to be red; so called from its red berry.) See *Rhus coriaria.*

Sumach, elm-leaved. See *Rhus coriaria.*

SU'MEN. (Arabian.) The lower or fat part of the belly.

SUN-DEW. See *Drosera rotundifolia.*

SUPER. 1. This term is applied, in chemistry and pharmacy, to several saline substances, in which there is an excess of one of its constituents beyond what is necessary to form the ordinary compound; as supersulphate of potassa, supercarbonate of soda, &c.

2. In anatomy, it regards situation; as *superscapularis, supergenualis.*

3. In physiology, it means an additional; as super foetation.

4. In medicine, it means excess; as superpurgation.

SUPERACE'TAS PLUMBI. See *Plumbi acetas.*

SUPERARSE'NIAS POTASSÆ. Superarseniate of potassa. A compound of potassa with excess of arsenic acid. It was called *Macquer's Arsenical Salt,* from its discoverer; and has been sometimes given in medicine, possessing similar properties to those of the white oxide of arsenic.

SUPE'RBUS. See *Rectus superior oculi.*

SUPERCI'LIUM. See *Eyebrow.*

SUPERCILIUM VENERIS. The milfoil. See *Achillea millefolium.*

SUPERFŒTATION. (*Superfœtatio;* from *super,* above or upon, and *fœtus,* a fœtus.) The impregnation of a woman already pregnant.

SUPERGEMINA'LIS. (From *super,* above, and *gemini,* the testicles.) The epididymis, or body above the testicles.

SUPERGENUA'LIS. (From *super,* above, and *genu,* the knee.) The patella, or knee-pan.

SUPERIMPREGNA'TIO. (*Superimpregnatio;* from *super,* above, and *impregnatio,* a conception.) Superfœtation.

SUPE'RIOR. Some muscles were so named from their relative situation.

SUPERIOR AURIS. See *Attollens aurem.*

SUPERLI'GULA. (From *super,* above, and *ligula,* a little tongue, the glottis.) The epiglottis.

SUPERPURGA'TIO. (From *super,* beyond, and *purgo,* to purge.) An excessive evacuation by stool.

SUPERSALT. See *Subsalt.*

SUPERSCAPULA'RIS. (From *super,* upon, and *scapula,* the shoulder-blade.) A muscle seated upon the scapula.

SUPERUS. Above: applied to the perianthium of flowers when placed above the germen; as in roses, and the genus Pyrus.

SUPINATION. (*Supinatio*; from *supinus*, placed upward.) The act of turning the palm of the hand upwards, by rotating the radius upon the ulna.

SUPINA'TOR. (From *supinus*, upwards.) A name given to those muscles which turn the hand upwards.

SUPINATOR BREVIS. See *Supinator radii brevis*.

SUPINATOR LONGUS. See *Supinator radii longus*.

SUPINATOR RADII BREVIS. A supinator muscle of the hand, situated on the forearm. *Supinator brevis, sive minor*, of Winslow; and *epicondylo-radial*, of Dumas. This small muscle, which is tendinous externally, is situated at the upper part of the forearm under the supinator longus, the extensor carpi radialis brevis, the extensor carpi ulnaris, the extensor digitorum communis, and the extensor minimi digiti.

It arises tendinous from the lower and anterior part of the outer condyle of the os humeri, and tendinous and fleshy from the outer edge and posterior surface of the ulna, adhering firmly to the ligament that joins the radius to that bone. From these origins its fibres descend forwards and inwards, and are inserted into the upper, inner, and anterior part of the radius around the cartilaginous surface, upon which slides the tendon of the biceps, and likewise into a ridge that runs downwards and outwards below this surface. It assists in the supination of the hand by rolling the radius outwards.

SUPINATOR RADII LONGUS. *Supinator longus*, of Albinus. *Supinator longus sive major*, of Winslow; and *humerosus radial*, of Dumas. A long flat muscle, covered by a very thin tendinous fascia, and situated immediately under the integuments along the outer convex surface of the radius. It arises, by very short tendinous fibres, from the anterior surface and outer ridge of the os humeri, about two or three inches above its external condyle, between the brachialis internus and the triceps brachii; and likewise from the anterior surface of the external intermuscular membrane, or ligament, as it is called. About the middle of the radius, its fleshy fibres terminate in a flat tendon, which is inserted into the inner side of the inferior extremity of the radius, near the root of its styloid process.

This muscle not only assists in rolling the radius outwards, and turning the palm of the hand upwards, on which account Riolanus first gave it the name of *supinator*, but it likewise assists in pronation, and in bending the forearm.

SUPPOSITO'RIUM. (From *sub*, under, and *pono*, to put.) A suppository, *i. e.* a substance to put into the rectum, there to remain and dissolve gradually.

Suppressed menses. See *Amenorrhœa*.

SUPPURATION. (*Suppuratio*; from *suppuro*, to suppurate.) That morbid action by which pus is deposited in inflammatory tumours. See *Pus*.

SUPRA. Above. This word before any other name, implies its situation being above it; as supra spinatus, above the spine of the scapula, &c.

SUPRA-COSTALES. See *Intercostal muscles*.

SUPRA-DECOMPOSITUS. See *Decompositus*.

SUPRA-SPINA'TUS. *Supra-spinatus seu super-scapularis*, of Cowper; and *sous-spino-scapulo-trochiterien*, of Dumas. A muscle of the arm first so named by Riolanus, from its situation. It is of considerable thickness, wider behind than before, and fills the whole of the cavity or fossa that is above the spine of the scapula. It arises fleshy from the whole of the base of the scapula that is above its spine, and likewise from the spine itself, and from the superior costa. Opposite to the basis of the coracoid process, it is found beginning to degenerate into a tendon, which is at first covered by fleshy fibres, and then passing under the acromion, adheres to the capsular ligament of the os humeri, and is inserted into the upper part of the large tuberosity at the head of the os humeri. This muscle is covered by a thin fascia, which adheres to the upper edge and superior part of the basis, as well as to the upper edge of the spine of the scapula. The principal use of the supra spinatus seems to be to assist in raising the arm upwards; at the same time, by drawing the capsular ligament upwards, it prevents it from being pinched between the head of the os humeri and that of the scapula. It may likewise serve to move the scapula upon the humerus.

324

SURA. (An Arabian word.) 1. The calf of the leg 2. The fibula.

SURCULUS. A term applied by botanists to the stem of mosses, or that part which bears the leaves. It is *simple*, in Polytricum; *branched*, in Minium androgynum; with *branches turned downward*, in Sphagnum palustre; *decumbent, creeping*, or *erect*.

SURDITAS. Deafness. See *Paracusis*.

SURFEIT. The consequence of excess in eating or drinking, or of something unwholesome or improper in the food. It consists in a heavy load or oppression of the stomach, with nausea, sickness, impeded perspiration, and at times eruptions on the skin.

SURGERY. *Chirurgia*. A branch of the healing art, having for its object the cure of external diseases.

SURTURBRAND. Fibrous brown coal, or bituminous wood, is so called in Iceland, where it occurs in great quantities.

SUS. The name of a genus of animals. Class, *Mammalia*; Order, *Belluæ*. The hog. The flesh called pork is considered a great delicacy, especially the young, and well fed, and is much used in most countries. Salted, it affords a harder food, still very nutritious to hard-working people, whose digestion is good.

SUS SCROFA. The systematic name of the hog, the fat of which is called lard.

Suspended animation. See *Resuscitation*.

SUSPENSO'RIUM. (From *suspendeo*, to hang.) A suspensory; a bag, or bandage, to suspend any part.

SUSPENSORIUM HEPATIS. The broad ligament of the liver.

SUSPENSORIUS TESTIS. The cremaster muscle of the testicle.

SUSU'RRUS. (From *susurro*, to murmur.) An imaginary sound in the ear.

SUTURE. (*Sutura*; from *suo*, to join together.) 1. In *surgery*, this term signifies the uniting the lips of a wound by sewing. *Clavata commissura*. A number of different kinds of sutures have been recommended by writers on surgery, but all of them are now reduced to two; namely, the *twisted*, and the *interrupted*, called also the *knotted suture*. The twisted suture is made in the following manner: having brought the divided parts nearly into contact, a pin is to be introduced from the outside inwards, and carried out through the opposite side to the same distance from the edge that it entered at on the former side; a firm wax ligature is then to be passed around it, making the figure of 8, by which the wounded parts are drawn gently into contact. The number of pins is to be determined by the extent of the wound; half an inch, or at most three quarters, is the proper distance between two pins. The interrupted suture is practised where a number of stitches is required, and the interruption is the only distance between the stitches.

2. In *anatomy*, the word suture is applied to the union of bones by means of dentiform margins, as in the bones of the cranium. See *Temporal, sphenoidal, zygomatic, transverse, coronal, lambdoidal*, and *sagittal sutures*.

3. In *botany*, it is applied to that part of a capsule, which is a kind of furrow on the external surface in which the valves are united. See *Capsula*.

SWALLOW-WORT. See *Asclepias vincetoxicum*.

SWAMMERDAM, JOHN, was born at Amsterdam, in 1637, and displayed an early predilection for natural history, particularly entomology. At Leyden, where he studied physic, he was distinguished by his skill and assiduity in anatomical experiments and the art of making preparations; and on taking his degree there, in 1667, he published a thesis on Respiration. At this time he began to practise his invention of injecting the vessels with ceraceous matter, from which anatomy has derived very important advantages. In the dissection of insects, he was singularly dexterous by the aid of instruments of his own invention. The Grand Duke of Tuscany invited him about this period to Florence on very liberal terms, but he declined the offer from aversion to a court-life, and to any religious restraints. In 1669 he published in his native language "A General History of Insects," afterward reprinted and translated into French and Latin, the latter with splendid figures. In 1672 another work appeared, entitled "Miraculum Naturæ," detailing the structure of the uterus; of which there were many subsequent editions. By intense application he became hypochondriacal and infatuated mysticism, so as to abandon all his scientific pursuits; and his constitution was worn out by his mortifications, so that he died in 1680. Several of his papers, which came long after into the hands of Boerhaave, were published under the title of "Biblia Naturæ;" in which the history of bees is particularly esteemed.

SWEAT. See *Perspiration.*

Sweet flag. See *Acorus calamus.*

Sweet marjoram. See *Origanum marjorana.*

Sweet navew. See *Brassica rapa.*

Sweet rush. See *Andropogon scœnanthus,* and *Acorus calamus.*

Sweet sultan. The *Centaurea moschata.*

Sweet willow. See *Myrica gale.*

SWIETEN, GERARD VAN, was born at Leyden, in 1700. From the loss of both his parents, his early education is said to have been somewhat neglected; but being sent at sixteen to the university of Louvain, he soon distinguished himself by his superior attainments. He then returned to his native place, and became a favourite pupil of the illustrious Boerhaave; and after studying seven years, took the degree of doctor in 1725; and so much had he profited by the instruction of that great master, as well as by his own unwearied researches, that he was immediately appointed to a medical professorship, which he occupied for many years with great reputation. At length, however, his success excited envy, and there being a law, which prohibited those not professing the religion of the State from holding any public appointment, Van Swieten, being a Roman Catholic, was obliged to resign his chair. He devoted the leisure thus acquired to the composition of his excellent Commentaries on the Aphorisms of Boerhaave: and while engaged in this work, he was invited by the Empress Maria Theresa to settle at Vienna, which he accepted in the year 1745, after stipulating, that he should be allowed to follow his usual mode of life, which was not well adapted for a court. The intellectual and moral endowments of this physician qualified him in every respect for conducting the medical school at Vienna; and that science in Germany was ultimately essentially benefitted by his exertions. He executed, during eight years, the office of professor with singular zeal; and having obtained the full confidence of his royal mistress, he was enabled to reform many abuses, and procure great advantages for the study of medicine in that city. His extensive erudition gained him the farther honour of being intrusted with the interests of learning in general in the Austrian dominions; he was appointed Imperial Librarian, President of the Censorship of Books, &c.; and also created a Baron of the Empire. He was likewise voluntarily enrolled in the list of almost all the distinguished literary societies of Europe. The inflexibility of his character led him to maintain a long opposition to small-pox inoculation. He died in 1772, and a statue was erected to his memory by the Empress at Vienna. His commentaries will always maintain their reputation, from the immense number of facts, well selected and well arranged, and the judicious summary of ancient and modern medical knowledge which they contain. He also published another useful work on the Diseases which prevail in Armies.

SWIETE'NIA. (Named after Van Swieten.) The name of a genus of plants. Class, *Decandria;* Order, *Monogynia.*

SWIETENIA MAHAGONI. The systematic name of the mahogany-tree. The bark of the wood of this tree is of a red colour internally; has an astringent bitter taste; and yields its active matter to water. It has been prepared as a substitute for Peruvian bark, and has been used as such with advantage. Dose, half a drachm.

SWINE-POX. See *Varicella.*

SWINESTONE. A variety of compact lucullite, a subspecies of limestone.

SWINGING. See *Æora.*

Sword-shaped. See *Lanceolatus.*

SYCO'MA. (From συκη, a fig.) *Sycosis.* A wart or excrescence resembling a fig on the eyelid, about the anus, or any other part.

SYDENHAM, THOMAS, was born at Winford-Eagle, in Dorsetshire, about the year 1624. He was entered at Oxford; but during the civil war, when that city was occupied by the royal party, he retired to

London. On this occasion, the illness of his brother brought him acquainted with Dr. Coxe, an eminent physician, who, finding Sydenham undecided as to the choice of his profession, persuaded him to study medicine on his return to Oxford. Accordingly, in 1648, he took the degree of bachelor of physic, and about the same period obtained a fellowship; then pursuing his studies a few years longer, he procured a doctor's degree from Cambridge, and settled as a physician in Westminster. The extensive practice which he is said to have enjoyed from 1660 to 1670, must be chiefly ascribed to the superior success of the means employed by him, which, being so different from those previously in use, became more readily a matter of notoriety; for, after the Restoration, his connexions could have contributed little to his advancement. He appears to have paid little attention to the prevailing medical doctrines, being early persuaded that the only mode of acquiring a correct knowledge of his art was to observe diligently the progress of diseases, whence the natural indications of cure might be derived; in which opinion he had the sanction of the celebrated Mr. Locke. It was to febrile diseases that he first applied this inductive method, and it cost him several years of anxious attention to satisfy himself as to the proper mode of treating them: the result of which he published in 1666, under the title of "Methodus curandi Febres," and again, nine years after, with additional remarks, suggested by subsequent experience. His writings are not altogether free from hypothesis; but he seems to have been little influenced by these in his practice; and by closely observing the operations of nature, and the effects of remedies, he was enabled to introduce very essential improvements. In small-pox especially, by checking the eruptive fever by means of cool air, and other antiphlogistic means, he ascertained that the eruption and consequent danger were greatly diminished; which plan applies likewise to other eruptive and febrile diseases, as has been since determined by general experience. His sagacity was also manifested in the correct histories which he has left of some diseases, as particularly small-pox, measles, gout, and hysteria. He was likewise very attentive to the varieties occurring, especially in febrile disorders at different seasons, or in different years; and was led to suppose these connected with a particular constitution of the air. He had been subject, for above thirty years, to gout, and stone in the kidney, which impaired his constitution, and at last terminated his life in 1689. After his death, a manual of practice, composed for his son, was published under the title of "Processus Integri in Morbis fere omnibus curandis." Sydenham ever maintained the character of a generous and public-spirited man; he conducted himself without that arrogance which too often accompanies original talent; and he has been universally acknowledged the first physician of his age. The numerous editions of his works, both singly and collectively, in almost every country of Europe, the deference paid to his authority, and the commendations bestowed upon him by almost all practical writers since, amply prove the solidity of his title to the high reputation attached to his name. The college of physicians, though he was only late in life admitted a licentiate, have subsequently placed his bust in their hall, near that of Harvey.

SY'LPHIUM. Assafœtida is so termed by some writers. See *Ferula assafœtida.*

SYLVANITE. Native tellurium.

Sylvius, digestive salt of. The muriate of potassa.

SY'LVIUS, FRANCIS DE LE BOE, was born at Hanau, in 1614. He took his degree at Basle, and then visited, for improvement, some of the chief universities in France and Germany. He settled first at his native place, but removed to Amsterdam, where he enjoyed a high reputation for several years, till he was called to Leyden, in 1658, to assume the office of first professor of medicine. He soon drew together, by his genius and eloquence, a numerous audience from all parts of Europe. He was one of the earliest advocates for Harvey's doctrine of the circulation of the blood and chiefly effected its reception into that school. But, on the other hand, he materially retarded the progress of medicine by a fanciful hypothesis, which attracted much notice, referring all diseases to chemical changes, producing an excess of acid, or of alkali. His works were chiefly controversial tracts, in which he defended his peculiar notions. He died in 1672.

SYLVIUS JAMES DU BOIS, was born at Amiens, in 1478. Having chosen the profession of physic, he studied diligently the writings of the ancients, especially Hippocrates and Galen, and was no less assiduous in the pursuit of other branches of medicine, particularly anatomy, pharmacy, and botany. Before taking a degree, he undertook a private course of lectures at Paris, in which he so distinguished himself, that in two years he collected a crowd of pupils from various parts of Europe; but the jealousy of the Parisian physicians obliged him to go to Montpelier, in 1520, for the purpose of graduation. His extreme parsimony, however, would not permit the necessary expenses; and he was at last successful in compromising his differences with the Parisian faculty. He subsequently continued his lectures with very great success; and in 1550 he was appointed professor of medicine at the royal college; but his death occurred five years afterward. His works were popular during the reign of the old school, but are now obsolete. As an anatomist, he merits great praise, having made various discoveries, notwithstanding the few opportunities he had of human dissection. He wrote with great violence against Vesalius, his pupil, because he had presumed to correct Galen.

SYMBLE'PHARUM. (From συν, with, and βλεφαρον, the eyelid.) A concretion of the eyelid to the globe of the eye. This chiefly happens in the superior, but very rarely in the inferior palpebra. The causes of this concretion are a bad conformation of the parts, or from ulcers of the cornea, the membrana conjunctiva, or internal superficies of the palpebræ, or imprudent scarifications, or burns, especially if the eye remains long closed. There are two species, the partial, or total; in the former, the adhesion is partial, in the latter, the membrana conjunctiva and cornea are concreted to the eyelid together.

SY'MBOLE. (From συμβαλλω, to knit together.) It is said either of the fitness of parts with one another, or of the consent between them by the intermediation of nerves, and the like.

SYMBOLO'GIA. (From συμβυλον, a sign, and λογος, a discourse.) The doctrine of the signs and symptoms of disease.

SYMMETRY. The exact and beautiful proportion of parts to one another.

SYMPATHETIC. *Sympatheticus.*
1. Relating to sympathy.
2. See *Intercostal nerve.*
Sympathetic nerve. See *Intercostal nerve.*

SYMPATHY. (*Sympathia*; from συμπασχω, to suffer together, to sympathize.) All the body is sympathetically connected together, and dependent, the one part upon the rest, constituting a general sympathy. But sometimes we find particular parts more intimately dependent upon each other than upon the rest of the body, constituting a particular sympathy. Action cannot be greatly increased in any one organ, without being diminished in some other; but certain parts are more apt to be affected by the derangement of particular organs than others; and it was the observance of this fact which gave foundation to the old and well known doctrine of sympathy, which was said to proceed "*tum ob communionem et similitudinem generis, tum ob viciniam.*" It may be thought that this position of action being diminished in one organ, by its increase, either in the rest or in some other part, is contradicted by the existence of general diseases or actions affecting the whole system. But in them we find, in the first place, that there is always some part more affected than the rest. This local affection is sometimes the first symptom, and affects the constitution in a secondary way, either by the irritation which it produces, or by an extension of the specific action. At other times the local affection is coeval with the general disease, and is called sympathetic. It is observed, in the second place, that as there is some part which is always more affected than the rest, so also is there some organ which has its action, in consequence of this, diminished lower than that of the rest of the system, and most commonly lower than its natural standard. From the extensive sympathy of the stomach with almost every part of the body, we find that this most frequently suffers, and has its action diminished in every disease, whether general or local, provided that the diseased action arises to any considerable degree. There are also other organs which may,

326

in like manner, suffer from their association or connexion with others which become diseased. Thus, for instance, we see, in the general disease called puerperal fever, that the action of the breasts is diminished by the increased inflammatory action of the uterus.

In consequence of this balance of action, or general connexion of the system, a sudden pain, consequent to violent action of any particular part, will so weaken the rest as to produce fainting, and occasionally death. But this dependence appears more evidently in what may be called the smaller systems of the body, or those parts which seem to be more intimately connected with each other than they are with the general system. Of this kind is the connexion of the breasts with the uterus of the female; of the urethra with the testicles of the male; of the stomach with the liver; and of the intestines with the stomach, and of this again with the brain; of the one extremity of the bone with the other; and of the body of the muscle with its insertion; of the skin with the parts below it.

These smaller systems, or circles, shall be treated regularly; but first it may be proper to observe, that these are not only intimately connected with themselves, but also with the general system, a universal sympathy being thus established.

That there is a very intimate connexion between the breasts and uterus has been long known; but it has not been very satisfactorily explained. Fallopius, and all the other authors, declare plainly that the sympathy is produced by an anastomosis of vessels: Bartholin adding that the child being born, the blood no longer goes to the uterus, but is directed to the breasts and changed into milk. But none of all those who talk of this derivation, assign any reasonable cause which may produce it.

In pregnancy, and at the menstrual periods, the uterus is active; but, when the child is delivered, the action of the uterus subsides, while the breasts in their turn become active, and secrete milk.

If, at this time, we should again produce action in the uterus, we diminish that of the breasts, and destroy the secretion of milk, as is well illustrated by the case of inflammation of the uterus, which is incident to lying-in women. When the uterus, at the cessation of the menses, ceases to be active, or to secrete, we often find that the breasts have an action excited in them, becoming slowly inflamed, and assuming a cancerous disposition. The uterus and breasts seem to be a set of glands balancing each other in the system, one only being naturally active, or secreting properly, at a time; and accordingly we seldom, if ever, find that when the uterus yields the menstrual discharge, the milk is secreted in perfection, during the continuance of this discharge, nor do we ever find them both inflamed at the same time.

The uterus has not only this connexion with the breasts, but it has also a very particular sympathy with the stomach, which again sympathizes with the brain; and thus we see how a disorder of the uterus may induce an extensive series of affections, each dependent on the other.

The organs of generation in the male form likewise a little system, in which all the parts exhibit this sympathy with each other. They likewise give us a very good instance of the association of action, or sympathy, in the common acceptation of that word.

Sympathy is divided into, first, the sympathy of equilibrium, in which one part is weakened by the increased action of another; and, secondly, the sympathy of association, in which two parts act together at the same time.

The sympathy of association is produced suddenly, and for a short time. The sympathy of equilibrium is produced more slowly, and continues to operate for a much longer time.

It is curious enough, that most, or at least many, of those organs, which seem to be connected by the sympathy of equilibrium, exhibit likewise more or less of the sympathy of association, when under the circumstances in which this can take place.

The sympathy of equilibrium is seen in the effects of inflammation of the end of the urethra on the testicle; which often diminishes its action, and produces a very disagreeable sensation of dulness, or, if this inflammation be suddenly diminished, the action of the testicle is as suddenly increased, and swelling takes place. The same is seen in the connexion of the urethra with the bladder and prostate gland, as is mentioned in all the dissertations on gonorrhœa. These parts likewise affect the stomach greatly, increased action in them weakening that organ much. This is seen in the effects of swelled testicle, or excessive venery, or inflamed bladder, and in a stone; all which weaken the stomach, and produce dyspepsia. The same remark applies to the kidney; vomiting and flatulence being produced by nephritis.

The sympathy of association, or an instance of sympathy in the common acceptation of the word, is likewise seen in the connexion between the glans and testicles in coition; but for this purpose, the action in the glans must be sudden, and of short duration; for, if continued long, weakness of the testicles, or diminished action, is induced. In those parts which exhibit this natural association of action, if the action of one part be suddenly and for a short time increased, the action of the sympathizing part will likewise be increased; as we see in the instance already given of coition; and likewise in paroxysms of the stone, in which the glans penis, after making water, becomes very painful.

But if the action be more slowly induced, and continued for a long time, then this association is set aside, by a stronger and more general principle of the equilibrium of action, and the sympathizing part is weakened. Hence violent inflammation of the end of the urethra produces a weakness and irritability of the bladder, dulness of the testicle, &c.

There is also an evident sympathy of equilibrium between the stomach and lower tract of intestines; which two portions may be said in general to balance each other in the abdomen. When the action of the intestines is increased in diarrhœa, the stomach is often weakened, and the patient tormented with nausea. This will be cured, not so easily by medicines taken into the stomach, as by anodyne clysters, which will abate the action of the intestines. When the intestines are inflamed, as in strangulated hernia, vomiting is a never-failing attendant.

When again the stomach is inflamed, the intestines are affected, and obstinate costiveness takes place; even in hysterical affections of the stomach, the intestines are often deranged. Injections of cold water frequently relieve these affections of the stomach, by their action on the intestines.

The liver and stomach are also connected with one another. When the liver is inflamed, or has its action increased, the stomach is weakened, and dyspeptic symptoms take place. When the stomach is weakened, as, for instance, by intoxication, then the action of the liver is increased, and a greater quantity than usual of bile is secreted. The same takes place in warm climates, where the stomach is much debilitated.

If the liver has its action thus frequently increased, it assumes a species of inflammation, or becomes, as it is called, scirrhous. This is exemplified in the habitual dram-drinkers, and in those who stay long in warm countries, and use freedoms with the stomach. The liver likewise sympathizes with the brain; for when this organ is injured, and its action much impaired, as in compression, inflammation and suppuration have been often known to take place in the liver.

Besides this connexion of the stomach with the liver, it is also very intimately dependent on the brain, being weakened when the action of the brain is increased; as we see in an inflammation of that organ. The brain again is affected with pain when the stomach is weakened by intoxication or other causes; and this pain will be often relieved by slowly renewing the action of the stomach by such stimuli as are natural to it, such as small quantities of soup frequently repeated. A slight increase of action in the stomach, at least if not of a morbid kind, affects the brain so as to produce sleep, diminishing its action. This we see in the effects of a full meal, and even of a draught of warm water. The stomach likewise sympathizes with the throat, squeamishness and anorexia being often produced by inflammation of the tonsils. This inflammation is frequently abated by restoring or increasing the action of the stomach. Hence the throat, in slight inflammation, is frequently easier after dinner; hence, likewise, the effects of emetics in cynanche.

The extremities of bones and muscles also sympathize in the same manner. When one end of a bone is inflamed, the action of the other is lessened, and pain is produced; for a painful sensation may result both from increased and diminished action. When the tendon of a muscle is inflamed, the body of that muscle often is pained, and *vice versa*.

Lastly, the external skin sympathizes with the parts below it. If it be inflamed, as in erysipelas, the parts immediately beneath are weakened, or have their natural action diminished. If this inflammation affect the face, or scalp, then the brain is injured; and headache, stupor, or delirium supervene. If it attack the skin of the abdomen, then the abdominal viscera are affected, and we have vomiting and purging, or obstinate costiveness, according to circumstances. This is illustrated by the disease of children, which is called by the women the bowel-hive, in which the skin is inflamed, as they suppose, from some morbid matter within.

If the internal parts be inflamed, the action of the surface is diminished, and, by increasing this action, we can lessen or remove the disease below; as we see daily proved by the good effects of blisters. When the stomach, intestines, or kidney have been very irritable, a sinapism has been known to act like a charm; and in the deep-seated inflammations of the breasts, bowels, or joints, no better remedy is known, after the use of the lancet, than blisters.

The utility of issues in diseases of the lungs, the liver, and the joints, is to be explained on the same principle. In these cases we find that issues do little good unless they be somewhat painful, or be in the state of healthy ulcers. An indolent flabby sore, however large the discharge (which is always thin, and accompanied with little action), does no good, but only adds to the misery of the patient. We may, however, err on the other hand, by making the issues too painful, or by keeping them active too long; for after they have removed the inflammatory disease below, they will still operate on these parts, lessening their action and preventing the healing process from going on properly. This is seen in cases of curvature of the spine, where, at first, the inflammation of the vertebra is diminished by the issues; but if they be kept long open after this is removed, they do harm. We often see the patient recover rapidly after his surgeon has healed the issue in despair, judging that it could do no farther service, but only increase the weakness of his patient.

It is a well-established fact, that when any particular action disappears suddenly from a part, it will often speedily affect that organ which sympathizes most with the part that was originally diseased. This is best seen in the inflammatory action, which, as practical writers have well observed, occasionally disappears quickly from the part first affected, and then shows itself in some other.

From the united testimony of all these facts, Mr. Burns, of Glasgow, maintains the doctrine just delivered, and proposes to introduce it into pathological reasonings. In the whole of the animal economy, we discover marks of the wisdom of the Creator, but perhaps in no part of it more than in this, of the existence of the sympathy of equilibrium; for, if a large part of the system were to have its action much increased, and all the other parts to continue acting in the same proportionate degree as formerly, the whole must be soon exhausted; (for increased action would require for its support an increased quantity of energy.) But upon this principle, when action is much increased in one part, it is to a certain degree diminished in some other, the general sum or degree of action in the body is thus less than it otherwise would be, and consequently the system suffers less.

SY'MPHYSIS. (From συν, together, and φυω, to grow.) Mediate connexion. A genus of the connexion of bones, in which they are united by means of an intervening body. It comprehends four species, viz. synchondrosis, syssarcosis, syneurosis, and syndesmosis.

SY'MPHYTUM. (From συμφυω, to unite: so called because it is supposed to unite and close the lips of wounds together.)

1. The name of a genus of plants in the Linnæan system. Class, *Pentandria*; Order, *Monogynia*.

2. The pharmacopœial name of the comfrey See *Symphytum officinale*.

SYMPHYTUM MACULOSUM. See *Pulmonaria officinalis*.

SYMPHYTUM MINUS. See *Prunella*.

SYMPHYTUM OFFICINALE. The systematic name of

the comfrey. *Consolida major.* This plant, *Symphy tum—foliis-ovatis lanceolatis decurrentibus,* is administered where the althæa cannot be obtained, its roots abounding with a viscid glutinous juice, whose virtues are similar to those of the althæa.

SYMPHYTUM PETRÆUM. See *Coris monspeliensis.*

SYNA'NCHE. See *Cynanche.*

SYNA'NCHICA. (From συναγχη, 'the quinsey: so called from its uses in that disease.) Quinseywort.

SYNARTHRO'SIS. (From συν, together, and αρθρον, a joint.) Immoveable connexion. A genus of connexion of bones, in which they are united together by an immoveable union. It has three species, viz. suture, harmony, and gomphosis.

SYNASTOMO'SIS. This is used in the same sense as *Anastomosis.*

SYNCHONDRO'SIS. (From συν, with, and χονδρος, a cartilage.) A species of symphysis, in which one bone is united with another by means of an intervening cartilage; as the vertebræ and the bones of the pubes.

SYNCHONDROTO'MIA. (From συνχονδρωσις, the symphysis of the pubes, and τεμνω, to cut.) The operation of dividing the symphysis of the pubes.

SY'NCHYSUS. (From συγχυω, to confound.) A solution of the vitreous humour into a fine attenuated aqueous fluid. In Cullen's Nosology, it is a variety of his species *caligo pupillæ.*

SYNCI'PITIS OSSA. See *Parietal bones.*

SY'NCIPUT. (*Synciput* vel *sinciput, itis.* n.) The forepart of the head or cranium.

SY'NCOPE. (From συν, with, and κοπ7ω, to cut, or strike down.) *Animi deliquium ; Leipothymia ; Defectio animi ; Dissolutio ; Exanimatio ; Asphyxia ; Virium lapsus ; Apopsychia ; Apsychia ; Ecchysis.* Fainting or swooning. A genus of disease in the Class *Neuroses,* and Order *Adynamiæ,* of Cullen, in which the respiration and action of the heart either cease, or become much weaker than usual, with paleness and coldness, arising from diminished energy of the brain, or from organic affections of the heart. Species : 1. *Syncope cardiaca,* the cardiac syncope, arising without a visible cause, and with violent palpitation of the heart, during the intervals, and depending generally on some organic affection of the heart or neighbouring vessels.

2. *Syncope occasionalis,* the exciting cause being manifest.

The disease is sometimes preceded by anxiety about the præcordia, a sense of fulness ascending from the stomach towards the head, vertigo or confusion of ideas, dimness of sight, and coldness of the extremities. The attacks are frequently attended with, or end in, vomiting, and sometimes in epileptic or other convulsions. The causes are sudden and violent emotions of the mind, pungent or disagreeable odours, derangement of the primæ viæ, debility from preceding disorders, loss of blood spontaneous or artificial, the operation of paracentesis, &c. During the paroxysm the nostrils are to be stimulated with some of the preparations of ammonia, or these may be exhibited internally, if the patient is capable of swallowing ; but when the disease has originated from large loss of blood, such stimulants must be used cautiously. When it is connected with a disordered state of the stomach, if an emetic can be given, or vomiting excited by irritating the fauces, it will probably afford relief. Sometimes sprinkling the face with cold water will recover the patient. And when there is reason for supposing an accumulation about the heart, the disease not having arisen from debilitating causes, a moderate abstraction of blood may be made with propriety. Between the fits we should endeavour to strengthen the constitution, where debility appears concerned in producing them, and the several exciting causes must be carefully guarded against. When organic affections of the heart, and parts connected with it, exist, all that can be done is, to palliate the attacks of fainting ; unless the primary disease can be removed, which is extremely rare.

SYNCOPE ANGINOSA. See *Angina pectoris.*

SYNDESMOLO'GIA. (From συνδεσμος, a ligament, and λογος, a discourse.) The doctrine of the ligaments.

SYNDESMO-PHARYNGEUS. See *Constrictor pharyngis medius.*

SYNDESMO'SIS. (From συνδεσμος, a ligament.) That species of symphysis or mediate connexion of

bones in which they are united by ligament, as the radius with the ulna.

SYNDE'SMUS. (From συνδεω, to bind together.) A ligament.

SYNE'CHIA. Σενεχια. A concretion of the iris with the cornea, or with the capsule of the crystalline lens. The proximate cause is adhesion of these parts, the consequence of inflammation. The remote causes are, a collapse of the cornea, a prolapse of the iris, a swelling or tumefied cataract, hypopium, or original formation. The species of this disorder are,

1. *Synechia anterior totalis,* or a concretion of the iris with the cornea. This species is known by inspecting the parts. The pupil in this species is dilated or coarctated, or it is found concreted ; from whence various lesions of vision.

2. *Synechia anterior partialis,* when only some part of the iris is accreted. This concretion is observed in one or many places ; from hence the pupil is variously disfigured, and an inordinate motion of the pupil is perceived.

3. *Synechia anterior composita,* when not only the whole iris, but also a prolapse of the crystalline lens, unites with the cornea.

4. *Synechia posterior totalis,* or a concretion of the whole uvea, with the ciliary processes and the capsule of the crystalline lens.

5. *Synechia posterior partialis,* when only some part of the capsule of the crystalline lens is concreted with the uvea and cornea. This accretion is simple, duplex, triplex, or in many places.

6. *Synechia complicata,* with an amaurosis, cataract mydriasis, myosis, or synizesis.

SYNEURO'SIS. (From συν, with, and νευρον, a nerve, because the ancients included membranes, ligaments, and tendons under the head of nerves.) A species of symphysis, in which one bone is united to another by means of an intervening membrane.

SYNGENESIA. (From συν, together, and γενεοις, generation.) The name of a class of plants, in the sexual system of Linnæus, consisting of plants in which the anthers are united into a tube, the filaments on which they are supported being mostly separate and distinct. The flowers are compound.

SYNIZE'SIS. A perfect concretion and coarctation of the pupil. It is known by the absence of the pupil, and a total loss of vision. The species are,

1. *Synizesis nativa,* with which infants are sometimes born. In this case, by an error of the first conformation of the pupil, there is no perforation ; it is very rarely found.

2. *Synizesis accidentalis,* a concretion of the pupil, from an inflammation or exulceration of the uvea or iris, or from a defect of the aqueous or vitreous humour.

3. *Synizesis,* from a secession of the iris or cornea. From whatever cause it may happen, the effect is certain, for the pupil contracts its diameter ; the longitudinal fibres, separated from the circle of the cornea, cannot resist the orbicular fibres : from hence the pupil is wholly or partially contracted.

4. *Synizesis complicata,* or that which is complicated with an amaurosis, synechia, or other occular disease. The amaurosis, or gutta serena, is known by the total absence of light to the retina. We can distinguish this not only by the pupil being closed, but likewise the eyelids ; for whether the eyelids be open or shut, all is darkness to the patient. The other complicated cases are known by viewing the eye, and considering the parts anatomically.

5. *Synizesis spuria,* is a closing of the pupil by mu cus, pus, or grumous blood.

SY'NOCHA. (From συνεχω, to continue.) *Febris synocha.* Inflammatory fever. A species of continued fever, characterized by increased heat ; pulse frequent, strong, hard ; urine high-coloured ; senses not impaired. This fever is so named from its being attended with symptoms denoting general inflammation in the system, by which we shall always be able readily to distinguish it from either the nervous or putrid. It makes its attack at all seasons of the year, but is most prevalent in the spring ; and it seizes persons of all ages and habits, but more particularly those in the vigour of life, with strong elastic fibres, and of a plethoric constitution. It is a species of fever almost peculiar to cold and tempe rate climates, being rarely, if ever, met with in very warm ones, except among Europeans lately arrived; and even then, the inflammatory stage is of very short duration, as it very soon assumes either the nervous or putrid type.

The exciting causes are sudden transitions from heat to cold, swallowing cold liquors, when the body is much heated by exercise, too free a use of vinous and spirituous liquors, great intemperance, violent passions of the mind, the sudden suppression of habitual evacuations, and the sudden repulsion of eruptions. It may be doubted if this fever ever originates from personal infection; but it is possible for it to appear as an epidemic among such as are of a robust habit, from a peculiar state of the atmosphere. It comes on with a sense of lassitude and inactivity, succeeded by vertigo, rigors, and pains over the whole body, but more particularly in the head and back; which symptoms are shortly followed by redness of the face and eyes, great restlessness, intense heat, and unquenchable thirst, oppression of breathing, and nausea. The skin is dry and parched; the tongue is of a scarlet colour at the sides, and furred with white in the centre; the urine is red and scanty; the body is costive; and there is a quickness, with a fulness and hardness in the pulse, not much affected by any pressure made on the artery. If the febrile symptoms run very high, and proper means are not used at an early period, stupor and delirium come on, the imagination becomes much disturbed and hurried, and the patient raves violently. The disease usually goes through its course in about fourteen days, and terminates in a crisis, either by diaphoresis, diarrhœa, hæmorrhage from the nose, or the deposite of a copious sediment in the urine; which crisis is usually preceded by some variation in the pulse.

Our judgment as to the termination of the disease must be formed from the violence of the attack, and the nature of the symptoms. If the fever runs high, or continues many days with stupor or delirium, the event may be doubtful; but if to these are added, picking at the bed-clothes, startings of the tendons, involuntary discharges by stool and urine, and hiccups, it will then certainly be fatal. On the contrary, if the febrile heat abates, the other symptoms moderate, and there is a tendency to a crisis, we may then expect a recovery. In a few instances, this fever has been known to terminate in mania.

On opening those who die of an inflammatory fever, an effusion is often perceived within the cranium, and now and then, topical affections of some of the viscera are to be observed.

The chief indication in synocha is to lessen the excessive vascular action by evacuations, and the antiphlogistic regimen. Of the former, by far the most important is blood-letting, which should be freely practised in this disease, making a large orifice into the vein, and taking from ten to twenty-four ounces of blood, according to the violence of the symptoms, and the strength of the patient. The disorder may sometimes be cut short at once by this active treatment in the beginning; but if it should continue urgent, and the strength of the pulse keep up, the repetition of it within more moderate limits will be from time to time advisable. Purging is next in efficacy, especially with those articles which produce copious serous discharges, and thoroughly clear out the intestines, as the saline cathartics, with infusion of senna, jalap with supertartrate of potassa, &c. As the disease advances, however, we must act less on this part, and attempt to promote the other discharges, particularly that by the skin: for which purpose calomel, antimonials, and the saline diaphoretics are to be exhibited. The antiphlogistic regimen consists in obviating stimuli of every kind, so far as this can be done safely; impressions on the senses, particularly the sight and hearing, bodily and mental exertion, &c. must be guarded against as much as possible. The diet should be of the most sparing kind; barley-water, or other mild liquid, with some acid, perhaps, added, or a little nitrate of potassa dissolved in it, taken in small quantities from time to time, chiefly to quench the thirst, and cool the body, will be the most proper; strictly interdicting animal food, fermented liquors, and the like. The stimulus of heat must be especially obviated by light clothing, or even exposing the body to the air, ventilating the apartment, sprinkling the floor with vinegar and water, &c. When the head is much affected, besides the general treatment, it will be proper to take blood locally, have the head shaved and cooled by some evaporating lotion, apply a blister to the neck, and, perhaps, stimulate the lower extremities. In like manner, any other organ being particularly pressed upon, may require additional means, which will be sufficiently understood by adverting to the several phlegmasiæ.

SY'NOCHUS. (From συνεχω, to continue.) A mixed fever. A species of continued fever, commencing with symptoms of synocha, and terminating in typhus; so that synocha and typhus, blended together in a slight degree, seem to constitute this species of fever, the former being apt to preponderate at its commencement, and the latter towards its termination.

Every thing which has a tendency to enervate the body, may be looked upon as a remote cause of this fever; and accordingly we find it often arising from great bodily fatigue, too great an indulgence in sensual pleasures, violent exertion, intemperance in drinking, and errors in diet, and now and then likewise from the suppression of some long-accustomed discharge. Certain passions of the mind (such as grief, fear, anxiety, and joy,) have been enumerated among the causes of fever, and in a few instances, it is probable, they may have given rise to it; but the concurrence of some other powers seems generally necessary to produce this effect. The most usual and universal cause of this fever is the application of cold to the body; and its morbid effect sseem to depend partly upon certain circumstances of the cold itself, and partly upon certain circumstances of the person to whom it is applied.

The circumstances which seem to give the application of cold due effect, are its degree of intensity, the length of time which it is applied; its being applied generally, or only in a current of air, its having a degree of moisture accompanying it, and its being a considerable or sudden change from heat to cold. The circumstances of persons rendering them more liable to be affected by cold, seem to be debility, induced either by great fatigue, or violent exertions, by long fasting, by the want of natural rest, by severe evacuations, by preceding disease, by errors in diet, by intemperance in drinking, by great sensuality, by too close an application to study, or giving way to grief, fear, or great anxiety, by depriving the body of part of its accustomed clothing, by exposing any one particular part of it, while the rest is kept of its usual warmth, or by exposing it generally or suddenly to cold when heated much beyond its usual temperature; these we may, therefore, look upon as so many causes giving an effect to cold which it otherwise might not have produced. Another frequent cause of fever seems to be breathing air contaminated by the vapours arising either directly or originally from the body of a person labouring under the disease. A peculiar matter is supposed to generate in the body of a person affected with fever, and this floating in the atmosphere, and being applied to one in health, will no doubt often cause fever to take place in him, which has induced many to suppose, that this infectious matter is produced in all fevers whatever, and that they are all, more or less, contagious.

The effluvia arising from the human body, if long confined to one place without being diffused in the atmosphere, will, it is well known, acquire a singular virulence, and will, if applied to the bodies of men become the cause of fever. Exhalations, arising from animal or vegetable substances in a state of putrefaction, have been looked upon as another general cause of fever: marshy or moist grounds, acted upon by heat for any length of time, usually send forth exhalations which prove a never-failing source of fever, but more particularly in warm climates. Various hypotheses have been maintained, with respect to the proximate cause of fever; some supposing it to be a lentor or viscidity prevailing in the mass of blood, and stagnating in the extreme vessels; others, that it is a noxious matter introduced into, or generated in, the body, and that the increased action of the heart and arteries is an effort of nature to expel the morbific matter; others, that it consisted in an increased secretion of bile; and others again, that it is to be attributed to a spasmodic constriction of the extreme vessels on the surface of the body; which last was the doctrine taught by the late Dr. Cullen.

An attack of this fever is generally marked by the patient's being seized with a considerable degree of languor, or sense of debility, together with a sluggishness in motion, and frequent yawning and stretching;

the face and extremities at the same time become pale, and the skin over the whole surface of the body appears constricted; he then perceives a sensation of cold in his back, passing from thence over his whole frame; and this sense of cold continuing to increase, tremors in the limbs and rigors of the body succeed.

With these there is a loss of appetite, want of taste in the mouth, slight pains in the head, back, and loins, small and frequent respirations. The sense of cold and its effects after a little time becomes less violent, and are alternated with flushings, and at last, going off altogether, they are succeeded by great heat diffused generally over the whole body; the face looks flushed, the skin is dry, as likewise the tongue; universal restlessness prevails, with a violent pain in the head, oppression at the chest, sickness at the stomach, and an inclination to vomit. There is likewise a great thirst and costiveness, and the pulse is full and frequent, beating, perhaps, 90 or 100 strokes in a minute. When the symptoms run very high, and there is a considerable determination of blood to the head, a delirium will arise. In this fever, as well as most others, there is generally an increase of symptoms towards evening.

If the disease is likely to prove fatal, either by its continuing a long time, or by the severity of its symptoms, then a starting of the tendons, picking at the bedclothes, involuntary discharges by urine and stool, coldness of the extremities, and hiccoughs, will be observed; where no such appearances take place, the disease will go through its course.

As a fever once produced will go on, although its cause be entirely removed, and as the continued or fresh application of a cause of fever neither will increase that which is already produced, nor occasion a new one; there can be no certainty as to the duration of fever; and it is only by attending to certain appearances or changes, which usually take place on the approach of a crisis, that we can form any opinion or decision. The symptoms pointing out the approach of a crisis are, the pulse becoming soft, moderate, and near its natural speed; the tongue losing its fur and becoming clean, with an abatement of thirst; the skin being covered with a gentle moisture, and feeling soft to the touch; the secretory organs performing their several offices; and the urine depositing flaky crystals of a dirty red colour, and becoming turbid on being allowed to stand any time.

Many physicians have been of opinion, that there is something in the nature of all acute diseases, except those of a putrid kind, which usually determines them to be of a certain duration, and, therefore, that these terminations, when salutary, happen at certain periods of the disease rather than at others, unless disturbed in their progress by an improper mode of treatment, or the arising of some accidental circumstance. These periods are known by the appellation of critical days; and from the time of Hippocrates down to the present, have been pretty generally admitted. The truth of them, Dr. Thomas thinks, can hardly be disputed, however they may be interrupted by various causes. A great number of phenomena show us, that both in the sound state and the diseased, nature has a tendency to observe certain periods; for instance, the vicissitudes of sleeping and watching occurring with such regularity to every one; the accurate periods that the menstrual flux observes, and the exact time of pregnancy in all viviparous animals, and many other such instances that might be adduced, all prove this law.

With respect to diseases, every one must have observed the definite periods which take place in regular intermittents, as well those universal as topical; in the course of true inflammation, which at the fourth, or at the farthest the seventh day, is resolved, or after this period changes into either abscess, gangrene, or scirrhus; in exanthematous eruptions, which, if they are favourable and regular, appear on a certain and definite day; for example, the small-pox about the fourth day. All these appear to be founded on immutable laws, according to which the motions of the body in health and in disease are governed.

The days on which it is supposed the termination of continued fevers principally happens, are the third, fifth, seventh, ninth, eleventh, fourteenth, seventeenth, and twentieth.

A simple continued fever terminates always by a regular crisis in the manner before mentioned, or from the febrile matter falling on some particular parts, it excites inflammation, abscess, eruption, or destroys the patient.

Great anxiety, loss of strength, intense heat, stupor, delirium, irregularity in the pulse, twitchings in the fingers and hands, picking at the bed-clothes, startings of the tendons, hiccoughs, involuntary evacuations by urine and stool, and such like symptoms, point out the certain approach of death.

On the contrary, when the senses remain clear and distinct, the febrile heat abates, the skin is soft and moist, the pulse becomes moderate and is regular, and the urine deposites flaky crystals, we may then expect a speedy and happy termination of the disease.

The usual appearances which are to be observed on dissection of those who die of this fever, are an effusion within the cranium, and topical affections perhaps of some viscera.

This disease being of a mixed nature, the treatment must be modified accordingly. In the beginning, the same plan is to be pursued as in synocha, except that we must be more sparing in the use of the lancet, in proportion as there is less power in the system, to maintain the increased action of the heart and arteries; although if any important part should be much affected, we must act more vigorously, to prevent its disorganization, and the consequent destruction of life. When the character of the disease is changed, the means proper will be such as are pointed out under the head of *Typhus.*

SYNO'VIA. (A term of no radical meaning, coined by Paracelsus.) An unctuous fluid secreted from certain glands in the joint in which it is contained. Its use is to lubricate the cartilaginous surfaces of the articulatory bones, and to facilitate their motions.

SYNOVIAL. *Synovialis.* Of or belonging to the synovia, or fluid of the joints.

SYNOVIAL GLANDS. *Glandulæ synoviales.* The assemblage of a fatty fimbriated structure within the cavities of some joints.

SYNTENO'SIS. (From συν, with, and τενων, a tendon.) A species of articulation where the bones are connected together by tendons.

SYNTE'XIS. (From συντηχω, to dissolve.) A marasmus or wasting of the body.

SY'NTHESIS. (From συντιθημι, to compose.) Combination. See *Analysis.*

SYNTHETI'SMUS. (From συνθεω, to concur.) The reduction of a fracture.

SYNULO'TICA. (From συνουλοω, to cicatrize.) Medicines which heal wounds.

SY'PHILIS. (The name of a shepherd, who fed the flocks of king Alcithous, who, proud of their number and beauty, insulted the sun; as a punishment for which, fable relates, that this disease was sent on earth; or from σιφλος, filthy.) *Lues venerea; Morbus gallicus; Aphrodisius morbus; Morbus indicus; Morbus neapolitanus; Patursa.* A genus of disease in the Class *Cachexia,* and Order *Impetigines,* of Cullen. Towards the close of the memorable fifteenth century, about the year 1494 or 1495, the inhabitants of Europe were greatly alarmed by the sudden appearance of this disease. The novelty of its symptoms, and the wonderful rapidity with which it was propagated throughout every part of the known world, soon made it an important object of medical inquiry.

In common language, it is said a person has syphilis or is poxed, when the venereal poison has been received into, or is diffused through the system, and there produces its peculiar effects, as ulcers of the mouth or fauces, spots, tetters, and ulcers of the skin, pains, swelling, and caries of the bones, &c. But as long as the effects of the poison are local and confined to or near the genitals, the disorder is not called syphilis, lues venerea, nor pox; but distinguished by some particular name, according to its different seat or appearance; such as gonorrhœa venerea, chancre, or bubo.

The venereal disease is always produced by a poison. Concerning the nature of this poison, we know no more than we do about that of the small-pox or any other contagion; we know only that it produces peculiar effects. The smallest particle of this poison is sufficient to bring on the most violent disorder over the whole body. It seems to spread and diffuse itself by a kind of fermentation and assimilation of matter; and, like other contagions, it requires some time after being applied to the human body, before it produces that effect. It is not known whether it has different degrees of acrimony and volatility, or whether it is always the same in its nature, varying only with regard to the particular part to which it is applied, or according to the different habit and constitution or particular idiosyncrasy of the person who receives the infection. We know that mercury possesses a certain and specific power of destroying the venereal virus; but we are quite uncertain whether it acts by a sedative, adstringent, or evacuant quality; or, which is not unlikely, by a chemical elective attraction whereby both substances uniting with one another are changed to a third, which is no more hurtful, but has some new properties entirely distinct from those which any of them had before they were united. The variolous miasma, we know, produces its effects in about twenty or twenty-four days after the infection is received from the atmosphere, and eight or ten days if by inoculation, but the venereal virus seems to keep no particular period. At some times, and, perhaps, in particular persons, Dr. Swediaur has seen chancres arise in the space of twelve hours, nay, in a still shorter time, indeed he mentions in a few minutes, after an impure coition; whereas in most cases, they make their appearance only in so many days. The generality of men feel the first symptoms of a clap between the second and fifth days after an impure coitus; but there are instances where they do not appear till after as many weeks or months. Dr. S. was consulted by a young man, who was seized with a violent discharge from the glans, along with a phimosis, but without any chancres, four weeks after coition; and during all the interval, he felt not the least symptom of the disease. Some years ago, a gentleman went out from London, in seemingly perfect health, to the East Indies; but on his arrival in that hot climate, after a voyage of four months, a violent clap broke out before he went on shore, though he could have received no infection during the voyage, as there was not a woman on board. There are instances which render it probable that the virus may lie four, five, or six weeks, and perhaps longer, on the surface of the genitals before it is absorbed; and were it not then to produce a chancre, might probably not be absorbed at all. We see daily examples, where common women communicate the infection to different men in the space of several weeks, while they themselves have not the least symptom of syphilis local or universal, the poison lying all that time in the vagina harmless, and generally without being absorbed. How long the venereal virus may lurk in the body itself, after it has been absorbed into the mass of blood, before it produces any sensible effect, is a matter of equal uncertainty. There is scarcely a practitioner who has not observed instances of its remaining harmless for weeks or even months in the body. Dr. Swediaur had a case, where, after lying dormant for half a year, it broke out with unequivocal symptoms. But the following instance, if it be depended upon, is still more extraordinary:

Some years ago, says the above writer, I was consulted by a gentleman about a sore throat, which I declared to be venereal. My patient was astonished; and assured me that for nine years past he had not had the least venereal complaint, nor had he any reason to believe he had since received any infection; but that he had been in the East Indies, where he was affected with a violent clap. On his return to Europe, being to appearance in good health, he married, and continued perfectly free of any such complaint ever since. By a mercurial course, however, the complaint for which he applied to me was completely removed. With regard to its effects, the venereal poison follows no constant rule; for though, in general, it affects first the throat, where it produces ulcerations, in others it exerts its virulence on the skin or bones. While the greatest part of mankind are thus easily affected by this poison, there are some few who seem to be altogether unsusceptible of the infection: as happens equally with the variolous contagion, though they go into infected places, and expose themselves to inoculation or every hazard by which the disease is generally communicated.

Some persons are more liable than others to be infected who are seemingly of the same habit; nay, the very same person seems to be more liable to be infected at one time than another, and those who have been once infected seem to be more liable to catch the infection a second time, than those who never were infected before with the disease. The climate, season, age, state of health, idiosyncrasy, are, perhaps, as in other diseases, the necessary predisposing causes. The same difference is observable in the progress made by the disease after the patient is infected. In some the progress is slow, and the disease appears scarcely to gain any ground; while in others it advances with the utmost rapidity, and speedily produces the most terrible symptoms. Whether the venereal poison can be abso.bed into the system, without a previous excoriation, or ulceration of the genitals, or some other parts of the surface of the body, is still a matter of doubt. Several cases, however, have occurred which render it highly probable, if not certain, that the poison really is now and then absorbed, without any previous excoriation or ulceration whatsoever, and thus produces buboes and other venereal symptoms in the body.

It has been asserted by the earliest and even by some late writers, that it may be caught by lying in the same bed or living in the same room with or after an infected person. What may have been the case at the commencement of the disease, cannot be said, but the most accurate observations and experiments which have been made upon the subject, do not confirm this to be the case in our times. Nor are nurses infected in the Lock-Hospital, where they live night and day with patients in all stages of the distemper. The fact seems to be, that patients in our times are apt to impose upon themselves, or upon physicians and surgeons, with regard to this matter; and the above opinion easily gains ground among the vulgar, especially in countries where people are more influenced by prejudices, superstition, servile situation in life, or other circumstances. Hence, we sometimes hear the most ridiculous accounts given in those countries by friars and common soldiers, of the manner by which they came to this disorder; such as piles, gravel, colics, contusions, fevers, little-houses, lying in suspected beds, or lying in bed with a suspected person, retention of the semen, coition with a woman in menstruation, the use of cider, bad wine, or beer, &c.

Another question undecided is, whether the venereal poison ever infects any fluid of our body, besides those of the mucous and lymphatic system. Does the venereal poison in an infected woman ever affect the milk, and consequently can the infection be conveyed to the infant by the milk alone, without any venereal ulcer on or about the nipples? It is equally a matter of uncertainty whether the venereal disease is ever conveyed from an infected father or mother, by coition, to the fœtus, provided their genitals are sound; or whether a child is ever affected with venereal symptoms in the uterus of an infected mother. Such infected infants as came under the observation of Dr. Swediaur, or of his friends, whose practice afforded them frequent opportunities of seeing new-born infants, seemed rather to militate against the opinion. Neither he nor any of them, have ever been able to observe ulcerations or other symptoms of a venereal kind upon newborn children; and such as make their appearance four, six, or eight, or more days afterward, on the genitals, anus, lips, mouth, &c. may rather be supposed to arise by infection during the passage from ulcers in the vagina of the mother, the skin of the infant being then nearly in as tender a state as the glans penis, or the labia; and this perhaps at the time when an absorption of the venereal poison might more easily take place without a previous excoriation, or ulceration of the skin. All the ways, therefore, by which we see, in our days, the venereal poison communicated from an unhealthy to a healthy person, may be reduced to the following heads:

1. By the coition of a healthy person with another who is infected with venereal disease of the genitals.

2. By the coition of a healthy person with another, apparently healthy, in whose genitals the poison lies concealed, without having yet produced any bad symptom. Thus, a woman who has perhaps received the infection from a man two or three days before, may during that time infect, and often does infect, the man or men who have to do with her afterward, without having any symptoms of the disease visible upon herself; and *vice versâ*, a man may infect a woman in the same manner. Such instances occur in practice every day.

3. By sucking; in this case the nipples of the wet

nurse may be infected by venereal ulcers in the mouth of the child: or, *vice versâ*, the nipples of the nurse being infected, will occasion venereal ulcers in the child's nose, mouth, or lips. It is uncertain, as mentioned above, whether the venereal poison was ever propagated by means of the milk from the breast.

4. By exposing to the contact of venereal poison any part of the surface of the body, by kissing, touching, &c. especially if the parts so exposed have been previously excoriated, wounded, or ulcerated by any cause whatever. In this manner we frequently see venereal ulcers arise in the scrotum and thighs; and there are some well-attested instances where the infection took place in the fingers of midwives or surgeons. Several instances are recorded of venereal ulcers in the nostrils, eyelids, and lips of persons who had touched their own genitals, or those of others, affected at the time with local venereal complaints, and then rubbed their nostrils, &c. with the fingers, without previously washing the hands. There was, a few years, ago in London, a melancholy example of a young lady, who, after having drawn a decayed tooth, and replaced it with one taken immediately from a young woman apparently in perfect health, was soon after affected with an ulcer in the mouth. The sore manifested symptoms of a venereal nature; but such was its obstinacy, that it resisted the most powerful mercurial remedies, terminating at last in a caries of the maxilla, with a most shocking erosion of the mouth and face, by which the unhappy patient was destroyed. During all this, however, we are informed that not the smallest venereal symptom was perceived in the woman from whom the sound tooth was procured.

5. By wounding any part of the body with a lancet or knife infected with the venereal virus. In this instance there is a similarity between the venereal poison and that of the small-pox. There are several examples of the latter being produced by bleeding with a lancet which had been previously employed for the purpose of inoculation, or of opening variolous pustules, without being properly cleaned afterward. In Moravia, in the year 1577, a number of persons who assembled in a house for bathing, had themselves, according to the custom of that time, scarified by the barber, were all of them infected with the venereal disease, and treated accordingly. Krato, the physician, and Jordan, who gave a description of this distemper, are both of opinion that it was communicated by means of the scarifying instrument. And Van Swieten relates several instances where the lues was communicated by a similar carelessness in cleaning the instrument used in bleeding or scarification.

The venereal poison applied to the urethra and vagina produce a clap. See *Gonorrhœa*. Coming into contact with other parts, it produces a chancre or bubo and constitutional symptoms. Chancre is the primary and immediate consequence of inoculation with true venereal matter in any of the ways which have been mentioned, and may arise in any part of the human body: but it generally shows itself in the pudenda, because the infecting medium is there first taken up in the one sex, and communicated by contact to the other. It is not, however, peculiar to these parts, for whenever the same kind of fluid is applied to a scratch on the hand, finger, lip, or nipple, the same consequence will follow. There can be no doubt but that the slightest abrasion possible, or breach of the cuticle, is sufficient to give a speedy admission to this destructive poison. A chancre makes its appearance with a slight inflammation which afterward ulcerates, or there arises a small pimple or pustule filled with a transparent fluid, which soon breaks and forms into a spreading ulcer. The period at which it makes its appearance after infection is very various, being most commonly in five or six days, but in some cases not till after the expiration of as many weeks. There is both a local and general predisposition to chancres: Jews and Mahommedans, from the constant exposure of the glans and loss of the prepuce, have the cuticle of the glans penis of much firmer texture than those who have not been circumcised; and they are, from this circumstance, much less subject to chancres than the rest of mankind. For the same reason they who, from the shortness of the prepuce, generally keep the glans uncovered, are not so liable to the diseases as those who have long narrow preputia; for persons thus formed constantly keep the surface of the glans and prepuce moist and tender,

and almost at every cohabitation are liable to abrasions and to excoriations.

There is an intermediate state of the venereal disease between a local and constitutional affection, which arises from the absorption of venereal matter from some surface to which it has been applied. The glands situated nearest the parts thus affected are apt to be come swelled and inflamed, so as to give rise to what is termed *bubo ;* and the parts of generation usually coming first in contact with the matter, so the glands in the groin generally afford this particular symptom. In most cases the venereal virus is absorbed from a chancre or an ulcer in the urethra; but instances have occurred where a bubo has arisen without either gonorrhœa or any kind of ulceration, and where the matter appears to have been absorbed, without any erosion of the skin or mucous membrane.

A bubo comes on with pain in the groin accompanied with some degree of hardness and swelling, and is at first about the size of a kidney bean, but continuing to increase, it at length becomes as large as an egg, occasions the person to experience some difficulty in walking, and is attended with a pulsation and throbbing in the tumour, and a great redness of the skin. In some cases the suppuration is quickly completed, in others it goes on very slow, and in others again the inflammatory appearances go off without any formation of pus. In a few instances the glans have been known to become scirrhous. The following are the characteristics of a venereal bubo. The swelling is usually confined to one gland, the colour of the skin where inflammation prevails is of a florid red, the pain is very acute, the progress from inflammation to suppuration and ulceration is generally very rapid, the suppuration is large in proportion to the size of the gland, and there is only one abscess.

A bubo is never attended with danger, where the inflamed gland proceeds on regularly to suppuration, but in particular cases it acquires an indolence after coming to a certain length, arising from a scrofulous taint, or by being combined with erysipelas it terminates in gangrene, and occasions a great loss of substance. This termination is, however, more frequently met with in hospitals than in private practice, and may partly be attributed to the contaminated state of the air of the wards wherein venereal patients are lodged.

A constitutional taint is the third form under which it has been mentioned, that the venereal poison is apt to show itself, and which always arises in consequence of the matter being absorbed and carried into the circulating mass of fluids. The absorption of it may, however, take place in three ways:

1st, It may be carried into the circulation, without producing any evident local effect on the part to which it was first applied.

2dly, It may take place in consequence of some local affection, such as either gonorrhœa, chancre, or bubo. And,

3dly, It may ensue from an application of the matter to a common sore or wound, similar to what happens in inoculating for the small-pox.

The most general way, however, in which a constitutional taint is produced, is by an absorption of the matter, either from a chancre or a bubo.

When venereal matter gets into the system, some symptoms of it may often be observed in the course of six or eight weeks, or probably sooner; but in some cases, it will continue in the circulating mass of fluids for many months before any visible signs of its effects are produced. The system being completely contaminated, it then occasions many local effects in different parts of the body, and shows itself under a variety of forms, many of which put on the appearance of a distinct disease. We may presume that this variety depends wholly on the difference of constitution, the different kind of parts affected, and the different state these parts were in at the time the matter or poison was applied.

The first symptoms usually show themselves on the skin and in the mouth or throat. When on the skin, reddish and brownish spots appear here and there on the surface, and eruptions of a copper colour are dispersed over different parts of the body, on the top of which there soon forms a thick scurf or scale. This scurf falls off after a short time, and is succeeded by another, and the same happening several times, and at length casting off deep scabs, an ulcer is formed which discharges an acrid fœtid matter. When the matter is secreted in the glands of the throat and mouth, the tongue will often be affected so as to occasion a thickness of speech, and the tonsils, palate, and uvula will become ulcerated so as to produce a soreness and difficulty of swallowing, and likewise a hoarseness in the voice. In a venereal ulcer of the tonsil, a portion of it seems as if it was dug out; it is, moreover, very foul, and has a thick, white matter adhering to it, which cannot be washed off. By these characteristic marks it may, in general, readily be distinguished from any other species of ulceration in these parts.

If the disease affects the eyes, obstinate inflammation, and sometimes ulceration, will also attack these organs.

The matter sometimes falls on deep-seated parts, such as the tendons, ligaments, and periosteum, and occasions hard, painful swellings to arise, known by the name of nodes.

When the disease is suffered to take its own course, and not counteracted by proper remedies, the patient will, in the course of time, be afflicted with severe pains, but more particularly in the night-time; his countenance will become sallow, his hair will fall off, he will lose his appetite, strength, and flesh, his rest will be much disturbed by night, and a small fever of the hectic kind will arise. The ulcers in the mouth and throat being likewise suffered to spread, and to occasion a caries of the bones of the palate, an opening will be made from the mouth of the nose; and the cartilages and bones of the nose being at length corroded away, this will sink on a level with the face. Some constitutions will bear up for a considerable time against the disease, while others again will soon sink under a general weakness and irritation produced by it. If the disorder is recent, and the constitution not impaired by other diseases, a perfect cure may easily be affected; but where it is of long standing, and accompanied with the symptoms of irritation which have been mentioned, the cure will prove tedious, and in many cases uncertain, as the constitution and strength of the patient may not admit of his going through a course of medicine sufficient to destroy the poison; or his health may be in such a state, as that only a very small quantity of mercury can be administered even at considerable intervals.

The general appearances to be observed on dissection of those who die of lues, are, caries of the bones, but more particularly those of the cranium, often communicating ulceration to the brain itself, together with enlargements and indurations of the lymphatic glands, scirrhus of several of the organs, particularly the liver and lungs, and exostoses of many of the hardest bones.

SYPHILIS INDICA. The yaws.

SYPHILIS POLONICA. A variety of venereal disease.

SYRIÆ OLEUM. A fragrant essential oil, obtained by distilling the canary balsam-plant, or moldavica.

Syrian herb mastich. See *Teucrium marum.*

SYRI'GMUS. See *Paracusis.*

SYRI'NGA. (From συριγξ, a pipe: so called because from its branches pipes were made after the removal of the pith.) The pipe-tree.

SYRI'NGMOS. See *Paracusis.*

SYRINGO'TOMUM. (From συριγξ, a fistula, and τεμνω, to cut.) An instrument to cut fistulas.

SY'RINX. (A Hebrew word.) A pipe. A syringe. A fistula.

SYRMAI'SMUS. (From συρμαιζω, to evacuate.) A gentle evacuation by vomit or stool.

SYRUP. See *Syrupus.*

Syrup of ginger. See *Syrupus zingiberis.*
Syrup of lemon. See *Syrupus limonum.*
Syrup of marsh-mallows. See *Syrupus altheæ.*
Syrup of mulberry. See *Syrupus mori.*
Syrup of orange. See *Syrupus aurantii.*
Syrup of poppy. See *Syrupus papaveris.*
Syrup of red poppy. See *Syrupus rhœados.*
Syrup of roses. See *Syrupus rosæ.*
Syrup of saffron. See *Syrupus croci.*
Syrup of senna. See *Syrupus sennæ.*
Syrup of Tolu. See *Syrupus tolutanus.*

SYRUPUS. (Serab, a potion, Arabian.) The name syrup is given to sugar dissolved in water; and in the present pharmacopœia this is termed simple syrup. See *Syrupus simplex.*

Syrups are generally made with the juice of vegetables or fruits, or by adding vegetable extracts or other substances. To keep syrups without fermenting, it is necessary that their temperature should be attended to, and kept as near 55° as possible. A good cellar will answer this purpose, for there are few summers in which the temperature of such a place rises to 60°.

SYRUPUS ACETI. Sugar and vinegar. A refrigerating syrup. See *Oxymel.*

SYRUPUS ALTHEÆ. Syrup of marsh-mallow. *Syrupus ex althæa. Syrupus de althæa.* Take of the fresh root of marsh-mallow, bruised, half a pound; refined sugar, two pounds; water, a gallon. Boil down the water with the marsh-mallow-root to half, and press out the liquor when cold. Set it by for 24 hours, that the feculencies may subside; then pour off the liquor, and having added the sugar, boil it down to a proper consistence. An emollient and demulcent; mostly given to allay tickling coughs, hoarseness, &c. in conjunction with other remedies.

SYRUPUS AURANTII. Syrup of orange. *Syrupus corticis aurantii. Syrupus e corticibus aurantiorum. Syrupus de cortice aurantiorum.* Take of fresh orange-peel, two ounces; boiling water, a pint; refined sugar, three pounds. Macerate the orange-peel in the water for 12 hours in a covered vessel; then pour off the liquor, and add the sugar. A pleasant bitter and stomachic.

SYRUPUS CARYOPHYLLI RUBRI. A warm and stimulating syrup.

SYRUPUS COLCHICI. An acrid and diuretic compound given in dropsies.

SYRUPUS CORTICIS AURANTII. See *Syrupus aurantii.*

SYRUPUS CROCI. Syrup of saffron. Take of saffron, an ounce; boiling water, a pound; refined sugar, two pounds and a half. Macerate the saffron in the water for 12 hours in a covered vessel, then strain the liquor, and add the sugar. This imparts a beautiful colour to liquids, and is sometimes employed as a cordial. Among the vulgar, syrup of saffron is in high esteem in measles, small-pox, &c.

SYRUPUS LIMONUM. Syrup of lemon. *Syrupus succi limonis. Syrupus e succo limonum. Syrupus e succo citrorum.* Take of lemon-juice, strained, a pint; refined sugar, two pounds. Dissolve the sugar in the lemon-juice in the manner directed for simple syrup. A very pleasant, cooling, and acid syrup which may be exhibited with advantage, in febrile and bilious affections.

SYRUPUS MORI. Syrup of mulberry. *Syrupus mororum.* Take of mulberry-juice, strained, a pint; refined sugar, two pounds. Dissolve the sugar in the mulberry-juice in the manner directed for simple syrup. Syrup of mulberries is very grateful and aperient, and may be given with such intentions to children.

SYRUPUS PAPAVERIS. *Syrupus papaveris albi. Syrupus e meconio. Syrupus de meconio, sive diacodium.* Take of capsules of white poppy, dried and bruised, the seeds being separated, 14 ounces; refined sugar, two pounds; boiling water, two gallons and a half. Macerate the capsules in the water for 24 hours, then boil it down by means of a water-bath to one gallon, and press out the liquor strongly. Boil down the liquor again, after being strained, to two pints, and strain it while hot. Set it by for 12 hours, that the feculencies may subside: then boil down the clear liquor to a pint, and add the sugar in the manner directed for simple syrup. It should be kept in stone bottles, and in a cellar. A useful anodyne preparation, which may be added with advantage to a vast variety of medicines against diseases of the bowels, coughs, &c.

SYRUPUS PAPAVERIS ERRATICI. See *Syrupus rhœados.*

SYRUPUS RHAMNI. Syrup of buckthorn. Take of the fresh juice of buckthorn-berries, four pints; ginger-root, sliced, allspice, powdered, of each half an ounce; refined sugar, three pounds and a half. Set by the juice for three days, that the feculencies may subside, and strain. To a pint of the clear juice add the ginger and allspice; then macerate in a gentle heat four hours, and strain; boil down what remains to one pint and a half, mix the liquors and add the sugar in the manner directed for simple syrup.

This preparation, in doses of three or four spoonfuls, operates as a brisk cathartic. The principal inconvenience attending it is, that it is very unpleasant, and occasions a thirst and dryness of the mouth and fauces, and sometimes violent gripes. These effects may be prevented by drinking liberally of water-gruel, or other warm liquids, during the operation.

SYRUPUS RHŒADOS. *Syrupus papaveris erratici. Syrupus de papavere erratico.* Syrup of red-poppy. Take of red-poppy petals, fresh, a pound; boiling water, a pint and two fluid ounces; refined sugar, two pounds and a half. Having heated the water in a water-bath, add gradually the red-poppy petals, frequently stirring them; then having removed the vessel, macerate for twelve hours; next press out the liquor, and set it by to settle; lastly, add the sugar as directed for simple syrup. This is a very mild anodyne, and used more for the colour, than for its medical properties.

SYRUPUS RIBIS NIGRI. Syrup of black currants. Aperient and diuretic qualities are attributed to this preparation.

SYRUPUS ROSÆ. Syrup of roses. *Syrupus rosarum solutivus. Syrupus e rosis siccis.* Take of damask-rose petals, dried, seven ounces; refined sugar, six pounds; boiling water, four pints. Macerate the rose-petals in the water for twelve hours, and strain; then evaporate the strained liquor, by means of a water-bath, to two pints and a half; then add the sugar in the manner described for simple syrup. A useful laxative for children. From ℥j. to ℥ss.

SYRUPUS RUBI IDÆI. Syrup of raspberry. A pleasant aperient syrup for children.

SYRUPUS SCILLITICUS. Expectorant and diuretic. See *Oxymel scillæ.*

SYRUPUS SENNÆ. Syrup of senna. Take of senna-leaves, two ounces; fennel-seed, bruised, an ounce; manna, three ounces; refined sugar, a pound; water, boiling, a pint. Macerate the senna-leaves and fennel-seeds in the water for an hour, with a gentle heat; strain the liquor, and mix with it the manna and sugar; then boil to the proper consistence. A useful purgative for children.

SYRUPUS SIMPLEX. *Syrupus.* Simple syrup. Take of refined sugar, two pounds and a half; water, a pint. Dissolve the sugar in the water in a water-bath, then set it aside for twenty-four hours; take off the scum;

and if there be any feculencies, pour off the clear liquor from them.

SYRUPUS TOLUTANUS. Syrup of Tolu. Take of balsam of Tolu, an ounce; water, boiling, a pint; refined sugar, two pounds. Boil the balsam in the water half an hour in a covered vessel, occasionally stirring it; strain the liquor when it is cold, and then add the sugar in the manner directed for simple syrup. A useful balsamic syrup, calculated to allay tickling coughs and hoarsenesses.

SYRUPUS VIOLÆ. A pleasant laxative for young children.

SYRUPUS ZINGIBERIS. Syrup of ginger. Take of ginger-root, sliced, two ounces; water, boiling, a pint; refined sugar, two pounds. Macerate the ginger-root in the water for twenty-four hours, and strain; then add the sugar in the manner directed for simple syrup A carminative and stomachic syrup. Dose from one to three drachms.

SYSPASIA. (From συσπαω, *contraho, convello.*) The name of a genus of diseases in Good's Nosology Class, *Neurotica;* Order, *Systatica.* Comatose spasm. It has three species, viz. *Syspasia convulsio, hysteria, epilepsia.*

SYSSARCO'SIS. (From συν, and σαρξ, flesh.) A species of union of bones, in which one bone is united to another by means of an intervening muscle. In this manner the os hyoides is connected with the sternum and other parts.

SYSTATICA. (From συνιστημι, *congredior, con socio.*) The name of an order of diseases in Class *Neurotica,* of Good's Nosology. Diseases affecting several, or all the sensorial powers simultaneously. Its genera are, *Agrypnia, Dysphonia, Antipathia, Cephalæa, Dinus, Syncope, Syspasia, Caries.*

System, absorbent. See *Absorbents* and *Lymphatics*
System, genital. The parts of generation.
System, nervous. See *Nerve.*
System of plants. See *Plants.*
System, vascular. The arteries and veins.

SY'STOLE. (From συςελλω, to contract.) The contraction of the heart.

SYSTREMMA. (From συστρεφω, *contorqueo,* to wind about, or twist.) The cramp.

T

T-BANDAGE. A bandage so named from its figure. It is principally used for supporting the dressings, after the operation for fistula in ano, in diseases of the perinæum, and those of the groins, anus, &c.

TABA'CUM. (From *Tobago,* the island from whence it was first brought.) Tobacco. See *Nicotiana.*

TABASHEER. The silica found in the hollow stem of the bamboo cane is so called. Its optical properties are peculiar.

TABE'LLA. (Diminutive of *tabula,* a table.) A lozenge.

TA'BES. (*Tabes, is,* f.; from *tabesco,* to consume or pine away.) A wasting of the body. A genus of disease in the Class, *Cachexiæ;* and Order, *Marcores,* of Cullen; characterized by emaciation and weakness, attended with hectic fever, but without any cough or spitting, which last symptoms distinguish it from phthisis. It has three species: 1. *Tabes purulenta,* from an ulcerous discharge: 2. *Tabes scrofulosa,* from a scrofulous habit: 3. *Tabes venenata,* from poison. See *Atrophy.*

TABES COXARIA. A wasting of the thigh and leg from an abscess, or other cause in the hip.

TABES DORSALIS. *Lordosis.* A wasting of the body, attended at first with pain in the back or loins, and afterward also in the neck and head, caused by a too early or a too frequent use of venery. Dr. Cullen makes it a variety of *atrophia inanitorum.* Hippocrates calls it *tabes ossis.*

TABES OSSIS SACRI. See *Tabes dorsalis.*

TABES PULMONALIS. See *Phthisis.*

TABES RENALIS. A wasting away of the body from an abscess of the kidney.

TABULAR SPAR. Table spar. Schaalstein of

Werner. Prismatic augite of Jameson. A mineral of a grayish white colour, found in primitive rocks at Orawicza.

TACAMAHACCA. (Indian.) See *Fagara octandra.*

TA'CTUS. See *Touch.*

TÆ'DA. (Δαιδα; from δαω, to burn.) A torch. A species of pine which burns like a torch. A medicated torch for fumigations.

TÆ'NIA. (Ταινια, a Hebrew word, signifying a fillet: the name of a worm, from its resemblance to a fillet or tape.) The tape-worm. A genus of intestinal worms; characterized by a long, flat, and jointed body. See *Worms.*

TAIL. See *Cauda.*

TALC. See *Talcum.*

TA'LCUM. (From *talk,* German.) Talc. Of this mineral, which is Jameson's sixth subspecies of rhomboidal mica, there are two kinds. 1. *Common talc,* of a greenish-white colour, greasy feel, breaks into curved plates or leaves, occurs in beds of mica slate, and clay slate, in several parts of Scotland. 2. *Indurated talc,* or *talc slate,* of a greenish-gray colour, found in Scotland, and abundantly on the Continent. It is used by carpenters, tailors, hat makers, and glaziers for drawing lines.

Talc is composed of pure magnesia mixed with near twice its weight of silex and less than its weight of alumine. The greenish foliaceous Venice talc was formerly used medicinally, as possessing antacid and aperient qualities.

Tallow. See *Fat.*

TA'LPA. (From τυφλος, blind.) *Talparia.* A mole. Also, a tumour resembling a mole in eating, and creeping under the skin.

TA′LUS. See *Astragalus*

TALCITE. Nacrite of Jameson. Earthly talc of Werner. A greenish-white, scaly mineral found in the mining district of Freyberg.

TAMALAPA′TRA. The Indian leaf is so termed by some authors. See *Laurus cassia.*

TAMARIND. See *Tamarindus.*

TAMARI′NDUS. (*Tamarindus, i*, m.; from *tamar*, or *tamarindi*, which is, in the Arabian language, a synonyme of the dactylus or date.) 1. The name of a genus of plants. Class, *Monadelphia*; Order, *Triandria.* The tamarind-tree.

2. The pharmacopœial name of the tamarind. See *Tamarindus indica.*

TAMARINDUS INDICA. The systematic name of the tamarind-tree. *Oxyphœnicon; Siliqua arabica; Balampulli; Tamaræa zecla; oxyphœnicia; Acacia indica.* The pulp of the tamarind, with the seeds, connected together by numerous tough strings or fibres, are brought to us freed from the outer shell, and commonly preserved in syrup. According to Long, tamarinds are prepared for exportation at Jamaica, in the following manner: "The fruit or pods are gathered in June, July, and August, when full ripe, which is known by their fragility or easy breaking on small pressure between the finger and thumb. The fruit taken out of the pod, and cleared from the shelly fragments, is placed in layers in a cask, and boiling syrup, just before begins to granulate, is poured in, till the cask is filled : the syrup pervades every part quite down to the bottom, and, when cool, the cask is headed for sale." The tamarind is employed as a laxative, and for abating thirst or heat in various inflammatory complaints, and for correcting putrid disorders especially of a bilious kind, in which the cathartic, antiseptic, and refrigerant qualities of the fruit have been found equally useful. When intended merely as a laxative, it may be of advantage (Dr. Woodville observes,) to join it with manna or purgatives of a sweet kind, by which its use is rendered safer and more effectual. Three drachms of the pulp are usually sufficient to open the body, but to prove moderately cathartic, one or two ounces are required. It is an ingredient in the *confectio cassiæ*, and *confectio sennæ.*

TAMARI′SCUS. See *Tamarix gallica.*

TA′MARIX. (*Tamarix, icis*, f.; from *Tamarik*, abstersion, Heb.: named from its properties of cleansing and purifying the blood.) The name of a genus of plants. Class, *Pentandria*; Order, *Digynia.* The tamarisk-tree.

TAMARIX GALLICA. The systematic name of the tamarisk-tree. *Tamariscus.* Tamarisk. The bark, wood, and leaves of this tree, were formerly employed medicinally, though seldom used at present. The former for its aperient and corroborant virtues in obstructions of the liver; the latter in icterus, hæmoptysis, and some affections of the skin.

TAME-POISON. See *Asclepias vincetoxicum.*

TANACE′TUM. (*Tanacetum, i*, n.; corrupted from *tanasia, athanasia*, the old name for tansy.) 1. The name of a genus of plants in the Linnæan system. Class, *Syngenesia*; Order, *Polygamia superflua.* Tansy.

2. The pharmacopœial name of the tansy. See *Tanacetum vulgare.*

TANACETUM BALSAMITA. The systematic name of the officinal alecost. *Balsamita mas; Balsamita major; Tanacetum hortense; Costus hortorum.* Costmary, or alecost. The plant which bears this name in the pharmacopœias, is the *Tanacetum balsamita; foliis ovatis, integris, serratis*, of Linnæus. A fragrant smelling herb, somewhat like that of mint; formerly esteemed as a corroborant, carminative, and emmenagogue.

TANACETUM HORTENSE. See *Balsamita mas.*

TANACETUM VULGARE. The systematic name of the common tansy. *Tanasia; Athanasia; Parthenium mas. Tanacetum—foliis bipinnatis incicis serratis*, of Linnæus. The leaves and flowers of tansy have a strong, not very disagreeable smell, and a bitter somewhat aromatic taste. The virtues of tansy are tonic, stomachic, anthelmintic, emmenagogue, and resolvent. It has been much used as a vermifuge; and testimonies of its efficacy are given by many respectable physicians. Not only the leaves, but the seeds have been employed with this intention, and substituted for those of santonicum. We are told by Dr. Clark, that in Scotland tansy was found to be of great service in various cases of gout; and Dr. Cullen, who afterward was informed of the effect it had produced upon those who had used the herb for this purpose, says, "I have known several who have taken it without any advantage, and some others who reported that they had been relieved from the frequency of their gout." Tansy is also recommended in the hysteria, especially when this disease is supposed to proceed from menstrual obstructions.

This plant may be given in powder to the quantity of a drachm or more for a dose; but it has been more commonly taken in infusion, or drank in tea.

TANA′SIA. See *Tanacetum.*

TANNIN. This, which is one of the immediate principles of vegetables, was first distinguished by Seguin from the gallic acid, with which it had been confounded under the name of the *astringent principle.* He gave it the name of tannin, from its use in the tanning of leather; which it effects by its characteristic property, that of forming with gelatin a tough insoluble matter.

It may be obtained from vegetables by macerating them in cold water; and precipitated from this solution, which contains likewise gallic acid and extractive matter, by hyperoxygenized muriate of tin. From this precipitate, immediately diffused in a large quantity of water, the oxide of tin may be separated by sulphuretted hydrogen gas, leaving the tannin in solution.

Professor Proust has since recommended another method, the precipitation of a decoction of galls by powdered carbonate of potassa, washing well the greenishgray flakes that fall down with cold water, and drying them in a stove. The precipitate grows brown in the air, becomes brittle and shining like a resin, and yet remains soluble in hot water. The tannin in this state, he says, is very pure.

Sir H. Davy, after making several experiments on different methods of ascertaining the quantity of tannin in astringent infusions, prefers for this purpose the common process of precipitating the tannin by gelatin; but he remarks, that the tannin of different vegetables requires different proportions of gelatin for its saturation; and that the quantity of precipitate obtained is influenced by the degree in which the solutions are con centrated.

Chenevix observed, that coffee-berries acquired by roasting the property of precipitating gelatin; and Hatchett has made a number of experiments, which show that an artificial tannin, or substance having its chief property, may be formed, by treating with nitric acid matters containing charcoal. It is remarkable that this tannin, when prepared from vegetable substances, as dry charcoal of wood, yields, on combustion, products analogous to those of animal matters. From his experiments it would seem, that tannin is, in reality, carbonaceous matter combined with oxygen; and the difference in the proportion of oxygen may occasion the differences in the tannin procured from different substances, that from catechu appearing to contain most.

Bouillon Lagrange asserts, that tannin, by absorbing oxygen, is converted into gallic acid.

It is not an unfrequent practice, to administer medicines containing tannin in cases of debility, and at the same time to prescribe gelatinous food as nutritious. But this is evidently improper, as the tannin, from its chemical properties, must render the gelatin indigestible.

TANSY. See *Tanacetum.*

Tansy, wild. See *Potentilla.*

TANTALUM. The metal, an account of which is given under the article columbic acid. See *Columbic acid* and *Columbium.*

TAPE-WORM. See *Tænia.*

TAPIOCA. See *Jatropha manihot.*

TAPPING. See *Paracentesis.*

TA′PSUS BARBATUS. See *Verbascum.*

TAR. See *Pinus sylvestris.*

Tar, Barbadoes. See *Petroleum barbadense.*

Tar-water. A once celebrated remedy, but now neglected more than it deserves. It is made by infusing tar in water, stirring it from time to time, and lastly pouring off the clear liquor now impregnated with the colour and virtues of the tar. It is drunk in many chronic affections, particularly of the lungs.

TARANTI′SMUS. (From *tarantula*, the animal, the bite of which is supposed to be cured only by music.)

The desire of dancing which is produced by the bite of the tarantula.

TARA'NTULA. (From *Taranta*, a city in Naples, where they abound.) A kind of venomous spider, whose bite is said to be cured by music.

TARA'XACUM. (From ταρασσω, to alter or change: because it alters the state of the blood.) See *Leontodon*.

TARA'XIS. (From ταρασσω, to disturb.) A slight inflammation of the eye.

TA'RCHON SYLVESTRIS. See *Achillea ptarmica.*

TARE. See *Ervum.*

TARRAS. *Terras.* A volcanic earth, used as a cement.

TARSI EXTENSOR MINOR. See *Plantaris.*

TA'RSUS. Ταρσος. 1. The instep, or that part of the foot which is between the leg and metatarsus: it is composed of seven bones, viz. the astragalus, os calcis, os naviculare, os cuboides, and three ossa cuneiformia.

2. The thin cartilage situated at the edges of the eyelids to preserve their firmness and shape.

TARTAR. See *Tartarum.*

Tartar cream of. The popular name of the pulverized supertartrate of potassa.

Tartar, emetic. See *Antimonium tartarizatum.*

Tartar, oil of. See *Potassæ subcarbonatis liquor.*

Tartar, regenerated. See *Potassæ acetas.*

Tartar, salt of. See *Potassæ subcarbonas.*

Tartar, soluble. See *Potassæ tartras.*

Tartar, spirit of. If the crystals of tartar be distilled by a strong heat, without any additional body, they furnish an empyreumatic acid, called the pyrotartareous acid, or spirit of tartar, and a very fœtid empyreumatic oil.

Tartar, vitriolated. See *Potassæ sulphas.*

TARTARIC ACID. *Acidum tartaricum; Sal essentiale tartari; Acidum tartari essentiale.* Tartareous acid. "The casks in which some kinds of wine are kept become incrusted with a hard substance, tinged with the colouring matter of the wine, and otherwise impure, which has long been known by the name of *argal*, or tartar, and distinguished into red and white according to its colour. This being purified by solution, filtration, and crystallization, was termed *cream*, or *crystals of tartar.* It was afterward discovered, that it consisted of a peculiar acid combined with potassa; and the supposition that it was formed during the fomentation of the wine, was disproved by Boerhaave, Neuman, and others, who showed that it existed ready formed in the juice of the grape. It has likewise been found in other fruits, particularly before they are too ripe; and in the tamarind, sumac, balm, carduus benedictus, and the roots of restharrow, germander, and sage. The separation of tartaric acid from this acidulous salt, is the first discovery of Scheele that is known. He saturated the superfluous acid, by adding chalk to a solution of the supertartrate in boiling water as long as any effervescence ensued, and expelled the acid from the precipitated tartrate of lime by means of the sulphuric. Or four parts of tartar may be boiled in twenty or twenty-four parts of water, and one part of sulphuric acid added gradually. By continuing the boiling, the sulphate of potassa will fall down. When the liquor is reduced to one-half, it is to be filtered; and if any more sulphate be deposited by continuing the boiling, the filtering must be repeated. When no more is thrown down, the liquor is to be evaporated to the consistence of a syrup; and thus crystals of tartaric acid, equal to half the weight of the tartar employed, will be obtained.

The tartaric acid may be procured in needly or laminated crystals, by evaporating a solution of it. Its taste is very acid and agreeable, so that it may supply the place of lemon-juice. It is very soluble in water. Burnt in an open fire, it leaves a coaly residuum; in close vessels it gives out carbonic acid and carburetted hydrogen gas. By distilling nitric acid off the crystals, they may be converted into oxalic acid, and the nitric acid passes to the state of nitrous.

To extract the whole acid from tartar, Thenard recommends, after saturating the redundant acid with chalk, to add muriate of lime to the supernatant neutral tartrate, by which means it is completely decomposed. The insoluble tartrate of lime being washed with abundance of water, is then to be treated with three-fifths of its weight of strong sulphuric acid, diluted previously with five parts of water. But Fourcroy's process, as

336

improved by Vauquelin, seems still better. Tartar is treated with quicklime and boiling water in the proportion, by the theory of equivalents, of 100 of tartar to 30 of dry lime, or 40 of the slaked. A caustic magma is obtained, which must be evaporated to dryness, and gently heated. On digesting this in water, a solution of caustic potassa is obtained, while tartrate of lime remains; from which the acid may be separated by the equivalent quantity of oil of vitriol.

According to Berzelius, tartaric acid is a compound of 3.807 hydrogen + 35.980 carbon + 60.213 oxygen = 100; to which result he shows that of Gay Lussac and Thenard to correspond, when allowance is made for a certain portion of water, which they had omitted to estimate. The analysis of tartrate of lead, gives 8.384 for the acid prime equivalent; and it may be made up of 3 hydrogen = 0.375   4.48

3 hydrogen	= 0.375	4.48
4 carbon	= 3.000	35.82
5 oxygen	= 5.000	59.70
	8.375	100.00

The crystallized acid is a compound of 8.375 acid + 1.125 water = 9.5; or, in 100 parts, 88.15 acid + 11.85 water.

The *tartrates*, in their decomposition by fire, comport themselves like all the other vegetable salts, except that those with excess of acid yield the smell of *caromel* when heated, and afford a certain quantity of the pyrotartaric acid. All the soluble neutral tartrates form, with tartaric acid, bitartrates of sparing solubility; while all the insoluble tartrates may be dissolved in an excess of their acid. Hence, by pouring gradually an excess of acid into barytes, strontites, and lime-waters, the precipitates formed at first cannot fail to disappear; while those obtained by an excess of the same acid, added to concentrated solutions of potassa, soda, or ammonia, and the neutral tartrates of these bases, as well as of magnesia and copper, must be permanent. The first are always flocculent; the second always crystalline; that of copper alone is in a greenish-white powder. It likewise follows, that the greater number of acids ought to disturb the solutions of the alkaline neutral tartrates, because they transform these salts into bitartrates; and, on the contrary, they ought to affect the solution of the neutral insoluble tartrates, which indeed always happens, unless the acid cannot dissolve the base of the tartrate. The order of apparent affinities of tartaric acid are, lime, barytes, strontites, potassa, soda, ammonia, and magnesia.

The tartrates of potassa, soda, and ammonia are not only susceptible of combining together, but also with the other tartrates, so as to form *double*, or *triple salts*. We may thus easily conceive why the tartrates of potassa, soda, and ammonia do not disturb the solutions of iron and manganese; and, on the other hand, disturb the solutions of the salts of barytes, strontites, lime, and lead. In the first case, double salts are formed, however small a quantity of tartrate shall have been employed; in the second, no double salt is formed, unless the tartrate be added in very great excess.

The *tartrates of lime* and barytes are white, pulverulent, and insoluble.

Tartrate *of strontian*, formed by the double decomposition of muriate of strontian and tartrate of potassa, according to Vauquelin, is soluble, crystallizable, and consists of 52.88 strontian, and 47.12 acid.

That of *magnesia* forms a gelatinous or gummy mass.

Tartrate of potassa, tartarized kali, and *vegetable salt*, of some, formerly called *soluble tartar*, because much more so than the supertartrate, crystallizes in oblong squares, bevelled at the extremities. It has a bitterish taste, and is decomposed by heat, as its solution is even by standing some time. It is used as a mild purgative.

The *supertartrate of potassa* is much used as a cooling and gently opening medicine, as well as in several chemical and pharmaceutical preparations. Dissolved in water, with the addition of a little sugar, and a slice or two of lemon-peel, it forms an agreeable cooling drink, by the name of *imperial:* and if an infusion of green balm be used, instead of water, it makes one of the pleasantest liquors of the kind with which we are acquainted. Mixed with an equal weight of nitre, and projected into a red-hot crucible, it detonates, and forms the *white flux;* treated in the same way, with half its weight of nitre, it forms the *black flux;* and simply mixed with nitre in various proportions, it is called *raw flux.* It is likewise used in dying, in hatmaking, in gilding, and in other arts.

The blanching of the crude tartar is aided by boiling its solution with one-twentieth of pipe-clay.

According to the analysis of Berzelius, it consists of 70.45 acid + 24.8 potassa + 4.75 water = 100; or,

2 primes acid,	= 16.75	70.30
1	: potassa, =	5.95	24.95
1	water, =	1.125	4.75
		23.825	100.00

60 parts of water dissolve 4 of bitartrate, at a boiling heat; and only 1 at 60° Fahr. It is quite insoluble in alkohol.

By saturating the superfluous acid, in this supertartrate, with soda, a triple salt is formed, which crystallizes in larger regular prisms of eight nearly equal sides, of a bitter taste, efflorescent, and soluble in about five parts of water. It consists, according to Vauquelin, of 54 parts tartrate of potassa and 46 tartrate of soda; and was once in much repute as a purgative, by the name of *Rochelle salt,* or *Sel de Seignette.*

The *tartrate of soda* is much less soluble than this triple salt, and crystallizes in slender needles or thin plates.

The *tartrate of ammonia* is a very soluble, bitter salt, and crystallizes easily. Its solution is spontaneously decomposable.

This too forms, with tartrate of potassa, a triple salt, the solution of which yields, by cooling, fine pyramidal or prismatic efflorescent crystals. Though both the neutral salts that compose it are bitter, this is not, but has a cooling taste.

Take of the supertartrate of potassa, two pounds and a half; three gallons of boiling-hot water; one pound of prepared chalk; one pound of sulphuric acid. Boil the cream of tartar in two gallons of the water, and gradually throw in the chalk, until all effervescence ceases; set the liquor aside, that the tartrate of lime may subside; pour off the liquor, and wash the tartrate of lime repeatedly with distilled water, until it is tasteless. The pour on it the sulphuric acid, diluted with the remaining gallon of boiling water, and set the whole aside for twenty-four hours, stirring it well now and then. Strain the liquor, and evaporate in a water-bath until crystals form. The virtues of this acid are antiseptic, refrigerant, and diuretic. It is used in acute fevers, scurvy, and hæmorrhage."—*Ure's Chem. Dict.*

TARTARINE. The name given by Kirwan to the vegetable alkali.

TA'RTARUM. (*Tartarum, i,* n.; from ταρʃαρος, infernal: because it is the sediment or dregs.) Tartar. 1. The concretion which fixes to the inside of hogsheads containing wine. It is alloyed with much extractive and colouring matter, from which it is purified by decoction with argillaceous earths and subsequent crystallization. By this means it becomes perfectly white, and shoots out crystals of tartar, consisting of a peculiar acid called acid of tartar, imperfectly saturated with potassa; it is therefore a supertartrate of that alkali, which, when powdered, is the cream of tartar of the shops. Its virtues are eccoprotic, diuretic, and refrigerant, and it is exhibited in abdominal physconia, dropsy, inflammatory and bilious fevers, dyspepsia from rancid or fat substances, bilious diarrhœa and colic, hæmorrhoids and obstipation.

2. A name heretofore given to many officinal preparations, containing the acid of tartar; but in consequence of recent changes in the chemical nomenclature, superseded by appellations more expressive of the respective compositions.

3. The name of the concretion which so frequently incrusts the teeth, and which is apparently phosphate of lime.

TARTARUM EMETICUM. See *Antimonium tartarizatum.*

TARTARUM REGENERATUM. See *Potassæ acetas.*

TARTARUM SOLUBILE. See *Potassæ tartras.*

TARTARUS AMMONIÆ. See *Tartras ammoniæ.*

TARTARUS CHALYBEATUS. See *Ferrum tartarizatum.*

TARTRAS. (*Tartras, atis,* m ; the tartaric being

F f f

its acid base.) A tartrate, or salt, formed by the combination of tartaric acid with salifiable bases; as tartrate of soda, potassa, &c.

TARTRAS AMMONIÆ. *Alkali volatile tartarizatum,* of Bergman. *Sal ammoniacum tartareum; Tartarus ammonia.* A salt composed of tartaric acid and ammonia; its virtues are diaphoretic, diuretic, and deobstruent. It is prescribed in fevers, atonic exanthemata, catarrh, arthritic and rheumatic arthrodynia, hysteric spasms, &c.

TARTRAS POTASSÆ. See *Potassæ tartras.*

TARTRAS POTASSÆ ACIDULUS. Cream of tartar. See *Potassa supertartras.*

TARTRAS POTASSÆ ACIDULUS FERRATUS. *Globuli martiales; Tartarus chalybeatus; Mars solubilis; Ferrum potabile.* Its virtues are adstringent. It is principally used externally in the form of fomentations or bath in contusions, distortions, and lux ations.

TARTRAS POTASSÆ ACIDULUS STIBIATUS. See *Antimonium tartarizatum.*

TARTRAS SODÆ. See *Soda tartarizata.*

TASTE. *Gustus.* " Savours are only the impression of certain bodies upon the organ of taste. Bodies which produce it are called *sapid.*

It has been supposed that the degree of sapidity of a body could be determined by that of its solubility; but certain bodies, which are insoluble, have a very strong taste, while other bodies very soluble have scarcely any. The sapidity appears to bear relation to the chemical nature of bodies, and to the peculiar efforts which they produce upon the animal economy.

Tastes are very numerous, and very variable. There have been numerous endeavours made to class them, though without complete success; they are better understood, however, than the odours, no doubt owing to the impressions received by the sense of taste being less fugitive than those received by the smell. Thus we are sufficiently understood, when we speak of a body having a taste that is *bitter, acid, sour, sweet,* &c.

There is a distinction of tastes which is sufficiently established, it being founded on the organization: that of agreeable and disagreeable. Animals establish it instinctively. This is the most important distinction; for those things which have an agreeable taste are generally useful for nutrition, while those whose savour is disagreeable, are, for the most part, hurtful.

Apparatus of taste.—The tongue is the principal organ of taste; however, the lips, the internal surface of the cheeks, the palate, the teeth, the *velum pendulum palati,* the *pharynx, œsophagus,* and even the stomach, are susceptible of receiving impressions by the contact of sapid bodies.

The salivary glands, of which the *excretory ducts* open into the mouth; the follicles which pour into it the *mucus,* which they secrete, have a powerful effect in forming the taste. Independently of the mucous follicles that the superior surface of the tongue presents, and which form upon it *fungous papillæ,* there are also little inequalities seen, one sort of which, very numerous, are called *villous papillæ;* the others, less numerous, and disposed on two rows on the sides of the tongue, are called *conical papillæ.*

All the nerves with which those parts are provided that are intended to receive the impressions of sapid bodies may be considered as belonging to the apparatus of taste. Thus the inferior maxillary nerves, many branches of the superior, among which it is necessary to notice the threads which proceed from the *spheno-palatine* ganglion, particularly the *naso-palatine* nerve of Scarpo, the nerve of the ninth pair, *glosso pharyngeus,* appear to be employed in the exercise of taste.

The lingual nerve of the fifth pair is that which anatomists consider the principal nerve of taste; and as a reason they say that its threads are continued into the *villous* and *conical papillæ* of the tongue.

Mechanism of taste.—For the full exercise of taste, the mucous membrane which covers the organs of it must be perfectly uninjured; it must be covered with *mucous fluid,* and the saliva must flow freely in the mouth. When the mouth becomes dry, the powers of taste cannot be excited.

It is also necessary that these liquids undergo no change: for if the mucous become thick, yellow, and the saliva acid, bitter, &c., the taste will be exerted but very imperfectly.

Some authors have assured us that the *papillæ* of

the tongue become really erect during the time that the taste is exerted. This assertion I believe to be entirely without foundation.

It is quite enough that a body be in contact with the organs of taste, for us to appreciate its savour immediately; but if it is solid, in most cases it is necessary to dissolve in the saliva to be tasted; this condition is not necessary for liquids and gases.

There appears to be a certain chemical action of sapid bodies upon the epidermis of the mucous membrane of the mouth; it is seen evidently at least in some, as vinegar, the mineral acids, a great number of salts, &c. In these different cases the colour of the epidermis is changed, and becomes white, yellow, &c. By the same causes, like effects are produced upon dead bodies. Perhaps to this sort of combination may be attributed the different kinds of impressions made by sapid bodies, as well as the variable duration of those impressions.

Hitherto no one has accounted for the faculty possessed by the teeth of being strongly influenced by certain sapid bodies. According to the researches of Miel, a distinguished dentist of Paris, this effect ought to be attributed to imbibition. The researches of Miel prove that the teeth imbibe very quickly liquids with which they are placed in contact. Different parts of the mouth appear to possess different degrees of sensibility for sapid bodies; for they act sometimes on the tongue, on the gums, on the teeth; at other times they have an exclusive action on the palate, on the pharynx, &c. Some bodies leave their taste a long time in the mouth; these are particularly the aromatic bodies. This *after-taste* is sometimes felt in the whole mouth, sometimes only in one part of it. Bitter bodies, for example, leave an impression in the pharynx: acids upon the lips and teeth: peppermint leaves an impression which exists both in the mouth and pharynx.

Tastes, to be completely known, ought to remain some time in the mouth; when they traverse it rapidly, they leave scarcely any impression; for this reason we swallow quickly those bodies which are disagreeable to us; on the contrary, we allow those that have an agreeable savour to remain a long time in the mouth.

When we taste a body which has a very strong and pertinacious taste, such as a vegetable acid, we become insensible to others which are feeble. This observation has been found valuable in medicine, in administering disagreeable drugs to the sick. We are capable of distinguishing a number of tastes at the same time, as also their different degrees of intensity; this is used by chemists, tasters of wine, &c. By this means we arrive sometimes at a tolerably exact knowledge of the chemical nature of bodies; but such delicacy of taste is not acquired until after long practice.

Is the lingual nerve that which is essential to taste? Nothing is known which can make us attribute this property entirely to it.

The choice of food depends entirely on the taste; joined to smell, it enables us to distinguish between substances that are hurtful and those that are useful. It is this sense which gives us the most correct knowledge of the composition of chemical bodies."

TA'XIS. An operation, by which those parts which have quitted their natural situation are replaced by the hand without the assistance of instruments, as in reducing hernia, &c.

TEA. See *Thea*.

TEAR. *Lachryma* The limpid fluid secreted by the lachrymal glands, and flowing on the surface of the eyes.

The organ which secretes this liquid is the lachrymal gland, one of which is situated in the external canthus of each orbit, and emits six or seven excretory ducts, which open on the internal surface of the upper eyelid above its tarsus, and pour forth the tears. The tears have mixed with them an arterious roscid vapour, which exhales from the internal surface of the eyelids, and external of the tunica conjunctiva, into the eye. Perhaps the aqueous humour also transudes through the pores of the cornea on the surface of the eye. A certain part of this aqueous fluid is dissipated in the air; but the greatest part, after having performed its office, is propelled by the orbicular muscle, which so closely constringes the eyelid to the ball of the eye as to leave no space between, unless in the internal angle, where the tears are collected. From this collection the tears are absorbed by the orifices of the puncta

lachrymalia; from thence they are propelled through the lachrymal canals, into the lachrymal sac, and flow through the ductus nasalis into the cavity of the nostrils, under the inferior concha nasalis. The *lachrymal sac* appears to be formed of longitudinal and transverse muscular fibres; and its three orifices furnished with small sphincters, as the spasmodic contriction of the puncta lachrymalia proves, if examined with a probe.

The tears have no smell but a saltish taste, as people who cry perceive. They are of a transparent colour and aqueous consistence.

The *quantity*, in its natural state, is just sufficient to moisten the surface of the eye and eyelids; but from sorrow, or any kind of stimulus applied to the surface of the eye, so great is the quantity of tears secreted that the puncta lachrymalia are unable to absorb them Thus the greatest part runs down from the internal angle of the eyelids, in the form of great and copious drops upon the cheeks. A great quantity also descends, through the lachrymal passages, into the nostrils; hence those who cry have an increased discharge from the nose.

Use of the tears.—1. They continually moisten the surface of the eye and eyelids, to prevent the pellucid cornea from drying and becoming opaque, or the eye from concreting with the eyelids. 2. They prevent that pain, which would otherwise arise from the friction of the eyelids against the bulb of the eye from continually winking. 3. They wash and clean away the dust of the atmosphere, or any thing acrid that has fallen into the eye. 4. Crying unloads the head of congestions.

TECTUS. Covered: applied as opposed to *nudus*, or naked; as to the seeds of the angiosperm plants.

TEETH. (*Dens*, a tooth; *quasi edens*, from *edo*, to eat.) Small bones fixed in the alveoli of the upper and under jaw. In early infancy Nature designs us for the softest aliment, so that the gums alone are then sufficient for the purpose of manducation; but as we advance in life, and require a different food, she wisely provides us with teeth. These are the hardest and whitest of our bones, and, at full maturity, we usually find thirty-two in both jaws; viz. sixteen above, and as many below. Their number varies indeed in different subjects; but it is seldom seen to exceed thirty-two, and it will very rarely be found to be less than twenty-eight.

Each tooth may be divided into two parts; viz. its body, or that part which appears above the gums; and its fangs or root, which is fixed into the socket. The boundary between these two, close to the edge of the gum, where there is usually a small circular depression, is called the neck of the tooth. The teeth of each jaw are commonly divided into three classes; but before each of these is treated of in particular, it will be right to say something of their general structure.

Every tooth is composed of its *cortex* or *enamel*, and its internal bony substances. The enamel, or, as it is sometimes called, the vitreous part of the tooth, is a very hard and compact substance, of a white colour, and peculiar to the teeth. It is found only upon the body of the tooth, covering the outside of the bony or internal substance. When broken it appears fibrous or striated; and all the striæ are directed from the circumference to the centre of the tooth. This enamel is thickest on the grinding surface, and on the cutting edges or points of the teeth, becoming gradually thinner as it approaches the neck, where it terminates insensibly. Some writers have described it as being vascular; but it is certain that no injection will ever reach this substance, that it receives no tinge from madder, and that it affords no appearance of a circulation of fluids. The bony part of a tooth resembles other bones in its structure, but is much harder than the most compact part of bones in general. It composes the inner part of the body and neck, and the whole of the root of the tooth. This part of a tooth, when completely formed, does not, like the other bones, receive a tinge from madder, nor do the minutest injections penetrate into its substance, although many writers have asserted the contrary. Mr. Hunter has been, therefore, induced to deny its being vascular, although he is aware that the teeth, like other bones, are liable to swellings, and that they are found anchylosed with their sockets. He supposes, however, that both these may be original formations; and, as the most convincing proof of their not being vascular, h? reasons from the analogy between them and other bones. He observes, for instance, that in a young animal that has been fed with madder, the parts of the teeth which were formed before it was put on madder diet will appear of their natural colour, but that such parts as were formed while the animal was taking the madder, will be of a red colour; whereas, in other bones, the hardest parts are susceptible of the dye, though more slowly than the parts which are growing. Again he tells us, that if you leave off feeding the animal with madder a considerable time before you kill it, you will find the above appearances still subsisting, with this addition, that all the parts of the teeth which were formed after leaving off the madder will be white. This experiment proves that a tooth once tinged does not lose its colour; whereas other bones do (though very slowly) return again to their natural appearance: and, as the dye in this case must be taken into the habit by absorbents, he is led to suspect that the teeth are without absorbents as well as other vessels. These arguments are very ingenious, but they are far from being satisfactory. The facts adduced by Mr. Hunter are capable of a different explanation from that which he has given them; and when other facts are added relative to the same subject, it will appear that this bony part of a tooth has a circulation through its substance, and even lymphatics, although, from the hardness of its structure, we are unable to demonstrate its vessels. The facts which may be adduced are, 1st, We find that a tooth recently drawn and transplanted into another socket, becomes as firmly fixed after a certain time, and preserves the same colour as the rest of the set; whereas a tooth that has been long drawn before it is transplanted, will never become fixed. Mr. Hunter, indeed, is aware of this objection, and refers the success of the transplantation, in the first instance, to the living principle possessed by the tooth, and which he thinks may exist independent of a circulation. But however applicable such a doctrine may be to zoophytes, it is suspected that it will not hold good in man, and others of the more perfect animals: and there does not appear to be any doubt but that, in the case of a transplanted tooth, there is a real union by vessels. 2dly, The swellings of the fangs of a tooth, which in many instances are known to be the effects of disease, and which are analogous to the swelling of other bones, are a clear proof of a similarity of structure, especially as we find them invested with a periosteum. 3dly, It is a curious fact, though as yet perhaps not generally known, that, in cases of phthisis pulmonalis, the teeth become of a milky whiteness, and, in some degree, transparent. Does not this prove them to have absorbents?

Each tooth has an inner cavity, which, beginning by a small opening at the point of the fang, becomes larger and terminates in the body of the tooth. This cavity is supplied with blood-vessels and nerves, which pass through the small hole in the root. In old people this hole sometimes closes, and the tooth becomes then insensible.

The teeth are invested with periosteum from their fangs to a little beyond their bony sockets, where it is attached to the gums. This membrane seems to be common to the tooth which it encloses, and to the sockets which it lines. The teeth are likewise secured in their sockets by a red substance called the gums, which every where covers the alveolar processes, and has as many perforations as there are teeth. The gums are exceedingly vascular, and have something like cartilaginous hardness and elasticity, but do not seem to have much sensibility. The gums of infants, which perform the offices of teeth, have a hard ridge extending through their whole length; but in old people, who have lost their teeth, this ridge is wanting. The three classes into which the teeth are commonly divided are, incisores, canini, and molares or grinders.

The incisores are the four teeth in the forepart of each jaw; they derive their name from their use in dividing and cutting the food in the manner of a wedge, and have each of them two surfaces, which meet in a sharp edge. Of these surfaces, the anterior one is convex, and the posterior one somewhat concave. In the upper jaw they are usually broader and thicker, especially the two middle ones, than those of the under jaw, over which they generally fall by being placed a little obliquely

The canini or cuspidati are the longest of all the teeth, deriving their name from their resemblance to a dog's tusk. There is one of these teeth on each side of the incisores, so that there are two in each jaw. They are the longest of all the teeth. Their fangs differ from that of the incisores only in being much larger, and their shape may be easily described to be that of an incisor with its edge worn off, so as to end in a narrow point instead of a thin edge. The canini not being calculated for dividing like the incisores, or for grinding, seem to be intended for laying hold of substances. Mr. Hunter remarks of these teeth, that we may trace in them a similarity in shape, situation, and use, from the most imperfect carnivorous animal, which we believe to be the human species, to the lion, which is the most perfectly carnivorous.

The molares or grinders, of which there are ten n each jaw, are so called, because from their size and figure they are calculated for grinding the food. The canini and incisores have only one fang, but the last three grinders in the under jaw have constantly two fangs, and the same teeth in the upper jaw three fangs. Sometimes these fangs are divided into two points near their base, and each of these points has, perhaps, been sometimes considered as a distinct fang. The grinders likewise differ from each other in their appearance. The first two on each side, which Mr. Hunter appears to have distinguished very properly by the name of bi-cuspides, seem to be of a middle nature between the incisores and grinders; they have in general only one root, and the body of the tooth terminates in two points, of which the anterior one is the highest, so that the tooth has in some measure the appearance of one of the canini. The two grinders beyond these, on each side, are much larger. Their body forms almost a square with rounded angles; and their grinding surface has commonly five points or protuberances, two of which are on the inner, and three on the outer part of the tooth. The last grinder is shorter and smaller than the rest, and, from its coming through the gums later than the rest, and sometimes not appearing till late in life, is called dens sapientiæ. The variation in the number of teeth usually depends on these dentes sapientiæ.

Having thus described the appearance of the teeth in the adult ; the manner of their formation and growth in the fœtus is next to be considered. We shall find that the alveolar process, which begins to be formed at a very early period, appears about the fourth month only as a shallow longitudinal groove, divided by sligh ridges into a number of intermediate depressions which are to be the future alveoli or sockets. These de pressions are at first filled with small pulpy substances included in a vascular membrane; and these pulpy substances are the rudiments of the teeth. As these advance in their growth, the alveolar processes become gradually more completely formed. The surface of the pulp first begins to harden: the ossification proceeding from one or more points, according to the kind of tooth that is to be formed. Thus in the incisores and canini, it begins from one point; in the bicuspides, from two points, corresponding with the future shape of those teeth; and in the molares from four or five points. As the ossification advances, the whole of the pulp is gradually covered with bone, excepting its under surface, and then the fang begins to be formed. Soon after the formation of this bony part, the tooth begins to be incrusted with its enamel; but in what manner this is deposited we are as yet unable to explain.—Perhaps the vascular membrane which encloses the pulp, may serve to secrete it. It gradually crystallizes upon the surface of the bony part, and continues to increase in thickness, especially at the points and basis of the tooth, till some time before the tooth begins to pass through the gum; and when this happens, the enamel seems to be as hard as it is afterward, so that the air does not appear to have the least effect in hardening it, as has been sometimes supposed. While the enamel is thus forming, the lower part of the pulp is gradually lengthened out and ossified, so as to form the fang. In those teeth which are to have more than one fang, the ossification begins at different parts of the pulp at one and the same time. In this manner are formed the incisores, the canini, and two molares on each side, making in the whole twenty teeth, in both jaws, which are sufficient for the purposes of manducation early in life As the fangs of the teeth are formed, their upper part is gradu ally pushed upwards, till at length, about the seventh, eighth, or ninth month after birth, the incisores, which are the first formed, begin to pass through the gum. The first that appears is generally in the lower jaw. The canini and molares not being formed so soon as the incisores, do not appear till about the twentieth or twenty-fourth month. Sometimes one of the canini, but more frequently one of the molares, appears first.

The danger to which children are exposed, during the time of dentition, arises from the pressure of the teeth in the gum, so as to irritate it, and excite pain and inflammation. The effect of this irritation is, that the gum wastes, and becomes gradually thinner at this part, till at length the tooth protrudes. In such cases, therefore, we may, with great propriety, assist nature by cutting the gum. These twenty teeth are called *temporary* or *milk* teeth, because they are all shed between the age of seven and fourteen, and are supplied by others of a firmer texture, with large fangs which remain till they become affected by disease, or fall out in old age, and are therefore called the *permanent* or *adult* teeth. The rudiments of these adult teeth begin to be formed at different periods. The pulp of the first adult incisor, and of the first adult grinder, may be perceived in a fœtus of seven or eight months, and the ossification begins in them about six months after birth. Soon after birth the second incisor, and canine tooth on each side, begin to be formed. About the fifth or sixth year the first bicuspis, and about the seventh the second bicuspi begin to ossify. These bicuspides are destined to replace the temporary grinders. All these permanent teeth are formed in a distinct set of alveoli; so that it is not by the growing of one tooth under another in the same socket, that the uppermost tooth is gradually pushed out, as is commonly imagined; but the temporary teeth, and those which are to succeed them, being placed in separate alveoli, the upper sockets gradually disappear, as the under ones increase in size, till at length the teeth they contain, having no longer any support, consequently fall out. But, besides these twenty teeth, which succeed the temporary ones, there are twelve others to be added to make up the number thirty-two. These twelve are three grinders on each side in both jaws; and in order to make room for this addition, we find the jaws grow as the teeth grow, so that they appear as completely filled with twenty teeth, as they are afterward with thirty-two. Hence, in children the face is flatter and rounder than in adults. The first adult grinder usually passes through the gum about the twelfth year; the second, which begins to be formed in the sixth or seventh year, cuts the gum about the seventeenth or eighteenth; and the third, or dens sapientiæ, which begins to be formed about the twelfth year, passes through the gum between the age of twenty and thirty. The dentes-sapientiæ have, in some instances, been cut at the age of forty, fifty, sixty, and even eighty years; and it sometimes happens, that they do not appear at all. Sometimes likewise it happens that a third set of teeth appear about the age of sixty or seventy. Diemerbroek tells us that he himself, at the age of fifty-six, had a fresh canine tooth in the place of one he had lost several years before; M. du Fay saw two incisores and wo canini cut the gum in a man aged eighty-four; Mr. Hunter has seen two foreteeth shoot up in the lower jaw of a very old person; and an account was lately published of a man who had a complete set of teeth at the age of sixty. Other instances of the same kind are to be met with in authors. The circumstance is curious, and from the time of life at which it takes place, and the return of the catamenia, which sometimes happens to women at the same age, it has been very ingeniously supposed, that there is some effort in nature to renew the body at that period.

The teeth are subject to a variety of *accidents*. Sometimes the gums become so affected as to occasion them to fall out, and the teeth themselves are frequently rendered carious by causes which have not hitherto been satisfactorily explained. The disease usually begins on that side of the tooth which is not exposed to pressure, and gradually advances till an opening is made into the cavity: as soon as the cavity is exposed, the tooth becomes liable to considerable pain, from the air coming into contact with the nerve. Besides these accidental means by which the teeth are occasionally affected, old age seldom fails to bring with it sure and natural causes for their removal. The alveoli fill up, and the teeth consequently fall out. The gums then

no longer meet in the forepart of the mouth, the chin projects forwards, and the face being rendered much shorter, the whole physiognomy appears considerably altered. Having thus described the formation, structure, growth, and decay of the teeth, it remains to speak of their uses; the chief of which we know to be in mastication. And here we cannot help observing the great variety in the structure of the human teeth, which fits us for such a variety of food, and which, when compared with the teeth given to other animals, may in some measure enable us to explain the nature of the aliment for which man is intended by Nature. Thus, in ruminating animals, we find incisores only in the lower jaw, for cutting the grass, and molares for grinding it; in graminivorous animals, we see molares alone; and in carnivorous animals, canine teeth for catching at their prey, and incisores and molares for cutting and dividing it. But, as man is not designed to catch and kill his prey with his teeth, we observe that our canini are shaped differently from the fangs of beasts of prey, in whom we find them either longer than the rest of the teeth, or curved. The incisores likewise are sharper in those animals than in man. Nor are the molares in the human subject similar to the molares of carnivorous animals; they are flatter in man than in these animals; and, in the latter, we likewise find them sharper at the edges, more calculated to cut and tear the food, and by their greater strength, capable of breaking the bones of animals. From these circumstances, therefore, we may consider man as partaking of the nature of these different classes; as approaching more to the carnivorous than to the herbivorous tribe of animals; but upon the whole, formed for a mixed aliment, and fitted equally to live upon flesh and upon vegetables. Those philosophers, therefore, who would confine a man wholly to vegetable food, do not seem to have studied nature. As the molares are the last teeth that are formed, so they are usually the first that fall out; this would seem to prove, that we require the same kind of aliment in old age as in infancy. Besides the use of the teeth in mastication, they likewise serve a secondary purpose, by assisting in the articulation of the voice.

TEETHING. See *Dentition* and *Teeth*.

TE'GULA HIBERNICA. See *Lapis hibernicus*.

TEGUMENTS. Under the term common integuments, anatomists comprehended the cuticle, rete mucosum, skin, and adipose membrane, as being the covering to every part of the body except the nails. See *Skin*.

TE'LA. A web of cloth. The cellular membrane is so called from its likeness to a fine web. See *Cellular membrane*.

TELA CELLULOSA. See *Cellular membrane*.

TELE'PHIUM. (Because it heals old ulcers, such as that of Telephus, made by Ulysses.) See *Sedum telephium*.

TELESIA. Sapphire.

TELLURETTED HYDROGEN. A combination of tellurium and hydrogen. To make this compound, hydrate of potassa and oxide of tellurium are ignited with charcoal, and the mixture acted on by dilute sulphuric acid, in a retort connected with a mercurial pneumatic apparatus. An elastic fluid is generated, consisting of hydrogen holding tellurium in solution. It is possessed of very singular properties. It is soluble in water, and forms a claret-coloured solution. It combines with the alkalies. It burns with a bluish flame, depositing oxide of tellurium. Its smell is very strong and peculiar, not unlike that of sulphuretted hydrogen. This elastic fluid was discovered by Sir H. Davy, in 1809.

TELLURIC ACID. *Acidum telluricum.* The oxide of tellurium combines with many of the metallic oxides, acting the part of an acid, and producing a class of compounds which have been called *tellurates*.

TELLU'RIUM. The name given by Klaproth to a metal extracted from several Transylvanian ores.

Pure tellurium is of a tin-white colour, verging to lead-gray, with a high metallic lustre; of a foliated fracture; and very brittle, so as to be easily pulverized. Its sp. gr. is 6.115. It melts before ignition, requiring little higher heat than lead, and less than antimony; and, according to Gmelin, is as volatile as arsenic. When cooled without agitation, its surface has a crystallized appearance. Before the blowpipe on charcoal, it burns with a vivid blue light, greenish on the edges and is dissipated in grayish-white vapours, of a pungent smell, which condense into a white oxide. This oxide heated on charcoal is reduced with a kind of explosion, and soon again volatilized. Heated in a glass retort, it fuses into a straw-coloured striated mass. It appears to contain about 16 per cent. of oxygen.

Tellurium is oxidized and dissolved by the principal acids. To sulphuric acid it gives a deep purple colour. Water separates it in black flocculi, and heat throws it down in a white precipitate.

With nitric acid it forms a colourless solution, which remains so when diluted, and affords slender dendritic crystals by evaporation.

The muriatic acid with a small portion of nitric, forms a transparent solution, from which water throws down a white submuriate. This may be redissolved almost wholly by repeated affusions of water. Alkohol likewise precipitates it.

Sulphuric acid, diluted with two or three parts of water, to which a little nitric acid has been added, dissolves a large portion of the metal, and the solution is not decomposed by water.

The alkalies throw down from its solutions a white precipitate, which is soluble in all the acids, and by an excess of the alkalies or their carbonates. They are not precipitated by prussiate of potassa. Tincture of galls gives a yellow flocculent precipitate with them. Tellurium is precipitated from them in a metallic state by zinc, iron, tin, and antimony.

Tellurium fused with an equal weight of sulphur, in a gentle heat, forms a lead-coloured striated sulphuret. Alkaline sulphurets precipitate it from its solutions of a brown or black colour. In this precipitate, either the metal or its oxide is combined with sulphur. Each of these sulphurets burns with a pale blue flame, and white smoke. Heated in a retort, part of the sulphur is sublimated, carrying up a little of the metal with it. It does not easily amalgamate with quicksilver.

TEMPERAMENTUM. (From *tempero*, to mix together.) The peculiar constitution of the humours. Temperaments have been variously distinguished: the division most generally received is into the sanguineous, phlegmatic, choleric, and melancholic.

TEMPERATURE. A definite degree of sensible heat, as measured by the thermometer. Thus we say, a high temperature, and a low temperature, to denote a manifest intensity of heat or cold; the temperature of boiling water, or 212° Fahr.; and a range of temperature, to designate the intermediate points of heat between two distant terms of thermometric indication.

TEMPLE. (*Tempora*, *um*, n.; and *tempus*, *oris*, n.) The lateral and flat parts of the head above the ears.

TEMPORAL. (*Temporalis*; from *tempus*.) Belonging to the temple.

TEMPORAL ARTERY. *Arteria temporalis.* A branch of the external carotid, which runs on the temples, and gives off the frontal artery.

TEMPORAL BONE. *Os temporis.* Two bones situated one on each side of the head, of a very irregular figure. They are usually divided into two parts, one of which, from the manner of its connexion with the neighbouring bones, is called *os squamosum*, and the other *os petrosum*, from its irregularity and hardness.

In both these parts there are processes and cavities to be described. Externally there are three processes; one anterior, called *zygomatic* process, which is stretched forwards to join with the os malæ, and thus forms the bony jugum under which the temporal muscle passes; one posterior, called the *mastoid* or *mamillary* process, from its resemblance to a nipple; and one inferior, called the *styloid* process, from its shape, which is said to resemble that of the ancient *stylus scriptorius*. In young subjects, this process is united with the bone by an intermediate cartilage, which, sometimes, even in adults, is not completely ossified. Three muscles have their origin from this process, and borrow half of their names from it, viz. stylo-glossus, stylo-hyoideus, and stylo-pharyngeus. Round the root of this process there is a particular rising of the os petrosum, which some writers describe as a process, and, from its appearance with the styloid, have named it *vaginalis*. Others describe the semicircular ridge of the meatus auditorius externus as a fifth process, to which they give the name of *auditory*. The depressions and cavities are, 1. A large fossa, which serves for the articulation of the lower jaw; it is situated between the zygomatic auditory and vaginal processes,

and is separated in its middle by a fissure, into which the ligament that secures the articulation of the lower jaw with this bone is fixed. The forepart of this cavity, which receives the condyle of the jaw, is covered with cartilage; the back part only with the periosteum. 2. A long fossa behind the mastoid process, where the digastric muscle has its origin. 3. The *meatus auditorius externus*, the name given to a large funnel-like canal that leads to the organ of hearing. 4. The *stylo-mastoid hole*, so called from its situation between the styloid and mastoid processes. It is likewise called the aqueduct of Fallopius, and affords a passage to the portio dura of the auditory, or seventh pair of nerves. 5. Below and on the forepart of the last foramen, we observe part of the jugular fossa, a thimble-like cavity, in which the beginning of the internal jugular vein is lodged. 6. Before and a little above this fossa is the orifice of a foramen, through which pass the internal carotid artery and two filaments of the intercostal nerve. This conduit runs first upward and then forward, forming a kind of elbow, and terminates at the end of the os petrosum. 7. At this part of the ossa temporum we observe the orifice of a canal which runs outwards and backwards in a horizontal direction, till it terminates in a cavity of the ear called tympanum. This canal, which in the recent subject is continued from the ear to the mouth, is called the *Eustachian tube*. 8. A small hole behind the mastoid process, which serves for the transmission of a vein to the lateral sinus. But this, like other foramina in the skull that serves only for the transmission of vessels, is neither uniform in its situation, nor to be met with in every subject. The internal surface of these bones may easily be divided into three parts. The first, uppermost, and largest is the squamous part, which is slightly concave from the impression of the brain. Its semicircular edge is sloping, so that the external lamella of the bone advances farther than the internal, and thus rests more securely on the parietal bones. The second and middlemost, which is the petrous part of the bone, forms a hard, craggy protuberance, nearly of a triangular shape. On its posterior side we observe a large foramen, which is the meatus auditorius internus; it receives the double nerve of the seventh pair, viz. the portio dura and portio mollis of that pair. About the middle of its anterior surface is a small foramen, which opens into the aqueduct of Fallopius, and receives a twig of the portio dura of the seventh pair of nerves. This foramen having been first described by Fallopius, and by him named *hiatus*, is sometimes called *hiatus Fallopii*. Besides these, we observe other smaller holes for the transmission of blood-vessels and nerves. Below this craggy protuberance is the third part, which, from its shape and connexion with the os occipitis by means of the lambdoidal suture, may be called the lambdoidal angle of the temporal bone. It is concave from the impression of the brain; it helps to form the posterior and inferior fossæ of the skull, and has a considerable furrow, in which is lodged part of the lateral sinus. The temporal bones differ a little in their structure from the other bones of the cranium. At their upper parts they are very thin, and almost without diploë, but below they have great strength and thickness. In the foetus, the thin upper part, and the lower craggy part, are separated by a cartilaginous substance; there is no appearance either of the mastoid or styloid processes, and, instead of a long funnel-like meatus auditorius externus, there is only a smooth bony ring within which the membrana tympani is fastened. Within the petrous part of these bones there are several cavities, processes, and bones, which belong altogether to the ear, do not enter into the formation of the cranium, and are described under the article *Ear*. The ossa temporum are connected by suture with the ossa parietalia, the os occipitis, the ossa malarum, and the os sphenoides, and are articulated with the lower jaw.

TEMPORALIS. (From *tempus*, the temple.) 1 See *Temporal*.

2. A muscle of the lower jaw, situated in the temple. *Arcardi-temporo-maxillaire*, of Dumas. *Crotaphites*, of Winslow. It arises fleshy from the lower, lateral, and anterior part of the parietal bone; from all the squamous portion of the temporal bone; from the lower and lateral part of the os frontis; from the posterior surface of the os malæ; from all the temporal pro-

cess of the sphenoid bone; and sometimes from a ridge at the lower part of this process. This latter portion, however, is often common to this muscle and the pterygoideus externus. It is of a semicircular shape, and its radiated fibres converge, so as to form a strong middle tendon, which passes under the jugum, and is inserted into the coronoid process of the lower jaw, to which it adheres on every side, but more particularly at its forepart, where the insertion is continued down to the body of the bone. This muscle is covered by a pretty strong fascia, which some writers have erroneously described as a part of the aponeurosis of the occipito-frontalis. This fascia adheres to the bones, round the whole circumference of the origin of the muscle, and, descending over it, is fixed below to the ridge where the zygomatic process begins, just above the meatus auditorius, to the upper edge of the zygomatic process itself, and anteriorly to the os malæ. This fascia serves as a defence to the muscles, and likewise gives origin to some of its fleshy fibres. The principal use of the temporal muscle is to draw the lower jaw upwards, as in the action of biting; and as it passes a little forwards to its insertion, it may at the same time pull the condyle a little backwards, though not so much as it would have done if its fibres had passed in a direct line from their origin to their insertion, because the posterior and lower part of the muscle passes over the root of the zygomatic process, as over a pulley.

TENDO. See *Muscle.*

TENDO ACHILLIS. See *Achillis tendo.*

TENDON. (From *tendo,* to stretch.) The white and glistening extremity of a muscle. See *Muscle.*

TENDRIL. See *Cirrus.*

TENE'SMUS. (From τεινω, to constringe: so called from the perception of a continual constriction or bound state of the part.) A continual inclination to go to stool, without a discharge.

TENNANTITE. A variety of gray copper ore found in Cornwall, in copper veins, that intersect granite and clay slate, associated with copper pyrites. It is of a lead-gray or iron black colour, and consists of copper, sulphur, arsenic, iron, and silica.

TE'NSOR. (From *tendo,* to stretch.) A muscle, the office of which is to extend the part to which it is fixed.

TENSOR PALATI. See *Circumflexus.*

TENSOR TYMPANI. *Internus auris,* of Douglas and Cowper. *Internus mallei,* of Winslow ; and *salpingomalleen,* of Dumas. A muscle of the ear, which pulls the malleus and the membrane of the tympanum towards the petrous portion of the temporal bone, by which the membrana tympani is made more concave and tense.

TENSOR VAGINÆ FEMORIS. *Fascialis. Membranosus,* of Douglas. *Membranus* vel *fascia lata,* of Cowper; and *Ilio aponeurosi-femoral,* of Dumas. *Musculus aponeurosis,* vel *fasciæ latæ,* of Winslow. A muscle situated on the outside of the thigh, which stretches the membranous fascia of the thigh, assists in the abduction of the thigh, and somewhat in its rotation inwards. It arises by a narrow, tendinous, and fleshy beginning from the external part of the anterior, superior, spinous process of the ilium, and is inserted a little below the great trochanter into the membranous fascia.

TENT. A roll of lint for dilating openings, sinuses, &c. See *Spongia præparata.*

TENTO'RIUM. A process of the dura mater, separating the cerebrum from the cerebellum. It extends from the internal horizontal spine of the occipital bone, directly forwards to the sella turcica of the sphenoid bone.

TEREBE'LLA. (Diminutive of *terebra,* a piercer or gimlet.) A trepan or instrument for sawing out circular portions of the skull. A trephine.

TEREBI'NTHINA. (From τερεβινθος, the turpentine-tree.) Turpentine, the produce of pine-trees. See *Turpentine.*

TEREBINTHINA ARGENTORATENSIS. Strasburg turpentine. This species is generally more transparent and less tenacious than either the Venice or Chio turpentines. It is of a yellowish-brown colour, and of a more agreeable smell than any of the turpentines, except the Chio. It is extracted in several parts of Germany, from the red and silver fir, by cutting out successively narrow strips of the bark. In some

places a resinous juice is collected from under the bark, called *Lachryma abiegna,* and *Oleum abietinum.*

TEREBINTHINA CANADENSIS. Canada turpentine. See *Pinus balsamea.*

TEREBINTHINA CHIA. The resin obtained from the *Pistacia terebinthus.*

TEREBINTHINA COMMUNIS. Common turpentine. See *Pinus sylvestris.*

TEREBINTHINA CYPRIA. Cyprus turpentine. See *Pistacia terebinthus.*

TEREBINTHINA VENETA. Venice turpentine: so called because we are supplied with it from the Venetians. See *Pinus larix.*

TEREBINTHINA VULGARIS. Common turpentine. The liquid resin of the Pinus sylvestris. See *Turpentine.*

TEREBINTHINÆ OLEUM. The oil distilled from the liquid resin of the Pinus sylvestris.

TE'RES. Round, cylindrical.

1. The name of some muscles and ligaments.

2. The name of the ascaris lumbricoides, or round worm, which infests the intestines. See *Worms.*

3. Applied to roots, stems, leaves, leafstalks, seeds, &c.

TERES LIGAMENTUM. The ligament at the bottom of the socket of the hip-joint.

TERES MAJOR. Riolanus, who was the first that distinguished this and the other muscles of the scapula by particular appellations, gave the name of *teres* to this and the following muscle, on account of their long and round shape. *Anguli-scapulo-humeral,* of Dumas This muscle, which is longer and thicker than the teres minor, is situated along the inferior costa of the scapula, and is in part covered by the deltoides.

It arises fleshy from the outer surface of the inferior angle of the scapula, (where it covers some part of the infra-spinatus and teres minor, with both which its fibres intermix,) and likewise from the lower and posterior half of the inferior costa of the scapula. Ascending obliquely towards the os humeri, it passes under the long head of the triceps brachii, and then becomes thinner and flatter to form a thin tendon of about an inch in breadth, and somewhat more in length, which runs immediately behind that of the latissimus dorsi, and is inserted along with it into the ridge at the inner side of the groove that lodges the long head of the biceps. These two tendons are included in the common capsula, besides which the tendon of this muscle adheres to the os humeri by two other capsulæ which we find placed one above the other.

This muscle assists in the rotatory muscle of the arm, and likewise in drawing it downwards and backwards; so that we may consider it as the congener of the latissimus dorsi.

TERES MINOR. *Marginisus-scapulo-trochiterien,* of Dumas. This muscle seems to have been first described by Fallopius. The teres minor is a thin fleshy muscle, situated along the inferior edge of the infraspinatus, and is in part covered by the posterior part of the deltoides.

It arises fleshy from all the convex edge of the inferior costa of the scapula; from thence it ascends obliquely upwards and forwards, and terminates in a flat tendon, which adheres to the lower and posterior part of the capsular ligament of the joint, and is inserted into the lower part of the great tuberosity of the os humeri, a little below the termination of the infra-spinatus.

The tendinous membrane, which is continued from the infra-spinatus, and spread over the teres minor, likewise forms a thin septum between the two muscles. In some subjects, however, they are so closely united, as to be with difficulty separated from each other. Some of the fibres of the teres minor are inter mixed with those of the teres major and subscapularis The uses of this muscle are similar to those of the infra-spinatus.

TE'RETRUM. (From τερεω, to pierce.) The trepan.

TERMINALIS. Terminal: applied to flower-stalk when it terminates a stem or branch ; as in *Centaurea scabiosa.*

TERMI'NTHUS. (From τερμινθος, the turpentine tree : so called from their resemblance to the fruit of the turpentine-tree.) *Albatis.* Black and ardent pustules, mostly attacking the legs of females.

TERNARY. Consisting of the number three, which

some chemical and mystical writers have made strange work with; but the most remarkable distinction of this kind, and the only one worth notice, is that of Hippocrates, who divides the parts of a human body into continentes, contenta, and impetum facientes, though the latter is resolvable into the mechanism of the two former, rather than any thing distinct in itself.

TERNATUS. Ternate: applied in botany to a leaf which consists of three leaflets, as that of the trefoil.

TERNUS. Ternate: applied to leaves, when there are three together; as in many of the plants of Chili and Peru, which seem particularly disposed to this arrangement, and in *Verbena triphylla.*

TE'RRA. See *Earth.*

TERRA CARIOSA. Rotten stone, a species of noneffervescent chalk, of a brown colour.

TERRA CATECHU. See *Acacia catechu.*

TERRA DAMNATA. See *Caput mortuum.*

TERRA FOLIATA TARTARI. The acetate of potassa.

TERRA JAPONICA. Japan earth. See *Acacia catechu.*

TERRA LEMNIA. See *Bole.*

TERRA LIVONICA. See *Bole.*

TERRA MARITA. The curcuma, or turmeric-root, is sometimes so called.

TERRA MORTUA. See *Caput mortuum.*

TERRA PONDEROSA. The heavy spar.

TERRA PONDEROSA SALITA. See *Murias barytæ.*

TERRA SIENNA. A brown ochre found at Sienna, in Italy, used in painting, both raw and burnt.

TERRA SIGILLATA. See *Bole.*

TERRA VERTE. An ore used in painting, which contains iron in some unknown state mixed with clay, and sometimes with chalk and pyrites.

TERRÆ OLEUM. See *Petroleum.*

TERREA ABSORBENTIA. Absorbent earths, distinguishable from other earthy and stony substances by their solubility in acids; as chalk, crabs' claws, oystershells, egg-shells, pearl, coral, &c.

TERRENUS. Terrene, earthy: applied to plants which grow in the earth only, in opposition to those which live only in water.

TE'RTHRA. (From τερθρον, a crane.) The middle and lateral parts of the neck.

TERTIAN. A third-day ague. See *Febris intermittens.*

Tertian ague. See *Febris intermittens.*

TERTIA'NA. See *Febris intermittens.*

TERTIANA DUPLEX. A tertian fever that returns every day; but the paroxysms are unequal, every other fit being alike.

TERTIANA DUPLICATA. A tertian fever returning every other day; but there are two paroxysms in one day.

TERTIANA FEBRIS. See *Febris intermittens.*

TERTIANA TRIPLEX. A tertian fever returning every day, every other day there are two paroxysms, and but one in the intermediate one.

TERTIANA'RIA. (From *tertiana*, a species of intermittent fever, which is said to be cured by this plant.) See *Scutellaria galericulata.*

TER'TIUM SAL. (From *tertius*, third.) A neutral salt, as being the product of an acid and an alkali, making a third body different from either.

TE'SSERA. (From τεσσαρα, four.) A four square bone. The cuboid bone.

TEST. Any reagent which, added to a substance, teaches us to discover its chemical nature or composition. See *Reagent.*

TE'STA. (*Quasi tosta*; from *torreo*, to burn.) 1. A shell. The oyster-shell.

2. In botany, it is the name of the skin which contains all the parts of a seed, as the embryo, the lobes, the vitellus, and albumen, and which gives shape to the seed, for the skin is perfectly formed while they are but a homogeneous liquid. The testa differs in thickness and texture in different plants. It is sometimes single, but more frequently lined with a finer and very delicate film, called by Gærtner *membrana*, as may be seen in a walnut, and the kernel of a peach, almond, or plum.—*Smith.*

TESTA PROBATRIX. A cupel or test. A pot for separating baser metals from gold and silver.

TESTA'DO. (From *testa*, a shell: because it is covered with a shell.)

1. A tortoise, also a snail.

2. An ulcer, which, like a snail, creeps under the skin.

TESTÆ PREPARATÆ. Prepared oyster-shells. Wash the shells, previously cleared of dirt, with boiling water, then prepare them as is directed with chalk.

TESTES CEREBRI. See *Tubercula quadrigemina.*

TESTICLE. See *Testis.*

Testicle, swelled. See *Orchitis.*

TESTI'CULUS. (*Testiculus*, diminutive of *testis.*) 1. A small testicle.

2. The *orchis* plant: so named from the resemblance of its roots to a testicle.

TESTICULUS CANINUS. See *Orchis mascula.*

TE'STIS. (*Testis, is*, m.; a witness, the *testes* being the witnesses of our manhood.) The testicle. Orchis. They are also called *didymi*, and by some *perin.* Two little oval bodies situated within the scrotum, and covered by a strong, white, and dense coat, called tunica albuginea. Each testicle is composed of small vessels, bent in a serpentine direction, arising from the spermatic artery, and convoluted into little heaps, separated from one another by cellular partitions. In each partition there is a duct receiving semen from the small vessels; and all the ducts constitute a net which is attached to the tunica albuginea. From this net-work twenty or more vessels arise, all of which are variously contorted, and, being reflected, ascend to the posterior margin of the testis, where they unite into one common duct, bent into serpentine windings, and forming a hard body called the *epididymis.* The spermatic arteries are branches of the aorta. The spermatic veins empty themselves into the vena cava and emulgent vein. The nerves of the testicle are branches of the lumbar and great intercostal nerve. The use of the testicle is to secrete the semen.

TETANIC. *Tetanicus.* Appertaining to tetanus or cramp.

TETANO'MATA. (From τετανοω, to smooth.) *Tetanothra.* Medicines which smooth the skin, and remove wrinkles.

TE'TANUS. (*Tetanus, i*, m.; from τεινω, to stretch.) Spasm with rigidity. *Convulsio indica; Holotonicos; Rigor nervosus.* A genus of disease in the Class *Neuroses*, and Order *Spasmi*, of Cullen; characterized by a spasmodic rigidity of almost the whole body. The varieties of tetanus are, 1. *Opisthotonos*, where the body is thrown back by spasmodic contractions of the muscles. 2. *Emprosthotonos*, the body being bent forwards. 3. *Trismus*, the locked jaw. Tetanus is often symptomatic of syphilis and worms.

These affections arise more frequently in warm climates than in cold ones, and are very apt to occur when much rain or moisture quickly succeeds excessively dry and sultry weather. They attack persons of all ages, sexes, temperaments, and complexions, but the male sex more frequently than the female, and those of a robust and vigorous constitution than those of a weak habit. An idea is entertained by many, Dr. Thomas observes, that negroes are more predisposed to attacks of tetanus than white people; they certainly are more frequently affected with it, but this circumstance does not arise from any constitutional predisposition, but from their being more exposed to punctures and wounds in the feet, by nails, splinters of wood, pieces of broken glass, &c. from usually going bare-footed.

Tetanic affections are occasioned either by exposure to cold, or by some irritation of the nerves, in consequence of local injury by puncture, incision, or laceration. Lacerated wounds of tendinous parts prove, in warm climates, a never-failing source of these complaints. In cold climates, as well as in warm, the locked jaw frequently arises in consequence of the amputation of a limb.

When the disease has arisen in consequence of a puncture, or any other external injury, the symptoms show themselves generally about the eighth day; bu when it proceeds from exposure to cold, they generally make their appearance much sooner.

In some instances it comes on suddenly, and with great violence; but it more usually makes its attack in a gradual manner; in which case, a slight stiffness is at first perceived in the back part of the neck, which, after a short time, becomes considerably increased, and at length renders the motion of the head both difficult and painful.

With the rigidity of the head there is likewise an uneasy sensation at the root of the tongue, together with some difficulty in swallowing, and a great tightness is perceived about the chest, with a pain at the extremity of the sternum, shooting into the back. A stiffness also takes place in the jaws, which soon increases to such a height, that the teeth become so closely set together, as not to admit of the smallest opening. This is what is termed the locked jaw, or *trismus*

In some cases, the spasmodic affection extends no further. In others the spasms at this stage of the disease, returning with great frequency become likewise more general, and now affect not only the muscles of the neck and jaws, but likewise those of the whole spine, so as to bend the trunk of the body very forcibly backwards, and this is what is named opisthotonos. Where the body is bent forwards the disease is called emprosthotonos.

During the whole course of the disorder, the abdominal muscles are violently affected with spasm, so that the belly is strongly retracted, and feels very hard, most obstinate costiveness prevails, and both the flexor and extensor muscles of the lower extremities are commonly affected at the same time so as to keep the limbs rigidly extended.

The flexors of the head and trunk become at length so strongly affected, as to balance the action of the extensor, and to keep the head and trunk so rigidly extended and straight, as to render it incapable of being moved in any direction. The arms, which were little affected before, are now likewise rigidly extended, the tongue also becomes affected with spasm, and, being convulsively darted out, is often much injured by the teeth at that moment snapping together. It is to this state of the disease that the term tetanus has been strictly applied.

The disorder continuing to advance, every organ of voluntary motion becomes affected; the eyes are rigid and immoveable, the countenance is hideously distorted, and expresses great distress; the strength is exhausted, and the pulse becomes irregular, and one universal spasm puts a period to a most miserable state of existence.

Attacks of tetanus are seldom attended with any fever, but always with violent pain, and the spasms do not continue for a constancy, but the muscles admit of some remission in their contraction, which is frequently renewed, especially if the patient makes the least attempt to speak, drink, or alter his position.

When tetanic affections arise in consequence of a wound, puncture, or laceration, in warm climates, Dr. Thomas observes, they are almost sure to prove fatal. The locked jaw in consequence of an amputation, likewise proves usually fatal. When these affections are produced by an exposure to cold, they may in most cases be removed by a timely use of proper remedies, although a considerable space will probably elapse before the patient will be able to recover his former strength.

On dissections of this disease, slight effusions within the cranium have been observed in a few instances: but in by far the greater number, nothing has been discovered, either in the brain, or any other organ.

The general indications are, 1. To remove any local irritation, which may appear to have excited the disease; 2. To lessen the general irritability, and spasmodic tendency; 3. To restore the tone of the system. If a thorn, or other extraneous substance, be lodged in any part, it must be extracted; any spicula of bone, which may have brought on the disease after amputation, should be removed; a punctured wound ought to be dilated, &c. Some have proposed dividing the nerve going to the part, or even amputating this, to cut off the irritation; others paralyzing the nerves by powerful sedatives, or destroying them by caustics; others again exciting a new action in the part by active stimulants; but the efficacy, and even propriety of such measures, is doubtful. To fulfil the second indication, various means have been proposed. The abstraction of blood, recommended by Dr. Rush, might perhaps appear advisable in a vigorous plethoric habit in the beginning of the disease, but it has generally proved of little utility, or even hurtful, and is rather contra-indicated by the state of the blood. Purging is a less questionable measure, as costiveness generally attends the disease, and in many cases it has appeared very beneficial, especially when calomel was employed. It has been found also, that a salivation, induced by mercury, has sometimes greatly relieved the disorder; but in other instances it has failed altogether. The remedy which has been oftenest employed, and with the most

decided advantage, is opium, and sometimes prodigious quantities of it have been exhibited; indeed, small doses are useless, and even large ones have only a temporary effect, so that they must be repeated, as the violence of the symptoms is renewed; and where the patient cannot swallow, it may be tried in glyster, or freely rubbed into the skin. Other sedative and antispasmodic remedies, have been occasionally resorted to, as hemlock, tobacco, musk, camphor &c. but for the most part with less satisfactory results. The warm-bath has sometimes proved a useful auxiliary in cold climates; but the cold-bath is much more relied upon, especially in the West Indies, usually in conjunction with the liberal use of opium. In Germany, alkaline baths, and the internal use of the same remedies, are stated to have been decidedly serviceable. Others have advised the large use of bark and wine, which seem, however, rather calculated to be preventives, or to fulfil the third indication; yet wine may be employed rather as nourishment, since in severe cases of the dis ease little else can be taken. Electricity seems too hazardous a remedy to be tried in a general affection, especially in the muscles of respiration; but if confined to the jaw, it may be useful in a mild form. At the period of convalescence the strength must be restored by suitable diet and medicines, the cold-bath, regular exercise, &c.; and removing the patient from the West Indies to a colder climate, till the health is fully established, would be a very proper precaution.

TETARTÆ'US. (Τεταρταιος, fourth.) A quartan fever.

TETRADYNAMIA. (From τεσσαρες, four, and δυναμις, power.) The name of a class of plants in the sexual system of Linnæus, containing hermaphrodite flowers, with six stamens, four of which are long, and two short.

TETRAGONUS. Quadrangular, square: applied to several parts of plants, as *Caulis tetragonus*, in that of the *Lamium album*, and a multitude of plants; *Folium tetragonium*, with four edges, or prominent angles, as that of *Iris tuberosa.*

TETRAGYNIA. (From τεσσαρες, four, and γυνη, a wife.) The name of an order of plants in several of the classes of the sexual system of Linnæus, con sisting of plants which, to the classic character, whatever it is, add the circumstance of having four pistils.

TETRAMY'RUM. (From τετρας, four, and μυρον, an ointment.) An ointment of four ingredients.

TETRANDRIA. (From τεσσαρες, four, and ανηρ, a husband.) The name of a class of plants in the sexual system of Linnæus. To it belong those which have hermaphrodite flowers with four stamina of equal length.

TETRANGU'RIA. (From τετρας four, and αγγος, a cup. so called because its fruit resembles a cup divided into four parts.) The citrul.

TETRAPETALOUS. Four-petalled: applied to the flower that consists of four single petals or leaves placed around the pistil.

TETRAPHA'RMACUM. (From τετρας, four, and φαρμακον, a drug.) A medicine composed of four ingredients.

TETRAPHYLLUS. (From τετρας, four, and φυλλον, a leaf.) Four-leaved.

TETTER. See *Herpes*.

TEU'CRIUM. (*Teucrium, ii*, n.; from *Teucer*, who discovered it.) The name of a genus of plants in the Linnæan system. Class, *Didynamia;* Order, *Gymnospermia.* The herb speedwell.

TEUCRIUM CAPITATUM. The systematic name of the poley mountain of Montpellier. *Polium montanum.* This plant bears the winter of our cli uate, and is generally substituted for the candy-species.

TEUCRIUM CHAMÆDRYS. The systematic name of the common germander. *Chamædrys; Chamædrys minor repens, vulgaris; Quercula calamandrina; Trissago; Chamædrops,* of Paulus Ægineta, and Ori basius. This plant, called creeping germander, smal germander, and English treacle; *Teucrium—foliis cuneiformi-ovatis, incisis, crenatis, petiolatis; floribus ternis; caulibus procumbentibus, subpilosis,* of Linnæus, has a moderately bitter and somewhat aromatic taste. It was in high repute among the ancients in in termittent fevers, rheumatism, and gout; and where an aromatic bitter is wanting, germander may be administered with success. The best time for gathering this herb is when the seeds are formed, and the tops are then preferable to the leaves. When dry, the dose is from 3 ss. to 3 j. Either water or spirit will extract their virtue; but the watery infusion is more bitter. This plant is an ingredient in the once celebrated powder called from the Duke of Portland, Portland powder.

TEUCRIUM CHAMÆPITYS. The systematic name of the ground-pine. *Chamæpitys; Arthetica; Arthretica; Ajuga; Abiga; Iva arthritica; Holocyron; Ionia; Sideritis.* Common ground-pine. This low hairy plant, *Teucrium—foliis trifidis, linearibus, integerrimis; floribus sessilibus, lateralibus, solitariis; caule diffuso,* of Linnæus, has a moderately bitter taste, and a resinous, not disagreeable smell, somewhat like that of the pine. The tops of leaves are recommended as aperients and corroborants of the nervous system, and said to be particularly serviceable in female obstructions and paralytic disorders.

TEUCRIUM CRETICUM. The systematic name of the poley mountain of Candy. *Polium creticum.* The tops and whole herb enter the antiquated compounds *mithridate* and *theriaca.* The plant is obtained from the island of Candy; has a moderately aromatic smell, and a nauseous bitter taste. It is placed among the aperients and corroborants.

TEUCRIUM IVA. *Chamæpitys moschata; Iva moschata monspeliensium; Chamæpitys anthyllus.* French ground-pine. It is weaker, but of similar virtues to Chamæpitys.

TEUCRIUM MARUM. The systematic name of the *Marum syriacum; Marum creticum; Majorana syriaca; Marum verum; Marum cortusi; Chæmedrys incana maritima;* Marum germander, or Syrian herb mastich. This shrub is the *Teucrium—foliis integerrimis ovatis acutis petiolatis, subtus tomentosis; floribus racemosis secundis,* of Linnæus. It grows plentifully in Greece, Egypt, Crete, and Syria. The leaves and younger branches, when recent, on being rubbed between the fingers, emit a volatile aromatic smell, which readily excites sneezing; to the taste they are bitterish, accompanied with a sensation of heat and acrimony. Judging from these sensible qualities of the plant, it may be supposed to possess very active powers. It is recommended as a stimulant aromatic, and deobstruent; and Linnæus, Rosenstein, and Bergius, speak highly of its utility. Dose, ten grains to half a drachm of the powdered leaves, given in wine. At present, however, marum is chiefly used as an errhine.

TEUCRIUM MONTANUM. The systematic name of the common poley mountain.

TEUCRIUM POLIUM. The systematic name of the golden poley mountain.

TEUCRIUM SCORDIUM. The systematic name of the *Scordium. Trissago palustris; Chamædrys palustris; Allium redolens.* Water germander. The leaves of this plant have a smell somewhat of the garlic kind, from which circumstance it is supposed to take its name. to the taste they are bitterish and slightly pungent. The plant was formerly in high estimation, but is now justly fallen into disuse, although recommended by some in antiseptic cataplasms and fomentations.

TEU'THRUM. Τευθρον. The herb polium. See *Teucrium polium.*

THA'LAMUS. (Θαλαμος; *Thalamus, i,* m. a bed.) A bed : the term applied to what is supposed to be the origin of the optic nerve, and to the receptacle of parts of fructification of plants. See *Receptaculum.*

THALAMUS NERVI OPTICI. Two bodies which form in part the optic nerve, placed near to each other, in appearance white, protruding at the base of the lateral ventricles, and running in their direction inwards, a little downwards, and upwards, are called the *Thalami nervorum opticorum.*

THALASSO'MELI. (From θαλασσα, the sea, and μελι, honey.) A medicine composed of sea-water and honey.

THALI'CTRUM. (*Thalictrum, ri,* n.; from θαλλω, to flourish.) 1. The name of a genus of plants in the Linnæan system. Class, *Polyandria;* Order, *Polygynia.*

2. The pharmacopœial name of the poor man's rhubarb. See *Thalictrum flavum.*

THALICTRUM FLAVUM. The systematic name of the poor man's rhubarb. The root of this plant is said to be aperient and stomachic, and to come very near in its virtues to rhubarb. It is a common plant in this country, but seldom used medicinally.

THALLITE. Epidote, or Pistacite.

THALLUS. (From θαλλος, an olive bud, or green bough; from θαλλω, to be verdant, to shoot forth, or spread abroad. A term applied by Acharius, for the frond or foliage of a lichen, whether that part be of a leafy, fibrous, scaly, or crustaceous nature.

THA'PSIA. (From *Thapsus,* the island where it was found.) The name of a genus of plants in the Linnæan system. Class, *Pentandria;* Order, *Digynia*

THAPSIA ASCLEPIAS. The deadly carrot. The root operates violently both upwards and downwards, and is not used in the present practice.

THA'PSUS. (From the island *Thapsus.*) The great white mullein, or cows' lungwort.

THE'A. Tea. The dried leaves of the tea-tree, of which there are two species, viz. 1. The *Thea nigra,* bohea, or black tea; and 2. The *viridis,* or green tea; both of which are natives of China or Japan, where they attain the height of five or six feet.

Great pains are taken in collecting the leaves *singly,* at three different times, viz. about the middle of February, in the beginning of March, and in April. Although some writers assert, that they are first exposed to the steam of boiling water, and then dried on copper plates; yet it is now understood that such leaves are simply dried on *iron* plates, suspended over a fire, till they become dry and shrivelled; when cool, they are packed in tin boxes to exclude the air, and in that state exported to Europe.

Teas are divided in Britain into three kinds of *green,* and five of *bohea.* The former class includes,

1. *Imperial* or *bloom tea,* having a large leaf, a faint smell, and being of a light green colour.

2. *Hyson,* which has small curled leaves, of a green shade inclining to blue.

3. *Singlo* tea, thus termed from the place where it is cultivated.

The boheas comprehend,

1. *Souchong,* which, on infusion, imparts a yellowish green colour.

2. *Camho,* a fine tea, emitting a fragrant violet smell, and yielding a pale shade; it receives its name from the province where it is reared.

3. *Pekoe tea* is known by the small white flowers that are mixed with it.

4. *Congo* has a larger leaf than the preceding variety, and yields a deeper tint to water; and,

5. *Common bohea,* the leaves of which are of a uniform green colour. There are besides other kinds of tea, sold under the names of *gunpowder tea,* &c. which differ from the preceding only in the minuteness of their leaves, and being dried with additional care.

The following interesting results of experiments on tea by Brande, have been published by him in his Journal.

One hundred parts of Tea.	Soluble in Water.	Soluble in Alkohol.	Precipit. with Jelly.	Inert Residue.
Green Hyson,.......... 14s. per lb.	41	44	31	56
Ditto, ... 12s.	34	43	29	57
Ditto, ... 10s.	36	43	26	57
Ditto, ... 8s.	36	42	25	58
Ditto, ... 7s.	31	41	24	59
Black Souchong, ... 12s.	35	36	28	64
Ditto, ... 10s.	34	37	28	63
Ditto, ... 8s.	37	35	28	63
Ditto, ... 7s.	36	35	24	64
Ditto, ... 6s.	35	31	23	65

Much has been said and written on the medicinal properties of tea; in its natural state it is a *narcotic* plant, on which account the Chinese refrain from its use till it has been divested of this property by keeping it at least for twelve months. If, however, good tea be drunk in moderate quantities, with sufficient milk and sugar, it invigorates the system, and produces a temporary exhilaration; but when taken too copiously, it is apt to occasion weakness, tremor, palsies, and various other symptoms arising from narcotic plants, while it contributes to aggravate hysterical and hypochondriacal complaints. Tea has also been supposed to possess considerable diuretic and sudorific virtues, which, however, depend more on the *quantity* of warm water employed as a vehicle, than the quantity of tea itself. Lastly, as infusions of these leaves are the safest refreshment after undergoing great bodily fatigue or mental exertion, they afford an agreeable beverage to those who are exposed to cold weather; at the same time tending to support and promote perspiration, which is otherwise liable to be impeded.

THEA GERMANICA. Fluellin or male speedwell. See *Veronica officinalis.*

THEBA'ICA. (*A Thebaide regione*, from the country about the ancient city of Thebes in Egypt, where it flourished) The Egyptian poppy.

THEBESII FORAMINA. The orifices of veins in the cavities of the heart.

THE'CA. (I rom τιθημι, to place.) A case, sheath, or box. 1. The canal of the vertebral column.

2. The capsule or dry fructification adhering to the apex of a frondose stem.

THECA VERTEBRALIS. The vertebral canal. See *Spine.*

THELY'PTERIS. (From θηλυς, female, and πτερις, fern.) The female fern.

THE'NAR See *Flexor brevis pollicis manus.*

THEOBRO MA. (*Theobroma, æ,* f.; from θεοι, the gods, and βρωμα, food: so called from the deliciousness of its fruit) The name of a genus of plants. Class, *Polyadelphia*; Order, *Decandria.*

THEOBROMA CACAO. The systematic name of the tree which affords cocoa and chocolate.

THEODO'RICUM. (From θεοι, the gods, and δωρον, a gift.) The pompous name of some antidotes.

THERAPEI'A. (From θεραπευω, to heal.) *Therapia.* The art of healing diseases. See *Therapeutica.*

THERAPEUTICA. (From Ξεραπευω, to cure.) *Therapia. Methodus medendi. Therapeutics.* That branch of medicine which treats of the operation of the different means employed for curing diseases, and of the application of these means.

THERI'ACA. (From Ξηρ, a viper, or venomous wild beast.) 1. Treacle, or molasses.

2. A medicine appropriated to the cure of the bites of venomous animals, or to resist poisons.

THERIACA ANDROMACHI. The Venice or Mithridate treacle; a composition of sixty-one ingredients, prepared, pulverized, and with honey formed into an electuary.

THERIACA COELESTIS. Liquid laudanum.

THERIACA COMMUNIS. Common treacle, or molasses.

THERIACA DAMOCRATIS. The same preparation as mithridate. See *Mithridatium.*

THERIACA EDINENSIS. Edinburgh theriaca. The Confectio opii.

THERIACA GERMANORUM. A rob of juniper-berries.

THERIACA LONDINENSIS. A cataplasm of cumminseed, bay-berries, germander, snake-root, cloves, and honey.

THERIACA RUSTICORUM. The roots of the common garlic were so called. See *Allium sativum.*

THERIO'MA. (From θηριοω, to rage like a wild beast.) A malignant ulcer.

THE'RMA. A warm-bath or spring. See *Mineral waters,* and Bath.

THERMOMETER. (*Thermometrum*; from θερμη, heat, and μετρον, a measure.) An instrument for measuring the degrees of heat. A thermometer is a hollow tube of glass, hermetically sealed, and blown at one end in the shape of a hollow globe. The bulb and part of the tube are filled with mercury, which is the only fluid that expands equally. When we immerse the bulb of the thermometer in a hot body, the mercury

expands, and of course *rises* in the tube; but when we plunge it into a cold body, the mercury contracts, and of course *falls* in the tube

The rising of the mercury indicates, therefore, an increase of heat; its falling, a diminution of it; and the quantity which it rises or falls, denotes the proportion of increase or diminution. To facilitate observation, the tube is divided into a number of equal parts, called degrees.

Further, if we plunge a thermometer ever so often into melting snow or ice, it will always stand at the same point. Hence we learn that *snow* or *ice* always begins to melt at the same temperature.

If we plunge a thermometer repeatedly into water kept boiling, we find that the mercury rises up to a certain point. This is therefore the point at which water always boils, provided the pressure of the atmosphere be the same.

There are four different thermometers used at present in Europe, differing from each other in the number of degrees into which the space between the freezing and boiling points is divided. These are Fahrenheit's, Reaumur's, Celsius's, and Delisle's.

The thermometer uniformly used in Britain, is Fahrenheit's; in this the freezing point is fixed at 32°—the boiling point, at 212° above 0°—or the part at which both the ascending and descending series of numbers commence.

In the thermometer which was first constructed by Reaumur, the scale is divided into a smaller number of degrees upon the same length, and contains not more than 80° between the freezing and the boiling points. The freezing point is fixed in this thermometer precisely at 0°, the term between the ascending and descending series of numbers. Again, 100 is the number of the degrees between the freezing and the boiling points in the scale of Celsius; which has been introduced into France, since the revolution, under the name of the Centigrade thermometer; and the freezing point is in this, as in the thermometer of Reaumur, fixed at 0°. One degree on the scale of Fahrenheit appears, from this account, to be equal to 4·9ths of a degree on that of Reaumur, and to 5·9ths of a degree on that of Celsius.

The space in Delisle's thermometer between the freezing and boiling points is divided into 150°, but the graduation begins at the boiling point, and increases towards the freezing point. The boiling point is marked 0, the freezing point 150. Hence 180 F. = 150 D., or 6 F. = 5 D. To reduce the degrees of Delisle's thermometer *under* the boiling point to those of Fahrenheit, we have F. = 212 — 6·5 D.; to reduce those *above* the boiling point F. = 212 + 6·5 D. Upon the knowledge of this proportion it is easy for the student to reduce the degrees of any of these thermometers into the degrees of any other of them.

Thieves-vinegar. See *Acetum aromaticum.*

THIGH. See *Femur.*

THIGH-BONE. See *Femur.*

THIRST. *Sitis.* The sensation by which we experience a desire to drink. It is variable according to individuals, and it is rarely uniform in the same person. Generally speaking, it consists of a feeling of dryness, of heat, and constriction, which reigns in the back part of the mouth, the pharynx, œsophagus, and sometimes the stomach. Though thirst continue but for a short time, these parts swell and become red, the mucous secretion ceases almost entirely; that of the follicles changes, becomes thick and tenacious; the flowing of the saliva diminishes, and its viscosity is sensibly augmented.

These phenomena are accompanied by a vague in quietude, by a general heat; the eyes become red, the mind is troubled, the motion of the blood is accelerated, the respiration becomes laborious, the mouth is frequently opened wide, in order to bring the external air into contact with the irritated parts, and thus to produce a momentary ease.

For the most part, the inclination to drink is developed, when by some cause, for example, heat and dryness of the atmosphere, the body has lost a great deal of fluid; but it appears under a great many different circumstances, such as having spoken long, having eaten certain sorts of food, or swallowed a substance which remains in the œsophagus, &c. The vicious habit of frequently drinking, and the desire of tasting some liquids, such as brandy, wine, &c., cause the developement for a feeling which has the greatest analogy with thirst.

There are people who never felt thirst, who drink from a sort of sympathy, but who could live a long time without thinking of it, or without suffering from the want of it; there are other persons in whom thirst is often renewed, and becomes so strong as to make them drink from forty to sixty pints of liquid in twenty-four hours; in this respect, great individual differences are remarked.

Thirst is an internal sensation, an instinctive feeling; it belongs essentially to the organization, and admits of no explanation.

THISTLE. See *Carduus.*

Thistle, carline. See *Carlina acaulis.*

Thistle, holy. See *Centaurea benedicta.*

Thistle, pine. See *Carlina gummifera.*

THLA'SPI. (*Thlaspi*, n.; indeclinable: from θλαω, to break; because its seed appears as if it were broken or bruised.) 1. The name of a genus of plants in the Linnæan system. Class, *Tetradynamia; * Order, *Siliculosa.*

2. The pharmaceutical name of the herb penny-cress. Two species of thlaspi are directed in some pharmacopœias for medicinal use:—the *Thlaspi arvense,* of Linnæus, or treacle mustard; and *Thlaspi campestre,* of Linnæus, or mithridate mustard. The seeds of both have an acrid biting taste, approaching to that of common mustard, with which they agree nearly in their pharmaceutic qualities. They have also an unpleasant flavour, somewhat of the garlic or onion kind.

THLASPI ARVENSE. The systematic name of the treacle mustard. See *Thlaspi.*

THLASPI CAMPESTRE. The systematic name of the mithridate mustard. See *Thlaspi.*

THORACIC. (*Thoracicus;* from *thorax,* the chest.) Belonging to the thorax, or chest.

THORACIC DUCT. *Ductus thoracicus: Ductus Pecquettii.* The trunk of the absorbents; of a serpentine form, and about the diameter of a crow-quill. It lies upon the dorsal vertebræ, between the aorta and vena azygos, and extends from the posterior opening of the diaphragm, to the angle formed by the union of the left subclavian and jugular veins, into which it opens and evacuates its contents. In this course, the thoracic duct receives the absorbent vessels from almost every part of the body.

THORAX. (*Thorax, acis,* f.; from θορεω, to leap: because in it the heart leaps.) The chest. That part of the body situated between the neck and the abdomen. The external parts of the thorax are, the common integuments, the breasts, various muscles, and the bones of the thorax. (See *Bone,* and *Respiration.*) The parts within the cavity of the thorax are, the pleura and its productions, the lungs, heart, thymus gland, œsophagus, thoracic duct, arch of the aorta, part of the vena cava, the vena azygos, the eighth pair of nerves, and part of the great intercostal nerve.

THORINA. An earth discovered in 1816 by Berzelius. He found it in small quantities in the gadolinite of Korarvet, and two new minerals which he calls the deutofluate of cerium, and the double fluate of cerium and yttria. It resembles zirconia.

To obtain it from those minerals that contain protoxide of cerium and yttria, we must first separate the oxide of iron by succinate of ammonia. The new earth, indeed, may, when alone, be precipitated by the succinates; but in the analytical experiments in which he has obtained it, it precipitated in so small a quantity along with iron, that he could not separate it from that oxide. The deutoxide of cerium is then precipitated by the sulphate of potassa; after which the yttria and the new earth are precipitated together by caustic ammonia Dissolve them in muriatic acid. Evaporate the solution to dryness, and pour boiling water on the residue, which will dissolve the greatest part of the yttria; but the undissolved residue still contains a portion of it. Dissolve it in muriatic or nitric acid, and evaporate it till it becomes as exactly neutral as possible. Then pour water upon it, and boil it for an instant. The new earth is precipitated, and the liquid contains disengaged acid. By saturating this liquid, and boiling it a second time, we obtain a new precipitate of the new earth.

This earth, when separated by the filter, has the appearance of a gelatinous, semitransparent mass. When

washed and dried, it becomes white, absorbs carbonic acid, and dissolves with effervescence in acids. Though calcined, it retains its white colour; and when the heat to which it has been exposed was only moderate, it dissolves readily in muriatic acid; but if the heat has been violent, it will not dissolve till it be digested in strong muriatic acid. This solution has a yellowish colour; but it becomes colourless when diluted with water, as is the case with glucina, yttria, and alumina. If it be mixed with yttria, it dissolves more readily after having been exposed to heat. The neutral solutions of this earth have a purely astringent taste, which is neither sweet, nor saline, nor bitter, nor metallic. In this property it differs from all other species of earths, except zirconia.

When dissolved in sulphuric acid with a slight excess of acid, and subjected to evaporation, it yields transparent crystals, which are not altered by exposure to the air, and which have a strong styptic taste.

This earth dissolves very easily in nitric acid; but after being heated to redness, it does not dissolve in it except by long boiling. The solution does not crystallize, but forms a mucilaginous mass, which becomes more liquid by exposure to the air, and which, when evaporated by a moderate heat, leaves a white, opaque mass, similar to enamel, in a great measure insoluble in water.

It dissolves in muriatic acid, in the same manner as in nitric acid. The solution does not crystallize. When evaporated by a moderate heat, it is converted into a syrupy mass, which does not deliquesce in the air, but dries, becomes white like enamel, and afterward dissolves only in very small quantity in water, leaving a subsalt undissolved; so that by spontaneous evaporation it lets the portion of muriatic acid escape to which it owed its solubility.

This earth combines with avidity with carbonic acid. The precipitates produced by caustic ammonia, or by boiling the neutral solutions of the earth in acids, absorb carbonic acid from the air in drying. The alkaline carbonates precipitate the earth combined with the whole of their carbonic acid.

The ferruginous prussiate of potassa poured into a solution of this earth, throws down a white precipitate, which is completely redissolved by muriatic acid.

Caustic potassa and ammonia have no action on this earth newly precipitated, not even at a boiling temperature.

The solution of carbonate of potassa, or carbonate of ammonia, dissolves a small quantity of it, which precipitates again when the liquid is supersaturated with an acid, and then neutralized by caustic ammonia; but this earth is much less soluble in the alkaline carbonates than any of the earths formerly known that dissolve in them.

Thorina differs from the other earths by the following properties:—From alumina, by its insolubility in hydrate of potassa; from glucina, by the same property; from yttria, by its purely astringent taste, without any sweetness, and by the property which its solutions possess of being precipitated by boiling when they do not contain too great an excess of acid. It differs from zirconia by the following properties:—1. After being heated to redness, it is still capable of being dissolved in acids 2. Sulphate of potassa does not precipitate it from its solutions, while it precipitates zirconia from solutions containing even a considerable excess of acid. 3. It is precipitated by oxalate of ammonia, which is not the case with zirconia. 4. Sulphate of thorina crystallizes readily, while sulphate of zirconia, supposing it free from alkali, forms, when dried, a gelatinous, transparent mass, without any trace of crystallization.

THORINUM. The supposed metallic basis of thorina, not hitherto extracted.

THORN. See *Prunus spinosa.*

Thorn, Ægyptian. See *Acacia vera.*

THORN-APPLE. See *Datura stramonium.*

[THOROUGHWORT. See *Eupatorium perfoliatum.* A.]

THROMBOSIS. (*Thrombosis, is,* f.; from θρομβος; The same as thrombus.

THRO'MBUS. (*Thrombus, i,* m.; from θροεω, to disturb.) A small tumour which sometimes arises after bleeding, from the blood escaping from the vein into the cellular structure surrounding it.

THRUSH See *Aphthæ.*

THRY'PTICA. (From θρυπτω, to break.) Medicines which are said to have the power of destroying stones in the bladder.

THULITE. A hard, peach-blossom coloured mineral, found at Souland, in Tellemark, in Norway.

THUMERSTONE. See *Axinite*.

THU'RIS CORTEX. The cascarilla and elutheria parks were so called. See *Croton cascarilla*.

THUS. (From θυω, to sacrifice: so called from its great use in sacrifices.) See *Juniperus lycia*, and *Pinus abies*.

THUS JUDÆORUM. See *Thymiama*.

THUS MASCULUM. See *Juniperus lycia*.

THUY'A. (From θυον, odour: so named from its fragrant smell.) *Thuja*. The name of a genus of plants. Class, *Monœcia*; Order, *Monadelphia*.

THUYA OCCIDENTALIS. The systematic name of the tree of life. *Arbor vitæ. Thuya—strobilis lævibus; squamis obtusis*, of Linnæus. The leaves and wood were formerly in high estimation as resolvents, sudorifics, and expectorants, and were given in phthisical affections, intermittent fevers, and dropsies.

THYLACI'TIS. (From θυλακος, a seed-vessel: so called from its large head.) The white garden poppy.

THY'MBRA. (A name borrowed from Dioscorides, whose real θυμβρα, however, is a species of *Saturcia*.) 1. The name of a genus of plants. Class, *Didynamia*; Order, *Gymnospermia*.

2. See *Satureia hortensis*.

THYMBRA HISPANICA. The name given by Tournefort to the common herb mastich. See *Thymus mastichina*.

THYME. See *Thymus*.

Thyme, lemon. See *Thymus serpyllum*.

Thyme, mother of. See *Thymus serpyllum*.

THYMELŒ'A. (From θυμος, thyme, and ελαια, an olive; the first alluding to the leaf, and the latter to the shape and oiliness of the fruit.) See *Daphne gnidium*.

THYMIA'MA. (From θυμα, an odour: so called from its odoriferous smell.) Muskwood. *Thus judæorum*. A bark in small brownish gray pieces, intermixed with bits of leaves, seeming as if the bark and leaves had been bruised and pressed together; brought from Syria, Cilicia, &c. and supposed to be the produce of the liquid storax-tree. This bark has an agreeable balsamic smell, approaching to that of liquid storax, and a sub-acrid bitterish taste, accompanied with some slight astringency.

THY'MIUM. (From θυμος, thyme; because it is of the colour of thyme.) A small wart upon the skin.

THYMOXA'LME. (From θυμος, thyme, οξυς, acid, and αλς, salt.) A composition of thyme, vinegar, and salt.

THY'MUS. (*Thymus, i*, m. Απο του θυμω, because it was used in faintings; or from θυμα, an odour, because of its fragrant smell.) 1. The name of a genus of plants in the Linnæan system. Class, *Didynamia*; Order, *Gymnospermia*. Thyme.

2. The pharmacopœial name of the common thyme. See *Thymus vulgaris*.

3. A small indolent carnous tubercle like a wart arising about the anus, or the pudenda, resembling the flowers of thyme, from whence it takes its name.

THYMUS CITRATUS. See *Thymus serpyllum*.

THYMUS CRETICUS. See *Satureia capitata*.

THYMUS GLAND. Θυμος. A gland of considerable size in the fœtus, situated in the anterior duplicature or space of the mediastinum, under the superior part of the sternum. An excretory duct has not yet been detected, but lymphatic vessels have been seen going from it to the thoracic duct. Its use is unknown.

THYMUS MASTICHINA. The systematic name of the common herb mastich. *Marum vulgare; Sampsuchus; Clinopodium mastichina gallorum; Thymbra hyspanica; Jaca indica*. A low shrubby plant, a native of Spain, which is employed as an errhine. It has a strong agreeable smell, like mastich. Its virtues are similar to those of the *Marum syriacum*, but less powerful.

THYMUS SERPYLLUM. The systematic name of the *Serpyllum; Serpillum; Gilarum; Serpyllum vulgare minus*. Wild or mother of thyme. *Thymus—floribus capitatis, caulibus repentibus, foliis planis obtusis basi ciliatis*, of Linnæus. This plant has the same sensible qualities as those of the garden thyme, but has a milder and rather more grateful flavour. Lemon thyme, the *Serpyllum citratum*, is merely a variety of

this plant. It is very pungent, and has a particularly grateful odour, approaching to that of lemons.

THYMUS VULGARIS. The systematic name of the common thyme. This herb, the *Thymus—erectus foliis revolutis ovatis, floribus verticillato spicatis*, of Linnæus, has an agreeable aromatic smell, and a warm pungent taste. Its virtues are said to be resolvent, em menagogue, tonic, and stomachic; yet there is no disease mentioned in which its use is particularly recom mended by any writer on the materia medica.

THYRO. Names compounded with this word belong to muscles which are attached to the thyroid car tilage; as,

THYRO ARYTÆNOIDEUS. A muscle situated about the glottis, which pulls the arytenoid cartilage forward nearer to the middle of the thyroid, and consequently shortens and relaxes the ligament of the larynx.

THYRO-HYOIDEUS. A muscle situated between the os hyoides and trunk, which pulls the os hyoides down wards, and the thyroid cartilage upwards.

THYRO-PHARYNGEUS. See *Constrictor pharyngis inferior*.

THYRO-PHARYNGO-STAPHILINUS. See *Palato pharyngeus*.

THYRO-STAPHILINUS. See *Palato pharyngeus*.

THYROID. (*Thyroideus*; from θυρεος, a shield, and ειδος, resemblance; from its supposed resemblance to a shield.) Resembling a shield.

THYROID CARTILAGE. *Cartilago thyroidea; Carti lago scutiformis*. Scutiform cartilage. The cartilage which is placed perpendicular to the cricoid cartilages of the larynx, constituting the anterior, superior, and largest part of the larynx. It is harder and more prominent in men than in women, in whom it forms the *pomum adami*.

THYROID GLAND. *Glandula thyroidea*. A large gland situated upon the cricoid cartilage, trachea, and horns of the thyroid cartilage. It is uncertain whether it be conglobate or conglomerate. Its excretory duct has never been detected, and its use is not yet known.

THYRSUS. (*Thyrsus, i*, m.; a young sprout.) In botany, a bunch, or dense and close pannicle, more or less of an ovate form. It is *oblong* in *Tussilago hybrida*, and *ovate* in *Tussilago petasites*.

TI'BIA. (*Tibia*, the hautboy; qu. *tubia*, from *tuba*, a tube: so called from its pipe-like shape.) *Focile majus; Arundo major; Fosilus;* and, from its resemblance to an old musical instrument, *Canna major; Canna-domestica cruris*. The largest bone of the leg. It is of a long, thick, and triangular shape, and is situated on the internal part of the leg. Its upper extremity is large, and flattened at its summit, where we observe two articulating surfaces, a little concave, and separated from each other by an intermediate irregular protuberance. Of these two cavities, the internal one is deepest, and of an oblong shape, while the external one is rounded, and more superficial. Each of these, in the recent subject, is covered by a cartilage, which extends to the intermediate protuberance, where it ter minates. These two little cavities receive the condyles of the os femoris, and the eminence between them is admitted into the cavity which is seen between the two condyles of that bone; so that this articulation affords a specimen of the complete ginglymus. Behind the intermediate protuberance, or tubercle, is a pretty deep depression, which serves for the attachment of a ligament, and likewise to separate the two cavities from each other. Under the edge of the external cavity is a circular flat surface, covered with cartilage, which serves for the articulation of the fibula; and at the forepart of the bone is a considerable tuberosity of an inch and a half in length, to which the strong ligament of the rotula is fixed.

The body of the tibia is smaller than its extremities, and, being of a triangular shape, affords three surfaces. Of these, the external one is broad, and slightly hollowed by muscles above and below; the internal surface is broad and flat, and the posterior surface is narrower than the other two, and nearly cylindrical. This last has a slight ridge running obliquely across it, from the outer side of the upper end of the bone to about one-third of its length downwards. A little below this we observe a passage for the medullary vessels, which is pretty considerable, and slants obliquely downwards. Of the three angles which separate these surfaces, the anterior one, from its sharpness, is called the *spinc* or *shin*. This ridge is not straight, but describes a figure like an Italic *f*, turning first inwards, then outwards, and lastly inwards again. The external angle is more rounded, and serves for the attachment of the interosseous ligament ; and the internal one is more rounded still by the pressure of muscles.

The tibia enlarges again at its lower extremity, and terminates in a pretty deep cavity, by which it is articulated with the uppermost bone of the foot. This cavity, in the recent subject, is lined with cartilage. Its internal side is formed into a considerable process, called *malleolus internus*, which, in its situation, resembles the styloid process of the radius. This process is broad, and of considerable thickness, and from its ligaments are extended to the foot. At its back part we find a groove, lined with a thin layer of cartilage, in which slide the tendons of the flexor digitorum longus, and of the tibialis posticus ; and a little behind this is a smaller groove, for the tendon of the flexor longus pollicis. On the side opposite to the malleolus internus, the cavity is interrupted, and immediately above it is a rough triangular depression, which is furnished with cartilage, and receives the lower end of the fibula.

The whole of this lower extremity of the bone seems to be turned somewhat outwards, so that the malleolus internus is situated more forwards than the inner border of the upper extremity of the bone.

In the fœtus, both ends of the tibia are cartilaginous, and become afterward epiphyses.

TIBIAL. (*Tibialis* ; from *tibia*, the bone of the leg, so called.) Belonging to the tibia.

TIBIAL ARTERY. *Arteria tibialis.* The two principal branches of the popliteal artery : the one proceeds forwards, and is called the *anterior tibial ;* the other backwards, and is called the *posterior tibial ;* of which he external tibial, the fibular, the external and internal plantar, and the plantal arch, are branches.

TIBIALIS. See *Tibial.*

TIBIALIS ANTICUS. *Tibio-sus-metatarsien,* of Dumas. A flexor muscle of the foot, situated on the leg, which bends the foot by drawing it upwards, and at the same time turns the toes inwards.

TIBIALIS GRACILIS See *Plantaris.*

TIBIALIS POSTICUS. *Tibio-tarsien,* of Dumas. A flexor muscle of the foot, situated on the leg, which extends the foot, and turns the toes inwards.

TIC DOULOUREUX. A painful affection of a nerve, so called from its sudden and momentary excruciating stroke. The more appropriate name is *neuralgia.* It mostly attacks the face, particularly that branch of the fifth pair, which comes out of the infraorbitary foramen.

TI'GLIA GRANA. See *Croton tiglium.*

TILBURY. A small town in Essex, celebrated for its fort. A mineral water is found at West Tilbury. It is an aperient and chalybeate now seldom used medicinally.

TILE ORE. A species of octohedral red copper ore.

TI'LIA. (*Tilia, æ,* f.; Πηελεα, *ulmus,* the elm-tree.) 1. The name of a genus of plants in the Linnæan system. Class, *Polyandria ;* Order, *Monogynia.*

2. The pharmacopœial name of the lime, or lindentree. See *Tilia europæa.*

TILIA EUROPÆA The systematic name of the lime-tree. The flowers of this tree are supposed to possess anodyne and antispasmodic virtues. They have a moderately strong smell, in which their virtue seems to consist, and abound with a strong mucilage. They are in high esteem in France. See *Tilia.*

TILLI GRANA. See *Croton tiglium.*

TI'LMUS. (From τιλλω, to pluck.) Floccitatio, or picking of bed-clothes, observable in the last stages of some disorders.

[TILTON, JAMES, M.D. was born in the county of Kent, in the state of Delaware, in June, 1745. His father, dying when he was very young, left him to the care of his mother, with very slender means. Notwithstanding this, he found means to study a profession, and obtained his degree of doctor in medicine from the University of Pennsylvania. He then commenced practice in his native State, and was successful in establishing himself, but the troubles of the revolution soon commenced, and in 1776 he joined the army of the United States as a surgeon, and was afterward promoted to the grade of hospital surgeon. After the successful termination of the revolutionary contest, when Dr. Tilton saw his country free and independent,

he once more retired to his native state, and recommenced the practice of his profession, which he continued for many years with distinguished reputation and abilities. In 1812, he had retired to his country-seat in the neighbourhood of Wilmington, when he was again called to take an active part in a new contest with our old enemy. After the declaration of war against Great Britain, Dr. Tilton was appointed Physician and Surgeon General of the United States Army, and continued to act in that capacity during the three years of the war.

As a physician Dr. Tilton was bold and decided ; he never temporized with disease. His remedies were few in number, but generally of an active kind. He died in May, 1822, nearly 77 years old. His publications were few, but valuable and useful. His friend, Dr. McLane, in a eulogy to his memory, gives the following summary of his character :

" In whatever view we may consider the character of Dr. Tilton, we shall find many traits to distinguish him from other men. He was in many respects an original ; wholly unlike most other men in person, countenance, manners, speech, gesture, and habits. His height was about six feet and a half, and his structure slender. Whether he walked or sat still ; whether in conversation or mute ; whether he ate, drank, or smoked ; whether in a grave mood or indulging in his loud laugh, all was in a style peculiar to himself, and most remarkable. For honesty and frankness he was proverbial ; in these important points he had few equals, certainly no superiors. His whole life afforded a luminous example of the effects of deep-rooted principles and moral rectitude upon the conduct of men ; and we have the fullest assurance to believe that he has reached those realms of peace and happiness, from which he can never be separated ; and has become the 'just man made perfect.' "—*Thach. Med. Biog.* A.]

TIMAC. The name of a root imported from the East Indies, which is said to possess diuretic virtues, and therefore exhibited in dropsies. It is not known from what plant it is obtained.

TIN. *Stannum. Jupiter* of the alchemists. It has been much doubted whether this metal is found native. In the opinion of Kirwan, there are sufficient authorities to determine the question in the affirmative. The *native oxide of tin,* or *tin stone,* occurs both massive and crystallized. Its colour is a dark brown, sometimes yellowish-gray. When crystallized, it is somewhat transparent. The *wood tin ore* is a variety of the native oxide, termed so from its fibrous texture. This variety has hitherto been found only in Cornwall. It occurs in fragments which are generally round, and its colour is brown, sometimes inclining to yellow. Tin is also found mineralized by sulphur, associated always with a portion of copper, and often of iron. This ore is called *tin pyrites.* Its colour is yellowish-gray. It has a metallic lustre, and a fibrous or lamellated texture ; sometimes it exhibits prismatic colours. Tin is comparatively a rare metal, as it is not found in great quantity any where but in Cornwall or Devonshire ; though it is likewise met with in the mines of Bohemia, Saxony, the island of Banca, the peninsula of Malacca, and in the East Indies.

Tin is a metal of a yellowish-white colour, considerably harder than lead, scarcely at all sonorous, very malleable, though not very tenacious. Under the hammer it is extended into leaves, called tin-foil, which are about one thousandth of an inch thick, and might easily be beaten to less than half that thickness, if the purposes of trade required it. Its specific gravity is 7.29. It melts at about the 442° of Fahrenheit's thermometer ; and by a continuance of the heat it is slowly converted into a white powder by oxidation. Like lead, it is brittle when heated almost to fusion, and exhibits a grained or fibrous texture if broken by the blow of a hammer. It may also be granulated by agitation at the time of its transition from the fluid to the solid state. The oxide of tin resists fusion more strongly than that of any other metal ; from which property it is useful to form an opaque white enamel when mixed with pure glass in fusion. The brightness of its surface, when scraped, soon goes off by exposure to the air ; but it is not subject to rust or corrosion by exposure to the weather.

To obtain pure tin, the metal should be boiled in nitric acid, and the oxide which falls down reduced by heat in contact with charcoal, in a covered crucible.

There are two definite combinations of tin and oxygen. The first or *protoxide* is gray : the second or *perozide* is white. The first is formed by heating tin in the air, or by dissolving tin in muriatic acid, and adding water of potassa to the solution while recent, and before it has been exposed to air. The precipitate, after being heated to whiteness to expel the water of the hydrate, is the pure protoxide. It is convertible into the peroxide by being boiled with dilute nitric acid, dried and ignited.

There are also two *chlorides* of tin. When tin is burned in chlorine, a very volatile clear liquor is formed, a non-conductor of electricity, and which, when mixed with a little water, becomes a solid crystalline substance, a true muriate of tin, containing the peroxide of the metal. This, which has been called the liquor of Libavius, may be also procured by heating together tin-filings and corrosive sublimate, or an amalgam of tin and corrosive sublimate. The other compound of tin and chlorine is a gray semitransparent crystalline solid. It may be procured by heating together an amalgam of tin and calomel. It dissolves in water, and forms a solution, which rapidly absorbs oxygen from the air, with deposition of peroxide of tin.

There are two *sulphurets* of tin. One may be made by fusing tin and sulphur together. It is of a bluish colour, and lamellated texture. It consists of 7.35 tin + 2 sulphur. The other sulphuret, or the bisulphuret, is made by heating together the peroxide of tin and sulphur. It is of a beautiful gold colour, and appears in fine flakes.

The salts of tin are characterized by the following general properties:—

1. Ferro-prussiate of potassa gives a white precipitate.
2. Hydrosulphuret of potassa, a brownish black with the protoxide ; and a golden yellow with the peroxide.
3. Galls do not affect the solutions of these salts.
4. Corrosive sublimate occasions a black precipitate with the protoxide salts ; a white with the peroxide.
5. A plate of lead frequently throws down metallic tin, or its oxide, from the saline solutions.
6. Muriate of gold gives, with the protoxide solutions, the purple precipitate of Cassius.
7. Muriate of platinum occasions an orange precipitate with the protoxide salts.

Concentrated sulphuric acid, assisted by heat, dissolves half its weight of tin, at the same time that sulphurous gas escapes in great plenty.

Nitric acid and tin combine together very rapidly without the assistance of heat.

The muriatic acid dissolves tin very readily, at the same time that it becomes of a darker colour, and ceases to emit fumes.

Aqua regia, consisting of two parts nitric and one muriatic acid, combines with tin with effervescence, and the developement of much heat.

The acetic acid scarcely acts upon tin. The operation of other acids upon this metal has been little inquired into. Phosphate, fluate, and borate of tin have been formed by precipitating the muriate with the respective neutral salts.

If the crystals of the saline combination of copper with the nitric acid be grossly powdered, moistened, nd rolled up in tinfoil, the salt deliquesces, nitrous fumes are emitted, the mass becomes hot, and suddenly takes fire. In this experiment, the rapid transition of the nitric acid to the tin is supposed to produce or develope heat enough to set fire to the nitric salts; but by what particular changes of capacity, has not been shown.

If small pieces of phosphorus be thrown on tin in fusion, it will take up from 15 to 20 per cent., and form a silvery white phosphuret of a foliated texture, and soft enough to be cut with a knife, though but little malleable. This phosphuret may be formed likewise by fusing tin filings with concrete phosphoric acid.

Tin unites with bismuth by fusion, and becomes harder and more brittle in proportion to the quantity of that metal added. With nickel it forms a white brilliant mass. It cannot easily be united in the direct way with arsenic, on account of the volatility of this metal ; but by heating it with the combination of the arsenical acid and potassa, the salt is partly decomposed ; and the tin combining with the acid, becomes converted into a brilliant brittle compound, of a plaited texture. It has been said, that all tin contains arsenic;

350

and that the crackling noise which is heard upon bending pieces of tin, is produced by this impurity; ou from the experiment of Bayen, this appears not to be the fact. Cobalt unites with tin by fusion, and forms a grained mixture of a colour slightly inclining to violet Zinc unites very well with tin, increasing its hardness and diminishing its ductility, in proportion as the quantity of zinc is greater.

This is one of the principal additions used in making pewter, which consists for the most part of tin.

Antimony forms a very brittle, hard mixture with tin Tungsten fused with twice its weight of tin, affords a brown spongy mass, which is somewhat ductile.

The uses of tin are very numerous, and so well known, that they scarcely need be pointed out. The tinning of iron and copper, the silvering of looking-glasses, and the fabrication of a great variety of vessels and utensils for domestic and other uses, are among the advantages derived from this metal.

TI'NCA. (*Tinca, æ,* f.; *quasi tincta :* so called, because it appears as if it were dyed.) The name of a genus of fishes. The tench.

TINCÆ os. The mouth of the uterus is so called by some writers from its resemblance to a tenche's mouth.

TINCAL. Crude borax, as it is imported from the East Indies in yellow greasy crystals. See *Borax*.

TINCTO'RIUS. (From *tingo,* to dye.) An epithet of a species of broom used by dyers. The genista tinctoria of Linnæus.

TINCTU'RA. (From *tingo,* to dye.) A tincture. A solution of any substance in spirit of wine. Rectified spirit of wine is the direct menstruum of the resins, and essential oils of vegetables, and totally extracts these active principles from sundry vegetable matters, which yield them to water not at all, or only in part. It dissolves likewise the sweet saccharine matter of vegetables, and generally those parts of animal bodies in which their peculiar smell and taste reside.

The virtues of many vegetables are extracted almost equally by water and rectified spirit ; but in the watery and spirituous tinctures of them there is this difference, that the active parts in the watery extractions are blended with a large proportion of inert gummy matter, on which their solubility in this menstruum in a great measure depends, while rectified spirit extracts them almost pure from gum. Hence, when the spirituous tinctures are mixed with watery liquors, a part of what the spirit had taken up from the subject generally separates and subsides, on account of its having been freed from that matter, which, being blended with it in the original vegetable, made it soluble in water. This, however, is not universal, for the active parts of some vegetables, when extracted by rectified spirits, are not precipitated by water, being almost soluble in both menstrua.

Rectified spirit may be tinged by vegetables of all colours, except blue. The leaves of plants, in general, will give out little of their natural colour to watery liquors, but communicate to spirit the whole of their green tincture, which for the most part proves elegant, though not very durable.

Fixed alkaline salts deepen the colour of spirituous tinctures ; and hence they have been supposed to promote the dissolving power of the menstruum, though this does not appear from experience. In the trials which have been made, no more was found to be taken up in the deep-coloured tinctures than in the paler ones, and often not so much. If the alkali be added after the extraction of the tincture, it will heighten the colour as much as when mixed with the ingredients at first. The addition of these salts in making tinctures is not only needless but prejudicial, as they generally injure the flavour of aromatics, and superadd a qua lity sometimes contrary to the intention of the medicine.

Volatile alkaline salts, in many cases, promote the action of the spirits. Acids generally weaken it; un less when the acid has been previously combined with the vinous spirit into a compound of new qualities, called dulcified spirit.

TINCTURA ALOES. Tincture of aloes. Take of the extract of spike aloe, powdered, half an ounce ; extract of liquorice, an ounce and a half ; water, a pint ; rectified spirit, four fluid ounces. Macerate in a sandbath until the extracts are dissolved, and then strain This preparation possesses stomachic and purgative qualities, but should never be given where there is a tendency to hæmorrhoids. In chlorotic cases and amenorrhœa, it is preferred to other purges. The dose is from half to a whole fluid ounce.

TINCTURA ALOES COMPOSITA. Compound tincture of aloes, formerly called *Elixir aloes ; Elixir proprietatis.* Take of extract of spiked aloe, powdered saffron, of each three ounces ; tincture of myrrh, two pints. Macerate for fourteen days, and strain. A more stimulating compound than the former. It is a useful application to old indolent ulcers. The dose is from half a fluid drachm to two.

TINCTURA ALOES VITRIOLATA. With the bitter infusion, a drachm or two of this elegant tincture is extremely serviceable against gouty and rheumatic affections of the stomach and bowels, and also in the weaknesses of those organs which frequently attend old age.

TINCTURA ASSAFŒTIDÆ. Tincture of assafœtida, formerly known by the name of *tinctura fœtida.* Take of assafœtida, four ounces ; rectified spirit, two pints. Macerate for fourteen days, and strain. Diluted with water, this is mostly given in all kinds of fits, by the vulgar. It is a useful preparation as an antispasmodic, especially in conjunction with sulphate of zinc. The dose is from half a fluid drachm to two.

TINCTURA AURANTII. Tincture of orange-peel, formerly *tinctura corticis aurantii.* Take of fresh orange-peel, three ounces ; proof spirit, two pints. Macerate for fourteen days, and strain. A mild and pleasant stomachic bitter.

TINCTURA BENZOINI COMPOSITA. Compound tincture of benzoin, formerly known by the names of *tinctura benzoes composita,* and *balsamum traumaticum.* Take of benzoin, three ounces ; thorax balsam, strained, two ounces ; balsam of Tolu, an ounce ; extract of spiked aloe, half an ounce ; rectified spirit, two pints. Macerate for fourteen days, and strain. This tincture is more generally applied externally to ulcers and wounds than given internally, though possessing expectorant, antispasmodic, and stimulating powers. Against coughs, spasmodic affections of the stomach and bowels, and diarrhœa, produced by ulcerations of those parts, it is a very excellent medicine. The dose, when given internally, is from half a fluid drachm to two.

TINCTURA CALUMBÆ. Tincture of calumba, formerly called *tinctura columbæ.* Take of calumba-root, sliced, two ounces and a half; proof spirit, two pints. Macerate for fourteen days, and strain. This tincture contains the active part of the root, and is generally given with the infusion of it, as a stomachic and adstringent.

TINCTURA CAMPHORÆ COMPOSITA. Compound tincture of camphor, formerly called *tinctura opii camphorata,* and *elixir paregoricum.* Take of camphor, two scruples ; opium, dried and powdered, benzoic acid, of each a drachm ; proof spirit, two pints. Macerate for fourteen days, and strain. The London college has changed the name of this preparation, because it was occasionally the source of mistakes under its old one, and tincture of opium was sometimes substituted for it. It differs also from the former preparation in the omission of the oil of aniseed, which was often complained of as disagreeable to the palate, and to which, as an addition, no increase of power could be affixed. The dose is from half a fluid drachm to half a fluid ounce.

TINCTURA CANTHARIDIS. Tincture of blistering fly. Formerly called *Tinctura lyttæ ; Tinctura cantharidum.* Take of blistering flies, bruised, three drachms; proof spirit, two pints. Macerate for fourteen days, and strain. In the last edition of the London Pharmacopœia, the colouring matter of the former preparation is omitted as useless, and the proportion of the fly increased. It is a very acrid, diuretic, and stimulating preparation, which should always be administered with great caution from its known action on the parts of generation. In chronic eruptions on the skin, and dropsical diseases of the aged, it is often very useful when other medicines have been inert. The dose is from half a fluid drachm to two.

TINCTURA CAPSICI. Tincture of capsicum. Take of capsicum-berries, an ounce ; proof spirit, two pints. Macerate for fourteen days, and strain.

TINCTURA CARDAMOMI. Tincture of cardamom. Take of cardamom-seeds, bruised, three ounces ; proof spirit, two pints. Macerate for fourteen days, and strain. A powerful stimulating carminative. In spasm of the stomach, an ounce, with some other diluted stimulant, is given with advantage. The dose may vary according to circumstances, from half a drachm to an ounce and upwards.

TINCTURA CARDAMOMI COMPOSITA. Compound tincture of cardamom, formerly called *tinctura stomachica.* Take of cardamom-seeds, carraway-seeds, cochineal of each, powdered, two drachms ; cinnamon-bark, bruised, half an ounce ; raisins, stoned, four ounces ; proof spirit, two pints. Macerate for fourteen days, and strain. A useful and elegant carminative and cordial. The dose from half a fluid drachm to half a fluid ounce and upwards.

TINCTURA CASCARILLÆ. Tincture of cascarilla. Take of cascarilla-bark, powdered, four ounces ; proof spirit, two pints. Macerate for fourteen days, and strain. A stimulating aromatic tonic, that may be exhibited in debility of the bowels and stomach, and in those cases of fever in which the Peruvian bark proves purgative. The dose from half a drachm to two drachms.

TINCTURA CASTOREI. Tincture of castor. Take of castor, powdered, two ounces ; rectified spirit, two pints. Macerate for seven days, and strain. A powerful stimulant and antispasmodic, mostly exhibited in hysterical affections in a dilute form. The dose is from half a fluid drachm to two.

TINCTURA CATECHU. Tincture of catechu, formerly known by the name *tinctura japonica.* Take of extract of catechu, three ounces ; cinnamon-bark, bruised, two ounces ; proof spirit, two pints. Macerate for fourteen days, and strain. An aromatic adstringent, mostly given in protracted diarrhœa. The dose is from half a fluid drachm to two.

TINCTURA CINCHONÆ. Tincture of cinchona. Formerly known by the name of *tinctura corticis peruviani simplex.* Take of lance-leaved cinchona-bark, powdered, seven ounces ; proof spirit, two pints. Macerate for fourteen days, and strain. The dose is from a fluid drachm to half a fluid ounce. For its virtues, see *Cinchona.*

TINCTURA CINCHONÆ AMMONIATA. Ammoniated tincture of cinchona. Volatile tincture of bark. Take of lance-leaved cinchona-bark, powdered, four ounces ; aromatic spirit of ammonia, two pints ; macerate for ten days, and strain.

TINCTURA CINCHONÆ COMPOSITA. Compound tincture of cinchona. Take of lance-leaved cinchona-bark, powdered, two ounces ; orange peel, dried, an ounce and a half; serpentary-root, bruised, three drachms ; saffron, a drachm ; cochineal, powdered, two scruples ; proof spirit, twenty fluid ounces. Macerate for fourteen days, and strain. The dose is from one fluid drachm to half a fluid ounce. For its virtues, see *Cinchona.*

TINCTURA CINNAMOMI. Tincture of cinnamon Formerly called *aqua cinnamomi fortis.* Take of cinnamon-bark, bruised, three ounces ; proof spirit, two pints. Macerate for fourteen days, and strain. The dose is from a fluid drachm to three or more.

TINCTURA CINNAMOMI COMPOSITA. Compound tincture of cinnamon. Formerly called *tinctura aromatica.* Take of cinnamon-bark, bruised, six drachms ; cardamom-seeds, bruised, three drachms ; long pepper, powdered, ginger-root, sliced, of each two drachms ; proof spirit, two pints. Macerate for fourteen days, and strain. The dose is from half a fluid drachm to two or more.

TINCTURA DIGITALIS. Tincture of fox-glove. Take of fox-glove leaves, dried, four ounces ; proof spirit, two pints. Macerate for fourteen days, and strain This tincture is introduced in the London Pharmacopœia as possessing the properties of the plant in a convenient, uniform, and permanent form; it is a saturated tincture, and in the same proportions has been long used in general practice. The dose is from ten to forty minims. For its virtues, see *Digitalis.*

TINCTURA FERRI ACETATIS. This preparation is directed in the Dublin Pharmacopœia, with acetate of potassa, two ounces ; sulphate of iron, one ounce ; and rectified spirit, two pints.

TINCTURA FERRI AMMONIATI. Tincture of ammoniated iron, formerly called *tinctura ferri ammoniacalis ; tinctura florum martialium ; tinctura martis mynsichti.* Take of ammoniated iron, four ounces ; proof spirit, a pint. Digest and strain. This is a most excellent chalybeate in all atonic affections, and may be given with cinchona in the cure of dropsical and other cachectic diseases. The dose is from half a fluid drachm to two.

TINCTURA FERRI MURIATIS. Tincture of muriate of iron. Formerly called *tinctura martis in spiritu salis; tinctura martis cum spiritu salis;* and lately known by the name of *tinctura ferri muriati.* Take of subcarbonate of iron, half a pound; muriatic acid, a pint; rectified spirit, three pints. Pour the acid upon the subcarbonate of iron in a glass vessel, and shake it occasionally for three days. Set it by that the fæces, if there be any, may subside; then pour off the solution, and add the spirit. Cline strongly recommends this in ischuria and many diseases of the kidneys and urinary passages. The dose is from ten to twenty drops. It is a good chalybeate, and serviceable against most diseases of debility without fever.

TINCTURA GENTIANÆ COMPOSITA. Compound tincture of gentian. Formerly called *tinctura amara.* Take of gentian-root, sliced, two ounces; orange-peel, dried, an ounce; cardamom-seeds, bruised, half an ounce; proof spirit, two pints. Macerate for fourteen days, with a gentle heat, and strain. The dose is from one fluid drachm to two. For its virtues, see *Gentiana.*

TINCTURA GUAIACI. Tincture of guaiacum. Take of guaiacum resin, powdered, half a pound; rectified spirit, two pints. Macerate for fourteen days, and strain. This tincture, which possesses all the active parts of this peculiar vegetable matter, is now first introduced into the London Pharmacopœia. The dose is from one fluid drachm to two. For its virtues, see *Guaiacum.*

TINCTURA GUAIACI AMMONIATA. Ammoniated tincture of guaiacum. Formerly called *tinctura guaiacina volatilis.* Take of guaiacum resin, powdered, four ounces; aromatic spirit of ammonia, a pint and a half. Macerate for fourteen days, and strain. The dose is from one fluid drachm to two.

TINCTURA HELLEBORI NIGRA. Tincture of black hellebore. Formerly called *tinctura melampodii.* "Take of black hellebore-root, sliced, four ounces; proof spirit, two pints. Macerate for fourteen days, and strain." The dose is from half to a whole fluid drachm. For its virtues, consult *Helleborus niger.*

TINCTURA HUMULI. Tincture of hop. Take of hops, five ounces; proof spirit, two pints. Macerate for fourteen days, and strain. Various modifications of the preparations of this bitter have lately been strongly recommended by Freke (Observations on Humulus Lupulus), and employed by many practitioners, who believe that it unites sedative and tonic powers, and thus forms a useful combination. The dose is from half to a whole fluid drachm. See *Humulus.*

TINCTURA HYOSCYAMI. Tincture of henbane. Take of henbane-leaves, dried, four ounces; proof spirit, two pints. Macerate for fourteen days, and strain. That the henbane itself is narcotic is abundantly proved, that the same power is also found in its tincture is also certain, but to produce the same effects requires a much larger dose. In some of the statements made to the College of Physicians of London, a different opinion has been given, and twenty-five drops have been considered as equivalent to twenty of tincture of opium: it does not produce costiveness, or the subsequent confusion of head which follows the use of opium, and will therefore be, even if its powers be weaker, of considerable use. The dose is from ten minims to one fluid drachm.

TINCTURA JALAPÆ. Tincture of jalap, formerly called *tinctura jalapii.* Take of jalap-root, powdered, eight ounces; proof spirit, two pints. Macerate for fourteen days, with a gentle heat, and strain. The dose is from one fluid drachm to half a fluid ounce. For its virtues, see *Convolvulus jalapa.*

TINCTURA KINO. Tincture of kino. Take of kino, powdered, three ounces; proof spirit, two pints. Macerate for fourteen days, and strain. All the astringency of kino is included in this preparation. The dose is from half a fluid drachm to two. See *Kino.*

TINCTURA LYTTÆ. See *Tinctura cantharidis.*

TINCTURA MYRRHÆ. Tincture of myrrh. Take of myrrh, bruised, four ounces; rectified spirit, two pints; water, a pint. Macerate for fourteen days, and strain. The dose is from half to a whole fluid drachm. For its virtues, see *Myrrha.*

TINCTURA OPII. Tincture of opium. Take of hard opium, powdered, two ounces and a half; proof spirit, two pints. Macerate for fourteen days and strain The dose is from ten minims, or twenty drops, to half a fluid drachm. For its virtues, see *Opium.*

TINCTURA RHEI. Tincture of rhubarb. Formerly known by the names of *Tinctura rhabarbari,* and *Tinctura rhabarbari spirituosa.* Take of rhubarb-root sliced, two ounces; cardamom-seeds, bruised, half an ounce; saffron, two drachms; proof spirit, two pints. Macerate for fourteen days, with a gentle heat, and strain. The dose is from half a fluid ounce to one and a half. For its virtues, see *Rheum.*

TINCTURA RHEI COMPOSITA. Compound tincture of rhubarb. Formerly called *Tinctura rhabarbari composita.* Take of rhubarb-root, sliced, two ounces; liquorice-root, bruised, half an ounce; ginger-root, sliced, saffron, of each two drachms; proof spirit, a pint; water, twelve fluid ounces. Macerate for fourteen days, with a gentle heat, and strain. This is a mild stomachic aperient. The dose is from half a fluid ounce to one and a half.

TINCTURA SCILLÆ. Tincture of squill. Take of squill-root, fresh dried, four ounces; proof spirit, two pints. Macerate for fourteen days, and strain. The virtues of this squill (see *Scilla*) reside in the tincture, which is administered in doses of from twenty drops to a fluid drachm.

TINCTURA SENNÆ. Tincture of senna. Formerly called *Elixir salutis.* Take of senna-leaves, three ounces; carraway-seeds, bruised, three drachms; cardamom-seeds, bruised, a drachm; raisins, stoned, four ounces; proof spirit, two pints. Macerate for fourteen days, with a gentle heat, and strain. A carminative, aperient, and purgative, in doses from two fluid drachms to a fluid ounce. See *Cassia senna.*

TINCTURA SERPENTARIÆ. Tincture of serpentary. Formerly called *Tinctura serpentariæ virginianæ.* Take of serpentary-root, three ounces; proof spirit, two pints. Macerate for fourteen days, and strain. This tincture possesses, in addition to the virtues of the spirit, those of the serpentaria. The dose is from half a fluid drachm to two. See *Aristolochia serpentaria.*

TINCTURA VALERIANÆ. Tincture of valerian. Formerly called *Tinctura valerianæ simplex.* Take of valerian-root, four ounces; proof spirit, two pints. Macerate for fourteen days, and strain. A useful antispasmodic in conjunction with others. The dose is from half a fluid drachm to two. See *Valeriana.*

TINCTURA VALERIANÆ AMMONIATA. Ammoniated tincture of valerian. Formerly called *Tinctura valerianæ volatilis.* Take of valerian-root, four ounces; aromatic spirit of ammonia, two pints. Macerate for fourteen days, and strain. A strong antispasmodic and stimulating tincture. The dose is from half a fluid drachm to two.

TINCTURA VERATRI. A very active alterative, recommended in the cure of epilepsy and cutaneous eruptions. Its administration requires great caution; the white hellebore being a powerful poison.

TINCTURA ZINGIBERIS. Tincture of ginger. Take of ginger-root, sliced, two ounces; proof spirit, two pints. Macerate for fourteen days, and strain. A stimulating carminative. The dose is from a fluid drachm to three.

Tincture. See *Tinctura.*

Tincture of assafœtida. See *Tinctura æssafœtidæ.*

Tincture of black hellebore. See *Tinctura hellebori nigri.*

Tincture of blistering fly. See *Tinctura lyttæ*

Tincture of calumba. See *Tinctura calumbæ.*

Tincture of capsicum. See *Tinctura capsici.*

Tincture of cardamom. See *Tinctura cardamomi*

Tincture of cascarilla. See *Tinctura cascarillæ*

Tincture of castor. See *Tinctura castorei.*

Tincture of catechu. See *Tinctura catechu.*

Tincture of cinchona. See *Tinctura cinchonæ.*

Tincture of cinnamon. See *Tinctura cinnamomi.*

Tincture of fox-glove. See *Tinctura digitalis.*

Tincture of guaiacum. See *Tinctura guaiaci.*

Tincture of guaiacum, ammoniated. See *Tinctura guaiaci ammoniata.*

Tincture of ginger. See *Tinctura zingiberis.*

Tincture of henbane. See *Tinctura hyoscyami.*

Tincture of hops. See *Tinctura humuli.*

Tincture of jalap. See *Tinctura jalapæ.*

Tincture of kino. See *Tinctura kino.*

Tincture of myrrh. See *Tinctura myrrhæ*

Tincture of opium. See *Tinctura opii.*
Tincture of orange-peel. See *Tinctura aurantii.*
Tincture of rhubarb. See *Tinctura rhei.*
Tincture of senna. See *Tinctura sennæ.*
Tincture of serpentary. See *Tinctura serpentariæ.*
Tincture of squills. See *Tinctura scillæ.*
Tincture of valerian. See *Tinctura valerianæ.*
Tincture of valerian, ammoniated. See *Tinctura valerianæ ammoniata.*
Tincture, compound, of aloes. See *Tinctura aloes composita.*
Tincture, compound, of benzoin. See *Tinctura benzoini composita.*
Tincture, compound, of camphor. See *Tinctura camphoræ composita.*
Tincture, compound, of cardamom. See *Tinctura cardamomi composita.*
Tincture, compound, of cinchona. See *Tinctura cinchonæ composita.*
Tincture, compound, of cinnamon. See *Tinctura cinnamomi composita.*
Tincture, compound, of gentian. See *Tincturæ gentianæ composita.*
Tincture, compound, of rhubarb. See *Tinctura rhei conposita.*

TI'NEA. (*Tinea;* from *teneo,* to hold.) *Tinea capitis.* The scald head: A genus of diseases in the Class *Locales,* and Order *Dialyses,* of Cullen; characterized by small ulcers at the root of the hairs of the head, which produce a friable white crust.

Tin-glass. See *Bismuth.*

TINNI'TUS. (*Tinnitus, us,* m. ; a ringing.) A ringing or tingling noise.

TINNITUS AURIUM. A noise like ringing or tingling in the ears. A species of paracusis. See *Paracusis.*

TISSUE. A term introduced by the French anatomists to express the textures which compose the different organs of animals. These have chemical and physical properties which it is important to study on the dead subject and in the living animal. We find in them almost all the physical qualities which are observed in inorganic bodies; different degrees of consistence from extreme hardness to fluidity, elasticity, transparency, refractiveness, &c. ; but we are particularly attracted by certain qualities which have been named the *properties of tissue.* These are the extensibility and contractility of tissue; the contractility *par racornissement,* from crispation. Independently of these physical qualities, the tissues have been studied in respect of their composition, and it has been found that some are principally composed of gelatine, others of albumen, others of phosphate of lime, others of fibrine, and so on. These various textures present also, in the living animal, certain phenomena which have not failed to attract the attention of physiologists.

TITANITES. A name given to certain ores of titanium which contain that metal in a state of oxide.

TITA'NIUM. This is a lately discovered metal. It was first noticed by Macgregor as existing in the state of an oxide mixed with iron, manganese, and silex, in a grayish-black sand found in the vale of Menachan, in Cornwall, and thence named menachanite, or oxide of titanium, combined with iron. It has since been discovered by Klaproth, in an ore named *titanite,* or oxide of titanium, combined with lime and silex. This ore is generally met with crystallized in four-sided prisms, not longer than a quarter of an inch. Its colour is a yellowish-red, or blackish-brown; it is opaque, and of an imperfect lustre. It breaks with a foliated, uneven, or conchoidal fracture. It exists also in an ore called red schorl, of Hungary, or red oxide of titanium. This ore, which is found generally crystallized in rectangular prisms, is of a brownish-red colour, of the specific gravity 4.2, and its texture foliated. In all these ores titanium exists in the state of an oxide.

Properties of titanium.—Titanium has been only obtained in very small agglutinated grains. It is of a red-yellow and crystalline texture, brittle, and extremely refractory. When broken with a hammer, while yet hot from its recent reduction, it shows a change of colours of purple, violet, and blue. In a very intense heat it is volatilized. Most of the acids have a striking action on this metal: though nitric acid has little effect upon it. It is very oxidable by the muriatic acid. It is not attacked by the alkalies. Nitro-muriatic acid converts it into a white powder. Sulphuric acid, when boiled upon it, is partly decomposed. It is one of the most infusible metals. It does not combine with sulphur, but it may be united to phosphorus. It does not alloy with copper, lead, or arsenic, but combines with iron.

Method of obtaining titanium.—It is extremely difficult to reduce the oxide of titanium to the metallic state. However, the experiments of Klaproth, Hecht, and Vauquelin have proved its reducibility. According to the two latter, one part of oxide of tetanium is to be melted with six of potassa; the mass, when cold, is to be dissolved in water. A white precipitate will be formed which is carbonate of titanium. This carbonate is then made into a paste with oil, and the mixture is put into a crucible filled with charcoal powder and a little alumine. The whole is then exposed for a few hours to the action of a strong heat. The metallic titanium will be found in the form of a blackish puffed-up substance, possessing a metallic appearance.

[A very curious ore of titanium, one of the newly discovered metals, has been found to exist in New-Jersey. A specimen of considerable size had been presented, several years ago, by Mr. Alber to Dr. Mitchill, as an ore of zinc. But it not appearing to him to be an ore of zinc, and indeed, his mind remaining rather uncertain as to what it truly was, he laid it aside in his cabinet, and at length furnished Professor Bruce with a part of it. This able mineralogist has not only made it a subject of experiment himself, but has taken the opinion of some of his chemical correspondents in Europe upon it; and it is their united opinion that it is composed chiefly of the oxide of titanium, combined with the other form of the metal, which, from its having been found in the valley of Menachan, in Cornwall, England, has been called Menachanite.

A further account of this remarkable substance is contained in a letter, from Professor Woodhouse to Senator Mitchill.

" The following experiments were performed upon the mineral found in New-Jersey, which I received from you in the year 1805, which was then supposed, by the person who presented it to you, to be an ore of zinc, and which Count Bournon has declared to be composed of iron and titanium.

" The specific gravity of this mineral is 5.28. When viewed, it has the appearance of black spots, the size of duck shot, surrounded by a red substance; and streaks of a white powder, (which is lithormarge,) are dispersed through it. Upon looking through a microscope, a crystal of titanium was seen adhering to it. One hundred grains of it, reduced to an impalpable powder, and exposed one hour to the intense heat of, an air furnace, lost fifteen grains in weight, and from a brown was turned to a black colour.

" One hundred grains of it, submitted to heat in the same manner with charcoal, produced a great number of small globules of pure iron. This metal can be separated from the powder by a magnet.

" One hundred grains of it, boiled in aqua regia, was totally soluble in this agent, which proves it contains no silex.

" The prussiate of potash, added to this solution, yielded a blue precipitate, which, when dried, weighed three hundred grains. Now, if we divide this sum by six, we shall have the quantity of metallic iron in the hundred grains of the ore, which is fifty.

" A portion of lime was thrown down from a solution of the mineral in aqua regia, by the oxalate of potash. Carbonate of ammonia, and a solution of potash produced a copious white and gelatinous precipitate.

" One hundred grains of it were mixed with six hundred of potash, and submitted to intense heat one hour, in a blacklead crucible. The part remaining in the crucible was powdered, boiled in water, and filtered. Upon adding a small portion of muriatic acid to the water, a white precipitate was thrown down, which was supposed to be the titanium. Upon collecting it, and mixing it with a small portion of spermaceti oil and charcoal, it was exposed to the heat of a blacksmith's forge, when nothing was obtained but a shining, heavy, black substance, of the appearance of glass.

" When the muriatic acid was added in excess to the filtered water obtained, by boiling the residue, which remained in the crucible, in water, no precipitate was produced, until a solution of potash was added to neutralize the acid.

" The solution of the mineral in nitric acid is astringent to the taste.

" " The ore appears to be composed of iron, titanium, lime, alumina, and no silicous earth."—*Med. Repos.*

From the above it appears that the ores of titanium are of very frequent occurrence within the United States. The locality of the specimens described, as far as could be ascertained, tend to confirm the opinion of Werner, as to titanium being one of the oldest of metals. Should this metal hereafter be applied extensively to the arts, it is presumed that the United States will be enabled to furnish any quantity required.—*Min. Jour.* A.]

TITHY'MALUS. (From τιθος, a dug, and μαλος, tender: so called from its smooth leaves and milky juice.) Spurge. Two plants are directed for medicinal purposes by this name. See *Euphorbia paralias,* and *Esula minor.*

TITHYMALUS CYPARISSIUS. See *Esula minor.*

TITHYMALYS PARALIOS. See *Euphorbia paralias.*

TITHYMELÆ'A. See *Daphne gnidium.*

TIT'LLICUM. (From *titillo,* to tickle: so called from its being easily tickled,) The arm-pit.

TOAD-FLAX. See *Antirrhinum linaria.*

TOBACCO. See *Nicotiana.*

Tobacco, English. See *Nicotiana rustica.*

Tobacco, Virginian. See *Nicotiana.*

TOE. *Digitus pedis.* The toes consist of three distinct bones disposed in rows, called phalanges, or rank of the toes. The great toe has but two phalanges; the others have three ranks of bones, which' have nothing particular, only the joints are made round and free, formed by a round head on one bone, and by a pretty deep hollow for receiving it, in the one above it.

TOFFANIA AQUA. (*Toffana;* or *Tophania;* the name of an infamous woman, who resided at Palermo, and afterward at Naples, who sold this poison.) See *Aquetta.*

Tolu balsam. See *Toluifera balsamum.*

TOLUI'FERA. (So called because it produces the balsam of Peru.) The name of a genus of plants in the Linnæan system. Class, *Decandria;* Order, *Monogynia.*

TOLUIFERA BALSAMUM. The systematic name of the tree which affords the Tolu balsam. *Balsamum tolutanum.* Balsam of Tolu. It grows in South America, in the province of Tolu, behind Carthagena, whence we are supplied with the balsam, which is brought to us in little gourd-shells. The balsam is obtained by making incisions into the bark of the tree, and is collected into spoons, which is made of black wax, from which it is poured into proper vessels. It thickens, and in time becomes concrete: it has a fragrant colour, and a warm, sweetish taste. It dissolves entirely in alkohol, and communicates its odour and taste to water, by boiling. It contains acid of benzoin. This is the mildest of all the balsams. It has been used as an expectorant; but its powers are very inconsiderable, and it is at present employed principally on account of its flavour, somewhat resembling that of lemons. It is directed, by the pharmacopœias, in the Syrupus solutanus, Tinctura tolutana, and Syrupus balsamicus.

TOLUTANUM BALSAMUM. See *Toluifera balsamum.*

TOMATUM. Love apple. See *Solanum lycopersicum.*

TOMBAC. A white alloy of copper with arsenic.

TOMBEI'UM. (From τεμνω, to cut.) An incision-knife.

TOMENTI'TIA. (From *tomentum,*a flock of wool: so called from its soft coat.) Cotton-weed.

TOMENTOSUS. Downy. Applied to stems, leaves, &c. as the stem of the Geranium rotundifolium.

TOME'NTUM. (*Tomentum, i, n.;* a flock of wool.)

1. This term is used in anatomy to the small vessels of the brain, which appear like wool.

2. In botany, a species of pubescence, very soft to the touch, of a white, or ferruginous colour, giving the surface a downy appearance, and so thick that they cannot be seen separately.

TOMENTUM CEREBRI. The small vessels that penetrate the cortical substance of the brain from the pia mater, which, when separated from the brain, and adhering to the pia mater, give it a flocky appearance.

TONGUE. *Lingua.* A soft, fleshy viscus, very

moveable in every direction, situated inferiorly in the cavity of the mouth, and constituting the organ of taste. It is divided into a base, body, and back, an inferior surface, and two lateral parts. It is composed of muscular fibres, covered by a nervous membrane, on which are a great number of nervous papillæ, particularly at the apex, and lateral parts, the rete mucosum, and epidermis. The arteries of the tongue are branches of the ranine and labial. The veins empty themselves into the great linguals, which proceed to the external jugular. The nerves come from the eighth, ninth, and fifth pair. The use of this organ is for chewing, swallowing, sucking, and tasting. See also *Taste.*

Tongue-shaped. See *Lingulatus.*

TONIC. (*Tonicus,* Τονικος; from τεινω, to pull or draw.) 1. A rigid contraction of the muscles, without relaxation, as in trismus, tetanus, &c. See *Tetanus.*

2. (From τονοω, to strengthen.) Medicines which increase the tone of the muscular fibre, such as vegetable bitters; also stimulants, astringents, &c.

TONSIL. (*Tonsillæ,* arum, f.) *Amygdala; Tola; Toles; Tolles.* An oblong, suboval gland, situated on each side of the fauces, and opening into the cavity of the mouth by twelve or more large excretory ducts

TOOTH. See *Teeth.*

TOOTHACHE. See *Odontalgia.*

Tooth-shaped. See *Dentatus.*

TOPAZ. According to Jameson this mineral species contains three subspecies common topaz, schorlite, and physalite.

Common topaz is of a wine-yellow colour, in granular crystallized concretions, harder than emerald. It comes from the Brazils, Siberia, Asia Minor, and Saxony. It forms an essential constituent of the topaz-rock.

TOPAZOLITE. A variety of precious garnet found at Mussa, in Piedmont.

TO'PHUS. (*Toph,* Hebrew.) A toph. *Epiporoma,* a soft swelling on a bone.) The concretion on the teeth or in the joints of gouty people. Also gravel.

TO'PICAL. (From τοπος, a place.) Medicines applied to a particular place.

TOPINA'RIA. A species of tumour in the skin of th*e* head.

TO'RCULAR. (From *torqueo,* to twist.) The tourniquet: a bandage to check hæmorrhages after wounds or amputations.

TORCULAR HEROPHILI. *Lechenon; Lenos.* The press of Herophilus. That place where the four sinuses of the dura mater meet together, first accurately described by Herophilus, the anatomist.

TORDY'LIUM. (*Tordylium, ii,* n. *Quasi tortilium;* from *torqueo,* to twist: so named from its tortuous branches, or from the neat orbicular figure of its seed, which seem as if artificially wrought or turned.) Che name of a genus of plants in the Linnæan system. Tlass, *Pentandria;* Order, *Digynia*

TORDYLIUM OFFICINALE. The systematic name of the officinale *seseli creticum.* The seeds are said to be diuretic.

TORMENTIL. See *Tormentilla.*

TORMENTI'LLA. (From *tormentum,* pain; because it was supposed to relieve pain in the teeth.) 1. The name of a genus of plants in the Linnæan system. Class, *Icosandria;* Order, *Monogynia.*

2. The pharmacopœial name of the upright stepfoil See *Tormentilla erecta.*

TORMENTILLA ERECTA. The systematic name of the upright stepfoil. *Heptaphyllum; Consolida rubra; Tormentilla—caule erectiusculo, foliis sessilibus,* of Linnæus. The root is the only part of the plant which is used medicinally; it has a strong styptic taste, but imparts no peculiar sapid flavour: it has been long held in estimation as a powerful astringent; and, as a proof of its efficacy in this way, it has been substituted for oak bark in the tanning of skins for leather. Tormentil is ordered in the *pulvis cretæ compositus,* of the London Pharmacopœia.

TO'RMINA. Severe pains.

TO'RPOR. A numbness, or deficient sensation.

TORTICO'LLIS. (From *torqueo,* to twist, and *collum,* the neck.) The wry neck.

TORTULOSUS. A little swelling out. Applied to the knotty pod of the *Rhaphanus sativus.*

TORTU'RA OSSIS. The locked jaw.

TOTA BONA. See *Chenopodium bonus henricus.*

TOUCH. *Tactus.* " By touch we are enabled to know the properties of bodies ; and as it is less subject to deception than the other senses, enabling us in certain cases to clear up errors into which the others have led us, it has been considered the first and the most excellent of all the senses ; but several of the advantages which have been attributed to it by physiologists and metaphysicians should be considerably limited.

We ought to distinguish *tact* from touch. *Tact* is, with some few exceptions, generally diffused through all our organs, and particularly over the cutaneous and mucous surfaces. It exists in all animals ; while touch is exerted evidently only by parts that are intended particularly for this use. It does not exist in all animals, and it is nothing else but *tact* united to muscular contractions directed by the will.

In the exercise of *tact,* we may be considered as passive, while we are essentially active in the exercise of *touch.*

Physical properties of bodies which employ the action of touch. Almost all the physical properties of bodies are susceptible of acting upon the organs of touch ; form, dimensions, different degrees of consistence, weight, temperature, locomotion, vibration, &c. are all so many circumstances that are exactly appreciated by the touch.

The organs destined to touch do not alone exercise this function ; so that in this respect the touch differs much from the other senses. As in most cases it is the skin which receives the tactile impressions produced by the bodies which surround us, it is necessary to say something of its structure.

The skin forms the envelope of the body ; it is lost in the mucous membranes at the entrance of all the cavities ; but it is improper to say that these membranes are a continuation of it.

The skin is formed principally by the *cutis vera,* a fibrous layer of various thickness, according to the part which it covers ; it adheres by a cellular tissue, more or less firm, at other times by fibrous attachments. The *cutis* is almost always separated from the subjacent parts by a layer of a greater or less thickness, which is of use in the exercise of touch.

The external side of the *cutis vera* is covered by the epidermis, a solid matter secreted by the skin. We ought not to consider the epidermis as a membrane ; it is a homogeneous layer, adherent by its internal face to the *chorion,* and full of a great number of holes, of which the one sort are for the passage of the hair, and the other for that of cutaneous perspiration ; they serve at the same time for the absorption which takes place by the skin. These last are called the pores of the skin.

It is necessary to notice, with regard to the epidermis, that it is void of feeling ; that it possesses none of the properties of life ; that it is not subject to putrefaction ; that it wears and is renewed continually ; that its thickness augments or lessens as it may be necessary : it is even said to be proof to the action of the digestive organs.

The connexion of the epidermis to the *cutis vera* is very close ; and yet it cannot be doubted that there is a particular layer between these two parts, in which certain particular phenomena take place. The organization of this layer is yet little known. Malpighi believed it to be formed of a particular mucus, the existence of which has been long admitted, and which bore the name of the corpus mucosum of Malpighi. Other authors have considered it, more justly, as a vascular net-work. Gall makes it similar to the gray matter which is seen in many parts of the brain.

Gantier, in examining attentively the external surface of the true skin, has noticed some small reddish projections, disposed in pairs ; they are easily perceived when the skin is laid bare by a blister. These little bodies are regularly disposed upon the palm of the hand, and on the sole of the foot. They are sensible, and are reproduced when they have been torn out. They appear to be essentially vascular. These bodies, without being understood, have been long called the *papillæ* of the skin. The epidermis is pierced by little holes, opposite their tops, through which small drops of sweat are seen to issue, when the skin is exposed to an elevated temperature. The skin contains a great number of sebaceous follicles ; it contains a great number of vessels and nerves, particularly at the

points where the sense of touch is more immediately exercised. The mode in which the nerves are terminated in the skin is totally unknown ; all that has been said of the cutaneous nervous papillæ is entirely hypothetical.

The exercise of tact and of touch is facilitated by the thinness of the *cutis vera,* by a gentle elevation of temperature, by an abundant cutaneous perspiration, as well as by a certain thickness and flexibility of the epidermis ; when the contrary dispositions exist, the tact and the touch are always more or less imperfect.

Mechanism of tact.—The mechanism of tact is extremely simple ; it is sufficient that bodies be in contact with the skin to furnish us with *data,* more or less exact, of their tactile properties. By tact we judge particularly of the temperature. When bodies deprive us of caloric, we call them cold ; when they yield it to us, we say they are hot ; and according to the quantity of caloric which they give or take, we determine their different degrees of heat or cold. The notions that we have of temperature are, nevertheless, far from being exactly in relation to the quantity of caloric that bodies yield to us, or take from us ; we join with it unawares a comparison with the temperature of the atmosphere, in such a manner that a body colder than ours, but hotter than the atmosphere, appears hot, though it really deprive us of caloric when we touch it. On this account, places which have a uniform temperature, such as cellars or wells, appear cold in summer, and hot in winter. The capacity also of bodies for caloric has a great influence upon us with regard to temperature ; as an example of this, we have only to notice the great difference of sensation produced by iron and wood, though the temperature of both be the same.

A body which is sufficiently hot to cause a chemical decomposition of our organs produces the sensation of burning. A body whose temperature is so low as to absorb quickly a great portion of the caloric of any part, produces a sensation of the same sort nearly : this may be proved in touching frozen mercury.

The bodies which have a chemical action upon the epidermis, those that dissolve it, as the caustic alkalies, and concentrated acids, produce an impression which is easy to be recognised, and by which these bodies may be known.

Every part of the skin is not endowed with the same sensibility ; so that the same body applied to different points of the skin in succession will produce a series of different impressions.

The mucous membranes possess great delicacy of tact. Every one knows the great sensibility of the lips, the tongue, of the conjunctiva, the pituitary membrane, of the mucous membrane, of the trachea, of the urethra, of the vagina, &c. The first contact of bodies, which are not destined naturally to touch these membranes, is painful at first, but this soon wears off.

Mechanism of touch.—In man, the hand is the principal organ of touch ; all the most suitable circumstances are united in it. The epidermis is thin, smooth, flexible ; the cutaneous perspiration abundant, as well as the oily secretion. The vascular eminences are more numerous there than any where else. The *cutis vera* has but little thickness ; it receives a great number of vessels and nerves ; it adheres to the subjacent *aponeuroses* by fibrous adhesions ; and it is sustained by a highly elastic cellular tissue. The extremities of the fingers possess all these properties in the highest degree : the motions of the hand are very numerous, and performed with facility, and it may be applied with ease to any body of whatsoever form.

As long as the hand remains immoveable at the surface of a body, it acts only as an organ of *tact.* To exercise *touch,* it must move, either by passing over the surface, to examine form, dimensions, &c., or to press it for the purpose of determining its consistence, elasticity, &c.

We use the whole hand to touch a body of considerable dimensions ; if, on the contrary, a body is very small, we employ only the points of the fingers. This delicacy of touch in the fingers has given man a great advantage over the animals. His touch is so delicate, that it has been considered the source of his intelligence.

From the highest antiquity the touch has been considered of more importance than any of the other senses ; it has been supposed the cause of human reason. This idea has continued to our times; it has been even remarkably extended in the writings of Condillac, of Buffon, and other modern physiologists. Buffon, in particular, gave such an importance to the touch, that he thought one man had little more ability than another, but only in so far as he had been in the habit of making use of his hands. He said it would be well to allow children the free use of their hands from the moment of their birth.

The touch does not really possess any prerogative over the other senses; and if in certain cases it assists the eye or the ear, it receives aid from them in others, and there is no reason to believe that it excites ideas in the brain of a higher order than those which are produced by the action of the other senses.

Of internal sensations.—All the organs, as well as the skin, possess the faculty of transmitting impressions to the brain, when they are touched by exterior bodies, or when they are compressed, bruised, &c. It may be said, that they generally possess *tact*. There must be an exception made of the bones, the tendons, the *aponeuroses*, the ligaments, &c.; which in a healthy state is insensible, and may be cut, burned, torn, without any thing being felt by the brain.

This important fact was not known to the ancients; they considered all the white parts as nervous, and attributed to them all those properties which we now know belong only to the nerves. These useful results, which have had a great influence upon the recent progress of surgery, we owe to Haller and his disciples.

All the organs are capable of transmitting spontaneously a great number of impressions to the brain without the intervention of any external cause. They are of three sorts. The first kind take place when it is necessary for the organs to act; they are called *wants, instinctive desires*. Such are hunger, thirst, the necessity of making water, of respiration, the venereal impulse, &c. The second sort take place during the action of the organs; they are frequently obscure, sometimes very violent. The impressions which accompany the different excretions, as of the *semen*, the *urine*, are of this number.

Such are also the impressions which inform us of our motions, of the periods of digestion:—even thought seems to belong to this kind of impression.

The third kind of internal sensations are developed when the organs have acted. To this kind belongs the feeling of fatigue, which is variable in the different sorts of functions.

The impressions which are felt in sickness ought to be added to these three sorts: these are much more numerous than the others. The study of them is absolutely necessary to the physician.

All those sensations which proceed from within, and which have no dependence upon the action of exterior bodies, have been collectively denominated *internal sensations, or feelings.*"—*Magendie's Physiology.*

TOUCH-ME-NOT. See *Noli me tangere.*

TOUCHSTONE. Lydian stone. A variety of flinty slate.

TOUCHWOOD. See *Agaricus.*

TOURMALINE. Rhomboidal tourmaline is divided into two subspecies, schorl and tourmaline. The latter mineral is of a green, brown, and red colour, in prismatic concretions, rolled pieces, but generally crystallized. It occurs in gneiss, mica slate, talc slate, &c.

TOURNEFORT, JOSEPH PITTON DE, was born at Aix, in Provence, in 1656. He was destined for the church, but a taste for natural knowledge led him, at his father's death, to change for the profession of physic. He therefore qualified himself thoroughly in anatomy, chemistry, and other branches of medical study, and likewise distinguished himself as an elegant writer and lecturer; but he displayed especially an ardent devotion to botany, which ever after made the chief object of his life. His zeal in this pursuit led him to encounter considerable danger in exploring the Alps, Pyrenees, &c. during several seasons, passing the intermediate winters at Montpellier; but he is said to have graduated at Orange. His merits as a botanist, soon became conspicuous at Paris, and the superintendence of the royal garden was resigned to him, by Fagon. In this school he soon drew together a crowd of students; but anxious for farther improvements, he travelled into the neighbouring countries, and thus greatly enriched his collections. He was admitted a member of the Academy of Sciences, and of the Me-

dical Faculty at Paris; and was likewise decorated with the Order of St. Michael. He published about the same period several botanical works, of which the principal is entitled, " Institutiones Rei Herbariæ." In the year 1700, he set out, under royal patronage, on a voyage to the Levant, with the view of investigating the plants of ancient writers, and making new discoveries; and on his return, after two years, he wrote a very interesting and valuable account of the expedition in French, which was not published, however, till after his death. This took place in 1708, in consequence of a hurt in the breast, which he received from a carriage. He left his collection of plants to the king, who bestowed in return a pension of a thousand livres on his nephew. Besides the botanical works published by him, he is said to have left several others in manuscript. One object, which had occupied much of his attention, was to determine the medical virtues of plants by a chemical analysis; but the loss of these labours is not to be regretted, as those of Geoffroy, on the same plan, turned out to be without any solid advantage. The elegance and facility of Tournefort's botanical method gained him many followers at first; but it has since been superseded by that of Linnæus, which is much more systematic and comprehensive. Still, however, it must be acknowledged, that the generic distinctions established by the former botanist, and most accurately delineated, have been the principal foundation of subsequent improvements.

TOURNIQUET. (French; from *tourner*, to turn.) An instrument used for stopping the flow of blood into a limb.

TOXICA'RIA. (*Toxicaria, æ,* f.; from τοξικον, a poison: so called from its poisonous quality.) The name of a plant.

TOXICARIA MACASSARIENSIS. An Indian poison obtained from a tree hitherto undescribed by any medical botanist, known by the name of Boas-upas: it is a native of Southern Asia. Concerning this plant, various and almost incredible particulars have been related, both in ancient and modern times; some of them true, others probably founded on superstition. Rumphius testifies that he had not met with any other more dreadful product from any vegetable. And he adds, that this poison, of which the Indians boast, was much more terrible to the Dutch than any warlike instrument. He likewise says, it is his opinion, that it is of the same natural order, if not of the same genus as the cestrum.

TOXICODE'NDRUM. (From τοξικον, a poison, and δενδρον, a tree.) The poison-tree, which is so noxious that no insects ever come near it. See *Rhus toxicodendron.*

TOXICOLOGY. (*Toxicologia;* from τοξον, an arrow or bow; because the darts of the ancients were usually besmeared with some poisonous substance; and λογος, a discourse.) A dissertation on poisons See *Poison.*

TO'XICUM. (From τοξον, an arrow, which was sometimes poisoned.) A deadly poison. See *Poison.*

TOXITE'SIA. The artemisia or mugwort.

TRABE'CULA. (*Trabecula,* a small beam.) This word is mostly applied by anatomists to the small medullary fibres of the brain, which constitute the commissures.

TRA'CHEA. (So called from its roughness; from τραχυς, rough.) The windpipe. The trachea is a cartilaginous and membranous canal, through which the air passes into the lungs. Its upper part, which is called the larynx, is composed of five cartilages. The uppermost and smallest of these cartilages is placed over the glottis or mouth of the larynx, and is called epiglottis, as closing the passage to the lungs in the act of swallowing. The sides of the larynx are composed of the two arytenoid cartilages, which are of a very complex figure, not easy to be described. The anterior and larger part of the larynx is made up of two cartilages, one of which is called thyroides or scutiformis, from its being shaped like a buckler: and the other *cricoides* or *annularis*, from its resembling a ring. Both these cartilages may be felt immediately under the skin, at the forepart of the thorax; and the thyroides, by its convexity, forms an eminence called the pomum adami, which is usually more considerable in the male than in the female subject.

All these cartilages are united to each other by means of very elastic ligamentous fibres; and are enabled by the assistance of their several muscles, to dilate or contract the passage of the larynx, and to perform that variety of motion which seems to point out the larynx as the principal organ of the voice; for when the air passes through a wound in the trachea, it produces little or no sound.

These cartilages are moistened by a mucus, which seems to be secreted by minute glands situated near them. The upper part of ,the trachea, and the oricoid and thyroid cartilages, are in some measure covered anteriorly by a considerable body, which is supposed to be of a glandular structure, and from its situation is called the thyroid gland, though its excretory duct has not yet been discovered, or its real use ascertained. The glottis is entirely covered by a very fine membrane, which is moistened by a constant supply of watery fluid. From the larynx the canal begins to take the name of trachea, or aspera arteria, and extends from thence as far down as the fourth or fifth vertebræ of the back, where it divides into two branches, which are the right and left bronchial tube. Each of these bronchia ramifies through the substance of that lobe of the lungs, to which it is distributed by an infinite number of branches, which are formed of cartilages separated from each other like those of the trachea, by an intervening membranous and ligamentary substance. Each of these cartilages is of an annular figure; and as they become gradually less and less in their diameter, the lower ones are in some measure received into those above them, when the lungs, after being inflated, gradually collapse by the air being pushed out from them in expiration. As the branches of the bronchia become more minute, their cartilages become more and more annular and membranous, till at length they become perfectly membranous, and at last become invisible. The trachea is furnished with fleshy or muscular fibres, some of which pass through its whole extent longitudinally, while the others are carried round it in a circular direction, so that by the contraction or relaxation of these fibres, it is enabled to shorten or lengthen itself, and likewise to dilate or contract the diameter of its passage. The trachea and its branches, in all their ramifications, are furnished with a great number of small glands which are lodged in their cellular substance, and discharge a mucous fluid on the inner surface of these tubes.

The cartilages of the trachea, by keeping it constantly open, afford a free passage to the air which we are obliged to be incessantly respiring; and its membranous part, by being capable of contraction or dilatation, enables us to receive and expel the air in a greater or less quantity, and with more or less velocity, as may be required in singing and declamation. This membranous structure of the trachea posteriorly, seems likewise to assist in the descent of the food, by preventing that impediment to its passage down the œsophagus, which might be expected, if the cartilages were complete rings. The trachea receives its arteries from the carotid and subclavian arteries, and its veins pass into the jugulars. Its nerves arise from the recurrent branch of the eighth pair, and from the cervical plexus.

TRACHELA'GRA. (*Trachelagra, æ*, f.; from τραχηλος, the throat, and αγρα, a seizure.) The gout in the neck.

TRACHE'LIUM. (*Trachelium, ii*, n.; from τραχηλος, the throat: so called from its efficacy in diseases of the throat.) The *Campanula trachelium*, of Linnæus, or herb throat-wort.

TRACHELO. (From τραχηλος, the neck.) Names compounded of this word belong to muscles, &c. which are attached to the neck; as *Trachelo-mastoideus*.

TRACHELOCE'LE. (From τραχεια, the windpipe, and κηλη, a tumour). A tumour upon the trachea. A bronchocele.

TRACHELO-MASTOIDEUS. A muscle situated on the neck, which assists the complexus, but pulls the head more to one side. It is the *complexus minor seu mastoideus lateralis*, of Winslow. *Trachelo-mastoidien*, of Dumas. It arises from the transverse processes of the five inferior cervical verterræ, where it is connected with the transversalis cervicis, and of the three superior dorsal, and it is inserted into the middle of the posterior part of the mastoid process.

TRACHELO'PHYMA. (From τραχηλος, the throat, and φυμα, a tumour.) A swelling of the bronchial gland.

TRACHE'LOS. (From τραχυς, rough; because of the rough cartilages.) The wind-pipe. See *Trachea*.

TRACHEOTOMY. (*Tracheotomia, æ*, f.; from τραχεια, the trachea, and τεμνω, to cut.) See *Bronchotomy*.

TRACHO'MA. (*Trachoma, atis*, n.; from τραχυς, rough.) An asperity in the internal superficies of the eyelid. The effects are a violent ophthalmia, and a severe pain, as often as the eyelid moves. The species are,

1. *Trachoma sabulosum*, from sand falling between the eye and the eyelid of persons travelling, blown by a high wind; this happens chiefly in sabulous situations, and may be prevented by spectacles for the purpose, or by guarding against the flights of sand by covering the eyes.

2. *Trachoma carunculosum*, which arises from caruncles, or fleshy verrucæ, growing in the internal superficies of the eyelid. This species of the trachoma is called morum palpebræ internæ, because the tuberculous internal superficies appears of a livid red like a mulberry. Others call these carunculæ pladorotes.

3. *Trachoma herpeticum*, which are hard pustules in the internal superficies of the eyelids. This is also called ficosis, and palpebra ficosa, from its resemblance to the granulated substances in a cut fig. With the Greeks, it is denominated atomablepharon, or proptoris.

TRACHYTE. A rock of igneous origin, principally composed of felspar. It has generally a porphyritic structure.

TRAGACANTH. See *Astragalus*.

TRAGACA'NTHA. (*Tragacantha, æ*, f.; from τραγος, a goat, and ακανθα, a thorn: so called from its pods resembling a goat's beard.) See *Astragalus tragacantha*.

TRA'GICUS. A proper muscle of the ear, which pulls the point of the tragus a little forward.

TRA'GIUM. (From τραγος, a goat: so named from its filthy smell.) 1. The name of a genus of plants. Class, *Pentandria*; Order, *Digynia*.

2. The bastard dittany, or *Dictamnus albus*.

TRAGO'CERUS. (From τραγος, a goat, and κερας, a horn; so named from the supposed resemblance of its leaves to the horn of a goat.) The aloe.

TRAGOPO'GON. (*Tragopogon, onis*, m.; from τραγος, a goat, and πωγων, a beard: so called because its downy seed, while enclosed in the calyx, resembles a goat's beard.) 1. The name of a genus of plants in the Linnæan system. Class, *Syngenesia*; Order, *Polygamia*.

2. The pharmacopœial name of the common goat's beard.

TRAGOPOGON PRATENSE. The systematic name of the common goat's beard. The young stems of this plant are eaten like asparagus, and are a pleasant and wholesome food. The root is also excellent, and was formerly used medicinally as a diuretic.

TRAGOPY'RUM. (*Tragopyrum, i*, n.; from τραγος, a goat, and πυρον, wheat: so named from its beard.) Buck-wheat.

TRAGO'RCHIS. (*Tragorchis, is*, m.; from τραγος, a goat, and ορχις, a testicle: so named from the supposed resemblance of its roots to the testicles of a goat.) A species of orchis.

TRAGORI'GANUM. (*Tragoriganum, i*, n.; from τραγος, a goat, and οριγανον, marjoram: so called because goats are fond of it.) A species of wild marjoram.

TRAGOSELI'NUM. (*Tragoselinum, i*, n.; from τραγος, a goat, and σελινον, parsley: named from its hairy coat like the beard of a goat.) The burnet saxifrage. See *Pimpinella saxifraga*.

TRA'GUS. (Τραγος. *Tragus, i*, m.; a goat: so called from its having numerous little hairs, or from its being hairy like the goat.) 1. *In anatomy.* A small cartilaginous eminence of the auricular or external ear, placed anteriorly, and connected to the anterior extremity of the helix. It is beset with numerous little hairs, defending, in some measure, the entrance of the external auditory passage.

2. *In botany.* This name has been variously applied, by Dioscorides, to meal or flour, and to a mari time shrub.

TRALLIAN. ALEXANDER, a learned and ingenious physician, who was born at Tralles, in Lydia, and flourished at Rome under the emperor Justinian, about the middle of the sixth century. Like Hippo crates, he travelled over various countries to improve his knowledge. Besides improving upon many of the compositions then employed, he invented several others: and particularly introduced the liberal use of the preparations of iron. He principally followed the practice of Hippocrates and Galen, but not indiscriminately. He appears, however, to have had too great faith in charms and amulets, which was the common error of the age in which he lived.

TRA'MIS. Τραμις. The line which divides the scrotum, and runs on to the anus. See *Raphe.*

TRANSFUSION. (*Transfusio;* from *transfundo,* to pour from one vessel into another.) The transmission of blood from one living animal to another by means of a canula. " Harvey was thirty years before he could get his discovery admitted, though the most evident proofs of it were every where perceptible; but as soon as the circulation was acknowledged, people's minds were seized with a sort of delirium: it was thought that the means of curing all diseases was found, and even of rendering man immortal. The cause of all our evils was attributed to the blood; in order to cure them, nothing more was necessary but to remove the bad blood, and to replace it by pure blood, drawn from a sound animal.

The first attempts were made upon animals, and they i: d complete success. A dog having lost a great part of its blood, received, by transfusion, that of a sheep, and it became well. Another dog, old and deaf, regained, by this means, the use of hearing, and seemed to recover its youth. A horse of twenty-six years having received in his veins the blood of four lambs, he recovered his strength.

Transfusion was soon attempted upon man. Denys and Emerez, the one a physician, the other a surgeon of Paris, were the first who ventured to try it. They introduced into the veins of a young man, an idiot, the blood of a calf, in greater quantity than that which had been drawn from them, and he appeared to recover his reason. A leprous person, and a quartan ague, were also cured by this means; and several other transfusions were made upon healthy persons without any disagreeable result.

However, some sad events happened, to calm the general enthusiasm caused by these repeated successes. The young idiot we mentioned fell into a state of madness a short time after the experiment. He was submitted a second time to the transfusion, and he was immediately seized with a *hæmaturia,* and died in a state of sleepiness and torpor. A young prince of the blood royal was also the victim of it. The parliament of Paris prohibited transfusion. A short time after, G. Riva, having, in Italy, performed the transfusion upon two individuals, who died of it, the pope prohibited it also.

From this period, transfusion has been regarded as useless, and even dangerous."

TRANSPARENCY. Diaphaneity. A quality in certain bodies, by which they give passage to the rays of light. It is opposed to opacity; hence *Cornea transparens,* and *Cornea opace.*

TRANSPIRATION. (*Transpiratio;* from *trans,* through, and *spiro,* to breathe.) See *Perspiration.*

TRANSUDATION. *Transudatio.* The passing through the cells or pores of any thing. The term should be distinguished from perspiration, which implies a function, by which the perspired fluid is secreted from the blood, whereas, by transudation, the blood or other fluid merely passes or oozes through unaltered.

TRANSVERSA'LIS. Transverse.

TRANSVERSALIS ABDOMINIS. A muscle situated on the anterior part of the abdomen: so named from its direction. It arises internally or posteriorly from the cartilages of the seven lower ribs, being there connected with the intercostals and diaphragm, also from the transverse process of the last vertebra of the back, from those of the four upper vertebræ of the loins, from the inner edge of the crista ilii, and from part of Poupart's ligament, and it is inserted into the inferior bone of the sternum, and almost all the length of the linea alba. Its use is to support and compress the abdominal viscera.

TRANSVERSALIS ANTICUS PRIMUS. See *Rectus capitis lateralis.*

TRANSVERSALIS CERVICIS. See *Longissimus dorsi.*

TRANSVERSALIS COLLI. A muscle, situated on the posterior part of the neck, which turns the neck obliquely backwards, and a little to one side.

TRANSVERSALIS DORSI. See *Multifidus spinæ.*

TRANSVERSALIS MAJOR COLLI. See *Longissimus dorsi.*

TRANSVERSALIS PEDIS. A muscle of the foot, which it contracts, by bringing the great toe and the two outermost toes nearer each other.

TRANSVERSE SUTURE. *Sutura transversalis.* This suture runs across the face, and sinks down into the orbits, joining the bones of the skull to the bones of the face; but with so many irregularities and interruptions, that it can scarcely be recognised as a suture.

TRANSVERSO-SPINALES. See *Multifidus spinæ.*

TRANSVERSUS AURIS. A muscle of the external ear, which draws the upper part of the concha towards the helix.

TRANSVERSUS PERINÆI. (*Musculus transversus perinæi.*) A muscle of the organs of generation which sustains and keeps the perinæum in its proper place.

TRANSVERSUS PERINÆI ALTER. *Prostaticus inferior,* of Winslow. A small muscle occasionally found accompanying the former.

TRAP. This term is derived from the Swedish word *trappa,* a stair. It is applied in geology to rocks principally characterized by the presence of hornblende and black iron clay.

TRAPA. (A term given by Linnæus, whose idea is certainly taken from the warlike instrument called caltrop, the tribulus of the ancients, which consisted of four iron radiated spikes, so placed, that one of them must always stand upwards, in order to wound the feet of the passengers. Such is the figure of the singular fruit of this genus; hence named by Tournefort, *tribuloides. Calcitrapa,* an old botanical term of similar meaning to *tribulus,* is compounded, perhaps, of *calco,* to tread or kick, and *τρεπω,* to turn, because the caltrops are continually kicked over if they fail of their intended mischief: here we have the immediate origin of *trapa.*) The name of a genus of plants, Class, *Tetrandria;* Order, *Monogynia.*

TRAPA NATANS. The systematic name of the plant which affords the nux aquatica. *Tribulus aquaticus.* Caltrops. The fruit is of a quadrangular and somewhat oval shape, including a nut of a sweet farinaceous flavour, somewhat like that of the chesnut, which is apt to constipate the bowels, and produce disease; however, it is said to be nutritious and demulcent, and to be useful in diarrhœas from abraded bowels, and against calculus. Likewise a poultice of these nuts is said to be efficacious in resolving hard and indolent tumours.

TRAPE'ZIUM. (A four-sided figure: so called from its shape.) The first bone of the second row of the carpus.

TRAPE'ZIUS. (From *τραπεζιος,* four-square: so named from its shape.) *Cucullaris.* A muscle situated immediately under the integuments of the posterior part of the neck and back. It arises by a thick round, and short tendon, from the lower part of a protuberance in the middle of the occipital bone backwards, and from the rough line that is extended from thence towards the mastoid process of the os temporis, and by a thin membranous tendon, which covers part of the complexus and splenius. It then runs downwards along the nape of the neck, and rises tendinous from the spinous processes of the two lowermost vertebræ of the neck, and from the spinous processes of all the vertebræ of the back, being inseparably united to its fellow, the whole length of its origin, by tendinous fibres, which, in the nape of the neck, form what is called *ligamentum colli,* or the cervical ligament. It is inserted fleshy into the broad and posterior half of the clavicle, tendinous and fleshy into one-half of the acromion, and into almost all the spine of the scapula.

This muscle serves to move the scapula in different directions. Its upper descending fibres pull it obliquely upwards; its middle transverse ones pull it directly backwards; its inferior fibres, which ascend obliquely upwards, draw it obliquely downwards and backwards.

The upper part of the muscle acts upon the neck and head, the latter of which it draws backwards, and turns upon its axis. It likewise concurs with other muscles in counteracting the flexion of the head forwards.

TRAPEZOI'DES OS The second bone of the

second row of the carpus: so called from its resemblance to the *trapezium*, or quadrilateral geometrical figure.

TRAUMATIC. (From τραυμα, a wound.) Any thing relating to a wound.

TRAVELLER'S JOY. See *Clematis vitalba*.

TREACLE. See *Theriaca*.

Treacle, mustard. See *Thlaspi*.

TREFOIL. (So called because the leaf is formed of three leaflets.) See *Trifolium*.

Trefoil marsh. See *Menyanthes trifoliata*.

TREMOLITE. A subspecies of straight edged augite. There are three kinds, the asbestous, common, and glassy.

TRE'MOR. An involuntary trembling.

TREPAN. *Trephine*. An instrument used by surgeons to remove a portion of bone from the skull.

TREPHINE. See *Trepan*.

TREW, CHRISTOPHER JAMES, was born at Lauffen, in Franconia, in 1695; and settled as a physician at Nuremberg, where he gained so much reputation, as to be made director of the academy "Naturæ Curiosorum." He also contributed much towards establishing a society under the title of "Commercium Literarium Noricum," for the advancement of medical and natural knowledge, which published some valuable memoirs. To these societies he communicated several papers, and he also published some splendid works in anatomy and botany. He died in 1769.

TRIANGULA'RIS. *Trigonus*. Triangular: a term very generally used in the different departments of science, to parts of animals, vegetables, minerals, &c., from their form. See *Caulis, Folium*, &c.

TRI'BULUS. (Τριβολος; from τριβω, to tear or injure: an instrument of war to be thrown in the way to annoy the enemy's horse: hence the name of an herb from its resemblance to this instrument.)

1. The name of a genus of plants. Class, *Decandria*; Order, *Monogynia*.

2. See *Trapa natans*.

TRIBULUS AQUATICUS. See *Trapa natans*.

TRICA. (*Trica, æ*, f.; from θριξ, τριχος, a hair: because they seem composed of a horse hair rolled, or partly folded, into a little, round, black head.) A term applied by Dr. Acharius to the black filaments, resembling a curled horse hair, in the *Gyrophora* and *Umbilicaria* of Hoffman.

TRICAUDA'LIS. (From *tres*, three, and *cauda*, a tail.) A muscle with three tails.

TRI'CEPS. (From *tres*, three, and *caput*, a head.) Three-headed.

TRICEPS ADDUCTOR FEMORIS. Under this appellation are comprehended three distinct muscles. See *Adductor brevis, longus*, and *magnus femoris*.

TRICEPS AURIS. See *Retrahentes auris*.

TRICEPS EXTENSOR CUBITI. This muscle, which occupies all the posterior part of the os humeri, is described as two distinct muscles by Douglas, and as three by Winslow. The upper part of its long head is covered by the deltoides: the rest of the muscle is situated immediately under the integuments.

It arises, as its name indicates, by three heads. The first, or long head, (the long head of the *biceps externus*, of Douglas; *anconeus major*, of Winslow, as it is called,) springs, by a flat tendon of an inch in breadth, from the anterior extremity of the inferior costa of the scapula, near its neck, and below the origin of the teres minor. The second head, (the short head of the *biceps externus*, of Douglas; *anconeus externus*, of Winslow,) arises by an acute, tendinous, and fleshy beginning, from the upper and outer part of the os humeri, at the bottom of its great tuberosity. The third head, (*brachialis externus* of Douglas; *anconeus internus*, of Winslow,) which is the shortest of the three, originates by an acute fleshy beginning, from the back part of the os humeri, behind the flat tendon of the latissimus dorsi. These three portions unite about the middle of the arm, so as to form one thick and powerful muscle, which adheres to the os humeri to within an inch of the elbow, where it begins to form a broad tendon, which, after adhering to the capsular ligament of the elbow, is inserted into the upper and outer part of the olecranon, and sends off a great number of fibres, which help to form the fascia on the outer part of the forearm. The use of this muscle is to extend the forearm.

TRICHIA. (From θριξ, a hair.) A disease of the hair. See *Trichoma*.

TRICHI'ASIS. (From θριξ, a hair.) *Trichosis*.

1. A disease of the eye-lashes, in which they are turned in towards the bulb of the eye.

2. A disease of the hair. See *Trichoma*.

TRICHI'SMUS. (From θριξ, a hair.) A species of fracture which appears like a hair, and is almost imperceptible.

TRICHO'MA. (From τριχες, the hair.) The plaited hair. See *Plica*.

TRICHOMANES. (From τριχες, hair, and μανος, thin, lax: so called because it resembles fine hair.) See *Asplenium trichomanes*.

TRICHOSIS. (Τριχωσις, *pilare malum;* from θριξ a hair.) Under this name Good makes a genus of disease in the Class *Eccritica*, Order *Acrotica*, of his Nosology. Morbid hair. It has eight species, viz. *Trichosis setosa, plica, hirsutus, distrix*. See *Plica*.

TRICHU'RIS. (From θριξ, a hair.) The long hairworm. See *Worms*.

TRICOCCUS. (From τρεις, three, and κοκκος, a grain.) Three-seeded.

TRICOCCÆ. The name of an order in Linnæus's Fragments of a Natural Method, consisting of those which have a triangular capsule with three seeds.

TRICUSPID. (*Tricuspis;* from *tres*, three, and *cuspis*, a point: so called from their being three-point ed.) Three-pointed.

TRICUSPID VALVE. The name of the valve in the right ventricle.

Trifoil, water. See *Menyanthes trifoliata*.

TRIFO'LIUM. (From *tres*, three, and *folium*, a leaf: so called because it has three leaves on each stalk.) The name of a genus of plants in the Linnæan system. Class, *Pentandria;* Order, *Monogynia*. Trefoil.

TRIFOLIUM ACETOSUM. The wood-sorrel was so called. See *Oxalis acetosella*.

TRIFOLIUM AQUATICUM. See *Menyanthes trifoliata*.

TRIFOLIUM ARVENSE. Hare's-foot trefoil.

TRIFOLIUM AUREUM. Herb trinity; noble liverwort.

TRIFOLIUM CABALLINUM. Melilotus.

TRIFOLIUM CÆRULEUM. Sweet trefoil.

TRIFOLIUM FALCATUM. The Auricula muris. See *Hieracium pilosella*.

TRIFOLIUM FIBRINUM. See *Menyanthes trifoliata*.

TRIFOLIUM HEPATICUM. See *Anemone hepatica*.

TRIFOLIUM MELILOTUS OFFICINALIS. The syste matic name of the officinal melilot; *Melilotus; Lotus sylvestris; Seratula campana; Trifolium caballinum; Coroda regia; Trifolium odoratum*. This plant has been said to be resolvent, emollient, anodyne, and to participate of the virtues of chamomile. Its taste is unpleasant, subacrid, subsaline, but not bitter; when fresh it has scarcely any smell; in drying, it acquires a pretty strong one of the aromatic kind, but not agreeable. The principal use of melilot has been in clysters, fomentations, and other external applications.

TRIFOLIUM ODORATUM. See *Trifolium melilotus officinalis*.

TRIFOLIUM PALUDOSUM. See *Menyanthes trifoliata*.

TRIGE'MINI. (*Trigeminus*, from *tres*, three, and *geminus*, double; three-fold.) *Nervi innominati*. The fifth pair of nerves, which arise from the crura of the cerebellum, and are divided within the cavity of the cranium into three branches, viz. the *orbital, superior*, and *inferior maxillary*. The orbital branch is divided into the frontal, lachrymal, and nasal nerves; the superior maxillary into the spheno-palatine, posterior alveolar, and infra-orbital nerves; and the inferior maxillary into two branches, the internal lingual, and one more properly called the inferior maxillary.

TRIGONE'LLA. (A diminutive of *trigona*, three-sided, alluding to its little triangular flower.) The name of a genus of plants. Class, *Diadelphia;* Order, *Decandria*.

TRIGONELLA FŒNUM GRÆCUM. The systematic name of the fœnugreek. *Fœnum græcum; Buceras; Ægoceras. Trigonella—leguminibus sessilibus strictis erectiusculis subfalcatis acuminatis, caule erecto* of Linnæus. A native of Montpellier. The seeds are brought to us from the southern parts of France and Germany; they have a strong disagreeable smell, and an unctuous farinaceous taste, accompanied with a slight bitterness. They are esteemed as assisting the formation of pus, in inflammatory tumours; and the meal, with that intention, is made into a poultice with milk.

TRIGONUS. See *Triangularis.*

TRIHILATÆ. (From *tres*, three, and *hilum*, the scar or external mark on the seed.) The name of a class of plants in Linnæus's Fragments of a Natural Method, consisting of plants, the seeds of which have the scar well marked; the style has three stigmas.

TRILOBUS. Three-lobed. Applied to parts of animals and plants which are so shaped.

TRINERVIS. Three-nerved. In botany, three-ribbed; as applied to leaves, &c.

TRINITA'TIS HERBA. See *Anemone hepatica.*

TRINITY-HERB. See *Anemone hepatica.*

["TRIOSTEUM. The *triosteum perfoliatum* is a native plant, the root of which is cathartic in the *dose* of thirty or thirty-five grains. It sometimes operates as an emetic in the same doses. The strength is somewhat impaired by keeping, so that the stock should be renewed every year."—*Big. Mat. Med.* A.]

TRIPARTITUS. Tripartite: divided into three.

TRIPA'STRUM APELLIDIS. *Tripastrum archimedis.* A surgical instrument for extending fractured limbs; so named because it resembled a machine invented by Apellides or Archimedes, for the launching of ships, and because it was worked with three cords.

TRIPHANE. See *Spodumene.*

TRIPHYLLUS. (From τρεις, three, and φυλλον, a leaf.) Three-leaved.

TRIPLINERVIS. Triply-ribbed: applied to a leaf, which has a pair of large ribs branching off from a main one above the base, which is the case in every species of sunflower, and the *Blakea triplinervis.*

TRIPOLI. Rottenstone. A grayish yellow-coloured mineral used for polishing.

TRIQUE'TRA. (*Triquetrus;* from *tres*, three.) *Ossicula wormiana.* The triangular-shaped bones, which are found mostly in the course of the lambdoidal suture of the skull.

TRIQUETRUS. Three-sided. Applied to some parts of plants; as the stems, flowerstalk, leaves, seeds, &c.

TRI'SMUS. (From τριζω, to gnash.) Locked jaw. Spastic rigidity of the under jaw. *Capistrum*, of Vogel. Dr. Cullen makes two species. 1. *Trismus nascentium*, attacking infants during the first two weeks from their birth. 2. *Trismus traumaticus*, attacking persons of all ages, and arising from cold or a wound. See *Tetanus.*

TRISSA'GO. (*Quasi tristago;* from *tristis*, sad: because it dispels sadness.) The common germander is sometimes so called. See *Teucrium chamædrys.*

TRISSAGO PALLUSTRIS. The water-germander was so called. See *Teucrium scordium.*

TRITÆO'PHYA. (From τιρ]αιος, tertian, and φυω, importing a like nature or original.) *Tritæus.* A fever much of a nature with a tertian, and taking its rise from it. Some call it a continued tertian. It is remittent or intermittent.

TRITÆOPHYA CAUSUS. The fever called *causus* by Hippocrates.

TRITÆ'US. See *Tritæophya.*

TRITICUM. (From *tero*, to thresh from the husk.) The name of a genus of plants. Class, *Triandria;* Order, *Digynia.* See *Wheat.*

TRITICUM REPENS. *Gramen caninum; Gramen Dioscoridis; Gramen repens; Loliaceum radice repente.* Dog's grass; Couch grass. A very common grass, the roots of which are agreeably sweet, and possess aperient properties. The expressed juice is recommended to be given largely.

TRITO'RIUM. (From *tritus*, beat small.) 1. A mortar.

2. A glass for separating the oil from the water in distilling.

TRITURATION. (*Trituratio;* from *tero*, to rub or grind.) *Tritura; Tritus.* The act of reducing a solid body into a subtile powder; as woods, barks, &c. It is performed mostly by the rotary motion of a pestle in metallic, glass, or Wedgewood mortars.

TROCAR. (Corrupted from *un trois quart*, French, *a three-quarters;* from the three sides with which the point is made.) The name of an instrument used in tapping for the dropsy.

TROCHA'NTER. (From τρεχω, to run: because the muscles inserted into them perform the office of running.) The name of two processes of the thigh-

bone, which are distinguished into the greater and less. See *Femur.*

TROCHI'SCUS. (Diminutive of τροχος, a wheel.) A troch or round tablet. Troches and lozenges are composed of powders made up with glutinous substances into little cakes, and afterward dried. This form is principally used for the more commodious exhibition of certain medicines, by fitting them to dissolve slowly in the mouth, so as to pass by degrees into the stomach; and hence these preparations have generally a considerable portion of sugar or other materials grateful to the palate. Some powders have likewise been reduced into troches, with a view to their preparation, though possibly for no very good reasons: for the moistening them, and afterward drying them in the air, must on this account be of greater injury, than any advantage arising from this form can counterbalance.

General rules for making troches:

1. If the mass proves so glutinous as to stick to the fingers in making up, the hands may be anointed with any sweet or aromatic oil; or else sprinkled with starch, or liquorice powder, or with flour.

2. In order to thoroughly dry the troches, put them on an inverted sieve, in a shady, airy place, and frequently turn them.

3. Troches are to be kept in glass vessels, or in earthen ones well glazed

TRO'CHLEA. (Τροχλεα, a pulley; from τρεχω, to run.) A kind of cartilaginous pulley, through which the tendon of one of the muscles of the eye passes.

TROCHLEA'RIS. See *Obliquus superior oculi.*

TROCHLEATO'RES. The fourth pair of nerves are so called, because they are inserted into the musculus trochearis of the eye. See *Pathetici.*

TROCHOI'DES. (From τροχος, a wheel, and ειδος, resemblance.) *Axea commissura.* A species of diarthrosis, or moveable connexion of bones, in which one bone rotates upon another; as the first cervical vertebra upon the odontoid process of the second.

TRONA. The African name for the native carbonate of soda found near Fezzan.

["The carbonate of soda, strictly so called, is found in the province of Sukena, two days' journey from Fezzan, in Africa. It appears in crusts, composed of minute crystals, at the foot of a mountain. It is there called *Trona*, and transported to Egypt, Tripoli, &c. This variety is also found near Buénos Ayres in considerable quantities, whence it has been transported to England. It there exists in stratified masses from two to six inches thick, resting on clay, which is strongly impregnated with common salt. It has a light yellowish-gray colour, a granular texture, is easily broken, and does not effloresce in the air."—*Cleav. Min.* A]

TRONCHIN, THEODORE, was born at Geneva in 1709, and went to study under Boerhaave, at Leyden, where he graduated in 1730. He then settled at Amsterdam, became a member of the College of Physicians, and an inspector of hospitals; and distinguished himself as a zealous promoter of inoculation. In 1754, he returned to Geneva, and ranked among the most eminent practitioners in Europe; a chair of medicine was instituted in his favour, and the Society of Pastors admitted him into their body. He was employed by the Duke of Orleans, and other persons of rank at Paris, to inoculate their children; and performed the same office for the Duke of Parma. In 1766, he accepted the appointment of principal physician to the Duke of Orleans; though he had previously declined an invitation from the Empress of Russia. His practice appears to have been simple and judicious, and his conduct marked by humanity and charity. He had little time for writing; but besides his inaugural dissertation, he published a treatise on the Colica Pictonum, in 1757, and contributed several articles to the Encyclopædia, and to the Memoirs of the Academy of Surgery: and to an edition of the works of Baillou he gave a Preface on the State of Medicine. He had the honour of being a member of the chief medical and scientific societies in Europe. His death happened in 1781.

TROPÆ'OLUM. (A diminutive of *tropæum*, or τρωπαιον, a warlike trophy. This fanciful but elegant name was chosen by Linnæus for this singular and striking genus, because he conceived the shield-like leaves and the brilliant flowers, shaped like golden helmets, pierced through and through, and stained with blood, might well justify such an allusion.) The name of a genus of plants. Class, *Octandria;* Order, *Mono-gynia.*

Tropæolum majus. The systematic name of the Indian cress. *Nasturtium indicum; Acriviola; Flos sanguineus monardi; Nasturtium peruvianum; Cardamindum minus.* Greater Indian cress, or Nasturtium. This plant is a native of Peru; it was first brought to France in 1684, and there called *La grande capucine.* In its recent state this plant, and more especially its flowers, have a smell and taste resembling those of water-cress; and the leaves, on being bruised in a mortar, emit a pungent odour, somewhat like that of horse-radish. By distillation with water, they impregnate the fluid in a considerable degree with the smell and flavour of the plant. Hence the antiscorbutic character of the nasturtium seems to be well founded, at least as far as we are able to judge from its sensible qualities: therefore, in all those cases where the warm and antiscorbutic vegetables are recommended, this plant may be occasionally adopted as a pleasant and effectual variety. Patients to whom the nauseous taste of scurvy-grass is intolerable, may find a grateful substitute in the nasturtium. The flowers are frequently used in salads, and the capsules are by many highly esteemed as a pickle. The flowers, in the warm summer months, about the time of sunset, have been observed to emit sparks like those of the electrical kind.

Trophis americana. Red fruited bucephalon. The fruit of the plant is a rough red berry, which is eaten in Jamaica, though not very pleasant.

TRUFFLE. See *Lycoperdon tuber.*

TRUNCATUS. Truncate. Used in botany. A truncate leaf is an abrupt one, which has the extremity cut off, as it were, by a transverse line; as in *Liriodendrum tulipifera,* and the petals of *Hura crepitans.*

TRUNCUS. (*Truncus, i,* m.) The trunk.

I. In *anatomy,* applied to the body strictly so called. It is divided into the *thorax* or chest, the *abdomen* or belly, and the *pelvis.*

II. In *botany,* that part of a plant which emerges from the root, and sustains all other parts. The genera of trunks are,

1. *Truncus:* applied to trees and shrubs, which are hick and woody

2. *Caulis:* the stem of herbs.

3. *Calmus:* the stem of grasses.

4. *Stipes:* the trunk of funguses, ferns, and palms.

5. *Scapus:* which is not a trunk, but a flower-stalk, emerging from the root.

[Truss. This is an instrument employed by surgeons to retain the intestines in their proper place, when they have been forced out of their natural position, forming the disease which is called a rupture or hernia. A hernia is reducible or not. When not reducible, it becomes a strangulated hernia, requiring a surgical operation, before the intestines can be restored to their proper position. When not strangulated, ruptures are liable to become so by accident, and hence trusses were invented to keep the intestines in their place, and if possible to cure the disease, by closing the opening through which the bowels protruded. Trusses have heretofore been considered as a palliative remedy, rather than the means of effecting a radical cure. This has arisen from the manner of constructing them; and although they sometimes effected the desired object, yet they more generally failed, because the pads of all the trusses heretofore applied, were made *convex.* The intention of this shape of the instrument was to press into the opening through which the gut descended, and to keep it well into its place; but while it had this effect, it tended to keep the opening from healing, and even to enlarge it. This evil was not fully remedied until Dr. Amos G. Hull, of New-York, turned his attention to the subject, and by his improvements in the construction of trusses, has rendered it certain that all recent ruptures, and those of children, may be permanently cured, and those of old people and of long standing may, in many cases, also be remedied. The pad of Dr. Hull's truss is *concave,* and not convex; and hence the raised circular margin, by proper adaptation, presses upon the sides of the hernial opening, and tends to close the aperture and cure the hernia.

The following particulars of this invention, and its application to the cure of hernia, we take from the New-York Medical and Physical Journal, vol. 4.

"The qualities we have united in the truss, are equally applicable to every species of hernia, and we can say, without the fear of contradiction, that the proportion of cures it has effected is altogether unparalleled. It may, perhaps, be an interesting inquiry to some, how this instrument produces its effects: and we think, after considering its construction, this question can be answered to the satisfaction of every rational mind. It will be observed, that this truss presents a concave surface to the rupture opening. The concavity of the plate is occupied by an elastic cushion, the resistance of which is sufficient to reduce the intruding intestine while it is prevented escaping to any consider able distance by the pressure of the metallic plate; which pressure being greatest at the circumference and diminishing towards the centre, tends constantly to approximate the hernial parietes, and afford them rest and mechanical support. It is therefore obvious that nothing is suffered to intervene between the lips of the opening, as is the case when the intestine protrudes, or a convex pad is applied, but a fair opportunity is presented for the fibres to recover their tone, or to heal, when any laceration has been produced by violence done to the parts. It is a law of the animal economy, particularly noticed by Dorsey, that all hollow parts of the body have a tendency to adapt themselves to their contents.

"For the cure of hernia, then, it is only necessary to remove every obstacle which counteracts this tendency This indication is certainly very far from being answered by the convex pad, and we think it can only be fulfilled by one which shall reduce the bowel without dilating the ring: with this view, we have applied the concave pad, which has more than answered our expectations, in preventing a descent of the gut, and in restoring the fibres, which it undoubtedly greatly facilitates by its constant and uniform pressure. But without investigating the *modus operandi,* it is sufficient for the patient, and for all practical purposes, for the physician to know, that with this instrument hernia may alway be secured. If applied in cases of umbilical or congenital hernia in children, it will, in every instance, remove the necessity of an operation. In cases of con genital hernia, it should be applied before adhesion takes place, but not until the testicle has made its descent. If this particular period should be more carefully observed by surgeons, and the application of the truss (instead of being abandoned to mechanics) receive a greater share of their attention, they might be instrumental in obviating much of the distress which has been entailed upon the world.

"The distinctive merits of this truss Dr. Hull sums up under the following heads:—

"*First.*—The concave internal surface of the rupture pad, from its pressure being greatest at the circumference, tends constantly to approximate the hernia! parietes, affording them rest and mechanical support.

"*Secondly.*—The combined hinge and pivot mode of connexion between the *spring* and *pad,* by means of a tenon and mortice, so constructed as to preserve a double hinge and limited joint, acting in every direc tion, thereby securing the uniform pressure of the spring on the pad, and sustaining the same nice coaptation of the pad and rupture opening, as well under the varied ordinary desultory muscular actions, as when the body is in a recumbent posture.

"*Thirdly.*—The graduating power and fixture of the pad to the spring, rendering, as will be readily perceived, the condition of the pad perfectly controllable, even to nameless minuteness. Also resulting from this mechanism, is the advantage of accommodating a large truss to a small person; hence the *facility of supplying, without disappointment, persons at a great distance*

"*Fourthly.*—The double inguinal truss, being simply the addition of another pad, attached to a short elastic metallic plate: this plate with its pad move on the main spring by the same power of adjustment and fixture as the first pad, the pressure of the pads being graduated at pleasure by an intervening cork wedge." A.]

TUBA. (From *tubus:* any hollow vessel.) 1. A tube.

2. In botany, the inferior part of a monopetalous corol. It is the cylindrical part which is enclosed in the calyx of the primrose. See *Corolla.*

Tuba eustachiana. *Tuba aristotelica; Aquæductus; Aquæductus fallopii; Meatus siccus; Palatinus ductus; Ductus auris palatinus.* The auditory tube The Eustachian tube, so called because it was first described by Eustachius, arises in each ear from the anterior extremity of the tympanum by means of a bony semi-canal; runs forwards and inwards, at the same time becoming gradually smaller; and after perforating the petrous portion of. the temporal bone, terminates in a passage, partly cartilaginous and partly membranous, narrow at the beginning, but becoming gradually larger, and ending in a pouch behind the soft palate. It is through this orifice that the pituitary membrane of the nose enters the tympanum. It is always open, and affords a free passage for the air into the tympanum; hence persons hear better with their mouth open.

TUBA FALLOPIANA. The Fallopian tube first described by Fallopius. The uterine tube. A canal included in two laminæ of the peritonæum, which arises at each side of the fundus of the uterus, passes transversely, and ends with its extremity turned downwards at the ovarium. Its use is to grasp the ovum, and convey the prolific vapour to it, and to conduct the fertilized ovum into the cavity of the uterus.

TUBER. (*Tuber, eris,* n.; from *tumeo,* to swell.) An old name for an excrescence.

1. In anatomy, applied to some parts which are rounded; as *tuber annulare,* &c.

2. In surgery, a knot or swelling in any part.

3. In botany, applied to a kind of round turgid root, as a turnip; hence these are called tuberose roots.

4. The name of a genus of plants in the Linnæan system. Class, *Cryptogamia;* Order, *Fungi.*

TUBER CIBARUM. The common truffle. See *Lycoperdon tuber.*

TUBERCULA QUADRIGEMINA. *Corpora quadrigemina; Eminentiæ quadrigeminæ; Natulæ.* Four white oval tubercles of the brain, two of which are situated on each side over the posterior orifice of the third ventricle and the aqueduct of Sylvius. The ancients called them nates and testes, from their supposed resemblance.

TUBE'RCULUM. (*Tuberculum, i,* n. diminutive of *tuber.*) A tubercle. In anatomy, applied to several elevations, and in morbid anatomy to a diseased structure, which consists of a solid roundish substance; as tubercles of the lungs, liver, &c.

In botany, it is applied to the hemispherical projections, as the fruit of the *Lichen caninus.*

TUBERCULUM ANNULARE. The commencement of the medulla oblongata.

TUBERCULUM LOWERI. An eminence in the right auricle of the heart where the two venæ cavæ meet: so called from Lower, who first described it.

TUBEROSUS. Tuberose, knobbed: applied to parts of plants. The root so called is of many kinds. The most genuine consists of fleshy knobs, various in form, connected by common stalks or fibres; as the potato, and Jerusalem artichoke.

TUBULARIS. Tubular. In Good's Nosology used to designate a species of purging, *diarrhœa tubularis,* in which membrane-like tubes pass with the motions.

TUBULOSUS. Tubulose. A leaf is so called which is hollow within, as that of the common onion. The florets of a compound flower are called *tubulosi,* tubular or cylindrical, to distinguish them from such as are ligulate, or riband-like.

TU'BULUS. A small tube or duct.

TUBULI LACTIFERI. The ducts or tubes in the nipple, through which the milk passes.

TUFT. See *Capitulum.*

TULP, NICHOLAS, was the son of an opulent merchant, and born at Amsterdam, in 1593. Having studied and graduated at Leyden, he settled in his native city, and rose to a high rank, not only in his profession, but also as a citizen. He was made burgomaster in 1652, and in that station resisted the invasion of Holland by Lewis XIV. twenty years after, and thus saved his country; on which occasion a medal was struck to his honour. He died in 1674. His three books of Medical Observations have been several times reprinted, and contain many valuable physiological remarks. He is said to have been among the first who observed the lacteal vessels.

TUMITE. See *Thummerstone.*

TU'MOUR. (*Tumor;* from *tumeo,* to swell.) A swelling.

TUMO'RES. Tumours. An order in the Class, *Locales,* of Cullen's Nosology, comprehending partial swellings without inflammation.

TUNBRIDGE. Tunbridge wells is a populous village in the county of Kent, which contains many chalybeate springs, all of which resemble each other very closely in their chemical properties. Two of these are chiefly used, which yield about a gallon in a minute, and therefore afford an abundant supply for the numerous invalids who yearly resort thither. The analysis of Tunbridge spring proves it to be a very pure water, as to the quantity of solid matter; and the saline contents (the iron excepted) are such as may be found in almost any water that is used as common drink. It is only as a chalybeate, and in the quantity of carbonic acid, that it differs from common water. Of this acid it contains one twenty-second of its bulk. The general operation of this chalybeate water is to increase the power of the secretory system in a gradual, uniform manner, and to impart tone and strength to all the functions; hence it is asserted to be of eminent service in irregular digestion, flatulency, in the incipient stages of those chronic disorders which are attended with great debility, in chlorosis, and numerous other complaints incident to the female sex. The prescribed method of using the Tunbridge water, observes Dr. Saunders, is judicious. The whole of the quantity daily used, is taken at about two or three intervals, beginning at eight o'clock in the morning, and finishing about noon. The dose at each time varies from about one to three quarters of a pint; according to the age, sex, and general constitution of the patient, and especially the duration of the course; for it is found that these waters lose much of their effect by long habit.

TUNGSTATE. *Tunistas.* A salt formed by the combination of the tungstic acid, with salifiable bases; as *tungstate of lime,* &c.

TUNGSTENUM. (*Tungsten,* Swed. ponderous stone.) A metal, never found but in combination, and by no means common. The substance known to mineralogists, under the name of tungsten, was, after some time, discovered to consist of lime, combined with the acid of this metal. This ore is now called *tungstate of lime,* and is exceedingly scarce. It has been found in Sweden and Germany, both in masses and crystallized, of a yellowish-white or gray colour. It has a sparry appearance, is shining, of a lamellated texture, and semitransparent. The same metallic acid is likewise found united to iron and manganese; it then forms the ore called Wolfram, or *tungstate of iron and manganese.* This ore occurs both massive and crystallized, and is found in Cornwall, Germany, France, and Spain. Its colour is brownish-black, and its texture foliated. It has a metallic lustre, and a lamellated texture; it is brittle and very heavy; it is found in solid masses, in the state of layers interspersed with quartz. These two substances are therefore ores of the same metal.

Properties.—Tungstenum appears of a steel-gray colour. Its specific gravity is about 17.6. It is one of the hardest metals, but it is exceedingly brittle; and it is said to be almost as infusible as platina. Heated in the air it becomes converted into a yellow pulverulent oxide, which becomes blue by a strong heat, or when exposed to light. Tungstenum combines with phosphorus and sulphur, and with silver, copper, iron, lead, tin, antimony, and bismuth; but it does not unite with gold and platina. It is not attacked by sulphuric, nitric, or muriatic acids; nitro-muriatic acid acts upon it very slightly. It is oxidizable and acidifiable by the nitrates and hyperoxymuriates. It colours the vitrified earths or the vitreous fluxes, of a blue or brown colour. It is not known what its action may be on water and different oxides. Its action on the alkalies is likewise unknown. It is not employed yet, but promises real utility, on account of its colouring property, as a basis for pigment, since the compounds it is said to form with vegetable colouring matter, afford colours so permanent, as not to be acted on by the most concentrated oxymuriatic acid, the great enemy of vegetable colours.

Methods of obtaining tungstenum.—The method of obtaining metallic tungstenum is a problem in chemistry Scheele, Bergman, and Gmelin did not succeed in their attempts to procure it. Klaproth tried to reduce the yellow oxide of this metal with a variety of combustible substances, but without success. Ruprecht and Tondy say they have obtained this metal by using combustible substances alone: and by a mixture of combustible and alkaline matter.

The following process is recommended by Richter, an ingenious German chemist.

Let equal parts of tungstic acid and dried blood be

exposed for some time to a red heat in a crucible; press the black powder which is formed into another smaller crucible, and expose it again to a violent heat in a forge, for at least half an hour. Tungstenum will then be found, according to this chemist, in its metallic state in the crucible. There are two oxides of tungstenum, the brown and the yellow, or tungstic acid.

TUNGSTIC ACID has been found only in two minerals; one of which, formerly called tungsten, is a tungstate of lime, and is very rare; the other, more common, is composed of tungstic acid, oxide of iron, and a little oxide of manganese. The acid is separated from the latter in the following way:—The wolfram cleared from its silicious *gangue*, and pulverized, is heated in a matrass with five or six times its weight of muriatic acid for half an hour. The oxides of iron and manganese being thus dissolved, we obtain the tungstic acid under the form of a yellow powder. After washing it repeatedly with water, it is then digested in an excess of liquid ammonia, heated, which dissolves it completely. The liquor is filtered and evaporated to dryness in a capsule. The dry residue being ignited, the ammonia flies off, and pure tungstic acid remains. If the whole of the wolfram has not been decomposed in this operation, it must be subjected to the muriatic acid again.

It is tasteless, and does not affect vegetable colours. The tungstates of the alkalies and magnesia are soluble and crystallizable, while the other earthy ones are insoluble, as well as those of the metallic oxides. The acid is composed of 100 parts metallic tungsten, and 25 or 26.4 oxygen.

TUNGSTOUS ACID. What has been thus called appears to be an oxide of tungsten.

Tunic of a seed. See *Arillus.*

TU'NICA. (*A tuendo corpore*, because it defends the body.) A membrane or covering; as the coats of the eye, &c.

TUNICA ACINIFORMIS. The uvea, or posterior lamella of the iris.

TUNICA ALBUGINEA OCULI. See *Adnata tunica.*

TUNICA ALBUGINEA TESTIS. See *Albuginea testis.*

TUNICA ARACHNOIDEA. See *Arachnoid membrane.*

TUNICA CELLULOSA RUYSCHII. The second coat of the intestines.

TUNICA CHOROIDEA. See *Choroid membrane.*

TUNICA CONJUNCTIVA. See *Conjunctive membrane.*

TUNICA CORNEA. See *Cornea.*

TUNICA FILAMENTOSA. The false or spongy chorion.

TUNICA RETINA. See *Retina.*

TUNICA VAGINALIS TESTIS. A continuation of the peritonæum through the inguinal ring, which loosely invests the testicle and spermatic cord. See *Testis.*

TUNICA VILLOSA. The villous, or inner folding coat of the intestines.

Turbeth mineral. See *Hydrargyrus vitriolatus.*

Turbeth-root. See *Convolvulus turpethum.*

TURBINATE, (*Turbinatus; from turbino*, to sharpen at the top, shaped like a sugar-loaf.) Shaped like a sugar-loaf.

TURBINATED BONES. The superior spongy portion of the ethmoid bone, and the inferior spongy bones, are so called by some writers. See *Spongiosa ossa.*

TURBINA'TUM. The pineal gland.

TURBINATUS.' Turbinate, or sugar-loaf form. Applied to the fig, &c.

Turbith. A cathartic eastern bark; a species of cicely.

Turkeystone. See *Whetslate.*

TURMERIC. See *Curcuma.*

TURNHOOF. A vulgar name of the ground-ivy. See *Glecoma hederacea.*

TURNIP. See *Brassica rapa.*

Turnip, French. See *Brassica rapa.*

TURNSOLE. See *Heliotropium.*

TURPENTINE. *Terebinthina.* There are many kinds of turpentine. Those employed medicinally are,

1. The Chian or Cyprus turpentine. See *Pistacia terebinthus.*

2. The common turpentine. See *Terebinthina communis.*

3. The Venice turpentine. See *Pinus larix.*

All these have been considered as hot, stimulating corroborants and detergents; qualities which they possess in common. They stimulate the primæ viæ, and prove laxative; when carried into the blood-vessels they excite the whole system, and thus prove service-

able in chronic rheumatism and paralysis. Turpentine readily passes off by urine, which it imbues with a peculiar odour; also by perspiration and by exhalation from the lungs; and to these respective effects are ascribed the virtues it possesses in gravelly complaints, scurvy, and pulmonic disorders. Turpentine is much used in gleets, and fluor albus, and in general with much success. The essential oil, in which the virtues of turpentine reside, is not only preferred for external use, as a rubefacient, but also internally as a diuretic and styptic; the latter of which qualities it possesses in a very high degree. Formerly, turpentine was much used as a digestive application to ulcers, &c.; but in the modern practice of surgery, it is almost wholly exploded.

Turpeth mineral. See *Hydrargyrus vitriolatus.*

TURPE'THUM. (From *Turpeth*, Indian turbeth.) See *Convolvulus turpethum.*

TURPETHUM MINERALE. See *Hydrargyrus vitriolatus.*

TURQUOIS. Calaite. A much-esteemed ornamental stone brought from Persia, of a smalt-blue and apple-green colour.

TURU'NDA. (*A terendo*, from its being rolled up.) A tent, or suppository.

TUSSILA'GO. (*Tussilago, inis*, f.; from *tussis*, a cough; because it relieves coughs.) 1. The name of a genus of plants in the Linnæan system. Class, *Syngenesia*; Order, *Polygamia superflua.*

2. The pharmacopœial name of the coltsfoot. See *Tussilago farfara.*

TUSSILAGO FARFARA. The systematic name of the *Bechium; Bechion; Calceum equinum; Chamæleuce; Filius antepatrem; Farfarella; Farfara; Tussilago vulgaris; Farfara bechium; Ungula caballina.* Coltsfoot. *Tussilago farfara—scapo unifloro imbricato, foliis subcordatis angulatis denticulatis.* The sensible qualities of this plant are very inconsiderable; it has a rough mucilaginous taste, but no remarkable smell. The leaves have always been esteemed as possessing demulcent and pectoral virtues; and hence they have been exhibited in pulmonary consumptions, coughs, asthmas, and catarrhal affections. It is used as tea, or given in the way of infusion with liquorice-root or honey.

TUSSILAGO PETASITES. The systematic name of the butter-bur.. *Petasites.* Pestilent-wort. The roots of this plant are recommended as aperient and alexipharmic, and promise, though now forgotten, to be of considerable activity. They have a strong smell, and a bitterish acrid taste, of the aromatic kind, but not agreeable.

TU'SSIS. A cough, a sonorous concussion of the breast, produced by the violent, and for the most part involuntary motion of the muscles of respiration. It is symptomatic of many diseases.

TUSSIS CONVULSIVA. See *Pertussis.*

TUSSIS EXANTHEMATICA. A cough attendant on an eruption.

TUSSIS FERINA. See *Pertussis.*

TUTENAG. 1 The Indian name for zinc.

2. A metallic compound brought from China.

TU'TIA. (Persian.) *Pompholyx; Cadmia.* Tutty. A gray oxide of zinc; it is generally formed by fusing brass or copper, mixed with blende, when it is incrusted in the chimneys of the furnace. Mixed with any common cerate, it is applied to the eye, in debilitated state, of the conjunctive membrane.

TUTIA PREPARATA. Prepared tutty is often put into collyria, to which it imparts an astringent virtue.

TUTTY. See *Tutia.*

TYLO'SIS. (From τυλος, a callus.) *Tyloma.* An induration of the margin of the eyelids.

TY'MPANI MEMBRANA. See *Membrana tympani.*

TYMPANI'TES. (From τυμπανον, a drum: so called because the belly is distended with wind, and sounds like a drum when struck.) Tympany. Drumbelly. An elastic distention of the abdomen, which sounds like a drum when struck, with costiveness and atrophy, but no fluctuation. Species: 1. *Tympanites intestinalis*, a lodgment of wind in the intestines, known by the discharge of wind giving relief.

2. *Tympanites abdominalis*, when the wind is in the cavity of the abdomen.

TY'MPANUM. (Τυμπανον. A drum.) The drum or barrel of the ear. The hollow part of the ear in which are lodged the bones of the ear. It begins behind the membrane of the tympanum, which terml nates the external auditory passage, and is surrounded by the petrous portion of the temporal bone. It terminates at the cochlea of the labyrinth, and has opening into it four foramina, viz. the orifices of the Eustachian tube and mastoid sinus, the fenestra ovalis, and rotunda. It contains the four ossicula auditus.

TY'PHA. (From τυφος, a lake; because it grows in marshy places.) The name of a genus of plants in the Linnæan system. The cat's tail.

TYPHA AROMATICA. See *Acorus calamus.*

TYPHA LATIFOLIA. The broad-leaved cat's tail, or bull-rush. The young shoots, cut before they reach the surface of the water, eat like asparagus when boiled.

TYPHOMA'NIA. (From τυφος, to burn, and μανια, delirium.) A complication of phrensy and lethargy with fever.

TY'PHUS. (From τυφος, stupor.) A species of continued fever, characterized by great debility, a tendency in the fluids to putrefaction and the ordinary symptoms of fever. It is to be readily distinguished from the inflammatory by the smallness of the pulse, and the sudden and great debility which ensues on its first attack; and, in its more advanced stage, by the petechiæ, or purple spots, which come out on various parts of the body, and the fœtid stools which are discharged; and it may be distinguished from a nervous fever by the great violence of all its symptoms on its first coming on.

The most general cause that gives rise to this disease, is contagion, applied either immediately from the body of a person labouring under it, or conveyed in clothes, or merchandise, &c.; but it may be occasioned by the effluvia arising from either animal or vegetable substances in a decayed or putrid state: and hence it is, that in low and marshy countries it is apt to be prevalent when intense and sultry heat quickly succeeds any great inundation. A want of proper cleanliness and confined air are likewise causes of this fever; hence it prevails in hospitals, jails, camps, and on board of ships, especially when such places are much crowded, and the strictest attention is not paid to a free ventilation and due cleanliness. A close state of the atmosphere, with damp weather, is likewise apt to give rise to putrid fever. Those of lax fibres, and who have been weakened by any previous debilitating cause, such as poor diet, long fasting, hard labour, continued want of sleep, &c. are most liable to it.

On the first coming of the disease, the person is seized with languor, dejection of spirits, amazing depression and loss of muscular strength, universal weariness and soreness, pains in the head, back, and extremities, and rigors; the eyes appear full, heavy, yellowish, and often a little inflamed; the temporal arteries throb violently, the tongue is dry and parched, respiration is commonly laborious, and interrupted with deep sighing; the breath is hot and offensive, the urine is crude and pale, the body is costive, and the pulse is usually quick, small, and hard, and now and then fluttering and unequal. Sometimes a great heat, load, and pain are felt at the pit of the stomach, and a vomiting of bilious matter ensues.

As the disease advances, the pulse increases in frequency (beating often from 100 to 130 in a minute); there is vast debility, a great heat and dryness in the skin, oppression at the breast, with anxiety, sighing, and moaning; the thirst is greatly increased; the tongue, mouth, lips, and teeth are covered over with a brown or black tenacious fur; the speech is inarticulate, and scarcely intelligible; the patient mutters much, and delirium ensues. The fever continuing to increase still more in violence, symptoms of putrefaction show themselves; the breath becomes highly offensive; the urine deposites a black and fœtid sediment; the stools are dark, offensive, and pass off insensibly; hæmorrhages issue from the gums, nostrils, mouth, and other parts of the body; livid spots or petechiæ appear on its surface; the pulse intermits and sinks; the extremities grow cold; hiccoughs ensue; and death at last closes the tragic scene.

When this fever does not terminate fatally, it generally begins, in cold climates, to diminish about the commencement of the third week, and goes off gradually towards the end of the fourth, without any very evident crisis; but in warm climates it seldom continues above a week or ten days, if so long.

Our opinion, as to the event, is to be formed by the degree of violence in the symptoms, particularly after petechiæ appear, although in some instances recoveries

have been effected under the most unpromising appearances. An abatement of febrile heat and thirst, a gentle moisture diffused equally over the whole surface of the body, loose stools, turbid urine, rising of the pulse, and the absence of delirium and stupor, may be regarded in a favourable light. On the contrary, petechia, with dark, offensive, and involuntary discharges by urine and stool, fœtid sweats, hæmorrhages, and hiccoughs, denote the almost certain dissolution of the patient.

The appearances usually perceived on dissection, are inflammations of the brain and viscera, but more particularly of the stomach and intestines, which are now and then found in a gangrenous state. In the muscular fibres there seems likewise a strong tendency to gangrene.

In the very early period of typhus fever, it is often possible, by active treatment, to cut short the disease at once; but where it has established itself more firmly, we can only employ palliative measures to diminish its violence, that it may run safely through its course. Among the most likely means of accomplishing the first object is an emetic; where the fever runs high, we may give antimonials in divided doses at short intervals till full vomiting is excited; or if there be less strength in the system, ipecacuanha in a full dose at once. Attention should next be paid to clear out the bowels by some sufficiently active form of medicine; and as the disease proceeds, we must keep up this function, and attempt to restore that of the skin, and the other secretions, as the best means of moderating the violence of vascular action. Some of the preparations of mercury, or if there be tolerable strength, those of antimony, assisted by the saline compounds, may be employed for this purpose. The general antiphlogistic regimen is to be observed in the early part of the disease, as explained under synocha. In cases where the skin is uniformly very hot and dry, the abstraction of caloric may be more actively made by means of the cold affusion, that is, throwing a quantity of cold water on the naked body of the patient; which measure has sometimes arrested the disease in its first stage; and when the power of the system is less, sponging the body occasionally with cold water, medicated, perhaps, with a little salt or vinegar, may be substituted as a milder proceeding. But where the evolution of heat is even deficient, such means would be highly improper; and it may be sometimes advisable to employ the tepid bath, to promote the operation of the diaphoretic medicines. If under the use of the measures already detailed, calculated to lessen the violence of vascular action, the vital powers should appear materially falling off, recourse must then be had to a more nutritious diet, with a moderate quantity of wine, and cordial, or tonic medicines. There is generally an aversion from animal food, whence the mucilaginous vegetable substances, as arrow-root, &c., rendered palatable by spice, or a little wine, or sometimes mixed with milk, may be directed, as nourishing and easy of digestion. If, however, there be no marked septic tendency, and the patient cloyed with these articles, the lighter animal preparations, as calves-foot jelly, veal broth, &c., may be allowed. The extent to which wine may be carried, must depend on the urgency of the case, and the previous habits of the individual; but it will commonly not be necessary to exceed half a pint, or a pint at most, in the twenty-four hours; and it should be given in divided portions, properly diluted, made, perhaps, into negus, whey, &c., according to the liking of the patient. The preference should always be given to that which is of the soundest quality, if agreeable: but where wine cannot be afforded, good malt liquor, or mustard whey, may be substituted. Some moderately stimulant medicines, as ammonia, aromatics, serpentaria, &c., may often be used with advantage, to assist in keeping up the circulation: also those of a tonic quality, as calumba, cusparia, cinchona, &c., occasionally in their lighter forms; but more especially the acids. These are, in several respects, useful; by promoting the secretions of the primæ viæ, &c., they quench thirst, remove irritation, and manifestly cool the body; and in the worst forms of typhus, where the putrescent tendency appears, they are particularly indicated from their antiseptic power; they are also decidedly tonic, and indeed those from the mineral kingdom powerfully so. These may be given freely as medicines, the carbonic acid also in the form of brisk fermenting liquors; and the native vegetable acids, as they exist in ripe fruits, being generally very grateful, may constitute a considerable part of the diet. In the mean time, to obviate the septic tendency, great attention should be paid to cleanliness and ventilation, and keeping the bowels regular by mild aperients, or clysters of an emollient or antiseptic nature: and where aphthæ appear, acidulated gargles should be directed. If the disease inclines more to the nervous form, with much mental anxiety, tremors, and other irregular affections of the muscles, or organs of sense, the antispasmodic medicines may be employed with more advantage, as æther, camphor, musk, &c., but particularly opium; which should be given in a full dose, sufficient to procure sleep, provided there be no appearances of determination of blood to the head; and it may be useful to call a greater portion of nervous energy to the lower extremities by the pediluvium, or other mode of applying warmth, or occasionally by sinapisms, not allowing these to produce vesication. But if there should be much increased vascular action in the brain, more active means will be required, even the local abstraction of blood, if the strength will permit; and it will

be always right to have the head shaved, and kept cool by some evaporating lotion, and a blister applied to the back of the neck. In like manner, other important parts may occasionally require local means of relief. Urgent vomiting may, perhaps, be checked by the effervescing mixture; a troublesome diarrhœa by small doses of opium, assisted by aromatics, chalk, and other astringents, or sometimes by small doses of ipecacuanha; profuse perspirations by the infusum rosæ, a cooling regimen, &c.

TYPHUS ÆGYPTIACUS. The plague of Egypt.
TYPHUS CARCERUM. The jail-fever.
TYPHUS CASTRENSIS. The camp-fever.
TYPHUS GRAVIOR. The most malignant species of typhus. See Typhus.
TYPHUS ICTERODES. Typhus with symptoms of jaundice. See Typhus.
TYPHUS MITIOR. The low-fever.
TYPHUS NERVOSUS. The nervous-fever.
TYPHUS PETECHIALIS. Typhus with purple spots
TYRI'ASIS. Τυριασις. A species of leprosy in which the skin may be easily withdrawn from the flesh.
TYRO'SIS. (From τυρόω, to coagulate.) A disorder of the stomach from milk curdled in it.

U

ULCER. (Ulcus, eris, n.; from ελκος, a sore.) A purulent solution of continuity of the soft parts of an animal body. Ulcers may arise from a variety of causes, as all those that produce inflammation, from wounds, specific irritation of the absorbents, from scurvy, cancer, the venereal or scrofulous virus, &c. The proximate or immediate cause is an increased action of the absorbents, and a specific action of the arteries, by which a fluid is separated from the blood upon the ulcerated surface. They are variously denominated; the following is the most frequent division:

1. The simple ulcer, which takes place generally from a superficial wound.
2. The sinuous, that runs under the integuments, and the orifice of which is narrow, but not callous.
3. The fistulous ulcer, or fistula, a deep ulcer with a narrow and callous orifice.
4. The fungous ulcer, the surface of which is covered with fungous flesh.
5. The gangrenous, which is livid, fœtid, and gangrenous.
6. The scorbutic, which depends on a scorbutic acrimony.
7. The venereal, arising from the venereal disease.
8. The cancerous ulcer, or open cancer. See Cancer.
9. The carious ulcer, depending upon a carious bone.
10. The inveterate ulcer, which is of long continuance, and resists the ordinary applications.
11. The scrofulous ulcer, known by its having arisen from indolent tumours, its discharging a viscid, glairy matter, and its indolent nature.

ULCERA SERPENTIA ORIS. See Aphtha.
Ulcerated sore throat. See Cynanche.
ULLA. The common diminutive ulla, or illa, is, according to Dr. Good, most probably derived from the Greek, υλη, ule or ile, materia, materies, of the matter, make, or nature of; thus, papula or papilla, of the matter or nature of pappus; lupula, of the matter or nature of lupus; pustula, of the matter or nature of pus; and so of many others.

ULMA'RIA. (From ulmus, the elm: so named because it has leaves like the elm.) See Spiræa ulmaria.
ULMIN. Dr. Thomson has given this temporary name to a very singular substance lately examined by Klaproth. It differs essentially from every other known body, and must therefore constitute a new and peculiar vegetable principle. It exuded spontaneously from the trunk of a species of elm, which Klaproth conjectures to be the ulmus nigra, and was sent to him from Palermo in 1802.

1. In its external characters it resembles gum. It was solid, hard, of a black colour, and had considerable

lustre. Its powder was brown. It dissolved readily in the mouth, and was insipid.

2. It dissolved speedily in a small quantity of water The solution was transparent, of a blackish-brown colour, and, even when very much concentrated by evaporation, was not in the least mucilaginous or ropy; nor did it answer as a paste. In this respect ulmin differs essentially from gum.

3. It was completely insoluble both in alkohol and æther. When alkohol was poured into the aqueous solution, the greater part of the ulmin precipitated in light brown flakes. The remainder was obtained by evaporation, and was not sensibly soluble in alkohol The alkohol by this treatment acquired a sharpish taste

4. When a few drops of nitric acid were added to the aqueous solution, it became gelatinous, lost its blackish-brown colour, and a light brown substance precipitated. The whole solution was slowly evaporated to dryness, and the reddish-brown powder which remained was treated with alkohol. The alkohol assumed a golden yellow colour; and, when evaporated, left a light brown, bitter, and sharp resinous substance.

5. Oxymuriatic acid produced precisely the same effects as nitric. Thus it appears that ulmin, by the addition of a little oxygen, is converted into a resinous substance. In this new state it is insoluble in water. This property is very singular. Hitherto the volatile oils were the only substances known to assume the form of resins. That a substance soluble in water should assume the resinous form with such facility, is very remarkable.

6. Ulmin when burned emitted little smoke or flame, and left a spongy but firm charcoal, which, when burned in the open air, left only a little carbonate of potassa behind.

U'LMUS. 1. The name of a genus of plants in the Linnæan system. Class, Pentandria; Order, Digynia.
2. The pharmacopœial name of the common elm See Ulmus campestris.
ULMUS CAMPESTRIS. The systematic name of the common elm. Ulmus—foliis duplicato-serratis, basi inæqualibus, of Linnæus. The inner tough bark of this tree, which is directed for use by the pharmacopœias, has no remarkable smell, but a bitterish taste, and abounds with a slimy juice, which has been recommended in nephritic cases, and externally as a useful application to burns. It is also highly recommended in some cutaneous affections allied to herpes and lepra. It is mostly exhibited in the form of decoction, by boiling four ounces in four pints of water to two pints; of which from four to eight ounces are given two or three times a day.

["**Ulmus fulva.** The *Ulmus fulva*, or slippery elm, inhabits the northern and western parts of the United States, from Canada to Pennsylvania. The inner bark of this tree is charged with a gummy substance in great quantity, so that if a small piece is chewed in the mouth, it almost instantly fills it with a thick, viscid mucilage. This bark, both in substance and decoction, is a valuable demulcent in dysentery, and in strangury, either produced by cantharides or resulting from other causes. Elm-bark has been used as food, and been found capable of supporting life in cases of emergency. Externally, it is employed as an emollient application, to promote suppuration, and to answer the different ends to which common poultices are applicable. For this purpose, either the green bark should be bruised, or the dried bark cut into shreds and boiled. Internally, it proves most palatable in the *infusion.*"—*Big. Mat. Med.* A.]

U'LNA. (From ωλενη, the ulna, or cubit.) *Cubitus.* The larger bone of the forearm. It is smaller and shorter than the os humeri, and becomes gradually smaller as it descends to the wrist. We may divide it into its upper and lower extremities, and its body or middle part. At its upper extremity are two considerable processes, of which the posterior one and largest is named *olecranon*, and the smaller and interior one the *coronoid* process. Between these two processes, the extremity of the bone is formed into a deep articulating cavity, which, from its semicircular shape, is called the *greater sigmoid cavity*, to distinguish it from another, which has been named the *less sigmoid cavity.* The *olecranon*, called also the *anconoid* process, begins by a considerable tuberosity, which is rough, and serves for the insertion of muscles, and terminates in a kind of hook, the concave surface of which moves upon the pulley of the os humeri. This process forms the point of the elbow. The *coronoid process* is sharper at its extremity than the olecranon, but is much smaller, and does not reach so high. In bending the arm, it is received into the fossa at the forepart of the pulley. At the external side of the coronoid process is the less sigmoid cavity, which is a small, semilunar articulating surface, lined with cartilage, on which the round head of the radius plays. At the forepart of the coronoid process we observe a small tuberosity, into which the tendon of the brachialis internus is inserted. The greater sigmoid cavity, the situation of which we just now mentioned, is divided into four surfaces by a prominent line which is intersected by a small sinuosity that serves for the lodgment of mucilaginous glands. The whole of this cavity is covered with cartilage. The body, or middle part of the ulna, is of a prismatic or triangular shape, so as to afford three surfaces and as many angles. The external and internal surfaces are flat and broad, especially the external one, and are separated by a sharp angle, which, from its situation, may be termed the internal angle. This internal angle, which is turned towards the radius, serves for the attachment of the ligament that connects the two bones, and which is therefore called the *interosseous* ligament. The posterior surface is convex, and corresponds with the olecranon. The borders, or angles, which separate it from the other two surfaces, are somewhat rounded. At about a third of the length of this bone from the top, in its forepart, we observe a channel for the passage of vessels. The lower extremity is smaller as it descends, nearly cylindrical, and slightly curved forwards and outwards. Just before it terminates, it contracts, so as to form a neck to the small head with which it ends. On the outside of this little head, answering to the olecranon, a small process, called the *styloid* process, stands out, from which a strong ligament is stretched to the wrist. The head has a rounded articulating surface, on its internal side, which is covered with cartilage, and received into a semilunar cavity formed at the lower end of the radius. Between it and the os cuneiforme, a moveable cartilage is interposed, which is continued from the cartilage that covers the lower end of the radius, and is connected by ligamentous fibres to the styloid process of the ulna. The ulna is articulated above with the lower end of the os humeri. This articulation is of the species called ginglymus; it is articulated also both above and below to the radius, and to the carpus at its lowest extremity. Its chief use seems to be to support and regulate the motions of the radius. In children, both extremities of this bone are first cartilaginous, and afterward epiphyses, before they are completely united to the rest of the bone.

ULNAR. (*Ulnaris;* from *ulna*, the bone so named.) Belonging to the ulna.

Ulnar artery. See *Cubital artery.*

Ulnar nerve. See *Cubital nerve.*

Ulna'ris externus. See *Extensor carpi ulnaris.*

Ulna'ris internus. See *Flexor carpi ulnaris.*

ULTRAMARINE. See *Lapis lazuli.*

UMBELLA. (*Umbella, æ,* f.; a little shade, or um brella.) An umbel; the rundle of some authors. A species of inflorescence in which several flower-stalks of rays, nearly equal in length, spread from one common centre, their summits forming a level, convex, or even globose surface, more rarely a concave one.

From the *insertion* of the umbel, it is distinguished into *pedunculate* and *sessile.* The former implies that the rays or flower-stalks come from one; and the latter, that the rays or stalkfets come, not from a common peduncle, but from the stem or branch of the plant; as in *Sium nodiflorum*, and *Prunus avium.*

From the *division* of the umbel it is said to be *simple*, when single-flowered; as in *Allium ursinum:* and *compound*, when each ray or stalk bears an *umbellula*, or partial umbel; as in the *Anethum fœniculum*

The *umbella involucrata* is supplied with involucra.

UMBELLULA. A partial or little umbel. See *Umbella.*

UMBER. An ore of iron.

UMBILI'CAL. (*Umbilicalis;* from *umbilicus*, the navel.) Of or belonging to the navel.

Umbilical cord. *Funis umbilicalis; Funiculus umbilicalis.* The navel-string. A cord-like substance of an intestinal form, about half a yard in length, that proceeds from the navel of the fœtus to the centre of the placenta. It is composed of a cutaneous sheath, cellular substance, one umbilical vein, and two umbilical arteries; the former conveys the blood to the child from the placenta, and the latter return it from the child to the placenta.

Umbilical hernia. See *Hernia umbilicalis.*

Umbilical region. *Regio umbilicalis.* The part of the abdominal parietes about two inches all round the navel.

UMBILI'CUS. The navel.

Umbilicus marinus. *Cotyledon marina; Andro sace; Acetabulum marinum; Androsace matthioli; Fungus petræus marinus.* A submarine production found on rocks and the shells of fishes, about the coast of Montpellier, &c. It is said to be, in the form of powder, a useful anthelmintic and diuretic.

UMBO. (The top of a buckler.) The knob or more prominent part in the centre of the hat or pileus of the fungus tribe.

Unceola elastica. This plant affords a juice which becomes an elastic gum. See *Caoutchouc.*

UNCIFORM. (*Unciformis;* from *uncus*, a hook, and *forma*, a likeness.) Hook-like: applied to bones, &c.

Unciform bone. The last bone of the second row of the carpus or wrist: so named from its hook-like process, which projects towards the palm of the hand, and gives origin to the great ligament by which the tendons of the wrist are bound down.

UNCINATUS. (From *uncus*, a hook.) Uncinate or hooked: applied to the stigma of the *Lantana.*

UNDERSTANDING. *Intellectus* See *Ideology.*

UNDULATUS. Undulated: applied to a leaf when the disk near the margin is waved obtusely up and down; as in *Reseda lutea.*

Unedo papyracea. See *Arbutus unedo.*

UNGUE'NTUM. (*Unguentum, i,* n.; from *ungo*, to anoint.) An ointment. The usual consistence of ointments is about that of butter. The following are among the best formulæ.

Unguentum apostolorum. *Dodeca pharmicum.* The apostles' ointment: so called because it has twelve ingredients in it exclusive of the oil and vinegar. Not used.

Unguentum cantharidis. *Unguentum lyttæ.* Ointment of the blistering-fly. Take of the blistering-fly, rubbed to a very fine powder, two ounces; distilled water, eight fluid ounces; resin cerate, eight ounces. Boil the water with the blistering-fly to one-half, and strain; mix the cerate with the liquor, and then let it evaporate to the proper consistence. This is some times used to keep a blister open, but the savine cerate is to be preferred

UNGUENTUM CETACEI. Ointment of spermaceti, formerly called *linimentum album*, and latterly, *unguentum spermaceti*. Take of spermaceti, six drachms; white wax, two drachms; olive oil, three fluid ounces. Having melted them together over a slow fire, constantly stir the mixture until it gets cold. A simple emollient ointment.

UNGUENTUM CICUTÆ. Hemlock ointment. Take of the fresh leaves of hemlock, and prepared hog's lard, of each four ounces. The hemlock is to be bruised in a marble mortar, after which the lard is to be added, and the two ingredients thoroughly incorporated by beating. They are then to be gently melted over the fire, and after being strained through a cloth, and the fibrous parts of the hemlock well pressed, the ointment is to be stirred till quite cold. To cancerous or scrofulous sores this ointment may be applied with a prospect of success.

UNGUENTUM ELEMI COMPOSITUM. Compound ointment of elemi, formerly called *linimentum arcæi*, and *unguentum e gummi elemi*. Take of elemi, a pound; common turpentine, ten ounces; prepared suet, two pounds; olive oil, two fluid ounces. Melt the elemi with the suet, then remove it from the fire, and immediately mix in the turpentine and oil, then strain the mixture through a linen cloth. Indolent ulcers, chilblains, chronic ulcers after burns, and indolent tumours are often removed by this ointment.

UNGUENTUM HYDRARGYRI FORTIUS. Strong mercurial ointment, formerly called *unguentum cœruleum fortius*. Take of purified mercury, two pounds; prepared lard, twenty-three ounces; prepared suet, an ounce. First rub the mercury with the suet and a little of the lard, until the globules disappear; then add the remainder of the lard, and mix. In very general use for mercurial frictions. It may be employed in almost all cases where mercury is indicated.

UNGUENTUM HYDRARGYRI MITIUS. Mild mercurial ointment, formerly called *unguentum cœruleum mitius*. Take of strong mercurial ointment, a pound; prepared lard, two pounds. Mix. Weaker than the former.

UNGUENTUM HYDRARGYRI NITRATIS. *Unguentum hydrargyri nitrati*. Ointment of nitrate of mercury. Take of purified mercury, an ounce; nitric acid, eleven fluid drachms; prepared lard, six ounces; olive oil, four fluid ounces. First dissolve the mercury in the acid, then, while the liquor is hot, mix it with the lard and oil melted together. A stimulating and detergent ointment. Tinea capitis, psorophthalmia, indolent tumours on the margin of the eyelid, and ulcers in the urethra, are cured by its application.

UNGUENTUM HYDRARGYRI NITRATIS MITIUS. Weaker only than the former.

UNGUENTUM HYDRARGYRI NITRICO-OXIDI. Ointment of nitric oxide of mercury. Take of nitric oxide of mercury, an ounce; white wax, two ounces; prepared lard, six ounces. Having melted together the wax and lard, add thereto the nitric oxide of mercury in very fine powder, and mix. A most excellent stimulating and escharotic ointment.

UNGUENTUM HYDRARGYRI PRÆCIPITATI ALBI. Ointment of white precipitate of mercury, formerly called *unguentum e mercurio præcipitato albo*, and latterly *unguentum calcis hydrargyri albæ*. Take of white precipitate of mercury, a drachm; prepared lard, an ounce and a half. Having melted the lard over a slow fire, add the precipitated mercury and mix. A useful ointment to destroy vermin in the head, and to assist in the removal of scald head, venereal ulcers of children, and cutaneous eruptions.

UNGUENTUM LYTTÆ. See *Unguentum cantharidis*.

UNGUENTUM OPHTHALMICUM. Ophthalmic ointment of Janin. Take of prepared hog's-lard, half an ounce; prepared tutty, Armenian bole, of each two drachms; white precipitate one drachm. Mix. This celebrated ointment may be used for the same diseases of the eye and eyelid as the ung. hydrarg. nitratis. It must be at first weakened with about twice its quantity of hog's-lard.

UNGUENTUM PICIS ARIDÆ. See *Unguentum resinæ nigræ*.

UNGUENTUM PICIS LIQUIDÆ. Tar ointment, formerly called *unguentum picis*; *unguentum e pice*. Take of tar, prepared suet, of each a pound. Melt them together, and strain the mixture through a linen cloth. This is applicable to cases of tinea capitis, and some eruptive complaints; also to some kinds of irritable sores.

UNGUENTUM RESINÆ FLAVÆ. Yellow basilicon is in general use as a stimulant and detersive; it is an elegant and useful form of applying the resin.

UNGUENTUM RESINÆ NIGRÆ. *Unguentum picis aridæ*. Pitch ointment, formerly called *unguentum basilicum nigrum*, vel *tetrapharmacum*. Take of pitch, yellow wax, yellow resin, of each nine ounces, olive oil, a pint. Melt them together, and strain the mixture through a linen cloth. This is useful for the same purposes as the tar ointment.

UNGUENTUM SAMBUCI. Elder ointment, formerly called *unguentum sambucinum*. Take of elder flowers, two pounds; prepared lard, two pounds. Boil the elder flowers in the lard until they become crisp, then strain the ointment through a linen cloth. A cooling and emollient preparation.

UNGUENTUM SULPHURIS. Sulphur ointment, formerly called *unguentum e sulphure*. Take of sublimed sulphur, three ounces; prepared lard, half a pound. Mix. The most effectual preparation to destroy the itch. It is also serviceable in the cure of other cutaneous eruptions.

UNGUENTUM SULPHURIS COMPOSITUM. Compound sulphur ointment. Take of sublimed sulphur, half a pound; white hellebore-root, powdered, two ounces; nitrate of potassa, a drachm; soft soap, half a pound; prepared lard, a pound and a half. Mix. This preparation is introduced into the last London Pharmacopœia as a more efficacious remedy for itch than common sulphur ointment. In the army, where it is generally used, the sulphur vivum, or native admixture of sulphur with various heterogeneous matters, is used instead of sublimed sulphur.

UNGUENTUM VERATRI. White hellebore ointment, formerly called *unguentum hellebori albi*. Take of white hellebore-root, powdered, two ounces: prepared lard, eight ounces: oil of lemons, twenty minims. Mix.

UNGUENTUM ZINCI. Zinc ointment. Take of the oxide of zinc, an ounce; prepared lard, six ounces. Mix. A very useful application to chronic ophthalmia and relaxed ulcers.

U'NGUIS. (*Unguis, is,* m.; from ονυξ, a hook.) 1. The nail. The nails are horny laminæ situated at the extremities of the fingers and toes; composed of coagulated albumen, and a little phosphate of lime.

2. An abscess or collection of pus between the lamellæ of the cornea transparens of the eye; so called from its resemblance to the lunated portion of the nail of the finger.

3. The lachrymal bone is named *os unguis*, from its resemblance to a nail of the finger.

4. In botany, *unguis*, or the claw: applied to the thin part of the petal of a polypetalous corolla.

U'NGULA CABALLINA. See *Tussilago*.

UNIFLORUS. Bearing one flower.

UNIO. (*Unio*, pl. *uniones*; from *unus*, one: so called because there is never more than one found in the same shell, or, according to others, for that many being found in one shell, not any one of them is like the other.) The pearl. See *Margarita*.

U'RACHUS. (From ουρον, urine, and εχω, to contain.) *Urinaculum*. The ligamentous cord that arises from the basis of the urinary bladder, along which it runs, and terminates in the umbilical cord. In the fœtuses of brute animals, which the ancients mostly dissected, it is a hollow tube, and conveys the urine to the allantoid membrane.

URA'GIUM. (From ουραγος, the hinder part of an army.) The apex or extreme point of the heart.

URANGLIMMER. Green mica. Chalcolite. An ore of uranium.

URANIS'CUS. (From ουρανος, the firmament: so called from its arch.) The palate.

URANITE. See *Uranium*.

URA'NIUM. Uranite This metal was discovered by Klaproth, in the year 1789. It exists combined with sulphur, and a portion of iron, lead, and silex, in the mineral termed *Pechblende*, or *oxide of uranium*. Combined with carbonic acid it forms the *chalcolite*, or *green mica*: and mixed with oxide of iron, it constitutes the *uranitic ochre*. It is always found in the state of an oxide with a greater or smaller portion of iron, or mineralized with sulphur and copper. The ores of uranium are of a blackish colour, inclining to a dark iron-gray, and of a moderate splendour; they are of a close texture, and when broken present a somewhat uneven, and in the smallest particles a conchoidal surface. They are found in the mines of Saxony.

Properties of uranium.—Uranium exhibits a mass of small metallic globules, agglutinated together. Its colour is a deep gray on the outside, in the inside it is a pale brown. It is very porous, and is so soft, that it may be scraped with a knife It has but little lustre. Its specific gravity is between eight and nine. It is more difficult to be fused than even manganese. When intensely heated with phosphate of soda and ammonia, or glacial phosphoric acid, it fuses with them into a grass-green glass. With soda or borax it melts only into a gray, opaque, scoriaceous bead. It is soluble in sulphuric, nitric, and muriatic acids. It combines with sulphur and phosphorus, and alloys with mercury. It has not yet been combined with other combustible bodies. It decomposes the nitric acid and becomes converted into a yellow oxide. The action of uranium alone upon water, &c. is still unknown, probably on account of its extreme scarcity.

Method of obtaining uranium.—In order to obtain uranium, the *pechblende* is first freed from sulphur by heat, and cleared from the adhering impurities as carefully as possible. It is then digested in nitric acid ; the metallic matter that it contains is thus completely dissolved, while part of the sulphur remains undissolved, and part of it is dissipated under the form of sulphuretted hydrogen gas. The solution is then precipitated by a carbonated alkali. The precipitate has a lemon-yellow colour when it is pure. This yellow carbonate is made into a paste with oil, and exposed to a violent heat, bedded in a crucible well lined with charcoal.

Klaproth obtained a metallic globule 28 grains in weight, by forming a ball of 50 grains of the yellow carbonate, with a little wax, and by exposing this ball in a crucible lined with charcoal to a heat equal to 170° of Wedgewood's pyrometer. Richter obtained in a single experiment 100 grains of this metal, which seemed to be free from all admixture. There are probably two oxides of uranium, the *protoxide*, which is a grayish black ; and the *peroxide*, which is yellow.

URANOCHRE. An ore of uranium.

URATE. *Uras.* A compound of uric or lithic acid, with a salifiable basis.

URCE'OLA. (From *urceolus*, a small pitcher : so named from its uses in scouring glazed vessels.) The herb feverfew.

UREA. A constituent of urine. The best process for preparing it is to evaporate urine to the consistence of syrup, taking care to regulate the heat towards the end of the evaporation ; to add very gradually to the syrup its volume of nitric acid (24° Baumé) of 1.20 ; to stir the mixture, and immerse it in a bath of iced water, to harden the crystals of the acidulous nitrate of urea which precipitate ; to wash these crystals with ice-cold water, to drain them, and press them between the folds of blotting paper. When we have thus separated the adhering heterogeneous matters, we redissolve the crystals in water, and add to them a sufficient quantity of carbonate of potassa, to neutralize the nitric acid. We must then evaporate the new liquor, at a gentle heat, almost to dryness, and treat the residuum with a very pure alkohol, which dissolves only the urea. On concentrating the alkoholic solution, the urea crystallizes.

The preceding is Thenard's process, which Dr. Prout has improved. He separates the nitrate of potassa by crystallization, makes the liquid urea into a paste with animal charcoal, digests this with cold water, filters, concentrates, then dissolves the new colourless urea in alkohol, and lastly, crystallizes.

Urea crystallizes in four-sided prisms, which are transparent and colourless, with a slight pearly lustre. It has a peculiar, but not urinous odour ; it does not affect litmus or turmeric papers ; it undergoes no change from the atmosphere, except a slight deliquescence in very damp weather. In a strong heat it melts, and is partly decomposed and partly sublimed without change. The spec. grav. of the crystals is about 1.35. It is very soluble in water. Alkohol, at the temperature of the atmosphere, dissolves about 20 per cent. ; and, when boiling, considerably more than its own weight, from which the urea separates, on cooling, in its crystalline form. The fixed alkalies and alkaline earths decom-

pose it. It unites with most of the metallic oxides, and forms crystalline compounds with the nitric and oxalic acids.

Urea has been recently analyzed by Dr. Prout and Berard. The following are its constituents :—

	per cent.	per cent.		per atom.
Hydrogen	10.80	6.66	2 =	2.5
Carbon	19.40	19.99	1 =	7.5
Oxygen	26.40	26.66	1 =	10.0
Azote	43.40	46.66	1 =	17.5
	100.00	100.00		37.5

Uric, or lithic acid, is a substance quite distinct from urea in its composition. This fact, according to Dr. Prout, explains, why an excess of urea generally accompanies the phosphoric diathesis, and not the lithic. He has several times seen urea as abundant in the urine of a person where the phosphoric diathesis prevailed, as to crystallize spontaneously on the addition of nitric acid, without being concentrated by evaporation.

As urea and uric acid, says Berard, are the most azotized of all animal substances, the secretion of urine appears to have for its object the separation of the excess of azote from the blood, as respiration separates from it the excess of carbon.

URE'DO. (From *uro*, to burn.) An itching or burning sensation of the skin, which accompanies many diseases. The nettle-rash is also so called.

URET. The compounds of simple inflammable bodies with each other, and with metals, are commonly designated by this word ; as sulph*uret* of phosphorus, carb*uret* of iron, &c. The terms *bisulphuret, bisulphate,* &c. applied to compounds, imply that they contain twice the quantity of sulphur, sulphuric acid, &c. existing in the respective sulphuret, sulphate, &c.

URE'TER. (*Ureter, eris,* m. ; from ουρον, urine.) The membranous canal which conveys the urine from the kidney to the urinary bladder. At its superior part it is considerably the largest, occupying the greatest portion of the pelvis of the kidney ; it then contracts to the size of a goose-quill, and descends over the psoas magnus muscle and large crural vessels into the pelvis, in which it perforates the urinary bladder very obliquely. Its internal surface is lubricated with mucus to defend it from the irritation of the urine in passing.

URETERI'TIS. (From ουρητηρ, the ureter.) An inflammation of the ureter.

URE'THRA. (From ουρον, the urine: because it is the canal through which the urine passes.) A membranous canal running from the neck of the bladder through the inferior part of the penis to the extremity of the glans penis, in which it opens by a longitudinal orifice, called *meatus urinarius.* In this course, it first passes through the prostate gland, which portion is distinguished by the name of the *prostatical urethra* ; it then becomes much dilated, and is known by the name of the *bulbous part,* in which is situated a cutaneous eminence called the *caput gallinaginis* or *verumontanum,* around which are ten or twelve orifices of the excretory ducts of the prostate gland, and two of the spermatic vessels. The remaining part of the urethra contains a number of triangular mouths, which are the *lacunæ,* or openings of the excretory ducts of the mucous glands of the urethra.

URETHRI'TIS. (From ουρηθρα, the urethra.) An inflammation in the urethra. See *Gonorrhœa.*

URE'TICA. (From ουρον, urine.) Medicines which promote a discharge of urine.

U'RIAS. (From ουρον, urine.) The urethra

URIC ACID. See *Lithic acid.*

URI'NA. See *Urine.*

URINA'CULUM. See *Urachus.*

URI'NÆ ARDOR. See *Dysuria.*

URINA'RIA. (From *urina,* urine: so named from its diuretic qualities.) The herb dandelion See *Leontodon taraxacum.*

URINARY. (*Urinarius ;* from *urina,* urine.) Appertaining to urine.

URINARY BLADDER. *Vesica urinaria.* The bladder is a membranous pouch, capable of dilatation and contraction, situated in the lower part of the abdomen, immediately behind the symphysis pubis, and opposite to the beginning of the rectum. Its figure is nearly that of a short oval. It is broader on the fore and back than on the lateral parts ; rounder above than below when empty; and broader below than above, when full. It is divided into the body, neck, and fundus, or upper part; the neck is a portion of the lower part, which is contracted by a sphincter muscle. This organ is made up of several coats; the upper, posterior, and lateral parts are covered by a reflection of the peritoneum, which is connected by cellular substance to the muscular coat. This is composed of several strata of fibres, the outermost of which are mostly longitudinal, the interior becoming gradually more transverse, connected together by reticular membrane. Under this is the cellular coat, which is nearly of the same structure with the tunica nervosa of the stomach. Winslow describes the internal or villous coat as somewhat granulated and glandular; but this has been disputed by subsequent anatomists. However, a mucous fluid is poured out continually from it, which defends it from the acrimony of the urine. Sometimes the internal surface is found very irregular, and full of rugæ, which appear to be occasioned merely by the strong contraction of the muscular fibres, and may be removed by distending it. The sphincter does not seem to be a distinct muscle, but merely formed by the transverse fibres being closely arranged about the neck. The urine is received from the ureters, which enter the posterior part of the bladder obliquely; and when a certain degree of distention has occurred, the muscular fibres are voluntarily exerted to expel it.

URINE. (*Urina*, *æ*, f. Ουρον; from *ορουω*, to rush out.) The saline liquid, secreted in the kidneys, and dropping down from them, guttatim, through the ureters, into the cavity of the urinary bladder. *The secretory organ* is composed of the arterious vessels of the cortical substance of the kidneys, from which the urine passes through the uriniferous tubuli and renal papillæ into the renal pelvis; whence it flows, drop by drop, through the ureters, into the cavity of the urinary bladder; where it is detained some hours, and at length, when *abundant*, eliminated through the urethra.

"Few of the apparatus of secretion are so complicated as that of the urine; it is composed of the two kidneys, of the *ureters*, of the bladder, and the *urethra*; besides, the abdominal muscles contribute to the action of these different parts, among which the kidneys alone form urine; the others serve in its transportation and expulsion.

Situated in the abdomen, upon the sides of the vertebral column, before the last false ribs and the *quadratus lumborum*, the kidneys are of small volume relatively to the quantity of fluid they secrete. They are generally surrounded with a great deal of fat. Their parenchyma is composed of two substances; the one exterior, vascular, or *cortical*, the other *tubular*, disposed in a certain number of cones, the base of which corresponds to the surface of the organ, and their summits unite in the membranous cavity called *pelvis*. Its cones appear formed by a great number of small hollow fibres, which are excretory canals of a particular kind, and which are generally filled with urine.

In respect of its volume, no organ receives so much blood as the kidney. The artery which is directed there is large, short, and proceeds immediately from the aorta; it has easy communication with the veins and the tubulous substance, as may easily be ascertained by means of the most coarse injections, which, being thrown into the renal artery, pass into the veins and into the pelvis, after having filled the cortical substance.

The filaments of the great sympathetic alone are distributed to the kidneys. The *calices*, pelvis, and ureter form together a canal which commences in the kidneys, where it embraces the top of the mammillary processes, and, placed at the sides of the vertebral column, it goes in the bottom of the pelvis to the bladder, where it terminates. This last organ is an extensible and contractile sac, intended to hold the fluid secreted by the kidneys, and which communicates with the exterior by a canal of considerable length in man, but very short in woman, called *urethra*.

The posterior extremity of the urethra is, only in man, surrounded by the *prostate* gland, which is considered by certain anatomists as a collection of mucous follicles. Two small glands placed before the anus pour a particular fluid into this canal. Two muscles, which descend from the pubis towards the rectum, pass upon the sides of the part of the bladder which ends in

the urethra, approach one another behind, and form a small arc which surrounds the neck of the bladder, and carries it more or less upwards.

If the pelvis is cut open in a living animal, the urine is seen to pass out slowly by the summits of the excretory cones. This liquid is deposited in the pelvis of the kidney, and then by little and little it enters into the *ureter*, through the whole length of which it passes. It thus arrives at the bladder, into which it penetrates by a constant exudation or dribbling.

A slight compression upon the uriniferous cones makes the urine pass out in considerable quantity: but instead of being limpid, as when it passes out naturally, it is muddy and thick. It appears then to be filtered by the hollow fibres of the tubular substance.

Neither the *pelvis* nor the *ureter* being contractile, probably the power which produces the motion of the urine is, on the one hand, that by which it is poured into the *pelvis*; and on the other, the pressure of the abdominal muscles, to which may be added, when we stand upright, the weight of the liquid.

Under the influence of these causes, the urine passes into the bladder, and slowly distends this organ, sometimes to a considerable degree; this accumulation being permitted by the extensibility of different organs.

How does the urine accumulate in the bladder? Why does it not flow immediately by the urethra? and why does it not flow back into the ureter? The answer is easy for the ureters. These conduits pass a considerable distance into the sides of the bladder. In proportion as the urine distends this organ, it flattens the ureters, and shuts them so much more firmly as it is more abundant. This takes place in the dead body as well as in the living; also, a liquid, or even air, injected into the bladder, by the urethra, never enters the ureters. It is, then, by a mechanism analagous to that of certain valves, that the urine does not return towards the kidneys.

It is not so easy to explain why the urine does not flow by the urethra. Several causes appear to contribute to this. The sides of this canal, particularly towards the bladder, have a continual tendency to contract, and to lessen the cavity; but this cause alone would be insufficient to resist the efforts of the urine to escape, when the bladder is full. In the dead body, in which the canal contracts nearly in the same manner, it has but a very weak resistance, and does not prevent the passage of the liquid outwards, though the bladder may be very little compressed.

The angle of the bladder with the urethra, when it is strongly distended, may also present an obstacle to the passage of the urine; but the principal cause, most probably, is the contraction of the elevating muscles of the anus, which, either by the disposition to contraction of the muscular fibres, or by their contraction under the influence of the brain, press the urethra upwards, compress its sides with more or less force against each other, and thus shut its posterior orifice.

Excretion of urine.—As soon as there is a certain quantity of urine in the bladder, we feel an inclination to discharge it. The mechanism of this expulsion deserves particular attention, and has not always been well understood.

If the urine is not always expelled, this ought not to be attributed to the want of contraction in the bladder, for this organ always tends to contract; but, by the influence of the causes that we have noticed, the internal orifice of the urethra resists with a force that the contraction of the bladder cannot surmount. The will produces this expulsion, 1st, by adding the contraction of the abdominal muscles to that of the bladder; 2dly by relaxing the *levatores ani*, which shut the urethra. The resistance of this canal being once overcome, the contraction of the bladder is sufficient for the complete expulsion of the urine it contained; but the action of the abdominal muscles may be added, and then the urine passes out with much greater force. We may also stop the flowing of the urine all at once, by contracting the levators of the anus.

The contraction of the bladder is not voluntary though by acting on the abdominal muscles, and the levators of the anus, we may cause it to contract when we choose.

The urine that remains in the urethra after the bladder is empty, is expelled by the contraction of the muscles of the perinæum, and particularly by that of the *acceleratores urinæ*.

Though the quantity of urine is very copious, and though it contains several proximate principles which are not found in the blood, and consequently a chemical action takes place in the kidneys, the secretion of the urine is nevertheless very rapid.

The physical properties of the urine are subject to great variations. If rhubarb or madder has been used, it becomes of a deep yellow, or blood red; if one has breathed an air charged with vapours of oil or turpentine, or if a little rosin has been swallowed, it takes a violet colour. The disagreeable odour that it takes by the use of asparagus, is well known.

Its chemical composition is not less variable. The more use that is made of watery beverages, the more considerable the total quantity and proportion of water becomes. If one drinks little, the contrary happens.

The uric acid becomes more abundant when the regimen is very substantial, and the exercise trifling. This acid diminishes, and may even disappear altogether, by the constant and exclusive use of unazotized food, such as sugar, gum, butter, oil, &c. Certain salts, carried into the stomach, even in small quantity, are found in a short time in the urine.

The extreme rapidity with which this translation takes place, has made it be supposed there is a direct communication between the stomach and the bladder. Even now there are considerable numbers of partisans in favour of this opinion.

It is not yet long since a direct canal from the stomach to the bladder was supposed to exist, but this passage has no existence. Others have supposed, without giving any proof, that the passage took place by the cellular tissue, by the anastomoses of the lymphatic vessels, &c.

Darwin having given to a friend several grains of nitrate of potassa, in half an hour he let blood of him, and collected his urine. The salt was found in the urine, but not in the blood. Brande made similar observations with prussiate of potassa. He concluded from it that the circulation is not the only means of communication between the stomach and the urinary organs, but without giving any explanation of the existing means. Sir Everard Home is also of this opinion.

I have made experiments in order to clear up this important question, and I have found, 1st, That whenever prussiate of potassa is injected into the veins, or absolved in the intestinal canal, or by a serous membrane, it very soon passes into the bladder, where it is easily recognised among the urine. 2dly, that if the quantity of prussiate injected is considerable, the tests can discover it in the blood; but if the quantity is small, its presence cannot be recognised by the usual means. 3dly, That the same result takes place by mixing the prussiate and blood together in a vessel. 4thly, That the same salt is recognised in all proportions in the urine. It is not extraordinary, then, that Darwin and Brande did not find in the blood the substance that they distinctly perceived in the urine.

With regard to the organs that transport the liquids of the stomach and intestines into the circulating system, it is evident, according to what we have said, in speaking of the chyliferous vessels, and the absorption of the veins, that these liquids are directly absorbed by the veins, and transported by them to the liver and the heart; so that the direction which these liquids follow, in order to reach the veins, is much shorter than is generally admitted, viz. by the lymphatic vessels, the mesenteric glands, and the thoracic duct."—*Magendie's Physiology.*

The urine of a healthy man is divided in general into,

1. *Crude,* or that which is emitted one or two hours after eating. This is for the most part aqueous, and often vitiated by some kinds of food.

2. *Cocted,* which is eliminated some hours after the digestion of the food, as that which is emitted in the morning after sleeping. This is generally in smaller quantity, thicker, more coloured, more acrid than at any other time. Of such cocted urine, the *colour* is usually citrine, and not unhandsome.

The *degree of heat* agrees with that of the blood. Hence in atmospheric air it is warmer, as is perceived if the hand be washed with urine. The *specific gravity* is greater than water, and that emitted in the morning is always heavier than at any other time. The *smell* of fresh urine is not disagreeable. The *taste* is saltish and nauseous. The *consistence* is somewhat thicker than water. The *quantity* depends on that of the liquid drink, its diuretic nature, and the temperature of the air.

Changes of urine in the air.—Preserved in an open vessel, it remains pellucid for some time, and at length there is perceived at the bottom a *nubecula,* or little cloud, consolidated as it were from the gluten. This nubecula increases by degrees, occupies all the urine, and renders it opaque. The natural smell is changed into a putrid *cadaverous* one; and the surface is now generally covered with a *cuticle,* composed of very minute crystals. At length, the urine regains its transparency, and the *colour* is changed from a yellow to a brown; the cadaverous smell passes into an *alkaline;* and a brown, grumous *sediment* falls to the bottom, filled with white particles, deliquescing in the air, and so conglutinated as to form, as it were, little soft calculi.

Thus *two sediments* are distinguishable in the urine; the *one* white and gelatinous, and separated in the beginning; the *other* brown and grumous, deposited by the urine when putrid.

Spontaneous degeneration.—Of all the fluids of the body, the urine first putrifies. In summer, after a few hours it becomes turbid, and sordidly black; then deposites a copious sediment, and exhales a fetor like that of putrid cancers, which at length becomes cadaverous. Putrid urine effervesces with acids, and, if distilled, gives off, before water, a urinous volatile spirit.

The properties of healthy urine are,

1. Urine reddens paper stained with turnsole and with the juice of radishes, and therefore contains an acid. This acid has been generally considered as the phosphoric, but Thenard has shown that in reality it is the *acetic.*

2. If a solution of ammonia be poured into fresh urine, a white powder precipitates, which has the properties of *phosphate of lime.*

3. If the phosphate of lime precipitated from urine be examined, a little magnesia will be found mixed with it. Fourcroy and Vauquelin have ascertained that this is owing to a little *phosphate of magnesia* which urine contains, and which is decomposed by the alkali employed to precipitate the phosphate of lime.

4. Proust informs us that *carbonic acid* exists in urine, and that its separation occasions the froth which appears during the evaporation of urine.

5. Proust has observed, that urine kept in new casks deposites small crystals, which effloresce in the air, and fall to powder. These crystals possess the properties of the *carbonate of lime.*

6. When fresh urine cools, it often lets fall a brick coloured precipitate, which Scheele first ascertained to be crystals of *uric acid.* All urine contains this acid, even when no sensible precipitate appears when it cools.

7. During intermitting fevers, and especially during diseases of the liver, a copious sediment of a brick-red colour is deposited from urine. This sediment contains the *rosacic acid* of Proust.

8. If fresh urine be evaporated to the consistence of a syrup, and muriatic acid be then poured into it, a precipitate appears which possesses the properties of *benzoic acid.*

9. When an infusion of tannin is dropped into urine, a white precipitate appears, having the properties of the combination of tannin and *albumen,* or gelatine. Their quantity in healthy urine is very small, often indeed not sensible. Cruickshanks found that the precipitate afforded by tannin in healthy urine amounted to 1-240th part of the weight of the urine.

10. If urine be evaporated by a slow fire to the consistence of a thick syrup, it assumes a deep brown colour, and exhales a fœtid ammoniacal odour. When allowed to cool, it concretes into a mass of crystals, composed of all the component parts of urine. If four times its weight of alkohol be poured into this mass, at intervals, and a slight heat be applied, the greatest part is dissolved. The alkohol which has acquired a brown colour is to be decanted off, and distilled in a retort in a sand heat till the mixture has boiled for some time, and acquired the consistence of a syrup. By this time the whole of the alkohol has passed off, and the matter, on cooling, crystallizes in quadrangular plates, which intersect each other. This substance is *urea,* which composes 9-20ths of the urine, provided the watery part be excluded. It is this substance which

characterizes urine, and constitutes it what it is, and to which the greater part of the very singular phenomena of urine are to be ascribed.

11. According to Fourcroy and Vauquelin, the colour of urine depends upon the urea; the greater the proportion of urea the deeper the colour. But Proust has detected a *resinous matter* in urine similar to the resin of bile, and to this substance he ascribes the colour of urine.

12. If urine be slowly evaporated to the consistence of a syrup, a number of crystals make their appearance on its surface; these possess the properties of the *muriate of soda*

13. The saline residuum which remains after the separation of urea from crystallized urine by means of alkohol, has been long known by the names of *fusible salt of urine*, and *microcosmic salt*. When these salts are examined, they are found to have the properties of phosphates. The rhomboidal prisms consist of *phosphate of ammonia* united to a little *phosphate of soda*, the rectangular tables, on the contrary, are phosphate of soda united to a small quantity of phosphate of ammonia; urine then contains *phosphate of soda*, and *phosphate of ammonia*.

14. When urine is cautiously evaporated a few cubic crystals are often deposited among the other salts; these crystals have the properties of *muriate of ammonia*.

15. When urine is boiled in a silver basin, it blackens the basin, and if the quantity of urine be large, small crusts of sulphuret of silver may be detached. Hence we see that urine contains *sulphur*.

Urine then contains the following substances:

1. Water.
2. Acetic acid.
3. Phosphate of lime.
4. Phosphate of magnesia.
5. Carbonic acid.
6. Carbonate of lime.
7. Uric acid.
8. Rosacic acid.
9. Benzoic acid.
10. Albumen.
11. Urea.
12. Resin
13. Muriate of soda.
14. Phosphate of soda.
15. Phosphate of ammonia.
16. Muriate of ammonia.
17. Sulphur.

According to Berzelius, healthy human urine is composed of, water 933, urea 30.10, sulphate of potassa 3.71, sulphate of soda 3.16, phosphate of soda 2.94, muriate of soda 4.45, sulphate of ammonia 1.65, muriate of ammonia 1.50, free acetic acid, with lactate of ammonia, animal matter soluble in alkohol, urea adhering to the preceding, altogether 17.14, earthy phosphates with a trace of fluate of lime 1.0, uric acid 1, mucus of the bladder 0.32, silica 0.03, in 1000.0

No liquor in the human body, however, is so variable, in respect to *quantity* and *quality*, as the urine; for it varies,

1. *In respect to age:* in the *fœtus* it is inodorous, insipid, and almost aqueous; but as the *infant* grows, it becomes more acrid and fœtid; and in *old age* more particularly so.

2. *In respect to drink:* it is secreted in greater quantity, and of a more pale colour, from cold and copious draughts. It becomes green from an infusion of Chinese tea.

3. *In respect to food:* from eating the heads of asparagus, or olives, it contracts a peculiar smell; from the fruit of the opuntia, it becomes red; and from fasting, turbid.

4. *In respect to medicines:* from the exhibition of rhubarb-root, it becomes yellow; from cassia-pulp, green; and from turpentine it acquires a violet odour.

5. *In respect to the time of the year:* in the winter the urine is more copious and aqueous; but in the summer, from the increased transpiration, it is more sparing, higher coloured, and so acrid that it sometimes occasions strangury. The climate induces the same difference.

6. *In respect of the muscular motion of the body:* it s secreted more sparingly, and concentrated by motion; and is more copiously diluted, and rendered more crude by rest.

7. *In respect of the affections of the mind:* thus fright makes the urine pale.

Use.—The urine is an excrementitious fluid, like lixivium, by which the human body is not only liberated from the superfluous water, but also from the superfluous salts, and animal earth; and is defended from corruption.

Lastly, the vis medicatrix naturæ sometimes elimi-

nates many morbid and acrid substances with the urine; as may be observed in fevers, dropsies, &c.

URINE, RETENTION OF. A want of the ordinary secretion of urine. In retention of urine there is none secreted: in a suppression, the urine is secreted but cannot be avoided.

Urine, suppression of. See *Ischuria.*

UROCRI'SIA. (From ουρον, urine, and κρινω, to judge. The judgment formed of diseases by the inspection of urine.

URORRHÆ'A. (From ουρον, the urine, and ρεω, to flow.) A discharge of the urine.

UROSCO'PIA. (From ουρον, the urine, and σκοπεω, to inspect.) Inspection of urine, that a judgment of diseases may be made from its appearance.

URSI'NA RADIX. The root of the plant called baldmoney. See *Æthusa meum.*

URSINE. *Ursinus.* Of or belonging to the bear.

URSUS. 1. The bear.

2. The name of a genus of animals. Class, *Mammalia;* Order, *Feræ.* It comprehends the several kinds of bears, the badger, and racoon.

URTI'CA. (*Ab urendo;* because it excites an itching and pustules like those produced by fire.) 1. The name of a genus of plants in the Linnæan system. Class, *Monœcia;* Order, *Tetrandria.* The nettle.

2. The pharmacopœial name of the common nettle See *Urtica dioica.*

URTICA DIOICA. The systematic name of the common stinging-nettle. This plant is well known, and though generally despised as a noxious weed, has been long used for medical, culinary, and economical purposes. The young shoots in the spring possess diuretic and antiscorbutic properties, and are with these intentions boiled and eaten instead of cabbage greens.

URTICA MORTUA. See *Lamium album.*

URTICA PILULIFERA. The systematic name of the pillbearing nettle. *Urtica romana.* The seed was formerly given against diseases of the chest, but is now deservedly forgotten. To raise an irritation in paralytic limbs, the fresh plant may be employed as producing a more permanent sting than the common nettle.

URTICA ROMANA. See *Urtica pilulifera.*

URTICA URENS. The systematic name of a less nettle than the dioica, and possessing similar virtues.

URTICA'RIA. (From *urtica*, a nettle.) *Febris urticata; Uredo; Purpura urticata; Scarlatina urtica.* The nettle-rash. A species of exanthematous fever, known by pyrexia and an eruption on the skin like that produced by the sting of the nettle. The little elevations, called the nettle-rash, often appear instantaneously, especially if the skin be rubbed or scratched, and seldom stay many hours in the same place, and sometimes not many minutes. No part of the body is exempt from them; and where many of them rise together, and continue an hour or two, the parts are often considerably swelled, which particularly happens in the arms, face, and hands. These eruptions will continue to infest the skin, sometimes in one place and sometimes in another, for one or two hours together, two or three times a day, or perhaps for the greatest part of twenty-four hours. In some constitutions they last only a few days, in others many months.

URTICA'TIO. (From *urtica*, a nettle.) The whipping a paralytic or benumbed limb with nettles, in order to restore its feeling.

U'SNEA. See *Lichen saxatilis.*

UTERA'RIA. (From *uterus*, the womb.) Medicines appropriated to diseases of the womb.

UTERINE. *Uterinus.* Appertaining to the uterus.

Uterine fury. See *Nymphomania.*

U'TERUS. Υστερα. *Matrix; Ager naturæ; Hystera; Metra; Utriculus.* The womb. A spongy receptacle resembling a compressed pear, situated in the cavity of the pelvis, above the vagina, and between the urinary bladder and rectum.

The form of the uterus resembles that of an oblong pear flattened, with the depressed sides placed towards the ossa pubis and sacrum; but, in the impregnated state, it becomes more oval, according to the degree of its distention. For the convenience of description, and for some practical purposes, the uterus is distinguished into three parts. The fundus, the body, and the cervix; the upper part is called the fundus, the lower the cervix; the space between them, the extent of which is undefined, the body. The uterus is about three inches in length, about two in breadth at the fundus, and one at the cervix. Its thickness is different at the fundus and cervix, being at the former usually rather less than half an inch, and at the latter somewhat more; and this thickness is preserved throughout pregnancy, chiefly by the enlargement of the veins and lymphatics; there being a smaller change in the size of the arteries. But there is so great a variety in the size and dimensions of the uterus in different women, independent of the states of virginity, marriage, or pregnancy, as to prevent any very accurate mensuration. The cavity of the uterus corresponds with the external form; that of the cervix leads from the os uteri, where it is very small, in a straight direction, to the fundus, where it is expanded into a triangular form, with two of the angles opposed to the entrance into the Fallopian tubes; and at the place of junction between the cervix and the body of the uterus, the cavity is smaller than it is in any other part. There is a swell or fulness of all the parts towards the cavity, which is sometimes distinguished by a prominent line running longitudinally through its middle. The villous coat of the vagina is reflected over the os uteri, and is continued into the membrane which lines the cavity of the uterus. The internal surface of the uterus is corrugated in a beautiful manner, but the rugæ, or wrinkles, which are longitudinal, lessen as they advance into the uterus, the fundus of which is smooth. In the intervals between the rugæ are small orifices, 'ike those in the vagina, which discharge a mucus, serving, besides other purposes, that of closing the os uteri very curiously and perfectly during pregnancy. The substance of the uterus, which is very firm, is composed of arteries, veins, lymphatics, nerves, and muscular fibres, curiously interwoven and connected together by cellular membrane. The muscular fibres are of a pale colour, and appear also in their texture somewhat different from muscular fibres in other parts of the body. The arteries of the uterus are the spermatic and hypogastric. The spermatic arteries arise from the anterior part of the aorta, a little below the emulgents, and sometimes from the emulgents. They pass over the psoæ muscles behind the peritonæum, enter between the two laminæ or duplicatures of the peritonæum which form the broad ligaments of the uterus, and proceed to the uterus, near the fundus of which they insinuate themselves; giving branches in their passage to the ovaria and Fallopian tubes. The hypogastric arteries are on each side a considerable branch of the internal iliacs. They pass to the sides of the body of the uterus, sending off a number of smaller branches, which dip into its substance. Some branches also are reflected upwards to the fundus uteri, which anastomose with the spermatic arteries, and others are reflected downwards, supplying the vagina. The veins which reconduct the blood from the uterus are very numerous, and their size in the unimpregnated state is proportioned to that of the arteries; but their enlargement during pregnancy is such, that the orifices of some of them, when divided, will admit even of the end of a small finger. The veins anastomose in the manner of the arteries which they accompany out of the uterus, and then, having the same names with the arteries, spermatic and hypogastric, the former proceeds to the vena cava on the right side, and on the left to the emulgent vein; and the latter to the internal iliac.

From the substance and surfaces of the uterus an infinite number of lymphatics arise, which follow th course of the hypogastric and spermatic blood-vessels. The first pass into the gland of the internal iliac plexus, and the other into the glands which are situated near the origin of the spermatic arteries. Of these Nuck first gave a delineation.

The uterus is supplied with nerves from the lower mesocolic plexus, and from two small flat circular ganglions, which are situated behind the rectum. These ganglions are joined by a number of small branches from the third and fourth sacral nerves. The ovaria derive their nerves from the renal plexus. By the great number of nerves, these parts are rendered very irritable, but it is by those branches which the uterus receives from the intercostal, that the intimate consent between it and various other parts is chiefly preserved. The muscular fibres of the uterus have been described in a very different manner by anatomists, some of whom have asserted that its substance was chiefly

muscular, with fibres running in transverse, orbicular or reticulated order, while others have contended that there were no muscular fibres whatever in the uterus. In the unimpregnated uterus, when boiled for the purpose of a more perfect examination, he former seems to be a true representation; and when the uterus is distended towards the latter part of pregnancy, these fibres are very thinly scattered; but they may be discovered in a circular direction, at the junction between the body and the cervix of the uterus, and surrounding the entrance of each Fallopian tube in a similar order. Yet it does not seem reasonable to attribute the time of labour to its muscular fibres only, if we are to judge of the power of a muscle by the number of fibres of which it is composed, unless it is presumed that those of the uterus are stronger than in common muscles. With respect to the glands of the uterus, none are discoverable dispersed through its substance upon the inner surface of the cervix; between the rugæ there are lacunæ which secrete mucus, and there are small follicles at the edge of the os uteri. These last are only observable in a state of pregnancy, when they are much enlarged. From the angles at the fundus of the uterus, two processes of an irregular round form originate, called from the name of the first describer, the *Fallopian tubes*. They are about three inches in length, and, becoming smaller in their progress from the uterus, have an uneven, fringed termination, called the fimbriæ. The canal which passes through these tubes is extremely small at their origin, but it is gradually enlarged, and terminates with a patulous orifice, the diameter of which is about one-third of an inch, surrounded by the fimbriæ. It is also lined by a very fine vascular membrane, formed into serpentine plicæ. Through this canal the communication between the uterus and ovaria is preserved. The Fallopian tubes are wrapped in duplicatures of the peritonæum, which are called the broad ligaments of the uterus; but a portion of their extremities, thus folded, hang loose on each side of the pelvis. From each lateral angle of the uterus, a little before and below the Fallopian tubes, the *round ligaments* arise, which are composed of arteries, veins, lymphatics, nerves, and a fibrous structure. These are connected together by cellular membrane, and the whole is much enlarged during pregnancy. They receive their outward covering from the peritonæum, and pass out of the pelvis through the ring of the external oblique muscle to the groin, where the vessels subdivide into small branches, and terminate at the mons veneris and contiguous parts. From the insertion of these ligaments into the groin, the reason appears why that part generally suffers in all the diseases and affections of the uterus, and why the inguinal glands are in women so often found in a morbid or enlarged state. The duplicatures of the peritonæum, in which the Fallopian tubes and ovaria are involved, are called the *broad ligaments* of the uterus. These prevent the entanglement of the parts, and are conductors of the vessels and nerves, as the mesentery is of those of the intestines. Both the round and broad ligaments alter their position during pregnancy, appearing to rise lower and more forward than in the unimpregnated state. Their use is supposed to be that of preventing the descent of the uterus, and to regulate its direction when it ascends into the cavity of the abdomen; but whether they answer these purposes may be much doubted. The use of the womb is for menstruation, conception, nutrition of the fœtus, and parturition. The uterus is liable to many diseases, the principal of which are retroversion and its falling down, hydatids, dropsy of the uterus, moles, polypes, ulceration, cancer, &c.

UTERUS, RETROVERSION OF. By the term retroversion, such a change of the position of the uterus is understood, that the fundus is turned backwards and downwards upon its cervix, between the vagina and rectum, and the os uteri is turned forwards to the pubis, and upwards, in proportion to the descent of the fundus, so that by an examination *per vaginam*, it cannot be felt, or not without difficulty, when the uterus is retroverted. By the same examination there may also be perceived a large round tumour, occupying the inferior part of the cavity of the pelvis, and pressing the vagina towards the pubes. By an examination *per anum*, the same tumour may be felt, pressing the rectum to the hollow of the sacrum, and if both these examinations are made at the same time, we may readily discover that the tumour is confined within the vagina and rectum. Besides the knowledge of the retroversion which may be gained by these examinations, it is found to be accompanied with other very distinguishing symptoms. There is in every case, together with extreme pain, a suppression of urine; and by the continuance of this distention of the bladder, the tumour formed by it in the abdomen often equals in size, and resembles in shape the uterus in the sixth or seventh months of pregnancy; but it is necessary to observe, that the suppression of urine is frequently absolute only before the retroversion of the uterus, or during the time it is retroverted; for when the retroversion is completed, there is often a discharge of urine, so as to prevent an increase of the distention of the bladder, though not in a sufficient quantity to remove it. There is also an obstinate constipation of the bowels, produced by the pressure of the retroverted uterus upon the rectum, which renders the injection of a clyster very difficult, or even impossible. But it appears that all the painful symptoms are chiefly in consequence of the suppression of urine; for none of those parts which are apt to sympathize in affections or diseases of the uterus are disturbed by its retroversion. The retroversion of the uterus has generally occurred about the third month of pregnancy, and sometimes after delivery it may likewise happen, where the uterus is, from any cause, enlarged to the size it acquires about the third month of pregnancy, but not with such facility as in the pregnant state, because the enlargement is then chiefly at the fundus. If the uterus is but little enlarged, or if it be enlarged beyond a certain time, it cannot well be retroverted; for, in the first case, should the cause of a retroversion exist, the weight at the fundus would be wanting to produce it; and in the latter the uterus would be raised above the projection of the sacrum, and supported by the spine.

UTRICA'RIA. (From *uter*, a bottle: so called from its appendages at the end of the leaves resembling bottles, to contain water.) A name of the *nepenthes*, or wonderful plant.

UTRI'CULUS. (Dim. of *uter*, a bottle: so called from its shape.) 1. The womb.

2. A little bladder. Applied by botanists to a species of capsule, which varies in thickness, never opens by any valve, and falls off with the seed. Sir J. Smith believes it never contains more than one seed, of which it is most commodiously, in botanical language, called an external coat, rather than a capsule. Gærtner applies it to Chænopodium and Clematis: in the former it seems to be pellicula; in the latter, testa.—*Smith.*

U'VA. (*Uva, æ,* f.; *Quasi uvida,* from its juice.) 1. An unripe grape.

2. A tumour on the eye resembling a grape.

Uva GRUINA. Crane-berries. The berries of the *Oxycoccos erythrocarpus.* They are brought from New-England, and are reckoned antiscorbutic.

Uva PASSA MAJOR. The raisin. See *Vitis vinifera*

Uva PASSA MINOR. The dried currant. See *Vitis corinthica.*

Uva URSI. Bear's whortle-berry. See *Arbutus uva ursi.*

U'VEA. (From *uva,* an unripe grape: so called because, in beasts, which the ancients chiefly dissected, it is like an unripe grape.) The posterior lamina of the iris. See *Choroid membrane.*

U'VULA. (Dim. of *uva,* a grape.) *Columella; Cion; Gargareon; Columna oris; Gurgulio; Interseptum.* The small conical fleshy substance hanging in the middle of the *velum pendulum palati,* over the root of the tongue. It is composed of the common membrane of the mouth, and a small muscle resembling a worm which arises from the union of the palatine bone, and descends to the tip of the uvula. It was called *Palato staphilinus,* by Douglas, and *Staphilinus epistaphilinus,* by Winslow. By its contraction, the uvula is raised up.

UVULA'RIA. (From *uvula;* because it cured diseases of the uvula.) See *Ruscus hypoglossum.*

V

VA'CCA. The cow. See *Milk.*

VACCA'RIA. (From *vacca,* a cow; because it is coveted by cows.) The herb cow's-basil.

VACCINATION. The insertion of the matter to produce the cow-pox. See *Variola vaccina.*

VACCINIA. See *Variola vaccina.*

VACCI'NIUM. (*Quasi baccinium,* from its berry.) The name of a genus of plants in the Linnæan system. Class, *Octandria;* Order, *Monogynia.*

VACCINIUM MYRTILLUS. The systematic name of the myrtle-berry. The berries which are directed in pharmacopœias by the name of *baccæ myrtillorum,* are the fruit of this plant. Prepared with vinegar and are esteemed as antiscorbutics, and when dry possess astringent virtues.

VACCINIUM OXYCOCCOS. The systematic name of the cranberry plant. *Oxycoccos palustris; Vaccinia palustris; Vitis idæa palustris.* Moor-berry. Cranberry. These berries are inserted in some pharmacopœias. They are about the size of our haws, and are pleasantly acid, and cooling, with which intention they are used medicinally in Sweden. In this country they are mostly preserved and made into tarts.

VACCINIUM VITIS IDÆA. The systematic name of the red whortleberry. *Vitis idæa.* The leaves of this plant, *vaccinium vitis idæa,* of Linnæus, are so adstringent as to be used in some places for tanning. They are said to mitigate the pain attendant on calculous diseases when given internally in the form of decoction. The ripe berries abound with a grateful acid juice; and are esteemed in Sweden as aperient, antiseptic, and refrigerant, and often given in putrid diseases.

VAGI'NA. *Vagina uteri.* The canal which leads from the external orifice of the female pudendum to the uterus. It is somewhat of a conical form, with the narrowest part downwards, and is described as being five or six inches in length, and about two in diameter. But it would be more proper to say, that it is capable of being extended to those dimensions; for in its common state, the os uteri is seldom found to be more than three inches from the external orifice, and the vagina is contracted as well as shortened. The vagina is composed of *two coats,* the first or innermost of which is villous, interspersed with many excretory ducts, and contracted into plicæ, or small transverse folds, particularly at the fore and back part, but, by child-bearing, these are lessened or obliterated. The second coat is composed of a firm membrane, in which muscular fibres are not distinctly observable, but which are endowed, to a certain degree, with contractile powers like a muscle. This is surrounded by cellular membrane, which connects it to the neighbouring parts. A portion of the upper and posterior part of the vagina is also covered by the peritonæum. The entrance of the vagina is constricted by muscular fibres, originating from the rami of the pubis, which run on each side of the pudendum, surrounding the posterior part, and executing an equivalent office, though they cannot be said to form a true sphincter.

The upper part of the vagina is connected to the circumference of the os uteri, but not in a straight line, so as to render the cavity of the uterus a continuation of that of the vagina. For the latter stretches beyond the former, and, being joined to the cervix, is reflected over the os uteri, which by this mode of union, is suspended with protuberant lips in the vagina, and permitted to change its position in various ways and directions. When, therefore, these parts are distended and unfolded at the time of labour, they are continued into each other, and there is no part which can be considered as the precise beginning of the uterus or termination of the vagina.

The diseases of the vagina are, first, such an abreviation and contraction as render it unfit for the uses for which it was designed: secondly, a cohesion of the sides in consequence of preceding ulceration: thirdly, cicatrices after an ulceration of the parts; fourthly, excrescences; fifthly, fluor albus. This abreviation and contraction of the vagina, which usually accompany each other, are produced by original defective formation, and they are seldom discovered before the time of marriage, the consummation of which they sometimes prevent. The curative intentions are to relax the parts by the use of emollient applications, and to dilate them to their proper size by sponge, or other tents, or, which are more effectual, by bougies gradually enlarged. But the circumstances which attend this disorder, are sometimes such as might lead us to form an erroneous opinion of the disease. A case of this kind, which was under Dr. Denman's care, from the strangury, from the heat of the parts, and the profuse and inflammatory discharge, was suspected to proceed from venereal infection; and with that opinion the patient had been put upon a course of medicine composed of quicksilver, for several weeks, without relief. When she applied to the Doctor, he prevailed upon her to submit to an examination, and found the vagina rigid, so much contracted as not to exceed half an inch in diameter, nor more than one inch and a half in length. The repeated, though fruitless attempts which had been made to complete the act of coition, had occasioned a considerable inflammation upon the parts, and all the suspicious appearances before mentioned. To remove the inflammation she was bled, took some gentle purgative medicines, used an emollient fomentation, and afterward some unctuous applications; she was also advised to live separate from her husband for some time. The inflammation being gone, tents of various sizes were introduced into the vagina, by which it was distended, though not very amply. She then returned to her husband, and in a few months became pregnant. Her labour, though slow, was not attended with any extraordinary difficulty. She was delivered of a full-sized child, and afterward suffered no inconvenience. Another kind of constriction of the external parts sometimes occurs, and which seems to be a mere spasm. By the violence or long continuance of a labour, by the morbid state of the constitution, or by the negligent and improper use of instruments, an inflammation of the external parts, or vagina, is sometimes produced in such a degree as to endanger a mortification. By careful management this consequence is usually prevented; but in some cases, when the constitution of the patient was prone to disease, the external parts have sloughed away, and in others, equal injury has been done to the vagina. But the effect of the inflammation is usually confined to the internal or villous coat, which is sometimes cast off wholly or partially. An ulcerated surface being thus left, when the disposition to heal has taken place, cicatrices have been formed of different kinds, according to the depth and extent of the ulceration, and there being no counteraction to the contractile state of the parts, the dimensions of the vagina become much reduced, or, if the ulceration should not be healed, and the contractibility of the parts continue to operate, the ulcerated surfaces, being brought together, may cohere, and the canal of the vagina be perfectly closed.

Cicatrices in the vagina very seldom become an impediment to the connexion between the sexes; when they do, the same kind of assistance is required as was recommended in the natural contraction or abbreviation of the part; they always give way to the pressure of the head of the child in the time of labour, though in many cases with great difficulty. Sometimes the appearances may mislead the judgment; for the above author was called to a woman in labour, who was thought to have become pregnant, though the hymen remained unbroken; but, on making very particular inquiry, he discovered that this was her second labour, and that the part, which, from its form and situation was supposed to be the hymen, with a small aperture, was a cicatrice, or unnatural contraction of the entrance into the vagina, consequent to an ulceration of the part after her former labour. Fungous excrescences arising from any part of the vagina or uterus, have been distinguished, though not very properly, by the general term polypus. See *Polypus*.

VAGINA OF NERVES. The outer covering of nerves. By some it is said to be a production of the pia mater only, and by others of the dura mater, because it agrees with it in tenacity, colour, and texture.

VAGINA OF TENDONS. A loose membranous sheath, formed by cellular membrane, investing the tendons, and containing an unctuous juice, which is secreted by the vessels of its internal surface. Ganglions are nothing more than an accumulation of this juice.

VAGINA'LIS TUNICA. See *Tunica vaginalis testis*.

VAGINANS. Sheathing; applied to parts of animals and plants, as the tunica vaginalis or testicle; to leaves which sheath the stem, or each other, as in grasses; and to the leafstalk of the *Canna indica*, which surrounds the stem like a sheath; hence *petiolus vaginans*.

VAGITUS. The cry of young children; also the distressing cry of persons under surgical operation.

VA'GUM, PAR. See *Par vagum*.

VALERIAN. See *Valeriana*.

Valerian, celtic. See *Valeriana celtica*.

Valerian, garden. See *Valeriana major*.

Valerian, great. See *Valeriana major*.

Valerian, less. See *Valeriana*.

VALERIA'NA. (From *Valerius*, who first particularly described it.) 1. The name of a genus of plants in the Linnæan system. Class, *Triandria*; Order, *Monogynia*. Valerian.

2. The pharmacopœial name of the wild valerian. See *Valeriana officinalis*.

VALERIANA CELTICA. The systematic name of the *Nardus celtica*. *Spica celtica dioscoridis*. Celtic nard. The root of this plant, a native of the Alps, has been recommended as a stomachic, carminative, and diuretic. At present it is only used in this country in the theriaca and mithridate, though its sensible qualities promise some considerable medicinal powers. It has a moderately strong smell, and a warm, bitterish, subacrid taste.

VALERIANA LOCUSTA. *Album olus.* Corn salad. This is cultivated in our gardens for an early salad. It is a wholesome, esculent plant, generally aperient and antiscorbutic.

VALERIANA MAJOR. See *Valeriana phu*.

VALERIANA MINOR. See *Valeriana officinalis*.

VALERIANA OFFICINALIS. The systematic name of the *Valeriana minor*. *Valeriana sylvestris; Leuco lachanum.* Officinal valerian; Wild valerian. *Valeriana—floribus triandris, foliis omnibus pinnatis*, of Linnæus. The root of this plant has been long extolled as an efficacious remedy in epilepsy, which caused it to be exhibited in a variety of other complaints termed nervous, in which it has been found highly serviceable. It is also in very general use as an antispasmodic, and is exhibited in convulsive hysterical diseases. A simple and volatile tincture are directed in the pharmacopœias.

VALERIANA PHU. The systematic name of the garden valerian. *Valeriana major.* The root of this plant is said to be efficacious in removing rheumatism, especially sciatica; and also inveterate epilepsies.

VALERIANA SYLVESTRIS. See *Valeriana officinalis*.

VA'LLUM. (From *vallus*, a hedge stake: so called from the regular trench-like disposition of the hairs.) The eyebrows.

VALSALVA, ANTON. MARIA, was born at Imola, in 1666, and placed at a proper age under Malpighi, at Bologna, where he applied so closely as to impair his health. He took his degree at the age of twenty-one, and connecting surgery with physic, acquired high reputation. He simplified the instruments in use, banished the practice of cauterizing the arteries after amputation, and employed manual operations in the cure of deafness. In 1697, he was chosen professor of anatomy in the university; and under his direction the school acquired great celebrity. among other distinguished pupils of his, Morgagni must be reckoned, whose chief work, "De Sedibus et Causis Morborum," contains many dissections by Valsalva. As he advanced in life he became corpulent and lethargic, and in 1723 was carried off by an apoplectic stroke. His museum was bequeathed to the institute of Bologna, and his surgical instruments to the Hospital for Incurables. The principal of his works is a treatise, "De Aure Humana;" and after his death, three of his dissertations on anatomical subjects were printed by Morgagni.

VALVA (*Valva*; from *valveo*, to fold up.) A thin and transparent membrane situated within certain vessels, as arteries, veins, and absorbents, the office of which appears to be to prevent the contents of the vessel from flowing back.

Valve of the colon. See *Intestine*.

Valve, semilunar. See *Semilunar valves*

Valve, tricuspid. See *Tricuspid valves.*

Valve, triglochin. See *Tricuspid valves.*

VA'LVULA. (From *valva*, a valve, of which it is a diminutive.) A little valve.

1. Applied to the valves of the venal and lymphatic system of animals.

2. In botany, to the parts or halves of a capsule, which split open when the seed is ripe.

VALVULA COLI. See *Intestine.*

VALVULA EUSTACHII. A membranous semilunar valve, which separates the right auricle from the inferior vena cava, first described by Eustachius.

VALVULA MITRALIS. See *Mitral valves.*

VALVULA SEMILUNARIS. See *Semilunar valves.*

VALVULA TRIGLOCHINIS. See *Tricuspid valves.*

VALVULA TULPII. See *Intestine.*

VALVULÆ CONNIVENTES. The semilunar folds formed of the villous coat of the intestinum duodenum, and jejunum. Their use appears to be to increase the internal surface of the intestines.

VANELLOE. See *Epidendrum vanilla.*

VANILLA. See *Epidendrum vanilla.*

VAPORA'RIUM. (From *vapor*, vapour.) A vapour-bath.

VAPRECULÆ. The name of an order of plants in Linnæus's Fragments of a Natural Method, consisting of such as are, and have a monophylous calyx, like a coloured corolla.

Varec. The French name for kelp.

VA'RIA. (From *varius*, changeable.) The small-pox; also small red pimples in the face.

VARICE'LLA. (Dim. of *varia*, the small-pox: so called from its being changeable.) *Variola lymphatica.* The chicken-pox. A genus of disease in the Class *Pyrexiæ*, and Order *Exanthemata*, of Cullen, known by moderate synocha, pimples bearing some resemblance to the small-pox, quickly forming pustules, which contain a fluid matter, but scarcely purulent, and after three or four days from their first appearance, desquamate.

VARICOCE'LE. (From *varix*, a distended vein, and κηλη, a tumour.) A swelling of the veins of the scrotum, or spermatic cord; hence it is divided into the *scrotal varicocele*, which is known by the appearance of livid and tumid veins on the scrotum; and *varicocele of the spermatic cord*, known by feeling hard vermiform vessels in the course of the spermatic cord. Varicocele mostly arises from excessive walking, running, jumping, wearing of trusses, and the like, producing at first a slight uneasiness in the part, which, of not remedied, continues advancing towards the loins.

VARIEGAT'US. Variegated: applied to an intermixture of colours; as in the leaves of some plants, *Mentha rotundifolia*, &c.

VARI'OLA. (From *varius*, changing colour, because it disfigures the skin.) The small-pox. A genus of disease in the Class *Pyrexiæ*, and Order *Exanthemata*, of Cullen, distinguished by synocha, eruption of red pimples on the third day, which on the eighth day contain pus, and afterward drying, fall off in crusts.

It is a disease of a very contagious nature, supposed to have been introduced into Europe from Arabia, and in which there arises a fever, that is succeeded by a number of little inflammations in the skin, which proceed to suppuration, the matter formed thereby being capable of producing the disorder in another person. It makes its attack on people of all ages, but the young of both sexes are more liable to it than those who are much advanced in life; and it may prevail at all seasons of the year, but is most prevalent in the spring and summer.

The small-pox is distinguished into the distinct and confluent, implying that in the former the eruptions are perfectly separate from each other, and that in the latter they run much into one another.

Both species are produced either by breathing air impregnated with the effluvia arising from the bodies of those who labour under the disease, or by the introduction of a small quantity of the variolous matter into the habit of inoculation; and it is probable, that the difference of the small-pox is not owing to any difference in the contagion, but depends on the state of the person to whom it is applied, or on certain circumstances concurring with the application of it.

A variety of opinions have been entertained respecting the effect of the variolous infection on the fœtus in utero: a sufficient number of instances, however, has

been recorded, to ascertain that the disease may be communicated from the mother to the child. In some cases, the body of the child, at its birth, has been covered with pustules, and the nature of the disease has been most satisfactorily ascertained by inoculating with matter taken from the pustules. In other cases, there has been no appearance of the disease at the birth, but an eruption and other symptoms of the disease have appeared so early, as to ascertain that the infection must have been received previously to the removal of the child from the uterus.

Four different states, or stages, are to be observed in the small-pox: first, the febrile; second, the eruptive; third, the maturative; and fourth, that of the declination or scabbing. When the disease has arisen naturally, and is of the distinct kind, the eruption is commonly preceded by a redness in the eyes, soreness in the throat, pains in the head, back, and loins, weariness and faintness, alternate fits of chilliness and heat, thirst, nausea, inclination to vomit, and a quick pulse. In some instances, these symptoms prevail in a high degree, and in others they are very moderate and trifling. In very young children, startings and convulsions are apt to take place a short time previous to the appearance of the eruption, always giving great alarm to those not conversant with the frequency of the occurrence.

About the third or fourth day from the first seizure, the eruption shows itself in little red spots on the face neck, and breast, and these continue to increase in number and size for three or four longer, at the end of which time they are to be observed dispersed over several parts of the body.

If the pustules are not very numerous, the febrile symptoms will generally go off on the appearance of the eruption, or then will become very moderate. It sometimes happens, that a number of little spots of an erysipelatous nature are interspersed among the pustules; but these generally go in again, as soon as the suppuration commences, which is usually about the fifth or sixth day, at which period, a small vesicle, containing an almost colourless fluid, may be observed upon the top of each pimple. Should the pustules be perfectly distinct and separate from each other, the suppuration will probably be completed about the eighth or ninth day, and they will then be filled with a thick yellow matter; but should they run much into each other, it will not be completed till some days later.

When the pustules are very thick and numerous on the face, it is apt about this time to become much swelled, and the eyelids to be closed up, previous to which, there usually arises a hoarseness, and difficulty of swallowing, accompanied with a considerable discharge of viscid saliva. About the eleventh day, the swelling of the face usually subsides, together with the affection of the fauces, and is succeeded by the same in the hands and feet, after which the pustules break, and discharge their contents: and then becoming dry, they fall in crusts, leaving the skin which they covered of a brown-red colour, which appearance continues for many days. In those cases where the pustules are large, and are late in becoming dry and falling off, they are very apt to leave pits behind them; but where they are small, suppurate quickly, and are few in number, they neither leave any marks behind them, nor do they occasion much affection of the system.

In the confluent small-pox, the fever which precedes the eruption is much more violent than in the distinct, being attended usually with great anxiety, heat, thirst, nausea, vomiting, and a frequent and contracted pulse, and often with coma or delirium. In infants, convulsive fits are apt to occur, which either prove fatal before any eruption appears, or they usher in a malignant species of the disease.

The eruption usually makes its appearance about the third day, being frequently preceded or attended with a rosy efflorescence, similar to what takes place in the measles; but the fever, although it suffers some slight remission on the coming out of the eruption, does not go off as in the distinct kind; on the contrary, it becomes increased after the fifth or sixth day, and continues considerable throughout the remainder of the disease.

As the eruption advances, the face, being thickly beset with pustules, becomes very much swelled, and the eyelids are closed up, so as to deprive the patient of sight, and a gentle salivation ensues, which towards the eleventh day, is so viscid as to be spit up with great difficulty. In children, a diarrhœa usually attends this stage of the disease instead of a salivation, which is to be met with only in adults. The vesicles on the top of the pimples are to be perceived sooner in the confluent small-pox than in the distinct; but they never rise to an eminence being usually flatted in; neither do they arrive to proper suppuration, as the fluid contained in them, instead of becoming yellow, turns to a brown colour.

About the tenth or eleventh day, the swelling of the face usually subsides, and then the hands and feet begin to puff up and swell, and about the same time the vesicles break, and pour out a liquor that forms into brown or black crusts, which, upon falling off, leave deep pits behind them that continue for life; and where the pustules have run much into each other, they then disfigure and scar the face very considerably.

Sometimes it happens that a putrescency of the fluids takes place at an early period of the disease, and shows itself in livid spots interspersed among the pustules, and by a discharge of blood by urine, stool, and from various parts of the body.

In the confluent small-pox, the fever which, perhaps, had suffered some slight remission from the time the eruption made its appearance to that of maturation, is often renewed with considerable violence at this last-mentioned period, which is what is called the secondary fever, and this is the most dangerous stage of the disease. It has been observed, even among the vulgar, that the small-pox is apt to appear immediately before or after the prevalence of the measles. Another curious observation has been made relating to the symptoms of these complaints, namely, that if, while a patient labours under the small-pox, he is seized with the measles, the course of the former is retarded till the eruption of the measles is finished. The measles appear, for instance, on the second day of the eruption of small-pox; the progress of this ceases, till the measles terminate by desquamation, and then it goes on in the usual way. Several cases are, however, recorded in the Medical and Physical Journal, as likewise in the third volume of the Medical Commentaries, in which a concurrence of the small-pox and measles took place without the progress of the former being retarded. The distinct small-pox is not attended with danger, except when it attacks pregnant women, or approaches nearly in its nature to that of the confluent; but this last is always accompanied with considerable risk, the degree of which is ever in proportion to the violence and permanence of the fever, the number of pustules on the face, and the disposition to putrescency which prevails.

When there is a great tendency this way, the disease usually proves fatal between the eighth and eleventh day, but, in some cases, death is protracted to the fourteenth or sixteenth. The confluent small-pox, although it may not prove immediately mortal, is very apt to induce various morbid affections.

Both kinds of small pox leave behind them a predisposition to inflammatory complaints, particularly to opthalmia and visceral inflammations, but more especially of the thorax; and they not unfrequently excite scrofula into action which might otherwise have lain dormant in the system.

The regular swelling of the hands and feet upon that of the face subsiding, and its continuance for the due time, may be regarded in a favourable light.

The dissections which have been made of confluent small-pox, have never discovered any pustules internally on the viscera. From them it also appears that variolous pustules never attack the cavities of the body, except those to which the air has free access, as the nose, mouth, trachea, the larger branches of the bronchia, and the outermost part of the meatus auditorius. In cases of prolapsus ani, they likewise frequently attack that part of the gut which is exposed to the air. They have usually shown the same morbid appearances inwardly, as are met with in putrid fever, where the disease has been of the malignant kind. Where the febrile symptoms have run high, and the head has been much affected with coma or delirium, the vessels of the brain appear, on removing the cranium and dura mater, more turgid, and filled with a darker coloured blood than usual, and a greater quantity of serous fluid is found, particularly towards the base of the brain. Under similar circumstances, the lungs have often a darker appearance, and their moisture is more copious than usual. When no inflammatory affection has supervened, they are most usually sound.

The treatment of small-pox will differ materially according to the species of the disease. In the distinct, ushered in by synochal pyrexia, it may be occasionally proper, in persons of a middle age, good constitution, and plethoric habit, to begin by taking away a moderate quantity of blood; the exhibition of an emetic will be generally advisable, provided there be no material tenderness of the stomach; the bowels must then be cleared, antimonial and other diaphoretics employed, and the antiphlogistic regimen strictly enforced. It is particularly useful in this disease during the eruptive fever to expose the patient freely to cold air, as taught by the celebrated Sydenham; and even the cold affusion may be proper, where there is much heat and redness of the skin, unless the lungs be weak. After the eruption has come out, the symptoms are usually so much mitigated, that little medical interference is necessary. But the confluent small-pox requires more management: after evacuating the primæ viæ, and employing other means to moderate the fever in the beginning, the several remedies adapted to support the strength and counteract the septic tendency, must be resorted to, as the disease advances, such as have been enumerated under typhus. The chief points of difference are, that bark may be more freely given to promote the process of suppuration, and opium to relieve the irritation in the skin; when the eruption has come out, it will be generally proper to direct a full dose of this remedy every night to procure rest, using proper precautions to obviate its confining the bowels, or determining to the head. Where alarming convulsions occur also, opium is the medicine chiefly to be relied upon, taking care subsequently to remove any source of irritation from the primæ viæ. Sometimes the tepid-bath may be useful under these circumstances, and favour the appearance of the eruption, where the skin is pale and cold, the pulse weak, &c. Where at a more advanced period the pustules flatten, and alarming symptoms follow, the most powerful cordial and antispasmodic remedies must be tried, as the confectio opii, æther, wine, &c. For the relief of the brain, or other important part, particularly affected, local means may be used, as in typhus. To prevent the eyes being injured, a cooling lotion may be applied, and blisters behind the ears, or even leeches to the temples.

VARIOLA VACCINA. *Vaccinia.* The cow-pox. Any pustulous disease affecting the cow, may be called the cow-pox: whether it arises from an over-distention of the udder, in consequence of a neglect in milking the cow, or from the sting of an insect, or any other cause. But the species which claims our particular attention, is that which was recommended to the world by Dr. Jenner, in the year 1798, as a substitute for the small-pox. This, which originates from the grease in the horse's heel, is called the *genuine cow-pox;* all other kinds are *spurious.*

That the vaccine fluid, fraught with such unspeakable benefits to mankind, derives its origin from this humble source, however it may mortify human pride, or medical vanity, is confirmed by the observations and experiments of competent judges. For proofs of this assertion, the reader may consult the works of Dr. Jenner; the Medical and Physical Journal; and a treatise on the subject by Dr. Loy, of which an analysis is given in the Annals of Medicine for the year 1801; and Mr. Ring's work on this disease, which contains the whole mass of evidence that has appeared concerning it.

The genuine cow-pox appears on the teats of the cow, in the form of vesicles, of a blue colour approaching to livid. These vesicles are elevated at the margin, and depressed at the centre. They are surrounded with inflammation. The fluid they contain is limpid. The animals are indisposed; and the secretion of milk is lessened. Solutions of the sulphates of zinc and copper are a speedy remedy for these pustules; otherwise they degenerate into ulcers, which are extremely troublesome. It must, however, be recollected, that much of the obstinacy attending these cases is owing to the friction of the pustules, in consequence of milking. It is probable, that a solution of the superacetate of lead would be preferable to irritating applications.

Similar effects are produced in the hands of the milkers, attended with febrile symptoms, and some-tunes with tumours in the axilla. Other parts, where the cuticle is abraded, or which are naturally destitute of that defence, are also liable to the same affection, provided active matter is applied. It even appears that, in some instances, pustules have been produced by the application of vaccine virus to the sound cuticle. One case of this kind may be found in a letter from Dr. Fowler, of Salisbury, to Dr. Pearson, published in the first work of Dr. Pearson on this subject.

The spurious cow-pox is white ; and another criterion is, that both in the brute animal and in the human subject, when infected with the casual cow-pox, the sores occasioned by the genuine species are more difficult to heal than those which are occasioned by the spurious kind. It is of the utmost importance to distinguish the genuine from the spurious sort, which is also, in some degree, infectious ; since a want of such discrimination would cause an idea of security against the small-pox, which might prove delusive.

Dr. Jenner has elucidated one point of the first importance, relative to the genuine cow-pox itself. It had frequently been observed, that when this disorder prevailed in a farm, some of the persons who contracted it by milking were rendered insusceptible of the small-pox, while others continued liable to that infection. This is owing to the different periods at which the disease was excited in the human subject; one person, who caught the disease while the virus was in an active state, is rendered secure from variolous contagion; while another, who received the infection of the cow pox when it had undergone a decomposition, is still susceptible of the small-pox. This uncertainty of the prevention, the value of which is beyond all calculation, is probably the reason why it was not before introduced into practice.

From the violent opposition which vaccine inoculation has met with, in consequence of certain apparent failures in the casual way, it may be doubted whether the public would ever have adopted the practice, had not this fallacy been detected by Dr. Jenner. To him also we are indebted for another discovery of the first importance ; namely, that the pustule excited in the human subject by vaccine matter, yields a fluid of a similar nature with that which was inserted. This experiment, so essential to the general propagation of the practice, and so happy in its result, was never before attempted. It was reserved to crown the labours of Dr. Jenner.

A considerable number of instances are on record, to prove that farriers and others who receive infection from the heel of a horse, are either partly or totally deprived of the susceptibility of the small-pox. When Dr. Jenner first published an account of his discoveries, this point was enveloped in some degree of obscurity. He then conceived, that the matter of grease was an imperfect preservative against the small-pox. This opinion was founded on the following circumstance : It had been remarked, that farriers either wholly escaped the small-pox, or had that distemper in a milder manner than other people. This, however, is easily reconcileable to reason, if we only suppose, that in some cases the infection is communicated when the virus possesses all its prophylactic virtue; and in others, when its specific quality is in some measure lost.

This variation in the effects produced by the virus of the horse, inclined Dr. Jenner to believe that it was modified, and underwent some peculiar alteration in the teats of the cow. He now concludes, that it is perfect when it excites the genuine disease in the cow ; yet a considerable advantage is derived from its being transferred to the latter animal, the nipples of which furnish a more obvious and a more abundant source of this inestimable fluid, than its original element the horse.

This theory, that the preservative against variolous contagion is perfect when it issues from the fountain-head, and comes immediately from the hands of Nature, is consonant with reason, and consistent with analogy. Thus, one obstacle more to the universal adoption of the practice is removed.

Another point respecting vaccine inoculation, which has been much controverted, is the permanency of its effect. Instances have been known where persons have escaped the small-pox for a number of years, and yet have ultimately proved not insusceptible of its infection. When such persons had previously undergone the vaccine disease, their apparent security was erroneously ascribed to that cause; but we have not even a shadow of proof, that the cow-pox possesses in the least degree the property of a temporary prophylactic, since it appears not even to retard the eruption of the small-pox, where previous infection has been received.

By this remark, it is not meant to be asserted, that it never supersedes or modifies the small-pox, for we have great reason to believe that such beneficial effects often flow from vaccination ; but where an eruption of the small-pox actually takes place after vaccine inoculation, the two diseases frequently co-exist, without retarding each other in the smallest degree. It is, therefore, contrary to all reason and analogy, to consider the cow-pox as a mere temporary preservative : it is nothing less than a perfect and permanent security against that terrible disease.

A number of cases are recorded by Dr. Jenner, and other authors, who have written on this subject, in which persons who have received the cow-pox by casual infection, twenty, thirty, forty, and fifty years before, still continued insusceptible of variolous contagion, in whatever form it was applied.

As the cow-pox destroys the susceptibility of the small-pox, so the small-pox destroys that of the cow-pox. To this general rule, however, a few exceptions are said to have occurred. Certain it is, that a pustule has now and then been excited by the insertion of vaccine virus, in those who have had the small-pox, and that this pustule has been known to yield to the genuine virus; but it is not equally certain that the pustule has been perfect in all respects. Possibly, it may have been defective in point of size or duration, in respect to its areola, or the limpidity of its contents. That such a pustule has, in some instances, yielded effectual virus, is admitted ; but this is no more than what has often happened, in cases where persons who have had the small-pox are a second time submitted to that infection in the same form.

The artificial cow-pox in the human subject is much milder than the casual disease; and incomparably milder than the small-pox, even under the form of inoculation. It neither requires medicine nor regimen it may be practised at any season of the year ; and, not being infectious by effluvia, one person may be inoculated without endangering the life of another.

This affection produces no pustulous eruptions When such attend vaccine inoculation, they are owing to some adventitious cause, such as the small-pox, which it is well known may co-exist with the cow-pox. The vaccine vesicle is confined to the parts where matter is inserted; it is, therefore, entirely a local and an inoculated disease. Nevertheless, it is certain, that eruptions of other kinds, in some instances, attend vaccine inoculation; such as a nettle-rash, or an eruption resembling a tooth-rash, but rather larger than what is commonly called by that name.

Among other singularities attending the cow-pox, the mildness of the disease, under the form of inoculation has been urged as an argument against the practice the cause appearing to ordinary comprehensions, inadequate to the effect. This, it must be allowed, is the best apology that can be offered for skepticism on that point; but it will weigh but little when put into the scale against actual observation, and incontrovertible fact. The efficacy of the cow-pox as a safeguard against the small-pox, rests, perhaps, on more extensive evidence, and a more solid foundation, than any other axiom in the whole circle of medical science.

That the cow-pox is not infectious by effluvia, is naturally concluded from its never being communicated from one person to another in the dairies; where the disease is casual, and appears under its worst form. The same inference may be drawn from its never spreading in a family, when only one person is inoculated at a time. To confirm this proposition more fully, the vaccine pustules have been ruptured, and persons who have never had the disorder have been suffered to inhale the effluvia several times a day, but to no purpose. This is no more than might be expected, in an affection where the pustulous appearance on the surface of the body is nearly local.

As to the constitutional indisposition, it is seldom considerable, unless there is a complication of this with some other distemper ; and whenever any unfavourable symptoms appear, they may in general be traced to some other cause. We have indeed great reason to believe, that no ill consequence ever arises from the cow-pox itself, unless from ignorance or neglect.

But notwithstanding the symptoms are so mild, they frequently occur at a very early period. A drowsiness, which is one of the most common attendants of the disease, is often remarked by the parents themselves, within forty-eight hours after the matter is inserted. In a majority of cases, a slight increase of heat is perceptible, together with an acceleration of the pulse, and other signs of pyrexia; but not in such a degree as to alarm the most timorous mother. Sometimes the patient is restless at nights; and now and then a case is met with, in which vomiting occurs, but in many cases, no constitutional indisposition can be perceived. Even then, the cow-pox has never failed to prove an effectual preservative against the small-pox, provided the pustule has been perfect.

This being the grand criterion of the security of the patient, too minute an attention cannot be paid to its rise, progress, and decline. The best mode of inoculating is by making a very small oblique puncture in the arm, near the insertion of the deltoid muscle, with the point of a lancet charged with fluid matter. In order to render infection more certain, the instrument may be charged again, and wiped upon the puncture.

In places where the patient is likely to be exposed to variolous contagion, it is advisable to inoculate in more places than one, but unless there is danger of catching the small-pox, it is better not to make more than one puncture in each arm, lest too much inflammation should ensue.

The vaccine fluid may be taken for inoculation as soon as it vesicle appears; but if the vesicle is punctured at a very early period, it is more apt to be injured. When virus is wanting for inoculating a considerable number, it is better to let the pustule remain untouched, till about the eighth day, by which time it has in general acquired a reasonable magnitude. After that day, if the pustule has made the usual progress, the matter begins to lose its virtue; but it may, in general, be used with safety, though with less certainty of producing infection, till the areola begins to be extensive.

The first sign of infection commonly appears on the third day. A small red spot, rather elevated, may be perceived at the place where the puncture was made. Sometimes, however, the mark of infection having succeeded is not visible till a much later period. It may be retarded, or even entirely prevented, by any other disorder, such as dentition, or any complaint attended with fever, or by extreme cold. Another frequent cause of a slow progress in the pustule, or a total failure of success, is debility. Sometimes it is impossible to discover any sign of infection for above a fortnight. In this respect the cow-pox is subject to the same laws, and liable to the same variation, as the small-pox.

When a considerable inflammation appears within two or three days after inoculation, there is reason to suspect that infection has not taken place; and if suppuration ensues, that suspicion ought, in general, to stand confirmed. Now and then, however, it happens, that after the spurious pustule, or more properly speaking, the phlegmon, has run its course, which is within a few days, a vesicle begins to appear, bearing every characteristic of the genuine vaccine disease, and yielding a limpid and efficient virus for future inoculations. In this case the patient is as perfectly secured from all danger of the small-pox, as if no festering of the puncture had preceded. The occurrence of such a case, though rare, is worthy to be recorded; because some practitioners have concluded a spurious pustule to be a certain proof of failure.

The areola commonly begins to be extensive on the ninth day, and to decline about the eleventh or twelfth. At this period also the pustule begins to dry; the first sign of which is a brown spot in the centre. In proportion as this increases the surrounding efflorescence decreases, till at length nothing remains but a circular scab, of a dark-brown mahogany colour, approaching to black. Sometimes it resembles the section of a tamarind-stone; and it often retains the depression in the centre, which characterizes this disease before exsiccation takes place.

Instances have been known, where the vaccine pustule, though regular, and perfect in all other respects, has been totally destitute of areola; at least, where neither the medical practitioner, on visiting the patient, nor the attendants, have remarked any appearance of that symptom. In these cases, the patient has proved as insusceptible of variolous infection, as if the surrounding efflorescence had covered the whole arm. It must, however, be confessed that we have no proof of the non-existence of an areola in these cases. It might have been trivial; it might have been transient; yet it might have been effectual. There is, however, greater reason to believe, that the surrounding efflorescence, though usually a concomitant circumstance, is not an essential requisite to the vaccine disease.

If by any accident the vesicle is ruptured, suppuration often ensues. In this case, more attention than ordinary ought to be paid to the progress, and to all the phenomena of the local affection; both on account of the uncertainty of success in the pustule, as a prophylactic, and the greater probability of tedious ulceration.

If there is room for the least doubt of the sufficiency of the first inoculation, a second ought to be performed without delay. This, if unnecessary, is seldom attended with inconvenience, and never with danger. Either no effect is produced, or a slight festering, which terminates in a few days. An exception occurs, but rarely, where a spurious, or perhaps, even a genuine pustule, takes place, in those persons who are known to have had the cow-pox or the small-pox already; but this cannot be the least cause of alarm to any one who knows the benign character of the distemper.

Various topical applications, both stimulant and sedative, have been recommended, in order to allay the violence of inflammation. If the operation for the insertion of matter is not unnecessarily severe, nor the pustule irritated by friction, or pressure, or other violence, no such applications are necessary. Nevertheless, if either the anxiety of the professional man, or the importunity of a tender parent, should demand a deviation from this general rule, any of the following remedies may be had recourse to. The pustule may be touched with very diluted sulphuric acid; which should be permitted to remain on the part half a minute, and then be washed off with a sponge dipped in cold water. This has been ignorantly, or artfully, called an escharotic; but any one who tries the application will soon discover, that its operation is mild and harmless.

To avoid cavil and misrepresentation, it is better to apply a saturnine lotion; compresses, dipped in such a lotion, may be applied at any time when inflammation runs high, and renewed as occasion requires.

If the pustule should chance to be broken, a drop of the liquor plumbi acetatis, undiluted, may be applied as an exsiccant; but if ulceration threatens to become obstinate, or extensive, a mild cataplasm is the best resource. In case the ulceration is only superficial, and not attended with immoderate inflammation, a bit of any adhesive plaster, spread on linen, will prove the most convenient dressing, and seldom fail of success. It will, in general, be unnecessary to renew it oftener than every other day.

These minute observations no one will despise, unless there be any person so ignorant as not to know that the care of the arm is almost the whole duty of the medical practitioner in vaccine inoculation; and that nothing disgusts the public so much against the practice, as a sore arm, and the ill consequences which, from a neglect of that symptom, too often ensue.

When fluid virus cannot be procured, it is necessary to be cautious how it is preserved in a dry state. The most improper mode is that of keeping it on a lancet; for the metal quickly rusts, and the vaccine matter becomes decomposed. This method, however, is as likely to succeed as any, when the matter is not to be kept above two or three days. If the virus be taken on glass, care must be taken not to dilute it much; otherwise it will probably fail.

Cotton thread is a very commodious vehicle. If it is intended to be sent to any considerable distance, it ought to be repeatedly dipped in the virus. No particular caution is necessary with regard to the exclusion of air; nevertheless, as it can be done with so little trouble, and is more satisfactory to those who receive the matter, it is better to comply with the practice. On this account it may be enclosed in a glass tube, or in a tobacco-pipe sealed at each end, or between two square bits of glass, which may, if necessary, be also charged with the matter, and wrapped in gold-beater's skin.

Nothing is more destructive to the efficacy of cow-pock matter than heat : on this account it must not be dried near the fire, nor kept in a warm place. The advantage of inserting it in a fluid state is so great, that it is to be wished every practitioner would endeavour to keep a constant supply for his own use, by inoculating his patients in succession, at such periods as are most likely to answer that purpose.

The rapidity with which this practice now spreads in various parts of the globe, justifies our cherishing a hope, that it will ere long extinguish that most dreadful pestilence, and perpetual bane of human felicity, the small-pox.

[Dr. Sylvanus Fansher of Middletown, in Connecticut, has devoted much time and attention to vaccination; and, in the following letter to Dr. Mitchill, proposes a method to hasten the progress of the vaccine vesicle.

"*Middletown, (Conn.) March,* 1828.

"DR. MITCHILL,

"Sir,—As you had the honour of announcing the happy tidings of the mild substitute for the small-pox in America, and as you once made honourable mention of my name relative to the art of preserving the vaccine virus, I therefore take the liberty to trouble you with the result of a series of experiments to hasten the progressive stages of the vaccine vesicle, which, I am induced to believe, promises to the world additional advantages from vaccination.

"During the earlier part of my vaccine practice, when persons came to me, with great concern, to know whether it would be too late to vaccinate a person, who had been exposed to the small-pox a week or more, and I have been under the painful necessity of expressing my fears that it would be too late ; I have, from past experience, often felt their *woes,* and sighed for a power that seemed to be denied to vaccinators or inoculators, which was, to be able to *force forward the vaccine process,* so as to hasten the constitutional affection at an earlier period than the well-known time for symptoms in either inoculation or vaccination.

"Having been an eye-witness of the extreme anguish of two fine children in 1803 and 1804, who applied too late for vaccination, I commenced making experiments to expedite vaccination, by various methods of inserting the virus. At length I found, that by making *broad punctures* on the body and shoulders, with active vaccine virus, I was able to produce an early pustule, and bring on the symptoms from 30 to 40 hours sooner than usual. And I am now able to produce above forty successful experiments to accelerate the vaccine process, substantiated by high medical authority. I write to you, Sir, because your sagacity and discernment will be the first to discover the usefulness of this improvement, and the first to detect error.

"I have the honour to be, &c.

"SYLVANUS FANSHER."

We may observe, from the above letter, that Dr. Fansher's method of hastening the vaccine process, by inserting the virus repeatedly by broad punctures on the body and shoulders, will probably prove efficacious. The ordinary mode of vaccination is, to introduce the smallest possible quantity of vaccine matter into the puncture; and hence it frequently happens, that the effect upon the constitution is so slight as to be hardly, or even not at all, perceptible. The consequence is, that cases of varioloid have sometimes occurred after vaccination, probably in cases in which it had not produced its proper influence on the system, or where that influence was insufficient. Dr. F.'s method will, doubtless, charge the system with the genuine disease, and prevent the after occurrence of varioloid, or variolus (small-pox). He thinks, however, that it will do more, and force the vaccine to outrun the small-pox, where exposure to infection has taken place. That it may do so, or at least that the effectual introduction of the vaccine may modify the small-pox, the following case, which a medical friend has reported to us, would seem to prove.

A child exposed to the influence of the natural small-pox was vaccinated, and four days after, the operation was repeated. On the eighth day from the first vaccination no appearance was observed of the progress of the kine-pock. Further vaccination was then con-sidered unnecessary and *too late,* and the parents were advised to have the child inoculated with the small-pox, which was preferable to having it in the natural way. Matter was taken from the brother, who had the small-pox very badly in the adjoining room, and inserted in the arm, near where the vaccine matter had been inserted. The pock rose on the arm, and to the surprise of the physician, the vaccine vesicle also rose, and they progressed together, modifying each other. The vaccine pock was smaller than usual, and went through its stages sooner than is common, though it had previously laid dormant, and appeared to have been put into activity by the small-pox. The small-pox was also modified, the pock were few, the sickness trifling, the confinement nothing ; and the child recovered before his brother, who was first taken. A.]

VA'RIUS. (From *varus,* unequal: so called from the irregularity of its shape.) The cuboid bone was formerly called os varium, from its irregular shape.

VA'RIX. (From *varus,* i. e. *obtortus.*) A dilatation of a vein. A genus of disease in the Class *Locales,* and Order *Tumores,* of Cullen ; known by a soft tumour on a vein which does not pulsate. Varicose veins mostly become serpentine, and often form a plexus of knots, especially in the groins and scrotum.

VAROLI, COSTANZO, was born at Bologna, in 1542, and became a professor of physic and surgery in his native city. At thirty, he was invited by Pope Gregory XIII. to settle at Rome as his first physician, and professor in the College of Sapienza. He was advancing in reputation by his anatomical discoveries, as well as in his practice, when a premature death cut him off in 1573. He was particularly distinguished in the Anatomy of the Brain, which he described in his Work " De Nervis Opticis, &c. :" and among the parts discovered, or more accurately demonstrated by him, was that formed by the union of the crura cerebri, and cerebelli, which has been since called the Pons Varolii, and which gives origin to several nerves. After his death, was published " De Resolutione Corporis Humani," an anatomical compendium, chiefly according to the ancients, but with several new observations.

VA'RUS. See *Ionthus.*

VAS. (*Vas, vasis,* n.; from *vasum :* hence in the plural, *vasa, orum ; a vescendo,* because they convey drink.) A vessel : applied to arteries, veins, ducts, &c.

VAS DEFERENS. A duct which arises from the epididymis, and passes through the inguinal ring in the spermatic cord into the cavity of the pelvis, and terminates in the vesicula seminalis. Its use is to convey the semen secreted in the testicle, and brought to it by the epididymis into the vesicula seminalis.

VA'SA BREVIA. The arteries which come from the spleen, and run along the large arch of the stomach to the diaphragm.

VASA VORTICOSA. The contorted vessels of the choroid membrane of the eye.

VA'STUS. (So called from its size.) A name given only to some muscles.

VASTUS EXTERNUS. A large, thick, and fleshy muscle, situated on the outer side of the thigh : it arises by a broad thick tendon, from the lower and anterior part of the great trochanter, and upper part of the linea aspera ; it likewise adheres by fleshy fibres, to the whole outer edge of that rough line. Its fibres descend obliquely forwards, and after it has run four or five inches downwards, we find it adhering to the anterior surface and outer side of the cruræus, with which it continues to be connected to the lower part of the thigh, where we see it terminating in a broad tendon, which is inserted into the upper part of the patella laterally, and it sends off an aponeurosis that adheres to the head of the tibia, and is continued down the leg.

VASTUS INTERNUS. This muscle, which is less considerable than the vastus externus, is situated at the inner side of the thigh, being separated from the preceding by the rectus.

It arises tendinous and fleshy from between the fore part of the os femoris, and the root of the less trochanter, below the insertion of the psoas magnus, and the iliacus internus ; and from all the inner side of the linea aspera. Like the vastus externus it is connected with the cruræus, but it continues longer fleshy than that muscle. A little above the knee we see its outer edge uniting with the inner edge of the rectus, after which it is inserted tendinous into the upper part and inner side of the patella, sending off an aponeurosis which adheres to the upper part of the tibia.

VEGETABLE. *Vegetabilis.* One of the three great divisions of nature. The most obvious difference between vegetables and animals is, that the latter are, in general, capable of conveying themselves from place to place; whereas vegetables, being fixed in the same place, absorb, by means of their roots and leaves, such support as is within their reach.

The nutrition or support of plants appears to require water, earth, light, and air. There are various experiments which have been instituted to show, that water is the only aliment which the root draws from the earth. Van Helmont planted a willow, weighing fifty pounds, in a certain quantity of earth covered with sheet-lead; he watered it for five years with distilled water; and at the end of that time the tree weighed one hundred and sixty-nine pounds three ounces, and the earth in which it had vegetated was found to have suffered a loss of no more than three ounces. Boyle repeated the same experiment upon a plant, which at the end of two years weighed fourteen pounds more, without the earth in which it had vegetated having lost any perceptible portion of its weight.

Duhamel and Bonnet supported plants with moss, and fed them with mere water: they observed, that the vegetation was of the most vigorous kind; and the naturalist of Geneva observes, that the flowers were more odoriferous, and the fruit of a higher flavour. Care was taken to change the supports before they could suffer any alteration. Tillet has likewise raised plants, more especially of the gramineous kind, in a similar manner, with this difference only, that his supports were pounded glass, or quartz in powder. Hales has observed, that a plant, which weighed three pounds, gained three ounces after a heavy dew. Do we not every day observe hyacinths and other bulbous plants, as well as gramineous plants, raised in saucers or bottles containing mere water? And Braconnot has lately found mustard-seed to germinate, grow, and produce plants, that came to maturity, flowered, and ripened their seed, in litharge, flowers of sulphur, and very small unglazed shot. The last appeared least favourable to the growth of the plants, apparently because their roots could not penetrate between it so easily.

All plants do not demand the same quantity of water; and nature has varied the organs of the several individuals conformably to the necessity of their being supplied with this food. Plants which transpire little, such as the mosses and the lichens, have no need of a considerable quantity of this fluid; and accordingly they are fixed upon dry rocks, and have scarcely any roots; but plants which require a larger quantity, have roots which extend to a great distance, and absorb humidity throughout their whole surface.

The leaves of plants have likewise the property of absorbing water, and of extracting from the atmosphere the same principle which the root draws from the earth. But plants which live in the water, and as it were swim in the element which serves them for food, have no need of roots; they receive the fluid at all their pores; and we accordingly find, that the fucus, the ulva, &c. have no roots whatever.

The dung which is mixed with earths, and decomposed, not only affords the alimentary principles we have spoken of, but likewise favours the growth of the plant by that constant and steady heat which its ulterior decomposition produces. Thus it is that Fabroni affirms his having observed the developement of leaves and flowers in that part of the tree only, which was in the vicinity of a heap of dung.

From the preceding circumstances it appears, that the influence of the earth in vegetation is almost totally confined to the conveyance of water, and probably the elastic products from putrefying substances, to the plant.

Vegetables cannot live without air. From the experiments of Priestley, Ingenhousz, and Sennebier, it is ascertained, that plants absorb the azotic part of the atmosphere; and this principle appears to be the cause of the fertility which arises from the use of putrefying matters in the form of manure. The carbonic acid is likewise absorbed by vegetables, when its quantity is small. If in large quantity, it is fatal to them. Chaptal has observed, that carbonic acid predominates in the fungus, and other subterraneous plants. But, by causing these vegetables, together with the

body upon which they were fixed, to pass, by imperceptible gradations, from an almost absolute darkness, into the light, the acid very nearly disappeared; the vegetable fibres being proportionally increased, at the same time that the resin and colouring principles were developed, which he ascribes to the oxygen of the same acid. Sennebier has observed, that the plants which he watered with water impregnated with carbonic acid, transpired an extraordinary quantity of oxygen, which likewise indicates a decomposition of the acid.

Light is almost absolutely necessary to plants. In the dark, they grow pale, languish, and die. The tendency of plants towards the light is remarkably seen in such vegetation as is effected in a chamber or place where the light is admitted on one side; for the plant never fails to grow in that direction. Whether the matter of light be condensed into the substance of plants, or whether it act merely as a stimulus or agent, without which the other requisite chemical processes cannot be effected, is uncertain.

It is ascertained, that the processes in plants serve, like those in animals, to produce a more equable temperature, which is for the most part above that of the atmosphere. Dr. Hunter, quoted by Chaptal, observed, by keeping a thermometer plunged in a hole made in a sound tree, that it constantly indicated a temperature several degrees above that of the atmosphere, when it was below the fifty-sixth division of Fahrenheit; whereas the vegetable heat, in hotter weather, was always several degrees below that of the atmosphere. The same philosopher has likewise observed, that the sap which, out of the tree, would freeze at 32°, did not freeze in the tree unless the cold were augmented 15° more.

The vegetable heat may increase or diminish by several causes, of the nature of disease; and it may even become perceptible to the touch in very cold weather, according to Buffon.

The principles of which vegetables are composed, if we pursue their analysis as far as our means have hitherto allowed, are chiefly carbon, hydrogen, and oxygen. Nitrogen is a constituent principle of several, but for the most part in small quantity. Potassa, soda, lime, magnesia, silex, alumina, sulphur, phosphorus, iron, manganese, and muriatic acid, have likewise been reckoned in the number; but some of these occur only occasionally, and chiefly in very small quantities; and are scarcely more entitled to be considered as belonging to them than gold, or some other substances, that have been occasionally procured from their decomposition.

The following are the principal products of vegetation:—

1. *Sugar.* Crystallizes. Soluble in water and alkohol. Taste sweet. Soluble in nitric acid, and yields oxalic acid.

2. *Sarcocol.* Does not crystallize. Soluble in water and alkohol. Taste bitter sweet. Soluble in nitric acid, and yields oxalic acid.

3. *Asparagin.* Crystallizes. Taste cooling and nauseous. Soluble in hot water. Insoluble in alkohol. Soluble in nitric acid, and converted into bitter principle and artificial tannin.

4. *Gum.* Does not crystallize. Taste insipid. Soluble in water, and forms mucilage. Insoluble in alkohol. Precipitated by silicated potassa. Soluble in nitric acid, and forms mucous and oxalic acids.

5. *Ulmin.* Does not crystallize. Taste insipid. Soluble in water, and does not form mucilage. Precipitated by nitric and oxymuriatic acids in the state of resin. Insoluble in alkohol.

6. *Inulin.* A white powder. Insoluble in cold water. Soluble in boiling water; but precipitates unaltered after the solution cools. Insoluble in alkohol. Soluble in nitric acid, and yields oxalic acid.

7. *Starch.* A white powder. Taste insipid. Insoluble in cold water. Soluble in hot water; opaque and glutinous. Precipitated by an infusion of nutgalls; precipitate redissolved by a heat of 120°. Insoluble in alkohol. Soluble in dilute nitric acid, and precipitated by alkohol. With nitric acid yields oxalic acid and a waxy matter.

8. *Indigo.* A blue powder. Taste insipid. Insoluble in water, alkohol, and æther. Soluble in sulphuric acid. Soluble in nitric acid, and converted into bitter principle and artificial tannin.

9. *Gluten.* Forms a ductile elastic mass with water. Partially soluble in water; precipitated by infusion of nutgalls and oxygenized muriatic acid. Soluble in acetic acid and muriatic acid. Insoluble in alkohol. By fermentation becomes viscid and adhesive, and then assumes the properties of cheese. Soluble in nitric acid, and yields oxalic acid.

10. *Albumen.* Soluble in cold water. Coagulated by heat, and becomes insoluble. Insoluble in alkohol. Precipitated by infusion of nutgalls. Soluble in nitric acid. Soon putrefies.

11. *Fibrin.* Tasteless. Insoluble in water and alkohol. Soluble in diluted alkalies, and in nitric acid. Soon putrefies.

12 *Gelatin.* Insipid. Soluble in water. Does not coagulate when heated. Precipitated by infusion of galls.

13. *Bitter principle.* Colour yellow or brown. Taste bitter. Equally soluble in water and alkohol. Soluble in nitric acid. Precipitated by nitrate of silver.

14. *Extractive.* Soluble in water and alkohol. Insoluble in æther. Precipitated by oxygenized muriatic acid, muriate of tin, and muriate of alumina; but not by gelatin. Dyes fawn colour.

15. *Tannin.* Taste astringent. Soluble in water and in alkohol of 0.810. Precipitated by gelatin, muriate of alumina, and muriate of tin.

16. *Fixed oils.* No smell. Insoluble in water and alkohol. Forms soaps with alkalies. Coagulated by earthy and metallic salts.

17. *Wax.* Insoluble in water. Soluble in alkohol, æther, and oils. Forms soap with alkalies. Fusible.

18. *Volatile oil.* Strong smell. Insoluble in water. Soluble in alkohol. Liquid. Volatile. Oily. By nitric acid inflamed, and converted into resinous substances.

19. *Camphor.* Strong odour. Crystallizes. Very little soluble in water. Soluble in alkohol, oils, acids. Insoluble in alkalies. Burns with a clear flame, and volatilizes before melting.

20. *Birdlime.* Viscid. Taste insipid. Insoluble in water. Partially soluble in alkohol. Very soluble in æther. Solution green.

21. *Resins.* Solid. Melt when heated. Insoluble in water. Soluble in alkohol, æther, and alkalies. Soluble in acetic acid. By nitric acid converted into artificial tannin.

22. *Guaiacum.* Possesses the characters of resins; but dissolves in nitric acid, and yields oxalic acid and no tannin.

23. *Balsams.* Possess the characters of the resins, but have a strong smell; when heated, benzoic acid sublimes. It sublimes also when they are dissolved in sulphuric acid. By nitric acid converted into artificial tannin.

24. *Caoutchouc.* Very elastic. Insoluble in water and alkohol. When steeped in æther, reduced to a pulp, which adheres to every thing. Fusible and remains liquid. Very combustible.

25. *Gum resins.* Form milky solutions with water, transparent with alkohol. Soluble in alkalies. With nitric acid converted into tannin. Strong smell. Brittle, opaque, infusible.

26. *Cotton.* Composed of fibres. Tasteless. Very combustible. Insoluble in water, alkohol, and æther. Soluble in alkalies. Yields oxalic acid to nitric acid.

27. *Suber.* Burns bright, and swells. Converted by nitric acid into suberic acid and wax. Partially soluble in water and alkohol.

28. *Wood.* Composed of fibres. Tasteless. Insoluble in water and alkohol. Soluble in weak alkaline lixivium. Precipitated by acids. Leaves much charcoal when distilled in a red heat. Soluble in nitric acid, and yields oxalic acid.

To the preceding we may add, emetin, fungin, hematin, nicotin, pollenin; the new vegetable alkalies, aconita, atropia, brucia, cicuta, datura, delphia, hyosciama, morphia, picrotoxia, strychnia, veratria; and the various vegetable acids.

Veil of mosses. See *Calyptra.*

VEIN. *Vena.* A long membranous canal, which continually becomes wider, does not pulsate, and returns the blood from the arteries to the heart. All veins originate from the extremities of arteries only, by anastomosis, and terminate in the auricles of the heart; *e. g.* the venæ cavæ in the right, and the pulmonary veins in the left auricle. They are composed like arteries, of three tunics, or coats, which are much more slender than in the arteries, and are supplied internally with semilunar membranes, or folds, called valves. Their use is to return the blood to the heart.

The blood is returned from every part of the body, except the lungs, into the right auricle, from three sources:

1. The *vena cava superior*, which brings it from the head, neck, thorax, and superior extremities.

2. The *vena cava inferior*, from the abdomen and inferior extremities.

3. The *coronary vein* receives it from the coronary arteries of the heart.

1. The *vena cava superior.* This vein terminates in the superior part of the right auricle, into which it evacuates the blood, from the *right* and *left subclavian vein*, and the *vena azygos.* The right and left subclavian veins receive the blood from the head and upper extremities, in the following manner. The veins of the fingers, called *digitals*, receive the blood from the digital arteries, and empty it into,

The *cephalic of the thumb*, which runs on the back of the hand along the thumb, and evacuates itself into the external radial.

The *salvatella*, which runs along the little finger, unites with the former, and empties its blood into the internal and external cubital veins. At the bend of the forearm are three veins, called the great cephalic, the basilic, and the median.

The *great cephalic* runs along the superior part of the forearm, and receives the blood from the external radial.

The *basilic* ascends on the under side, and receives the blood from the *external* and *internal cubital veins*, and some branches which accompany the brachial artery, called *venæ satellites.*

The *median* is situated in the middle of the forearm, and arises from the union of several branches. These three veins all unite above the bend of the arm, and form,

The *brachial vein*, which receives all their blood, and is continued into the axilla, where it is called,

The *axillary vein.* This receives also the blood from the scapula, and superior and inferior parts of the chest, by the *superior* and *inferior thoracic vein*, the *vena muscularis*, and the *scapularis.*

The axillary vein then passes under the clavicle, where it is called the *subclavian*, which unites with the external and internal jugular veins, and the vertebral vein which brings the blood from the vertebral sinuses; it receives also the blood from the *mediastinal, pericardiac, diaphragmatic, thymic, internal mammary*, and *laryngeal* veins, and then unites with its fellow, to form the vena cava superior, or, as it is sometimes called, *vena cava descendens.*

The blood from the external and internal parts of the head and face is returned in the following manner into the external and internal jugulars, which terminate in the subclavians.

The *frontal, angular, temporal, auricular, sublingual*, and *occipital* veins, receive the blood from the parts after which they are named; these all converge to each side of the neck, and form a trunk, called the *external jugular vein.*

The blood from the brain, cerebellum, medulla oblongata, and membranes of these parts, is received into the lateral sinuses, or vein of the dura mater, one of which empties its blood through the foramen lacerum in basi cranii on each side into the *internal jugular*, which descends in the neck by the carotid arteries, receives the blood from the *thyroideal* and *internal maxillary veins*, and empties itself into the subclavians within the thorax.

The vena azygos receives the blood from the *bronchial, superior œsophageal, vertebral*, and *intercostal veins*, and empties it into the superior cava.

2. *Vena cava inferior.* The vena cava inferior is the trunk of all the abdominal veins and those of the lower extremities, from which parts the blood is returned in the following manner. The veins of the toes, called the *digital veins*, receive the blood from the digital arteries, and form on the back of the foot three branches, one on the great toe, called the *cephalic*, another which runs along the little toe, called the *vena saphena*, and a third on the back of the foot, *veno dorsalis pedis*; and those on the sole of the foot evacuate themselves into the *plantar veins.*

The three veins on the upper part of the foot coming

together above the ankle, form the *anterior tibial;* and the plantar veins with a branch from the calf of the leg, called the *sural vein,* from the *posterior tibial;* a branch also ascends in the direction of the fibula, called the *peroneal vein.* These three branches unite before the ham, into one branch, the *subpopliteal vein,* which ascends through the ham, carrying all the blood from the foot: it then proceeds upon the anterior part of the thigh, where it is termed the *crural* or *femoral vein,* receives several muscular branches, and passes under Poupart's ligament into the cavity of the pelvis, where it is called the *external iliac.*

The arteries which are distributed about the pelvis evacuate their blood into the *external hæmorrhoidal veins,* the *hypogastric veins,* the *internal pudendal,* the *vena magna ipsius penis,* and *obturatory veins,* all of which unite in the pelvis, and form the *internal iliac vein.*

The external iliac vein receives the blood from the external pudendal veins, and then unites with the internal iliac at the last vertebra of the loins; after which it forms with its fellow the *vena cava inferior* or *ascendens,* which ascends on the right side of the spine, receiving the blood from the *sacral, lumbar, emulgent, right spermatic veins,* and the *vena cava hepatica;* and having arrived at the diaphragm, it passes through the right foramen, and enters the right auricle of the heart, into which it evacuates all the blood from the abdominal viscera and lower extremities.

Vena cava hepatica. This vein ramifies in the substance of the liver, and brings the blood into the vena cava inferior from the branches of the *vena portæ,* a great vein which carries the blood from the abdominal viscera into the substance of the liver. The trunk of this vein, about the fissure of the liver in which it is situated, is *divided* into the hepatic and abdominal portions. The *abdominal portion* is composed of the *splenic, meseraic,* and *internal hæmorrhoidal veins.* These three venous branches carry all the blood from the stomach, spleen, pancreas, omentum, mesentery, gall-bladder, and the small and large intestines, into the *sinus* of the vena portæ. The *hepatic portion* of the vena portæ enters the substance of the liver, divides into innumerable ramifications, which secrete the bile, and the superfluous blood passes into corresponding branches of the *vena cava hepatica.*

The *action of the veins.* Veins do not pulsate; the blood which they receive from the arteries flows through them very slowly, and is conveyed to the right auricle of the heart, by the contractility of their coats, the pressure of the blood from the arteries, called the *vis a tergo,* the contraction of the muscles, and respiration; and it is prevented from going backward in the vein by the valves, of which there are a great number.

Veinless leaf. See *Avenius.*

Veiny leaf. See *Venosus.*

VEJUCA DU GUACO. A plant which has the power of curing and preventing the bite of venomous serpents.

VELAME'NTUM BOMBYCINUM. The interior soft membrane of the intestines.

VE'LUM. A veil.

VELUM PENDULUM PALATI. *Velum; Velum palatinum.* The soft palate. The soft part of the palate, which forms two arches, affixed laterally to the tongue and pharynx.

VELUM PUPILLÆ. See *Membrana pupillaris.*

VENA. (From *venio,* to come; because the blood comes through it.) A vein. See *Vein.*

VENA AZYGOS. See *Azygos vena.*

VENA MEDINENSIS. See *Medinensis vena.*

VENA PORTÆ. (*Vena portæ, à portando;* because through it things are carried.) *Vena portarum.* The great vein, situated at the entrance of the liver, which receives the blood from the abdominal viscera, and carries it into the substance of the liver. It is distinguished into the *hepatic* and *abdominal* portion; the former is ramified through the substance of the liver, and carries the blood destined for the formation of the bile, which is returned by branches to the trunk of the vena cava; the latter is composed of three branches; viz. the splenic, mesenteric, and internal hæmorrhoidal veins. See *Vein.*

VENÆ LACTEÆ. The lacteal absorbents were so called. See *Lacteals.*

VENEREAL. (*Venereus; from Venus,* because it belongs to acts of venery.) Of or belonging to the sexual intercourse.

Venereal disease. See *Gonorrhœa* and *Syphilis.*

VENOSUS. Veiny. Applied by botanists to a leaf which has the vessels, by which it is nourished, branched, subdivided, and more or less prominent, forming a network over either or both its surfaces; as in Cratægus, Pyrolus terminalis, &c.

VE'NTER. A term formerly applied to the larger circumscribed cavities of the body, as the abdomen and thorax.

VENTRICLE. (*Ventriculus:* from *venter.*) A term given by anatomists to the cavities of the brain and heart. See *Cerebrum,* and *Heart.*

VENTRI'CULUS PULMONARIS. The right ventricle of the heart.

VENTRICULUS SUCCENTURIATUS. That portion of the duodenum, which is surrounded by the peritoneum, is sometimes so large as to resemble a second stomach, and is so called by some writers.

VENTRILOQUISM. *Gastriloquism. Engastrimythus.* The formation of the voice within the mouth in such a way, as to imitate other voices than that which is natural to the person, and so as not to be seen to move the lips. Nothing is more easy to man than to imitate the different sounds he hears: this in fact he performs in many circumstances. Many persons imitate perfectly the voice and pronunciation of others, actors, for example. Hunters imitate the different cries of the game, and thus succeed in decoying it into their nets.

This faculty of imitating the different sounds, has given rise to the art called ventriloquism; but the persons who exercise this art, have no organization different from that of other men; they require only to have the organs of voice and speech very perfect, in order that they may readily produce the necessary sounds.

The basis of this art is easily understood. We have found by experience, instinctively, that sounds are changed by many causes: for example, that they become feeble, less distinct, and that their expression changes, according as they are more distant from us; a man who is at the bottom of a well wishes to speak to persons who are at the top; but his voice will not reach their ears until it has received certain modifications, which depend upon the distance and the form of the tube through which it passes.

If a person remark these modifications with care, and endeavour to imitate them, he will produce acoustic illusions, which would be equally deceiving to the ear as the observation of objects through a magnifying glass is to the eye. The error will be complete if he employ those deceptions which are necessary to distract the attention.

These illusions will be numerous in proportion to the talents of the performer: but we must not imagine that a ventriloquist produces vocal sounds, and articulates differently from other people. His voice is formed in the ordinary manner; only he is capable of modifying, according to his pleasure, the volume, the expression, &c. of it; and with regard to the words that he pronounces without moving his lips, he takes care to choose those into which no labial consonants enter, otherwise he would be obliged to move his lips. This art is, in certain respects, for the ear what painting is for the eye.

VE'NUS. Copper was formerly so called by the chemists.

VERATRIA. Veratrine. A new vegetable alkali, discovered lately by Pelletier and Caventou, in the *veratrum sabatilla,* or cevadilla, the *veratrum album,* or white hellebore, and the *colchicum autumnale,* or meadow saffron.

The seeds of cevadilla, after being freed from an unctuous and acrid matter by æther, were digested in boiling alkohol. As this infusion cooled, a little wax was deposited; and the liquid being evaporated to an extract, redissolved in water, and again concentrated by evaporation, parted with its colouring matter. Acetate of lead was now poured into the solution, and an abundant yellow precipitate fell, leaving the fluid nearly colourless. The excess of lead was thrown down by sulphuretted hydrogen, and the filtered liquor being concentrated by evaporation, was treated with magnesia, and again filtered. The precipitate, boiled in alkohol, gave a solution, which, on evaporation, left a pulverulent matter, extremely bitter, and with decidedly alkaline characters. It was at first yellow, but by solution in alkohol, and precipitation by water, was obtained in a fine white powder.

The precipitate by the acetate of lead, gave, on examination, gallic acid; and hence it is concluded, that the new alkali existed in the seed as a gallate.

Veratria was found in the other plants above mentioned. It is white, pulverulent, has no odour, but excites violent sneezing. It is very acrid, but not bitter. It produced violent vomiting in very small doses, and, according to some experiments, a few grains may cause death. It is very little soluble in cold water. Boiling water dissolves about 1-1000th part, and becomes acrid to the taste. It is very soluble in alkohol, and rather less soluble in æther.

VERATRINE. See *Veratria.*

VERA'TRUM. 1. The name of a genus of plants in the Linnæan system. Class, *Polygamia;* Order, *Monœcia.*

2. The pharmacopœial name of white hellebore. See *Veratrum album.*

VERATRUM ALBUM. *Helleborus albus; Elleborum album.* White hellebore, or veratrum. *Veratrum—racemo supra-decomposito, corollis erectis,* of Linnæus. This plant is a native of Italy, Switzerland, Austria, and Russia. Every part of the plant is extremely acrid and poisonous. The dried root has no particular smell, but a durable, nauseous, and bitter taste, burning the mouth and fauces: when powdered, and applied to issues, or ulcers, it produces griping and purging; if snuffed up the nose, it proves a violent sternutatory. Gesner made an infusion of half an ounce of this root with two ounces of water; of this he took two drachms, which produced great heat about the scapulæ and in the face and head, as well as the tongue and throat, followed by singultus, which continued till vomiting was excited. Bergius also experienced very distressing symptoms, upon tasting this infusion. The root, taken in large doses, discovers such acrimony, and operates by the stomach and rectum with such violence, that blood is usually discharged; it likewise acts very powerfully upon the nervous system, producing great anxiety, tremors, vertigo, syncope, aphonia, interrupted respiration, sinking of the pulse, convulsions, spasms, and death. Upon opening those who have died of the effects of this poison, the stomach discovered marks of inflammation, with corrosions of its internal coat. The ancients exhibited this active medicine in maniacal cases, and it is said with success. The experience of Greding is somewhat similar: out of twenty-eight cases, in which he exhibited the bark of the root collected in the spring, five were cured. In almost every case that he relates, the medicine acted more or less upon all the excretions; vomiting and purging were very generally produced, and the matter thrown off the stomach was constantly mixed with bile; a florid redness frequently appeared on the face, and various cutaneous efflorescences upon the body; and, in some, pleuritic symptoms, with fever, supervened, so as to require bleeding; nor were the more alarming affections of spasms and convulsions unfrequent. Critical evacuations were also very evident; many sweating profusely, in some the urine was considerably increased, in others the saliva and mucous discharges: the uterine obstructions, of long duration, were often removed by its use. Veratrum has likewise been found useful in epilepsy, and other convulsive complaints: but the diseases in which its efficacy seems least equivocal, are those of the skin, as itch, and different prurient eruptions, herpes, morbus pediculosus, lepra, scrofula, &c.; and in many of these it has been successfully employed both internally and externally, As a powerful stimulant and irritating medicine, its use has been resorted to in desperate cases only, and even then it ought first to be exhibited in very small doses, as a grain, and in a diluted state, and to be gradually increased, according to the effects, which are generally of an alarming nature. The active ingredient of this plant is an alkali lately detected. See *Veratria.*

VERATRUM NIGRUM. See *Helleborus niger.*

VERATRUM SABADILLA. *Cevadilla hispanorum; Sevadilla; Sabadilla; Hordeum causticum; Canis interfector.* Indian caustic barley. The plant whose seeds are thus denominated, is a species of *veratrum:* they are powerfully caustic, and are administered with very great success as a vermifuge. They are also diuretic and emetic. The dose to a child, from two to four years old, is two grains; from hence to eight, five grains; from eight to twelve, ten grains. A new alkali has been detected in the seeds of this plant. See *Veratria.*

[VERATRUM VIRIDE. See *American hellebore.* A.]

VERBA'SCUM. (*Quasi barbascum,* from its hairy coat.) 1. The name of a genus of plants in the Linnæan system. Class, *Pentandria;* Order, *Monogynia.*

2. The pharmacopœial name of the yellow and black mullein.

VERBASCUM NIGRUM. The systematic name of the black mullein. *Candela regia; Tapsus barbatus; Candelaria; Lanaria.* The *Verbascum nigrum,* and *Verbascum thapsus* appear to be ordered indifferently by this name in the pharmacopœias. The flowers, leaves, and roots, are used occasionally as mild astringents. The leaves possess a roughish taste, and promise to be of service in diarrhœas and other debilitated states of the intestines.

VERBASCUM THAPSUS. The systematic name of the yellow mullein. See *Verbascum nigrum.*

VERBE'NA. (*Quasi herbena;* a name of distinction for all herbs used in sacred rites.) Vervain. 1. The name of a genus of plants in the Linnæan system. Class, *Decandria;* Order, *Monogynia.*

2. The pharmacopœial name of the vervain. See *Verbena officinalis.*

VERBENA FŒMINA. The hedge mustard is sometimes so called. See *Erysimum alliaria.*

VERBENA OFFICINALIS. The systematic name of *Verbenaca; Peristerium; Hierobotane; Herba sacra.* Vervain. This plant is destitute of odour, and to the taste manifests but a slight degree of bitterness and astringency. In former times the verbena seems to have been held sacred, and was employed in celebrating the sacrificial rites; and with a view to this, more than the natural power of the plant, it was worn suspended about the neck as an amulet. This practice, thus founded on superstition, was, however, in process of time, adopted in medicine; and, therefore, to obtain its virtues more effectually, the vervain was directed to be bruised before it was appended to the neck; and of its good effects thus used for inveterate headaches, Forestus relates a remarkable instance. In still later times it has been employed in the way of cataplasm, by which we are told the most severe and obstinate cases of cephalalgia have been cured, for which we have the authorities of Etmuller, Hartman, and more especially De Haën. Notwithstanding these testimonies in favour of the vervain, it has deservedly fallen into disuse in Britain; nor has the pamphlet of Mr. Morley, written professedly to recommend its use in scrofulous affections, had the effect of restoring its medical character. This gentleman directs the root of vervain to be tied with a yard of white satin riband round the neck, where it is to remain till the patient recovers. He also has recourse to infusions and ointments prepared from the leaves of the plant, and occasionally calls in aid the most active medicines of the materia medica.

VERDIGRIS. *Ærugo.* An impure subacetate of copper. It is prepared by stratifying copper plates with the husks of grapes, after the expression of their juice, and when they have been kept for some time imperfectly exposed to the air, in an apartment warm but not too dry, so as to pass to a state of fermentation, whence a quantity of vinegar is formed. The copper plates are placed in jars in strata, with the husks thus prepared, which are covered. At the end of twelve, fifteen, or twenty days, these are opened: the plates have an efflorescence on their surface of a green colour and silky lustre: they are repeatedly moistened with water; and at length a crust of verdigris is formed, which is scraped off by a knife, is put into bags, and dried by exposure of these to the air and sun. It is of a green colour, with a slight tint of blue.

In this preparation the copper is oxidized, probably by the atmospheric air, aided by the affinity of the acetic acid; and a portion of this acid remains in combination with the oxide, not sufficient, however, to produce its saturation. When acted on by water, the acid, with such a portion of oxide as it can retain in solution, are dissolved, and the remaining oxide is left undissolved. From this analysis of it by the action of water, Proust inferred that it consists of 43 of acetate of copper, 27 of black oxide of copper, and 30 of water;

h a water not being accidental, but existing in it in ntimate combination.

Verdigris is used as a pigment in some of the processes of dying, and in surgery it is externally applied as a mild detergent in cleansing foul ulcers, or other open wounds. On account of its virulent properties, it ought not to be used as a medicine without professional advice; and in case any portion of this poison be accidentally swallowed, emetics should be first given, and afterward cold water, gently alkalized, ought to be drunk in abundance.

VERHEYEN, PHILIP, was born in 1648 at Ves-bronck, in the county of Waes, and assumed the clerical profession; but an inflammation of his leg having rendered amputation necessary, he was determined afterward to study medicine. He accordingly graduated and settled at Louvain, where he was nominated professor of anatomy in 1689, and four years after of surgery also. His application was indefatigable, so that he attained distinguished eminence, and attached to his school a great number of disciples. His celebrity was principally the result of a work, entitled, "Anatomia Corporis Humani," which passed through many editions and improvements, and superseded the compendium of Bartholine. He published also a Compendium of Medicine, a Treatise on Fevers, &c.

VERJUICE. An acid liquor prepared from grapes or apples, that are unfit to be converted into wine or cider. It is also made from crabs. It is principally used in sauces and ragouts, though it sometimes forms an ingredient in medicinal compounds.

VERMICULA'RIS. (From vermis, a worm.) Vermicular: shaped like, or having the properties of, a worm. Applied very generally in natural history.

VERMIFORM. (Vermiformis; from vermis, a worm, and forma, resemblance.) Worm-like.

VERMIFORM PROCESS. Protuberantia vermiformis. The substance which unites the two hemispheres of the cerebellum like a ring, forming a process. It is called vermiform, from its resemblance to the contortions of worms.

VERMIFUGE. (Vermifugus; from vermis, a worm, and fugo, to drive away.) See Anthelmintic.

VERMILION. See Cinnabar.

VE'RMIS. A worm. See Worm.

VERMIS MORDICANS. Vermis repens. A species of herpetic eruption on the skin.

VERMIS TERRESTRIS. See Earth-worm.

VERNATIO. (From ver, the spring.) This term is applied, like foliatus, to the manner in which the leaves are folded or wrapped up, and expanded in the spring. See Germ.

VERNEY, GUICHARD-JOSEPH DU, was the son of a physician at Tours, and born in 1648. After studying at Avignon, he removed, at nineteen, to Paris, where he acquired high reputation as an anatomical lecturer. He was admitted, nine years after, into the Academy of Sciences, whose memoirs he enriched by his researches in natural history. In 1679 he was nominated professor of anatomy at the Royal Gardens. His work on the Organ of Hearing appeared about four years after, and was translated into various languages. He continued the pursuit of natural history with great ardour, and even to the detriment of his health, yet he was enabled, by a good constitution, to reach his eighty-second year. He bequeathed his valuable anatomical preparations to the academy. After his death, a treatise on the Diseases of the Bones was published from his manuscripts; and subsequently various other papers, under the title of "Œuvres Anatomique."

VERO'NICA. 1. The name of a genus of plants in the Linnæan system. Class, Diandria; Order, Monogynia. Speedwell.

2. The pharmacopœial name of the male veronica. See Veronica officinalis.

VERONICA BECCABUNGA. Beccabunga; Anagallis cquatica; Laver germanicum; Veronica aquatica; Cepæa. Water-pimpernel and brooklime. The plant which bears these names, is the Veronica—racemis lateralibus, foliis ovatis planis, caule repente, of Linnæus. It was formerly considered of much use in several diseases, and was applied externally to wounds and ulcers: but if it have any peculiar efficacy, it is to be derived from its antiscorbutic virtue. As a mild refrigerant juice, it is preferred where an acrimonious

state of the fluids prevails, indicated by prurient eruptions upon the skin, or in what has been called the hot scurvy. To derive much advantage from it, the juice ought to be taken in large quantities, or the fresh plant eaten as food.

VERONICA OFFICINALIS. The systematic name of the plant which is called in the pharmacopœias Veronica mas; Thea germanica; Betonica pauli; Cha mædrys spuria. Veronica—spicis lateralibus pedunculatis; foliis oppositis; caule procumbente, of Linnæus, is not unfrequent on dry barren grounds and heath, as that of Hampstead, flowering in June and July. This plant was formerly used as a pectoral against coughs and asthmatic affections, but it is now justly forgotten.

[VERONICA VIRGINICA. This is a tall native plant, differing from the rest of its family in habit, and considered by Nuttall and some other botanists as a separate genus. Its root is very bitter, and somewhat nauseous. It sometimes operates as a cathartic, in the dose of a scruple; but in several trials which I have made with it, I have found it uncertain in this respect. Big. Mat. Med. A.]

VERRICULA'RIS TUNICA. The retina of the eye.

VERRUCA. 1. A wart, or thickening and induration of the cuticle which is raised up in different forms, mostly of the size of a lentil, or flat pea.

2. In botany, applied to a small round prominence on the inferior surface of the funguses.

VERRUCA'RIA. (From Verruca, a wart: because it was supposed to destroy warts.) The Heliotropium europæum, or turnsole.

VERRUCOSUS. Warty: applied to such appearances on vegetables, as on the stem of the Euonymus verrucosus; and to the appearance on the gourd-seed vessel, as in the Cucurbita verrucosa. See Pepo.

VE'RTEBRA. (Vertebra, æ, f.; from verto, to turn.) The spine is a long bony column, which extends from the head to the lower part of the trunk, and is composed of irregular bones, which are called vertebræ.

The spine may be considered as being composed of two irregular pyramids, which are united to each other in that part of the loins where the last of the lumbar vertebræ is united to the os sacrum.

The vertebræ, which form the upper and longest pyramid, are called true vertebræ: and those which compose the lower pyramid, or the os sacrum and coccyx, are termed false vertebræ, because they do not in every thing resemble the others, and particularly because, in the adult state, they become perfectly immoveable, while the upper ones continue to be capable of motion. For it is upon the bones of the spine that the body turns, and their name has its derivation from the Latin verb verto, to turn, as observed above.

The true vertebræ, from their situations with respect to the neck, back, and loins, are divided into three classes, of cervical, dorsal, and lumbar vertebræ. We will first consider the general structure of all these, and then separately describe their different classes.

In each of the vertebræ, as in other bones, we may remark the body of the bone, its process and cavities. The body may be compared to part of a cylinder cut off transversely; convex before, and concave behind, where it makes part of the cavity of the spine.

Each vertebra has commonly seven processes. The first of these is the spinous process, which is placed at the back part of the vertebra, and gives the name of spine to the whole of this bony canal. Two others are called transverse processes, from their situation with respect to the spine, and are placed on each side of the spinous process. The four others, which are called oblique processes, are much smaller than the other three. There are two of these on the upper and two on the lower part of each vertebra, rising from near the basis of the transverse processes. They are sometimes called articular processes, because they are articulated with each other; that is, the two superior processes of one vertebra are articulated with the two inferior processes of the vertebra above it; and they are called oblique processes, from their situation with respect to the processes with which they are articulated. These oblique processes are articulated to each other by a species of ginglymus, and each process is covered at its articulation with cartilage.

There is in every vertebra, between its body and apophyses, a foramen, large enough to admit a finger. These foramina correspond with each other through all the vertebræ, and form a long bony conduit, for the lodgment of the spinal marrow.

Besides this great hole, there are four notches on each side of every vertebræ, between the oblique processes and the body of the vertebra. Two of these notches are at the upper, and two at the lower part of the bone. Each of the inferior notches, meeting with one of the superior notches of the vertebra below it, forms a foramen; while the superior notches do the same with the inferior notches of the vertebra above it. These four foramina form passages for blood-vessels, and for the nerves that pass out of the spine.

The vertebræ are united together by means of a substance, compressible like cork, which forms a kind of partition between the several vertebræ. This intervertebral substance seems, in the fœtus, to approach nearly to the nature of ligaments; in the adult it has a great resemblance to cartilage. When cut horizontally, it appears to consist of concentrical curved fibres: externally, it is firmest and hardest; internally, it becomes thinner and softer, till at length, in the centre, we find it in the form of a mucous substance, which facilitates the motion of the spine.

Genga, an Italian anatomist, long ago observed, that the change which takes place in these intervertebral cartilages, (as they are usually called,) in advanced life, occasions the decrease in stature, and the stooping forwards, which are usually to be observed in old people. The cartilages then become shrivelled, and consequently lose, in a great measure, their elasticity. But, besides this gradual effect of old age, these cartilages are subject to a temporary diminution, from the weight of the body in an erect posture, so that people who have been long standing, or who have carried a considerable weight, are found to be shorter than when they have been long in bed. Hence we are taller in the morning than at night. This fact, though seemingly obvious, was not ascertained till of late years. The difference in such cases depends on the age and size of the subject; in tall, young people, it will be nearly an inch; but in older, or shorter persons, it will be less considerable.

Besides the connexion of the several vertebræ, by means of these cartilages, there are likewise many strong ligaments, which unite the bones of the spine to each other. Some of these ligaments are external, and others internal. Among the external ligaments, we observe one which is common to all the vertebræ, extending, in a longitudinal direction, from the forepart of the body or the second vertebra of the neck, over all the other vertebræ, and becoming broader as it descends towards the os sacrum, where it becomes thinner, and gradually disappears. This external longitudinal ligament, if we may so call it, is strengthened by other shorter ligamentous fibres, which pass from one vertebra to another, throughout the whole spine. The internal ligament, the fibres of which, like the external one, are spread in a longitudinal direction, is extended over the back part of the bodies of the vertebræ, where they help to form the cavity of the spine, and reaches from the foramen of the occipital bone to the os sacrum.

We may venture to remark, that all the vertebræ diminish in density and firmness of texture, in proportion as they increase in size, so that the lower vertebræ, though larger, are not so heavy in proportion as those above them. In consequence of this mode of structure, the size of the vertebræ is increased without adding to their weight; and this is an object of no little importance in a part of the body, which, besides flexibility and suppleness, seems to require lightness as one of its essential properties.

In the fœtus, at the ordinary time of birth, each vertebra is found to be composed of three bony pieces, connected by cartilages which afterward ossify. One of these pieces is the body of the bone; the other two are the posterior and lateral portions, which form the foramen for the medulla spinalis. The oblique processes are at that time complete, and the transverse processes beginning to be formed, but the spinous processes are totally wanting.

The cervical vertebræ are seven in number; their bodies are smaller and of a firmer texture than the other bones of the spine. The transverse processes of these vertebræ are short, and forked for the lodgment of muscles; and, at the bottom of each of these processes, there is a foramen, for the passage of the cer-

vical artery and vein. The spinous process of each of these vertebræ is likewise shorter than the other vertebræ, and forked at its extremity; by which means it allows a more convenient insertion to the muscles of the neck. Their oblique processes are more deserving of that name than either those of the dorsal or lumbar vertebræ. The uppermost of these processes are slightly concave, and the lowermost slightly convex. This may suffice for a general description of these vertebræ; but the first, second, and seventh deserve to be spoken of more particularly. The first, which is called *Atlas*, from its supporting the head, differs from all the other vertebræ of the spine. It forms a kind of bony ring, which may be divided into its anterior and posterior arches, and its lateral portions. Of these, the anterior arch is the smallest and flattest; at the middle of its convex forepart we observe a small tubercle which is here what the body is in the other vertebræ. To this tubercle a ligament is attached, which helps to strengthen the articulation of the spine with the os occipitis. The back part of this anterior portion is concave, and covered with cartilage, where it receives the odontoid process of the second vertebra. The posterior portion of the vertebra, or, more properly speaking, the posterior arch, is larger than the anterior one. Instead of a spinous process, we observe a rising, or tubercle, larger than that which we have just now described, on the forepart of the bone. The lateral portions of the vertebra project, so as to form what are called the transverse processes, one on each side, which are longer and larger than the transverse processes of the other vertebræ. They terminate in a roundish tubercle, the end of which has a slight bend downwards. Like the other transverse processes, they are perforated at their basis, for the passage of the cervical artery. But, besides these transverse processes, we observe, both on the superior and inferior surface of these lateral portions of the first vertebra, an articulating surface, covered with cartilage, answering to the oblique processes in the other vertebræ. The uppermost of these are oblong, and slightly concave, and their external edges rise somewhat higher than their internal brims. They receive the condyloid processes of the os occipitis, with which they are articulated by a species of gingly mus. The lowermost articulating surfaces, or the inferior oblique processes, as they are called, are large, concave, and circular, and are formed for receiving the superior oblique processes of the second vertebra; so that the atlas differs from the rest of the cervical vertebræ in receiving the bones, with which it is articulated both above and below. In the fœtus we find this vertebra composed of five, instead of three pieces, as in the other vertebræ. One of these is the anterior arch; the other four are the posterior arch and the sides, each of the latter being composed of two pieces. The transverse process, on each side, remains long in a state of epiphysis with respect to the rest of the bone.

The second vertebra is called *dentatus*, from the process on the upper part of its body, which has been, though perhaps improperly, compared to a tooth. This process, which is the most remarkable part of the vertebra, is of a cylindrical shape, slightly flattened, however, behind and before. Anteriorly, it has a convex, smooth, articulating surface, where it is received by the atlas, as we observed in our description of that vertebra. It is by means of this articulation that the rotatory motion of the head is performed; the articulation of the os occipitis with the superior oblique processes of the first vertebra, allowing only a certain degree of motion backwards and forwards, so that when we turn the face either to the right or left, the atlas moves upon this odontoid process of the second vertebra. But as the face cannot turn a quarter of a circle, that is, to the shoulder, upon this vertebra alone, without being liable to injure the medulla spinalis, we find that all the cervical vertebræ concur in this rotary motion, when it is in any considerable degree; and indeed we see many strong ligamentous fibres arising from the sides of the odontoid process, and passing over the first vertebra, to the os occipitis, which not only strengthen the articulation of these bones with each other, but serve to regulate and limit their motion. It is on this account that the name of *moderators* has sometimes been given to these ligaments. The transverse processes of the vertebra *dentata* are short, inclined downwards, and forked at their extremities. Its spinous process is short and thick. Its superior oblique processes are slightly convex, and somewhat larger than the articulating surfaces of the first vertebra, by which mechanism the motion of that bone upon this second vertebra is performed with greater safety. Its inferior oblique processes have nothing singular in their structure.

The seventh vertebra of the neck differs from the rest chiefly in having its spino us process of a greater length, so that, upon this account, it has been sometimes called *vertebra prominens.*

The dorsal vertebræ, which are twelve in number, are of a middle size, between the cervical and lumbar vertebræ; the upper ones gradually losing their resemblance to those of the neck, and the lower ones coming nearer to those of the loins. The bodies of these vertebræ are more flattened at their sides, more convex before, and more concave behind, than the other bones of the spine. Their upper and lower surfaces are horizontal. At their sides we observe two depressions, one at their upper, and the other at their lower edge, which, united with similar depressions in the vertebræ above and below, form articulating surfaces, covered with cartilage, in which the heads of the ribs are received. These depressions, however, are not exactly alike in all the dorsal vertebræ; for we find the head of the first rib articulated solely with the first of these vertebræ, which has therefore the whole of the superior articulating surface within itself, independent of the vertebra above it. We may likewise observe a similarity in this respect in the eleventh and twelfth of the dorsal vertebræ, with which the eleventh and twelfth ribs are articulated separately. Their spinous processes are long, flattened at the sides, divided at their upper and back part into two surfaces by a middle ridge, which is received by a small groove in the inner part of the spinous process immediately above it, and connected to it by a ligament. These spinous processes are terminated by a kind of round tubercle, which slopes considerably downwards, except in the three lowermost vertebræ, where they are shorter and more erect. Their transverse processes are of considerable length and thickness, and are turned obliquely backwards. Anteriorly, they have an articulating surface, for receiving the tuberosity of the ribs, except in the eleventh and twelfth of the dorsal vertebræ to which the ribs are articulated by their heads only. In the last of these vertebræ the transverse processes are very short and thick, because otherwise they would be apt to strike against the lowermost ribs, when we bend the body to either side.

The *lumbar vertebræ,* the lowest of the true vertebræ, are five in number. They are larger than the dorsal vertebræ. Their bodies are extremely prominent, and nearly of a circular form at their forepart; posteriorly they are concave. Their intermediate cartilages are of considerable thickness, especially anteriorly, by which means the curvature of the spine forwards, towards the abdomen, in this part, is greatly assisted. Their spinous processes are short and thick, of considerable breadth, erect, and terminated by a kind of tuberosity. Their oblique processes are of considerable thickness; the superior ones are concave, and turned inwards; the inferior ones convex, and turned outwards. Their transverse processes are thin and long, except in the first and last vertebra, where they are much shorter, that the lateral motions of the trunk might not be impeded. The inferior surface of all these vertebræ is slightly oblique, so that the forepart of the body of each is somewhat thicker than its hind-part; but this is more particularly observable in the lowermost vertebra, which is connected with the os sacrum. Many anatomists describe the os sacrum and the os coccygis when considering the bones of the spine, while others regard them as belonging more properly to the pelvis. These bones the reader may consult. It now remains to notice the uses of the spine. We find the spinal marrow lodged in this bony canal, secure from external injury. It defends the thoracic and abdominal viscera, and forms a pillar which supports the head, and gives a general firmness to the whole trunk.

To give it a firm basis, we find the bodies of the vertebræ gradually increasing in breadth as they descend; and to fit it for a variety of motion, it is composed of a great number of joints, with an intermediate elastic substance, so that to great firmness there is added a perfect flexibility.

We have already observed, that the lowermost and largest vertebræ are not so heavy in proportion as those above them; their bodies being more spongy, excepting at their circumference, where they are more immediately exposed to pressure; so that nature seems every where endeavouring to relieve us of an unnecessary weight of bone. But behind, where the spinal marrow is more exposed to injury, we find the processes composed of very hard bone; and the spinous processes are in general placed over each other in a slanting direction, so that a pointed instrument cannot easily get between them, excepting in the neck, where they are almost perpendicular, and leave a greater space between them. Hence, in some countries, it is usual to kill cattle by thrusting a pointed instrument between the occiput and the atlas, or between the atlas and the second vertebra. Besides these uses of the vertebræ in defending the spinal marrow, and in articulating the several vertebræ, as is the case with the oblique processes, we shall find that they all serve to form a greater surface for the lodgment of muscles, and to enable the latter to act more powerfully on the trunk, by affording them a lever of considerable length.

In the neck, we see the spine projecting somewhat forward, to support the head, which, without this assistance, would require a greater number of muscles. Through the whole length of the thorax it is carried in a curved direction backwards, and thus adds considerably to the cavity of the chest, and consequently affords more room to the lungs, heart, and large blood-vessels. In the loins, the spine again projects forwards, in a direction with the centre of gravity, by which means the body is easily kept in an erect posture; for otherwise we should be liable to fall forwards. But, at its inferior part, it again recedes backwards, and helps to form a cavity called the pelvis, in which the urinary bladder, intestinum rectum, and other viscera, are placed.

In a part of the body that is composed of so great a number of bones, and constructed for such a variety of motion, as the spine is, luxation is more to be expected than fracture; and this is very wisely guarded against in every direction, by the many processes that are to be found, in each vertebra, and by the cartilages, ligaments, and other means of connexion, which we have described as uniting them together.

VERTEBRAL. *Vertebralis.* Appertaining to the vertebræ, or bones of the spine.

Vertebral artery. *Arteria vertebralis.* A branch of the subclavian, proceeding through the vertebræ to within the cranium, where, with its fellow, it forms the basilary artery, the internal auditory, and the posterior artery of the dura mater.

VE'RTEX. *(Vertex, icis, m.; from verto.)* The crown of the head. The os verticis is the parietal bone.

Verticalia ossa. See *Parietal bones.*

VERTICALIS. Vertical. Perpendicular. Applied to leaves which have both sides at right angles with the horizon; as in Lactuca scariola.

VERTICELLUS. A whorl. The name of a species of inflorescence, in which the flowers surround the stem in a sort of ring.

From the *insertion* of the flowers, the *vesture,* and *distance* of the verticellus, it is called,

1. *Pedunculatus;* as in *Milissa officinalis.*
2. *Sessilis,* in *Mentha arvensis.*
3. *Dimidiatus,* going half round; as in *Ballota disticha.*
4. *Nudus,* without floral or other leaf; as in *Salvia verticilata.*
5. *Bracteatus,* in *Ballota nigra.*
6. *Distans,* in *Salvia indica.*
7. *Confertus,* when crowded together.

Ve'rticis os. See *Parietal bones.*

VERTI'GO. Giddiness.

VERVAIN. See *Verbena officinalis.*

Vervain, female. See *Erysimum alliaria.*

VESA'LIUS, Andrew, was born at Brussels about the year 1514. After pursuing his studies at different universities, and serving for two years professionally with the imperial army, he settled at Padua, and taught anatomy with great applause, which he subsequently continued at some other schools in Italy. In 1544, he became physician to Charles V., and resided chiefly at the imperial court. About twenty years after, in the midst of his professional career, an extraordinary circumstance occurred, which was the cause of his ruin Being summoned to examine the body of a Spanish gentleman, and having begun the operation too precipitately, the heart was observed to palpitate ; in consequence of which, he was accused before the Inquisition: but the interposition of Philip II. procured him to be merely enjoined to make a pilgrimage to the Holy Land. While at Jerusalem, he was invited to the anatomical chair at Padua ; but on his return, the ship was wrecked on the coast of Zante, where he soon after died. Vesalius has been represented as the first person who rescued anatomy from the slavery imposed upon it by deference to ancient opinions, and led the way to modern improvements. His first publication of note was a set of Anatomical Tables, which was soon followed by his great work "De Corporis Humani Fabrica," printed at Basil in 1543, and often since in several countries. The earliest impressions of the plates were most valued, but the explanations were made subsequently more correct. In a treatise " De Radicis Chinæ Usu," he severely criticised the errors of Galen, which engaged him in a controversy with Fallopius. His medical and surgical writings are not held in much estimation.

VESA'NIÆ. (The plural of vesania ; from vesanas, a madman.) The fourth order in the Class Neuroses, of Cullen's nosological arrangement ; comprehending diseases in which the judgment is impaired, without either coma or pyrexia.

VESI'CA. (Diminutive of vas, a vessel.) A bladder.

VESICA FELLIS. The gall-bladder. See Gall-bladder.

VESICA URINARIA. The urinary bladder. See Urinary bladder.

VESICATORY. (Vesicatorius ; from vesica, a bladder : because it raises a bladder.) See Epispastic.

VESICLE. (Vesicula ; a diminutive of vesica, a bladder.) An elevation of the cuticle, containing a transparent watery fluid.

VESI'CULA. See Vesicle.

VESICULA FELLIS. The gall-bladder.

VESICULÆ DIVÆ BARBARÆ. The confluent small-pox.

VESICULÆ GINGIVARUM. The thrush.

VESICULÆ PULMONALES. The air-cells which compose the greatest part of the lungs, and are situated at the termination of the bronchia.

VESICULÆ SEMINALES. Two membranous receptacles, situated on the back part of the bladder, above its neck. The excretory ducts are called ejaculatory ducts. They proceed to the urethra, into which they open by a peculiar orifice at the top of the verumontanum. They have vessels and nerves from the neighbouring parts, and are well supplied with absorbent vessels, which proceed to the lymphatic glands about the loins. The use of the vesiculæ seminales is to receive the semen brought into them by the vasa deferentia, to retain, somewhat inspissate, and to excern it sub coitu into the urethra, from whence it is propelled into the vagina uteri.

Vesicular fever. See Pemphigus.

VESTI'BULUM. A round cavity of the internal ear, between the cochlea and semicircular canals, in which are an oval opening communicating with the cavity of the tympanum, and the orifices of the semicircular canals. It is within this cavity and the semicircular canals, that the new apparatus discovered by the celebrated neurologist Scarpa, lies. He has demonstrated membranous tubes, collected loosely by cellular texture, within the bony semicircular canals, each of which is dilated in the cavity of the vestibule into an ampulla ; it is upon these ampullæ, which communicate by means of an alveus communis, that branches of the portio mollis are expanded.

VESUVIAN. Idocrase of Haüy. A subspecies of pyramidal garnet of a green or brown colour, found in great abundance in unaltered ejected rocks in the vicinity of Vesuvius. At Naples it is cut into ring stones.

VETO'NICA CORDI. See Betonica.

VEXILLUM. (Vexillum, i, n. ; a banner or standard.) The standard, or large uppermost petal at the back of a papilionaceous flower.

VIA. A way or passage. Used in anatomy. See Primæ viæ.

VI'BEX. (Vibex, icis, plu. Vibices.) The large purple spot which appears under the skin in certain malignant fevers.

VIBRI'SSÆ. (Vibrissa ; from vibro, to quaver.) Hairs growing in the nostrils. See Capillus.

VIBURNUM LANTANA. Liburnum. The pliant mealy tree. The berries are considered as adstringent.

VICHY. The name of a town in France, in the neighbourhood of which is a tepid mineral spring. On account of its chalybeate and alkaline ingredients, it is taken internally, being reputed to be of great service in bilious colics, diarrhœas, and in disorders of the stomach, especially such as arise from a relaxed or debilitated state of that organ.

These waters are likewise very useful when employed as a tepid-bath, particularly in rheumatism, sciatica, gout, &c. By combining the internal use with the external application, they have often effected a cure where other remedies had failed to afford relief.

VI'CIA. (Viscia, an old Latin name, derived by some etymologists from Vincio, to bind together, as the various species of this genus twine, with their tendrils, round other plants.) The name of a genus of plants in the Linnæan system. Class, Diadelphia ; Order, Decandria.

VICIA FABA. The systematic name of the common bean-plant. It is a native of Egypt. There are many varieties. Beans are very wholesome and nutritious to those whose stomachs are strong, and accustomed to the coarser modes of living. In delicate stomachs they produce flatulency, dyspepsia, cardialgia, &c. especially when old. See Legumina.

VICTORIA'LIS LONGA. See Allium victorialis.

VIEUSSENS, RAYMOND, was born at a village in Rovergne, graduated at Montpellier, and in 1671 was chosen physician to the hospital of St. Eloy. The result of his anatomical researches in this situation was published under the title of Neurology, and gained him great reputation. His name became known at court, and Mad. de Montpensier made him her physician. After her death he returned to Montpellier, and directed his attention to chemistry ; and having found an acid in the caput mortuum of the blood, he made this the groundwork of a new medical theory. In advanced life, his writings were multiplied without augmenting his reputation. He died in 1726.

VIGILANCE. Pervigilium. Vigilance, when attended by anxiety, pain in the head, loss of appetite, and diminution of strength, is by Sauvages and Sagar considered as a genus of disease, and is called Agrypnia.

VILLOSUS. Villous, shaggy : applied in anatomy to a velvet-like arrangement of fibres or vessels, as the villous coat of the intestines : and in botany to the stem of the Cineraria integrifolia, and to other parts of plants ; as the receptacle of the Artemisia absynthium.

VILLUS. A species of hairy pubescens of plants, consisting of soft, slender, upright, short, and scarcely conspicuous, and for the most part white hair-like filaments.

VI'NCA. (From vincio, to bind : because of its usefulness in making bands.) The name of a genus of plants in the Linnæan system. Class, Pentandria ; Order, Monogynia.

VINCA MINOR. The systematic name of the less periwinkle. Vinca pervinca ; Clematis daphnoides major. It possesses bitter and adstringent virtues, and is said to be efficacious in stopping nasal hæmorrhages when bruised and put into the nose. Boiled, it forms a useful adstringent gargle in common sore throat, and it is given by some in phthisical complaints.

VINCA PERVINCA. See Vinca minor.

VINCETO'XICUM. (From vinco, to overcome, and toxicum, poison : so named from its supposed virtue of resisting and expelling poison.) See Asclepias vincetoxicum.

VINE. See Vitis.

Vine, white. See Bryonia alba.

Vine, wild. See Bryonia alba.

VINEGAR. See Acetum.

Vinegar, aromatic. See Acetum aromaticum.

Vinegar, distilled. See Acetum.

Vinegar, spirits of. See Acetum.

Vinegar of squills. See Acetum scillæ.

Vinegar, thieves'. See Acetum aromaticum.

VI'NUM. See Wine.

VINUM ALOES. Wine of aloes. Formerly known by the names of Tinctura hieræ, and Tinctura sacra Take of extract of spiked aloe, eight ounces ; canella-bark, two ounces ; wine, six pints ; proof spirits, two pints. Rub the aloes into powder with white sand, previously cleansed from any impurities ; rub the canella-bark also into powder ; and after having mixed these powders together, pour on the wine and spirit. Macerate for fourteen days occasionally shaking the mixture, and afterward strain. A stomachic purgative, calculated for the aged and phlegmatic, who are not troubled with the piles. The dose is from a half to a whole fluid ounce.

VINUM ANTIMONII. In small doses this proves alterative and diaphoretic, and a large dose emetic; in which last intention it is the common emetic for children.

VINUM ANTIMONII TARTARIZATI. See *Antimonium tartarizatum.*

VINUM FERRI. Wine of iron, formerly called *Vinum chalybeatum.* Take of iron filings, two ounces; wine, two pints. Mix, and set the mixture by for a month, occasionally shaking it; then filter it through paper. For its virtues, see *Ferrum tartarizatum.*

VINUM IPECACUANHÆ. Wine of ipecacuanha. Take of ipecacuanha-root, bruised, two ounces; wine, two pints. Macerate for fourteen days, and strain. The dose, when used as an emetic, is from two fluid drachms to half a fluid ounce.

VINUM OPII. Wine of opium, formerly known by the names of *Laudanum liquidum sydenhami,* and *Tinctura thebaica.* Take of extract of opium, an ounce; cinnamon-bark, bruised, cloves, bruised, of each a drachm; wine, a pint. Macerate for eight days, and strain. See *Opium.*

VINUM VERATRI. Wine of white hellebore. Take of white hellebore-root, sliced, eight ounces; wine, two pints and a half; macerate for fourteen days, and strain. See *Veratrum.*

VI'OLA. (From Ιον; because it was first found in Ionia.) 1. The name of a genus of plants in the Linnæan system. Class, *Syngenesia ;* Order, *Monogynia.* The violet.

2. The pharmacopœial name of the sweet violet. See *Viola odorata.*

VIOLA CANINA. The dog-violet. The root of this plant possesses the power of vomiting and purging the bowels; with which intention a scruple of the dried root must be exhibited. It appears, though neglected in this country, worthy the attention of physicians.

VIOLA IPECACUANHA. The plant which was supposed to afford the ipecacuanha root.

VIOLA LUTEA. See *Cheiranthus cheiri.*

VIOLA ODORATA. The systematic name of the sweet violet. *Viola—acaulis, foliis cordatis, stolonibus repentibus,* of Linnæus. The recent flowers of his plant are received into the catalogues of the materia medica. They have an agreeable sweet smell, and a mucilaginous bitterish taste. Their virtues are purgative or laxative, and by some they are said to possess an anodyne and pectoral quality. The officinal preparation of this flower is a syrup, which, to young children, answers the purpose of a purgative; it is also of considerable utility in many chemical inquiries, to detect an acid or an alkali; the former changing the blue colour to a red, and the latter to a green.

VIOLA PALUSTRIS. See *Pinguicula.*

[VIOLA PEDATA. The violets are generally mucilaginous plants, and employed as demulcents in catarrh and strangury. Some of them are allied to ipecacuanha, and contain *emetin* in their substance. The *viola pedata,* a native species retained in the pharmacopœia, is considered a useful expectorant and lubricating medicine in pulmonary complaints, and is given in syrup or decoction. *Big. Mat. Med.* A.]

VIOLA TRICOLOR. Harts-ease. Pansies. This well-known beautiful little plant grows in corn-fields, waste and cultivated grounds, flowering all the summer months. It varies much by cultivation; and by the vivid colouring of its flowers often becomes extremely beautiful in gardens, where it is distinguished by various names. To the taste, this plant in its recent state is extremely glutinous, or mucilaginous, accompanied with the common herbaceous flavour and roughness. By distillation with water, according to Haase, it affords a small quantity of odorous essential oil, of a somewhat acrid taste. The dried herb yields about half its weight of watery extract, the fresh plant about one-eighth. Though many of the old writers on the materia medica represent this plant as a powerful medicine in epilepsy, asthma, ulcers, scabies, and cutaneous complaints, yet the viola tricolor owes its present character as a medicine to the modern authorities of Starck, Metzger, Haase, and others, especially as a

remedy for the crusta lactea. For this purpose, a handful of the fresh herb, or half a drachm of it dried, boiled two hours in milk, is to be strained and taken night and morning. Bread, with this decoction, is also to be formed into a poultice, and applied to the part. By this treatment, it has been observed, that the eruption during the first eight days, increases, and that the urine, when the medicine succeeds, has an odour similar to that of cats; but on continuing the plant a sufficient time, this smell goes off, the scabs disappear; and the skin recovers its natural purity. Instances of the successful exhibition of this medicine, as cited by these authors, are very numerous, indeed this remedy, under their management, seems rarely, if ever, to have failed. It appears, however, that Mursinna, Akermann, and Henning were less fortunate in the employment of this plant: the last of whom declares, that in the different cutaneous disorders in which he used it, no benefit was derived. Haase, who administered this species of violet in various forms and large doses, extended its use to many chronic disorders; and from the great number of cases in which it proved successful, we are desirous of recommending it to a farther trial in this country.

It is remarkable that Bergius speaks of this plant as a useful mucilaginous purgative, and takes no notice of its efficacy in the crustea lactea, or in any other disease.

VIOLA'RIA. See *Viola.*

VIOLET. See *Viola odorata.*

Violet, dog. See *Viola canina.*

VIPER. See *Vipera.*

VIPER-GRASS. See *Scorzoner .*

VI'PERA. (*Quod vi pariat :* because it was thought that its young eat through the mother's bowels.) The viper or adder. See *Coluber berus.*

VIPERA'RIA. See *Aristolochia serpentaria.*

VIPERI'NA. (From *viperá,* a snake: so called from the serpentine appearance of its roots.) See *Aristolochia serpentaria.*

VIPERINA VIRGINIANA. See *Aristolochia serpentaria.*

VI'RGA AUREA. See *Solidago virga aurea.*

VIRGA'TA SUTURA. The sagittal suture of the skull

VIRGIN'S BOWER. See *Clematis recta.*

Virgin's milk. A solution of gum-benzoin.

VIRGINA'LE CLAUSTRUM. The hymen.

Virginian snake-root. See *Aristolochia virginiana.*

Virginian tobacco. See *Nicotiana.*

VI'RUS. See *Contagion.*

VIS. Power. In physiology, applied to vital power and its effects: hence *vis vitæ, vis insita, vis irritabilis, vis nervia,* &c.

VIS CONSERVATRIX. See *Vis medicatrix naturæ.*

VIS ELASTICA. Elasticity.

VIS INERTIÆ. The propensity to rest inherent in nature.

VIS INSITA. This property is defined by Haller to be that power by which a muscle, when wounded, touched, or irritated, contracts, independent of the will of the animal that is the object of the experiment, and without its feeling pain. See *Irritability.*

VIS MEDICATRIX NATURÆ. *Vis conservatrix.* A term employed by physicians to express that healing power in an animated body, by which, when diseased, the body is enabled to regain its healthy actions.

VIS MORTUA. That property by which a muscle after the death of the animal, or a muscle, immediately after having been cut out from a living body, contracts.

VIS NERVOSA. This property is considered by Whytt to be another power of the muscles by which they act when excited by the nerves.

VIS PLASTICA. That facility of formation which spontaneously operates in animals.

VIS A TERGO. Any impulsive power.

VIS VITÆ. The natural power of the animal machine in preserving life.

From the most remote antiquity, philosophers were persuaded that a great part of the phenomena peculiar to living bodies, did not follow the same course, nor obey the same laws, as the phenomena proper to brute matter.

To these phenomena of living bodies, a particular cause has been assigned, which has received different denominations. Hippocrates bestows on it the appellation of *physis,* or nature; Aristotle calls it the *moving* or *generating principle;* Kaw Boerhaave, the *impetum faciens;* Van Helmont, *archæa;* Stahi, the *soul;* others, the *vis insita, vis vitæ, vital force,* &c.

VISCIDITY. (*Viciditas;* from *viscus.*) Viscosity: glutinous, sticky, like the bird-lime.

VISCIDUS. Viscid. 1 Of the nature of ropy pulp of the *viscum,* or missletoe In general use to imply viscidity in fluids, &c

2. See *Lentor.*

VI'SCUM. (*Viscum, i,* n.; and *Viscus, i,* m. Derived from the Greek, ἰξος, altered by the Æolians into βίσκος.) 1. The fruit of the misletoe. See *Viscum album.*

2. The name of a genus of parasitical plants in the Linnæan system. Class *Diœcia;* Order, *Tetrandria.*

Viscum album. *Viscus guercinus.* Misletoe. This singular parasitical plant most commonly grows on apple-trees, also on the pear, hawthorn, service, oak, hazel, maple, ash, lime-tree, willow, elm, hornbean, &c. It is supposed to be propagated by birds, especially by the field-fare and thrush, which feed upon its berries, the seeds of which pass through the bowels unchanged; and along with the excrement adhere to the branches of trees where they vegetate.

The misletoe of the oak has, from the times of the ancient Druids, been always preferred to that produced on other trees; but it is now well known that the *viscus quercus* differs in no respect from others.

This plant is the ἰξ of the Greeks, and was in former times thought to possess many medicinal virtues; however, we learn but little concerning its efficacy from the ancient writers on the Materia Medica, nor will it be deemed necessary to state the extraordinary powers ascribed to the misletoe by the crafty designs of Druidical knavery. Both the leaves and branches of the plant have very little smell, and a very weak taste of the nauseous kind. In distillation they impregnate water with their faint unpleasant smell, but yield no essential oil. Extracts made from them by water, are bitterish, roughish, and subsaline. The spirituous extract of the wood has the greatest austerity, and that of the leaves the greatest bitterness. The berries abound with an extremely tenacious and most ungrateful sweet mucilage.

The *viscus quercus* obtained great reputation for the cure of epilepsy; and a case of this disease, of a woman of quality, in which it proved remarkably successful, is mentioned by Boyle. Some years afterward its use was strongly recommended in various convulsive disorders by Colbach, who has related several instances of its good effects. He administered it in substance in doses of half a drachm, or a drachm, of the wood or leaves, or an infusion of an ounce. This author was followed by others, who have not only given testimony of the efficacy of the misletoe in different convulsive affections, but also in those complaints denominated nervous, in which it was supposed to act in the character of a tonic. But all that has been written in favour of this remedy, which is certainly well deserving of notice, has not prevented it from falling into general neglect; and the colleges of London and Edinburgh have, perhaps not without reason, expunged it from their catalogues of the Materia Medica.

VI'SCUS. (*Viscus, eris,* n.; plural, *viscera.*) 1. Any organ or part which has an appropriate use, as the viscera of the abdomen, &c.

2. (*Viscus, i,* m.) The name of the misletoe. See *Viscum album.*

VISION. (*Visus, ûs,* m.) The function which enables us to perceive the magnitude, figure, colour, distance, &c. of bodies. The organs which compose the apparatus of vision enter into action under the influence of a particular excitant, or stimulus, called *light.*

We perceive bodies, we take cognizance of many of their properties, though they are often at a great distance;—there must then be between them and our eye some intermediate agent; this intermediate substance we denominate *light.* Light is an excessively subtle fluid, which emanates from those bodies called *luminous,* as the sun, the fixed stars, bodies in a state of ignition, phosphorescence, &c. Light is composed of atoms which move with a prodigious rapidity, since they pass through about eighty thousand leagues of space in a second.

A series of atoms, or particles, which succeed each other in a right line without interruption are denominated a *ray of light.* The atoms which compose every ray of light are separated by intervals, that are considerable in proportion to their mass; which circumstances permit a considerable number of rays to cross each other in the same point, without their particles coming in contact.

The light that proceeds from luminous bodies forms diverging cones, which would prolong themselves in definitely, did they meet with no obstacles. Philosophers have from thence concluded, that the intensity of light in any place, is always in an inverse ratio to the square of the distance of the luminous bodies from which it proceeds. The cones that are formed by the light in passing from luminous bodies, are, in general, called pencils of light, or pencils of rays, and the bodies through which the light moves are designated by the name of *media.*

When light happens to come in contact with cer_n bodies that are called opaque, it is repulsed, and its direction is modified according to the disposition of those bodies.—The change that light suffers in its course is, in this case, called *reflection.* The study of reflection constitutes that part of physics, which is named *catoptrics.*

Certain bodies allow the light to pass through them; for instance glass: they are said to be *transparent.* In passing through these bodies, light suffers a certain change which is called *refraction.* As the mechanism of vision rests entirely upon the principle of refraction, the examination of these becomes, therefore, a matter of importance.

The point where a ray of light enters into a medium is called the point of immersion; and that where it goes out is called the point of emergence.

If the ray comes in contact with a medium in a line perpendicular to its surface, the ray then continues its direction without any change; but if its direction is oblique to the surface of the medium, the ray is then turned out of its course, and appears broken at the point of immersion.

The *angle of incidence* is that which the incident ray makes with a perpendicular line drawn over the point of immersion upon the surface of the medium, and the *angle of refraction* is that which the broken ray makes with the perpendicular.

If the ray of light pass from a rare medium into one more dense, it inclines towards the perpendicular at the point of contact; but it declines from it if it pass from a dense medium into one that is rarer. The same phenomenon takes place, but in a contrary direction, when the ray enters into the first medium; this takes place in such a manner, that if the two surfaces of the medium traversed by the ray are parallel to each other, the ray in passing into the surrounding medium, will take a direction parallel to that of the incident ray.

Bodies refract the light in proportion to their density and combustibility. Thus, of two bodies of equal density, one of which being composed of more combustible elements than the other, the refractive power of the first will be greater than that of the second.

All transparent bodies refract at the same time that they reflect the light. On account of this property these bodies are capable of being used as a sort of mirror. When their density is very inconsiderable, such as that of the air, they are not visible unless their mass be considerable.

The form of a refractive body has no influence upon its refractive power; but it modifies the disposition of the refracted rays in respect to each other. In fact, the perpendiculars to the surfaces of the body, approaching or receding according to the form of the body, the refracting rays should at the same time approach or recede.

When, by the effort of a refractive body, the rays tend towards each other, the point where they unite is called *the focus of the refractive body.* Bodies of a lenticular form are those which present principally this phenomenon.

A refractive body, with parallel surfaces, does not change the direction of the rays, but it inclines them towards its axis by a sort of *transportation.* A refractive body of two convex sides does not possess a greater refractive power than a body convex on one side, and plane on the other; but the point behind it in which the rays are united is much nearer.

The discovery of the action of refractive bodies upon light has not been an object of simple curiosity; it has led to the construction of ingenious instruments, by means of which the sphere of human vision has been extended to an extraordinary degree.

Apparatus of vision.—The apparatus of vision is composed of three distinct parts.

The *first* modifies the light.

The *second* receives the impression of that fluid.

The *third* transmits this impression to the brain.

The apparatus of vision is of an extremely delicate texture, capable of being deranged by the least accident. Nature has also placed before this apparatus a series of organs, the use of which is to protect and maintain it in those conditions necessary to the perfect exercise of its functions. Those protecting parts are the eyebrows, the eyelids, and the *secreting* and *excreting* apparatus of the tears.

The eyebrows, which are peculiar to man, are formed,

1. By *hair*, of a variable colour.

2. By the *skin*.

3. By *sebaceous* follicles placed at the root of every hair.

4. By *muscles* destined for their various motions, viz. the frontal portion of the occipito-frontalis, the superior edge of the orbicularis palpebrarum, the supercilium.

5. Numerous *vessels*.

6. *Nerves.*

The eye is composed of parts which have very different uses in the production of vision. They may be distinguished into refractive, and non-refractive.

The refractive parts are:

A. The *transparent cornea*, a refractive body, convex and concave, which, in its transparency, its form, and its insertion, pretty much resembles the glass that is placed before the face of a watch.

B. The *aqueous humour* which fills the chambers of the eye; a liquid which is not purely aqueous, as its name indicates, but is essentially composed of water, and of a little albumen.

C. The *crystalline humour*, which is improperly compared to a lens. The comparison would be exact, were it merely for the form; but it is defective in regard to structure. The crystalline is composed of concentric layers, the hardness of which increases from the surface to the centre, and which probably possesses different refractive powers. The crystalline is, besides, surrounded by a membrane, which has a great effect upon vision, as experience teaches us. A lens is homogeneous in all its parts; at its surface, as in every point of its substance; it possesses every where the same refractive power. However, it is necessary to remark that the curve of the anterior surface of the crystalline is very far from being similar to that of the posterior aspect. This last belongs to a sphere, of which the diameter is much less than that of the sphere to which the curve of the anterior surface belongs. Until now it has been understood that the crystalline was composed mostly of albumen; but according to a new analysis of Berzelius, it does not contain any: it is formed almost entirely of water, and of a peculiar matter that has a great analogy, in its chemical properties, to the colouring matter of the blood.

D. Behind the crystalline is the *vitreous humour*, so called because of its resemblance to melted glass.

Each of the parts which we have noticed is enveloped by a very thin membrane, which is transparent like the part that it covers: thus, before the cornea is the conjunctiva; behind it is the membrane of the aqueous humour, which lines all the anterior chamber of the eye; that is, the anterior surface of the iris, and the posterior surface of the cornea.

The crystalline is surrounded by the crystalline capsule, which adheres by its circumference to the membrane that covers the vitreous humour. This, in passing from the circumference of the crystalline upon the anterior and posterior surfaces of this part, leaves between an interval which has been called the *canal goudronné.*

The vitreous humour is also surrounded by a membrane called *hyaloid*. This membrane does not alone contain this humour, it is sent down among it, and separating, forms it into cells. The details of anatomy with regard to the disposition of the cells, have not hitherto added any thing to what is known of the use of the vitreous humour.

The eye is not only composed of parts that are refractive, but it is composed also of membranes which have each a particular use; these are:—

A. The *sclerotic*, the exterior envelope of the eye, which is a membrane of a fibrous nature; it is thick and resisting, and its use is evidently to protect the interior parts of the organ; it serves besides as a point of insertion for many muscles that move the eye.

B. The *choroid*, a vascular and nervous membrane, formed by two distinct plates; it is impregnated with a dark matter which is very important to vision.

C. The *iris*, which is seen behind the transparent cornea, is differently coloured in different individuals; it is pierced in the centre by an opening called the *pupil*, which dilates or contracts according to certain circumstances which we shall notice. The iris adheres outwardly, and by its circumference, to the sclerotic, by a cellular tissue of a particular nature, which is called the *ciliary*, or *iridian* ligament. There are, behind the iris, a great number of white lines arranged in the manner of rays, which would unite at the centre of the iris, if they were sufficiently prolonged: these are the *ciliary processes.*

Neither the use nor the structure of these bodies has been properly determined: they are believed by some to be nervous, by others to be muscular, while others think them glandular, or vascular. The truth is, their real structure is not understood.

The colour of the iris depends on its structure, which is variable, and on that of the dark layer of its posterior surface, the colour of which shines through the iris. For instance, the tissue of the iris is nearly white in blue eyes; in this case the dark colour behind appears almost alone, and determines the colour of the eyes.

Anatomists differ about the nature of the tissue of the iris: some think it entirely like that of the choroid, essentially composed of vessels and of nerves; others have imagined they saw a great many muscular fibres in it; others consider this membrane a tissue *sui generis;* and others confound it with the *erectile* structure. Edwards has shown that the iris is formed by four layers very easy to be distinguished, two of which are a continuation of the laminæ of the choroid; a third belongs to the membrane of the aqueous humour; and a fourth forms the proper tissue of the iris.

Between the choroid and the hyaloid there exists a membrane essentially nervous. This membrane, known by the name of the *retina*, is almost transparent; it presents a slight opacity, and a tint feebly inclining to *lilac;* it is composed of the expansion of the threads which compose the optic nerve.

The eye receives a great number of vessels, the *ciliary arteries and veins*, and many nerves, the greater part of which come from the *ophthalmic ganglion.*

The *optic nerve* preserves the communication between the brain and the eye.

Mechanism of vision.—In order the better to explain the action of light in the eye, let us suppose a luminous cone commencing in a point placed in the prolongation of the *anterior-posterior axis* of the eye. We see that only the light which falls upon the cornea can be useful for vision; that which falls on the white of the eye, the eyelids and eyelashes, contributes nothing; it is reflected by those parts differently according to their colour. The cornea itself does not receive the light on its whole extent; for it is generally covered in part by the border of the eyelids.

The cornea having a fine polish on its surface, as soon as the light reaches it, part of it is reflected, which contributes to form the brilliancy of the eye. The same reflected light forms the images which one sees behind the cornea. In this case the cornea acts as a convex mirror. The form of the cornea indicates the influence it should have upon the light which enters the eye: on account of its thickness, it only causes the rays to converge a little towards the axis of the pencil; in other words it increases the intensity of the light which penetrates into the anterior chamber.

The rays, in traversing the cornea, pass from a more rare to a denser medium; consequently they ought to converge from the perpendicular towards the point of contact. If, on entering into the anterior chamber, they passed out again, they would diverge as much from the perpendicular as they had converged before; and would, therefore, assume their former divergence; but as they enter into the aqueous humour, which is a medium more refractive than air—they incline less from the perpendicular, and consequently diverge less than if they had passed back into the air.

Of all the light transmitted to the anterior chamber, only that which passes the pupil can be of use to vision; all that which falls upon the iris is reflected, returns through the cornea, and exhibits the colour of the iris.

In traversing the posterior chamber the light undergoes no new modification, as it proceeds always in the same medium (the aqueous humour).

It is in traversing the crystalline that light undergoes the most important modification. Philosophers compare the action of this body to that of a lens, the use of which would be to assemble all the rays of any cone of light upon a certain point of the retina. But as the crystalline is very far from being like a lens, we merely mention this opinion, which is generally received, to remark that it merits a fresh investigation. Every thing positive which can be said on the subject is, that the crystalline ought to increase the intensity of the light which is directed towards the bottom of the eye, with an energy proportionate to the convexity of its posterior surface. It may be added, that the light which passes near the circumference of the crystalline is probably reflected in a different manner from that which passes through the centre; and that therefore the contraction and dilatation of the pupil ought to possess an influence upon the mechanism of vision, which deserves the attention of philosophers.

The whole of the light which arrives at the anterior surface of the crystalline, does not penetrate into the vitreous body; it is partly reflected. One part of this reflected light traverses the aqueous humour and the cornea, and contributes to form the brilliancy of the eye; another falls upon the posterior surface of the iris, and is absorbed by the dark matter found there.

It is probable that something of this sort happens at every one of the strata or layers which forms the crystalline.

The vitreous body possesses a less refractive power than the crystalline, consequently the rays of light which, after having passed the crystalline, penetrate into the vitreous body, diverge from the perpendicular at the point of contact. Its use then, with regard to the direction of the rays in the eye, is to increase their convergence. It might be said, that in order to produce the same result, nature had only to render the crystalline a little more refractive; but the vitreous humour has another most essential use, which is, to give a larger extent to the retina, and thus to increase the field of vision.

What we said about a cone of light, commencing in a point placed in the prolongation of the anterio-posterior axis of the eye, must be repeated for every luminous cone commencing in other points, and directed towards the eye; with this difference, that, in the first case, the light tends to unite at the centre of the retina; while the light of the other cones tends to unite in different points, according to that form which they commence. Thus the luminous cones commencing from below, unite at the upper part of the retina, while those that come from above, unite at the lower part of this membrane. The other rays follow a direction analogous; so that there will be formed at the bottom of the eye an exact representation of every body placed before it, with this difference, that the images will be inverted, or in a position contrary to that of the objects they represent.

This result is ascertained by different means. For this purpose, eyes, constructed artificially of glass, which represent the transparent cornea, and the crystalline; and of water, which represents the aqueous and vitreous humours, have long been employed.

Motions of the iris.—Some say that the pupil varies its dimensions according to the distance of the object. This fact has not been sufficiently demonstrated; hitherto the influence of the intensity of light is the only thing that has been correctly observed.

The choroid is of use to vision, principally by the dark matter with which it is impregnated, and which absorbs the light immediately after it has traversed the retina. One may consider, as a confirmation of this opinion, what happens to some individuals in whom some parts of this membrane become *varicose:* the dilated vessels throw off the darker matter which covered them, and every time that the image of the object falls upon the point of the retina corresponding to these vessels, the object appears spotted with red.

The state of vision in Albino men and animals, in which the choroid and the iris are not coloured black, supports still more this assertion; vision is extremely imperfect in them: during the day, they can scarcely see sufficiently to go about. Mariotte, Lecat, and others, have allowed to the choroid the faculty of perceiving light. This idea is completely without proof.

We know very little, that is certain, of the ciliary processes. They are generally supposed *contractile;* but some think that they are destined to the motions of the iris, while others imagine they are intended to bring forward the crystalline.

The rays of light have now reached the retina, which receives the impression of light when it is within certain limits of intensity. A very feeble light is not felt by the retina; too strong a light hurts it, and renders it unfit for action.

When the retina receives too strong a light, the impression is called *dazzling;* the retina is then incapable for some time of feeling the presence of the light. This happens when one looks at the sun. After having been long in the dark, even a very feeble light produces dazzling.—When the light is exceedingly weak, and the eye made to observe objects narrowly, the retina becomes fatigued, there follows a painful feeling in the orbit, and also in the head.

A light, of which the intensity is not very strong, but which acts for a certain time upon a determined point of the retina, renders it at last insensible in this point. When we look for some time at a white spot upon a black ground, and afterward carry the eye to a white ground, we seem to perceive a black spot; this happens because the retina has become insensible in the point which was formerly fatigued by the white light. In the same manner, after the retina has been some time without acting in one of its points while the others have acted, the point which has been in repose becomes of an extreme sensibility, and on this account objects seem as if they were spotted. In this manner it is explained, why, after having looked a long time at a red spot, white bodies appear as if spotted with green: in this case, the retina has become insensible to the red rays, and we know that a ray of white light, from which the red is subtracted, produces the sensation of green.

The same sort of phenomena happens when we have looked long at a red body, or one of any other colour, and afterward look at white, or differently coloured bodies.—We perceive with facility the *direction* of the light received by the retina. We believe instinctively that light proceeds in a right line, and that this line is the prolongation of that according to which the light penetrated into the cornea. Therefore, whenever the light has been modified in its direction, before reaching the eye, the retina gives us nothing certain. Optical illusions proceed principally from this cause.

The retina can receive at the same time impressions in every point of its extent, but the sensations which result from them are incorrect. It may be affected by the image of one or two objects only, though a much greater number be impressed on it; the vision is then much more defined.

The central part of the membrane appears to possess much more sensibility than the rest of its extent; we therefore make the image fall on this part when we wish to examine an object with attention.

Does the light act upon the retina by simple contact only, or must it traverse this membrane? The presence of the choroid in the eye, or rather the dark matter which covers it, renders this second opinion the most probable.

That part of the retina which corresponds with the centre of the optic nerve, has been said to be insensible to the impression of light. I know nothing which can directly prove this assertion.

There is no doubt that the optic nerve transmits to the brain, in an instant, the impression that the light makes on the retina; but by what mechanism we are entirely ignorant. The manner in which the two optic nerves are confounded upon the *sphenoid bone*, ought, doubtless to have a considerable influence upon the transmission of the impressions received by the eyes;—but this is also a point upon which it is difficult to form any probable conjecture.

Notwithstanding what has been said at different periods, as well as the late efforts of Gall, to prove that we see with only one eye at a time, there seems sufficient proof not only that the two eyes concur at the same time in the production of vision, but that it is absolutely necessary this should be so, for certain most important operations of this function. There are however certain cases in which it is more convenient to employ only one eye; for instance, when it is necessary to understand perfectly the *direction* of the light, or the *situation* of any body relative to us. Thus we shut one eye to take aim with a gun, or to place a number of bodies upon a level in a right line.

Another case in which it is advantageous to employ only one eye is, when the two organs are unequal, either in refractive power or insensibility. For the same reason we shut one eye when we employ a telescope. But, except in these particular cases, it is of the utmost importance to employ both eyes at once. The following experiment proves that both eyes see the same object at the same time.

Receive the image of the sun upon a plane in a dark chamber; put before your eyes too thick glasses, each of which presents one of the prismatic colours. If your eyes are good and both equally strong, the image of the sun will appear of a dirty white, whatever be the colour of the glasses employed. If one of your eyes is much stronger than the other, the image of the sun will be seen of the same colour as the glass which is before the strongest eye.

One object produces then really two impressions while the brain perceives only one. To produce this the motions of the two eyes must be in unison. If, after a disease, the movement of the eyes are no longer regular, we receive two impressions from the same object, which constitutes *strabismus*, or squinting. We may also, at pleasure, receive two impressions from one body; for that purpose, it is only necessary to derange the harmony of the two eyes.

Estimation of the distance of objects.—Vision is produced essentially by the action of light upon the retina, and yet we always consider the bodies from which light proceeds as being the cause of it, though they are often placed at a considerable distance. This result can be produced only by an intellectual operation.

We judge differently of the distance of bodies according to the degree of that distance; we judge correctly when they are near us, but it is not the same when they are at a short distance; our judgment is then often incorrect: but when they are at a great distance, we are constantly deceived. The united action of the two eyes is absolutely necessary to determine exactly the distance, as the following experiment proves.

Suspend a ring by a thread, and fix a hook to the end of a long rod, of a size that will easily pass the ring; stand at a convenient distance, and try to introduce the hook: in using both eyes, you may succeed with ease in every attempt you make; but if you shut one eye, and then endeavour to pass the hook through, you will not succeed any longer; the hook will go either too far or else not far enough, and it will only be after trying repeatedly that it will be got through. Those persons whose eyes are very unequal in their power, are sure to fail in this experiment, even when they use them both.

When a person loses an eye by accident, it is sometimes a whole year before he can judge correctly of the distance of a body placed near him. Those who have only one eye, determine distance, for the most part, very incorrectly. The size of the object, the intensity of the light that proceeds from it, the presence of intermediate bodies, &c. have a great influence upon our just estimation of distance.

We judge most correctly of objects that are placed upon a level with our bodies. Thus, when we look from the top of a tower at the objects below, they appear much less than they would if they were placed at the same distance, on the same plane with ourselves. Hence the necessity of giving a considerable volume to objects that are intended to be placed on the tops of buildings, and which are to be seen from a distance. The smaller the dimensions of an object are, the nearer it ought to be to the eye, in order to be distinctly seen. What is called the distinct point of view is also very

variable. A horse is seen very distinctly at six yards, but a bird could not be distinctly seen at the same distance. If we wish to examine the hair or the feathers of those animals, the eye requires to be much nearer. However, the same object may be seen distinctly at different distances; for example, it is quite the same to many persons whether they place the book that they are reading at one or two feet of distance from the eye. The intensity of the light which illuminates an object, has a considerable effect upon the distance at which it can be distinctly seen.

Estimation of the size of bodies.—The manner in which we arrive at a just determination of the size of bodies, depends more upon knowledge and habit than upon the action of the apparatus of vision. We form our judgment relative to the dimensions of bodies, from the size of the image which is formed in the eye, from the intensity of the light which proceeds from the object, from the distance at which we think it is placed, and, above all, from the habit of seeing such objects. We therefore judge with difficulty of the size of a body that we see for the first time, when we cannot appreciate the distance. A mountain which we see at a distance for the first time, appears generally much less than it really is; we think it is near us when it is very far away.

Beyond a distance somewhat considerable, we are so completely deceived, that judgment is unable to correct us. Objects appear to us infinitely less than they really are: as happens with the celestial bodies.

Estimation of the motion of bodies.—We judge of the motion of a body by that of its image upon the retina, by the variations of the size of this image, or, which is the same thing, by the change of the direction of the light which arrives at the eye.

In order that we may be able to follow the motion of a body, it ought not to be displaced too rapidly, for we could not then perceive it; this happens with bodies projected by the force of gunpowder, particularly when they pass near us. When they move at a distance from us, the light comes from them to the eye for a much longer space of time, because the field of view is much greater, and we can see them with more facility. We ought to be ourselves at rest, in order to judge correctly of the motions of bodies.

When bodies are at a considerable distance from us, we cannot easily perceive their motions to or from us. In this case, we judge of the motion of the body, only by the variation of the size of its image. Now this variation being infinitely small, because the body is at a great distance, it is very difficult, and frequently impossible, for us to estimate its motion. Generally we perceive with great difficulty, sometimes we cannot perceive at all, the motion of a body which moves extremely slow; this may be on account of the slowness of its own motion, as in the case of the hand of a watch, or it may be the result of the slow motion of the image, which happens with the stars, and objects very far from us.

Of optical illusions.—After what we have just said, of the manner in which we estimate the distance, the size, and the motion of bodies, we may easily see that we are often deceived by sight. These deceptions are known in Physics, and in Physiology, by the name of optical illusions. Generally we judge pretty well of bodies placed near us; but we are most commonly deceived with regard to those that are distant. Those illusions which happen to us with regard to objects that are near us, are the result, sometimes of the reflection, sometimes of the refraction, of light before it reaches the eye; and sometimes of the law that we establish instinctively; namely, that light proceeds always in right lines.

We must refer to this cause those illusions occasioned by mirrors: objects are seen in plane mirrors at the same distance behind them, as the mirrors are distant from the eye. To this cause may be attributed also the apparent increase, or diminution of bodies seen through a glass. If the glass make the rays converge, the body will appear greater; if it cause them to diverge, the body will appear less. These glasses produce still another illusion; objects appear surrounded by the colours of the solar spectrum, because their surfaces not being parallel, they decompose light in the manner of the prism.

We are constantly deceived by objects at a distance, in a manner that we cannot prevent, because those deceptions result from certain laws which govern the animal economy. An object seems near us in proportion as its image occupies a greater space upon the retina; or in proportion to the intensity of the light which proceeds from it.

Of two objects of a different volume, equally illuminated and placed at the same distance, the greatest will appear the nearest, should circumstances be such as to admit of the distance being justly estimated. Of two objects of equal volume, placed at an equal distance from the eye, but unequally illuminated, the brightest will appear the nearest; it would be the same, if the objects were at unequal distances, as can be easily seen in looking at a string of lamps: if there happen to be one of them brighter than the rest, it will appear the nearest, while that which is really the nearest will appear the farthest, if it is the least bright. An object seen without any intermedium, always appears nearer than when there happens to be between it and the eye, some body that may have an influence upon the estimation that we make of its distance.

When a bright object strikes the eye, while all the objects around it are obscured, it appears much nearer than it really is; a light in the night produces this effect.

Objects appear always small in proportion as they are distant; thus, the trees in a long alley, appear so much smaller, and so much nearer together, in proportion as they are farther from us. It is by observing these illusions, and the laws of the animal economy, upon which they are founded, that art has been enabled to imitate them. The art of painting, in certain cases, merely transfers to the canvass those optical errors into which we most habitually fall.

The construction of optical instruments is also founded upon these principles: some of them augment the intensity of the light, which proceeds from the objects observed; others cause it to diverge, or converge, in order to increase or diminish their apparent volume, &c.

By the constant exercise of the sense of sight, we are enabled to get over many optical illusions, as will be proved by the curious history of the blind youth, spoken of by Cheselden. This celebrated surgeon, by a surgical operation, generally said to be that for cataract, but, more probably, it was a division of the *membrana pupillaris*, procured sight to a very intelligent person who was born blind: and he observed the manner in which this sense was developed in this young man. "When he saw the light for the first time, he knew so little how to judge of distances, that he believed the objects which he saw touched his eyes (and this was his expression) as the things which he felt touched his skin. The objects which were most pleasant to him were those whose form was regular and smooth, though he had no idea of their form, nor could he tell why they pleased him better than the others. During the time of his blindness he had such an imperfect idea of colours, that he was then able to distinguish, by a very strong light, that they had not left an impression sufficient by which he could again recognise them. Indeed, when he saw them, he said the colours he then saw were not the same as those he had seen formerly; he did not know the form of any object; nor could he distinguish one object from another, however different their figure or size might be: when objects were shown to him which he had known formerly by the touch, he looked at them with attention, and observed them carefully in order to know them again; but as he had too many objects to retain at once, he forgot the greater part of them, and when he first learned, as he said, to see and to know objects, he forgot a thousand for one that he recollected. It was two months before he discovered that pictures represent solid bodies; until that time he had considered them as planes and surfaces differently coloured, and diversified by a variety of shades; but when he began to conceive that these pictures represented solid bodies, in touching the canvass of a picture with his hand he expected to find in reality something solid upon it, and he was much astonished when, upon touching those parts which seemed round and unequal, he found them flat, and smooth like the rest; he asked, which was the sense that deceived him,—the sight or the touch? There was shown to him a little portrait of his father, which was in the case of his mother's watch he said, that he knew very well it was the resemblance of his father; but he asked, with great astonishment, how it was possible for so large a visage to be kept in so small a space, as that appeared to him as impossible as that a bushel should be contained in a pint. He could not support much light at first, and every object seemed very large to him; but after he had seen larger things he considered the first smaller: he thought there was nothing beyond the limits of his sight. The same operation was performed on the other eye about a year after the first, and it succeeded equally well. At first he saw objects with his second eye much larger than with the other, but not so large, however, as he had seen them with the first eye; and when he looked at the same object with both eyes at once, he said that it appeared twice as large as with the first eye; but he did not see double, at least it could not be ascertained that he saw objects double, after he had got the sight of the second eye."

This observation is not singular; there exists a number of others, and they have all given results nearly alike. The conclusion that may be drawn from it is, that the exact manner in which we determine the distance, size, and form of objects, is the result of habit, or, which is the same thing, of the education of the sense of sight.

Vision, defective. See *Dysopia.*

VI'SUS. See *Vision.*

VISUS DEFIGURATIS. See *Metamorphopsia.*

VITA. (*Vita, æ,* f.; *à vivendo.*) See *Life.*

VITÆ ARBOR. See *Arbor vitæ.*

VITÆ LIGNUM. See *Guaiacum.*

Vital actions. See *Vital functions.*

Vital air. See *Oxygen.*

Vital force. See *Vis vitæ.*

Vital functions. See *Function.*

Vital principle. See *Life.*

VITA'LBA. See *Clematis recta.*

VITELLUS. (*Vitellus, i,* m.; from *vita,* life; because the life of the chick is in it.)

1. The yelk of an egg.

2. In botany applied by Gærtner to that part of a seed which is very firmly and inseparably connected with the embryo, yet never rising out of the integuments of the seed in germination, but absorbed, like the albumen, for the nourishment of the embryo. If the albumen be present, the vitellus is always situated between it and the embryo, and yet is constantly distinct from the former. It is esteemed by Gærtner to compose the bulk of the seed in the fusci, mosses, and ferns. In the natural order of grasses, the vitellus forms a scale betwen the embryo and the albumen. Sir J. Smith thinks the vitellus is nothing else than a subterraneous cotyledon. See *Albumen.*

VI'TEX. (From *vieo,* to bind.) The name of a genus of plants in the Linnæan system. Class, *Didynamia;* Order, *Angiospermia.*

VITEX AGNUS CASTUS. The systematic name of the *Agnus castus; Elæagnon.* The chaste tree. *Vitex —foliis digitatis, serratis, spicis verticillatis,* of Linnæus. The seeds are the medicinal part, which have, when fresh, a fragrant smell, and an acrid aromatic taste. Formerly they were celebrated as anaphrodisiacs; but experience does not discover in them any degree of such virtue, and some have described to them an opposite one. They are now fallen into disuse.

VI'TI SALTUS. See *Chorea.*

VITILI'GO. (*Vitiligo, inis,* f.; from *vitio,* to infect.) See *Alphus.*

VI'TIS. 1. The name of a genus of plants in the Linnæan system. Class, *Pentandria;* Order, *Monogynia.*

2. The pharmacopœial name of the grape. See *Vitis vinifera.*

VITIS ALBA. See *Bryonia alba.*

VITIS CORINTHICA. The dried fruit of this tree is the *Uva passa minor; Passa corinthiaca.* The virtues of the currant are similar to those of the raisin. See *Vitis vinifera.*

VITIS IDÆA. See *Vaccinium.*

VITIS SYLVESTRIS. White bryony.

VITIS VINIFERA. The systematic name of the grape tree. *Vitis—foliis lobatis sinuatis nudis,* of Linnæus. Vine leaves and the tendrils have an adstringent taste, and were formerly used in diarrhœas, hæmorrhages, and other disorders requiring refrigerant and styptic medicines. The juice or sap of the vine called lachryma, has been recommended in calculous disorders: and it is said to be an excellent application to weak eyes and specks of the cornea. The unripe fruit has a harsh, rough, sour taste; its expressed juice, called verjuice, was formerly much esteemed, but is now superseded by the juice of lemons; for external use, however, particularly in bruises and pains, verjuice is still employed, and considered to be a very useful application. The dried fruit is termed *Uva passa major*. *Passula major*, the raisin. Raisins are prepared by immersing the fresh fruit into a solution of alkaline salt and soap-ley, made boiling hot, to which is added some olive oil, and a small quantity of common salt, and afterward drying them in the shade. They are used as agreeable, lubricating, acescent sweets in pectoral decoctions, and for obtunding the acrimony in other medicines, and rendering them grateful to the palate and stomach. They are directed in the *decoctum hordei compositum, tinctura sennæ,* and *tinctura cardamomi composita.* See also *Wine* and *Acetum.*

VITRA'RIA. The pellitory of the wall.

VITREOUS. (*Vitreus;* from *vitrum*, glass: so named from its transparency.) Glassy: applied to parts of the body.

VITREOUS HUMOUR. *Humor vitreus.* The pellucid body which fills the whole bulb of the eye behind the crystalline lens. The vitreous substance is composed of small cells which communicate with each other, and are distended with a transparent fluid.

VITRIOL. See *Vitriolum.*
Vitriol, acid of. See *Sulphuric acid.*
Vitriol, blue. See *Cupri sulphas.*
Vitriol, green. See *Ferri sulphas.*
Vitriol, Roman. See *Cupri sulphas.*
Vitriol, sweet, spirit of. See *Spiritus ætheris sulphurici.*
Vitriol, white. See *Zinci sulphas.*
Vitriolated kali. See *Potassæ sulphas.*

VITRI'OLUM. (From *vitrum*, glass: so called from its likeness to glass. Hollandus says this word is fictitious, and composed from the initials of the following sentence: *Vade in terram rimando, invenies, optimum lapidem veram medicinam.*) *Calcadinum; Calcatar; Calcotar; Calcanthos; Calcanthum; Calcitea.* Vitriol, or sulphate of iron. See *Ferri sulphas.*

VITRIOLUM ALBUM. See *Zinci sulphas.*
VITRIOLUM CŒRULEUM. See *Cupri sulphas.*
VITRIOLUM ROMANUM. See *Cupri sulphas.*
VITRIOLUM VIRIDE. See *Ferri sulphas.*

VI'TRUM. (*Vitrum, i,* n.) Glass.

VITRUM ANTIMONII. Glass of antimony. Antimony first calcined, then fused in a crucible.

VITRUM ANTIMONII CERATUM. A diaphoretic compound exhibited in the cure of dysenteries arising from checked perspiration.

VITRUM HYPOCLEPTICUM. A funnel to separate oil from water.

VIVERRA. The name of a genus of animals in the Order *Feræ*, of the Linnæan classification.

VIVERRA CIVETTA. The systematic name of the ash-coloured weazel, which, with the following species, affords the perfume called civet.

VIVERRA ZIBETHA. The systematic name of the civet-cat. See *Civetta.*

VIVUM. A name variously applied: to mercury, because it moves about as if it were alive; hence *argentum vivum :* to lime, because when moisture is added it cracks and swells, as if alive.

VOICE. *Vox.* By *voice* we understand the sound which is produced in the larynx, at the instant when the air traverses this organ, either to enter or go out of the *trachea.*

In order to understand the mechanism by which the voice is produced and modified, we must say something of the manner in which sound is produced, in which it is propagated and modified in wind instruments, particularly those that have most analogy with the organ of voice.

A wind instrument is generally formed of a tube, either straight or bent, in which, by various processes, the air is made to vibrate.

Wind instruments are of two sorts: the one sort are called *mouth* instruments, the other sort *reed* instruments.

In the mouth instruments (the horn, trumpet, trombone, flageolet, flute, organ,) the column of air contained in the tube is the sonorous body. The air must be caused to vibrate in it in order to produce sounds.

For this purpose, the means employed are variable, according to the sort of instrument. The length, the width, the form of the tube, the openings in its sides, or its extremities, the power of the vibrations, and the manner in which they are excited, are the causes or the various sounds of this sort of instruments. The nature of the matter which forms the sounds has no influence but upon the tone.

The reed instruments are the most necessary to be known, for the organ of the voice is of this kind. Their theory is, unfortunately, much more imperfect than that of the other sort. In this sort of instruments, (the clarionet, hautboy, bassoon, voice organ, &c) we ought to distinguish between the reed, or *anche*, and the body of the tube. Their mechanism is essentially different.

A reed is always formed of one, and sometimes of two, thin plates, susceptible of a rapid motion, the alternate vibrations of which are intended to intercept and permit, *by turns*, the passage of a current of air. For this reason, the sounds which they produce do not follow the same laws as the sounds formed by elastic plates, with one end fixed, and the other free, which produce sonorous undulations in the open air. In the reed instruments, the reed alone produces and modifies the sound. If the plate is long, the motions are long, slow, and consequently the sounds are grave. On the contrary, a short plate produces acute sounds, because the alternations of transmission and interception of the current of air are more rapid.

When a number of different sounds are intended to be produced by a reed, it is necessary to vary the length of the plate. The bassoon and clarionet players do this when they wish to produce different sounds on the same instrument. We add, as an important circumstance, that the greater or less elevation of sound produced by the instrument, partly depends on the elasticity, the weight, and the form of the little tongue, or plate, and on the force of the current of air. If all these elements are not the same, the length being invariable, the tone will be different.

A reed is never employed alone; it is always fitted to a tube through which the wind passes that has been blown into the reed, and which ought, on this account, to be open at the two extremities. The tube has no influence upon the tone of the music; it acts only upon the intensity, the *timbre*, and upon the power of making the reed *speak.*

Apparatus of voice.—The larynx ought properly to be considered as the organ of voice.

The size of the larynx varies according to age and sex. It is placed at the anterior part of the neck where a small projection is seen, between the tongue and the trachea. It is small in children and women, greater in young men, and still larger in adult age.

The larynx not only produces the voice, but it is also the agent of its principal modifications; on which account, a perfect knowledge of the anatomy of this organ is indispensably necessary to a perfect knowledge of the mechanism of voice. As we cannot enter here into all the details of the structure of the larynx, we will only touch upon such as are most necessary to be known, many of which are not yet well understood.

Four cartilages and three fibro-cartilages enter into the composition of the larynx, and form the skeleton of it. The cartilages are the *cricoid*, the *thyroid*, and the two *arytænoid.* The *thyroid* joins with the *cricoid* by the extremity of its two inferior *horns.* In the living state, the *thyroid* is fixed with respect to the *cricoid*, which is contrary to what is generally supposed. Every *arytænoid* cartilage is articulated with the *cricoid* by means of a surface, which is oblong, and concave in a transverse direction. The *cricoid* presents a surface which is similarly disposed to that of the *arytænoid*, with this difference, that it is convex in the same direction in which the other is concave. Round the articulation there is a *synovial capsule*, firm before and behind, and moveable without and within. Before the articulation is the *thyro-arytænoid* ligament; behind is a strong ligamentous band that might be called *crico-arytænoid*, on account of the manner in which it is fixed.

Thus disposed, the articulation admits only of lateral movements of the *arytænoid* upon the *cricoid* cartilage. No movement forward or backward can take place, nor a certain movement up and down, mentioned in anatomical books which none of the muscles is so disposed as to produce. This articulation ought to be considered as a simple lateral *ginglymus*. The fibro cartilages of the larynx are the *epiglottis*, and two small bodies that are found above the top of the *arytænoid* cartilages, and that have been called by Santorini, *capitula cartilaginum arytænoidearum.*

There are a great many muscles attached to the larynx. These muscles are called external : they are intended to move the whole organ, either in carrying it up or down, backward or forward, &c. The larynx has also other muscles, whose use is to give a movement to the different parts in respect of each other. These muscles have been called internal. They are,

1st, The *crico-thyroid*, the use of which is not, as has hitherto been believed, to lower the thyroid upon the cricoid cartilage, but, on the contrary, to raise the cricoid towards the thyroid cartilage, or in making it pass a little below its inferior edge.

2d, The muscles *crico-arytænoideus posterior*, and the *crico-arytænoideus lateralis*, the use of which is to draw outwards the arytænoid cartilages, in separating them from one another.

3d, The *arytænoid* muscle, which draws the arytænoid cartilages together.

4th, The *thyro-arytænoideus*, a knowledge of which is more important than that of all the muscles of the larynx, because its vibrations produce the vocal sound. This muscle forms the lips of the *glottis*, and the inferior, superior, and lateral sides of the ventricles of the larynx.

5th, Lastly, the muscles of the *epiglottis*, which are the *thyro-epiglottideus*, the *arytæno-epiglottideus*, and some fibres that may be considered as the vestige of the *glosso-epiglottideus* muscle that exists in some animals, whose contraction has an influence upon the position of the *epiglottis.*

The larynx is covered within by a *mucous membrane*. This membrane, in passing from the epiglottis to the arytænoid and thyroid cartilages, forms two folds, called 'ateral ligaments of the epiglottis. They concur in the 'ormation of the superior and inferior ligaments of the glottis.

In the substance of the epiglottis, and behind it, are found a great number of *mucous follicles*, and some *mucous glands.* Within the mass of the ligaments of the epiglottis, there exists a collection of those bodies that have been very improperly called *arytænoid glands.*

Between the epiglottis behind, and the os hyoides and thyroid cartilage before, there is seen a considerable quantity of the adipose *cellular tissue*, which is very *elastic*, and similar to that which exists near certain articulations. There has been no use assigned to this body. Dr. Magendie believes it serves to facilitate the frequent movements of the thyroid cartilage upon the posterior face of the os hyoides, and to keep the epiglottis separated from the upper part of this bone, while, at the same time, it provides it with a very elastic support, favourable to the action of the *fibrocartilages* in the production of the voice, or in deglutition.

The *vessels* of the larynx present nothing remarkable. It is not so with the nerves of this organ. Their distribution merits a careful examination. There are four of these nerves, the *superior laryngeal* and the *inferior.*

The *recurrent nerve* is distributed to the posterior crico-arytænoid, to the lateral crico-arytænoid, and thyro-arytænoid. None of the ramifications of this nerve go to the arytænoid, or to the crico-thyroid, muscles. On the contrary, the superior nerve of the larynx goes to the arytænoid muscle, which it provides with a considerable branch and to the crico-thyroid, to which it gives a small filament, more remarkable for the distance it proceeds than for its size. In certain cases this filament does not exist. The external branch of the nerve of the larynx is then of a larger size. The remainder of the filaments of the laryngeal nerves are distributed to the epiglottis, and to the mucous membrane which covers the entrance of the larynx. This part possesses an extraordinary sensibility.

The interval which separates the thyro-arytænoid muscles, and the arytænoid cartilages, is called *glottis.* In the dead body, the glottis presents the appearance of a longitudinal slit of about eight or ten lines long, and two or three wide ; it is wider behind than before. Here the two sides meet at the point of their insertion

into the *thyroid* cartilage. The posterior extremity of the glottis is formed by the *arytænoid* muscles.

If the arytænoid cartilages are brought together so as to touch on their internal faces, the glottis is diminished nearly a third of its length. It then presents a slit which is from five to six lines long, and from half a line to a line long. The sides of this slit are called the *lips of the glottis.* They present a sharp edge turned upward and inward. They are essentially formed by the arytænoid muscle, and by the ligament of the same name, which, as an *aponeurosis*, covers the muscle to which it adheres strongly, and which, being itself covered by the mucous membrane, forms the thinnest parts or edge of the *lip.* These lips of the glottis vibrate in the production of the voice; they might be called the *human reed.* Above the inferior ligaments of the glottis are the *ventricles of the larynx*, the cavity of which is larger than it seems at first sight. The superior, inferior, and external sides of it are formed by the thyro-arytænoid muscle, turned upon itself. The extremity, or anterior side, is formed by the thyroid cartilage. By means of these ventricles, the lips of the glottis are completely isolated upon their upper side.

Above the opening of the ventricles we see two bodies, which, in their manner of being disposed, have a great deal of analogy with the vocal chords, and which form a sort of second glottis above the first. These bodies are called the *superior ligaments of the glottis.* They are formed by the superior edge of the thyro-ary tænoid muscle, a little adipose cellular tissue, and the mucous membrane of the larynx, which covers them before penetrating into the ventricles. These observations are easily made upon the larynx of dead bodies. The glottis of a living person has never been examined, at least there has been nothing written on this subject; but when those of animals, as of dogs, are examined, they contract and enlarge alternately. The arytænoid cartilages are directed outwards when the air penetrates into the lungs ; and in the instant when the air passes out, they come close together.

Mechanism of the Production of Voice.—If we take the trachea and the larynx of an animal or of a man, and blow air strongly into the trachea, directing it towards the larynx, there is no sound produced, but only a slight noise, resulting from the pressure of the air against the sides of the larynx. If, in blowing, we bring together the arytænoid cartilages, so that they may touch upon their internal face, a sound will be produced, something like the voice of the animal to which the larynx used in the experiment belongs.

The sound will be dull or sharp, according as the cartilages are pressed more or less forcibly together : its intensity will be more or less, according to the intensity of the air. It is easily seen, in this experiment, that the sound is produced by the vibrations of the inferior ligament of the glottis.

Both man and the animals are deprived of voice by making an opening below the larynx. The voice is reproduced if the opening is closed mechanically. Dr Magendie knows a person who has been in this situation for four years. He cannot speak without pressing a cravat strongly against a fistulous opening in the larynx. The same thing takes place when the larynx is opened below the inferior ligaments of the glottis.

But if a wound exists above the glottis, if the epiglottis and its muscles are affected, if the superior ligament of the glottis, even if the superior aspect of the arytænoid cartilages are injured, the voice continues.

Lastly, the glottis of an animal being laid bare in the instant that it cries, shows very well that voice is produced by the vibrations of the vocal chords, or lips of the glottis. This is enough to prove, beyond all doubt, that the voice is formed in the glottis by the motion of its inferior ligaments.

This fact being established, is it possible, on physical principles, to account for the formation of the voice ? The following explanation appears the most probable. The air being pressed from the lungs, proceeds in a pipe of considerable size. This pipe very soon becomes contracted, and the air is forced to pass through a narrow slit, the two sides of which are vibrating plates, which permit and intercept the air, I ke the plates of reeds, and which ought, in the same manner, by these alternations, to produce sonorous undulations in the transmitted current of air.

But, in blowing into the trachea of a dead body, why does it not produce a sound like that of the human voice ? Why is the palsied state of the internal muscles of this organ followed by the loss of the voice ? Why, in a word, is an act of the will necessary to produce the vocal sound ? The answer to this is not difficult. The ligaments of the glottis have not the faculty of vibrating like plates of reeds, except the thyro-arytænoid muscles are contracted; and, therefore, in every case in which the muscles are not contracted, the voice will not be produced

Experiments performed on animals are perfectly in unison with this doctrine. Divide the two recurrent nerves, and the voice will cease. If only one is cut, the voice will be only half lost.

Dr. Magendie, however, has seen a number of animals, in which the two recurrent nerves had been cut, cry very loud when they suffered severe pain. These sounds were very similar to the sounds that would be produced mechanically with the larynx of the animal when dead, by blowing into the trachea, and bringing together the arytænoid cartilages. This phenomenon is easily understood by the distribution of the nerves of the larynx. The recurrents being cut, the thyro-arytænoid muscles do not contract, and thence results the loss of voice; but the arytænoid muscle, that receives its nerves from the superior laryngeal, contracts, and brings together, in the instant of a strong expiration, the arytænoid cartilages, and the slit of the glottis becomes sufficiently narrow for the air to throw the thyro-arytænoid muscles, though they are not contracted, into vibration.

Intensity or volume of the voice. The intensity of the voice, like that of all other sounds, depends upon the extent of the vibrations.

The vibrations of the *vocal chords* will be in proportion to the force with which the air is expelled from the breast; and the longer the chords are, that is, the more voluminous the larynx is, the more considerable will be the extent of the vibrations. A strong person, with a large chest, and a larynx of large dimensions, presents the most advantageous condition for the intensity of the voice. If such a person becomes sick, his voice, on account of his weakness, loses much of its intensity, because it is no longer expelled with the same force from the chest.

Children, women, and eunuchs, whose larynx is proportionably less than that of a man in adult age, have also much less intensity of voice.

In the ordinary production of the voice, it results from the simultaneous motions of the two sides of the glottis. Were one of these sides to lose the faculty of causing the air to vibrate, the voice would lose, necessarily, half its intensity, the force of expiration being the same. This may be proved in cutting one of the recurrent nerves of a dog, or in paying attention to the voice of a person who has had a complete attack of *hemiplegia.*

Tone of the voice.—Every individual has a particular tone of voice by which he is known: there is also a particular tone which belongs to the different sexes and age. The tone of the voice presents an infinite number of modifications. Upon what circumstances do these depend ? This is unknown. The feminine tone, however, which is found in children and eunuchs, generally agrees with the state of the cartilages of the larynx. On the contrary, the masculine tone which women sometimes possess, appears to be connected with the state of these cartilages, and particularly with that of the thyroids. Tone is a modification of sound, of which philosophers have by no means given an exact explanation.

Of the extent of the voice.—The sounds which the human larynx is capable of producing are very numerous. Many celebrated authors have endeavoured to explain the manner of their formation; but they have rather given us comparisons than explanations.

We have examined the reed of the organ of voice; we shall now consider the tube that the vocal sound traverses after having been produced. In proceeding from below upwards, the tube is composed, 1st, of the interval between the epiglottis before, its lateral ligaments upon the sides, and of the posterior side of the pharynx; 2dly, of the pharynx behind, and laterally, and of the most posterior part of the base of the tongue before; 3dly, sometimes of the mouth, and sometimes of the nasal cavities; at other times, of these two cavities together.

This tube, capable of being prolonged or shortened,

of being made wider or narrower; being susceptible of assuming an infinite variety of forms, ought to be very capable of performing all the functions of the body of a reed instrument;—that is, to be capable of harmonizing with the larynx, and of thus favouring the production of the numerous tones of which the voice is susceptible; of increasing the intensity of the vocal sound, by taking a conical form, with the base outwards; of giving a roundness and agreeableness to the sound, by suitably exposing its exterior opening, or by almost entirely shutting it, &c.

Until the influence of the tube of reed instruments has been determined with precision, it is evident that we can form only probable conjectures respecting the influence of the tube of the organ of voice. In this respect we can make only a small number of observations, which relate particularly to the most apparent phenomena.

A. The larynx is raised in the production of acute sounds; it is lowered, on the contrary, in the formation of those that are grave; consequently, the vocal tube is shortened in the first case, and lengthened in the second.

We suppose that a short tube is more favourable to the transmission of acute sounds, while a long one is more so for those that are grave. The tube changes its length at the same time that it changes its breadth; and this is remarkable, as we have seen above that the breadth of the tube has a great influence upon its facility of transmitting sounds.

When the larynx descends, that is, when the vocal tube is prolonged, the thyroid cartilage descends, and removes from the os hyoides the whole height of the thyro-hyoid membrane. By this separation the gland of the epiglottis is carried forward, and places itself in the cavity of the posterior aspect of the os hyoides; this gland draws after it the epiglottis: from this results a considerable enlargement of the inferior part of the vocal tube.

The contrary phenomenon happens when the larynx is raised. The thyroid cartilage then rises, and becomes engaged behind the os hyoides, by displacing and pushing backward the epiglottid gland; this pushes the epiglottis, and the vocal tube is much contracted. By imitating the motion upon the dead body, we may easily ascertain that the narrowing may proceed to five-sixths of the breadth of the tube. Now, we adapt a large tube to a reed for the purpose of producing grave sounds; on the contrary, it is a narrow tube which is generally employed for the purpose of transmitting acute sounds. We can then, to a certain degree, account for the utility of the changes of breadth which take place in the inferior part of the vocal tube.

B. The presence of the ventricles of the larynx immediately above the inferior ligaments of the glottis, appears intended to isolate those ligaments, so that they may vibrate freely in the air. When foreign bodies enter the ventricles, or when a false membrane, or mucosities are formed, the voice is generally extinguished, or much weakened.

C. From its form, its position, its elasticity; from the motions which its muscles impress upon it, the epiglottis appears to belong essentially to the apparatus of the voice; but what are its uses ? We have already seen that it contributes powerfully to the narrowing of the vocal tube; it may be supposed that it has a more important function.

D. The vocal tube has visibly an influence upon the intensity of the voice. The most intense sounds which the voice can produce, cause the mouth to be opened very wide, the tongue to be drawn a little back, and the velum of the palate raised into a horizontal position, and to become elastic, closing all communication with the nostrils.

In this case the pharynx and the mouth evidently perform the office of a speaking trumpet, that is to say they represent very exactly a tube with a reed, which increases in wideness outwards, the effect of which is to augment the intensity of the sound produced by the reed. If the mouth is in part closed, the lips carried forward and turned towards each other, the sound will acquire rotundity, and an agreeable expression; but it will lose part of its intensity: this result is easily explained after what we have said of the influence of the form of tubes in reed instruments.

For the same reasons, whenever the vocal sound

passes into the nose, it will become dull, for the form of the cavities of the nose is well fitted for diminishing the intensity of sounds. If the mouth and nose are shut at the same time, no sound can be produced.

E. We have seen, in considering the production of voice, that a great number of modifications relative to expression arise from changes of the thickness, and of the elasticity of the lips of the glottis. The tube may produce a number of others, according to its different degrees of length or breadth; according to its form, the contraction of the pharynx, the position of the tongue, or of the velum of the palate; according as the sound passes wholly or in part through the mouth, or the nose, or both together; according to the individual disposition of the mouth or nose; the existence or non-existence of teeth; the size of the tongue, &c.; the expression of the voice is continually modified according to all these circumstances. For example, whenever the sound traverses the nasal cavities, it becomes disagreeably nasal.

Those persons are mistaken, who think that the intensity of vocal sound may be augmented by repercussion, in passing through the nasal cavities; these cavities produce quite a contrary effect. Whenever the voice is introduced into them, from whatever cause, it becomes dull.

F. Besides the numerous modifications which the tube of the vocal organ causes in the intensity and the expression of the voice, in alternately permitting or intercepting its productions: there is another very important kind of modification produced by it. By means of this the vocal sound is divided into very small portions, each possessing a distinct character, because each of them is produced by a distinct motion of the tube. This sort of influence of the vocal tube is called the *faculty of articulating*, which presents, besides, an infinite variety of individual differences suitable to the peculiar organization of the vocal tube.

We have hitherto treated of the human voice in a general manner; we now proceed to speak of its principal modifications; namely, the cry or native voice; the voice properly so called, or acquired voice; speech, or articulate voice; singing, or *appreciable* voice.

The cry, or native voice.—The cry is a sound which cannot be appreciated; it is, like all those sounds produced by the larynx, susceptible of variation in tone, intensity, and expression. The cry is easily distinguished from all other vocal sounds; but as its character depends upon the expression, it is impossible to account physically for the difference between it and the latter. Whatever is the condition of man, or whatever his age, he is capable of crying. The new-born child, the idiot, the person deaf from birth, the savage, the civilized, the decrepit old man, all are capable of producing cries. We ought, then, to consider the cry as particularly attached to organization; indeed, we may be convinced of this in examining its uses.

By the cry we express vivid sensations, whether they proceed from without or within; whether they are agreeable or painful:—there are cries of pleasure and of pain. By the cry we express our most simple instinctive wants, the natural passions. There is a cry of fury, another of fear, &c.

The social wants and passions, not being an indispensable consequence of organization, and the state of civilization being necessary for their development, they have no peculiar cry. The cry comprehends, generally, the most intense sounds that the organ of voice can produce; its expression has often something in it which offends the ear, and it has a strong action upon those who are near it.

By means of the cry, important relations are established among mankind. The cry of joy inclines to joy; the cry of pain excites pity; the cry produced by terror causes fear, even in those at a distance, &c. This sort of language is found in most animals; it is almost the only language which has been given them; the song of birds ought to be considered as a modification of their cry.

Acquired voice, or voice properly so called.—In the usual state of man, that is, when he lives in society, and when he is possessed of the faculty of hearing, he knows, from earliest youth, that mankind utter sounds which are not cries he very soon finds that he can produce the same sort of sounds with his larynx, and immediately, what is called *acquired voice*, is developed in him, by the effect of imitation, and the advantages he derives from it. A deaf child cannot make any remark with regard to sound, and, therefore, he never acquires it. There seems to be no difference between the voice and the cry, except in intensity and expression, for it is likewise formed of inappreciable sounds, or of sounds whose intervals are not exactly distinguished by the ear.

Since the voice is the consequence of hearing, and of an intellectual process, it cannot be developed if those circumstances, by which it is produced, do not exist. In fact, children born deaf, who have never had any idea of sound; idiots, that establish no relation between the sounds which they hear, and those which their larynx can produce, have no voice, though the vocal apparatus of both may be fit to form and modify sounds as well as that of individuals perfectly formed. For the same reason those whom we improperly term *savages*, because they have been found wandering in forests since their infancy, can have no voice; the understanding not being developed in a solitary state, but only in social life.

The expression, the intensity, the tone of the voice, are susceptible of numerous modifications on the part of the larynx; the vocal tube also exerts a powerful influence upon the voice: speech and singing are only modifications of the social voice.

Modifications of the voice by age.—The larynx is in proportion very small in the fœtus, and the new-born infant; its small volume forms a contrast with that of the os hyoides, with the tongue and other organs of deglutition, which are already much developed. Besides, it is round, and the thyroid cartilage forms no projection in the neck.

The lips of the glottis, the ventricles, the superior ligaments, are very short in proportion to what they become afterward; for the thyroid cartilage not being much developed, they consequently occupy a small space. The cartilages are flexible, and have not nearly the solidity which they possess afterward.

The larynx preserves these characters almost till puberty; at this period a general revolution takes place in the economy. The development of the genital organs determines a sudden increase in the nutrition of many of the organs, of which that of the voice is one.

The greatest activity of nutrition is first remarked in the muscles; afterward, but more slowly, it is seen in the cartilages: the general form of the larynx is then modified; the thyroid cartilage becomes developed in its anterior part, it forms a projection in the neck, and greater in the male than in the female. From this circumstance results a considerable prolongation of the lips of the glottis, or thyro-arytænoid muscles; and this phenomenon is much more worthy of remark than the general increase of the glottis which happens at the same time.

Though these changes in the larynx are rapid, they do not happen all at once; sometimes it is six or eight months before they terminate.

After puberty the larynx does not suffer any other remarkable changes; its volume and the projection of the thyroid cartilage continue to increase, and become more strongly marked. The cartilages become partially ossified in manhood.

In old age the ossification of the cartilages continues, and becomes almost complete; the epiglottic gland diminishes considerably, and the internal muscles, but those particularly that form the lips of the glottis, diminish in volume, assume a colour less deep, and lose their elasticity; in a word, they take the same modifications as the muscular system in general.

The production of voice, as it supposes the passage of air to and from the lungs to take place, cannot exist in the fœtus, plunged as it is in the *liquor amnii;* but the child is capable of producing very acute sounds at the instant of birth.

Vagitus is the name that is given to this voice, or cry of children, by which they express their wants and feelings. We must recollect that this is the object of the cry.

Towards the end of the first year, the child begins to form sounds that are easily distinguished from the *vagitus.* These sounds, at first vague and irregular, very soon become more distinct and connected; nurses then begin to make them pronounce the most simple words, and afterward, those that are more complicated.

The pronunciation of children has very little resemblance to that of adults; but there is also a great difference between them. In children, the teeth have not yet quitted their alveoli; the tongue is comparatively very large; when the lips are closed they are larger than is necessary for covering anteriorly the gums; the nasal cavities are not much developed, &c.

Children advance only by degrees, and in proportion as their organs of pronunciation approach those of the adult, to articulate exactly the different combinations of letters. They are not capable of forming appreciable sounds, or of singing, until long after they have acquired the faculty of speech. This sort of sounds is the voice properly so called, or acquired : they could not exist in the child were it deaf. They ought not to be considered as a modification of the vagitus.

Until the period of puberty, the larynx remains proportionably very small, as well as the lips of the glottis : the voice is also composed entirely of acute sounds. It is physically impossible that the larynx should produce grave ones.

At puberty, particularly in males, the voice undergoes a remarkable modification : it acquires in a few days, often all at once, a gravity, and a dull or deaf expression, that it was far from having before.

It sinks in general about an octave. The voice of a young man is said to *moult*, according to the common expression. In certain cases the voice is almost entirely lost for some weeks; it frequently contracts a marked hoarseness. Sometimes it happens that the young man produces involuntarily a very acute sound when he wishes to produce a grave one; it is then scarcely possible for him to produce appreciable sounds, or to sing true.

This state of things continues sometimes nearly a year, after which the voice becomes more clear, and remains so during life: but some individuals lose entirely, during the *moulting* of the voice, the faculty of singing; others, who having a fine extensive voice before the *moulting*, have afterward only a very ordinary one.

The gravity that the voice acquires depends evidently upon the developement of the larynx, and particularly on the prolongation of the lips of the glottis. As these parts cannot stretch backward, they come forward : it is also at this time that the larynx projects in the neck, and the *pomum adami* appears. In the female, the lips of the glottis do not present at puberty this increase in breadth; the voice also generally remains acute.

The voice generally preserves the same characters until after adult age; at least the modifications that it undergoes in the interval are but inconsiderable, and affect principally the expression, and the volume. Towards the beginning of old age, the voice changes anew, its expression alters, and its extent diminishes: singing is more difficult, the sounds become noisy, and their production painful and fatiguing. The organs of pronunciation being changed by the effect of age, the teeth become shorter, and frequently being lost, the pronunciation is sensibly changed. All these phenomena are more noted in confirmed old age. The voice is weak, shaking, and broken ; singing has the same characters which depend on impaired muscular contraction. Speech also undergoes remarkable modifications ; the slowness of the motions of the tongue, the want of the teeth, the lips proportionably longer, &c. necessarily influence the pronunciation."—*Magendie's Physiology.*

VOLA'TICUS. (*Volaticus ;* from *volo*, to fly.) Volatile; that goeth or flieth, as it were, away suddenly.

VOLATILE. See *Volaticus.*

Volatile alkali. See *Ammonia.*

Volatile caustic, alkali. See *Ammonia.*

VOLATILITY. The properties of bodies by which they are disposed to assume the vaporous or elastic state, and quit the vessels in which they are placed.

VOLCANITE. See *Augite.*

VOLSE'LLA. A probang, or instrument to remove bodies sticking in the throat.

VOLUBILIS. Twining. Botanists apply it to stems which twine round other plants by their own spiral form, either from left to right, supposing the observer in the centre (or, in other words, according to the apparent motions of the sun); as in *Tamus communis*, and the honeysuckle . or from right to left contrary to

the sun, as with *Convolvulus sæpium*, the French bean, &c.

VOLVA. (*Volva, æ,* f. ; from *valva*.) The wrapper or covering of the fungous tribe, of a membranous texture, concealing their parts of fructification, and in due time bursting all round, forming a ring upon the stalk, as in *Agaricus campestris.* Such is the original meaning of this term, as explained by Linnæus; but it has become more generally used by Linnæus himself for the fleshy external covering of some other fungi, which is scarcely raised out of the ground, and enfolds the whole plant when young. It is *simple, double,* or *stellated,* very much cut; as in *Lycopodium stellatum.*

VOLVULUS. (From *volvo*, to roll up.) The iliac passion, or inflammation in the bowels, called twisting of the guts. See *Iliac passion.*

VOLVULUS TERRESTRIS. Small bind-weed. The Convolvulus minor.

VO'MER. Named from its great resemblance to a ploughshare. It is a slender thin bone, separating the nostrils from each other, consisting of two plates much compressed together, very dense and strong, yet so thin as to be transparent; these two plates seem at every edge to separate from each other, and thus a groove is formed at every side.—1. This groove on the upper edge, or, as it may be called, its base, is wide, and receives into it the projecting points of the ethmoid and sphenoid bones, and thus it stands very firmly and securely on the skull, and capable of resisting blows of considerable violence.—2. The groove, upon the lower part, is narrower, and receives the rising line in the middle of the palate plate, where the bones join to form the palate suture. At the forepart it is united by a ragged surface, and by something like a groove, to the middle cartilage of the nose, and as the vomer receives the other bones into its grooves, it is, as it were, locked in on all sides, receiving support and strength from each, but more particularly from the thick and strong membrane which covers the whole, and which is so continuous as to resemble a periosteum, or rather a continued ligament, from its strength; thus the slender vomer possesses sufficient strength to avert from it all those evils which must inevitably have occurred, had it been less wisely or less strongly constructed.

VO'MICA. (From *vomo*, to spit up; because it discharges a sanies.) An abscess of the lungs.

VOMITING, *Vomitio.* A forcible ejection of food, or any other substance from the stomach, through the œsophagus and mouth.

"That internal sensation which announces the ne cessity of vomiting is called *nausea ;* it consists of a general uneasiness, with a feeling of dizziness in the head, or in the epigastric region: the lower lip trembles, and the saliva flows in abundance. Instantly, and involuntarily, convulsive contractions of the abdominal muscles, and at the same time, of the diaphragm, succeed to this state; the first are not very intense, but those that follow are more so; they at last become such, that the matters contained in the stomach surmount the resistance of the *cardia*, and are thus darted, as it were, into the œsophagus and mouth; the same effect is produced many times in succession; it ceases for a time, and begins again after some interval.

At the instant that the matters driven from the stomach traverse the pharynx and the mouth, the glottis shuts, the *velum* of the palate rises, and becomes horizontal, as in deglutition; nevertheless, every time that one vomits, a certain quantity of liquid is introduced either into the larynx, or the nasal canals.

Vomiting was long believed to depend upon the rapid convulsive contraction of the stomach; but it has been shown, by a series of experiments, that, in the process, this viscus is nearly passive ; and that the true agents of vomiting are, on the one hand, the diaphragm, and, on the other, the large abdominal muscles.

In the ordinary state, the diaphragm and the muscles of the abdomen co-operate in vomiting; but each of them can, nevertheless, produce it separately. Thus, an animal still vomits, though the diaphragm has been rendered immoveable by cutting the diaphragmatic nerves; it vomits the same, though the whole abdominal muscles have been taken away by the knife, with the precaution of leaving the linea alba and the peritonæum untouched."

Vomiting of blood. See *Hæmatemesis.*

VO'MITUS CRUENTUS. See *Hæmatemesis.*

Voracious appetite. See *Bulimia.*

Vox abscissa. Hoarseness, and also a loss of voice.

Vulga'go. The asarabacca was so called. See *Asarum.*

VULNERA'RIA. (From *vulnus,* a wound.) Medicines which heal wounds. An herb named from its use in healing wounds.

Vulneraria aqua. Arquebusade.

VU'LNUS. A wound.

Vulnus sclopeticum. A gun-shot wound.

VULPENITE. A mineral of a grayish-white colour, found along with granular foliated limestone, at Vulpino, in Italy.

VU'LVA. (*Quasi valva,* the aperture to the womb, or *quasi volva,* because the fœtus is wrapped up in it., The pudendum muliebre, or parts of generation proper to women; also a foramen in the brain.

VULVA'RIA. (From *vulva,* the womb; so named from its smell, or use in disorders of the womb.) Stinking orach. See *Chenopodium vulvaria.*

W

WACKE. A mineral substance intermediate between clay and basalt.

WADD. A name of plumbago.

Wadd, black. An ore of manganese: so called in Derbyshire.

WAKE ROBIN. See *Arum.*

WALL-FLOWER. See *Cheiranthus cheiri.*

WALL-PELLITORY. See *Parietaria.*

WALL-PEPPER. See *Sedum acre.*

WALNUT. See *Juglans.*

WALTHER, Augustine Frederic, a physician, was appointed, in 1723, professor of anatomy and surgery at Leyden. Several of his dissertations on anatomical subjects are commended, and have been reprinted by Haller. The best of his larger pieces is "De Lingua Humana Libellus," in quarto. As a botanist he published a Catalogue of the Plants in his own garden, and a work on the Structure of Plants. He died about the year 1746.

WALTON. A town, near Tewkesbury in Gloucestershire, where there is a mineral spring, containing a small portion of iron dissolved in fixed air; of absorbent earth combined with hepatic air; of vitriolated magnesia, and muriated mineral alkali; but the proportions of these constituent parts have not been accurately ascertained. Walton water is chiefly efficacious in obstructions and other affections of the glands.

[WARREN, Dr. Joseph, was born in Roxbury, near Boston, in 1741. He was a distinguished physician and patriot of the American Revolution, and was killed early in the contest, at the battle of Bunker's Hill, June 17, 1775. The following is from Thacher's Life of Warren:

"The calmness and indifference of the veteran ' in clouds of dust and seas of blood,' can only be acquired by long acquaintance with the trade of death; but the heights of Charlestown will bear eternal testimony, how suddenly in the cause of freedom the peaceful citizen can become the invincible warrior; stung by oppression, he springs forward from his tranquil pursuits, undaunted by opposition and undismayed by danger, to fight even to death for the defence of his rights. Parents, wives, children, and country, all the hallowed properties of existence, are to him the talisman that takes fear from his heart and nerves his arm to victory. In the requiem over those who have fallen in the cause of their country, which ' Time, with his own eternal lips shall sing,' the praises of Warren shall be distinctly heard.

The blood of those patriots who have fallen in defence of republics has often ' cried from the ground,' against the ingratitude of the country for which it was shed. No monument was reared to their fame; no record of their virtues written; no fostering hand extended to their offspring; but they and their deeds were neglected and forgotten. Towards Warren there was no ingratitude,—our country is free from this stain. Congress were the guardians of his honours, and remembered that his children were unprotected orphans. Within a year after his death, Congress passed the following resolution:

'That a monument be erected to the memory of General Warren, in the town of Boston, with the following inscription:—

'In Honour of JOSEPH WARREN, Major-General of Massachusetts Bay. He devoted his life to the liberties of his country; and in bravely defending them, fell an early victim in the battle of bunker hill,

June 17, 1775. The Congress of the United States, as an acknowledgment of his services and distinguished merit, have erected this monument to his memory."

It was resolved, likewise, ' That the eldest son of General Warren should be educated from that time at the expense of the United States.' On the first of July, 1780, Congress, recognising these former resolutions, further resolved, ' That it should be recommended to the executive of Massachusetts Bay, to make provision for the maintenance and education of his three younger children; and that Congress would defray the expense to the amount of the half-pay of a major-general; to commence at the time of his death, and continue till the youngest of the children should be of age.' The part of the resolutions relating to the educating of the children, was carried into effect accordingly. The monument is not yet erected, but it is not too late. The shade of Warren will not repine at this neglect, while the ashes of Washington repose without gravestone or epitaph." *Thach. Med. Biog.* A.]

WATER. *Aqua.* This fluid is so well known, as scarcely to require any definition.

It is transparent, without colour, smell, or taste; in a very slight degree compressible; when pure, not liable to spontaneous change; liquid in the common temperature of our atmosphere, assuming the solid form at 32° Fahrenheit, and the gaseous at 212°, but returning unaltered to its liquid state on resuming any degree of heat between these points: capable of dissolving a greater number of natural bodies than any other fluid whatever, and especially those known by the name of the saline; performing the most important functions in the vegetable and animal kingdoms, and entering largely into their composition as a constituent part.

"Native water is seldom, if ever, found perfectly pure. The waters that flow within or upon the surface of the earth, contain various earthy, saline, metallic, vegetable, or animal particles, according to the substances over or through which they pass. Rain and snow waters are much purer than these, although they also contain whatever floats in the air, or has been exhaled along with the watery vapours.

The purity of water may be known by the following marks or properties of pure water:—

1. Pure water is lighter than water that is not pure.

2. Pure water is more fluid than water that is not pure.

3. It has no colour, smell, or taste.

4. It wets more easily than the waters containing metallic and earthy salts, called hard waters, and feels softer when touched.

5. Soap, or a solution of soap in alkohol, mixes easily and perfectly with it.

6. It is not rendered turbid by adding to it a solution of gold in aqua regia, or a solution of silver, or of lead, or of mercury, in nitric acid, or a solution of acetate of lead in water.

Water was, till modern times, considered as an elementary or simple substance.

Previous to the month of October, 1776, the celebrated Macquer, assisted by Sigaud de la Fond, made an experiment by burning hydrogen gas in a bottle, without explosion, and holding a white china saucer over the flame. His intention appears to have been that of ascertaining whether any fuliginous smoke was produced, and he observes, that the saucer remained perfectly clean and white, but was moistened with perceptible drops of a clear fluid, resembling water; and which, in fact, appeared to him and his assistant to be nothing but pure water. He does not say whether any test was applied to ascertain this purity, neither does he make any remark on the fact.

In the month of September, 1777, Bucquet and Lavoisier, not being acquainted with the fact which is incidentally and concisely mentioned by Macquer, made an experiment to discover what is produced by he combustion of hydrogen. They fired five or six pints of hydrogen in an open and wide-mouthed bottle, and instantly poured two ounces of lime-water through the flame, agitating the bottle during the time the combustion lasted. The result of this experiment showed, that carbonic acid was not produced.

Before the month of April, 1781, Mr. John Warltire, encouraged by Dr. Priestley, fired a mixture of common air and hydrogen gas in a close copper vessel, and found its weight diminished. Dr. Priestley, likewise, before the same period, fired a like mixture of hydrogen and oxygen gas in a closed glass vessel, Mr. Warltire being present. The inside of the vessel, though clean and dry before, became dewy, and was lined with a sooty substance. These experiments were afterward repeated by Mr. Cavendish and Dr. Priestley; and it was found, that the diminution of weight did not take place, neither was the sooty matter perceived. These circumstances, therefore, must have arisen from some imperfection in the apparatus or materials with which the former experiments were made.

It was the summer of the year 1781, that Mr. Henry Cavendish was busied in examining what becomes of the air lost by combustion, and made those valuable experiments which were read before the Royal Society on the 15th of January, 1784. He burned 500,000 grain measures of hydrogen gas, with about two and a half times the quantity of common air, and by causing the burned air to pass through a glass tube eight feet in length, 135 grains of pure water were condensed. He also exploded a mixture of 19,500 grain measures of oxygen gas, and 37,000 of hydrogen, in a close vessel. The condensed liquor was found to contain a small portion of nitric acid, when the mixture of the air was such, that the burned air still contained a considerable portion of oxygen. In this case it may be presumed, that some of the oxygen combines with a portion of nitrogen present.

In the mean time, Lavoisier continued his researches, and during the winter of 1781-1782, together with Gingembre, he filled a bottle of six pints with hydrogen, which being fired, and two ounces of lime-water poured in, was instantly stopped with a cork, through which a flexible tube communicating with a vessel of oxygen was passed. The inflammation ceased, except at the orifice of the tube, through which the oxygen was pressed, where a beautiful flame appeared. The combustion continued a considerable time, during which the lime-water was agitated in the bottle. Neither this, nor the same experiment repeated with pure water, and with a weak solution of alkali instead of lime-water, afforded the information sought after, for these substances were not at all altered.

The inference of Mr. Warltire, respecting the moisture on the inside of the glass in which Dr. Priestley first fired hydrogen and common air, was, that these airs, by combustion, deposited the moisture they contained. Mr. Watt, however, inferred from these experiments, that water is a compound of the burned airs, which have given out their latent heat by combustion; and communicated his sentiments to Dr. Priestley in a letter dated April 26, 1783.

It does not appear, that the composition of water was known or admitted in France, till the summer of 1783, when Lavoisier and De la Place, on the 24th of June, repeated the experiment of burning hydrogen and oxygen in a glass vessel over mercury, in a still greater quantity than had been burned by Mr. Cavendish. The result was nearly five gross of pure water. Monge made a similar experiment at Paris nearly at the same time, or perhaps before.

This assiduous and accurate philosopher then proceeded, in conjunction with Meusnier, to pass the steam of water through a red-hot iron tube, and found that the iron was oxydized, and hydrogen disengaged; and the steam of water being passed over a variety of other combustible or oxidable substances produced

similar results, the water disappearing and hydrogen being disengaged. These capital experiments were accounted for by Lavoisier, by supposing the water to be decomposed into its component parts, oxygen and hydrogen, the former of which unites with the ignited hydrogen, while the latter is disengaged.

The grand experiment of the composition of water by Fourcroy, Vauquelin, and Seguin, was begun on Wednesday, May 13, 1790, and was finished on Friday, the 22d of the same month. The combustion was kept up 185 hours with little interruption, during which time the machine was not quitted for a moment. The experimenters alternately refreshed themselves when fatigued, by lying for a few hours on mattresses in the laboratory.

To obtain the hydrogen, 1. Zinc was melted and rubbed into a powder in a very hot mortar. 2. This metal was dissolved in concentrated sulphuric acid diluted with seven parts of water. The air procured was made to pass through caustic alkali. To obtain the oxygen, two pounds and a half of crystallized hyperoxymuriate of potassa were distilled, and the air was transferred through caustic alkali.

The volume of hydrogen employed was 25963.568 cubic inches, and the weight was 1039.358 grains.

The volume of oxygen was 12570.942, and the weight was 6209.869 grains.

The total weight of both elastic fluids was 7249.227.

The weight of water obtained was 7244 grains, or 12 ounces 4 gros 45 grains.

The weight of water which should have been obtained was 12 ounces 4 gros 49.227 grains.

The deficit was 4.227 grains.

The quantity of azotic air before the experiment was 415.256 cubic inches, and at the close of it 467. The excess after the experiment was consequently 51.744 cubic inches. This augmentation is to be attributed, the academicians think, to the small quantity of atmospheric air in the cylinders of the gasometers at the time the other airs were introduced. These additional 51 cubic inches could not arise from the hydrogen, for experiment showed, that it contained no azotic air. Some addition of this last fluid, the experimenters think, cannot be avoided, on account of the construction of the machine.

The water being examined, was found to be as pure as distilled water. Its specific gravity to distilled water was as 18671 : 18670.

The decomposition of water is most elegantly effected by electricity.

The composition of water is best demonstrated by exploding 2 volumes of hydrogen and 1 of oxygen, in the eudiometer. They disappear totally, and pure water results. A cubic inch of this liquid, at 60° weighs 252.52 grains, consisting of

    28.06 grains hydrogen, and
    224.46   oxygen.

The bulk of the former gas is 1325 cubic inches.
That of the latter is   662
                                   ____
                                   1987
                                   ____

Hence there is a condensation of nearly two thousand volumes into one; and one volume of water contains 662 volumes of oxygen. The prime equivalent of water is 1.125; composed of a prime of oxygen = 1.0 + a prime of hydrogen = 0.125; or 9 parts by weight of water, consisting of 8 oxygen + 1 hydrogen."

The simple waters are the following:

1. Distilled water. This is the lightest of all others, containing neither solid nor gaseous substances in solution, is perfectly void of taste and smell, colourless and beautifully transparent, has a soft feel, and wets the fingers more readily than any other. It mixes uniformly with soap into a smooth opaline mixture, but may be added to a solution of soap in spirit of wine without injuring its transparency. The clearness of distilled water is not impaired by the most delicate chemical reagents, such as lime-water, a solution of barytes in any acid, nitrated silver, or acid of sugar. When evaporated in a silver vessel it leaves no residuum; if preserved from access of foreign matter floating in the air, it may be kept for ages unaltered in vessels upon which it has no action, as it does not possess within itself the power of decomposition. As it freezes exactly at 32° of Fahrenheit, and boils at 212° under the atmospherical pressure of 29.8 inches

these points are made use of as the standard ones for thermometrical division; and its specific weight being always the same under the mean pressure and temperature, it is employed for the comparative standard of specific gravity.

Pure distilled water can only be procured from water which contains no volatile matters that will rise in distillation, and continue still in union with the vapour when condensed. Many substances are volatile during distillation, but most of the gases, such as common air, carbonic acid, and the like, are incapable of uniting with water at a high temperature: other bodies, however, such as vegetable essential oil, and, in general, much of that which gives the peculiar odour to vegetable and animal matter, will remain in water after distillation. So the steam of many animal and vegetable decoctions has a certain flavour which distinguishes it from pure water; and the aqueous exhalation from living bodies, which is a kind of distillation, has a similar impregnation.

To obtain distilled water perfectly pure, much stress was laid by former chemists on repeating the process a great number of times; but it was found by Lavoisier, that rain water once distilled, rejecting the first and last products, was as pure a water as could be procured by any subsequent distillations.

Distilled water appears to possess a higher power than any other as a resolvent of all animal and vegetable matter, and these it holds in solution as little as possible altered from the state in which they existed in the body that yielded them. Hence the great practical utility of that kind of chemical analysis which presents the proximate constituent parts of these bodies, and which is effected particularly by the assistance of pure water. On the other hand, a saline, earthy, or otherwise impure water, will alter the texture of some of the parts, impair their solubility, produce material changes on the colouring matter, and become a less accurate analyzer on account of the admixture of foreign contents.

Distilled water is seldom employed to any extent in the preparation of food, or in manufactures, on account of the trouble of procuring it in large quantities; but for preparing a great number of medicines, and in almost every one of the nicer chemical processes that are carried on in the liquid way, this water is an essential requisite. The only cases in which it has been used largely as an article of drink, have been in those important trials made of the practicability of procuring it by condensing the steam of sea water by means of a simple apparatus adapted to a ship's boiler; and these have fully shown the ease with which a large quantity of fresh water, of the purest kind, may be had at sea, at a moderate expense, whereby one of the most distressing of all wants may be relieved. There are one or two circumstances which seem to show that water, when not already loaded with foreign matter, may become a solvent for concretions in urinary passages. At least, we know that very material advantage has been derived in these cases from very pure natural springs, and hence a course of distilled water has been recommended as a fair subject of experiment.

2. *Rain water*, the next in purity to distilled water, is that which has undergone a natural distillation from the earth, and is condensed in the form of rain. This is a water so nearly approaching to absolute purity as probably to be equal to distilled water for every purpose except in the nicer chemical experiments. The foreign contents of rain water appear to vary according to the state of the air through which it falls. The heterogeneous atmosphere of a smoky town will give some impregnation to rain as it passes through, and this, though it may not be at once perceptible on chemical examination, will yet render it liable to spontaneous change; and hence, rain water, if long kept, especially in hot climates, acquires a strong smell, becomes full of animalcula, and in some degree putrid. According to Margraaff, the constant foreign contents of rain water appear to be some traces of the muriatic and nitric acids; but as this water is always very soft, it is admirably adapted for dissolving soap, or for the solution of alimentary or colouring matter, and it is accordingly used largely for these purposes. The specific gravity of rain water is so nearly the same as that of distilled water, that it requires the most delicate instruments to ascertain the difference. Rain, that

falls in towns, acquires a small quantity of lime and calcareous matter from the mortar and plaster of the houses.

3. *Ice* and *snow water*. This equals rain water in purity, and, when fresh melted, contains no air, which is expelled during freezing. In cold climates and in high latitudes, thawed snow forms the constant drink of the inhabitants during winter; and the vast masses of ice which float on the polar seas afford an abundant supply to the mariner. It is well known, that in a weak brine, exposed to a moderate freezing cold, it is only the watery part that congeals, leaving the unfrozen liquor proportionably stronger of the salt. The same happens with a dilute solution of vegetable acids, with fermented liquors, and the like; and advantage is taken of this property to reduce the saline part to a more concentrated form. Snow water has long lain under the imputation of occasioning those strumous swellings in the neck which deform the inhabitants of many of the Alpine valleys; but this opinion is not supported by any well-authenticated, indisputable facts, and is rendered still more improbable, if not entirely overturned, by the frequency of the disease in Sumatra, where ice and snow are never seen, and its being quite unknown in Chili and in Thibet, though the rivers of these countries are chiefly supplied by the melting of the snow, with which the mountains are covered.

4. *Spring water.* Under this comprehensive class are included all waters that spring from some depth beneath the soil, and are used at the fountain head, or at least before they have run any considerable distance exposed to the air. It is obvious that spring water will be as various in its contents as the substances that compose the soil through which it flows. When the ingredients are not such as to give any peculiar medical or sensible properties, and the water is used for common purposes, it is distinguished as a hard or soft spring, sweet or brackish, clear or turbid, and the like. Ordinary springs insensibly pass into mineral springs, as their foreign contents become more notable and un common; though sometimes waters have acquired great medical reputation from mere purity.

By far the greater number of springs are cold; but as they take their origin at some depth from the surface, and below the influence of the external atmosphere, their temperature is, in general, pretty uniform during every vicissitude of season, and always several degrees higher than the freezing point. Others, again, arise constantly hot, or with a temperature always exceeding the summer heat; and the warmth possessed by the water is entirely independent of that of the atmosphere, and varies little, winter or summer.

One of the principal inconveniences in almost every spring water, is its hardness, owing to the presence of earthy salts, which, in by far the greater number of cases, are only the insipid substances, chalk, and selenite, which do not impair the taste of the water; while the air which it contains, and its grateful coolness, render it a most agreeable, and generally a perfectly innocent drink; though sometimes, in weak stomachs, it is apt to occasion an uneasy sense of weight in that organ, followed by a degree of dyspepsia. The quantity of earthy salts varies considerably; but, in general, it appears that the proportion of five grains of these in the pint will constitute a hard water, unfit for washing with soap, and for many other purposes of household use in manufactures. The water of deep wells is always, *ceteris paribus*, much harder than that of springs which overflow their channel; for much agitation and exposure to air produce a gradual deposition of the calcareous earth; and hence spring water often incrusts to a considerable thickness the inside of any kind of tube through which it flows, as it arises from the earth. The specific gravity of these waters is also, in general, greater than that of any other kind of water, that of the sea excepted. Springs that overflow their channel, and form to themselves a limited bed, pass insensibly into the state of stream or river water, and become thereby altered in some of their chemical properties.

5. *River water.*—This is in general much softer and more free from earthy salts than the last, but contains less air of any kind: for, by the agitation of a long current, and in most cases a great increase of temperature, it loses common air and carbonic acid, and, with this last, much of the lime which it held in solution. The specific gravity thereby becomes less, the taste not so harsh, but less fresh and agreeable, and out of a hard

spring is often made a stream of sufficient purity for most of the purposes where a soft water is required. Some streams, however, that arise from a clean silicious rock, and flow in a sandy or stony bed, are from the outset remarkably pure. Such are the mountain lakes and rivulets in the rocky districts of Wales, the source of the beautiful waters of the Dee, and numberless other rivers that flow through the hollow of every valley. Switzerland has long been celebrated for the purity and excellence of its waters, which pour in copious streams from the mountains, and give rise to some of the finest rivers in Europe. An excellent observer and naturalist, the illustrious Haller, thus speaks of the Swiss waters:—"Vulgaribus aquis Helvetia super omnes fere Europæ regiones excellit. Nusquam liquidas illas aquas et crystalli simillimas se mihi obtulisse memini postquam ex Helvetia excessi. Ex scopulis enim nostræ per puros silices percolatæ nulla terra vitiantur." Some of them never freeze in the severest winter, the cause of which is probably, as Haller conjectures, that they spring at once out of a subterraneous reservoir so deep as to be out of the reach of frost; and during their short course, when exposed to day, they have not time to be cooled down from 53°, their original temperature, to below the freezing point.

Some river waters, however, that do not take their rise from a rocky soil, and are indeed at first considerably charged with foreign matter, during a long course, even over a rich cultivated plain, become remarkably pure as to saline contents, but often fouled with mud, and vegetable or animal exuviæ, which are rather suspended than held in true solution. Such is that of the Thames, which, taken up at London at low water, is a very soft and good water, and, after rest and filtration, it holds but a very small portion of any thing that could prove noxious or impede any manufacture. It is also excellently fitted for sea-store; but it here undergoes a remarkable spontaneous change. No water carried to sea becomes putrid sooner than that of the Thames. When a cask is opened after being kept a month or two, a quantity of inflammable air escapes, and the water is so black and offensive as scarcely to be borne. Upon racking it off, however, into large earthen vessels (oil jars are commonly used for the purpose), and exposing it to the air, it gradually deposites a quantity of black slimy mud, becomes clear as crystal, and remarkably sweet and palatable. The Seine has as high a reputation in France, and appears from accurate experiments to be a river of great purity. It might be expected that a river which has passed by a large town, and received all its impurities, and been used by numerous dyers, tanners, hatters, and the like, that crowd to its banks for the convenience of plenty of water, should thereby acquire such a foulness as to be very perceptible to chemical examination for a considerable distance below the town; but it appears, from the most accurate examination, that where the stream is at all considerable, these kinds of impurity have but little influence in permanently altering the quality of the water, especially as they are for the most part only suspended, and not truly dissolved; and, therefore, mere rest, and especially filtration, will restore the water to its original purity. Probably, therefore, the most accurate chemist would find it difficult to distinguish water taken up at London from that procured at Hampton Court, after each has been purified by simple filtration.

6. *Stagnated waters.*—The waters that present the greatest impurities to the senses, are those of stagnant pools, and low marshy countries. They are filled with the remains of animal and vegetable matter undergoing decomposition, and, during that process, becoming in part soluble in water, thereby affording a rich nutriment to the succession of living plants and insects which is supplying the place of those that perish. From the want of sufficient agitation in these waters, vegetation goes on undisturbed, and the surface becomes covered with conferva and other aquatic plants; and as these standing waters are in general shallow, they receive the full influence of the sun, which further promotes all the changes that are going on within them. The taste is generally vapid, and destitute of that freshness and agreeable coolness which distinguish spring water. However, it should be remarked, that stagnant waters are generally soft, and many of the impurities are only suspended, and therefore separable by filtration; and perhaps the unpalatableness of this drink has caused it to be in worse credit than it de-

serves, on the score of salubrity. The decidedly noxious effects produced by the air of marshes and stagnant pools, have been often supposed to extend to the internal use of these waters; and often, especially in hot climates, a residence near these places has been as much condemned on the one account as on the other; and, in like manner, an improvement in health has been as much attributed to a change of water as of air.

WATER-BRASH. See *Pyrosis*.
Water-cress. See *Sisymbrium nasturtium*.
Water-dock. See *Rumex hydrolapathum*.
Water-flag, yellow. See *Iris pseudacorus*.
Water-germander. See *Teucrium scordium*.
Water-hemp. See *Eupatorium*.
Water-lily, white. See *Nymphæa alba*.
Water-lily, yellow. See *Nymphæa lutea*.
Water-parsnip. See *Sium nodiflorum*.
Water-pepper. See *Polygonum hydropiper*.
Water-zizania. See *Zizania aquatica*.
Waters, mineral. See *Mineral waters*.

WAVELITE. (So named after Dr. Wavell, who first discovered it at Barnstable, in Devonshire.) A mineral of a grayish-white colour, composed of alumina, 70; lime, 1.4; water, 26.2; as hard as fluor spar.

WAX. See *Cera*.

WEDEL, George Wolffgang, was born in 1645, at Golzan in Lusatia, and graduated at Jena in 1667; where, after a temporary exercise of his profession at Gotha, he became medical professor; in which station he continued with reputation for almost half a century. He combined with his skill in medicine a considerable acquaintance with mathematics and philology, as well as with the oriental and classical languages. He was an associate to the Academy Naturæ Curiosorum, and to the Royal Society of Berlin, physician to several German sovereigns, a count palatine, and an imperial counsellor. Notwithstanding these high offices and numerous engagements, he was attentive to the poor, and assiduous in his literary labours. He is celebrated for his pharmaceutical knowledge, and his elegance of prescription, so that many of his compositions have been adopted in dispensatories. Of his works, besides his academical dissertations, the principal are "Opiologia;" "Pharmacia in Artis formam redacta;" "De Medicamentorum Facultatibus;" "De Morbis Infantum;" and "Exercitationes Medico-Philologicæ."

WELD. Woald. The *Reseda luteola* of Linnæus, which is used as a yellow dye.

WEPFER, John James, was born in 1620, at Schaffhausen, and after visiting several universities in Italy, graduated at Basil, and settled in his native place. His reputation was extensive there and in Germany, and he attained, by his dissections and experiments, a high rank among those who have contributed to improve medical science. In 1658, he published a celebrated work, entitled "Observationes Anatomicæ," &c., since often reprinted with the title of "Historia Apoplecticorum." In an epistle "De Dubiis Anatomicis," he asserted the entire glandular structure of the liver, prior to Malpighi. Another valuable work is called "Cicutæ Aquaticæ Historia et Noxæ." His constitution was injured by attendance, at an advanced age, on the duke of Wurtemburg, and the imperial army under his command; and he was carried off by a dropsy in 1695. His papers were published by two of his grandsons, in a work entitled "Observationes Medico-Practicæ," &c. To the Ephemerides Naturæ Curiosorum he made several valuable communications, being a member of that society.

WERNERITE. Foliated scapolite.

WHARTON, Thomas, was born in Yorkshire in 1610, and educated at Cambridge. He afterward became a private tutor at Oxford: but on the commencement of the civil wars, he removed to London, and engaged in the practice of physic. On the surrender of Oxford to the parliament in 1646, he obtained a doctor's degree there, became a member of the College of Physicians in London, and got into considerable practice. In 1652, he read lectures on the glands before the College; and he afterward published a work on that subject, entitled "Adenographia." The descriptions cannot be relied upon, being chiefly taken from brutes; yet there are some useful observations on the diseases of those organs. His name has been affixed to the salivary ducts on the side of the tongue.

WHEAT. *Triticum.* The seeds of the *Triticum*

hibernum, and *æstivum*, of Linnæus, are so termed. It is to these plants, therefore, we are indebted for our bread, and the various kinds of pastry. Wheat is first ground between mill-stones, and then sifted to obtain its farina or flour. The flour of wheat may be separated into its three constituent parts, in the following manner. The flour is to be kneaded into a paste with water in an earthen vessel, and the water continue pouring upon it from a cock; this liquid, as it falls upon the paste, takes up from it a very fine white powder, by means of which it acquires the colour and consistency of milk. This process is to be continued till the water run off clear, when the flour will be separated into three distinct parts: 1. A gray elastic matter that sticks to the hand, and on account of its properties has gained the name of the glutinous, or vegeto-animal part. 2. A white powder which falls to the bottom of the water, and is the *fæculum* or starch. 3. A matter which remains dissolved in the water, and seems to be a sort of mucilaginous extract.

Flour, from whatever species of corn obtained, is likewise disposed to vinous fermentation, on account of its saccharine contents. The aptitude for fermentation of these mealy seeds increases if they be first converted into malt; insomuch as by this process, the gluten which forms the germ is separated, and the starchy part appears to be converted into saccharine matter. The making of malt, for which purpose barley and wheat are generally chosen, is as follows: The grains are put in the malting tub, and immersed in cold water, in a temperate and warm season, changing this fluid several times, especially in hot weather, and they are thus kept soaking till they be sufficiently soft to the touch. Upon this they are piled up in heaps on a roomy, clean, airy floor, where, by the heat spontaneously taking place, the vegetation begins, and the grains germinate. To cause the germination to go on uniformly, the heaps are frequently turned. In this state the vegetation is suffered to continue till the germs have about two-thirds or three-fourths of the length of the corn. It is carried too far when the leafy germs have begun to sprout.

For this reason, limits are set to the germination by drying the malt, which is effected by transferring it to the kiln, or by spreading it about in spacious airy lofts. Dried in the last way, it is called air-dried malt; in the first, kiln-malt. In drying this latter, care must be taken that it does not receive a burned smell, or be in part converted into coal.

From this malt, beer is made by extraction with water and fermentation.

With this view, a quantity of malt freed from its germs, and sufficient for one intended brewing, is coarsely bruised by grinding, and in the mash-tub first well mixed with some cold, then scalded with hot water, drawn upon it from the boiler. It is afterward strongly and uniformly stirred. When the whole mass has stood quietly for a certain time, the extract, (mash,) or sweetwort, is brought into the boiler, and the malt remaining in the tub is once more extracted by infusion with hot water.

This second extract, treated in like manner, is added to the first, and both are boiled together.

This clear decoction is now drawn off, and called boiled wort. To make the beer more fit for digestion, and at the same time to deprive it of its too great and unpleasant sweetness, the wort is mixed with a decoction of hops, or else these are boiled with it. After which it ought to be quickly cooled, to prevent its transition into acetous fermentation, which would ensue if it were kept too long in a high temperature.

On this account the wort is transferred into the cooler, where it is exposed with a large surface to cold air, and from this to the fermenting tub, that by addition of a sufficient portion of recent yest it may begin to ferment. When this fermentation has proceeded to a due degree, and the yest ceases to rise, the beer is conveyed into casks placed in cool cellars, where it finishes its fermentation, and where it is well kept and preserved, under the name of barrelled beer, with the precaution of filling up occasionally the vacancy caused in the vessels by evaporation; or the beer is bottled before it has done fermenting, and the bottles are stopped a little before the fermentation is completely over. By so doing the bottled beer is rendered sparkling. In this state it frequently bursts the bottles, by the disengagement of the carbonic acid gas which it

contains, and it strongly froths, like champaign, when brought into contact with air on being poured into another vessel.

Beer well prepared should be limpid and clear, possess a due quantity of spirit, and excite no disagreeable sweet taste, and contain no disengaged acid. By these properties it is a species of vinous beverage, and is distinguished from wine in the strict sense, and other liquors of that kind, by the much greater quantity of mucilaginous matter which it has received by extraction from the malted grains, but which also makes it more nourishing. Brown beer derives its colour from malt strongly roasted in the kiln, and its bitterish taste from the hops. Pale beer is brewed from malt dried in the air, or but slightly roasted, with but little or no hops at all. See *Beer*.

Wheat, buck. See *Polygonum fagopyrum*.

Wheat, eastern buck. See *Polygonum divaricatum*.

Wheat, Indian. See *Zea mays*.

WHEAT, TURKEY. The Turkey wheat is a native of America, where it is much cultivated, as it is also in some parts of Europe, especially in Italy and Germany. There are many varieties, which differ in the colour of the grain, and are frequently raised in our gardens by way of curiosity, whereby the plant is well known. It is the chief bread-corn in some of the southern parts of America, but since the introduction of rice into Carolina, it is but little used in the northern colonies. It makes a main part too of the food of the poor people in Italy and Germany. This is the sort of wheat mentioned in the book of Ruth, where it is said that Boaz treated Ruth with parched ears of corn dipped in vinegar. This method of eating the roasted ears of Turkey wheat is still practised in the East; they gather in the ears when about half ripe, and having scorched them to their minds, eat them with as much satisfaction as we do the best flour-bread.

In several parts of South America they parch the ripe corn, never making it into bread, but grinding it between two stones, mix it with water in a calabash, and so eat it. The Indians make a sort of drink from this grain, which they call *bici*. This liquor is very windy and intoxicating, and has nearly the taste of sour small beer: but they do not use it in common, being too lazy to make it often, and therefore it is chiefly kept for the celebration of feasts and weddings, at which times they mostly get intolerably drunk with it. The manner of making this precious beverage, is to steep a parcel of corn in a vessel of water, till it grows sour, then the old women being provided with calabashes for the purpose, chew some grains of the corn in their mouths, and spitting it into the calabashes, empty them, spittle and all, into the sour liquor, having previously drawn off the latter into another vessel.

The chewed grain soon raises a fermentation, and when this ceases, the liquor is let off from the dregs, and set by till wanted. In some of the islands in the South Sea, where each individual is his own lawgiver, it is no uncommon thing for a near relation to excuse a murderer for a good drunken bout of ciri.

[Turkey wheat is the Indian corn of America. It makes a rich, wholesome, and nutritious bread-corn, and may be cooked in a greater variety of ways than any other grain. Dr. Hooper is mistaken in supposing it is but little used in the northern parts of the United States (formerly colonies). There is not a farm or plantation in any part of the country without a portion planted in Indian corn. A portion of Indian meal mixed with wheat or rye flour, improves the bread made in that way. A.]

WHET-SLATE. A greenish gray-coloured mineral, used to sharpen steel instruments.

WHEY. The fluid part of milk which remains after the curd has been separated. It contains a saccharine matter, some butter, and a small portion of cheese.

WHISKEY. A dilute alkohol obtained by distilling malt.

[Whiskey is obtained in this country from rye, Indian corn, potatoes, &c. It is a spirit which, when concentrated by repeated distillation, produces alkohol, and may be obtained from various fruits, roots, seeds, &c. See *Fruits, affording spirit*. A.]

WHISPERING. A lowness of speech, caused by uttering the words so feebly, as not to produce any vibration of the larynx.

White-swelling. See *Arthropuosis*, and *Hydarthrus*

WHITES. See *Leucorrhœa.*
WHITING. See *Gadus.*
Whortleberry, bears'. See *Arbutus uva ursi.*
Whortleberry, red. See *Vaccinium vitis idæa.*

WHYTT, ROBERT, was born in 1714, at Edinburgh, where he studied physic, and after visiting the medical schools at London, Paris, and Leyden, settled in the exercise of his profession, became a fellow, then president of the college, and chairman of the Institutions of Medicine in that university. As a medical practitioner and teacher, and also as a writer, he acquired deserved celebrity. The first of his publications was an "Essay on the Vital and other involuntary Motions of Animals," 1751, in which he opposed the Stahlian Theory, and ascribed them to the operation of stimuli. Four years after, his "Physiological Essays" appeared, in which he supposes the circulation assisted by an oscillatory motion of the minute vessels, and treats of sensibility and irritability. He also wrote on the Use of Lime-water in Calculous Complaints; and on Nervous Diseases; and contributed likewise some papers to the Edinburgh Essays. The Observations on Hydrocephalus, were published after his death, which occurred in 1766, after labouring long under a complication of chronic complaints.

WIDOW-WAIL. See *Daphne mezereum.*
Wild carrot. See *Daucus sylvestris.*
Wild cucumber. See *Momordica elaterium.*
[*Wild hoarhound.* See *Eupatorium teucrium.*
Wild lettuce. See *Lactuca virosa.* A.]
Wild navew. See *Brassica napus.*

WILLIS, THOMAS, was born in Wiltshire, about the year 1621, and entered at Oxford, with a view to the clerical profession; but he afterward changed to physic, took his bachelor's degree in 1646, and commenced practice at the university. He distinguished himself by his steady attachment to the church of England, and also by his love of science, so that he became one of the first members of that philosophical society at Oxford, which laid the foundation of the Royal Society of London. He was ambitious of excelling as a chemist, and published, in 1659, a treatise on Fermentation, and another on Fever, with a Dissertation on the Urine. After the Restoration he was appointed to the Sedleian professorship of Natural Philosophy, and received his doctor's degree. In 1664, he published his celebrated work "Cerebri Anatome," with a description of the nerves; which was followed, after three years, by his "Pathologia Cerebri et Nervosi Generis," in which he treats of Convulsive Diseases, and the Scurvy. In the mean time he had settled in London, and being nominated a physician in ordinary to the king, was advancing to the first rank in practice. His next publication was on Hysteria and Hypochondriasis. In 1672, he produced another work, "De Anima Brutorum;" which he supposed like the vital principle in man of a corporeal nature. The year following he began to print his "Pharmaceutice Rationalis," which he did not live to complete, being carried off by a pleurisy in his fifty-fourth year. His works engaged great attention at first, and are still admired, though modern improvements have diminished their value. They are written in an elegant Latin style.

WILLOW. See *Salix.*
Willow, crack. See *Salix fragilis.*
Willow, sweet. See *Myrica gale.*
Willow, white. See *Salix fragilis.*
Willow-herb. See *Lythrum salicaria.*
Willow-herb, rosebay. See *Epilobium angustifolium.*
Willow-leaved oak. See *Quercus phellos.*

WINE. *Vinum.* "Chemists give the name of wine in general to all liquors that have become spirituous by fermentation. Thus cider, beer, hydromel or mead, and other similar liquors, are wines.

The principles and theory of the fermentation which produces these liquors are essentially the same.

All those nutritive, vegetable, and animal matters which contain sugar ready formed, are susceptible of the spirituous fermentation. Thus wine may be made of all the juices of plants, the sap of trees, the infusions and decoctions of farinaceous vegetables, the milk of frugiverous animals; and, lastly, it may be made of all ripe succulent fruits; but all these substances are not equally proper to be changed into a good and generous wine.

As the production of alkohol is the result of the spi-

rituous fermentation, that wine may be considered as essentially the best, which contains most alkohol. But of all substances susceptible of the spirituous fermentation, none is capable of being converted into so good wine, as the juice of the grapes of France, or of other countries that are nearly in the same latitude, or in the same temperature. The grapes of hotter countries, and even those of the southern provinces of France, do indeed furnish wines that have a more agreeable, that is, more of a saccharine taste; but these wines, though they are sufficiently strong, are not so spirituous as those of the provinces near the middle of France: at least from these latter wines the best vinegar and brandy are made. As an example, therefore, of spirituous fermentation in general, we shall describe the method of making wine from the juice of the grapes of France.

This juice, when newly expressed, and before it has begun to ferment, is called *must*, and in common language sweet wine. It is turbid, has an agreeable and very saccharine taste. It is very laxative; and when drunk too freely, or by persons disposed to diarrhœas, it is apt to occasion these disorders. Its consistence is somewhat less fluid than that of water, and it becomes almost of a pitchy thickness when dried.

When the must is pressed from the grapes, and but into a proper vessel and place, with a temperature between fifty-five and sixty degrees, very sensible effects are produced in it, in a shorter or longer time according to the nature of the liquor, and the exposure of the place. It then swells, and is so rarefied, that it frequently overflows the vessel containing it, if this be nearly full. An intestine motion is excited among its parts, accompanied with a small hissing noise and evident ebullition. The bubbles rise to the surface, and at the same time is disengaged a quantity of carbonic acid of such purity, and so subtle and dangerous, that it is capable of killing instantly men and animals exposed to it in a place where the air is not renewed. The skins, stones, and other grosser matters of the grapes, are buoyed up by the particles of disengaged air that adhere to their surface, are variously agitated, and are raised in form of a scum, or soft and spongy crust, that covers the whole liquor. During the fermentation, this crust is frequently raised, and broken by the air disengaged from the liquor which forces its way through it; afterward the crust subsides, and becomes entire as before.

These effects continue while the fermentation is brisk, and at last gradually cease: then the crust, being no longer supported, falls in pieces to the bottom of the liquor. At this time, if we would have a strong and generous wine, all sensible fermentation must be stopped. This is done by putting the wine into close vessels, and carrying these into a cellar or other cool place.

After this first operation, an interval of repose takes place, as is indicated by the cessation of the sensible effects of the spirituous fermentation; and thus enables us to preserve a liquor no less agreeable in its taste, than useful for its reviving and nutritive qualities, when drunk moderately.

If we examine the wine produced by this first fermentation, we shall find, that it differs entirely and essentially from the juice of grapes before fermentation. Its sweet and saccharine taste is changed into one that is very different, though still agreeable, and somewhat spirituous and piquant. It has not the laxative quality of must, but affects the head, and occasions, as is well known, drunkenness. Lastly, if it be distilled, it yields, instead of the insipid water obtained from must by distillation with the heat of boiling water, a volatile, spirituous, and inflammable liquor, called spirit of wine, or alkohol. This spirit is consequently a new being, produced by the kind of fermentation, called the vinous or spirituous.

When any liquor undergoes the spirituous fermentation, all its parts seem not to ferment at the same time, otherwise the fermentation would probably be very quickly completed, and the appearances would be much more striking: hence, in a liquor much disposed to fermentation, this motion is more quick and simultaneous than in another liquor less disposed. Experience has shown, that a wine, the fermentation of which is very slow and tedious, is never good or very spirituous; and therefore, when the weather is too cold, the fermentation is usually accelerated by heating the place in which) the wine is made. A proposal has been made by a person very intelligent in economical affairs, to apply a greater than the usual heat to accelerate the fermentation of the wine, in those years in which grapes have not been sufficiently ripened, and when the juice is not sufficiently disposed to fermentation.

A too hasty and violent fermentation is perhaps also hurtful, from the dissipation and loss of some of the spirit; but of this we are not certain. However, we may distinguish, in the ordinary method of making wines of grapes, two periods in the fermentation, the first of which lasts during the appearance of the sensible effects above mentioned, in which the greatest number of fermentable particles ferment. After this first effort of fermentation, these effects sensibly diminish, and ought to be stopped, for reasons hereafter to be mentioned. The fermentative motion of the liquors then ceases. The heterogeneous parts that were suspended in the wines by this motion, and render it muddy, are separated and form a sediment, called the lees; after which the wine becomes clear; but though the operation is then considered as finished, and the fermentation apparently ceases, it does not really cease; and it ought to be continued in some degree, if we would have good wine.

In this new wine a part of the liquor probably remains that has not fermented, and which afterward ferments, but so very slowly, that none of the sensible effects produced in the first fermentation are here perceived. The fermentation, therefore, still continues in the wine, during a longer or shorter time, although in an imperceptible manner; and this is the second period of the spirituous fermentation, which may be called the imperceptible fermentation. We may easily perceive that the effect of this imperceptible fermentation is the gradual increase of the quantity of alkohol. It has also another effect no less advantageous, namely, the separation of the acid salt called tartar from the wine. This matter is, therefore, a second sediment, that is formed in the wine, and adheres to the sides of the containing vessels. As the taste of tartar is harsh and disagreeable, it is evident that the wine, which by means of the insensible fermentation has acquired more alkohol, and has disengaged itself of the greater part of its tartar, ought to be much better and more agreeable; and for this reason chiefly old wine is universally preferable to new wine.

But insensible fermentation can only ripen and meliorate the wine, if the sensible fermentation have regularly proceeded, and been stopped in due time. We know certainly that if a sufficient time have not been allowed for the first period of the fermentation, the unfermented matter that remains, being in too large a quantity, will then ferment in the bottles, or close vessels, in which the wine is put, and will occasion effects in so much more sensible, as the first fermentation shall have been sooner interrupted : hence these wines are always turbid, emit bubbles, and sometimes break the bottles from the large quantity of air disengaged during the fermentation.

We have an instance of these effects in the wine of Champaign, and in others of the same kind. The sensible fermentation of these wines is interrupted, or rather suppressed, that they may have this sparkling quality. It is well known that these wines make the corks fly out of the bottles; that they sparkle and froth when they are poured into glasses; and lastly, that they have a taste much more lively and more piquant than wines that do not sparkle; but this sparkling quality, and all the effects depending on it, are only caused by a considerable quantity of carbonic acid gas, which is disengaged during the confined fermentation that the wine has undergone in close vessels. This air, not having an opportunity of escaping, and of being dissipated as fast as it is disengaged, and being interposed between all the parts of the wine, combines in some measure with them, and adheres in the same manner as it does to certain mineral waters, in which it produces nearly the same effects. When this air is entirely disengaged from these wines, they no longer sparkle, they lose their piquancy of taste, become mild, and even almost insipid.

Such are the qualities that wine acquires in time, when its first fermentation has not continued sufficiently long. These qualities are given purposely to certain kinds of wine, to indulge taste or caprice; but such wines are supposed to be unfit for daily use.

Wines for daily use ought to have undergone so completely the sensible fermentation, that the succeeding fermentation shall be insensible, or at least exceedingly little perceived. Wine, in which the first fermentation has been too far advanced, is liable to worse inconveniences than that in which the first fermentation has been too quickly suppressed; for every insensible liquor is, from its nature, in a continual intestine motion, more or less strong according to circumstances from the first instant of the spirituous fermentation, till it is completely purified: hence, from the time of the completion of the spirituous fermentation, or even before, the wine begins to undergo the acid or acetous fermentation. This acid fermentation is very slow and insensible, when the wine is included in very close vessels, and in a cool place; but it gradually advances, so that in a certain time the wine, instead of being improved, becomes at last sour. This evil cannot be remedied; because the fermentation may advance, but cannot be reverted.

Wine-merchants, therefore, when their wines become sour, can only conceal or absorb this acidity by certain substances, as by alkalies and absorbent earths. But these substances give to wine a dark-greenish colour, and a taste which, though not acid, is somewhat disagreeable. Besides, calcareous earths accelerate considerably the total destruction and putrefaction of the wine. Oxides of lead, having the property of forming with the acid of vinegar a salt of an agreeable saccharine taste, which does not alter the colour of the wine, and which besides has the advantage of stopping fermentation and putrefaction, might be very well employed to remedy the acidity of wine, if lead and all its preparations were not pernicious to health, as they occasion most terrible colics, and even death, when taken internally. We cannot believe that any wine-merchant, knowing the evil consequences of lead, should, for the sake of gain, employ it for the purpose mentioned ; but if there be any such persons, they must be considered as the poisoners and murderers of the public. At Alicant, where very sweet wines are made, it is the practice to mix a little lime with the grapes before they are pressed. This, however, can only neutralize the acid already existing in the grape.

If wine contain litharge, or any other oxide of lead, it may be discovered by evaporating some pints of it to dryness, and melting the residuum in a crucible, at the bottom of which a small button of lead may be found after the fusion: but an easier and more expeditious proof is by pouring into the wine some liquid sulphuret. If the precipitate occasioned by this addition of the sulphuret be white, or only coloured by the wine, we may know that no lead is contained in it; but if the precipitate be dark coloured, brown, or blackish, we may conclude, that it contains lead or iron.

The only substances that cannot absorb or destroy, but cover and render supportable the sharpness of wine, without any inconvenience, are, sugar, honey, and other saccharine alimentary matters; but they can succeed only when the wine is very little acid, and when an exceeding small quantity only of these substances is sufficient to produce the desired effect ; otherwise the wine would have a sweetish, tart, and not agreeable taste.

From what is here said concerning the acescency of wine, we may conclude that when this accident happens, it cannot by any good method be remedied and that nothing remains to be done with sour wine but to sell it to vinegar-makers, as all honest wine-merchants do.

As the *must* of the grape contains a greater proportion of tartar than our currant or gooseberry juices do, Dr. Ure has been accustomed, for many years, to recommend, in his lectures, the addition of a small portion of that salt to our *must*, to make it ferment into a more genuine wine. Dr. M'Culloch has lately prescribed the same addition in his popular treatise on the art of making wine.

The following is Brande's valuable table of the quantity of spirit in different kinds of wine :—

		Proportion of spirit per cent. by measure.
1. Lissa		26.47
Ditto		24.35
	Average	25.41
2. Raisin wine		26.40
Ditto		25.77

Raisin wine	23.20
Average	25.12
3. Marsala	26.30
Ditto	25.05
Average	25.09
4. Madeira	24.42
Ditto	23.93
Ditto (Sircial)	21.40
Ditto	19.24
Average	22.27
5. Currant wine	20.55
6. Sherry	19.81
Ditto	19.83
Ditto	18.79
Ditto	18.25
Average	19.17
7. Teneriffe	19.79
8. Colares	19.75
9. Lachryma Christi	19.70
10. Constantia, white	19.75
11. Ditto, red	18.92
12. Lisbon	18.94
13. Malaga (1666)	18.94
14. Bucellas	18.49
15. Red Madeira	22.30
Ditto	18.40
Average	20.35
16. Cape Muschat	18.25
17. Cape Madeira	22.94
Ditto	20.50
Ditto	18.11
Average	20.51
18. Grape wine	18.11
19. Calcavella	19.20
Ditto	18.10
Average	18.65
20. Vidonia	19.25
21. Alba Flora	17.26
22. Malaga	17.26
23. White Hermitage	17.43
24. Rousillon	19.00
Ditto	17.26
Average	18.13
25. Claret	17.11
Ditto	16.32
Ditto	14.08
Ditto	12.91
Average	15.10
26. Malmsey Madeira	16.40
27. Lunel	15.52
28. Sheraaz	15.52
29. Syracuse	15.28
30. Sauterne	14.22
31. Burgundy	16.60
Ditto	15.22
Ditto	14.53
Ditto	11.95
Average	14.57
32. Hock	14.37
Ditto	13.00
Ditto (old in cask)	8.88
Average	12.08
33. Nice	14.63
34. Barsac	13.86
35. Tent	13.30
36. Champaign (still)	13.80
Ditto (sparkling)	12.80
Ditto (red)	12.56
Ditto (ditto)	11.30
Average	12.61
37. Red Hermitage	12.32
38. Vin de Grave	13.94
Ditto	12.80
Average	13.37
39. Frontignac	12.79
40. Cote Rotie	12.32
41. Gooseberry wine	11.84
42. Orange wine—average of six samples made by a London manufacturer	11.26
43. Tokay	9.88
44. Elder wine	9.87
45. Cider, highest average	9.87
Ditto, lowest ditto	5.21
46. Perry, average of four samples	7.26
47. Mead	7.32
48. Ale (Burton)	8.88

Ditto (Edinburgh)	6.20
Ditto (Dorchester)	5.56
Average	6.87
49. Brown Stout	6.80
50. London Porter (average)	4.20
51. Ditto small beer (ditto)	1.28
52. Brandy	53.39
53. Rum	53.68
54. Gin	51.60
55. Scotch whiskey	54.32
56. Irish ditto	53.90

The wines principally used in medicine are, the *vinum album hispanicum*, or sherry, *vinum canarium* canary or sack wine, the *vinum rhenanum*, or Rhenish wine, and the *vinum rubrum*, or port wine. These differ from each other in the proportion of their con stituent principles, and particularly in that of alkohol, which they contain. The qualities of wines depend not only upon the difference of the grapes, as containing more or less of saccharine juice and the acid matter which accompanies it, but also upon circumstances attending the process of fermentation. New wines are liable to a strong degree of acescency when taken into the stomach, and thereby occasion much flatulency and eructations of acid matter; heartburn and violent pains in the stomach from spasms are also often produced; and the acid matter, by passing into the intestines and mixing with the bile, is apt to occasion colics or excite diarrhœas. Sweet wines are likewise more disposed to become acescent in the stomach than others; but as the quantity of alkohol which they contain is more considerable than appears sensibly to the taste, their acescency is thereby in a great measure counteracted. Red port, and most of the red wines, have an astringent quality, by which they strengthen the stomach, and prove useful in restraining immoderate evacuations; on the contrary, those which are of an acid nature, as Rhenish, pass freely by the kidneys, and gently loosen the belly. But this, and perhaps all the thin or weak wines, though of an agreeable flavour, yet as containing little alkohol, are readily disposed to become acid in the stomach, and thereby to aggravate all arthritic and calculous complaints, as well as to produce the effects of new wine. The general effects of wine are, to stimulate the stomach, exhilarate the spirits, warm the habit, quicken the circulation, promote perspiration, and, in large quantities, to prove intoxicating, and powerfully sedative. In many disorders, wine is universally admitted to be of important service, and especially in fevers of the typhus kind, or of a putrid tendency; in which it is found to raise the pulse, support the strength, promote a diaphoresis, and to resist putrefaction; and in many cases it proves of more immediate advantage than the Peruvian bark. Delirium, which is the consequence of excessive irritability, and a defective state of nervous energy, is often entirely removed by the free use of wine. It is also a well-founded observation, that those who indulge in the use of wine are less subject to fevers of the ma lignant and intermittent kind. In the putrid sore throat, in the small-pox, when attended with great debility and symptoms of putridity, in gangrenes, and in the plague, wine is to be considered as a principal remedy; and in almost all cases of languor, and of great prostration of strength, wine is experienced to be a more grateful and efficacious cordial than can be furnished from the whole class of aromatics.

WING. See *Ala*.

WINSLOW, James Benignus, was born in 1669, in the isle of Funen, and having studied a year under Borrichius, was sent with a pension from the king of Denmark, to seek improvement in the principal universities of Europe. In 1698, he became a pupil of the celebrated Duverney, at Paris, where he was induced to abjure the Protestant religion; and the patronage of Bossuet, who converted him, procured for him the degree of doctor in 1705. He afterward read lectures of anatomy and surgery at the Royal Gardens; and in 1743 was promoted to the professorship in that institution. In the mean time, he communicated several papers on anatomical and physiological subjects to the Academy of Sciences, by whom, as well as by the Royal Society of Berlin, he was admitted an associate His great work, mentioned by Haller as superseding all former compositions of anatomy, and entitled " Exposition Anatomique de la Structure du Corps Humain," first appeared at Paris in 1732, 4to. It was frequently reprinted, and translated into various languages; and is still regarded as of standard authority. It was intended as a plan of a larger work, which, however, he did not finish. He reached the advanced age of ninety-one.

Winter-bark. See *Winteranus cortex.*

Winter-cherry. See *Physalis alkekengi.*

WINTE'RA. (Named after Captain Winter, who brought the bark from the straits of Magellan in 1579, and introduced it to the knowledge of physicians as useful in scurvy, &c.)

WINTERA AROMATICA. The systematic name of the winter-bark tree. The bark is called *Cortex winteranus; Cortex magellanicus; Cortex canellæ albæ;* and the tree, *Winteranus spurius; Canella cubana; Winterania canella,* and *Winteria aromatica—pedunculis aggregatis terminalibus, pistalis quatuor,* of Linnæus. It is a native of the West Indies. The bark is brought into Europe in long quills, somewhat thicker than cinnamon. Their taste is moderately warm, aromatic, and bitterish, and of an agreeable smell somewhat resembling that of cloves. Canella alba has been supposed to possess considerable medicinal powers in the cure of scurvy and some other complaints. It is now merely considered as a useful and cheap aromatic, and is chiefly employed for the purpose of correcting and rendering less disagreeable the more powerful and nauseous drugs; with which view it is used in the *tinctura amara, vinum amarum, vinum rhœi,* &c. of the Edinburgh Pharmacopœia.

WINTERANUS CORTEX. See *Wintera aromatica.*

WINTERA'NUS SPURIUS. See *Canella alba.*

[WINTER GREEN See *Pyrola umbellata.* A.]

WISEMAN, RICHARD, was first known as a surgeon in the civil wars of Charles I., and accompanied Prince Charles, when a fugitive, in France, Holland, and Flanders. He served for three years in the Spanish navy, and, returning with the prince to Scotland, was made prisoner in the battle of Worcester. After his liberation in 1652, he settled in London. When Charles II. was restored, he became eminent in his profession, and was made one of the sergeant-surgeons to the king. In 1676, he appears, from the preface to his works, to have been a sufferer by ill health for twenty years: but the time of his death is not known. The result of his experience was given in "Several Surgical Treatises on Tumours, Ulcers, Diseases of the Anus, Scrofula, Wounds, Gunshot Wounds, Fractures and Luxations, and Syphilis." He seems to have given a faithful account of more than six hundred cases, recording his failures as well as his cures. He advocated the efficacy of the royal touch in scrofula, though the fallacy is evident even from his own narration. His writings have long been regarded as standard authority.

WITHERING, WILLIAM, was born in 1741, and finished his medical education at Edinburgh, where he took his degree at twenty-five. From Stafford, where he first settled and married, he removed to Birmingham, and speedily obtained a very extensive practice by his skill and assiduity, without neglecting his scientific pursuits, which were chiefly in botany and chemistry. He was author of several valuable publications: "A Botanical Arrangement of British Plants," which appeared at first in 1776, in two volumes, 8vo., but progressively increased to four; a translation of Bergman's "Sciagraphia Regni Mineralis;" and some chemical and mineralogical papers contributed to the Royal Society, of which he was a fellow. "Account of the Scarlet Fever, &c.;" "Account of the Foxglove," with Practical Remarks on the Dropsy and other Diseases, published in 1785. His lungs being weak, he found it necessary, in the winter of 1793, to go to Lisbon, and afterward to relax from his professional exertions. His death occurred in 1799.

WITHERITE. See *Heavy-spar.*

WOAD. See *Isatis tinctoria.*

WOLFRAM. An ore of tungsten.

WOLF'S-BANE. See *Aconitum napellus.*

WOMB. See *Uterus.*

Womb, inflammation of. See *Hysteritis.*

Wood-louse. See *Oniscus asellus.*

Wood-sorrel. See *Oxalis acetosella.*

Wood-stone. See *Hornstone.*

WOODVILLE, WILLIAM, was born at Cockermouth in 1752. After serving a short apprenticeship to an apothecary he graduated at Edinburgh in 1775.

Then passing some time on the Continent, he settled near his native place, and practised there for five or six years. He next came to London, and was soon appointed a physician to the Middlesex Dispensary. In 1790, he published the first part, which was afterward completed in four quarto volumes, of a highly valuable work, entitled "Medical Botany." The following year he was elected physician to the Small-pox Hospital; and in executing the duties of that office he displayed the highest zeal. He gave a manifest proof of his attention to the subject, by publishing in 1796 the first part of a "History of the Small-pox in Great Britain, &c.;" but the discovery of vaccination superseded the necessity of completing that work. Dr. Woodville was duly impressed with the importance of what had been announced by Dr. Jenner; but feeling a proper degree of skepticism at first, he was anxious to investigate the practice fully, before he gave it his sanction. Unfortunately he was led into an error at the outset, by not keeping in recollection, that the atmosphere of the hospital was loaded with variolous contagion, whence some unpleasant results appeared; but this being suggested to him, he was induced, on more mature consideration, strenuously to advocate the practice of vaccination; and by the excellent opportunities he enjoyed, he contributed very materially to its rapid success. He died in 1805.

WOODWARD, JOHN, was born in Derbyshire in 1664, and put apprentice to some trade in London; but evincing an ardour for science, Dr. Barwick took him into his family, and for four years instructed him in medicine and anatomy; after which he procured him the medical professorship at Gresham College He published about this time an essay towards a Natural History of the Earth, which, though executed without sufficient preparation, procured his election into the Royal Society. In 1695, he was created M.D. by Archbishop Tenison, and the year after obtained the same degree from Cambridge; whence he was admitted into the College of Physicians as a fellow, in 1702. He however pursued his inquiries into natural history and antiquities for some time with great zeal. In 1718, he published a work entitled "The State of Physic and of Diseases," containing some fanciful theories, which were ably confuted by Dr. Freind, both ludicrously and seriously. He died at Gresham College in 1727, bequeathing his personal property to the University of Cambridge, for the endowment of an annual lectureship, on some subject taken from his own writings. Soon after his death, a catalogue of his fossils was published in 1737, his "Select Cases and Consultations in Physic," containing some valuable observations. He supposed the vital principle to reside not in the nerves, but in the blood, and other parts of the body; and he made many experiments to establish the vis insita of muscles.

Woody nightshade. See *Solanum dulcamara.*

WORL. See *Verticillus.*

WORM. *Vermis.* There are several kinds of animals which infest the human body. Their usual division is into those which inhabit only the intestinal canal, as the ascarides, &c.; and those which are found in other parts, as hydatids, &c. Such is the nature and office of the human stomach and intestines, that insects and worms, or their ovula, may not unfrequently be conveyed into that canal with those things that are continually taken as food; but such insects, or worms, do not live long, and seldom, if ever, generate in a situation so different from their natural one. Besides these, there are worms that are never found in any other situation than the human stomach or intestines, and which there generate and produce their species. Thus it appears that the human stomach and intestines are the seat for animalcula, which are translated from their natural situation, and also for worms proper to them, which live in no other situation.

First Class. This contains those which are generated and nourished in the human intestinal canal, and which there propagate their species.

Second Class, comprehends those insects or worms that accidentally enter the human primæ viæ ab extra, and which never propagate their species in that canal, but are soon eliminated from the body. Such are several species of *Scarabæi,* the *Lumbricus terrestris* the *Fasciola,* the *Gordius intestinalis,* and others The second class belongs to the province of natural history. The consideration of the first class belongs to the physician, which, from the variety it affords, may be divided into different orders, genera, and species.

Order I. Round worms.
Genus I. Intestinal ascarides.
Character. Body round, head obtuse, and furnished with three vesicles.
Species 1. *Ascaris lumbricoides.* The long round worm, or lumbricoid ascaris.
Character. When full grown, a foot in length. Mouth triangular.
2. *Ascaris vermicularis.* The thread or maw-worm.
Character. When full grown, half an inch in length. Tail terminates in a fine point.
Genus II. Intestinal trichurides.
Character. Body round, tail three times the length of the body, head without vesicles.
Species. *Trichuris vulgaris.* The trichuris, or long thread-worm.
Character. The head furnished with a proboscis.
Order II. The flat worms.
Genus I. Intestinal tape-worm.
Character. Body flat and jointed.
Species 1. *Tænia osculis marginalibus.* The long tape-worm.
Character. The oscula are situated upon the margin of the joints.
2. *Tænia osculis superficialibus.* The broad tape-worm.
Character. The oscula are placed upon the flattened surface.

These worms were all known to the ancients, the trichuris only excepted, and are mentioned in the works of Hippocrates, Galen, Celsus, Paulus Ægineta, and Pliny.

When worms are generated in the intestines, they often produce the following symptoms, viz. variable appetite, fœtid breath, acrid eructations and pains in the stomach, grinding of the teeth during sleep, picking of the nose, paleness of the countenance; sometimes dizziness, hardness and fulness of the belly; slimy stools, with occasional griping pains, more particularly about the navel, heat and itching about the anus; short dry cough; emaciation of the body; slow fever, with evening exacerbations and irregular pulse, and sometimes convulsive fits.

Worm-bark. See *Geoffræa jamaicensis.*
Worm-grass, perennial. See *Spigelia.*
Worm, Guinea. See *Dracunculus.*
Worm, ring. See *Herpes.*
WORMSEED. See *Artemisia santonica.*
WORMWOOD. See *Artemisia absinthium.*
Wormwood, common. See *Artemisia absinthium.*
Wormwood, mountain. See *Artemisia glacialis.* —

Wormwood, Roman. See *Artemisia absinthium.*
Wormwood, sea. See *Artemisia maritima.*
Wormwood, Tartarian. See *Artemisia santonica.*
WORT. An infusion of malt. This has been found useful in the cure of the scurvy. Dr. Macbride, in his very ingenious experimental essays, having laid down as a principle, "that the cure of the scurvy depends on the fermentative quality in the remedies made use of," was led to inquire after a substance capable of being preserved during a long sea-voyage, and yet containing materials by which a fermentation might occasionally be excited in the bowels. Such a one appeared to him to be found in malt, which is well known to be the grain of barley, brought suddenly to a germinating state by heat and moisture, and then dried, whereby its saccharine principle is developed, and rendered easy of extraction by watery liquors. The sweet infusion of this he proposed to give as a dietic article to scorbutic persons, expecting that it would ferment in their bowels, and give out its fixed air, by the antiseptic powers of which the strong tendency to putrefaction in this disease might be corrected.

It was some time before a fair trial of this purposed remedy could be obtained; and different reports were made concerning it. By some cases, however, published in a postscript of the second edition of the doctor's work in 1767, it appears that scorbutic complaints of the most dangerous kind have actually been cured at sea by the use of wort. Its general effects were to keep the patient's bowels open, and to prove highly nutritious and strengthening. It sometimes purged too much, but this effect was easily obviated by the tinctura thebaica. Other unquestionable cases of its success in this disease are to be seen in the London Medical Essays and Inquiries.

The use of wort has hence been adopted in other cases where a strong and putrid disposition in the fluids appeared to prevail, as in cancerous and phagedenic ulcers; and instances are published, in the fourth volume of the work above mentioned, of its remarkable good effects in these cases.

As the efficacy of the malt infusion depends upon its producing changes in the whole mass of fluids, it is obvious that it must be taken in large quantities for a considerable length of time, and rather as an article of diet than medicine. From one to four pints daily have generally been directed. The proportion recommended in preparing it, is one measure of ground malt to three equal measures of boiling water. The mixture must be well stirred, and left to stand, covered, three or four hours. It should be made fresh every day.
WOUNDWORT. See *Laserpitium chironium*
WRAPPER. See *Valva*
WRIST. See *Carpus.*

X

XALA'PPA. (From the province of Xalappa, in New Spain, whence it comes.) Jalap.

XA'NTHIUM. (From ξανθος, yellow: so named because it is said to make the hair yellow.) The name of a genus of plants in the Linnæan system. Class, *Monœcia*; Order, *Pentandria.* The less burdock.

XANTHIUM STRUMARIUM. The systematic name of the less burdock. This herb of Linnæus was once esteemed in the cure of scrofula, but, like most other remedies against this disease, proves ineffectual. The seeds are administered internally in some countries against erysipelas.

[*Xanthoxylum fraxineum.* See *Prickly-ash.* A.]
XERA'SIA. (From ξηρος, dry.) An excessive tenuity, or softness of the hairs, similar to down.

XEROCOLLY'RIUM. (From ξηρος, dry, and κολλυριον a collyrium.) A dry collyrium.

XEROMY'RUM. (From ξηρος, dry, and μυρον, an ointment.) A dry ointment.

XEROPHTHA'LMIA. (Ξηρος, dry, and οφθαλμια, an inflammation of the eye.) A dry inflammation of the eye without discharge.

XI'PHIUM. (From ξιφος, a sword: so named from the sword-like shape of its leaves.) Spurgewort.

XIPHOID. (*Xiphoides;* from ξιφος, a sword, and ειδος, likeness.) A term given by anatomists to par's which had some resemblance to an ancient sword, as the xiphoid cartilage.

Xiphoid cartilage. See *Cartilago ensiformis*
XYLOA'LOES. See *Lignum aloes.*
XYLOBA'LSAMUM. See *Amyris gileadensis.*

Y

YAM. See *Dioscorea.*

YANOLITE. See *Axinite.*

YARROW. See *Achillea millefolium.*

YAWS. 1. The African name for raspberry.

2. The name of a disease which resembles a raspberry. See *Frambæsia.*

Yayama. The Brazilian name of the pine-apple.

YELLOW EARTH. An ochre yellow-coloured mineral, found in Upper Lusatia.

Yellow fever. See *Febris continua.*

Yellow saunders. See *Santalum album.*

YENITE. See *Lievrite.*

YEST. See *Fermentum.*

Yoked leaf. See *Conjugatus.*

YOLK. See *Vitellus.*

Yorkshire sanicle. See *Pinguicula.*

YPSILOGLO'SSUS, (From υψιλοειδες, the ypsiloid bone, and γλωσσα, the tongue.) A muscle originating in the os hyoides, and terminating in the tongue.

YPSILOI'DES. (From υ, the Greek letter, called ypsilon, and ειδος, a likeness.) The os hyoides: so named from its likeness to the Greek letter ypsilon.

YTTRIA. This is a new earth discovered in 1794, by Professor Gadolin, in a stone from Ytterby, in Sweden.

It may be obtained most readily by fusing the gadolinite with two parts of caustic potassa, washing the mass with boiling water, and filtering the liquor, which is of a fine green. This liquor is to be evaporated, til no more oxide of manganese falls down from it in a black powder; after which the liquid is to be saturated with nitric acid. At the same time digest the sediment that was not dissolved, in very dilute nitric acid, which will dissolve the earth with much heat, leaving the silex, and the highly oxided iron, undissolved. Mix the two liquors, evaporate them to dryness, redissolve and filter, which will separate any silex or oxide of iron that may have been left. A few drops of a solution of carbonate of potassa will separate any lime that may be present, and a cautious addition of hydrosulphuret of potassa will throw down the oxide of manganese that may have been left; but if too much be employed, it will throw down the yttria likewise. Lastly, the yttria is to be precipitated by pure ammonia, well washed and dried.

Yttria is perfectly white, when not contaminated with oxide of manganese, from which it is not easily freed. Its specific gravity is 4.842. It has neither taste nor smell. It is infusible alone; but with borax melts into a transparent glass, or opaque white, if the borax were in excess. It is insoluble in water, and in caustic fixed alkalies; but it dissolves in carbonate of ammonia, though it requires five or six times as much as glucine. It is soluble in most of the acids. The oxalic acid, or oxalate of ammonia, forms precipitates in its solutions perfectly resembling the muriate of silver. Prussiate of potassa, crystallized and redissolved in water, throws it down in white grains; phosphate of soda, in white gelatinous flakes; infusion of galls, in brown flocks.

Some chemists are inclined to consider yttria rather as a metallic than as an earthy substance : their reasons are, its specific gravity, its forming coloured salts, and its property of oxygenizing muriatic acid after it has undergone a long calcination.

When yttria is treated with potassium in the same manner as the other earths, similar results are obtained; the potassium becomes potassa, and the earth gains appearances of metallization; so that it is scarcely to be doubted, says Sir H. Davy, that yttria consists of inflammable matter, metallic in its nature, combined with oxygen. The salts of yttria have the following general characters :—

1. Many of them are insoluble in water.

2. Precipitates are occasioned in those which dissolve, by phosphate of soda, carbonate of soda, oxalate of ammonia, tartrate of potassa, and ferroprussiate of potassa.

3. If we except the sweet-tasted soluble sulphate of yttria, the other salts of this earth resemble those with the base of lime in their solubility.

YTTRO-CERITE. A mineral of a reddish, grayish white, and a violet-blue colour, consisting of oxide of cerium, yttria, lime, and fluoric acid, found hitherto only at Finbo, in Sweden.

YTTRO-TANTALITE. An ore of tantalum, from which the columbic acid is procured.

YUCCA. (*Yucca, Yuca,* or *Iucca,* of the original inhabitants of America.) The name of a genus of plants in the Linnæan system. Class, *Hexandria;* Order, *Monogynia.*

YUCCA GLORIOSA. See *Adam's needle.*

Z

ZA'CCHARUM. See *Saccharum.*

ZACCHIA, PAOLO, an eminent physician, was born at Rome in 1585, and became distinguished by his learning and accomplishments, as well as by his professional skill. He was physician to Pope Innocent X., and celebrated among his contemporaries by various publications, of which the principal is entitled, "Quæstiones Medico-legales," and has been often reprinted. He was also the author, in Italian, of two esteemed works, on the Lent diet, and on hypochondriacal affections. He died in 1659.

ZA'FFRAN. (Arabian.) Saffron.

ZAFFRE. Saffre. The residuum of cobalt after the sulphur, arsenic, and other volatile matters of this mineral have been expelled by calcination.

ZAI'BAC. (Arabian.) Quicksilver.

ZA'RZA. An ancient and provincial name of the sarsaparilla.

ZE'A. (*Zea, æ,* f. : a name borrowed from the ancient Greeks, whose ζεια appears to have been some kind of *Triticum* or *Hordeum,* agreeing with this genus only as being a grain cultivated for the use of man.) The maize.

ZEA MAYS. The systematic name of the Indian wheat-plant, the common maize, or Indian corn, a native of America and cultivated in Italy and several parts of Europe, for its grain, which is ground for the same purposes as our wheat, to which it is very little inferior.

ZEDOA'RIA. 1. The name of a genus of plants in the Linnæan system. Class, *Monandria;* Order, *Monogynia.* Zedoary.

2. The pharmacopœial name of a *Kæmpfera.* See *Kæmpfera rotunda.*

ZEDOARIA LONGA. The long roots of the *Kæmpfera rotunda,* of Linnæus.

ZEDOARIA ROTUNDA. The round root of the zedoary plant. See *Kæmpfera rotunda.*

ZEDOARY. See *Zedoaria.*

ZEINE. A yellow substance, having the appearance of wax, obtained from maize or Indian corn.

ZEOLITE. The name of a very extensive mineral genus, containing the following species:

1. Dodecahedral zeolite, or leucite.

2. Hexahedral zeolite, or analcime.

3. Rhomboidal zeolite, chabasite, or chabasie

4. Pyramidal zeolite, or cross stone.

5. Diprismatic zeolite, or laumonite.

6. Prismatic zeolite, or mesotype, divided into three subspecies : natrolite ; mealy zeolite, of a white colour, of various shades ; and fibrous zeolite, of which there are two kinds.

a. The *acicular*, or *needle zeolite*, the mesotype of Haüy. This is of a grayish, yellowish, or reddish-white colour. It is found in Scotland.

b. Common fibrous zeolite, of a white colour.

7. Prismatoidal zeolite, or stilbite, comprehending,

a. Foliated zeolite, stilbite of Haüy of a white and red colour, beautiful specimens of which are found in Stirlingshire.

b. Radiated zeolite, of a yellowish-white, or grayish-white colour.

8. Axifrangible zeolite, or apophyllite.

ZE′RNA. An ulcerated impetigo.

ZERO. The commencement of a scale marked 0: thus we say, the zero of Fahrenheit, which is 32° below the melting point of ice ; the zero of the centigrade scale, which coincides with the freezing of water. The absolute zero is the imaginary point in the scale of temperature, when the whole heat is exhausted: the term of absolute cold or privation of caloric.

ZI′BETHUM. (From *Zobeth*, Arabian.) *Civetta.* Civet. A soft, unctuous, odoriferous substance, about the consistence of honey or butter, of a whitish, yellowish, or brownish colour, sometimes blackish, contained in some excretory follicles near the anus of the *Viverra zibetha*, of Linnæus. It has a grateful smell when diluted, and an unctuous subacrid taste, and possesses stimulating, nervine, and antispasmodic virtues.

ZIMMERMAN, JOHN GEORGE, was born in 1728, at Brug, in the canton of Bern, and studied medicine under Haller at Gottingen, where he took his degree at 23. Having married a relation of Haller, at Bern, he settled as a physician in his native town ; the retirement of which gave him an opportunity of composing many pieces in prose and verse, and particularly a sketch of his popular work " On Solitude." His treatise " On the Experience of Medicine," appeared *in* 1763, and three years after, that on dysentery. In 1768, he accepted the post of physician to the king of England for Hanover, whither he removed. Here the accumulation of business tended in some measure to allay the irritability of his temper ; and being obliged about three years after, to put himself under the care of a surgeon at Berlin for some local complaint, the notice that was taken of him, even by the king, contributed much to improve his health and spirits, and of course his happiness. Having lost his first wife, he formed a second matrimonial connexion in 1782 ; which helped much to alleviate the afflictions to which he was afterward exposed. In 1786 he was sent for to attend the great Frederick in his last illness : and he published an account of the conversations which he had with that celebrated prince. He was led, too, to defend the character of Frederick against the censures of Count de Mirabeau, which suffered him to severe criticisms. His political and religious principles induced him also to attack those societies which paved the way to the French revolution ; and he advised the Emperor Leopold to suppress them by force ; and having laid an unavowed publication to the charge of a particular person, he subjected himself to a prosecution for a libel. His mind had arrived to such a state of irritation, that the approach of the French towards Hanover almost subverted his reason ; he abstained from food, and died absolutely worn out in 1795.

ZIMOME. See *Gluten*, *vegetable*.

ZINC. (*Zincum*, a German word.) A metal found in nature combined with oxygen, carbonic acid, and sulphuric acid ; and mineralized by sulphur. Native oxide of zinc is commonly called *calamine*. It occurs in a loose, and in a compact form, amorphous, of a white, gray, yellow, or brown colour, without lustre, or transparency. Combined with carbonic acid, it is called *vitreous zinc ore*, or *native carbonate of zinc*. It is found in solid masses, sometimes in six-sided compressed prisms, both ends being covered with pentagons. Its colour is generally grayish inclining to black. It is often transparent. *Sulphate of zinc* is found efflorescent in the form of stalactites, or in rhombs. *Sulphuret of zinc*, or *blende*, is the most abundant ore. It is

found of various colours ; brown, yellow, hyacinth black, &c., and with various degrees of lustre and transparency. This zinc ore is contaminated with iron, lead, argillaceous and silicious earths, &c. It occurs both in amorphous masses and crystallized in a diversity of polygonal figures.

It is of a bluish-white colour, somewhat brighter than lead ; of considerable hardness, and so malleable as not to be broken with the hammer, though it cannot be much extended in this way. It is very easily extended by the rollers of the flatting mill. Its sp. gr. is from 6.9 to 7.2. In a temperature between 210° and 300° of F., it has so much ductility that it can be drawn into wire, as well as laminated.

When broken by bending, its texture appears as if composed of cubical grains. On account of its imperfect malleability, it is difficult to reduce it into small parts by filing or hammering ; but it may be granulated, like the malleable metals, by pouring it, when fused, into cold water ; or, if it be heated nearly to melting, it is then sufficiently brittle to be pulverized.

It melts long before ignition, at about the 700th degree of Fahrenheit's thermometer ; and, soon after it becomes red-hot, it burns with a dazzling brighter than of a bluish or yellowish tinge, and is oxidized with such rapidity, that it flies up in the form of white flowers, called the *flowers of zinc*, or *philosophical wool*. These are generated so plentifully, that the access of air is soon intercepted ; and the combustion ceases, unless the matter be stirred, and a considerable heat kept up. The white oxide of zinc is not volatile, but is driven up merely by the force of the combustion. When it is again urged by a strong heat, it becomes converted into a clear yellow glass. If zinc be heated in closed vessels, it rises without decomposition.

When zinc is burned in chlorine, a solid substance is formed of a whitish-gray colour, and semitransparent. This is the only chloride of zinc, as there is only one oxide of the metal. It may likewise be made by heating together zinc filings and corrosive sublimate. It is as soft as wax, fuses at a temperature a little above 212°, and rises in the gaseous form at a heat much below ignition. Its taste is intensely acrid, and it corrodes the skin. It acts upon water, and dissolves in it, producing much heat ; and its solution decomposed, by an alkali, affords the white hydrated oxide of zinc. This chloride has been called *butter of zinc*, and *muriate of zinc*.

Blende is the native sulphuret of zinc. The two bodies are difficult to combine artificially. The salts of zinc possess the following general characters :—

1. They generally yield colourless solutions with water.

2. Ferroprussiate of potassa, hydrosulphuret of potassa, hydriodate of potassa, sulphuretted hydrogen, and alkalies, occasion white precipitates.

3. Infusion of gall produces no precipitate.

The diluted *sulphuric acid* dissolves zinc: at the same time that the temperature of the solvent is increased, and much hydrogen escapes, an undissolved residue is left, which has been supposed to consist of plumbago. Proust, however, says, that it is a mixture of arsenic, lead, and copper. As the combination of the sulphuric acid and the oxide proceeds, the temperature diminishes, and the sulphate of zinc, which is more soluble in hot than cold water, begins to separate, and disturb the transparency of the fluid. If more water be added, the salt may be obtained in fine prismatic four-sided crystals. The white vitriol, or copperas, usually sold, is crystallized hastily, in the same manner as loaf-sugar, which on this account it resembles in appearance ; it is slightly efflorescent. The white oxide of zinc is soluble in the sulphuric acid, and forms the same salt as is afforded by zinc itself.

The hydrogen gas that is extricated from water by the action of sulphuric acid, carries up with it a portion of zinc, which is apparently dissolved in it ; but this is deposited spontaneously, at least in part, if not wholly, by standing. It burns with a brighter flame than common hydrogen.

Sulphate of zinc is prepared in the large way from some varieties of the native sulphuret. The ore is roasted, wetted with water, and exposed to the air. The sulphur attracts oxygen, and is converted into sulphuric acid ; and the metal, being at the same time oxidized, combines with the acid. After some time, the sulphate is extracted by solution in water; and the solution being evaporated to dryness, the mass is run into moulds. Thus the white vitriol of the shops generally contains a small portion of iron, and sometimes of lead.

Sulphurous acid dissolves zinc, and sulphuretted hydrogen is evolved. The solution, by exposure to the air, deposites needly crystals, which, according to Fourcroy and Vauquelin, are sulphuretted sulphite of zinc. By dissolving oxide of zinc in sulphurous acid, the pure sulphite is obtained. This is soluble, and crystallizable.

Diluted *nitric acid* combines rapidly with zinc, and produces much heat, at the same time that a large quantity of nitrous air flies off. The solution is very caustic, and affords crystals by evaporation and cooling, which slightly detonate upon hot coals, and leave oxide of zinc behind. This salt is deliquescent.

Muriatic acid acts very strongly upon zinc, and disengages much hydrogen; the solution, when evaporated, does not afford crystals, but becomes gelatinous. By a strong heat it is partly decomposed, a portion of the acid being expelled, and part of the muriate sublimes and condenses in a congeries of prisms.

Phosphoric acid dissolves zinc. The phosphate does not crystallize, but becomes gelatinous, and may be fused by a strong heat. The concrete phosphoric acid heated with zinc filings is decomposed.

Fluoric acid likewise dissolves zinc.

The *boracic acid* digested with zinc becomes milky; and if a solution of borax be added to a solution of muriate or nitrate of zinc, an insoluble borate of zinc is thrown down.

A solution of *carbonic acid* in water dissolves a small quantity of zinc, and more readily its oxide. If the solution be exposed to the air, a thin iridescent pellicle forms on its surface.

The *acetic acid* readily dissolves zinc, and yields by evaporation crystals of acetate of zinc, forming rhomboidal or hexagonal plates. These are not altered by exposure to the air, are soluble in water, and burn with a blue flame.

The *succinic acid* dissolves zinc with effervescence, and the solution yields long, slender, foliated crystals.

Zinc is readily dissolved in *benzoic acid*, and the solution yields needle-shaped crystals, which are soluble both in water and in alkohol. Heat decomposes them by volatilizing their acid.

The *oxalic acid* attacks zinc with a violent effervescence, and a white powder soon subsides, which is oxalate of zinc. If oxalic acid be dropped into a solution of sulphate, nitrate, or muriate of zinc, the same salt is precipitated; it being scarcely soluble in water unless an excess of acid be present. It contains seventy-five per cent. of metal.

The *tartaric acid* likewise dissolves zinc with effervescence, and forms a salt difficult of solution in water.

The *citric acid* attacks zinc with effervescence, and small brilliant crystals of citrate of zinc are gradually deposited, which are insoluble in water. Their taste is styptic and metallic, and they are composed of equal parts of the acid and of oxide of zinc.

The *malic acid* dissolves zinc, and affords beautiful crystals by evaporation.

Lactic acid acts upon zinc with effervescence, and produces a crystallizable salt.

The *metallic acids* likewise combine with zinc. If arsenic acid be poured on it, an effervescence takes place, arsenical hydrogen gas is emitted, and a black powder falls down, which is arsenic in the metallic state, the zinc having deprived a portion of the arsenic, as well as the water, of its oxygen. If one part of zinc filings, and two parts of dry arsenic acid be distilled in a retort, a violent detonation takes place when the retort becomes red, occasioned by the sudden absorption of the oxygen of the acid by the zinc. The arseniate of zinc may be precipitated by pouring arsenic acid into the solution of acetate of zinc, or by mixing a solution of an alkaline arseniate with that of sulphate of zinc. It is a white powder, insoluble in water.

By a similar process zinc may be combined with the molybdic acid, and with the oxide of tungsten, the tungstic acid of some, with both of which it forms a white insoluble compound; and with the chromic acid, the result of which compound is equally insoluble, but of an orange-red colour.

Zinc likewise forms some triple salts. Thus, if the white oxide of zinc be boiled in a solution of muriate of ammonia, a considerable portion is dissolved; and though part of the oxide is again deposited as the solution cools, some of it remains combined with the acid and alkali in the solution, and is not precipitable either by pure alkalies or their carbonates. This triple salt does not crystallize.

If the acidulous tartrate of potassa be boiled in water with zinc filings, a triple compound will be formed, which is very soluble in water, but not easily crystallized. This, like the preceding, cannot be precipitated from its solution either by pure or carbonated alkalies.

A triple sulphate of zinc and iron may be formed by mixing together the sulphates of iron and of zinc dissolved in water, or by dissolving iron and zinc in dilute sulphuric acid. This salt crystallizes in rhomboids, which nearly resemble the sulphate of zinc in figure, but are of a pale green-colour. In taste, and in degree of solubility, it differs little from the sulphate of zinc. It contains a much larger proportion of zinc than of iron.

A triple sulphate of zinc and cobalt, as first noticed by Link, may be obtained by digesting zaffre in a solution of sulphate of zinc. On evaporation, large quadrilateral prisms are obtained, which effloresce on exposure to the air.

Zinc is precipitated from acids by the soluble earths and the alkalies : the latter redissolve the precipitate, if they be added in excess.

Zinc decomposes, or alters, the neutral sulphates in the dry way. When fused with sulphate of potassa, it converts that salt into a sulphuret: the zinc at the same time being oxidized, and partly dissolved in the sulphuret. When pulverized zinc is added to fused nitre, or projected together with that salt into a red-hot crucible, a very violent detonation takes place; insomuch that it is necessary for the operator to be careful in using only small quantities, lest the burning matter should be thrown about. The zinc is oxidized, and part of the oxide combines with the alkali, with which it forms a compound soluble in water.

Zinc decomposes common salt, and also sal ammoniac, by combining with the muriatic acid. The filings of zinc likewise decompose alum, when boiled in a solution of that salt, probably by combining with its excess of acid.

Zinc may be combined with phosphorus, by projecting small pieces of phosphorus on the zinc melted in a crucible, the zinc being covered with a little resin, to prevent its oxidation. Phosphuret of zinc is white, with a shade of bluish-gray, has a metallic lustre, and is a little malleable. When zinc and phosphorus are exposed to heat in a retort, a red sublimate rises, and likewise a bluish sublimate in needly crystals with a metallic lustre. If zinc and phosphoric acid be heated together, with or without a little charcoal, needly crystals are sublimed, of a silvery-white colour. All these, according to Pelletier, are phosphuretted oxides of zinc.

Most of the metallic combinations of zinc have been already treated of. It forms a brittle compound with antimony; and its effects on manganese, tungsten, and molybdena, have not yet been ascertained.

Zinc, vitriolated. See *Zinci sulphas.*

Zi'nci acetas. See *Acetas zinci.*

Zinci oxidum. *Zincum calcinatum.* Oxide of zinc. Flowers of zinc. *Nihil album; Lana philosophorum.* "Throw gradually little pieces of zinc into a large deep crucible placed obliquely and made of a white heat, another crucible being placed over it, so that the zinc may be exposed to the air, and that it may be frequently stirred with an iron spatula; take out directly the oxide, which is formed from time to time; then pass the white and lighter part of it through a sieve. Lastly, pour water upon this, that a very fine powder may be formed, in the same manner as chalk is directed to be prepared." The properties of this oxide are analogous to those of the sulphate, (except that it is hardly active enough to excite vomiting,) if given in larger doses: but it is more precarious in its effects; and chiefly used at present as an external astringent

Zinci sulphas. *Zincum vitriolatum. Vitriolum album.* Sulphate of zinc. White vitriol. This occurs native, but not sufficiently pure for medical use. It is thus prepared in the pharmacopœia. "Take of zinc, broken to little pieces, three ounces; sulphuric acid, by weight, five ounces: water, four pints. Mix them in a glass vessel, and when the effervescence is over, filter the solution through paper; then boil it down, till a pellicle appears, and set it by to crystallize." This preparation is given internally in the dose of from Ɔj to Ʒss, as a vomit. In small doses it cures dropsies, intermitting headaches, and some nervous diseases; and is a powerful antispasmodic and tonic. A solution of white vitriol is also used to remove gleets, gonorrhœas, and for cleaning foul ulcers, having an astringent or stimulant effect, according to its strength.

ZI'NCUM. See *Zinc.*

ZINCUM CALCINATUM. See *Zinci oxidum.*

ZINCUM VITRIOLATUM. See *Zinci sulphas.*

ZINCUM VITRIOLATUM PURIFICATUM. See *Zinci sulphas.*

ZINGI. An ancient name of the stellated aniseed. See *Illicium anisatum.*

ZI'NGIBER. (*Zingiberis, is,* f. *Zingiber, eris,* n. *Zingiberi;* indec. Ζιγγιβερις, of Dioscorides, a name which the Greeks seem to have taken from the Arabians, when they got the plant.) The name of a genus of plants, according to Roscoe. Class, *Monandria;* Order, *Monogynia.*

ZINGIBER ALBUM. Ginger-root when deprived of its radicles and sordes.

ZINGIBER COMMUNE. See *Zingiber officinale.*

ZINGIBER NIGRUM. The root of the *zingiber officinale* is so called when suffered to dry with its radicles and the sordes which usually hang to it.

ZINGIBER OFFICINALE. The systematic name of the ginger-plant. *Zingiber album; Zingiber nigrum; Zingiber commune; Zinziber; Amomum zingiber,* of Linnæus. The white and black ginger are both the produce of the same plant, the difference depending upon the mode of preparing them. Ginger is generally considered as an aromatic, and less pungent and heating to the system than might be expected from its effects upon the organ of taste. It is used as an antispasmodic and carminative. The cases in which it is more immediately serviceable are flatulent colics, debility, and laxity of the stomach and intestines; and in torpid and phlegmatic constitutions to excite brisker vascular action. It is seldom given but in combination with other medicines. In the pharmacopœias it is directed in the form of a syrup and condiment, and in many compositions ordered as a subsidiary ingredient.

ZINN, JOHN GODFREY, was born in 1726, studied under Haller at Gottingen, and became botanical professor in that university. His first experiments were undertaken to ascertain the sensibility of different parts of the brain; he then proceeded to the examination of the eye, on which he published a work in much estimation. The result of his botanical labours appeared in several papers, and in a catalogue of the plants about Gottingen, arranged according to the plan of his preceptor. He died prematurely in 1758. He was a member of several learned societies.

ZI'NZIBER. See *Zingiber.*

ZIRCONIA. Zircon. An earth discovered in the year 1793, by Klaproth of Berlin, in the Zircon or Jargon, a gem first brought from the island of Ceylon, but also found in France, Spain, and other parts of Europe. Its colour is either gray, greenish, yellowish, reddish-brown, or purple. It has little lustre, and is nearly opaque. Zircon is likewise found in another gem called the hyacinth. This stone is of a yellowish-red colour, mixed with brown. It possesses lustre and transparency. To obtain it, the stone should be calcined and thrown into cold water, to render it friable, and then powdered in an agate mortar. Mix the powder with nine parts of pure potassa, and project the mixture by spoonfuls into a red-hot crucible, taking care that each portion is fused before another is added. Keep the whole in fusion, with an increased heat, for an hour and a half. When cold, break the crucible, separate its contents, powder and boil in water, to dissolve the alkali. Wash the insoluble part; dissolve in muriatic acid; heat the solution, that the silex may fall down; and precipitate the zircon by caustic fixed alkali. Or the zircon may be precipitated by carbonate of soda, and the carbonic acid expelled by heat.

New process for preparing pure zirconia.—Powder the zircons very fine, mix them with two parts of pure potassa, and heat them red-hot in a silver crucible, for an hour. Treat the substance obtained with distilled water, pour it on a filter, and wash the insoluble part well; it will be a compound of zirconia,

silex, potassa, and oxide of iron. Dissolve it in muriatic acid, and evaporate to dryness, to separate the silex. Redissolve the muriates of zirconia and iron in water; and to separate the zirconia which adheres to the silex, wash it with weak muriatic acid, and add this to the solution. Filter the fluid, and precipitate the zirconia and iron by pure ammonia; wash the precipitates well, and then treat the hydrates with oxalic acid, boiling them well together, that the acid may act on the iron, retaining it in solution, while an insoluble oxalate of zirconia is formed. It is then to be filtered, and the oxalate washed, until no iron can be detected in the water that passes. The earthy oxalate is, when dry, of an opaline colour. After being well washed, it is to be decomposed by heat in a platinum crucible.

Thus obtained, the zirconia is perfectly pure, but is not affected by acids. It must be reacted on by potassa as before, and then washed until the alkali is removed. Afterward dissolve it in muriatic acid, and precipitate by ammonia. The hydrate thrown down, when well washed, is perfectly pure, and easily soluble in acids.

Zircon is a fine white powder, without taste or smell, but somewhat harsh to the touch. It is insoluble in water; yet if slowly dried, it coalesces into a semitransparent yellowish mass, like gum-arabic, which retains one-third its weight of water. It unites with all the acids. It is insoluble in pure alkalies; but the alkaline carbonates dissolve it. Heated with the blowpipe, it does not melt, but emits a yellowish phosphoric light. Heated in a crucible of charcoal, bedded in charcoal powder, placed in a stone crucible, and exposed to a good forge fire for some hours, it undergoes a pasty fusion, which unites its particles into a gray opaque mass, not truly vitreous, but more resembling porcelain. In this state it is sufficiently hard to strike fire with steel, and scratch glass; and is of the specific gravity of 4.3.

There is the same evidence for believing that zirconia is a compound of a metal and oxygen, as that afforded by the action of potassium on the other earths. The alkaline metal, when brought into contact with zirconia ignited to whiteness, is, for the most part, converted into potassa, and dark particles, which, when examined by a magnifying glass, appear metallic in some parts, of a chocolate-brown in others, are found diffused through the potassa and the decompounded earth.

According to Sir H. Davy, 4.66 is the prime equivalent of zirconium on the oxygen scale, and 5.66 that of zirconia.

ZIZA'NIA. (An ancient name, ζιζανιον, of the Greeks, synonymous with *infelix lolium,* of the Latins.) The name of a genus of plants in the Linnæan system. Class, *Monœcia;* Order, *Hexandria.*

ZIZANIA AQUATICA. The systematic name of a reed, the grain of which is much esteemed in Jamaica and Virginia. The Indians are exceedingly fond of it, and account it more delicious than rice.

[The zizania aquatica is a native of most of the northern parts of the United States, but it has disappeared in the settled and cultivated parts of the country. It is now principally found on the streams and shoal waters of the north-western lakes and rivers, where it grows spontaneously in the water, like rice in the southern states. During seed-time, the aborigines of the country collect it for food; which they use by parching with fire, and then pounding with a stone. The meal thus produced tastes much like parched Indian corn. The plant is the *Fausse avoine,* or false oats of the French Canadians. The grain is black, and from half an inch to an inch in length, with much of the appearance, when growing, of oats or rice. A.]

ZI'ZYPHUS. The jujubes were formerly so called. See *Rhamnus zizyphus.*

ZOISITE. A subspecies of prismatic augite, which is divided into two kinds:

1. *Common zoisite,* of a yellowish-gray colour, found in Corinthia.

2. *Friable zoisite,* of a reddish colour, which comes also from Corinthia.

ZO'NA. (From ζωννυμι, to surround.) The shingles. See *Erysipelas.*

ZOOLOGY. (*Zoologia;* from ζωον, an animal, and λογος, a discourse.) That part of natural history which treats of animals.

ZOONIC ACID. In the liquid procured by distillation from animal substances, which had been supposed to contain only carbonate of ammonia and an oil. Berthollet imagined he had discovered a peculiar acid, to which he gave the name of zoonic. Thenard, however, has demonstrated that it is merely acetic acid combined with animal matter

ZOONO'MIA. (From ζωον, an animal, and νομος, a law.) The laws of organic life.

ZOOPHYTE. (*Zoophyte, i, n.*; from ζωον, an animal, and φυτον, a plant.) A kind of intermediate body, supposed to partake both of the nature of an animal and a vegetable. In the Linnæan system, *zoophytes* constitute an order of the Class *Vermes*.

ZOOTOMY. (*Zootomia;* from ζωον, an animal, and τεμνω, to cut.) The dissection of animals.

ZO'STER. (From ζωννυμι, to gird.) A kind of erysipelas which goes round the body like a girdle.

Zu'CHAR. (Arabian.) Sugar.

ZUMATE. A compound of the zumic acid, with a salifiable basis.

ZUMIC ACID. (*Acidum zumicum,* from ζυμη, leaven.) An acid produced from vegetable substances which have undergone the acetous fermentation. Its claim to be considered as a distinct compound is doubtful. See *Nanceic acid.*

ZUNDERERZ. Tinder ore. An ore of silver.

ZYGO'MA. (From ζυγος, a yoke: because it transmits the tendon of the temporal muscle like a yoke.) The cavity under the zygomatic process of the temporal bone, and os malæ.

ZYGOMATIC. (*Zygomaticus;* from *zygoma.*) Belonging to the zygoma.

ZYGOMATIC PROCESS. An apophysis of the os jugale, and another of the temporal bone, are so called.

ZYGOMATIC SUTURE. *Sutura zygomatica.* The union of the zygomatic process of the temporal bone to the cheek bone.

ZYGOMATICUS MAJOR. This muscle arises from the cheek bone near the zygomatic suture, taking a direction downwards and inwards to the angle of the mouth. It is a long slender muscle, which ends by mixing its fibres with the orbicularis oris, and the depressor of the lip.

ZYGOMATICUS MINOR. This muscle arises a little higher up than the zygomaticus major, upon the cheek bone, but nearer the nose; it is much more slender than that muscle, and is often wanting. It is the zygomatic muscle that marks the face with that line which extends from the cheek bone to the corner of the mouth, which is particularly distinguishable in some persons. The zygomatic muscles pull the angles of the mouth up as in laughter, and from, in this way, rendering the face distorted, it has obtained the name of distortor oris. The strong action of this muscle is more particularly seen in laughter, rage, or grinning.

ZYTHO'GALA. Ζυθογαλα. Beer and milk, which make together what we commonly call *posset-drink,* a term often to be met with in Sydenham.

ZZ. The ancients signify *Myrrh* by these two letters, from ζμυρνη, a name for it common among them. They have also been used for *Zingiber.*

THE END

APPENDIX.

[THE following obsolete terms have been omitted in the body of the work, but to preserve Dr. Hooper's Dictionary perfect, they are inserted in the present place and form.]

A'ABAM. An obsolete term used by some ancient alchemists for lead.

A'BANET. (Hebrew. The girdle worn by the Jewish priests.) A girdle-like bandage.

ABA'RTAMEN. Lead.

A'BAS. An Arabian term for the scald-head, and also for epilepsy.

ABO'IT. An Arabic term for white lead.

A'BRIC. An Arabic term for sulphur.

ABSTRACTI'TIUS. (From *abstraho*, to draw away.) An obsolete term formerly applied to any native spirit, not produced by fermentation. •

ACA'CA. (Ακακος ; from *a*, neg., and κακος, bad.) Formerly applied to those diseases, which are rather troublesome than dangerous.

ACA'LAI. (Arabian.) Common salt.

ACA'LCUM. Tin.

ACA'NOR. (Hebrew.) A furnace.

ACA'ZDIR. Tin.

A'CCIB. An obsolete term for lead.

A'CESIS. (From ακεομαι, to cure.) 1. A remedy or cure.

2. The herb water-sage ; so called from its supposed healing qualities.

ACE'STORIS. (From ακεομαι, to cure.) It strictly signifies a female physician, and is used for a midwife.

ACHMA'DIUM. Antimony.

A'CHNE. An obsolete term applied to
1. Chaff.
2. Scum or froth of the sea.
3. A white mucus in the fauces, thrown up from the lungs, like froth.
4. A whitish mucilage in the eyes of those who have fevers, according to Hippocrates.
5. It signifies also lint.

ACONI'TUM. (*Aconitum, i, m.* Of this name various derivations are given by etymologists ; as, ακοιη, a *whetstone* or *rock*, because it is usually found in barren and rocky places: ακονιτος, *a*, neg., and κονις, *dust ;* because it grows without earth, or on barren situations ; agreeable to Ovid's description, " Quæ quia nascuntur dura vivacia caute, Agrestes aconita vocant:" ακοναω, te *sharpen* ; because it was used in medicine intended to quicken the sight: ακων, ακη, a *dart ;* because they poison darts therewith : or, ακονιζομαι, to accelerate ; for it hastens death.) Aconite. 1. A genus of plants in the Linnæan system, all the species of which have powerful effects on the human body. Class, *Polyandria ;* Order, *Trigynia.*

2. The pharmacopœial name of the common, or blue wolf's-bane. See *Aconitum napellies.*

ACO'NIUM. A little mortar.

ACORI'TES. (From ακορον, galangal.) *Acorites vinum.* A wine mentioned by Dioscorides, made with galangal, liquorice, &c. infused with wine.

ACORTINUS. A lupin.

A'CRA. (An Arabian word.) *Acrai.*
1. Excessive venereal appetite.
2. The time of menstruation.

ACTON. A village four miles from London, where is a well that affords a purging water. This is one of the strongest purging waters near London: and has been drank in the quantity of from one to three pints in a morning, against scorbutic and cutaneous affections. This medical spring is no longer resorted to by the public.

ADAICES. Sal-ammoniac.

ADAMITUM. See *Adamita.*

ADARI'GES. An ammoniacal salt.

A'DEC. Sour milk, or buttermilk.

ADIATHOROSUS. A spirit distilled from tartar Obsolete.

ADIBAT. Mercury.

A'DICE. Αδικη. A nettle.

ADI'RIGE. Ammoniacal salt.

A'DOC. Milk.

A'DRAM. Fossil salt.

AEI'GLUCES. (From αει, always, and γλυκυς, sweet.) A sweetish wine, or must.

Æ'ON. The spinal marrow.

ÆONE'SIS. A washing or sprinkling the whole body.

ÆSCHROMYTHE'SIS. The obscene language of the delirious.

ÆSECA'VUM. Brass.

ÆSTA'TES. Freckles in the face ; sunburnings.

ÆTAS CREPITA. See *Age.*

ÆTAS VIRILIS. See *Age.*

Æ'THNA. A chemical furnace.

Æ'THOCES. *Ætholices.* Superficial pustules in the skin, raised by heat, as boils, fiery pustules.

ÆTHYA. A mortar.

Æ'TTIOI PHLEBES. Eagle veins. The veins which pass through the temples to the head, were so called formerly by Rufus Ephesius.

ÆTOLIUM. See *Ætocion.*

A'FFION. An Arabic name for opium.

A'FFIUM. An Arabic name for opium.

AGERA'TUS LAPIS. (*Ageratus,* common.) A stone used by cobblers

A'GES. (From αγης, wicked : so called because it is generally the instrument of wicked acts.) The palm of the hand.

A'GIS. The thigh or femur.

A'GMA. *Agme.* A fracture.

AGO'CE. 1 The deduction or reasoning upon diseases from their symptoms and appearances.

2. The order, state, or tenour of a disease or body.

AGO'STOS. (From αγω, to bring, or lead.) That part of the arm from the elbow to the fingers ; also the palm or hollow of the hand.

AGRE'STA. (Αγριος, wild.) 1. The immature fruit of the vine.

2. Verjuice, which is made from the wild apple.

AGRE'STEN. Common tartar

AGUIA. (From *a*, priv., and γυιον, a member.) Paralytic weakness of a limb. Where the use of the members is defective or lost.

A'GUL. *Alhagi.* An Arabian name for the Syrian thorn. The leaves are purgative

AGYION. See *Aguia.*

AGY'RTÆ. (From αγυρτς, a crowd of people, or a mob; or from αγειρω, to gather together.) It formerly expressed certain strollers, who pretended to strange things from supernatural assistances; it was afterward applied to all illiterate dabblers in medicine. Now obsolete.

AHALOTH. The Hebrew name of Lignum aloes. See *Lignum aloes.*

AHAME'LLA. See *Achmella.*

AHO'VAI THEVETICLUSH. A chesnut-like fruit of Brazil, of a poisonous nature.

AHU'SAL. Orpiment.

AI'LMAD. Antimony.

AI'TMAD. Antimony.

AJURA'RAT. Lead.

ALA'BARI. Lead.

A'LACAR. Sal ammoniac.

A'LAFI. *Alafor. Alafort.* Alcaline.

A'LAMAD. *Alamed.* Antimony.

ALA'MBIC. Mercury.

ALAPOU'LI. See *Bilimbi.*

ALASALET. *Alaset.* Ammoniacum.

ALASI. *Alafor.* An alcaline salt.

ALA'STROB. Lead.

A'LATAN. Litharge.

ALAU'RAT. Nitre.

ALBADAL. An Arabic name for the sesamoid bone of the first joint of the great toe.

ALBAGE'NZI. *Albagiazi.* Arabic names for the os sacrum.

ALBA'RA. (Chaldean.) The white leprosy.

ALBARAS. 1. Arsenic.

2. A white pustule.

A'LBERAS. (Arabian.) White pustules on the face: also, staphisagria, because its juice was said to remove these pustules.

ALBE'STON. Quicklime.

A'LBETAD. Galbanum.

A'LBI SUBLIMATI. Muriated mercury.

A'LBIMEC. Orpiment. See *Arsenic.*

A'LBOR. Urine.

ALBO'REA. Quicksilver.

A'LBOT. A crucible.

ALBO'TAI. Turpentine.

A'LBOTAR. Turpentine.

A'LBOTAT. White lead.

A'LBOTIM. Turpentine.

A'LBOTIS. A cutaneous phlegmon or boil.

ALBUHAR. White lead.

A'LCEBAR. See *Lignum aloes.*

A'LCEBRIS VIVUM. This signifies, according to Rulandus, Sulphur vivum.

A'LCHABRIC. Sulphur vivum.

A'LCHACHIL. Rosemary.

A'LCHARITH. Quicksilver.

A'LCHIBRIC. Sulphur.

A'LCHIEN. This word occurs in the Theatrum Chemicum, and seems to signify that power in nature by which all corruption and generation are effected

ALCHIMELEC. (Hebrew.) The Egyptian melilot.

A'LCHLYS. A speck on the pupil of the eye, somewhat obscuring vision.

A'LCHUTE. The mulberry.

A'LCIMAD. Antimony.

A'LCOB. Sal ammoniac.

ALCO'CALUM. Most probably the Indian name of the artichoke.

A'LCOFOL. Antimony.

A'LCOLA. (Hebrew.) 1. The thrush.

2. Paracelsus gives this name to tartar, or excrement of urine, whether it appears as sand, mucilage, &c.

ALCOLI'TA. Urine.

ALCO'NE. Brass.

A'LCOR. Æs ustum.

A'LCTE. The name of a plant mentioned by Hippocrates, supposed to be the elder.

ALCU'BRITH. Sulphur.

ALEARA. A cucurbit.

ALE'BRIA. (From *alo,* to nourish.) An obsolete term for that which is nourishing.

A'LEC. *Alech.* Vitriol.

ALE'CHARITH. Mercury.

ALEI'MMA. (From αλειφω, to anoint.) An ointment.

ALE'MZADAR. Sal ammoniac.

ALE'MZADAT. Sal ammoniac.

ALFA'CTA. Distillation.

A'LFADAS. *Alfides.* Cerusse.

ALFA'SRA. *Alphesara.* Arabic terms for the vine.

ALFA'TIDE. Sal ammoniac.

A'LFOL. Sal ammoniac.

A'LFUSA. Tutty.

A'LGALI. A catheter. Also nitre.

A'LGARAH. See *Anchilops.*

ALGE'RIÆ. *Algirie.* Lime.

A'LGEROTH. See *Algaroth.*

A'LGIBIC. Sulphur vivum.

ALGUADA. A white leprous eruption.

ALINDE'SIS. (Αλινδησις; from αλινδουμαι, to be d about.) A bodily exercise which seems to be rolling on the ground, or rather in the dust, after being anointed with oil. Hippocrates says it hath nearly the same effect as wrestling.

ALIPÆ'NOS. (From *a,* neg. and λιπαινω, to be fat.) *Alipænum; Alipantos.* An external remedy, without fat or moisture.

ALIPE. Remedies for wounds in the cheek, to prevent inflammation.

ALI'STELIS. (From αλς, the sea.) Sal ammoniac.

ALKAFI'AL. Antimony.

A'LKANT. Quicksilver.

ALKA'NTHUM. Arsenic.

ALKASA. A crucible.

ALKE'RVA. (Arabian.) Castor oil.

A'LKI PLUMBI. Supposed to be the sugar or acetate of lead.

A'LKOSOR. Camphire.

ALKSOAL. A crucible.

ALKYMIA. Powder of basilisk.

A'LLABOR. Lead.

A'LLICAR. Vinegar.

ALLI'COA. Petroleum.

ALLIGATU'RA. A ligature or bandage

ALLIO'TICUM. (From αλλιοω, to alter, or vary.) An alterative medicine, consisting of various antiscorbutics.—*Galen.*

ALLO'CHOOS. (From αλλος, another, and χεω, to pour.) Hippocrates uses this word to mean delirious.

A'LMAGRA. *Bolum cuprum.* 1. Red earth, or ochre, used by the ancients as an astringent.

2. Rulandus says it is the same as *Lotio.*

3. In the Theatrum Chemicum, it is a name for the white sulphur of the alchemists.

ALMARA'NDA. *Almakis.* Litharge.

ALMA'RCAB. An Arabic word for litharge of silver.

ALMARCA'RIDA. Litharge of silver.

ALMA'RGEN. *Almarago.* Coral.

ALMARKASI'TA. Mercury.

ALMA'RTAK. Powder of litharge.

ALMATA'TICA. Copper.

ALMEAILE'TU. A word used by Avicenna, to express a preternatural heat less than that of fever and which may continue after a fever.

ALMECA'SITE. *Almechasite.* Copper

ALMI'SA. Musk.

ALMIZA'DAR. Sal ammoniac.

ALMIZA'DIR. Verdigris.

A'LNEC. Tin.

A'LNERIC. Sulphur vivum.

A'LOHAR. (Arabian.) *Alohoc.* Mercury.

ALO'MBA. (Arabian.) *Alooc.* Lead.

ALPHABE'TUM CHEMICUM. Raymond Lully hath given the world this alphabet, but to what end is difficult to say:

A *significat Deum.*

B ———— *Mercurium.*

C ———— *Salis petram.*

D ———— *Vitriolum.*

E ———— *Menstruale.*

F ———— *Lunam claram.*

G ———— *Mercurium nostrum.*

H ———— *Salem purum.*

I ———— *Compositum lunæ.*

K ———— *Compositum solis.*

L ———— *Terram compositi lunæ.*

M ———— *Aquam compositi lunæ.*

N ———— *Ærem compositi lunæ.*

O ———— *Terram compositi solis.*

P ———— *Aquam compositi solis.*

Q ———— *Ærem compositi solis.*

R ———— *Ignem compositi solis.*

S ———— *Lapidem album.*

T ———— *Medicinam corporis rubei.*

U ———— *Calorem fumi secreti.*

X ———— *Ignem siccum cineris.*

Y ———— *Calorem balnei.*

Z ———— *Separationem liquorum.*

Z ———— *Alembicum cum cucurbitâ.*

A'LPHANIC. *Alphenic.* An Arabian word, signifying tender, for barley-sugar, or sugar-candy.

A'LRACHAS. Lead.

ALRA'TICA. An Arabic word used by Albucasis, to signify a partial or a total imperforation of the vagina.

ALSA'MACH. An Arabic name for the great hole in the os petrosum.

A'LTAFOR. Camphire.

ALTHA'NACA. *Althanaca.* Orpiment.

ALTHEBE'GIUM. An Arabian name for a sort of swelling, such as is observed in cachectic and leucophlegmatic habits.

ALTIHIT. So Avicenna calls the *Laserpitium* of the ancients.

A'LUD. Arabian aloes.

ALUSAR. Manna.

ALZE'MAFOR. Cinnabar.

A'MBE. (Αμβη, the edge of a rock; from αμβαινω, to ascend.) An old chirurgical machine for reducing dislocations of the shoulder, and so called, because its extremity projects like the prominence of a rock. Its invention is imputed to Hippocrates. The ambe is the most ancient mechanical contrivance for the above purpose, but is not used at present

A MBELA. (Arabian.) The cornered hazel-nut, the bark of which is purgative.

A'MBULO. (From αμβαλλω, to cast forth.) *Flatus furiosus.* A periodical flatulent disease caused, according to Michaelis, by vapours shooting through various parts of the body.

AMY'CTICA. (From αμυσσω, to vellicate.) Medicines which stimulate and vellicate the skin, according to Cælius Aurelianus.

ANA'TRIS. Mercury. *Ruland.*

A'NERIC. *Anerit.* Sulphur vivum.

ANTARIS. Mercury.

ANTI'ADES. (From αν]ιαω, to meet.) 1. The tonsils are so called because they answer one another. 2. The mumps.—*Nic Piso.*

ARCHIMA'GIA. (From αρχη, the chief, and *magaa,* the Arabian for meditation.) Chemistry, as being the chief of sciences.

A'RFAR. *Arsag.* Arsenic.--*Ruland,* &c.

A SSAC. (Arabian.) Gum ammoniacum.

A'SSALA. The nutmeg.

A'SSANUS. The name of an old weight, consisting of two drachms.

A'SUAR. Indian myrobalans, or purging nut.

A'SUGAR. Verdigris.

ASU'OLI. Soot.

A'TAC. Nitre.

ATA'XIR. (Arabian.) 1. A tenesmus. 2. A disease of the eyes.

ATA'XMIR. (Arabian.) Removal of preternatural hair growing under the natural ones of the eyelids.

A'TEBRAS. A chemical subliming vessel.

ATHA'NOR. (Arabian.) A chemical digesting furnace.

ATHENA. A plaster in much repute among the ancients.

ATHENATO'RIUM. A thick glass cover formerly used for chemical purposes.

ATHENIO'NIS CATAPOTIUM. The name of a pill in Celsus's writings.

ATHENI'PPON. *Athenippum.* The name of a collyrium.

ATHO'NOR. (Arabian.) A chemical furnace.

ATI'NCAR. (Arabian.) Borax.

ATRAME'NTUM SUTORIUM. A name of green vitriol.

AURUS BRAZILIENSIS. An obsolete name of the *Calamus aromaticus.*

AUTOLITHO'TOMUS. (From αυτος, himself, λιθος, a stone, and τεμνω, to cut.) One who cuts himself for the stone.

AVA'NSIS. *Avante.* Indigestion.

BA'IAC. White lead.

BA'RAC. (From *borak,* Arabian, splendid.) *Barach panis.* Nitre.

BA'RAS. (Arabian.) In M. A. Severinus, it is synonymous with Alphus, or Leuce.

BARA'THRUM. (Arabian.) Any cavity or hollow place.

BARBA'RIA. *Barbaricum.* An obsolete term formerly applied to rhubarb.

BARO'PTIS. A black stone, said to be an antidote to venomous bites.

BAUDA. A vessel for distillation was formerly so called.

BAU'RACH. (Arab. *Bourach.*) A name formerly applied to nitre, borax, soda, and many other salts.

BDE'LLUS. (From βδεω, to break wind.) A discharge of wind by the anus.

BDELY'GMIA. (From βδεω, to break wind.) Any filthy and nauseous odour.

BELLU'TTA TSJAMPACAM. (Indian.) A tree of Malabar, to which many virtues are attributed.

BELU'ZZAR. *Beluzaar.* The Chaldee word for antidote.

BE'NATH. (Arabian.) Small pustules produced by sweatings in the night.

BERE'DRIAS. An ointment.

BERNA'RVI. An electuary.

BERRIO'NIS. A name of black resin.

BERY'TION. (From Berytus, its inventor.) A collyrium described by Galen.

BES. An eight ounce measure.

BESA'CHAR. A sponge.

BES'ASA. Formerly applied to wild rue.

BESEASE. An old name for mace.

BESE'NNA. (An Arabian word.) *Muscarum fungus.* Probably a sponge, which is the nidus of some sorts of flies.

BEZOAS. An obsolete chemical epithet.

BLA'NCA MULIERUM. White lead.

BO'SA. An Egyptian word for an inebriating mass, made of the meal of darnel, hempseed, and water.

BO'SMOROS. (From βοσκω, to eat, and μορος, a part; because it is divided for food by the mill.) *Bosporas.* A species of meal.

BO'THOR. (Arabian.) Tumours; pimples in the face: also the small-pox or measles.

BO'TIA. A name given to scrofula.

BO'TIN. A name for turpentine.

BO'TIUM. *Boetum.* 1. A bronchocele. 2. Indurated bronchial glands.

BOTOTHI'NUM. The most evident symptom of disease.

BO'TUS. *Botia. Botus barbatus.* A cucurbit of the chemists.

BRA'CIUM. Copper. Verdigris.

BURAC. (An Arabian word.) Borax, or any kind of salt.

C, in the chemical alphabet, means nitre.

CA'LCATON. White arsenic. Troches of arsenic. An obsolete term.

CALCE'NA. *Culcenonius ; Calcetus.* Paracelsus uses these words to express the tartarous matter in the blood ; or that the blood is impregnated with the tartarous principles.

CALCHOI'DES. (From χαλιξ, a chalk stone, and ειδος, form.) An obsolete name of the cuneiform bones

CALCIDI'CIUM. The name of a medicine in which arsenic is an ingredient.

CALCITA'RI. Alkaline salt.

CALCITE'A. Vitriol.

CALCITEO'SA. Litharge.

CA'LCITHOS. Verdigris.

CALCITRE'A. Vitriol.

CA'LCOTAR. Vitriol.

CA'RABE. See *Capyridion.*

CA'RABE. (Persian) Amber.

CHI'BUR. Sulphur.

DIAMI'SYOS. (From δια, and μισυ, misy.) A com position in which misy is an ingredient.

DYSRA'CHITIS. The name of a plaster.

EBEL. The seeds of sage, or of juniper.

EBE'SMECII. Quicksilver.

EBSEMECH. Quicksilver.

ECCATHA'RTICA. (From εκκαθαιρω, to purge outwards.) According to Gorræus, eccathartics are medicines which open the pores of the skin ; but in general they are understood to be deobstruent. Sometimes expectorants are thus called, and also purgatives. An obsolete term.

EDES. Amber.

EDE'SSENUM. An eye-water of tragacanth, gum arabic, opium, &c.

E'DETZ. Amber.

E'DIC. *Edich ; Eder.* Iron.

E'DRA. A fracture; also the lower part of the rectum.

E'FFIDES. Ceruss.

ELA'NULA. Alum.

E'LAQUIR. Red vitriol.

E'LAS MARIS. Burnt lead.

ELE'RSNA. An old term for black lead.

ELE'SMATIS. An old term for burnt lead.

ENS MARTIS. An oxide of iron.

ENS PRIMUM SOLARE. Antimony.

ENS VENERIS. The muriate of copper.

FUMUS ALBUS. Mercury.

FUMUS CITRINUS. Sulphur.

FUMUS DUPLEX. Sulphur and mercury.

FUMUS RUBENS. Orpiment.

GE'NIPI. A term of barbarous origin applied to two plants.

GE'RYON. Quicksilver.

ILEI'DOS. In the Spagyric language, it is the ele mentary air.

LA'RBASON. Antimony.

SATANUS DEVORANS. Antimony

SATHE. The penis.

N C R

'07